a LANGE medical book

SYMPTOM TO DIAGNOSIS

An Evidence-Based Guide

Third Edition

Scott D. C. Stern, MD, FACP
Professor of Medicine
Clinical Director of Clinical Pathophysiology and Therapeutics
University of Chicago
Pritzker School of Medicine
Chicago, Illinois

Adam S. Cifu, MD, FACP
Professor of Medicine
Co-Director, Junior Clerkship in Medicine
University of Chicago
Pritzker School of Medicine
Chicago, Illinois

Diane Altkorn, MD, FACP
Professor of Medicine
Director, Senior Student Clerkships in Medicine
University of Chicago
Pritzker School of Medicine
Chicago, Illinois

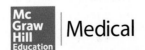

Medical

New York   Chicago   San Francisco   Athens   London   Madrid   Mexico City
Milan   New Delhi   San Juan   Seoul   Singapore   Sydney   Toronto

Symptom to Diagnosis: An Evidence-Based Guide, Third Edition

Copyright © 2015 by McGraw-Hill Education. All rights reserved. Printed in China. Except as permitted under the United States Copyright Act of 1976, no part of this publication may be reproduced or distributed in any form or by any means, or stored in a data base or retrieval system, without the prior written permission of the publisher.

4 5 6 7 8 9 0   DSS   19 18 17 16

ISBN 978-0-07-180344-1
MHID 0-07-180344-0
ISSN 1556-2719

This book was set in Adobe Garamond Pro by Cenveo® Publisher Services.
The editors were Harriet Lebowitz and Sarah Henry.
The production supervisor was Catherine Saggese.
The copyeditor was Jennifer Bernstein.
Project management was provided by Anupriya Tyagi at Cenveo Publisher Services.
The text designer was Eve Siegel.
RR Donnelley/China was printer and binder.

This book is printed on acid-free paper.

McGraw-Hill books are available at special quantity discounts to use as premiums and sales promotions, or for use in corporate training programs. To contact a representative, please visit the Contact Us pages at www.mhprofessional.com.

International Edition ISBN 978-1-25-925253-2; MHID 1-25-925253-1. Copyright © 2015. Exclusive rights by McGraw-Hill Education, for manufacture and export. This book cannot be re-exported from the country to which it is consigned by McGraw-Hill Education. The International Edition is not available in North America.

In memory of Kim Michele Stern
Scott Stern

For Sarah, Ben, and Amelia
Adam Cifu

In memory of my father, Robert Seidman
Diane Altkorn

Contents

Contributing Authors

Jean-Luc Benoit, MD
Associate Professor of Medicine
Section of Infectious Diseases and Global Health
University of Chicago
Chicago, Illinois
AIDS/HIV Infection

Philip Hoffman, MD
Professor of Medicine
Section of Hematology-Oncology
University of Chicago
Chicago, Illinois
Bleeding Disorders
(Coauthored with Diane Altkorn)

Matthew Kalscheur, MD
Cardiovascular Medicine Fellow
University of Wisconsin Hospital and Clinics
Madison, Wisconsin
Hypotension
(Coauthored with Scott Stern)

Wei Wei Lee, MD
Assistant Professor of Medicine
Section of General Medicine
University of Chicago
Chicago, Illinois
Sore Throat
(Coauthored with Adam Cifu)

Amber Pincavage, MD
Assistant Professor of Medicine
Section of General Medicine
University of Chicago
Chicago, Illinois
Dysuria
(Coauthored with Adam Cifu)

Elizabeth Schulwolf, MD
Assistant Professor of Medicine
Division of Hospital Medicine
Loyola University Medical Center
Maywood, Illinois
Screening and Health Maintenance
(Coauthored with Diane Altkorn)

Sachin Shah, MD
Assistant Professor of Medicine
Section of General Medicine
University of Chicago
Chicago, Illinois
Hematuria
(Coauthored with Diane Altkorn)

Sarah Stein, MD
Associate Professor of Medicine
Section of Dermatology
University of Chicago
Chicago, Illinois
Rash
(Coauthored with Adam Cifu)

Preface

Our goal in creating *Symptom to Diagnosis* was to develop an interesting, practical, and informative approach to teaching the diagnostic process in internal medicine. Interesting, because real patient cases are integrated within each chapter, complementing what can otherwise be dry and soporific. Informative, because *Symptom to Diagnosis* articulates the most difficult process in becoming a physician: making an accurate diagnosis. Many other textbooks describe *diseases*, but fail to characterize the process that leads from patient presentation to diagnosis. Although students can, and often do, learn this process through intuition and experience without direct instruction, we believe that diagnostic reasoning is a difficult task that can be deciphered and made easier for students. Furthermore, in many books the description of the disease is oversimplified, and the available evidence on the predictive value of symptoms, signs, and diagnostic test results is not included. Teaching based on the classic presentation often fails to help less experienced physicians recognize the common, but atypical presentation. This oversight, combined with a lack of knowledge of test characteristics, often leads to prematurely dismissing diagnoses.

Symptom to Diagnosis aims to help students and residents learn internal medicine and focuses on the challenging task of diagnosis. Using the framework and terminology presented in Chapter 1, each chapter addresses one common complaint, such as chest pain. The chapter begins with a case and an explanation of a way to frame, or organize, the differential diagnosis. As the case progresses, clinical reasoning is clearly articulated. The differential diagnosis for that particular case is summarized in tables that delineate the clinical clues and important tests for the leading diagnostic hypothesis and important alternative diagnostic hypotheses. As the chapter progresses, the pertinent diseases are reviewed. Just as in real life, the case unfolds in a stepwise fashion as tests are performed and diagnoses are confirmed or refuted. Readers are continually engaged by a series of questions that direct the evaluation. Each chapter contains several cases and includes a diagnostic algorithm.

Symptom to Diagnosis can be used in three ways. First, it is designed to be read in its entirety to guide the reader through a third-year medicine clerkship. We used the Core Medicine Clerkship Curriculum Guide of the Society of General Internal Medicine/Clerkship Directors in Internal Medicine to select the symptoms and diseases we included, and we are confident that the text does an excellent job teaching the basics of internal medicine. Second, it is perfect for learning about a particular problem by studying an individual chapter. Focusing on one chapter will provide the reader with a comprehensive approach to the problem being addressed: a framework for the differential diagnosis, an opportunity to work through several interesting cases, and a review of pertinent diseases. Third, *Symptom to Diagnosis* is well suited to reviewing specific diseases through the use of the index to identify information on a particular disorder of immediate interest.

Our approach to the discussion of a particular disease is different than most other texts. Not only is the information bulleted to make it concise and readable, but the discussion of each disease is divided into 4 sections. The *Textbook Presentation*, which serves as a concise statement of the common, or classic, presentation of that particular disease, is the first part. The next section, *Disease Highlights*, reviews the most pertinent epidemiologic and pathophysiologic information. The third part, *Evidence-Based Diagnosis*, reviews the accuracy of the history, physical exam, and laboratory and radiologic tests for that specific disease. Whenever possible, we have listed the sensitivities, specificities, and likelihood ratios for these findings and test results. This section allows us to point out the findings that help "rule in" or "rule out" the various diseases. History and physical exam findings so highly specific that they point directly to a particular diagnosis are indicated with the following "fingerprint" icon:

$$\overset{\triangle}{\text{FP}} = \text{fingerprint}$$

We also often suggest a test of choice. It is this part of the book in particular that separates this text from many others. In the final section, *Treatment*, we review the basics of therapy for the disease being considered. Recognizing that treatment evolves at a rapid pace, we have chosen to limit our discussion to the fundamentals of therapy rather than details that would become quickly out of date.

The third edition differs from the second in several ways. First, there are five new chapters—Bleeding Disorders, Dysuria, Hematuria, Hypotension, and Sore Throat. Second, we have more clearly articulated the process of working from patient-level data (signs, symptoms, and laboratory tests) to an accurate diagnosis. This process includes greater use of algorithms, often very early in the chapters.

For generations the approach to diagnosis has been learned through apprenticeship and intuition. Diseases have been described in detail, but the approach to diagnosis has not been formalized. In *Symptom to Diagnosis* we feel we have succeeded in articulating this science and art and, at the same time, made the text interesting to read.

Scott D. C. Stern, MD
Adam S. Cifu, MD
Diane Altkorn, MD

Acknowledgments

We would like to thank our coauthors, who now number eight, for their hard work in expanding this text. We are grateful for the support of Harriet Lebowitz and James Shanahan at McGraw-Hill, who have helped us throughout this process and believed in our vision. Thanks to Jennifer Bernstein for her meticulous copyediting. Finally, our patients deserve special praise, for sharing their lives with us, trusting us, and forgiving us when our limited faculties err, as they inevitably do. It is for them that we practice our art.

Scott Stern: I would like to thank a few of the many people who have contributed to this project either directly or indirectly. First I would like to thank my wife Laura, whose untiring support throughout the last 32 years of our lives and during this project, made this work possible. Other members of my family have also been very supportive including my children Michael, David, and Elena; my parents Suzanne Black and Robert Stern; and my grandmother, Elsie Clamage. Two mentors deserve special mention. David Sischy shared his tremendous clinical wisdom and insights with me over 10 wonderful years that we worked together. David is the best diagnostician I have met and taught me more about clinical medicine than anyone else in my career. I remain in his debt. I would also like to note my appreciation to my late advisor, Dr. John Ultmann. Dr. Ultmann demonstrated the art of compassion in his dealings with patients on a day-to-day basis on a busy hematology-oncology service in 1983.

Adam Cifu: Excellent mentors are hard to find. I have been fortunate to find great ones throughout my life and career.

My parents gave me every opportunity imaginable. Claude Wintner taught me the importance of organization, dedication, and focus, and gave me a model of a gifted educator. Olaf Andersen nurtured my interest in science and guided my entry into medicine. Carol Bates showed me what it means to be a specialist in general medicine and a clinician educator. My family, Sarah, Ben, and Amelia, always remind me of what is most important. Thank you.

Diane Altkorn: I want to thank the students and house officers at the University of Chicago for helping me to continually examine and refine my thinking about clinical medicine and how to practice and teach it. I have been fortunate to have many wonderful mentors and teachers. I particularly want to mention Dr. Steven MacBride, who first taught me clinical reasoning and influenced me to become a general internist and clinician educator. As a resident and junior faculty member, I had the privilege of being part of Dr. Arthur Rubenstein's Department of Medicine at the University of Chicago. Dr. Rubenstein's commitment to excellence in all aspects of medicine is a standard to which I will always aspire. His kind encouragement and helpful advice have been invaluable in my professional development. Finally, I am grateful for my family. My parents have provided lifelong support and encouragement. My husband, Bob, is eternally patient and supportive of everything I do. And without my children Danny and Emily, my life would be incomplete.

I have a patient with a problem. How do I figure out the possible causes?

THE DIAGNOSTIC PROCESS

Constructing a differential diagnosis, choosing diagnostic tests, and interpreting the results are key skills for all physicians. The diagnostic process, often called clinical reasoning, is complex, and errors in reasoning are thought to account for 17% of all adverse events. Diagnostic errors can occur due to faulty knowledge, faulty data gathering, and faulty information processing. While this chapter will focus on the reasoning process, remember that the data you acquire through your history and physical exam, sometimes accompanied by preliminary laboratory tests, form the basis for your initial clinical impression. Even with flawless reasoning, your final diagnosis will be wrong if you do not start with accurate data. You must have well developed interviewing and physical examination skills.

Clinicians often use a combination of 2 reasoning processes: non-analytical/intuitive and analytical. The intuitive process is rapid and consists of an unconscious match to examples stored in memory, while the analytical process is slow, logical, and rule-based. Clinicians should be aware of common biases in clinical reasoning (Table 1-1) and reflect upon their reasoning processes, looking for potential errors. This chapter breaks down the reasoning process into a series of steps that can help you work through large differential diagnoses, avoid biases, and retrospectively identify sources of error when your diagnosis is wrong.

A MODEL FOR CLINICAL REASONING (Figure 1-1)

Step 1: Identify the Problem

Be certain you understand what the patient is telling you. Sometimes "I'm tired" means "I become short of breath when I walk" and at other times means "My muscles are weak." Construct a complete problem list consisting of the chief complaint, other acute symptoms and physical exam abnormalities, chronic active problems (such as diabetes or hypertension), and important past problems (such as history of bowel obstruction or cancer). Problems that are likely to be related, such as shortness of breath and chest pain, should be grouped together. It is necessary to accurately identify the problem every time you evaluate a patient.

Step 2: Frame the Differential Diagnosis

The differential diagnosis should be framed in a way that **facilitates recall.** It might be possible to memorize long lists of causes, or differential diagnoses, for various problems. However, doing so would not necessarily lead to a useful organization of differentials that helps you remember or use them. Instead, it is preferable to use some kind of *problem-specific framework* to organize differentials into subcategories that are easier to remember and often clinically useful. Problem-specific frameworks can be **anatomic,** a framework often used for chest pain; **organ/system,** used for symptoms with very broad differentials like fatigue; **physiologic;** or based on **pivotal points** (defined below). Each chapter in *Symptom to Diagnosis* begins with a problem-specific framework for the differential. Using such frameworks has been shown to improve the diagnostic accuracy of medical students.

Step 3: Organize the Differential Diagnosis

Structuring the differential diagnosis into **clinically useful subgroups** can enable you to systematically work through the differential diagnosis. Sometimes the framework that is easiest to remember, such as grouping causes of dyspnea as cardiac or pulmonary, does not facilitate reasoning. Then, reorganizing the differential in a way that helps you understand the order in which to consider various diagnoses is necessary. The most clinically useful differentials are organized using pivotal points, one of a pair of opposing descriptors that compare and contrast diagnoses, or clinical characteristics. Examples include old versus new headache, unilateral versus bilateral edema, and right lower quadrant pain versus epigastric pain. When pivotal points are used to frame the differential in the first place, it is not necessary to reorganize the differential.

You can frame and reorganize the differential yourself or find a source that does so in a way that makes sense to you. Each chapter in *Symptom to Diagnosis* contains a diagnostic algorithm that uses pivotal points to highlight logical reasoning pathways for each symptom. Steps 2 and 3 need to be done only once for each problem you encounter; with experience, you will develop a repertoire of logically framed differentials and structured diagnostic approaches.

Step 4: Limit the Differential Diagnosis

Since every disease in a differential may not be relevant to an individual patient, using **pivotal points** to create a **patient-specific** differential diagnosis can help narrow the list. Extracting pivotal points from the history and physical exam enables the clinician to limit a large, complete differential diagnosis to a more focused set of diagnoses pertinent to that particular patient. This step, and steps 5 through 9, should be included in your clinical reasoning for all patients.

Table 1-1. Common biases in clinical reasoning.

Name of Bias	Description
Availability	Considering easily remembered diagnoses more likely irrespective of prevalence
Base rate neglect	Pursuing "zebras"
Representativeness	Ignoring atypical features that are inconsistent with the favored diagnosis
Confirmation bias	Seeking data to confirm, rather than refute the initial hypothesis
Premature closure	Stopping the diagnostic process too soon

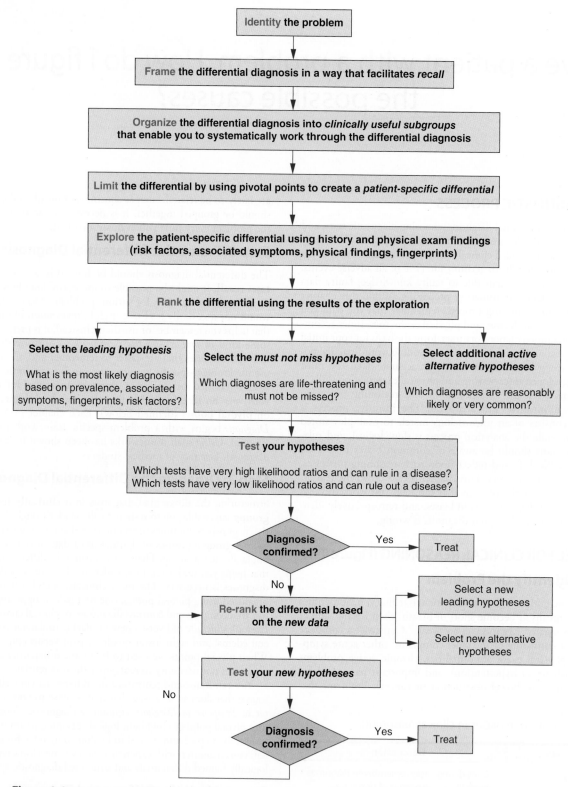

Figure 1-1. A model for clinical reasoning.

Step 5: Explore Possible Diagnoses Using History and Physical Exam Findings

The next step is to look for *clinical clues* that point toward the most likely diagnosis. Does the patient have risk factors for a particular diagnosis? Does the patient's description of the symptom suggest a likely cause? What have you observed on physical exam? *Focus on the positive—positive findings on history or physical exam are important* (65% of positive findings have a specificity > 80% and 43% of positive findings have a specificity > 90%). One-third have an LR+ > 5, and 16% have an LR+ > 10. Some very specific findings strongly suggest a specific diagnosis because they are rarely seen in patients without the disease, just as fingerprints point to a specific person because they are not seen in more than 1 individual. Such "fingerprint" findings will be marked with the symbol "FP" throughout the book. On the other hand, *do not be fooled by the negative; "classic" findings, especially individual findings, are often absent.* Only 21% of negative findings have a sensitivity > 80%, and only 11% of > 90%; just 7% have an LR– of < 0.1.

Step 6: Rank the Differential Diagnosis

Rank the differential diagnosis using the results obtained in Step 5. Even in a limited differential, not all diagnoses are equally likely or equally important. There are 4 approaches to ranking, or prioritizing, the differential diagnosis for a given problem: possibilistic, probabilistic, prognostic, and pragmatic.

A. **Possibilistic approach:** Consider all known causes equally likely and simultaneously test for all of them. This is not a useful approach.

B. **Probabilistic approach:** Consider first those disorders that are more likely; that is, those with the highest **pretest probability,** the probability that a disease is present before further testing is done.

C. **Prognostic approach:** Consider the most serious diagnoses first.

D. **Pragmatic approach:** Consider the diagnoses most responsive to treatment first.

Clearly there are limitations to each of these individual approaches. Experienced clinicians simultaneously integrate probabilistic, prognostic, and pragmatic approaches when reorganizing and prioritizing a differential diagnosis in order to decide when testing is necessary and which test to order (Table 1-2). Clinicians use their knowledge of pivotal points; "fingerprints"; risk factors; typical or "textbook" presentations of disease; the variability of disease presentation; and prevalence and prognosis to select a leading hypothesis, must not miss hypotheses, and other active alternative hypotheses.

Step 7: Test Your Hypotheses

Sometimes you are certain about the diagnosis based on the initial data and proceed to treatment. Most of the time, however, you require additional data to confirm your diagnostic hypotheses; in other words, you need to order diagnostic tests. Whenever you do so, you should understand how much the test will change the probability the patient has the disease in question.

Step 8: Re-rank the Differential Based on New Data

Remember, ruling out a disease is usually not enough; you must also determine the cause of the patient's symptom. For example, you may have eliminated myocardial infarction (MI) as a cause of chest pain, but you still need to determine whether the pain is due to gastroesophageal reflux, muscle strain, aortic dissection, etc. Whenever you have not made a diagnosis, or when you encounter data that conflict with your original hypotheses, go back to the complete differential diagnosis and reprioritize it, taking the new data into consideration. Failure to reconsider the possibilities is called premature closure (see Table 1-1), one of the most common diagnostic errors made by clinicians.

Step 9: Test the New Hypotheses

Repeat the process until a diagnosis is reached.

CONSTRUCTING A DIFFERENTIAL DIAGNOSIS

Step 1: Identify the Problem

Table 1-2. Ranking the differential diagnosis.

Diagnostic Hypotheses	Testing Implications
Leading Hypothesis	
• The most likely diagnosis based on prevalence, demographics, risk factors, symptoms and signs	Choose tests to confirm this disease • High specificity • High LR+
Active Alternatives	
• Diagnoses that are life-threatening—**must not miss** diagnoses	Choose tests to exclude these diseases • High sensitivity • Very low LR–
• Diagnoses with high prevalence—**most common** diagnoses	
• Diagnoses that are reasonably likely based on demographics, risk factors, symptoms and signs	
Other Hypotheses	
• Not excluded	Do not test for these diseases initially • Test later if the leading hypothesis and active alternatives are disproved
• Not serious, treatable, or likely enough to be tested for initially	
Excluded Hypotheses	
• Diagnoses disproved based on demographics, risk factors, symptoms and signs	No further testing necessary

PATIENT 1

Mrs. S is a 58-year-old woman who comes to an urgent care clinic complaining of painful swelling of her left calf that has lasted for 2 days. She feels slightly feverish but has no other symptoms such as chest pain, shortness of breath, or abdominal pain. She has been completely healthy except for hypertension, osteoarthritis of her knees, and a cholecystectomy, with no history of other medical problems, surgeries, or fractures. Her only medication is hydrochlorothiazide. She had a normal pelvic exam and Pap smear 1 month ago. Physical exam shows that the circumference of her left calf is 3.5 cm greater than her right calf, and there is 1+ pitting edema. The left calf is uniformly red and very tender, and there is slight tenderness along the popliteal vein and medial left thigh. There is a healing cut on her left foot. Her temperature is 37.7°C. The rest of her exam is normal.

What is Mrs. S's problem list?

Problem lists should begin with the acute problems, followed by chronic active problems, ending with inactive problems. Mrs. S's problems are (1) painful left leg edema with erythema, (2) hypertension, (3) osteoarthritis of the knees, and (4) status post cholecystectomy.

Step 2: Frame the Differential Diagnosis

How do you frame the differential diagnosis for edema?

As discussed in Chapter 17, Edema, the problem-specific organization of the full differential diagnosis starts with the distribution of the edema: generalized versus unilateral and limb versus localized. The causes of edema are fairly distinct for each of these subcategories. For instance, heart failure and chronic kidney disease cause generalized not unilateral edema.

Step 3: Organize the Differential Diagnosis

Since the edema differential is framed using the pivotal point of edema distribution, it is not necessary to organize it—step 3 has already been done.

Step 4: Limit the Differential Diagnosis

 What are the pivotal points in Mrs. S's presentation? How would you limit the differential?

Mrs. S has **acute unilateral leg** edema, a pivotal point that leads to a limited portion of the edema differential.

Diagnostic possibilities are now narrowed to a distinct subset of diseases that can be organized using an anatomic framework:

A. Skin: Stasis dermatitis

B. Soft tissue: Cellulitis

C. Calf veins: Distal deep venous thrombosis (DVT)

D. Knee: Ruptured Baker cyst

E. Thigh veins: Proximal DVT

F. Pelvis: Mass causing lymphatic obstruction

Step 5: Use History and Physical Exam Findings to Explore Possible Diagnoses

Consider the risk factors for each of the diagnostic possibilities as well as their associated symptoms and signs. For example, venous insufficiency is a risk factor for stasis dermatitis, and there may be hemosiderin staining along the malleolar surface on physical exam. Cellulitis often follows skin injury, and physical exam shows erythema and tenderness. DVT is more frequent in patients with underlying malignancy or recent immobilization, and there may be shortness of breath if the clot has embolized.

Step 6: Rank the Differential Diagnosis

 What are the important clinical clues in Mrs. S's presentation? How would you rank and prioritize the limited differential? What is your leading hypothesis? What are your active alternatives?

Mrs. S has a constellation of symptoms and signs supporting the diagnosis of cellulitis as the leading hypothesis: fever; an entry site for infection on her foot; and a red, tender, swollen leg. Even without risk factors for DVT, the active alternatives are proximal and calf DVT, being both common and "must not miss" diagnoses. If cellulitis and DVT are not present, ruptured Baker cyst and a pelvic mass should be considered. Finally, stasis dermatitis is excluded in a patient without a history of chronic leg swelling.

 How certain are you that Mrs. S has cellulitis? Should you treat her with antibiotics? How certain are you that she does not have DVT? Should you test for DVT?

THE ROLE OF DIAGNOSTIC TESTING

Step 7: Test Your Hypotheses

 I have a leading hypothesis and an active alternative—how do I know if I need to do a test or if I should start treatment?

Once you have generated a leading hypothesis, with or without active alternatives, you need to decide whether you need further information before proceeding to treatment or before excluding other diagnoses. One way to think about this is in terms of certainty: how certain are you that your hypothesis is correct, and how much more certain do you need to be before starting treatment? Another way to think about this is in terms of **probability:** is **your pretest probability** of disease high enough or low enough that you do not need any further information from a test?

Determine the Pretest Probability

There are several ways to determine the pretest probability of your leading hypothesis and most important (often most serious) active alternatives: use a validated clinical decision rule (CDR), use prevalence data regarding the causes/etiologies of a symptom, and use your overall clinical impression.

A. Use a validated CDR

1. Investigators construct a list of potential predictors of a disease, and then examine a group of patients to determine whether the predictors and the disease are present.

   a. Logistic regression is then used to determine which predictors are most powerful and which can be omitted.

   b. The model is then validated by applying it in other patient populations.

   c. To simplify use, the clinical predictors in the model are often assigned point values, and different point totals correspond to different pretest probabilities.

2. CDRs are infrequently available but are the most precise way of estimating pretest probability.

3. If you can find a validated CDR, you can come up with an exact number (or a small range of numbers) for your pretest probability.

B. Use information about the prevalence of etiologies for a symptom.

1. You can sometimes find this information in textbooks or review articles.

2. You can find studies providing this information by searching the symptom in question, combined with the term "differential diagnosis."

3. It is important to assess the quality of the studies you find before using the data. Guyatt's *Users' Guides to the Medical Literature* provides criteria for evaluating articles about differential diagnosis and disease frequency.

C. Use your overall clinical impression.

1. This is a combination of what you know about disease prevalence and the match between the expected history and physical with that of the patient, mixed with your clinical experience, and the ever elusive attribute "clinical judgment."

2. This is just as imprecise as it sounds, and it has been shown that physicians are disproportionately influenced by their most recent clinical experience.

3. Nevertheless, it has also been shown that the overall clinical impression of *experienced* clinicians has significant predictive value.

4. Clinicians generally categorize pretest probability as low, moderate, or high. This rather vague categorization is still helpful. Do not get distracted thinking a number is necessary.

Consider the Potential Harms

Consider the potential harms of both a missed diagnosis and the treatment.

A. It is very harmful to miss certain diagnoses, such as MI or pulmonary embolism, while it is not so harmful to miss others, such as mild carpal tunnel syndrome. You need to be very certain that life-threatening diseases are not present (that is, have a very low pretest probability), before excluding them without testing.

B. Some treatments, such as thrombolytics, are more harmful than others, such as oral antibiotics; you need to be very certain that potentially harmful treatments are needed (that is, the pretest probability is very high) before prescribing them without testing.

THE THRESHOLD MODEL: CONCEPTUALIZING PROBABILITIES

The ends of the bar in the threshold model represent 0% and 100% pretest probability. The **treatment threshold** is the probability above which the diagnosis is so likely you would treat the patient without further testing. The **test threshold** is the probability below which the diagnosis is so unlikely it is excluded without further testing (Figure 1-2).

For example, consider Ms. A, a 19-year-old woman, who complains of 30 seconds of sharp right-sided chest pain after lifting a heavy box. The pretest probability of cardiac ischemia is so low that no further testing is necessary (Figure 1-3).

Now consider Mr. B, a 60-year-old man, who smokes and has diabetes, hypertension, and 15 minutes of crushing substernal chest pain accompanied by nausea and diaphoresis, with an ECG showing ST-segment elevations in the anterior leads. The pretest probability of an acute MI is so high you would treat without further testing, such as measuring cardiac enzymes (Figure 1-4).

Diagnostic tests are necessary when the pretest probability of disease is in the middle, above the test threshold and below the treatment threshold. A really useful test shifts the probability of disease so much that the **posttest probability** (the probability of disease after the test is done) crosses one of the thresholds (Figure 1-5).

You are unable to find much information about estimating the pretest probability of cellulitis. You consider the potential risk of starting antibiotics to be low, and your overall clinical impression is that the pretest probability of cellulitis is high enough to cross the treatment threshold, so you start antibiotics.

You consider the pretest probability of DVT to be low, but not so low you can exclude it without testing, especially given the potential seriousness of this diagnostic possibility. You are able to find a CDR that helps you quantify the pretest probability, and calculate that her pretest probability is 17% (see Chapter 15).

You have read that duplex ultrasonography is the best noninvasive test for DVT. How good is it? Will a negative test rule out DVT?

Figure 1-2. The threshold model.

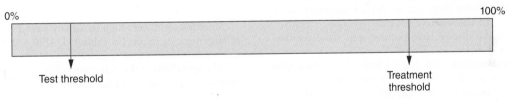

Figure 1-3. Ms. A's threshold model.

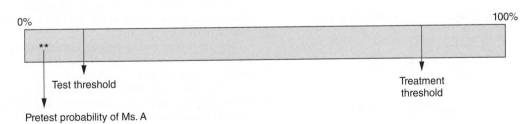

Figure 1-4. Mr. B's threshold model.

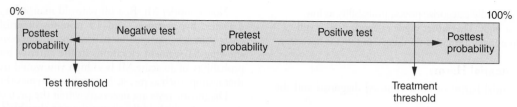

Figure 1-5. The role of diagnostic testing.

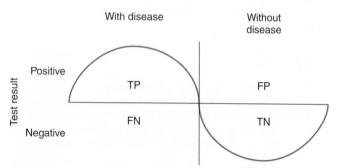

Figure 1-6. A perfect diagnostic test.

UNDERSTANDING TEST RESULTS

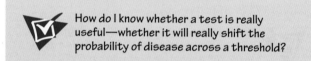

How do I know whether a test is really useful—whether it will really shift the probability of disease across a threshold?

A perfect diagnostic test would always be positive in patients with the disease and would always be negative in patients without the disease (Figure 1-6). Since there are no perfect diagnostic tests, some patients with the disease have negative tests (false-negative), and some without the disease have positive tests (false-positive) (Figure 1-7).

The **test characteristics** help you to know how often false results occur. They are determined by performing the test in patients known to have or not have the disease, and recording the distribution of results (Table 1-3).

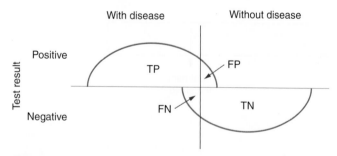

Figure 1-7. A pictorial representation of test characteristics.

Table 1-3. Test characteristics.

	Disease Present	**Disease Absent**
Test positive	True-positives	False-positives
Test negative	False-negatives	True-negatives

Table 1-4. Results for calculating the test characteristics of duplex ultrasonography.

	Proximal DVT Present	**Proximal DVT Absent**
Abnormal duplex US	TP = 86 patients	FP = 2 patients
Normal duplex US	FN = 4 patients	TN = 108 patients
	Total number of patients with DVT = 90	Total number of patients without DVT = 110

DVT, distal deep venous thrombosis ; FN, false-negative; FP, false-positive; TN, true-negative; TP, true-positive; US, ultrasound.

Table 1-4 shows the test characteristics of duplex ultrasonography for the diagnosis of proximal DVT, based on a hypothetical group of 200 patients, 90 of whom have DVT.

The **sensitivity** is the percentage of patients with DVT who have a true-positive (TP) test result:

Sensitivity = TP/total number of patients with DVT = 86/90 = 0.96 = 96%

Since tests with very high sensitivity have a very low percentage of false-negative results (in Table 1-4, 4/90 = 0.04 = 4%), a negative result is likely a true negative.

The **specificity** is the percentage of patients without DVT who have a true-negative (TN) test result:

Specificity = TN/total number of patients without DVT = 108/110 = 0.98 = 98%

Since tests with very high specificity have a low percentage of false-positive results (in Table 1-4, 2/110 = 0.02 = 2%), a positive result is likely a true positive.

The sensitivity and specificity are important attributes of a test, but they do not tell you whether the test result will change your pretest probability enough to move beyond the test or treatment thresholds; the shift in probability depends on the interactions between sensitivity, specificity, and pretest probability. The **likelihood ratio (LR),** the likelihood that a given test result would occur in a patient with the disease compared with the likelihood that the same result would occur in a patient without the disease, enables you to calculate how much the probability will shift.

The positive likelihood ratio (LR+) tells you how likely it is that a result is a true-positive (TP), rather than a false-positive (FP):

$$\textbf{LR+} = \frac{\text{TP/total with DVT}}{\text{FP/total without DVT}} = \frac{\%\text{TP}}{\%\text{FP}} = \frac{\textbf{sensitivity}}{1 - \textbf{specificity}} = \frac{0.96}{0.02} = 48$$

Positive LRs that are significantly above 1 indicate that a true-positive is much more likely than a false-positive, pushing you

0%   100%

Small LR−   Small LR+

Pretest
probability

Very small LR− (< 0.1)   Big LR+ (>10)

Test threshold   Treatment
threshold

Figure 1-8. Incorporating likelihood ratios (LRs) into the threshold model.

across the treatment threshold. An LR+ > 10 causes a large shift in disease probability; in general, tests with LR+ > 10 are very useful for ruling in disease. An LR+ between 5 and 10 causes a moderate shift in probability, and tests with these LRs are somewhat useful. "Fingerprints," findings that often rule in a disease, have very high positive LRs.

The negative likelihood ratio (LR−) tells you how likely it is that a result is a false-negative (FN), rather than a true-negative (TN):

$$LR- = \frac{FN/total\ with\ DVT}{TN/total\ without\ DVT} = \frac{\%FN}{\%TN} = \frac{1 - sensitivity}{specificity} = \frac{0.04}{0.98} = 0.04$$

Negative LRs that are significantly less than 1 indicate that a false-negative is much less likely than a true-negative, pushing you below the test threshold. An LR− less than 0.1 causes a large shift in disease probability; in general, tests with LR− less than 0.1 are very useful for ruling out disease. An LR− between 0.1 and 0.5 causes a moderate shift in probability, and tests with these LRs are somewhat useful.

The closer the LR is to 1, the less useful the test; tests with a LR = 1 do not change probability at all and are useless. The threshold model in Figure 1-8 incorporates LRs and illustrates how tests can change disease probability.

When you have a specific pretest probability, you can use the LR to calculate an exact posttest probability (see Box, Calculating an Exact Posttest Probability and Figure 1-9, Likelihood Ratio Nomogram). Table 1-5 shows some examples of how much LRs of different magnitudes change the pretest probability.

If you are using descriptive pretest probability terms such as low, moderate, and high, you can use LRs as follows:

A. A test with an LR− of 0.1 or less will rule out a disease of low or moderate pretest probability.

B. A test with an LR+ of 10 or greater will rule in a disease of moderate or high probability.

C. **Beware if the test result is the opposite of what you expected!**

1. If your pretest probability is high, a negative test rarely rules out the disease, no matter what the LR− is.

2. If you pretest probability is low, a positive test rarely rules in the disease, no matter what the LR+ is.

3. *In these situations, you need to perform another test.*

Mrs. S has a normal duplex ultrasound scan. Since your pretest probability was moderate and the LR− is < 0.1, proximal DVT has been ruled out. Since duplex ultrasound is less sensitive for distal than for proximal DVT, clinical follow-up is particularly important. Some clinicians repeat the duplex

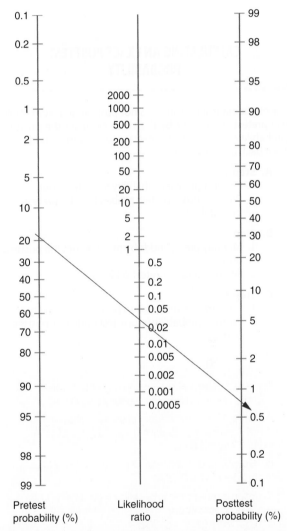

Figure 1-9. Likelihood ratio nomogram. Find the patient's pretest probability on the left, and then draw a line through the likelihood ratio for the test to find the patient's posttest probability.

ultrasound after 1 week to confirm the absence of DVT, and some clinicians order a D-dimer assay. When she returns for reexamination after 2 days, her leg looks much better, with minimal erythema, no edema, and no tenderness. The clinical response confirms your diagnosis of cellulitis, and no further diagnostic testing is necessary. (See Chapter 15 for a full discussion of the diagnostic approach to lower extremity DVT.)

Table 1-5. Calculating posttest probabilities using likelihood ratios (LRs) and pretest probabilities.

	Pretest Probability y = 5%	Pretest Probability y = 10%	Pretest Probability y = 20%	Pretest Probability y = 30%	Pretest Probability y = 50%	Pretest Probability y = 70%
LR = 10	34%	53%	71%	81%	91%	96%
LR = 3	14%	25%	43%	56%	75%	88%
LR = 1	5%	10%	20%	30%	50%	70%
LR = 0.3	1.5%	3.2%	7%	11%	23%	41%
LR = 0.1	0.5%	1%	2.5%	4%	9%	19%

CALCULATING AN EXACT POSTTEST PROBABILITY

For mathematical reasons, it is not possible to just multiply the pretest probability by the LR to calculate the posttest probability. Instead, it is necessary to convert to odds and then back to probability.

A. Step 1
1. Convert pretest probability to pretest odds.
2. Pretest odds = pretest probability/(1 − pretest probability).

B. Step 2
1. Multiply pretest odds by the LR to get the posttest odds.
2. Posttest odds = pretest odds × LR.

C. Step 3
1. Convert posttest odds to posttest probability.
2. Posttest probability = posttest odds/(1 + posttest odds).

For Mrs. S, the pretest probability of DVT was 17%, and the LR− for duplex ultrasound was 0.04.

A. Step 1: pretest odds = pretest probability/ (1 − pretest probability) = 0.17/(1 − 0.17) = 0.17/0.83 = 0.2

B. Step 2: posttest odds = pretest odds × LR = 0.2 × 0.04 = 0.008

C. Step 3: posttest probability = posttest odds/ (1 + posttest odds) = 0.008/(1 + 0.008) = 0.008/1.008 = 0.008

So Mrs. S's posttest probability of proximal DVT is 0.8%.

REFERENCES

Bowen JL. Educational strategies to promote clinical diagnostic reasoning. N Engl J Med. 2006;355:2217–25.

Coderre S, Jenkins D, McLaughlin K. Qualitative differences in knowledge structure are associated with diagnostic performance in medical students. Adv in Health Sci Educ. 2009;14:677–84.

Croskerry P. From mindless to mindful practice—cognitive bias and clinical decision making. N Engl J Med. 2013;368:2445–8.

Graber ML, Franklin N, Gordon R. Diagnostic error in internal medicine. Arch Intern Med. 2005;165:1493–9.

Guyatt G, Rennie D, Cook D. *Users Guides to the Medical Literature*, 2nd ed. McGraw Hill/JAMA. 2008.

Norman G, Eva K. Diagnostic error and clinical reasoning. Med Educ. 2010; 44:94–100.

Richardson WS, Wilson MC, Guyatt GH, Cook DJ, Nishikawa J; for the Evidence-Based Medicine Working Group. Users' Guides to the Medical Literature: XV. How to use an article about disease probability for differential diagnosis. JAMA. 1999;281:1214–9.

Sanders L. *Every Patient Tells a Story*. New York: Broadway Books; 2009.

2

I have a healthy patient. How do I determine which screening tests to order?

PATITENT

Mr. S is a healthy 45-year-old white man who wants to be "checked for everything."

How do you know when it is worthwhile to screen for a disease? Where do you find information on screening guidelines? How do you interpret screening guidelines?

It seems intuitive that it is best to prevent a disease from occurring at all and next best to diagnose and treat it early. However, there are risks and benefits to every intervention, and it is especially important to make sure an intervention is not going to harm a healthy individual. This chapter focuses on understanding the reasoning behind current screening practices.

A. Screening can be used to identify an unrecognized disease or risk factor in a seemingly well person.

B. Screening can be accomplished by collecting a thorough history, performing a physical examination, or obtaining laboratory tests.

C. Examples of screening include mammography and cholesterol testing.

  1. Mammography can detect unrecognized, asymptomatic breast cancer.

  2. Cholesterol testing can be used

    a. To identify high-risk individuals who do not yet have coronary disease (called primary prevention by clinicians).

    b. To prevent complications in patients with known coronary disease (called secondary prevention by clinicians, not actually screening).

D. The following criteria are helpful in determining whether screening for a disease is worthwhile:

  1. The burden of disease must be sufficient to warrant screening.

    a. Screen only for conditions that cause severe disease, disability, or death.

    b. Consider prevalence of target disease and ability to identify high-risk group since the yield of screening is higher in high-risk groups.

  2. The test used for screening must be of high quality.

    a. Screening tests should accurately detect the target disease when it is asymptomatic.

    b. Screening tests should have high sensitivity and specificity.

    c. Test results should be reproducible in a variety of settings.

    d. Screening tests must be safe and acceptable to patients.

    e. Ideally, screening tests should be simple and shown to be cost effective.

  3. There should be evidence that screening reduces morbidity or mortality.

    a. There must be effective treatment for the target disease.

    b. Early detection followed by treatment must improve survival compared with detection and treatment at the usual time of presentation; in other words, people in whom the condition was diagnosed by screening should have better health outcomes than those in whom the condition was diagnosed clinically.

    c. The benefits of screening must outweigh any adverse effects of the screening test, treatment, or impact of early diagnosis.

    d. Ideally, benefits and harms are evaluated through a randomized trial of screening (Figure 2-1).

      (1) The best outcome to measure is either all-cause mortality or disease-specific mortality, such as breast cancer or prostate cancer mortality.

      (2) Outcomes such as cancer stage distribution (ie, whether there are more or fewer early-stage cancers found) and length of survival after diagnosis can be misleading because of lead time and length time biases.

        (a) Lead time bias: If early treatment is not more effective than later treatment, the duration of time

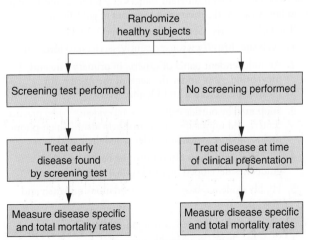

Figure 2-1. Design for a randomized trial of screening.

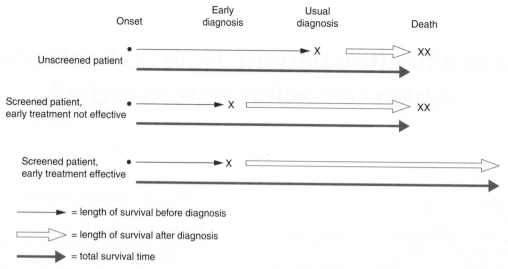

Figure 2-2. Lead time bias. (The total survival times for the unscreened patient and the screened patient in whom early treatment is not effective are the same. The total survival time for the screened patient in whom early treatment is effective is lengthened.)

the individual lives with the disease is longer, but the mortality rate is the same (Figure 2-2).

(b) Length time bias: Cancers that progress rapidly from onset to symptoms are less likely to be detected by screening than slow-growing cancers, so that screening tends to identify a group with a better prognosis.

e. Often, screening decisions are made based on less direct evidence, such as cohort or case-control studies. Given the biases inherent in these study designs, this is suboptimal and has led to the institution of screening programs that provide no benefit.

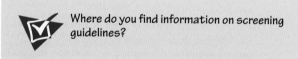 **Where do you find information on screening guidelines?**

Because of the complexity and rapid evolution of the evidence underlying screening recommendations, most physicians rely on published guidelines to inform them about screening decisions. Guidelines are developed and updated by a variety of organizations. It is important to be familiar with different sources of guidelines and to understand how to access the most recent versions of guidelines.

A. The US Preventive Services Task Force (USPSTF)

1. Web site: http://www.uspreventiveservicestaskforce.org/
2. An independent panel of experts in primary care and prevention, now under the aegis of the Agency for Healthcare Research and Quality (AHRQ)
3. Supported by outside experts, several evidence-based practice centers, and university centers that help identify high-priority topics, produce systematic reviews, and draft guidelines.
4. USPSTF guidelines often form the basis of clinical guidelines developed by professional societies.
5. Highly evidence-based recommendations on when and how to screen

B. The National Guideline Clearinghouse (NGC)

1. Web site: http://www.guideline.gov/
2. A public resource for evidence-based clinical practice guidelines

3. Sponsored by the AHRQ and US Department of Health and Human Services
4. A way to access and compare a variety of guidelines, including those written by USPSTF, professional societies, and other private organizations

C. Professional/specialty societies

1. Often do their own independent reviews and issue their own guidelines regarding relevant diseases
2. Specific guidelines generally available through the society Web site or the NGC
3. Examples include
   a. Specialty societies (eg, American College of Physicians [internal medicine], American College of Obstetrics and Gynecology, American College of Surgery)
   b. Subspecialty societies (eg, American Thoracic Society, American College of Rheumatology, American Urologic Association, American College of Gastroenterology, American College of Cardiology)
   c. Others (eg, American Cancer Society, American Diabetes Association, National Osteoporosis Foundation, American Heart Association)

 How do you interpret screening guidelines?

The USPSTF has developed a standardized system and vocabulary for evaluating the quality of the evidence addressing screening questions and for grading recommendations. The recommendation grade is based on a combination of the quality of the underlying evidence and an assessment of the size of the benefit. This general approach is often adopted by other organizations that make screening recommendations.

A. USPSTF levels of certainty regarding net benefit

1. High: Consistent results from well-designed studies in representative primary care populations that assess the effects of the preventive service on health outcomes; it is unlikely that these conclusions will change based on future studies.

2. Moderate: Evidence sufficient to determine the effects of the preventive service on health outcomes, but methodologic issues such as limited generalizability, inconsistent findings, or inadequate size or number of studies exist; these conclusions could change based on future studies.

3. Low: Insufficient evidence to assess effects on health outcomes, due to limited number or size of studies, flaws in study designs, inconsistency of findings, lack of generalizability.

B. Grades of recommendations

1. Grade A: The USPSTF recommends this service. There is high certainty that the net benefit is substantial.

2. Grade B: The USPSTF recommends this service. There is high certainty that the net benefit is moderate or there is moderate certainty that the net benefit is moderate to substantial.

3. Grade C: The USPSTF recommends selectively offering or providing this service to individual patients based on professional judgment and patient preferences. There is at least moderate certainty that the net benefit is small.

4. Grade D: The USPSTF recommends against the service. There is moderate or high certainty that the service has no net benefit or that the harms outweigh the benefits.

5. Grade I statement: The USPSTF concludes that the current evidence is insufficient to assess the balance of benefits and harms of the service. Evidence is lacking, of poor quality, or conflicting, and the balance of benefits and harms cannot be determined.

Mr. S feels fine and has no medical history. He takes no medications, does not smoke currently, and drinks occasionally. However, he did smoke occasionally in college, and he estimates he smoked a total of 2–3 packs of cigarettes over 4 years. He exercises regularly by cycling 50–100 miles/week. His family history is notable for high cholesterol, hypertension, and a cerebrovascular accident (CVA) in his father; his mother was diagnosed with colon cancer at age 54. His physical exam shows a BP of 120/80 mm Hg and pulse of 56 bpm. His body mass index (BMI) is 22 kg/m². HEENT, neck, cardiac, pulmonary, abdominal, and extremity exams are normal. He refuses a rectal exam. Mr. S shows you a list of tests he wants done, derived from research he has done on the Internet: lipid panel, prostate-specific antigen (PSA), chest radiograph, and fecal occult blood test (FOBT). In addition, he shows you a letter from a company offering "vascular screening" with ultrasounds of the carotids and aorta and wants to know if he should have those tests done.

 Should Mr. S be screened for prostate cancer with a PSA?

Prostate Cancer Screening

A. What is the burden of disease?

1. 240,000 new diagnoses of prostate cancer in 2011, with approximately 34,000 deaths

2. Second leading cause of cancer death in men in the United States

3. Lifetime risk of a prostate cancer diagnosis is about 15.9%; the lifetime risk of death is about 2.8%; autopsy studies suggest that 70% of men over age 70 have occult prostate cancer that did not impact their health status.

B. Is it possible to identify a high-risk group that might especially benefit from screening?

1. Older age increases the likelihood of prostate cancer but decreases the likelihood of death from prostate cancer (due to increased mortality from other causes).

   a. 200 cases/100,000 white men aged 50–59 compared with 900/100,000 men older than 70 years

   b. Mortality from untreated prostate cancer is 22–23% in men under the age of 71, 12% in men between the ages of 71 and 81, and only 4% in men older than 81 years.

2. African American race

   a. Higher prostate cancer incidence than white men: 217.5 vs 134.5 cases per 100,000

   b. Higher prostate cancer mortality than white men: 56.1 vs 23.4 deaths per 100,000

3. Family history: Relative risk of about 2 for men with a first-degree relative with prostate cancer; relative risk about 5 if 2 first-degree relatives affected.

C. What is the quality of the screening test?

1. Digital rectal exam (DRE)

   a. Sensitivity 59%

   b. Specificity unknown, but possibly as high as 94%; reproducibility poor

   c. Positive predictive value: 5–30%

   d. Neither sensitive nor specific enough to be used as a screening test, although may add to cancer detection when combined with PSA

2. PSA

   a. For a PSA ≥ 4.0 ng/mL, sensitivity is 68–80%, specificity 60–70%.

   b. Positive predictive values (PPVs) vary with PSA level.

      (1) For a PSA of 4–10 ng/mL, the PPV is about 25%.

      (2) For a PSA > 10 ng/mL, the PPV is 42–64%.

   c. Prostate cancer is found in some men even with very low PSA levels.

      (1) PSA ≤ 0.5 ng/mL: cancer in 6.6% of men, 12% of which was high grade

      (2) PSA 0.6–1.0 ng/mL: cancer in 10%

      (3) PSA 1.1–2.0 ng/mL: cancer in 17%

      (4) PSA 2.1–3.0 ng/mL: cancer in 24%, 19% of which was high grade

   d. PSA velocity (rate of change in PSA), PSA density (PSA per volume of prostate tissue measured on transrectal ultrasound or MRI), and free PSA (ratio of unbound to total PSA) are purported to increase PSA accuracy, but data are insufficient to recommend their use.

D. Does screening reduce morbidity or mortality?

1. Two large randomized controlled trials of PSA screening found lower grade cancers in the screened group.

2. The Prostate Lung Colorectal and Ovarian (PLCO) trial of 76,693 American men aged 55–74 years

   a. Annual PSA for 6 years and DRE for 4 years; 97% follow up at 7 years, 67% at 10 years

b. 50% of control group screened outside of trial, biasing the results against a positive effect of screening

c. Increased frequency of diagnosis, but no difference in prostate cancer mortality

3. European trial of 182,000 men aged 50–74 years

  a. PSA every 4 years; median follow-up 9 years

  b. Relative risk of prostate cancer death in screened group = 0.8 (95% CI, 0.67–0.98); absolute risk reduction = 0.7

  c. To prevent 1 prostate cancer death, 1410 patients would need to be screened and 48 cases diagnosed.

  d. In a separate analysis of just the Swedish patients in the trial, who were screened every 2 years, the relative risk of prostate cancer death was 0.56 (95% CI, 0.39–0.82), with an absolute risk reduction of 0.4; the number needed to screen was 293 and to diagnose was 12.

4. To compare benefits and risks of screening, consider 1000 men aged 55–69 screened with a PSA every 1–4 years.

  a. Prostate cancer will be diagnosed in 110.

  b. 100–120 will have at least 1 false-positive PSA requiring a biopsy.

  c. Erectile dysfunction due to treatment will develop in 29.

  d. Urinary incontinence due to treatment will develop in 18.

  e. 1 prostate cancer death will be avoided; without screening, 5 would die of prostate cancer; with screening, 4 would die of prostate cancer.

E. What are the current guidelines?

1. USPSTF (2012)

  a. Recommends against PSA screening for prostate cancer

  b. Grade D recommendation

2. American Cancer Society (2012)

  a. Asymptomatic men ≥ 50 years of age, with at least a 10-year life expectancy, should receive information on the issues regarding prostate cancer screening and then participate in informed decision making. Prostate cancer screening should not be done without an informed decision-making process.

  b. Men in higher risk groups should receive this information before age 50.

3. American College of Physicians (2012)

  a. Clinicians should inform men aged 50–69 years of the limited potential benefits and substantial harm of prostate cancer screening, and screen only those men who express a clear preference for screening.

  b. Clinicians should not screen average risk men under the age of 50, men over the age of 69, or men with a life expectancy of less than 10–15 years.

  c. Talking points to be used in discussions with patients can be found in Qaseem A et al (2012).

F. Table 2-1 summarizes information on staging, testing, histology, prognosis, and treatment of prostate cancer.

Table 2-1. Prostate cancer.

Staging	Stage	Definition
	I	Tumor confined within the prostate (T1–2); Gleason[1] ≤ 6; PSA < 10
	IIA	Tumor confined within the prostate (T1–2); Gleason[1] ≤ 7; PSA < 20
	IIB	Tumor confined within the prostate (T1–2); Gleason[1] ≥ 8; PSA ≥ 20
	III	Tumor extends through the prostate capsule and can invade seminal vesicle (T3); any Gleason[1] and any PSA
	IV	Tumor invades structures other than the seminal vesicles (T4) **or** any regional lymph node involvement **or** any distant metastasis

Commonly used tests	For diagnosis: Ultrasound-guided transrectal biopsy	For staging: Abdominal/pelvic CT scan Bone scan PSA

Histology
Adenocarcinoma (95%)
Small cell tumors
Intralobular acinar carcinoma
Ductal carcinoma
Clear cell carcinoma
Mucinous carcinoma

Prognosis
100% 5-year survival for tumors confined to the prostate
28.7% 5-year survival for metastatic disease
Most men die of other diseases, rather than the prostate cancer

Treatment
Stage 1
- Watchful waiting
- Radical prostatectomy
- External-beam radiation therapy (EBRT)
- Implantation of radiation seeds directly into prostate

Stage 2
- Same options as Stage 1
- Additional option of adding hormonal therapy to EBRT

Stage 3
- Same as stage 2
- Consider orchiectomy as method to reduce hormonal stimulation of the cancer

Stage 4
- Palliative radiation or transurethral resection of the prostate
- Hormonal therapies
- Bisphosphonates

[1]Gleason score: Gleason scoring for adenocarcinomas ranges from grade 1 (well-differentiated) to grade 5 (very poorly differentiated). The tumor is assigned a grade based on predominant histology and the second most predominant histology. These 2 numbers are scored yielding a total from 2 to 10. Example, predominant histology is well differentiated with areas of very poorly differentiated is reported as 1+5=8. PSA, prostate-specific antigen.

You review the small potential benefit and significant potential harms of screening with Mr. S, also pointing out that none of the guidelines recommend even discussing PSA testing before age 50 in white men without an affected first-degree relative.

 Should Mr. S be screened for colorectal cancer with fecal occult blood testing?

Colon Cancer Screening

A. What is the burden of disease?

1. Third most common cancer in the United States and second leading cause of death from cancer

2. About 102,900 diagnoses in 2010, with about 51,000 deaths each year

3. Americans have a 5% lifetime risk of developing colorectal cancer; 90% of cases occur after age 50

4. 80–95% of colorectal cancers arise from adenomatous polyps

   a. 10% of polyps > 1 cm become malignant in 10 years; 25% do so after 20 years

   b. Adenomas found in 40% of adults by age 60

   c. Advanced adenomas, defined as those ≥ 10 mm or having high-grade dysplasia or a villous component, are the most likely to develop into carcinoma.

B. Is it possible to identify a high-risk group that might especially benefit from screening? (Tables 2-2 and 2-3)

1. 20% of colorectal cancers occur in patients with specific risk factors.

   a. History of either colorectal cancer or adenomatous polyps in a first-degree relative, especially if diagnosed before age 60

   b. Personal history of adenomatous polyps

   c. Long-standing ulcerative colitis

2. 6% occur in patients with rare genetic syndromes, such as familial polyposis or hereditary nonpolyposis colorectal cancer (HNPCC).

   a. Colorectal cancer develops in 80% of patients with HNPCC by age 50 years.

Table 2-2. Questions that help identify patients at high risk for colorectal cancer.

Has the patient had colorectal cancer or an adenomatous polyp?
Does the patient have an illness, such as inflammatory bowel disease, that increases the risk of colorectal cancer?
Has colorectal cancer or an adenomatous polyp been diagnosed in a family member? 　Was it a first-degree relative (parent, sibling, or child)? 　At what age was the cancer or polyp first diagnosed? 　How many first-degree relatives have been diagnosed?

Table 2-3. Magnitude of risk for colorectal cancer.

Risk Factor	Approximate Relative Risk of Colorectal Cancer
None	Baseline risk = 5%
One first-degree relative with colon cancer	2–3
Two first-degree relatives with colon cancer	3–4
First-degree relative aged ≤ 50 at cancer diagnosis	3–4
One second- or third-degree relative with colon cancer	1.5
Two second-degree relatives with colon cancer	2–3
One first-degree relative > age 60 with an adenoma	1.8
One first-degree relative < age 60 with an adenoma	2.6

   b. The mutation associated with HNPCC also increases the risk of cancer of the uterus, ovary, ureter, renal pelvis, stomach, small bowel, and bile duct.

   c. Familial polyposis patients have diffuse colonic polyps at an early age, and colorectal cancer will develop without intervention.

3. The remaining colorectal cancers occur sporadically.

C. What is the quality of the screening test?

1. Guaiac-based FOBT

   a. Two distinct samples of 3 different stools are applied to 6 test card panels.

   b. If Hgb is present, a blue color appears when hydrogen peroxide is added.

   c. False-negative tests can occur if the patient has ingested > 250 mg of vitamin C, and false-positive tests occur with use of aspirin, nonsteroidal antiinflammatory drugs (NSAIDs), and ingestion of red meat.

   d. "Low sensitivity" tests, such as Hemocult II have a sensitivity of 25–38% and specificity of 98%.

   e. "High sensitivity" tests, such as Hemoccult SENSA, have a sensitivity of 64–80% and specificity of 87–90%.

   f. Annual screening detected 49% of cancers; biannual screening detected 27–39% of cancers.

   g. A single panel test after a DRE has a sensitivity of 9% and should never be considered an adequate screening test for colorectal cancer.

2. Immunochemical FOBT

   a. Requires 1–2 stool samples instead of 3; optimal interval for screening is not known.

   b. Several qualitative immunochemical FOBT tests are available in the United States; in general, they are more sensitive than guaiac-based FOBT with similar specificities; quantitative testing is not available in the United States.

3. Flexible sigmoidoscopy

   a. Examines approximately the first 60 cm of the colon; patients with polyps are referred for a full colonoscopy.

   b. Only 20–30% of proximal cancers are associated with a distal adenoma.

   c. However, sigmoidoscopy has been found to identify 66% of men with significant findings in the colon, assuming finding a polyp triggers a full colonoscopy; only 55% of lesions in women would be identified because cancers in women are more often proximal.

   d. Detects 7 cancers and about 60 large (> 1 cm) polyps/1000 examinations

   e. Bowel perforation rate is 0.88/1000 sigmoidoscopies

   f. Serious complication rate (deaths or events requiring hospital admission) 3.4/10,000 procedures

4. Combined FOBT and sigmoidoscopy

   a. 7 additional cancers/1000 examinations compared with sigmoidoscopy alone

   b. Did not improve yield at initial screening exam

5. Colonoscopy

   a. Miss rate of 5% for cancers, 2% for adenomas ≥ 1 cm, 13% for adenomas 6–9 mm, and 25% for those < 5 mm (based on studies of tandem colonoscopies by 2 examiners)

   b. Complication rates

      (1) Major complications (perforation or bleeding) is 1/1000 procedures

      (2) Perforation rate is 0.6/1000 procedures, with the risk being 4 times higher if polypectomy is performed.

      (3) Bleeding occurs in 8.7/1000 colonoscopies with polypectomy.

6. Double-contrast barium enema

   a. Sensitivity = 48%

   b. Specificity = 85%

   c. Perforation rate = 1/25,000

7. CT colonography

   a. CT scanning with 2- and 3-dimensional image display

   b. Requires same bowel preparation as colonoscopy

   c. A small rectal catheter is inserted for air insufflation, but no sedation is required.

   d. Sensitivity for cancer = 96%

   e. Sensitivity for polyps ≥ 10 mm = 85–93%, with specificity 97%

   f. Sensitivity for polyps 6–9 mm = 70–86%, with specificity 86–93%

D. Does screening reduce morbidity or mortality?

1. Guaiac-based FOBT

   a. 3 large randomized trials show reduced colorectal cancer mortality.

   b. Relative risk reduction of colorectal cancer death: 15–33%

   c. Number needed to screen = 217 for annual screening, 344–1250 for biennial screening

2. Flexible sigmoidoscopy

   a. A meta-analysis of five randomized trials showed that the relative risk of colorectal cancer mortality was 0.72 in the screened group.

   b. The PLCO Screening Trial randomized nearly 155,000 persons aged 55–74 to sigmoidoscopy every 3–5 years or to usual care. The relative risk of colorectal cancer mortality was 0.74 in the screened group (absolute reduction from 3.9 to 2.9 colorectal cancer deaths/10,000 person years).

3. Combination guaiac-based FOBT and sigmoidoscopy

   a. In 1 randomized trial, more cancers were found with the combination of guaiac-based FOBT and sigmoidoscopy vs guaiac-based FOBT alone.

   b. Colorectal cancer mortality was not an endpoint.

4. Colonoscopy

   a. No randomized trial data

   b. 1 case-control study showed lower incidence of colon cancer (OR = 0.47) and lower colorectal cancer mortality (OR = 0.43).

   c. A 2009 case-control study found a reduction in death for colorectal cancers in the left colon (OR = 0.33) but not the right colon (OR = 0.99); other case-control studies have found similar reductions in both left- and right-sided late-stage cancers.

   d. Generally assumed that the mortality reductions seen in the FOBT trials is actually due to the follow-up colonoscopies.

5. Double-contrast barium enema: no outcome data available

6. CT colonography

   a. No randomized trial data available

   b. 1 nonrandomized study showed that rates of detection of advanced adenomas + cancers were similar in patients screened with CT colonography (3.2%) compared with conventional colonoscopy (3.4%).

7. Potential harms of screening include the complication rates noted previously, complications of sedation used for colonoscopy, radiation exposure, and patient discomfort.

E. What are the current guidelines?

1. USPSTF (2008)

   a. Strongly recommends screening average risk men and women beginning at age 50 years and continuing to age 75 years, using FOBT, sigmoidoscopy, or colonoscopy

      (1) Grade A recommendation

      (2) Insufficient data to assess the benefits and harms of CT colonography and fecal DNA testing as screening modalities (I recommendation)

   b. Recommends against routine screening in adults age 76–85 years (C recommendation)

   c. Recommends against screening in adults older than age 85 years (D recommendation)

2. American Cancer Society (2008)

   a. Begin screening at age 50

   b. Acceptable strategies include annual FOBT alone (either guaiac based or immunochemical), annual FOBT plus sigmoidoscopy every 5 years, sigmoidoscopy alone every 5 years, colonoscopy every 10 years, CT colonography every 5 years, or double-contrast barium enema every 5 years.

   c. Imaging procedures that can detect both adenomatous polyps and cancer are preferred over stool tests that primarily detect cancer.

Table 2-4. Colonoscopic surveillance of polyps found at the baseline exam.

Pathology	Recommended Surveillance Interval (years)
< 10 mm hyperplastic polyps	10
1–2 small (< 10 mm) tubular adenomas	5–10
Sessile serrated polyp(s) < 10 mm	5
3–10 tubular adenomas > 10 adenomas ≥ 1 large (≥ 10 mm) tubular adenoma or sessile serrated polyp ≥ 1 villous adenomas Adenoma with high-grade dysplasia	3

3. American College of Gastroenterology (2009)

   a. Begin screening at age 50 in average risk adults and at age 45 in African-Americans; repeat every 10 years.

   b. Begin screening at age 40, repeating every 5 years, (or 10 years younger than the age of the youngest affected relative) in adults with

      (1) 1 first-degree relative with colorectal cancer or an advanced adenoma (≥ 1 cm, high-grade dysplasia, villous elements) diagnosed at < 60 years of age.

      (2) 2 first-degree relatives with colorectal cancer or advanced adenomas at any age.

   c. Colonoscopy is the preferred method; flexible sigmoidoscopy, CT colonography, and stool tests are acceptable alternatives.

   d. Surveillance after polypectomy (Table 2-4)

F. Table 2-5 summarizes information on staging, testing, histology, prognosis, and treatment of colon cancer.

You explain to Mr. S that because colon cancer was diagnosed in his mother when she was 54 years old, his risk of developing colon cancer during his lifetime is increased from about 6% to somewhere between 12% and 18%. Although fecal occult blood testing alone is an acceptable screening strategy for low-risk individuals, all of the expert guidelines recommend screening colonoscopy for patients with his risk profile.

 Should Mr. S be screened for hyperlipidemia with a lipid panel?

Cholesterol Screening

A. What is the burden of disease?

   1. Coronary heart disease (CHD) is the leading cause of death in the United States.

   2. Overall costs of CHD and stroke in 2003 estimated to be > $50 billion.

Table 2-5. Colon cancer.

Staging	Stage	Definition
	Stage 0	Confined to the innermost layer of the colon (carcinoma in situ)
	Stage I	Cancer is in the inner layers of the colon
	Stage II	Cancer has spread through the muscularis mucosa
	Stage III	Cancer has metastasized to the lymph nodes
	Stage IV	Distant metastasis
Commonly used tests	**For diagnosis:** Colonoscopy	**For staging:** Abdominal/pelvic CT scan
Histology	Adenocarcinoma (> 90%) • Well differentiated (10%) • Moderately differentiated (70%) • Poorly differentiated (20%) Mucinous adenocarcinoma Signet ring adenocarcinoma Medullary carcinoma	
Prognosis	Overall 1-year survival is 84% Overall 5-year survival is 64% Stage 1 5-year survival is 90% Stage IV 5-year survival is 12%	
Treatment	Local resection or polypectomy for stage 0 Resection of involved colon for stages I–II Resection of involved colon possibly followed by chemotherapy for stage III Resection of the involved colon and isolated metastases when possible, often followed by chemotherapy for stage IV	

3. Lifetime risk of a CHD event, calculated at age 40 years, is 49% for men and 32% for women; nearly one-third of CHD events are attributable to total cholesterol > 200 mg/dL.

B. Is it possible to identify a high-risk group that might especially benefit from screening?

   1. The low-density lipoprotein (LDL) and high-density lipoprotein (HDL) levels themselves are independent risk factors for CHD, with the increased risk being continuous and linear.

      a. For every 38 mg/dL increase in LDL above 118 mg/dL, the relative risk for CHD is 1.42 in men and 1.37 in women.

      b. For every 15.5 mg/dL increase in HDL above 40 mg/dL in men, the relative risk for CHD is 0.64.

      c. For every 15.5 mg/dL increase in HDL above 51 mg/dL in women, the relative risk for CHD is 0.69.

      d. Total cholesterol–HDL ratio

         (1) In men, a ratio ≥ 6.4 was associated with a 2–14% greater risk than predicted from total cholesterol or LDL alone.

         (2) In women, a ratio ≥ 5.6 was associated with a 25–45% greater risk than predicted from total cholesterol or LDL alone.

   2. Patients with established atherosclerotic cardiovascular disease (ASCVD), defined as acute coronary syndrome, a history

of myocardial infarction, stable angina, coronary or other arterial revascularization, stroke, transient ischemic attack, or peripheral arterial disease, are in the highest risk category.

3. Patients without established ASCVD should have a global risk score calculated.

 a. The American College of Cardiology/American Heart Association (ACC/AHA) 2013 guidelines recommend the Pooled Cohort Equations, a new risk assessment tool that estimates the 10-year risk of a first ASCVD event, defined as nonfatal myocardial infarction or coronary heart disease death or fatal or nonfatal stroke.

 (1) Derived and validated in non-Hispanic whites and non-Hispanic African Americans

 (2) Can use the equations developed for non-Hispanic whites in other populations, although risk assessments may not be as accurate

 (3) Found at http://my.americanheart.org/cvriskcalculator

 b. The Framingham Risk Score is another commonly used calculator available at http://cvdrisk.nhlbi.nih.gov/calculator.asp.

 (1) Validated in populations over age 40

 (2) Unclear if it can be used in conjunction with the new ACC/AHA guidelines described below.

C. What is the quality of the screening test?

1. Total cholesterol and HDL are minimally affected by eating and can be measured in fasting or nonfasting individuals.

2. Triglycerides may be increased 20–30% by eating and must be measured in the fasting state.

3. LDL can be directly measured but is most commonly estimated using the following equation, which is valid only when the fasting triglycerides are less than 400 mg/dL: total cholesterol − (triglycerides/5 + HDL) = LDL.

4. Total cholesterol may vary by 6% in day-to-day measurements, with HDL varying as much as 7.5%; clinicians should obtain 2 measurements before starting therapy.

D. Does screening reduce morbidity or mortality?

1. In meta-analyses of primary prevention studies of statin drug therapy, including only patients without established coronary artery disease,

 a. All cause mortality is reduced by 14%, with a number needed to treat over 5 years of 138.

 b. Total cardiovascular disease events are reduced by 25%, with a number needed to treat over 5 years of 49.

 c. CHD events are reduced by 27%, with a number needed to treat over 5 years of 88.

2. No evidence that diet therapy reduces CHD events in primary prevention populations.

 a. Maximum expected cholesterol reduction with diet therapy is 10–20%.

 b. Most trials achieve an average reduction of about 5%.

E. What are the current guidelines?

1. USPSTF (2008)

 a. Screen all men at age 35 and women with risk factors at age 45.

 (1) Grade A recommendation

 (2) Good evidence that screening can identify asymptomatic people at increased risk for coronary

artery disease and that lipid-lowering drug therapy decreases the incidence of CHD.

 b. Screen men aged 20–35 and women aged 20–45 if other risk factors are present.

 (1) Grade B recommendation

 (2) Other risk factors include diabetes, family history of cardiovascular disease before age 50 in male relatives or age 60 in female relatives, family history suggestive of familial hyperlipidemia, obesity (BMI ≥ 30 kg/m²), presence of multiple other risk factors (eg, hypertension, smoking).

 c. No recommendation regarding screening younger adults without risk factors (grade C recommendation).

 d. Screening should include measurement of total cholesterol and HDL.

 e. Optimal screening interval unclear

2. ACC/AHA (2013)

 a. The ACC/AHA issued updated risk assessment guidelines in 2013 for patients *without* ASCVD.

 (1) Adults aged 20–79 should be assessed every 4–6 years for traditional ASCVD risk factors: total and HDL cholesterol, systolic BP, use of antihypertensive therapy, diabetes, current smoking.

 (2) Adults aged 40–79 should have an assessment of ASCVD risk every 4–6 years, using the Pooled Cohort Equations.

 (3) In selected individuals in whom there is uncertainty regarding initiation of pharmacologic therapy based on the Pooled Cohort Equations assessment, one can consider additional risk factors:

 (i) Family history of premature cardiovascular disease (first-degree male relative < 55 years of age; first-degree female relative < 65 years of age)

 (ii) High sensitivity C-reactive protein ≥ 2 mg/L

 (iii) Coronary artery calcium score ≥ 300 Agatston units or ≥ 75th percentile for age, sex, and ethnicity

 (iv) Ankle-brachial index < 0.9

 b. The 2013 treatment guidelines are summarized in Chapter 23, Hypertension.

3. American College of Physicians (2012)

 a. Screen all men ≥ 35 years of age and all women ≥ 45 years of age with a fasting lipid panel.

 b. Screen at an earlier age in patients with multiple risk factors, including obesity, or family history of premature coronary artery disease (clinical CHD before the age of 55 in a parent or grandparent).

 c. Repeat lipid screening every 5 years, or when the patient's risk factor profile changes

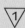

You agree with Mr. S that a fasting lipid panel is an important screening test to do for men over 45, even in the absence of other risk factors.

 Should Mr. S have a screening chest radiograph?

Lung Cancer Screening

A. What is the burden of disease?

1. Lung cancer is leading cause of cancer death in both men and women.

2. About 160,000 deaths from lung cancer in 2012, more than the number of deaths from breast, prostate, and colon cancer combined.

3. Prognosis of non-stage I lung cancers is poor.

B. Is it possible to identify a high-risk group that might especially benefit from screening?

1. Cigarette smoking is responsible for about 85% of lung cancers.

   a. Compared with nonsmokers, relative risk of developing lung cancer is about 20.

   b. A 65-year-old who has smoked 1 pack/day for 50 years has a 10% risk of developing lung cancer over the next 10 years.

   c. A 75-year-old who has smoked 2 packs/day for 50 years has a 15% risk.

2. Other risk factors include family history of lung cancer and exposure to asbestos, nickel, arsenic, haloethers, polycyclic aromatic hydrocarbons, and environmental cigarette smoke.

C. What is the quality of the screening test?

1. Chest radiograph: sensitivity = 60%, specificity = 94%

2. CT scan: sensitivity = 94%, specificity = 73%

D. Does screening reduce morbidity or mortality?

1. 6 randomized trials of chest radiography, with or without sputum cytology, failed to demonstrate a decrease in lung cancer mortality; all were limited by the control population undergoing some screening.

2. National Lung Screening Trial (NLST)

   a. Over 53,000 *asymptomatic* subjects aged 55–74 with ≥ 30 pack year smoking history; former smokers must have quit within the past 15 years

   b. Exclusions: previous lung cancer, other cancer within the last 5 years, CT scan within the last 18 months, metallic implants in the chest or back, home oxygen use, pneumonia, or other acute upper respiratory tract infection treated with antibiotics within the last 12 weeks

   c. Randomized to 3 annual screenings with low-dose CT scan or single view posteroanterior chest film; an abnormal screen was defined as a nodule ≥ 4 mm

   d. Lung cancer–specific mortality was significantly reduced in the low-dose CT group.

      (1) CT group lung cancer mortality rate = 1.3%, compared to 1.6% in the chest film group

      (2) Relative risk reduction = 20%; absolute risk reduction of 3 lung cancer deaths per 1000 patients screened with CT; number needed to screen to prevent 1 lung cancer death = 320

   e. Nearly 40% of participants had at least 1 positive CT result; 96% of these were false positives. Most false-positive results were resolved by follow-up CT scans, although some patients required biopsies.

E. What are the current guidelines?

1. USPSTF (2013)

   a. Annual screening with low-dose CT in adults ages 55–80 who have a 30 pack-year smoking history and currently smoke or have quit within the past 15 years.

   b. Screening should be discontinued once a person has not smoked for 15 years or develops a health problem substantially limiting life expectancy or ability to have curative lung surgery.

   c. Grade B recommendation

2. American College of Chest Physicians, American Cancer Society, and American Society of Clinical Oncology (2012): discuss screening with patients who meet the NLST eligibility criteria described above

F. Table 2-6 summarizes information on staging, testing, histology, prognosis, and treatment of lung cancer.

You explain to Mr. S that there have been no studies showing that screening chest radiographs reduce lung cancer deaths in smokers, much less in nonsmokers. You add that he does not meet NLST criteria and so should not be screened for lung cancer.

 Should Mr. S be screened for abdominal aortic aneurysm and carotid artery stenosis with ultrasonography?

Abdominal Aortic Aneurysm (AAA) Screening

A. What is the burden of disease?

1. 4–8% of older men and 0.5–1.5% of older women have an AAA.

2. AAA accounts for about 9000 deaths per year in the United States.

   a. 1-year rupture rates are 9% for AAAs 5.5–5.9 cm, 10% for 6–6.9 cm, and 33% for AAAs ≥ 7 cm.

   b. Only 10–25% of patients with ruptured AAA survive to hospital discharge.

B. Is it possible to identify a high-risk group that might especially benefit from screening?

1. Age > 65, ever smoking (≥ 100 lifetime cigarettes), male sex, and family history are the strongest risk factors for an AAA > 4.0 cm.

   a. The OR increases by 1.7 for each 7-year age interval.

   b. Current or past smoking increases the risk of AAA by 3–5.

   c. The prevalence of AAA increases more rapidly with age in ever smokers than in never smokers.

   d. The prevalence of AAA > 4 cm in never smokers is < 1% for all ages.

   e. The OR is 1.94 for a positive family history.

   f. The OR is ~1.3–1.5 for history of coronary artery disease, hypercholesterolemia, or cerebrovascular disease.

   g. The OR is 0.53 for black persons and 0.52 for patients with diabetes.

C. What is the quality of the screening test?

1. Ultrasonography has a sensitivity of 95% and specificity of 100% for the detection of AAA, defined as an infrarenal aortic diameter > 3.0 cm.

2. One-time screening is sufficient since cohort studies of repeated screening have shown that over 10 years, the incident rate for new AAAs is 4%, with no AAAs of > 4.0 cm found.

3. Abdominal palpation is not reliable.

Table 2-6. Lung cancer.

Staging	Stage	Definition
	IA (T1N0M0)	Tumor size ≤ 3 cm surrounded by lung parenchyma; no evidence of bronchial invasion
	IB (T2N0M0)	Tumors > 3 cm or any size that invades visceral pleura or main bronchus
	IIA (T1N1M0)	Tumor size ≤ 3 cm with involvement of peribronchial or hilar lymph nodes
	IIB (T2N1M0 and T3 N0 M0)	Tumor size > 3 cm with involvement of peribronchial or hilar lymph nodes
	IIIA (T3N1M0 and T1,2,3 N2 M0)	Tumors with localized, circumscribed extrapulmonary extension with involvement of peribronchial or hilar nodes **or** any tumor with involvement of ipsilateral mediastinal and subcarinal nodes
	IIIB (T4 any N, M0; any T3 M0)	Extensive extrapulmonary tumor invasion of mediastinal structures
	Stage IV	Any distant metastasis
Commonly used tests	**For diagnosis:** Biopsy methods • Bronchoscopy • Mediastinoscopy • Anterior mediastinotomy	**For staging:** CT scan to the level of the adrenal glands (sensitivity 51%, specificity 86% for mediastinal nodes) Positron emission tomography (sensitivity 74%, specificity 85% for mediastinal nodes)
Histology	Small cell (20–25%) Non–small cell • Squamous (25%) • Adenocarcinoma (40%) • Large cell adenocarcinoma (10%)	
Prognosis	Based on stage at diagnosis Overall 5-year survival is 16% because only 15% are diagnosed at a localized stage when the overall survival is 52%	
Treatment	Resection for local disease Adjuvant chemotherapy after resection for stages IIA–IIIA Chemotherapy + radiation for nonresectable stage III Chemotherapy + palliative care for stage IV	

D. Does screening reduce morbidity or mortality?

1. A meta-analysis of 4 randomized controlled trials of screening for AAA in men showed a reduction in mortality from AAA, with a pooled OR of 0.57 (95% CI, 0.45–0.74).

   a. Overall in-hospital mortality for open AAA repair is 4.2%; lower mortality is seen in high volume centers performing > 35 procedures/year (3% mortality vs 5.5% in low volume centers) and when vascular surgeons perform the repair (2.2% for vascular surgeons, 4.0% for cardiac surgeons, 5.5% for general surgeons).

   b. 30-day postoperative mortality is higher with open repair than with endovascular repair (2% absolute risk increase, number needed to harm = 50). There are no differences in long-term all-cause mortality or cardiovascular mortality, or in rates of stroke; therefore, endovascular repair is preferred.

2. There was no reduction in all cause mortality, or in AAA-specific mortality in women.

E. What are the current guidelines?

1. USPSTF (2005)

   a. One-time screening by ultrasonography in men age 65–75 who have ever smoked

   b. Grade B recommendation, based on good evidence of decreased AAA-specific mortality with screening

2. Society of Vascular Surgery (2009)

   a. One-time screening for all men over 65 (at 55 if family history is positive)

   b. One-time screening for women over 65 who have smoked or have a positive family history

Carotid Artery Stenosis (CAS) Screening

A. What is the burden of disease?

1. The estimated prevalence of significant CAS (60–99%) in the general population is about 1%.

2. The contribution of significant CAS to morbidity or mortality from stroke is not known, nor is the natural progression of asymptomatic CAS.

B. Is it possible to identify a high-risk group that might especially benefit from screening?

1. CAS is more prevalent in patients with hypertension or heart disease and in those who smoke.

2. There are no risk assessment tools that reliably identify patients with clinically important CAS.

C. What is the quality of the screening test?

1. For the detection of > 70% stenosis, carotid duplex ultrasonography has a sensitivity of 86–90% and a specificity of 87–94%.

2. For the detection of > 60% stenosis, the sensitivity is 94% and the specificity is 92%.

3. There is some variability in measurements done in different laboratories.

4. Screening for bruits on physical exam has poor reliability and sensitivity.

D. Does screening reduce morbidity or mortality?

1. There have been 2 randomized controlled trials of carotid endarterectomy for asymptomatic CAS, both of which showed about a 5% absolute reduction in stroke or perioperative death in the surgical group (~5.5–6.5%), compared with the medically treated group (~11–12%); the absolute risk reduction for disabling stroke was about 2.5%.

   a. These results may not be generalizable due to the highly selected participants and surgeons.

   b. The medical treatment was not well defined and did not include current standard care, such as aggressive control of BP and lipids.

2. All abnormal ultrasounds need to be confirmed by digital subtraction angiography, which has a stroke rate of 1%, or by magnetic resonance angiography or CT angiography, both of which are < 100% accurate.

3. 30-day perioperative stroke or death rates in asymptomatic patients range from 1.6% to 3.7%, with rates for women at the higher end of the range; in some states, rates are as high as 6%.

4. The perioperative myocardial infarction rate is 0.7–1.1%, going up to 3.3% in patients with more comorbidities.

E. What are the current guidelines?

1. USPSTF (2007)

   a. Recommends against screening for asymptomatic CAS in the general adult population

   b. Grade D recommendation, based on moderate certainty that the benefits of screening do not outweigh the harms.

2. The American Heart Association and the American Stroke Association (2011) do not recommend population-based screening.

3. Other societies, including the American College of Cardiology, the American College of Radiology, and the Society for Vascular Surgery do not recommend routine screening, although do recommend screening patients with bruits and to consider screening in patients with known atherosclerotic disease.

You explain to Mr. S that he should not invest in the "vascular screening." Screening for CAS is not recommended for the general population, and since he is younger than 65 years with a minimal history of smoking, he does not need to be screened for AAA.

Mr. S has a second list for his wife, a 42-year-old similarly healthy woman who is scheduled to see you next: lipid panel, bone mineral density (BMD), Pap smear, and mammogram.

Mrs. S also has no medical history, except for 2 normal vaginal deliveries, the first at age 25. Her menses are regular. She does not smoke or drink, and she jogs regularly. She had 1 sexual partner before Mr. S and has been monogamous for 20 years. Her family history is negative, except for osteoporosis in her mother and grandmother. She has had a normal Pap smear every year since her first child was born. She weighs 125 pounds, her BP is 105/70 mm Hg, and her general physical exam, including breast exam, is entirely normal.

 Should Mrs. S be screened for cervical cancer with a Pap smear?

Cervical Cancer Screening

A. What is the burden of disease?

1. About 12,200 new cases of cervical cancer and 4210 cervical cancer–related deaths in the United States in 2010

2. Incidence rates vary by race/ethnicity: 11.1 per 100,000 in Hispanic women; 10 per 100,000 in black women; 7.4/100,000 in white women; 7.3/100,000 in Asian women

3. Rates are considerably higher in countries where cytologic screening is not widely available; worldwide, cervical cancer is the second most common cancer in women and the most common cause of mortality from gynecologic malignancy.

4. Women with preinvasive lesions have a 5-year survival of nearly 100%, with a 92% 5-year survival for early-stage invasive cancer; only 13% survive distant disease.

B. Is it possible to identify a high-risk group that might especially benefit from screening?

1. 93–100% of squamous cell cervical cancers contain DNA from high-risk human papillomavirus (HPV) strains.

   a. Low- and high-risk subtypes

   b. Cervix especially vulnerable to infection during adolescence when squamous metaplasia is most active.

   c. Most infections cleared by the immune system in 1–2 years without producing neoplastic changes.

      (1) 90% of low-risk subtypes resolve over 5 years

      (2) 70% of high-risk subtypes resolve

   d. Women older than 30 years with HPV are more likely to have high-grade lesions or cancer than women younger than 30 with HPV.

2. Early-onset of intercourse (before age 17) and a greater number of lifetime sexual partners (> 2) are risk factors for acquiring HPV.

3. Cigarette smoking increases risk by 2- to 4-fold.

4. Immunocompromise and other sexually transmitted infections, such as herpes and HIV, also increase risk.

5. In utero exposure to diethylstilbestrol and previous treatment for high-grade lesions are also risk factors for cervical cancer.

C. What is the quality of the screening test?

1. Interpretation of Pap smears: the Bethesda Classification of Cervical Cytology

   a. Negative for intraepithelial lesion or malignancy

   b. Epithelial cell abnormalities: squamous cells

      (1) Atypical squamous cells (ASC)

         (a) ASC-US: of undetermined significance

         (b) ASC-H: cannot exclude high-grade squamous intraepithelial lesion

(2) Low-grade squamous intraepithelial lesion

    (a) Cellular changes consistent with HPV

    (b) Same as mild dysplasia, histologic diagnosis of cervical intraepithelial neoplasia (CIN) 1

(3) High-grade squamous intraepithelial lesion

    (a) Same as moderate/severe dysplasia, histologic diagnosis of CIN 2, CIN 3, CIS (carcinoma in situ)

    (b) Should indicate if invasion suspected

(4) Squamous cell carcinoma

  c. Epithelial cell abnormalities: glandular cells

    (1) Atypical (endocervical, endometrial, or glandular)

    (2) Atypical, favors neoplastic

    (3) Endocervical adenocarcinoma in situ

    (4) Adenocarcinoma

2. Pap smear techniques

  a. Conventional Pap smear: cervical cells are spread on a glass slide and treated with a fixative by the examiner

  b. Liquid-based cytology: cervical cells are suspended in a vial of liquid preservative by the examiner, followed by debris removal and placement onto a slide in the laboratory

3. HPV testing

  a. A cervical specimen is placed into a transport medium or into the liquid preservative used for the liquid-based cytology Pap smear method.

  b. Specific RNA probes are added that combine with oncogenic DNA, and the DNA-RNA hybrids are detected by antibodies.

4. Test characteristics of conventional and liquid-based cytology are the same.

  a. Sensitivity for high-grade squamous intraepithelial lesion is ~ 56%; for low-grade squamous intraepithelial lesion, ~ 77%.

  b. Specificity for high-grade squamous intraepithelial lesion is ~ 97%; for low-grade squamous intraepithelial lesion, ~ 80%.

5. HPV testing is more sensitive but less specific for the detection of CIN 2 and CIN 3; false-positive rates are higher in women under 35 years of age.

D. Does screening reduce morbidity or mortality?

  1. No randomized trial data demonstrate a reduction in cervical cancer mortality with screening.

  2. Many observational studies show a decrease in both the incidence of cervical cancer (60–90%) and cervical cancer mortality (20–60%).

  3. Many cervical cancers in the United States occur in women who have never been screened; modeling studies suggest than screening such women would reduce cervical cancer mortality by 74%.

  4. Screening intervals are based on a combination of randomized trial data and modeling studies.

E. What are the current guidelines?

  1. USPSTF (2012)

    a. Recommends screening women aged 21–65 with cytology (Pap smear) every 3 years; women aged 30–65 can be screened every 5 years with a combination of cytology and HPV testing (Grade A recommendation)

    b. Recommends against screening women older than 65 *with a history of adequate recent screening,* who are not otherwise at high risk

      (1) Grade D recommendation

      (2) Adequate screening is defined as 3 consecutive negative cytology results or 2 consecutive negative HPV results within 10 years of the cessation of screening, with the most recent test occurring within 5 years.

    c. Recommends against routine screening women who have had a total hysterectomy and no history of CIN 2, CIN 3, or cervical cancer (Grade D recommendation)

    d. Recommends against screening in women younger than 21 years (Grade D recommendation)

    e. Recommends against HPV testing in women younger than 30 years (Grade D recommendation)

  2. American Cancer Society (2012) guidelines are similar to the guidelines of USPSTF.

You explain to Mrs. S that the combination of her sexual history and her history of 12 normal Pap smears in a row puts her at extremely low risk for cervical cancer. You point out that all expert guidelines consider it acceptable to perform Pap smears every 3 years in women with her history.

 Should Mrs. S be screened for breast cancer with a mammogram?

Breast Cancer Screening

A. What is the burden of disease?

  1. Most frequently diagnosed cancer in women

  2. The overall lifetime risk of developing breast cancer is 12%

  3. The 10-year risk at age 40 is 1.5%; at age 50, it is 2.4%; at age 60 it is 3.5%

  4. In 2008, 182,460 cases of invasive cancer and 67,770 cases of in situ cancer were diagnosed, with 40,480 deaths.

B. Is it possible to identify a high-risk group that might especially benefit from screening?

  1. Women who have a *BRCA1/BRCA2* mutation are a special high-risk group, with a relative risk of developing breast cancer of 10.0–32.0; certain family history patterns are associated with an increased likelihood of *BRCA* mutations.

    a. For women of Ashkenazi Jewish descent: Any first-degree relative or 2 second-degree relatives on the same side of the family with breast or ovarian cancer

    b. For all other women:

      (1) 2 first-degree relatives with breast cancer, at least 1 of whom was diagnosed at age 50 or younger

      (2) 3 or more first- or second-degree relatives with breast cancer

      (3) Both breast and ovarian cancer among first- and second-degree relatives

      (4) A first-degree relative with bilateral breast cancer

      (5) 2 or more first- or second-degree relatives with ovarian cancer

Table 2-7. Magnitude of risk for breast cancer.

Risk Factor	Approximate Relative Risk of Breast Cancer
50-year-old woman with no additional risk factors	10-year risk = 2.4%
BRCA1/BRCA2	10–32
Therapeutic radiation to the chest at age < 30 years	7.0–17.0
High breast density on mammography	5.0
Atypical ductal or lobular hyperplasia or lobular carcinoma in situ on previous biopsy	4.0
Mother or sister with breast or ovarian cancer	1.5–2.0
Postmenopausal obesity	1.2–1.9
Age at first birth > 30 years	1.2–1.7
White race	1.1–1.5
Age at menarche < 12 years or age at menopause > 55 years	1.2–1.3
Current use of hormone replacement therapy	1.2
> 2 drinks/day	1.2

(6) A first- or second-degree relative with both breast and ovarian cancer

(7) Breast cancer in a male relative

2. Otherwise, age is the strongest risk factor (relative risk = 18 for women aged 70–74 compared with women aged 30–34).

3. Other risk factors are listed in Table 2-7.

4. Protective factors include > 16 months of breastfeeding, 5 or more pregnancies, exercise, postmenopausal BMI < 23 kg/m², oophorectomy before age 35.

5. A Breast Cancer Risk Assessment Tool has been developed.

   a. Available at http://www.cancer.gov/bcrisktool/

   b. Uses statistical methods applied to data from the Breast Cancer Detection and Demonstration Project, a mammography screening project conducted in the 1970s, to assess breast cancer risk

C. What is the quality of the screening test?

1. Digital and film mammography have similar overall test characteristics, but digital mammography is more sensitive in women under age 50 years, premenopausal women, and those with dense breasts.

   a. Overall sensitivity of digital = 70%; overall sensitivity of film = 66%; specificity 92% for both

   b. For women under 50 years of age, digital sensitivity = 78%, film sensitivity = 51%

2. About 23% of women have at least 1 false-positive mammogram requiring additional evaluation (additional imaging or biopsy).

3. The false-positive rate tends to be higher in younger women and those taking hormone replacement therapy due to increased breast density.

D. Does screening reduce morbidity or mortality?

1. Table 2-8 summarizes the results of meta-analyses of randomized trials of screening mammography.

2. Potential harms include anxiety about testing, overdiagnosis, radiation exposure, and false-positive mammograms.

   a. The rate of overdiagnosis (finding cancers that would never have become clinically significant) is unclear, with estimates ranging from 1% to 32%.

   b. There is a small risk of radiation-induced breast cancer (86 cancers and 11 deaths per 100,000 persons screened annually from age 40 to age 55 and then biennially).

3. Meta-analyses of trials of breast self-examination (randomized and nonrandomized) show no effect on breast cancer mortality.

E. What are the current guidelines?

1. USPSTF (2009)

   a. Recommends against routine screening in women aged 40–49 years (Grade C recommendation; should decide in context of patient's values and risk level)

   b. Screen women aged 50–74 every 2 years

      (1) Grade B recommendation

      (2) The 2-year interval is based on observations that reductions in breast cancer mortality were similar in studies using 18- to 33-month screening intervals and 12-month screening intervals; additionally, decision analyses using statistical models found that biannual screening resulted in 2 additional deaths/1000 women screened compared to annual screening.

   c. Current evidence is insufficient to assess benefits and harms of screening women aged 75 years or older (I statement).

   d. Recommends against teaching breast self-examination (D recommendation); evidence is insufficient regarding clinical breast exam (I statement).

2. American Cancer Society (2013)

   a. Begin annual mammography at age 40

Table 2-8. Efficacy of breast cancer screening.

Age	RR Breast Cancer Death (95% CI)	Number Needed to Invite to Screening to Prevent 1 Breast Cancer Death[1]	False-Positive Rate per 1000 Women Screened
40–49	0.85 (0.75–0.96)	1904	97.8
50–59	0.86 (0.75–0.99)	1339	86.6
60–69	0.68 (0.54–0.87)	377	79.0
70–79	1.12 (0.73–1.72)	NA	68.8

[1]Compliance with screening was 75–85%, so the number needed to screen to prevent 1 death would be 15–25% lower.
CI, confidence interval; RR, relative risk.

b. Clinical breast exam every 3 years from ages 20–39 and annually beginning at age 40

3. American College of Obstetrics and Gynecology (2009)

a. Mammography every 1–2 years beginning at age 40; annually beginning at age 50

b. Clinical breast exam annually beginning at age 20

F. Table 2-9 summarizes information on staging, testing, histology, prognosis, and treatment of breast cancer.

You explain to Mrs. S that in women with no factors that increase the risk of breast cancer, the chance that she will have a false-positive mammogram is much larger than the chance a breast cancer will be found. Whether she should be screened prior to age 50 depends on her personal risk tolerance.

 Should Mrs. S be screened for osteoporosis?

Osteoporosis Screening

A. What is the burden of disease?

1. In the United States, about 12 million people over the age of 50 have osteoporosis.

2. Osteoporotic fracture will occur in 50% of postmenopausal women.

a. Hip fracture will occur in 15%, which is associated with loss of independence in up to 60% of patients and excess mortality of 10–20% within 1 year.

b. Vertebral deformity will develop in 25%.

B. Is it possible to identify a high-risk group that might especially benefit from screening?

1. Low BMD itself is the strongest risk factor for fracture.

2. Increasing age is the strongest risk factor for low BMD; other risk factors include low body weight (< 132 pounds), lack of hormone replacement therapy use, family history of osteoporosis, personal history of fracture, ethnic group (white, Asian, Hispanic), current smoking, 3 or more alcoholic drinks/day, long-term corticosteroid use (≥ 5 mg of prednisone daily for ≥ 3 months).

3. The WHO Fracture Risk Algorithm (FRAX) calculates the 10-year probability of hip or major osteoporotic fracture using femoral neck BMD and clinical risk factors (available at http://www.shef.ac.uk/FRAX/).

a. Although the full FRAX algorithm incorporates femoral neck BMD, it is possible to input just clinical risk factors to estimate the patient's clinical risk.

b. Using just clinical risk factors, a 65-year-old woman with no additional positive answers has a 9.3% 10-year risk for any osteoporotic fracture.

C. What is the quality of the screening test?

1. Background

a. Can measure bone density with a variety of methods (dual-energy x-ray absorptiometry, single-energy x-ray absorptiometry, ultrasonography, quantitative CT) at a variety of sites (hip, lumbar spine, heel, forearm)

b. Current bone density is compared with peak predicated bone density and then reported as number of SD above or below peak predicted bone density.

c. Osteoporosis is defined as a bone density "T score" at least 2.5 SD below peak predicted bone density (T score = −2.5 or more negative).

d. Osteopenia is defined as a T score between −1.0 and −2.5.

e. Normal is within 1 SD of peak predicted bone density.

2. Dual-energy x-ray bone absorptiometry is the gold standard test.

a. Has been shown to be a strong predictor of hip fracture risk; femoral neck is best site to measure.

b. The relative risk of hip fracture is 2.5 for each decrease of 1 SD in bone density at the femoral neck.

c. The relative risk of vertebral fracture is 1.9 for each decrease of 1 SD in bone density at the femoral neck.

3. There are limited data regarding the optimal interval between screening exams.

a. One study found that a repeat bone density 8 years after the initial test did not improve fracture risk prediction when compared with the initial test.

b. Another study stratified patients by baseline bone density and then determined the estimated time interval for 10% of women in each cohort to develop osteoporosis or an osteoporotic fracture.

(1) For women with a normal BMD (T score, −1.0 or higher), the interval was 16 years.

(2) For women with mild osteopenia (T score, −1.01 to −1.49), the interval was 17 years.

(3) For women with moderate osteopenia (T score, −1.50 to −1.99), the interval was 5 years; for those with advanced osteopenia (T score, −2.0 to −2.49), the interval was 1 year.

D. Does screening reduce morbidity or mortality?

1. No studies of the effectiveness of screening in reducing osteoporotic fractures

2. Many studies show treatment substantially reduces fracture risk.

3. Potential harms of screening include misinterpretation of test results, increasing anxiety in patients, side effects of medications, and cost.

4. If 10,000 women aged 65–69 are screened, assuming a 12% prevalence of osteoporosis and that treatment reduces vertebral fracture by 50% and hip fracture by 66%

a. The number needed to screen to prevent 1 vertebral fracture over 5 years is 233 and to prevent 1 hip fracture is 556.

b. In women aged 60–64 (osteoporosis prevalence 6.5%), the number needed to screen for vertebral fracture is 435 and for hip fracture is 1000; in women aged 75–79 (osteoporosis prevalence 28%), the number needed to screen for vertebral fracture is 96 and for hip fracture is 238.

E. What are the current guidelines?

1. USPSTF (2011)

a. Screen for osteoporosis in women aged 65 years or older and in younger women with a similar risk (> 9.3% 10-year risk based on the FRAX calculator).

(1) Grade B recommendation

(2) Good evidence that the risk of osteoporosis increases with age, that bone density measurements accurately predict fracture risk, and that treating asymptomatic women reduces fracture risk.

Table 2-9. Breast cancer.

Staging	Stage	Definition
	Stage 0	Carcinoma in situ, including DCIS, LCIS, and Paget disease only involving the nipple
	Stage IA	Tumor size ≤ 2 cm and localized to the breast
	Stage IB	Tumor size ≤ 2 cm and focus of breast cancer cells < 2 mm is found in the lymph nodes
	Stage IIA	Tumor size ≤ 2 cm and a focus breast cancer cells > 2 mm is found in 1–3 axillary lymph nodes or in lymph nodes near the breast bone **or** tumor is > 2 cm and < 5 cm and has not spread to the lymph nodes
	Stage IIB	Tumor is > 2 cm and < 5 cm and a focus breast cancer cells < 2 mm is found in the lymph nodes **or** tumor is > 2 cm and < 5 cm and cancer has spread to 1–3 axillary lymph nodes or to lymph nodes near the breast bone **or** tumor is > 5 cm and has not spread to lymph nodes
	Stage IIIA	Tumor is any size and cancer is found in 4–9 axillary lymph nodes or in lymph nodes near the breast bone **or** > 5 cm and a focus breast cancer cells < 2 mm is found in the lymph nodes **or** > 5 cm and cancer has spread to 1–3 axillary lymph nodes or to lymph nodes near the breast bone
	Stage IIIB	Tumor is any size and has spread to the chest wall or skin of the breast and ulcerated and can have spread to 9 axillary lymph nodes or lymph nodes near the breast bone
	Stage IIIC	Tumor is any size and has spread to the chest wall or skin of the breast and ulcerated and can have spread to ≥ 10 axillary lymph nodes or lymph nodes near the breast bone or supraclavicular lymph nodes
	Stage IV	Any distant metastasis
Commonly used tests	**For diagnosis:** Biopsy methods • Fine-needle aspiration (sampling with a thin needle) • Core biopsy (sampling with a wide needle • Incisional (part of mass is removed) • Excisional (all of mass is removed)	**For staging:** Sentinel lymph node biopsy • Performed at the time of surgery • A radioactive blue dye is injected into the lymphatic system near the tumor • The first node to take up dye is removed and analyzed microscopically • If positive, other nodes may be removed
Histology	Noninvasive • DCIS Invasive • Ductal (76%) • Lobular (10–15%): often multiple and bilateral • Medullary • Inflammatory: dermal lymphatic invasion with skin changes (peau d'orange) • Paget disease of the nipple	
Prognosis	Based on the stage at the time of diagnosis Overall 5-year survival is 90% 5-year survival for localized breast cancer is 98% 5-year survival for stage IV is 24%	
Treatment	Surgery • Approach determined by tumor size, patient preference • Lumpectomy • Segmental mastectomy • Total mastectomy • Modified radical mastectomy • Breast reconstruction at time of surgery or later Radiation therapy • After lumpectomy and sometimes mastectomy Hormonal therapy • Works best in cancers with estrogen/progesterone receptors • Aromatase inhibitors such as exemestane, anastrozole • Selective estrogen response modifiers such as tamoxifen Trastuzumab (Herceptin) for *HER2/neu* positive cancers Chemotherapy indicated based on stage and biomarker profile	

DCIS, ductal carcinoma in situ; LCIS, lobular carcinoma in situ.

b. Current evidence is insufficient to assess the balance of risk and benefits of screening in men (I recommendation).

2. National Osteoporosis Foundation (NOF) (2013)

a. Screen women age 65 and older and men age 70 and older.

b. Screen postmenopausal women and men age 50–69 based on risk factor profile.

You agree with Mrs. S that she is at increased risk for osteoporosis, but you explain that her 10-year risk is quite low, based on the FRAX calculator. There is no indication for BMD testing at this time. You discuss the importance of maintaining adequate calcium and vitamin D intake (1200 mg daily of calcium and 800–1000 international units daily of vitamin D).

CASE RESOLUTION

Based on your discussion, Mr. S decides to forego the chest radiograph and PSA level. He agrees to be scheduled for a fasting lipid panel and a colonoscopy.

You discuss with Mrs. S that she has no additional risk factors for coronary disease, and expert guidelines disagree about when to start screening for hyperlipidemia in low-risk women.

Mrs. S opts to have a mammogram but is happy to let a Pap smear and lipid panel wait a couple of years. She leaves with a handout about the role of calcium and vitamin D intake in the prevention and treatment of osteoporosis.

Table 2-10 summarizes numbers needed to screen for commonly used tests.

Table 2-10. Numbers needed to screen (NNS).

Disease	Test	Population	NNS
AAA	Ultrasonography	Ever smoking men, age 65–74	500 to prevent 1 AAA specific death over 5 years
Osteoporosis	DEXA	Women 75–79	238 to prevent 1 hip fracture; 96 to prevent 1 vertebral fracture
		Women 65–69	556 to prevent 1 hip fracture over 5 years; 233 to prevent 1 vertebral fracture
		Women 60–64	1000 to prevent 1 hip fracture; 435 to prevent 1 vertebral fracture
Breast cancer	Mammography	Women 60–69	320 to prevent 1 breast cancer death over 14 years
		Women 50–59	1138 to prevent 1 breast cancer death over 14 years
		Women 40–49	1618 to prevent 1 breast cancer death over 14 years
Colorectal cancer	Fecal occult blood testing	Annual screening, patients over 50	217 to prevent 1 colorectal cancer death
		Biennial screening	344–1250 to prevent 1 colorectal cancer death
Lung cancer	Low-dose CT	Asymptomatic persons aged 55–74 with ≥ 30 pack year smoking history; former smokers must have quit within the past 15 years	320 to prevent 1 lung cancer death
Prostate cancer	PSA	Men 55–69	1410 to prevent 1 prostate cancer death

AAA, abdominal aortic aneurysm; DEXA, dual-energy x-ray bone absorptiometry; PSA, prostate-specific antigen.

REFERENCES

Aberle DR, DeMello S, Berg CD et al. Results of the two incidence screenings in the National Lung Screening Trial. N Engl J Med. 2013;369:920–31.

Boiselle PM. Computed tomography screening for lung cancer. JAMA. 2013;309: 1163–70.

Greenland P, Alpert JS, Beller GA et al. 2010 ACCF/AHA guideline for assessment of cardiovascular risk in asymptomatic adults: a report of the American College of Cardiology Foundation/American Heart Association Task Force on Practice Guidelines. J Am Coll Cardiol. 2010;56:e50–103.

Hoffman RM. Screening for prostate cancer. N Engl J Med. 2011;365:2013–9.

Nelson HD, Maney EM, Dana T et al. Screening for osteoporosis: an update for the U.S. Preventive Services Task Force. Ann Intern Med. 2010;153:99–111.

Nelson HD, Tyne K, Naik A et al. Screening for breast cancer: an update for the U.S. Preventive Services Task Force. Ann Intern Med. 2009;151:727–37.

Porter N. Screening for dyslipidemia. (accessed 9/10/13) http://pier.acponline.org/physicians/screening/s367/s367.html.

Qaseem A, Barry MJ, Denberg TD et al. Screening for prostate cancer: a guidance statement from the Clinical Guidelines Committee of the American College of Physicians. Ann Intern Med. 2012;158:761–69.

Qaseem A, Denberg TD, Hopkins RH et al. Screening for colorectal cancer: a guidance statement from the American College of Physicians. Ann Intern Med. 2010;156:378–86.

Smith RA, Brooks D, Cokkinides V et al. Cancer screening in the United States, 2013: a review of current American Cancer Society guidelines, current issues in cancer screening, and new guidance on cervical cancer screening and lung cancer screening. CA Cancer J Clin. 2013;63:88–105.

U. S. Preventive Services Task Force. (accessed 9/10/13) http://www.uspreventiveservicestaskforce.org/index.html.

Warner E. Breast cancer screening. N Engl J Med. 2011;365:1025–32.

I have a patient with abdominal pain. How do I determine the cause?

CHIEF COMPLAINT

PATIENT 1

Mr. C is a 22-year-old man who complains of diffuse abdominal pain.

What is the differential diagnosis of abdominal pain? How would you frame the differential?

CONSTRUCTING A DIFFERENTIAL DIAGNOSIS

Abdominal pain is the most common cause for hospital admission in the United States. Diagnoses range from benign entities (eg, irritable bowel syndrome [IBS]) to life-threatening diseases (eg, ruptured abdominal aortic aneurysms [AAAs]). The first pivotal step in diagnosing abdominal pain is to identify the **location** of the pain. The differential diagnosis can then be limited to a subset of conditions that cause pain in that particular quadrant of the abdomen (Figure 3-1).

Several other pivotal points can help narrow the differential diagnosis including (1) the time course of the pain, (2) peritoneal findings on exam, (3) unexplained hypotension, and (4) abdominal distention. Each of these is reviewed below.

The time course of the pain is a pivotal feature. Some diseases present subacutely/chronically over weeks to months or years (eg, IBS) whereas others present acutely, within hours to days of onset (eg, appendicitis). In patients with their first episode of acute severe abdominal pain, a variety of life-threatening, must not miss diagnoses must be considered (eg, AAA). Many of these diseases that cause acute abdominal pain cannot recur because patients are either treated or die of complications (eg, AAA, acute appendicitis, splenic rupture.) Since prior episodes are incompatible with many of these diagnoses, a history of such prior episodes narrows the differential diagnosis. Therefore, the differential diagnosis of abdominal pain can be organized based on whether patients are presenting with their first episode of acute abdominal pain, a recurrent episode of acute abdominal pain, or chronic/subacute abdominal pain. Table 3-1 outlines the typical time course associated with different diseases causing abdominal pain. See Table 3-2 for a summary of abdominal pain organized by location, time course, and clinical clues.

Peritoneal findings of rebound tenderness, rigidity, and guarding are pivotal features and suggest an intra-abdominal catastrophe. Typical causes include AAA, bowel infarction (due to bowel obstruction or acute mesenteric ischemia), bowel perforation (due to appendicitis, peptic ulcer disease [PUD], diverticulitis), pancreatitis, or pelvic inflammatory disease (PID).

Unexplained hypotension is yet another potential pivotal clue. While many patients with abdominal pain experience hypotension due to dehydration from nausea, vomiting, or poor oral intake, some patients with abdominal pain present with *unexplained* hypotension. Unexplained hypotension can suggest sepsis, retroperitoneal hemorrhage, or other diseases. Table 3-3 lists diseases associated with abdominal pain and unexplained hypotension.

Orthostatic vital signs should be taken in patients with abdominal pain. They may provide invaluable diagnostic and therapeutic information.

The final pivotal finding is significant abdominal distention, which may develop from excess air or fluid in the abdomen. Excess air may occur with bowel obstruction or bowel perforation (free air). Excess fluid may be seen in patients with ascites or hemorrhage. Percussion and shifting dullness can usually distinguish excess air from fluid in such patients. Table 3-4 lists the diagnostic considerations in patients with abdominal distention.

Other important historical points include factors that make the pain better or worse (eg, eating), radiation of the pain, and associated symptoms (nausea, vomiting, anorexia, inability to pass stool and flatus, melena, hematochezia, change in color of the urine or stool, fever, chills, weight loss, altered bowel habits, orthostatic symptoms, urinary symptoms) or prior abdominal surgeries (increasing the risk of small bowel obstruction [SBO]). Pulmonary symptoms or a cardiac history can be clues to pneumonia or myocardial infarction presenting as abdominal pain. In women, sexual and menstrual histories are important. The patient should be asked about alcohol consumption as well as prescription and over-the-counter medications.

A few final points about the physical exam are worth emphasizing. First, vital signs are just that, vital. Hypotension, fever, tachypnea, and tachycardia are critical clinical clues that must not be overlooked. The HEENT exam should look for pallor or icterus. Jaundice suggests either hepatitis or biliary disease. Careful heart and lung exams can suggest pneumonia or other extra-abdominal causes of abdominal pain.

The physical exam of a patient with abdominal pain includes more than just the abdominal exam.

Of course, the abdominal exam is key. Inspection assesses for distention as noted above. Auscultation evaluates whether bowel sounds are present. Absent bowel sounds may suggest an intra-abdominal catastrophe; high-pitched tinkling sounds and rushes suggest an intestinal obstruction. Palpation should be performed last. *It is useful to distract the patient by continuing to talk with him or her during abdominal palpation. This allows the examiner to get a*

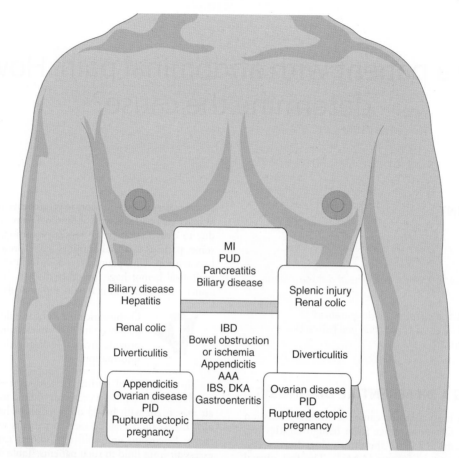

AAA, abdominal aortic aneurysm; DKA, diabetic ketoacidosis; IBD, inflammatory bowel disease; IBS, irritable bowel syndrome; MI, myocardial infarction; PID, pelvic inflammatory disease; PUD, peptic ulcer disease.

Figure 3-1. The differential diagnosis of abdominal pain by location.

Table 3-1. Differential diagnoses in abdominal pain organized by time course.

Acute Abdominal Pain		Subacute/Chronic Abdominal Pain
First episode	**Recurrent episode**	
AAA	Biliary disease	Chronic mesenteric ischemia
Acute mesenteric ischemia	DKA	IBD
Appendicitis	Diverticulitis	IBS
Biliary disease	Nephrolithiasis	Hepatitis
Diverticulitis	Pancreatitis	PUD
DKA	PID	
Ectopic pregnancy	Small or large bowel obstruction	
Gastroenteritis		
Ischemic colitis		
Myocardial infarction		
Ovarian torsion		
Nephrolithiasis		
Pancreatitis		
Peritonitis (from ruptured PUD, diverticulitis, etc)		
PID		
Small or large bowel obstruction		
Splenic rupture		

AAA, abdominal aortic aneurysm; DKA, diabetic ketoacidosis; IBD, inflammatory bowel disease; IBS, irritable bowel syndrome; PID, pelvic inflammatory disease; PUD, peptic ulcer disease.

Table 3-2. Summary table of abdominal pain by location, time course, and clinical clues

Location	Differential Diagnosis	Acute 1 X	Acute > 1 X	Chronic	Unexplained Hypotension	Clinical Clues
Right upper quadrant	Biliary disease	✓	✓		✓¹	Postprandial or nocturnal pain Dark urine
	Hepatitis			✓		Alcohol use Injection drug use Jaundice
	Pancreatitis	✓	✓	✓	✓¹	Alcohol use Gallstones
	Renal colic: (Usually flank pain)	✓	✓			Hematuria (usually microscopic) Severe pain
Left upper quadrant	Renal colic: (Usually flank pain)	✓	✓			Hematuria (usually microscopic) Severe pain
	Splenic infarct or rupture	✓			✓	Endocarditis Trauma Shoulder pain
Epigastrium	Biliary disease	✓	✓		✓¹	Postprandial or nocturnal pain Dark urine
	Pancreatitis	✓	✓	✓	✓¹	Worse supine History of alcohol abuse or gallstones
	Peptic ulcer			✓	✓²	Melena History of NSAID use
Diffuse periumbilical	AAA	✓			✓	Smoking Male gender Hypotension, syncope or pulsatile abdominal mass
	Appendicitis	✓			✓¹	Migration and progression
	Acute mesenteric ischemia	✓			✓¹	History of AF Heart failure Valvular heart disease Catheterization Pain out of proportion to exam
	Bowel obstruction	✓				Inability to pass stool or flatus Prior surgery
	Chronic mesenteric ischemia			✓		PVD or CVD Pain brought on by food Weight loss
	Gastroenteritis	✓				Diarrhea Travel history
	Inflammatory bowel disease			✓		Family history Hematochezia Weight loss
	Irritable bowel syndrome			✓		Intermittent diarrhea or constipation
	Splenic rupture	✓			✓	Trauma
Right lower quadrant	Appendicitis				✓¹	Migration and progression
	Ectopic pregnancy	✓			✓	Sexually active woman in child bearing years
	Ovarian torsion	✓				
	PID	✓	✓		✓¹	Sexually active woman Vaginal discharge Cervical motion tenderness
Left lower quadrant	Diverticulitis	✓	✓		✓¹	Diarrhea Fever
	Ectopic pregnancy	✓			✓	Sexually active woman in child bearing years
	Ovarian torsion	✓				
	PID	✓	✓		✓¹	Sexually active woman Vaginal discharge Cervical motion tenderness

¹If associated with sepsis.
²If associated with hemorrhage.
AAA, abdominal aortic aneurysm; AF, atrial fibrillation; CVD, cardiovascular disease; NSAIDs, nonsteroidal antiinflammatory drugs; PID, pelvic inflammatory disease; PVD, peripheral vascular disease.

Table 3-3. Differential diagnoses in patients with abdominal pain and unexplained hypotension.

Mechanism of Hypotension	Differential Diagnosis
Intra-abdominal hemorrhage	Abdominal aortic aneurysm Ruptured ectopic pregnancy Splenic rupture
Sepsis	Acute mesenteric ischemia Appendicitis Ascending cholangitis Bowel obstruction (with infarction) Cholecystitis Diverticulitis Inflammatory bowel disease Ischemic colitis Nephrolithiasis (if accompanied by ascending infection) Pancreatitis Pelvic inflammatory disease Peptic ulcer disease (with perforation) Spontaneous bacterial peritonitis
Other	Adrenal insufficiency Diabetic ketoacidosis Myocardial infarction

Table 3-4. Differential diagnosis in patients with abdominal pain and distention.

Air		Fluid	
Free air	Luminal air	Ascites	Hemorrhage
Appendicitis Bowel infarction (SBO, AMI) Diverticulitis PUD (with perforation)	LBO SBO	Pancreatitis SBP	AAA Ruptured ectopic pregnancy Ruptured spleen

AAA, abdominal aortic aneurysm; AMI, acute mesenteric ischemia; LBO, large bowel obstruction; SBO, small bowel obstruction; SBP, spontaneous bacterial peritonitis.

better appreciation of the location and severity of maximal tenderness. The clinician should palpate the painful area last. The rectal exam should be performed, and the stool tested for occult blood. Finally, the pelvic exam should be performed in adult women and the testicular exam in men.

Mr. C felt well until the onset of pain several hours ago. He reports that the pain is a pressure-like sensation in the mid/upper abdomen, which is not particularly severe. He had never had this symptom before. He reports no fever, nausea, vomiting, or diarrhea. His appetite is diminished, and he has not had a bowel movement since the onset of pain. He reports no history of urinary symptoms such as frequency, dysuria, or hematuria. His past medical history is unremarkable. On physical exam, his vital signs are temperature, 37.0°C; RR, 16 breaths per minute; BP, 110/72 mm Hg; and pulse, 85 bpm. His cardiac and pulmonary exams are normal. Abdominal exam reveals a flat abdomen with hypoactive but positive bowel sounds. He has no rebound or guarding; although he has some mild diffuse tenderness, he has no focal or marked tenderness. There is no hepatosplenomegaly. Rectal exam is nontender, and stool is guaiac negative.

 At this point, what is the leading hypothesis, what are the active alternatives, and is there a must not miss diagnosis? Given this differential diagnosis, what tests should be ordered?

RANKING THE DIFFERENTIAL DIAGNOSIS

The patient's history is not particularly suggestive of any diagnosis. The first pivotal point determines the location of the pain. Mr. C's pain is in the mid/upper abdomen, which limits the differential diagnosis. Common causes of mid/upper abdominal pain include appendicitis, IBS, PUD, pancreatitis, inflammatory bowel disease (IBD), SBO, or large bowel obstruction (LBO), AAA, diabetic ketoacidosis, and gastroenteritis (Figure 3-1). Several of these diagnoses are very unlikely and need not be considered further. AAA would be exceptionally rare in this age group and gastroenteritis is very unlikely in the absence of either vomiting or diarrhea. The lack of a history of diabetes would make diabetic ketoacidosis unlikely unless this was the initial presentation. A simple blood sugar could help exclude this diagnosis. Other pivotal points in patients with abdominal pain include its time course (see Table 3-1), and if present, unexplained hypotension or abdominal distention (see Tables 3-3 and 3-4). The patient reports that this is an acute episode that has not occurred previously. This makes IBD and IBS very unlikely, focusing attention on the remaining possibilities of appendicitis, PUD, pancreatitis, and bowel obstruction. Since appendicitis should always be considered in young, otherwise healthy patients with unexplained abdominal pain, this is the leading hypothesis (Table 3-5). He has neither unexplained hypotension nor distention to help focus the differential diagnosis further.

Table 3-5. Diagnostic hypotheses for Mr. C.

Diagnostic Hypothesis	Demographics, Risk Factors, Symptoms and Signs	Important Tests
Leading Hypothesis		
Appendicitis	Migration of pain from periumbilical region to right lower quadrant	Clinical exam CT scan
Active Alternatives-Most Common		
Peptic ulcer	NSAID use *Helicobacter pylori* infection Melena Pain relieved by eating	EGD Urea breath test for *H pylori*
Pancreatitis	Alcohol abuse Gallstones	Serum lipase
Active Alternatives-Must Not Miss		
Early bowel obstruction	Prior abdominal surgery Inability to pass stool or flatus Nausea, vomiting	Abdominal radiographs, CT scan Small bowel study Barium enema

EGD, esophagogastroduodenoscopy; NSAID, nonsteroidal antiinflammatory drug.

Mr. C reports no history of nonsteroidal antiinflammatory drug (NSAID), aspirin, or alcohol ingestion. He has no known gallstones and no prior history of abdominal surgery. He reports that he is passing flatus and denies vomiting.

 Is the clinical information sufficient to make a diagnosis? If not, what other information do you need?

Leading Hypothesis: Appendicitis

Textbook Presentation

The classic presentation of appendicitis is abdominal pain that is initially diffuse and then intensifies and migrates toward the right lower quadrant (RLQ) to McBurney point (1.5–2 inches from the anterior superior iliac crest toward umbilicus). Patients often complain of bloating and anorexia.

Disease Highlights

A. Appendicitis is one of the most common causes of an acute abdomen, with a 7% lifetime occurrence rate.

B. It develops secondary to obstruction of the appendiceal orifice with secondary mucus accumulation, swelling, ischemia, necrosis, and perforation.

C. Initially, the pain is poorly localized. However, progressive inflammation eventually involves the parietal peritoneum, resulting in pain localized to the RLQ.

D. The risk of perforation increases steadily with age (ages 10–40, 10%; age 60, 30%; and age > 75, 50%).

Evidence-Based Diagnosis

A. The classic presentation of nausea and vomiting with pain migration from the periumbilical area to the RLQ is present in only 50–65% of patients.

B. RLQ pain is the most useful clinical finding; LR+, 7.3–8.5; LR–, 0.0–0.3

C. Most individual clinical findings have a low sensitivity for appendicitis making it difficult to rule out the diagnosis.
   1. In 1 study, guarding was completely absent in 22% of patients, and rebound was completely absent in 16% of patients with appendicitis.
   2. Fever was present in only 40% of patients with perforated appendices.

 Fever, severe tenderness, guarding, and rebound may be absent in patients with appendicitis.

D. Nonetheless, certain findings increase the likelihood of appendicitis when present (ie, rebound, guarding) (Table 3-6).

E. Symptoms are different in octogenerians than in patients aged 60–79 years.
   1. The duration of symptoms is longer prior to evaluation (48 vs 24 hours).
   2. They are less likely to report pain that migrated to the RLQ (29% vs 49%).

F. History is particularly important in women to differentiate other causes of RLQ pain (eg, PID, ruptured ectopic pregnancy, ovarian torsion, and ruptured ovarian cyst). The most useful clinical clues that suggest PID include the following:
   1. History of PID
   2. Vaginal discharge
   3. Cervical motion tenderness on pelvic exam

 Rule out ectopic pregnancy in women of childbearing age who complain of abdominal pain by testing urine for beta-HCG.

G. WBC
   1. The WBC has low discriminatory value for diagnosing acute appendicitis. One meta-analysis reported a LR+ of 2.46, LR– of 0.26 for a WBC > 10,000 /mcL.
   2. Very low WBCs (< 7000/mcL) and very high WBCs (> 17,000/mcL) substantially decrease or increase the

Table 3-6. Classic clinical and laboratory findings in appendicitis.

Finding	Sensitivity	Specificity	LR+	LR–
Clinical findings				
Guarding (moderate to severe)	46%	92%	5.5	0.59
Rebound (moderate to severe)	61%	82%	3.5	0.47
Vomiting	49%	76%	2.0	0.7
Pain migration to RLQ	54%	63%	1.5	0.7
RLQ tenderness	89–100%	12–59%	1.1–2.2	0–0.2
Fever > 38.1°C	15–67%	85%	1	1
Laboratory findings				
WBC > 7000/mcL	98%	21%	1.2	0.1
WBC > 11,000/mcL	76%	74%	2.9	0.3
WBC > 17,000/mcL	15%	98%	7.5	0.9

RLQ, right lower quadrant; WBC, white blood cell.

likelihood of appendicitis respectively (see Table 3-6). Moderate elevations are less predictive.

3. A low WBC does not exclude appendicitis in patients who have severe rebound or guarding; 80% of such patients had appendicitis even when WBC was < 8000/mcL.

 The WBC is not reliably elevated in patients with acute appendicitis.

H. C-reactive protein (CRP) levels are not highly diagnostic. For CRP > 10 mg/L, LR+ is 2.0 and LR– is 0.32.

I. One paper suggested that the combination of an elevated WBC (> 10,000/mcL) and an elevated CRP (> 12 mg/L) suggest appendicitis; LR+, 8.2 (both present); LR– 0.05 (both absent)

J. Urinalysis may be misleading and reveal pyuria and hematuria due to bladder inflammation from an adjacent appendicitis.

K. Plain radiography is useful only to detect free air or signs of another process (ie, SBO).

L. CT scanning is an accurate imaging method that is helpful when the diagnosis is uncertain.

1. Noncontrast CT scanning

   a. 92.7% sensitive, 96% specific; LR+, 24; LR–, 0.08

   b. IV and oral contrast may increase sensitivity further

2. A meta-analysis compared CT use with clinical evaluation alone

   a. CT scanning lowered the rate of unnecessary surgery compared with clinical evaluation alone from 16.7% to 8.6% (P < 0.001).

   b. The 2 randomized controlled trials within the meta-analysis showed similar reductions in unnecessary surgery in patients undergoing CT vs clinical evaluation without CT (2.6% vs 13.9% and 6.7% vs 27%).

3. CT scanning has also been demonstrated to lower overall costs.

M. Ultrasonography: 78% sensitive, 83% specific; LR+, 4.5; LR–, 0.27

N. Clinical decision rules: Scoring systems to predict appendicitis have been developed (eg, the Alvarado score). However validation studies have documented a high rate of appendicitis even among patients with low scores.

O. Pregnancy

1. Although inferior to CT, ultrasonography is recommended due to the risk of radiation to the fetus.

2. Indeterminate studies in the third trimester are common.

3. Unenhanced MRI

   a. An alternative option for patients with indeterminate ultrasound; sensitivity, 91%; specificity, 98%; LR+, 45; LR– 0.09

   b. Gadolinium is a pregnancy category C drug and is not advised.

4. Surgical and gynecologic consultation are suggested.

Treatment

A. Observation is critical.

B. Monitor urinary output and vital signs.

C. IV fluid resuscitation

D. Broad-spectrum antibiotics, including gram-negative and anaerobic coverage

E. Urgent appendectomy is recommended. Trials of medical therapy (antibiotics and observation without surgery) have demonstrated both a high rate of recurrence and complications.

MAKING A DIAGNOSIS

Mr. C's symptoms are consistent with—but certainly not diagnostic of—appendicitis. He has no risk factors for any of the alternative diagnoses of pancreatitis, PUD, or bowel obstruction (alcohol use, NSAID ingestion, or prior abdominal surgery, respectively). Diagnostic options include obtaining a CBC (always done but clearly of limited value), continued observation and reexamination, surgical consultation, and obtaining a CT scan. Given the lack of evidence for any of the less concerning possibilities you remain concerned that the patient has early appendicitis. You elect to observe the patient, obtain a CBC and lipase, order a CT scan and ask for a surgical consult.

 Frequent clinical observations are exceptionally useful when evaluating a patient with possible appendicitis.

 The CBC reveals a WBC of 8700/mcL (86% neutrophils, 0% bands) and a HCT of 44%. The lipase is normal. On reexamination the patient complains that the pain is now more severe in the RLQ. On exam, he is moderately tender but still without rebound or guarding.

The migration of pain to the RLQ is suggestive of appendicitis. Less likely considerations might include Crohn ileitis as well as diverticulitis or colon cancer (both unlikely in this age group). If the patient were a woman, PID and ovarian pathology (ruptured ectopic pregnancy, ovarian torsion, or ruptured ovarian cyst) would also need to be considered.

 Diffuse abdominal pain that subsequently localizes and becomes more constant, suggests parietal peritoneal inflammation.

 The CT scan reveals a hypodense fluid collection on the right side inferior to the cecum. An appendolith is seen. The interpretation is possible appendiceal perforation versus Crohn disease.

CASE RESOLUTION

 The patient's symptom complex, particularly the pain's migration, localization, and intensification are highly suggestive of appendicitis. CT findings make this diagnosis likely. At this point, surgical exploration is appropriate.

The patient undergoes surgery and purulent material is found in the peritoneal cavity. A necrotic appendix is removed, and the peritoneal cavity is irrigated. The patient is treated with broad-spectrum antibiotics and does well postoperatively.

CHIEF COMPLAINT

PATIENT 2

Ms. R is a 50-year-old woman who comes to the office complaining of abdominal pain. The patient reports that she has been having "episodes" or "attacks" of abdominal pain over the last month, with about 3 "attacks" during this time. She reports that the attacks of pain are in the epigastrium, last up to 4 hours, and often awaken her at night. The pain is described as a severe cramping-like sensation that is very intense and steady for hours. Occasionally, the pain radiates to the right back. The pain is associated with emesis. She reports that the color of her urine and stool are normal. On physical exam, her vital signs are stable. She is afebrile. On HEENT exam, she is anicteric. Her lungs are clear, and cardiac exam is unremarkable. Abdominal exam is soft with only mild epigastric discomfort to deep palpation. Murphy sign (tenderness in the right upper quadrant [RUQ] with palpation during inspiration) is negative. Rectal exam reveals guaiac-negative stool.

> At this point, what is the leading hypothesis, what are the active alternatives, and is there a must not miss diagnosis? Given this differential diagnosis, what tests should be ordered?

RANKING THE DIFFERENTIAL DIAGNOSIS

The first pivotal feature of Ms. R's abdominal pain is its epigastric location. Common causes of epigastric pain include PUD, biliary colic, and pancreatitis (Figure 3-1). The second pivotal feature of Ms. R's abdominal pain is its time course, with multiple acute episodes. Many diseases cause well-defined recurrent discrete episodes of abdominal pain (Table 3-1) but of these, only pancreatitis and biliary colic tend to occur in the epigastrium. PUD is a common cause of epigastric abdominal pain and obviously needs to be considered. However, the pain in PUD is typically more chronic than acute, and not typically discrete or so severe, making this a less likely possibility. Ms. R does not have other pivotal clues such as unexplained hypotension or abdominal distention that could focus the differential. The final clinical clue is the severe crampy quality of the pain. Severe intense crampy abdominal pain ("colicky") suggests obstruction of a hollow viscera, which can be caused by biliary, bowel, or ureteral obstruction (due to biliary obstruction, bowel obstruction, or nephrolithiasis, respectively). Taken together, the epigastric location, multiple discrete episodes, quality and intensity of the pain, biliary colic is the leading hypothesis. Table 3-7 lists the differential diagnosis.

2

Ms. R reports no history of alcohol binging, NSAID use, or known PUD. The pain does not improve with food or antacids. The pain is not relieved by defecation.

> Is the clinical information sufficient to make a diagnosis? If not, what other information do you need?

Table 3-7. Diagnostic hypotheses for Ms. R.

Diagnostic Hypotheses	Demographics, Risk Factors, Symptoms and Signs	Important Tests
Leading Hypothesis		
Biliary colic	Episodic and crampy pain may radiate to back	Ultrasonography
Active Alternatives—Most Common		
Peptic ulcer disease	NSAID use *Helicobacter pylori* infection Melena Pain relieved by eating or by antacids	EGD Urea breath test for *H pylori*, stool antigen assay
Pancreatitis	Alcohol abuse Gallstones	Serum lipase

EGD, esophagogastroduodenoscopy; NSAID, nonsteroidal antiinflammatory drug.

Leading Hypothesis: Biliary Colic

Textbook Presentation

Gallstone disease may present as incidentally discovered asymptomatic cholelithiasis, biliary colic, cholecystitis, cholangitis, or pancreatitis. The pattern depends on the location of the stone and its chronicity (Figure 3-2). Biliary colic typically presents with episodes of intense abdominal pain that begin 1 hour or more after eating and commonly wake patients from sleep. The pain is usually located in the RUQ, although epigastric pain is also common. The pain may radiate to the back and may be associated with nausea and vomiting. The pain usually lasts for more than 30 minutes and may last for hours.

Disease Highlights

A. Asymptomatic cholelithiasis

  1. Predisposing factors

    a. Increasing age is the predominant risk factor. The prevalence is 8% in patients older than 40 years and 20% in those older than 60 years (Figure 3-3).

    b. Obesity

    c. Gender: women are affected more than men (risk increases during pregnancy)

    d. Gallbladder stasis (due to rapid weight loss, which may occur in patients on very low calorie diets, on total parenteral nutrition, and after surgery)

    e. Other less common risk factors include family history, Crohn disease, and hemolytic anemias (eg, thalassemia, sickle cell disease) which can lead to increased bilirubin excretion and bilirubin stones.

  2. Cholecystectomy not advised for patients with asymptomatic cholelithiasis.

> Make sure the gallstones are *causing the pain* before advising cholecystectomy.

  3. Annual risk of biliary colic developing in patients with asymptomatic gallstones is 1–4%.

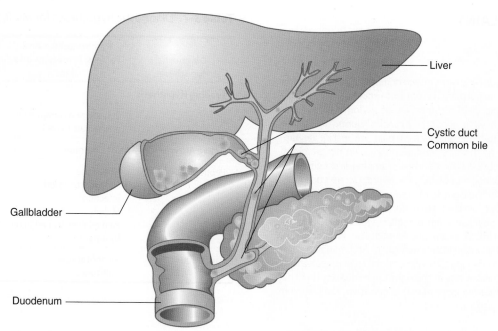

Figure 3-2. Calculi may lodge in several locations. In the cystic duct, they may cause biliary colic or cholecystitis. In the common bile duct, they may cause cholangitis and/or pancreatitis.

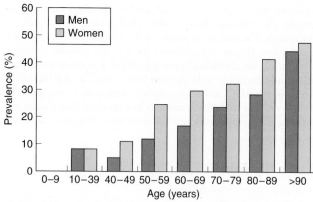

Figure 3-3. Prevalence of asymptomatic gallstones by age. (Reproduced with permission from Bateson MC. Gallbladder disease. BMJ. 1999;318:1745–8.)

B. Biliary colic

1. Occurs when a gallstone becomes lodged in the cystic duct and the gallbladder contracts against the obstruction.

2. Presents as one of the classic visceral obstructive syndromes with severe, constant, and crampy waves of pain that incapacitate the patient.

3. Characterized by episodes of pain with pain-free intervals of weeks to years.

4. Pain begins 1–4 hours after eating or may awaken the patient during the night. May be precipitated by fatty meals.

5. The pain is usually associated with nausea and vomiting.

6. The pain usually lasts < 2–4 hours. An episode that lasts longer than 4–6 hours and is accompanied by fever or marked tenderness suggests cholecystitis has developed.

7. Resolution occurs if the stone comes out of the gallbladder neck. The intense pain improves fairly rapidly, although mild discomfort may persist for 1 to 2 days.

8. Prognosis

   a. Biliary colic recurs in 50% of symptomatic patients.

   b. Acute cholecystitis develops if the stone remains lodged in the cystic duct.

   c. Complications (eg, pancreatitis, acute cholecystitis, or ascending cholangitis) occur in 25% of patients who have experienced biliary colic.

9. Colic occasionally develops in patients without stones secondary to sphincter of Oddi dysfunction or scarring leading to obstruction.

Evidence-Based Diagnosis

A. Pain may localize to the RUQ (54% of patients), epigastrium (34% of patients) or may present as a band-like pain across the entire upper abdomen, or rarely in the mid-abdomen. Pain may radiate to back, right scapula, right flank, or chest.

B. Laboratory tests (liver function tests [LFTs]), lipase, urinalysis) are normal in uncomplicated biliary colic. Abnormalities suggest other diagnoses or complications (eg, stone migration into the common bile duct [CBD]).

C. Ultrasonography is the test of choice; sensitivity 89%, specificity 97%, LR+ 30, LR– 0.11 (CT scan is only 79% sensitive.)

D. Endoscopic ultrasound (EUS) is 100% sensitive and is useful in patients with a negative transabdominal ultrasound but in whom biliary colic is still strongly suspected.

Treatment

A. Cholecystectomy is recommended.

B. Lithotripsy is not advised.

C. Dissolution therapies (eg, ursodiol) are reserved for nonsurgical candidates.

MAKING A DIAGNOSIS

Ms. R's history suggests biliary colic. You order an ultrasound of the RUQ.

A RUQ ultrasound reveals multiple small gallstones within the gallbladder. The CBD is normal, and no other abnormalities are seen. A serum lipase and LFTs are normal, and urea breath test for *Helicobacter pylori* is negative.

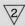
Have you crossed a diagnostic threshold for the leading hypothesis, biliary colic? Have you ruled out the active alternatives? Do other tests need to be done to exclude the alternative diagnoses?

Alternative Diagnosis: PUD

See Chapter 32, Unintentional Weight Loss.

Alternative Diagnosis: Acute Pancreatitis (see below)

CASE RESOLUTION

Ms. R discussed her case with her primary care physician and surgeon. Both agree that her symptom complex and ultrasound suggest biliary colic. Furthermore, there was no evidence of any of the alternative diagnoses. The normal lipase effectively rules out pancreatitis, and the combination of no NSAIDs and a negative urea breath test for *H pylori* makes PUD very unlikely. They recommend surgery, which she schedules for the end of the summer.

FOLLOW-UP

Ms. R returns 3 weeks later (and prior to her scheduled surgery) in acute distress. She reports that her pain began last evening, is in the same location as her previous bouts of pain, but unlike her previous episodes, the pain has persisted. She is very uncomfortable. She reports that her urine has changed color and is now quite dark, "like tea." In addition, she complains of "teeth chattering" chills. On physical exam, Ms. R is febrile (38.5°C). Her other vital signs are stable. Sclera are anicteric and cardiac and pulmonary exams are all completely normal. Abdominal exam reveals moderate tenderness in the epigastrium and RUQ. Murphy sign is positive.

At this point, what is the leading hypothesis, what are the active alternatives, and is there a must not miss diagnosis? Given this differential diagnosis, what tests should be ordered?

RANKING THE DIFFERENTIAL DIAGNOSIS

This episode of abdominal pain raises several possibilities. The first is that the current symptom complex is in some way related to her known cholelithiasis. The persistent pain suggests either cholecystitis (due to a stone lodged in the cystic duct), choledocholithiasis, ascending cholangitis, or pancreatitis. Of note, her dark urine is a pivotal clinical clue. Both hematuria and bilirubinuria can cause dark urine. Bilirubinuria only occurs in patients with conjugated hyperbilirubinemia which, in turn, is due to either CBD obstruction or hepatitis. In Ms. R, the preexistent biliary colic, persistent RUQ pain, and dark urine make the most likely diagnosis CBD obstruction due to migration of a stone into the CBD (choledocholithiasis) (Figure 3-2). On the other hand, in cholecystitis, only the cystic duct is obstructed. The CBD is unobstructed and therefore cholecystitis does not cause hyperbilirubinemia, bilirubinuria, dark urine, or significant increases in ALT (SGPT) or AST (SGOT). Finally, Ms. R's fever suggests that the CBD obstruction has been complicated by ascending infection and taken together suggests ascending cholangitis, a life-threatening condition (Figure 3-4).

Dark urine suggests bilirubinuria and may precede icterus.

Rigors (defined as visible shaking or teeth chattering chills) suggests bacteremia and should increase the suspicion of a life-threatening bacterial infection.

Other considerations include hepatitis or pancreatitis (which may be caused by concomitant pancreatic duct obstruction). While hepatitis can cause RUQ pain, hyperbilirubinemia, and bilirubinuria, it would also require giving Ms. R another unrelated diagnosis and is therefore less likely. Table 3-8 lists the differential diagnosis.

Laboratory results include WBC 17,000/mcL (84% neutrophils, 10% bands). HCT is 38%; lipase, 17 units/L (nl 11–65 units/L); alkaline phosphatase, 467 units/L (nl 30–120); bilirubin, 4.2 mg/dL; conjugated bilirubin, 3.0 mg/dL (nl 0 – 0.3); GGT, 246 units/L (nl 8–35); ALT, 100 units/L (nl 15–59). Ultrasound shows sludge and stones within the gallbladder. No CBD dilatation or CBD stone is seen. Blood cultures are ordered and you initiate broad-spectrum IV antibiotics (ie, piperacillin/tazobactam).

Is the clinical information sufficient to make a diagnosis of ascending cholangitis? If not, what other information do you need?

Leading Hypothesis: Choledocholithiasis & Ascending Cholangitis

Textbook Presentation

Patients typically have some form of biliary obstruction (biliary colic, acute cholecystitis or gallstone pancreatitis). The presence of pain, fever, and jaundice suggest ascending cholangitis is present.

Disease Highlights

A. 5–20% of patients with symptomatic gallstones have stones within the CBD (choledocholithiasis).

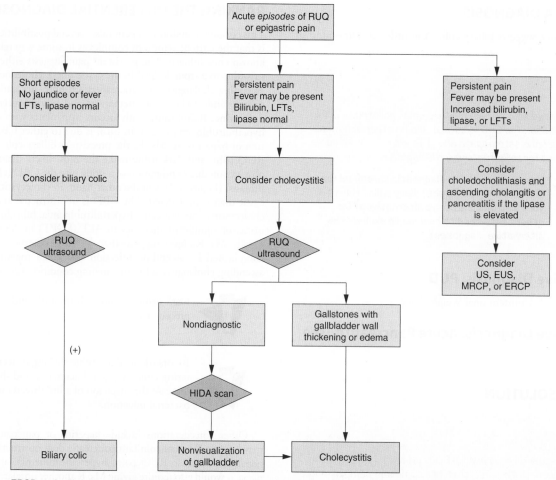

ERCP, endoscopic retrograde cholangiopancreatography; EUS, endoscopic ultrasound; HIDA, hepatobiliary iminodiacetic acid; LFTs, liver function tests; MRCP, magnetic resonance, cholangiopancreatography; RUQ, right upper quadrant; US, ultrasound.

Figure 3-4. Diagnostic approach: biliary disease.

Table 3-8. Diagnostic hypotheses for Ms. R on follow-up.

Diagnostic Hypothesis	Demographics, Risk Factors, Symptoms and Signs	Important Tests
Leading Hypothesis		
Ascending cholangitis	RUQ or epigastric pain Dark urine Fever Rigors	Ultrasound Endoscopic ultrasound ERCP MRCP CBC ALT, AST, bilirubin Blood cultures
Active Alternatives—Most Common		
Acute cholecystitis	RUQ pain Fever	Ultrasound
Pancreatitis	Alcohol abuse Gallstones	Serum lipase Ultrasound
Hepatitis	Alcohol abuse Injection drug use RUQ pain Nausea Dark urine	Elevated ALT and AST Viral serologies

ALT, alanine transaminase; AST, aspartate transaminase; CBC, complete blood cell; ERCP, endoscopic retrograde cholangiopancreatography; MRCP, magnetic resonance cholangiopancreatography; RUQ, right upper quadrant.

B. Patients with choledocholithiasis may be asymptomatic.

C. Complications of choledocholithiasis may be the presenting manifestations.

  1. Obstruction and jaundice may be present.

  2. Fever, jaundice, and leukocytosis may be present due to ascending infection from the duodenum (ascending cholangitis). Ascending cholangitis may also occur when the CBD is obstructed due to tumors or strictures.

  3. Pancreatitis may occur if there is concomitant obstruction of the pancreatic duct.

Evidence-Based Diagnosis

A. Ascending cholangitis

  1. Clinical findings in patients with cholangitis include jaundice, 79%; temperature ≥ 38.0 °C, 77%; and RUQ pain, 68%. In various studies 42–75% of patients had all 3 (Charcot triad).

  2. There is leukocytosis in 73% of patients and elevated alkaline phosphatase and bilirubin in 91% and 87%, respectively.

  3. 74% of patients are bacteremic

 Bacteremia is exceptionally common in ascending cholangitis. Antibiotics should be administered promptly to patients in whom this diagnosis is suspected.

Table 3-9. Test characteristics for choledocholithiasis.

Finding	Sensitivity	Specificity	LR+	LR−
Cholangitis	11%	99%	18.3	0.93
Jaundice	36%	97%	10.1	0.69
Dilated CBD on ultrasound	42%	96%	6.9	0.77
Elevated alkaline phosphatase	57%	86%	2.6	0.65
Elevated amylase	11%	95%	1.5	0.99

CBD, common bile duct.
Modified, with permission, from Paul A, Millat B, et al. Diagnosis and treatment of common bile duct stones. Surg Endosc. 1998;12:856–64.

B. Choledocholithiasis

1. Any of the following suggests choledocholithiasis and warrants CBD evaluation (Table 3-9):

    a. Cholangitis

    b. Jaundice

    c. Dilated CBD on ultrasound

    d. Elevated alkaline phosphatase

    e. Elevated amylase or lipase

2. CBD stones are present in 5–8% of patients without any of the aforementioned risk factors.

3. Transabdominal ultrasound is noninvasive but *not* consistently sensitive for choledocholithiasis as opposed to its performance in cholelithiasis (sensitivity 25–81%, specificity 88–91%). A dilated CBD is seen in only 25% of patients.

4. Endoscopic retrograde cholangiopancreatography (ERCP), magnetic resonance cholangiopancreatography (MRCP), and EUS are highly accurate in detecting CBD stones. These techniques share high sensitivity (90–100%) and specificity (90–100%).

    a. ERCP

    (1) Invasive procedure that allows direct cannulation of CBD *and* relieves obstruction via simultaneous stone extraction and sphincterotomy

    (2) > 90% sensitive, 99% specific for diagnosis

    (3) Requires sedation

    (4) Complicated by pancreatitis in 1–5% of patients

    (5) Preferred procedure in patients with a high pretest probability of CBD stones particularly those with jaundice and fever in whom ERCP can also permit stone extraction

    (6) In patients less likely to have a CBD stone (ie, those with cholelithiasis and isolated elevation in alkaline phosphatase), a less invasive test (eg, MRCP or EUS) is an appropriate initial study.

    b. MRCP

    (1) Noninvasive scan visualizes CBD and adjacent structures

    (2) Highly accurate for CBD stones: 90–100% sensitive, 88–100% specific

    c. EUS

    (1) Both sensitive (94–99%) and specific (94–95%) for CBD stones.

    (2) One study reported that EUS was more sensitive than ERCP (97% vs 67%).

    (3) A normal EUS or MRCP would obviate the need for a more invasive ERCP.

    (4) EUS followed by selective ERCP in patients with documented CBD stones is an appropriate strategy in patients with suspected choledocholithiasis without cholangitis. Reserving ERCP for the subset of patients with *documented* choledocholithiasis decreased the need for ERCP by 67% and the complication rate by 12% compared with performing ERCP in all patients with suspected choledocholithiasis.

    d. CT scanning is only 75% sensitive for choledocholithiasis. Two studies suggest that multidetector CT using iotroxate (which is excreted in the biliary system) is highly accurate for choledocholithiasis (85–96% sensitive, 88–94% specific).

    e. Summary: The ASGE recommends the following based on the risk of choledocholithiasis:

    (1) High-risk patients (> 50% risk): ERCP is recommended in patients with

        (a) Suspected ascending cholangitis

        (b) Documented CBD stones

        (c) Bilirubin > 4 mg/dL

        (d) Bilirubin levels of 1.8–4 mg/dL and dilated CBDs

    (2) Moderate-risk patients (10–50% risk): MRCP or EUS is recommended followed by selective ERCP in patients with *documented* choledocholithiasis.

        (a) Patients with dilated CBD on ultrasound

        (b) Elevated bilirubin levels (1.8–4 mg/dL)

        (c) Gallstone-associated pancreatitis

        (d) Elevated LFTs

        (e) Age > 55 years

        (f) An alternative approach is laparoscopic cholecystectomy with intraoperative cholangiogram and postoperative ERCP in patients with choledocholithiasis.

    (3) Low-risk patients (< 10% risk): In patients with gallstone disease and none of the aforementioned risk factors, laparoscopic cholecystectomy without other preoperative CBD evaluation is recommended.

Treatment

A. Ascending cholangitis

1. Blood cultures, IV broad-spectrum antibiotics, and IV hydration should begin immediately

2. Biliary drainage with ERCP should be performed urgently in patients with moderate to severe disease.

3. Biliary drainage with ERCP should be performed

    a. Emergently in patients with persistent pain, hypotension, altered mental status, persistent high fever, WBC ≥ 20,000/mcL, and bilirubin ≥ 10 mg/dL

    b. Electively in more stable patients

4. If ERCP is unavailable, percutaneous transhepatic drainage or surgical decompression can be used.

B. In patients who have choledocholithiasis without ascending cholangitis, CBD stones can be removed via intraoperative CBD exploration or ERCP.

C. Cholecystectomy

MAKING A DIAGNOSIS

Neither dilation of the CBD nor CBD stone can be seen on ultrasound (but is only 25% sensitive). You still suspect choledocholithiasis because of the jaundice and increased transaminases.

Twenty-four hours later, blood cultures are positive for *Escherichia coli* (consistent with ascending cholangitis).

Have you crossed a diagnostic threshold for the leading hypothesis, ascending cholangitis? Have you ruled out the active alternatives? Do other tests need to be done to exclude the alternative diagnoses?

Alternative Diagnosis: Acute Hepatitis

See Chapter 26, Jaundice & Abnormal Liver Enzymes.

Alternative Diagnosis: Acute Cholecystitis

Textbook Presentation

Typical symptoms of acute cholecystitis include *persistent* RUQ or epigastric pain, fever, nausea, and vomiting.

Disease Highlights

A. Secondary to prolonged cystic duct obstruction (> 4–6 hours)

B. Persistent obstruction results in increasing gallbladder inflammation and pain. Necrosis, infection, and gangrene may occur.

C. Jaundice and marked elevation of liver enzymes are seen only if the stone migrates into the CBD and causes obstruction.

Evidence-Based Diagnosis

A. No clinical finding is sufficiently sensitive to rule out cholecystitis.
  1. Fever: present in 0–35% of patients
  2. Murphy sign
     a. Sensitivity, 65%; specificity, 87%
     b. LR+ = 5.0, LR– = 0.4

B. Laboratory findings
  1. Leukocytosis (> 10,000/mcL) is present in 52–63% of patients.
  2. Cholecystitis does *not* typically cause significant increases in lipase or LFTs. Such findings suggest complications of pancreatitis and choledocholithiasis.

C. Ultrasound (by radiologists)
  1. Test of choice due to speed, cost, ability to image adjacent organs and lack of radiation.
  2. Sensitivity, 88%; specificity, 80%, LR+, 4.4; LR–, 0.15
  3. Cholelithiasis is usually present (84–99%) but is not in and of itself diagnostic of acute cholecystitis.
  4. Additional findings that suggest acute cholecystitis include gallstones *with* gallbladder wall thickening, pericholecystic fluid, sonographic Murphy sign, or gallbladder enlargement > 5 cm. However, more specific findings may be less sensitive (27–38%).
  5. If ultrasound is normal, and clinical suspicion is high, consider HIDA (see below).

D. Bedside ultrasound by trained non-radiologists
  1. Used with increasing frequency in emergency departments
  2. One study reported good accuracy when performed by emergency department physicians with 5 hours of training; sensitivity, 91%; specificity, 66%; LR+, 2.7; LR–, 0.14.
  3. Abnormal results should be confirmed with formal ultrasonography.
  4. Normal results are probably adequate to rule out cholecystitis in patients with low pretest probabilities but not in those for whom there is a higher suspicion of acute cholecystitis.

E. Cholescintigraphy (HIDA) scans
  1. Radioisotope is excreted by the liver into the biliary system. In normal patients, the gallbladder concentrates the isotope and is visualized.
  2. Nonvisualization of the gallbladder suggests cystic duct obstruction and is highly specific for acute cholecystitis (97% sensitive, 90% specific).
  3. Nonvisualization can also be seen in prolonged fasting, hepatitis, alcohol abuse, and prior biliary sphincterotomy.
  4. Useful when the pretest probability is high, due to persistent pain, and the ultrasound is nondiagnostic (ie, the ultrasound demonstrates stones within the gallbladder) but no clear evidence of cholecystitis is seen (eg, no stones within the cystic duct nor evidence of gallbladder wall thickening or pericholecystic fluid).
  5. Visualization of the gallbladder essentially excludes acute cholecystitis.

F. A diagnostic algorithm is shown in Figure 3-4.

Treatment

Patients with acute cholecystitis should be admitted, administered parenteral antibiotics, and undergo cholecystectomy. The precise timing of surgery (early vs delayed) is controversial.

Alternative Diagnosis: Acute Pancreatitis

Textbook Presentation

Patients with acute pancreatitis often complain of a constant and boring abdominal pain of moderate to severe intensity that develops in the epigastrium and may radiate to the back. Associated symptoms may include nausea, vomiting, low-grade fever, and abdominal distention.

Disease Highlights

A. Etiology
  1. Alcohol abuse (typically binge drinking) and choledocholithiasis (with concomitant obstruction of pancreatic outflow) cause 80% of acute pancreatitis cases.
  2. 15–25% of cases are idiopathic, many of which may be due to microlithiasis or sphincter of Oddi dysfunction.
     a. 34–67% of patients with idiopathic pancreatitis were found to have small gallstones on EUS or ERCP.
     b. Sphincter of Oddi dysfunction may be particularly common in patients with prior cholecystectomy.
  3. Post ERCP
  4. Drugs commonly associated with pancreatitis include azathioprine, didanosine, estrogens, furosemide, hydrochlorothiazide, L-asparaginase, metronidazole, opioids, pentamidine, sulfonamides, corticosteroids, tamoxifen, tetracycline, valproate, and many others.

5. Less common causes include trauma, marked hypertriglyceridemia (> 1000 mg/dL), hypercalcemia, ischemia, HIV infection, other infection, pancreatic carcinoma, pancreatic divisum, autoimmune pancreatitis, cystic fibrosis, and organ transplantation.

6. Regardless of the inciting event, trypsinogen is activated to trypsin, which activates other pancreatic enzymes resulting in pancreatic autodigestion and inflammation (which may become systemic and lethal). Interleukins contribute to the inflammation.

B. Complications may be local or systemic. Severe, potentially fatal pancreatitis develops in about 20% of patients.

1. Local complications

   a. Pancreatic pseudocyst

   b. Pancreatic necrosis

   c. Infections

   (1) Bacterial translocation from the bowel with resultant local and systemic infection

   (2) Infected pancreatic pseudocyst (abscess)

   (3) Infected pancreatic necrosis

   (4) Ascending cholangitis (in patients with gallstone-associated pancreatitis [GAP])

2. Systemic complications

   a. Hyperglycemia

   b. Hypocalcemia

   c. Acute respiratory distress syndrome

   d. Acute kidney injury

   e. Disseminated intravascular coagulation

3. Death

   a. Usually occurs in patients with infected pancreatic necrosis and in patients in whom multiple organ dysfunction develops.

   b. Several predictive scores have been developed including the Ranson criteria as well as the Glasgow and Apache II scores. All use similar variables that increase the likelihood of organ failure, including increased age and elevated WBC, BUN, glucose, or lactate dehydrogenase. Hypoxia and hypocalcemia are also associated with an increased risk.

   c. Hemoconcentration (HCT ≥ 50%) on admission predicts severe pancreatitis; LR+ 7.5 (vs 0.4 for patients with HCT ≤ 45%).

   d. CRP > 150 mg/L at 48 hours can also predict severe pancreatitis; sensitivity, 85–86%; specificity, 74–87%; LR+, 3.2–6.6; LR–, 0.16–0.2

Evidence-Based Diagnosis

A. History and physical

1. Low-grade fevers (< 38.3°C) are common (60%).

2. Pain may radiate to the back (50%) and may be exacerbated in the supine position.

3. Nausea and vomiting are usually present (75%).

4. Rebound is rare on presentation; guarding is common (50%).

5. Periumbilical bruising (Cullen sign) is rare.

6. Retroperitoneal bleeding from pancreatitis or a variety of other causes (including ruptured AAA) can lead to flank bruising (Grey Turner sign), which is rare, but can be a valuable clue when present.

B. Laboratory studies

1. Lipase

   a. 94% sensitive, 96% specific; LR+ = 23, LR– = .06

   b. Remains elevated longer than serum amylase

   c. Marked elevations suggest pancreatitis secondary to gallstones.

2. Amylase

   a. Less sensitive and specific than lipase

   b. Should not be routinely ordered if lipase available

3. LFTs

   a. Studies suggest that *significant* elevations of the bilirubin, alkaline phosphatase, ALT, or AST in patients with pancreatitis suggest etiology secondary to gallstones (GAP). These enzymes increase due to concomitant obstruction of the CBD.

   (1) ALT or AST elevations > 100 IU/L suggest GAP (sensitivity ≈ 55%, specificity ≈ 93%; LR+ 8–9)

   (2) AST levels < 50 IU/L make GAP unlikely (sensitivity 90%, specificity 68%; LR– 0.15).

   (3) 10% of patients with GAP have normal levels of alkaline phosphatase, bilirubin, AST, and ALT.

   b. Patients with GAP have high risk of recurrent pancreatitis and require cholecystectomy.

4. Imaging: A variety of imaging techniques can be used in patients with acute pancreatitis.

   a. Plain radiography is useful to rule out free air or SBO.

   b. Transabdominal ultrasound is noninvasive and should be performed in *all* patients with pancreatitis to determine if they have gallstones or CBD dilatation suggesting GAP.

   c. CT scanning is 87–90% sensitive and 90–92% specific for the diagnosis of acute pancreatitis but insensitive for determining whether or not patients have GAP.

   (1) Should be performed when the diagnosis is unclear or complications are suspected (pseudocysts or pancreatic necrosis)

   (2) Pancreatic necrosis should be suspected in patients with severe pancreatitis, when signs of sepsis are present, and in patients who do not improve in the first 72 hours.

   (3) IV contrast is required to demonstrate necrosis.

5. Detecting GAP

   a. GAP should be suspected in any patient with pancreatitis that is not clearly secondary to alcohol.

   b. Neither transabdominal ultrasound nor CT is sensitive at detecting choledocholithiasis (21% and 40%, respectively).

   c. MRCP is highly accurate for choledocholithiasis (80–94% sensitive) as are EUS and ERCP (≈ 96–98% sensitive).

   d. ERCP

   (1) Can cause pancreatitis and is therefore limited to patients with persistent obstruction or cholangitis.

   (2) Its use in patients with severe pancreatitis is controversial.

   e. Preoperatively, patients with GAP should have CBD evaluation with ERCP, MRCP, or EUS. A reasonable option in such patients is EUS followed by ERCP if stones are identified.

6. Imaging in idiopathic pancreatitis
    a. One study suggested EUS is superior to MRCP (except in patients with prior cholecystectomy).
    b. EUS more commonly discovered microlithiasis and sludge (suggesting GAP) than MRCP.
    c. Sensitivity of EUS is 88–96%, compared with 24% of MRCP.
7. Calcium and triglycerides should be ordered to exclude less common causes of acute pancreatitis.
8. Figure 3-5 outlines an approach to evaluation of pancreatitis.

Treatment

A. Vital signs, orthostatic BPs, and urinary output should be carefully monitored to assess intravascular volume.
B. IV fluid is critical to maintain appropriate BP and urinary output (> 0.5 mL/kg/h).

1. One study demonstrated lactated Ringers was superior to normal saline with a significant reduction in the incidence of systemic inflammatory response syndrome at 24 hours (absolute risk reduction ≈ 15%, NNT = 6.7).
2. Lactated Ringers should be avoided in patients with hypercalcemia.
C. No oral intake
D. Opioids for pain relief
E. Nasogastric tube if recurrent vomiting
F. Oxygen, electrolyte, and glucose monitoring
G. ICU admission for severe pancreatitis
H. *Prophylactic* antibiotics for patients with pancreatic necrosis are controversial.
I. If infection is suspected (due to increasing fever, leukocytosis or deterioration) evaluate with fine-needle aspiration and culture. If infection is confirmed, broad-spectrum antibiotics should be administered and surgical debridement considered.

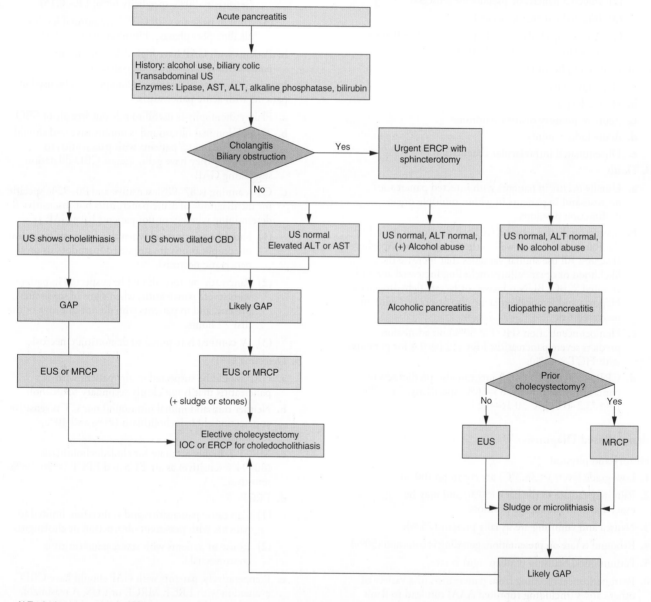

ALT, alanine transaminase; AST, aspartate transaminase; CBD, common bile duct; EUS, endoscopic ultrasound; GAP, gallstone pancreatitis; IOC, intraoperative cholangiogram; MRCP, magnetic resonance cholangiopancreatography; US, ultrasound.

Figure 3-5. Evaluation of pancreatitis.

J. ERCP and sphincterotomy (see above)

K. GAP: Cholecystectomy and ERCP/sphincterotomy

1. Surgery during the index admission is superior to delayed surgery or ERCP with sphincterotomy (ERCP/S) decreasing the rate of recurrent acute pancreatitis and other biliary events.

2. Recurrent GAP was seen in 1.7% of patients receiving surgery during their index admission vs 5.3% of patients having delayed ERCP/S and 13.2% in patients without surgery.

3. CBD evaluation (with intraoperative cholangiogram, MRCP, or EUS) is also required to ensure that the CBD is clear of stones.

L. Alcohol abstinence

M. Nutrition

1. Enteral feeding is superior to parenteral feeding and has been shown to decrease mortality.

2. Enteral feeding avoids a variety of IV catheter–related complications and decreases gut bacterial translocation, which may contribute to infection.

3. Jejunal feeding tubes are preferred.

Alternative Diagnosis: Chronic Pancreatitis

See Chapter 32, Unintentional Weight Loss.

CASE RESOLUTION

An ERCP demonstrates multiple small stones within the CBD, which are extracted. Ms. R underwent cholecystectomy and recovered without incident.

CHIEF COMPLAINT

PATIENT 3

Mr. J is a previously healthy 63-year-old man with severe abdominal pain for 48 hours. The pain is periumbilical with severe crampy exacerbations that last for several minutes and then subside. He notes loud intestinal noises (borborygmi) during the periods of increased pain. The pain is associated with nausea and vomiting. He denies diarrhea. He reports decreased appetite with no oral intake in the last 48 hours. He denies having this pain previously.

At this point, what is the leading hypothesis, what are the active alternatives, and is there a must not miss diagnosis? Given this differential diagnosis, what tests should be ordered?

RANKING THE DIFFERENTIAL DIAGNOSIS

The first pivotal point for Mr. J's abdominal pain is its periumbilical location. A variety of diseases present with pain in this location, including AAA, appendicitis (early), bowel ischemia, bowel obstruction, diabetic ketoacidosis, gastroenteritis, IBS, and IBD (Figure 3-1). The second useful pivotal point to consider is the time course of Mr. J's abdominal pain (Table 3-1). This allows us to further limit the differential diagnosis to those diseases causing *acute* periumbilical pain. Many of the aforementioned diseases cause acute pain, but not typically IBS and IBD. Furthermore, diabetic ketoacidosis is unlikely (unless this is his presentation of diabetes). Gastroenteritis is also unlikely given the absence of diarrhea and the severity of the pain. Finally, Mr. J's severe crampy abdominal pain suggests some type of visceral obstruction. The syndromes associated with pain of this quality include ureteral obstruction secondary to kidney stones, biliary obstruction, or intestinal obstruction (large or small bowel). The associated nausea and vomiting can be seen with any of those diseases. However, the combination of the location of the pain and the loud intestinal sounds that accompany the pain makes bowel obstruction the leading hypothesis. It will also be important to determine if he has unexplained hypotension or abdominal distention during his exam. Table 3-10 lists the differential diagnoses for Mr. J.

Table 3-10. Diagnostic hypotheses for Mr. J.

Diagnostic Hypothesis	Demographics, Risk Factors, Symptoms and Signs	Important Tests
Leading Hypothesis		
Bowel obstruction	Inability to pass stool or flatus Nausea, vomiting Prior abdominal surgery or altered bowel habits Hematochezia Abdominal distention, hyperactive bowel sounds (with tinkling) or hypoactive bowel sounds	Abdominal radiographs CT scan
Active Alternatives—Must Not Miss		
AAA	Smoking history Orthostatic hypotension Pulsatile abdominal mass Decreased lower extremity pulses	Abdominal CT scan
Appendicitis	Migration of pain from periumbilical region to right lower quadrant	Clinical exam CT scan
Bowel ischemia: Acute mesenteric ischemia	Atrial fibrillation, valvular heart disease, heart failure, hypercoagulable state Abrupt onset pain. Pain out of proportion to exam	CT angiography
Bowel ischemia: Ischemic colitis	Age > 60, vascular disease, hypotension (due to MI, sepsis), hematochezia, diarrhea	Colonoscopy

AAA, abdominal aortic aneurysm; MI, myocardial infarction.

Three weeks ago, Mr. J noted a small amount of blood on the stool. He reports no other change in bowel habits until 4 days ago. Since that time, he has been constipated and has not passed stool or flatus. He has no prior history of intra-abdominal surgeries, hernias, or diverticulitis. He has no history of smoking and states that the pain does not radiate to his back. There is no prior history of atrial fibrillation, valvular heart disease or known hypercoagulable state. On physical exam, he is intermittently very uncomfortable with episodes of severe diffuse cramping pain. Vital signs reveal orthostatic hypotension: supine BP, 110/75 mm Hg; pulse, 90 bpm; upright BP, 85/50 mm Hg; pulse, 125 bpm; temperature, 37.0°C; RR, 18 breaths per minute. He is anicteric. Cardiac and lung exams are unremarkable. On abdominal inspection there is prominent distention. Auscultation shows intermittent rushes. Percussion is tympanitic and on palpation there is mild diffuse tenderness to exam without rebound or guarding. Stool is brown and heme positive.

The constipation, absence of flatus, and rushing bowel sounds further increase the suspicion of bowel obstruction. The tympanitic abdominal distention is a pivotal finding suggesting accumulation of air in the abdomen, in this case most likely due to obstruction. Most cases of SBO are due to adhesions from prior surgery. Mr. J's negative surgical history makes SBO less unlikely. However, the hematochezia raises the possibility of a malignant obstruction and large bowel obstruction. The orthostatic hypotension is most likely due to dehydration from the vomiting and lack of oral intake and does not in and of itself suggest intra-abdominal hemorrhage from an AAA.

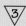

Laboratory findings are WBC 10,000/mcL (70% neutrophils, 0% bands); HCT, 41%. Electrolytes: Na, 141 mEq/L; K, 3.0 mEq/L; HCO₃, 32 mEq/L; Cl, 99 mEq/L; BUN, 45 mg/dL; creatinine 1.0 mg/dL. An abdominal upright radiograph is shown Figure 3-6.

Is the clinical information sufficient to make a diagnosis? If not, what other information do you need?

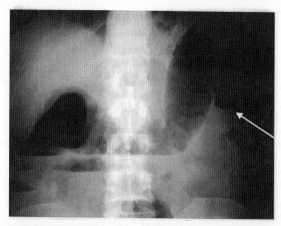

Figure 3-6. Plain radiography reveals grossly distended ascending colon, multiple air-fluid levels and an abrupt termination of air in the transverse colon (arrow) suggestive of large bowel obstruction.

Leading Hypothesis: Large Bowel Obstruction (LBO)

Textbook Presentation

Bowel obstruction presents with waves of severe crampy abdominal pain that the patient finds incapacitating. Vomiting is common. The pain is often diffuse and poorly localized. Initially, the patient may have several bowel movements as the bowel *distal* to the obstruction is emptied in the first 12–24 hours. Bowel sounds are hyperactive early in the course. Abdominal distention is often present. (Distention is less prominent in proximal SBOs.) At first, the pain is intermittent; later, the pain often becomes more constant, bowel sounds may diminish and become absent, constipation progresses and the patient becomes unable to pass flatus. If bowel infarction occurs, focal tenderness and peritoneal findings may be seen.

 In patients with abdominal pain, the absence of bowel movements or flatus suggests bowel obstruction.

Disease Highlights

A. Bowel obstruction accounts for 4% of patients with abdominal pain.

B. LBO accounts for 20% of all bowel obstructions.

C. Etiology: cancer (53%), sigmoid or cecal volvulus (17%), diverticular disease (12%), extrinsic compression from metastatic cancer (6%), other (12%) (adhesions rarely cause LBO)

Evidence-Based Diagnosis

A. History and physical exam in LBO and SBO (Table 3-11)

1. None of the expected clinical findings are very sensitive.

   a. Vomiting, 75%

   b. Abdominal distention, 63%

2. Certain findings are fairly specific.

   a. Constipation, 95%; LR+, 8.8

    b. Prior abdominal surgery, 94%; LR+, 11.5

   c. Abdominal distention, 89%; LR+, 5.7

Table 3-11. Test characteristics for predicting bowel obstruction.

Finding	Sensitivity	Specificity	LR+	LR−
Visible peristalsis	6%	99.7%	20	0.94
Prior abdominal surgery	69%	94%	11.5	0.33
Constipation	44%	95%	8.8	0.59
Abdominal distention	63%	89%	5.7	0.42
Increased bowel sounds	40%	89%	3.6	0.67
Reduced bowel sounds	23%	93%	3.3	0.83
Colicky pain	31%	89%	2.8	0.78
Vomiting	75%	65%	2.1	0.38

Modified, with permission, from Böhmer H. Simple Data from History and Physical Examination Help to Exclude Bowel Obstruction and to Avoid Radiographic Studies in Patients with Acute Abdominal Pain. *Eur J Surg* 1998;164:777.

3. Certain combinations are insensitive (27–48%) but highly specific.

a. Distention associated with any of the following highly suggestive (LR+ ≈ 10): increased bowel sounds, vomiting, constipation, or prior surgery

b. Increased bowel sounds with prior surgery or vomiting also very suggestive of obstruction (LR+ of 11 and 8, respectively)

B. A CBC and electrolytes should be obtained: Anion gap acidosis suggests bowel infarction or sepsis.

> Marked leukocytosis, left shift or anion gap acidosis in a patient with bowel obstruction is a *late* finding and suggests bowel infarction.

C. Plain radiography may show air-fluid levels and distention of large bowel (> 6 cm).
  1. 84% sensitive, 72% specific for presence of LBO (not etiology)
  2. Small bowel distention also occurs if ileocecal valve is incompetent.

D. Barium enema (water soluble) or colonoscopy
  1. Barium enema is highly accurate for LBO.
     a. 96% sensitive, 98% specific
     b. LR+ 48, LR– 0.04
  2. Can determine etiology preoperatively (if patient stable)
  3. Can exclude acute colonic pseudo-obstruction (distention of the cecum and colon without mechanical obstruction)
  4. Colonoscopy can decompress pseudo-obstruction and prevent cecal perforation.

E. CT scan is also accurate in the diagnosis of LBO.
  1. 91% sensitive, 91% specific
  2. LR+ 10.1, LR– 0.1

Treatment of LBO

A. Aggressive rehydration and monitoring of urinary output is vital.

B. Broad-spectrum antibiotics advised: 39% of patients have microorganisms in the mesenteric nodes.

C. Surgery, stents, and balloon dilatation have been used. Consultation is advised.

D. For patients with sigmoid volvulus, and no evidence of infarction, sigmoidoscopy allows decompression and elective surgery at a later date to prevent recurrence.
  1. Emergent indications for surgery: perforation or ischemia
  2. Nonemergent indications for surgery: increasing distention, failure to resolve

MAKING A DIAGNOSIS

After reviewing the plain films, you order a barium enema.

Have you crossed a diagnostic threshold for the leading hypothesis, large bowel obstruction? Have you ruled out the active alternatives? Do other tests need to be done to exclude the alternative diagnoses?

Alternative Diagnosis: SBO

Textbook Presentation

The presentation is similar to that for LBO with the exception that patients are more likely to have a history of prior abdominal surgery.

Disease Highlights

A. Bowel obstruction accounts for 4% of patients with abdominal pain.

B. SBO accounts for 80% of all bowel obstructions.

C. Etiology
  1. Postsurgical adhesions, 70%
  2. Malignant tumor, 10–20%
     a. Usually metastatic
     b. However, 39% of SBOs in patients with a prior malignancy are due to adhesions or benign causes.
  3. Hernia (ventral, inguinal, or internal), 10%
  4. IBD (with stricture), 5%
  5. Radiation
  6. Less common causes of SBO include gallstones, bezoars, and intussusception.

D. SBOs may be partial or complete.
  1. Complete SBO
     a. 20–40% progress to strangulation and infarction. Strangulation may occur secondary to mesenteric twisting cutting off the blood supply or due to increasing intraluminal pressure directly compromising perfusion.
     b. Clinical signs do *not* allow for identification of strangulation prior to infarction: Fever, leukocytosis, and metabolic acidosis are late signs of strangulation and suggest infarction.
     c. 50–75% of patients admitted for SBO require surgery
  2. Partial SBO
     a. Rarely progresses to strangulation or infarction
     b. Characterized by continuing ability to pass stool or flatus (> 6–12 hours after symptom onset) or passage of contrast into cecum
     c. Resolves spontaneously (without surgery) in 60–85% of patients

Evidence-Based Diagnosis

A. Ideally, tests for SBO should identify obstruction *and* ischemia or infarction, if present (since ischemia and infarction are indications for emergent surgery rather than further observation.) Unfortunately, even tests that successfully predict SBO do not reliably determine whether there is ischemia and infarction.

B. See test characteristics of history and physical exam under LBO.

C. Physical exam findings are insensitive at predicting infarction. However, localized tenderness, rebound, or guarding would all suggest infarction is present.

D. WBC may be normal even in presence of ischemia.

E. Plain radiographs may show ≥ 2 air-fluid levels or dilated loops of bowel proximal to obstruction (> 2.5 cm diameter of small bowel).
  1. Sensitivity for obstruction 59–93%, specificity 83%
  2. Rarely determines etiology
  3. Complete obstruction is unlikely in patients with air in the colon or rectum.

F. Bedside ultrasound

    1. Can show dilated bowel (≥ 25 mm) proximal to normal or collapsed distal bowel.

    2. One study demonstrated excellent accuracy: sensitivity, 91%; specificity, 84%; LR+, 5.7; LR−, 0.11

    3. Superior to plain films (18% sensitive, 56% specific; LR+, 0.41; LR−, 1.5)

G. CT scanning

    1. Sensitivity for determining high-grade obstruction is 80–93%.

        a. Obstruction is suggested by a transition point between bowel proximal to the obstruction, which is dilated, and bowel distal to the obstruction, which is collapsed.

        b. CT scanning should be performed prior to nasogastric suction, which may decompress the proximal small bowel and thereby decreases the sensitivity of the CT scan for SBO.

    2. May delineate etiology of obstruction

    3. Test of choice to diagnose SBO (not ischemia)

    4. Not reliably sensitive at determining the presence of ischemia and infarction (and the need for immediate surgery). Different studies have reported sensitivities ranging from 15% to 100% (specificity 85–94%).

 The absence of CT signs of ischemia in patients with SBO does not in fact rule out ischemia.

    5. CT scan only 48% sensitive for partial SBO

H. Gastrografin small bowel series

    1. Diagnosis

        a. Accurate in the diagnosis of SBO and useful to predict nonoperative resolution

        b. 97% sensitive, 96% specific. (Spontaneous resolution is likely in patients in whom contrast reaches the colon.)

        c. Unlike CT scanning, small bowel series cannot delineate etiology of SBO or demonstrate ischemic changes.

    2. Therapy

        a. Gastrografin is hyperosmolar and draws fluid into bowel lumen, potentially dilating bowel.

        b. Randomized trials of patients with presumed adhesive SBO demonstrate reduced odds of surgical intervention in patients receiving gastrografin compared to controls (0.44–0.87).

Treatment

A. Fluid resuscitation

    1. IV rehydration is important to correct the prominent intravascular dehydration from decreased oral intake, vomiting, *and* third spacing of fluid within the bowel.

    2. Monitor vital signs, orthostasis, and urinary output carefully.

B. Careful, frequent observation and repeated physical exam over the first 12–24 hours

C. Nasogastric suction

D. Broad-spectrum antibiotics (59% of patients have bacterial translocation to mesenteric lymph nodes)

E. Frequent plain radiographs and CBC

F. Indications for surgery include any of the following:

    1. Signs of ischemia (increased pain, fever, tenderness, peritoneal findings, acidosis, or worsening leukocytosis)

    2. CT findings of infarction

    3. SBO secondary to hernia

    4. SBO clearly not secondary to adhesion (no prior surgery)

    5. Some clinicians recommend surgery when bowel obstruction fails to resolve in 24 hours. Others suggest a small bowel study.

Alternative Diagnosis: Ischemic Bowel Secondary to Acute Mesenteric Ischemia or Ischemic Colitis

Ischemic Bowel

Three distinct clinical subtypes of ischemic bowel include chronic mesenteric ischemia (chronic small bowel ischemia), acute mesenteric ischemia (acute ischemia of small bowel), ischemic colitis (ischemia of the large bowel). Chronic mesenteric ischemia is discussed at the end of the chapter.

1. Acute Mesenteric Ischemia

Textbook Presentation

Acute mesenteric ischemia is a life-threatening condition that virtually always presents with the abrupt onset of acute severe abdominal pain that is typically out of proportion to a relatively benign physical exam. Acute mesenteric ischemia usually occurs in patients with risk factors for systemic embolization (eg, atrial fibrillation) or arterial thrombosis. Unexplained metabolic acidosis can be an important clue.

Disease Highlights

A. Etiology: Usually due to superior mesenteric artery or celiac artery embolism (50%). Other causes include thrombosis (15–25%), low flow states without obstruction (15–30%) (nonobstructive mesenteric ischemia), and mesenteric venous thrombosis (5%).

    1. Embolism

        a. Risk factors include atrial fibrillation, acute myocardial infarction, valvular heart disease, heart failure, ventricular aneurysms, angiography of abdominal aorta, and hypercoagulable states.

        b. The onset is often sudden without prior symptoms.

    2. Thrombosis

        a. Usually occurs in patients with atherosclerotic disease of the involved artery.

        b. Approximately half of such patients have a prior history of chronic mesenteric ischemia with intestinal angina.

    3. Nonobstructive mesenteric ischemia

        a. May have an insidious onset

        b. Often occurs in elderly patients with mesenteric atherosclerotic disease and superimposed hypotension (due to myocardial infarction, heart failure, dialysis, or sepsis). Alpha-agonists, digoxin, and beta-blockers may also increase the risk of nonobstructive mesenteric ischemia.

        c. Also seen in critically ill patients after cardiopulmonary bypass or other major surgery

        d. Other causes include cocaine use and following endurance exercise activities (eg, marathon, cycling).

4. Mesenteric venous thrombosis is often secondary to portal hypertension, hypercoagulable states, and intra-abdominal inflammation.

B. Patients have acute abdominal pain that is often out of proportion to their abdominal exam. If left untreated, bowel infarction and peritoneal findings will develop.

C. Incidence: 0.1–0.3% of hospital admissions

D. Mortality is high at 30–82%.

Evidence-Based Diagnosis

A. Common presenting symptoms are abdominal pain (94%), nausea (56%), vomiting (38%), and diarrhea (31%).

B. 50% of patients have a prior history of intestinal angina.

C. The WBC is abnormal in 90% of patients and often markedly elevated (mean WBC 21.4 × 10⁹/mL).

D. Lactate level was elevated in 77–89% of patients (mean 3.3 mmol/L [normal < 2.0 mmol/L]).

 A normal lactate level does not rule out acute mesenteric ischemia.

E. Plain abdominal radiographs may reveal thickening of bowel loops or thumbprinting but are insensitive (40%).

F. Doppler ultrasonography is insensitive due to bowel distention.

G. Standard CT scanning may demonstrate superior mesenteric artery occlusion or findings suggesting ischemic and necrosis such as segmental bowel wall thickening or pneumatosis but is insensitive (64%). One study reported 100% sensitivity but patients were studied 3 days after symptom onset, when infarction may have been easier to demonstrate.

H. CT angiography is very accurate (89–96% sensitive, 97–98% specific), rapidly available and fast. It is increasingly used as the initial study prior to angiography. Magnetic resonance angiography has also been used.

I. Catheter angiography is the gold standard and can also be therapeutic. However, it is invasive, time consuming, and may not be available on an emergent basis.

Treatment

A. Emergent revascularization (via thromboembolectomy, thrombolysis, vascular bypass or angioplasty) and surgical resection of necrotic bowel are the mainstays of therapy. Prompt surgical intervention (< 12 hours) reduces mortality compared with delayed intervention (> 12 hours) (14% vs 75%).

B. Broad-spectrum antibiotics

C. Volume resuscitation

D. Preoperative and postoperative anticoagulation to prevent thrombus propagation

E. For patients with nonobstructive mesenteric ischemia, improved perfusion is paramount.

F. Intra-arterial papaverine improves mesenteric blood flow by reducing reactive mesenteric arteriolar vasoconstriction.

2. Ischemic Colitis

Textbook Presentation

Ischemic colitis typically presents with left-sided abdominal pain. Patients frequently have bloody or maroon stools or diarrhea. Profuse bleeding is unusual.

Disease Highlights

A. The most common form of intestinal ischemia

B. Usually due to nonocclusive decrease in colonic perfusion

C. Distribution: Typically involves the watershed areas of the colon, most commonly the splenic flexure, descending colon, and rectosigmoid junction. Right colonic involvement occurs occasionally. Rectal involvement is rare and points to other diseases.

D. Precipitating events may include hypotension, myocardial infarction, sepsis, heart failure, or cardiac or aortic surgery but is usually not identified.

E. Uncommon causes include vasculitis, hypercoagulable states, vasoconstrictors, cocaine, vascular surgery, drugs (eg, alosetron), and long-distance running or bicycling (presumably due to shunting and hypoperfusion).

Evidence-Based Diagnosis

A. Abdominal pain (not usually severe) is reported by 68–84% of patients.

B. Hematochezia is a helpful diagnostic clue when present but not diagnostic when absent. Sensitivity 46%, specificity 90.9%; LR+ 5.1, LR−, 0.6

C. Diarrhea is seen in approximately 40% of patients.

D. Abdominal tenderness is common (81%), but rebound tenderness is rare (15%).

E. Risk factors that increase the likelihood of ischemic colitis include age > 60 years, hemodialysis, cardiovascular disease, hypertension, diabetes mellitus, hypoalbuminemia, and medications that induce constipation.

F. Features that distinguish acute mesenteric ischemia (small bowel) from ischemic colitis are summarized in Table 3-12.

G. Colonoscopy (without preparation) is the preferred test to evaluate ischemic colitis.

H. Plain radiographs rarely demonstrate free air (perforation) or thumbprinting (specific for ischemia).

Table 3-12. Features that distinguish ischemic colitis from acute mesenteric ischemia.

Ischemic Colitis	Acute Mesenteric Ischemia
Usually due to nonocclusive decrease in colonic perfusion	Usually due to acute arterial occlusion of SMA or celiac artery
Precipitating cause often not identified	Precipitating cause typical (MI, atrial fibrillation etc)
Patients are usually not severely ill	Patients appear severely ill
Abdominal pain usually mild	Abdominal pain usually severe
Abdominal tenderness usually present	Abdominal tenderness not prominent early
Hematochezia common	Hematochezia uncommon until very late
Colonoscopy procedure of choice, angiography not usually indicated	Angiography indicated

MI, myocardial infarction; SMA, superior mesenteric artery.

I. Ultrasound may show segmental circumferential thickening a long segment (>10cm) of the splenic flexure or sigmoid with sudden transition from abnormal to normal areas. Color flow is absent or greatly diminished in 80% of cases, helping distinguish this from IBD in which flow is increased.

J. CT scanning may demonstrate segmental circumferential wall thickening (which is nonspecific) or be normal.

K. Vascular studies are usually normal and not indicated except in the unusual case of isolated right-sided ischemic colitis.

Treatment

A. Therapy is primarily supportive, with bowel rest, IV hydration, and broad-spectrum antibiotics.

B. Colonic infarction occurs in a small percentage of patients (15–20%) and requires segmental resection.

C. Indications for surgery include peritonitis, sepsis, free air on plain radiographs, clinical deterioration (persistent fever, increasing leukocytosis, lactic acidosis), or strictures.

CASE RESOLUTION

The barium enema reveals an obstructive apple core lesion in the sigmoid colon suggestive of carcinoma of the colon. Mr. J underwent surgical exploration, which confirmed an obstructing colonic mass. The mass was resected and a colostomy created. Pathologic evaluation revealed adenocarcinoma of the colon.

CHIEF COMPLAINT

PATIENT

Mr. L is a 65-year-old man who arrives in the emergency department complaining of 1 hour of excruciating constant diffuse periumbilical abdominal pain radiating to his flank. He has never had pain like this before. He has suffered 1 episode of vomiting and feels light headed. The emesis was yellow. He has moved his bowels once this morning. There is no change in his bowel habits, melena, or hematochezia. Nothing seems to make the pain better or worse. He was without any pain until this morning. His past medical history is remarkable for hypertension and tobacco use. On physical exam, he is diaphoretic and in obvious acute distress. Vital signs are BP, 110/65 mm Hg; pulse, 90 bpm; temperature, 37.0°C; RR, 20 breaths per minute. HEENT, cardiac, and pulmonary exams are all within normal limits. Abdominal exam reveals moderate diffuse tenderness, without rebound or guarding. Bowel sounds are present and hypoactive. Stool is guaiac negative.

 At this point, what is the leading hypothesis, what are the active alternatives, and is there a must not miss diagnosis? Given this differential diagnosis, what tests should be ordered?

RANKING THE DIFFERENTIAL DIAGNOSIS

Mr. L has diffuse abdominal pain, which is also acute and severe. This focuses the differential diagnosis on AAA, appendicitis, bowel obstruction, bowel ischemia, diabetic ketoacidosis, nephrolithiasis, and pancreatitis. The hyperacute onset and severity are most suggestive of AAA, bowel ischemia, nephrolithiasis, and pancreatitis. The radiation to the flank increases the likelihood of AAA, nephrolithiasis, and pancreatitis. Clearly, AAA is a must not miss diagnosis. Less likely possibilities would be diverticulitis with rupture, which can cause severe sudden onset of pain, although the pain is more often in the left lower quadrant (LLQ) than diffuse. Table 3-13 lists the differential diagnoses for Mr. L.

Table 3-13. Diagnostic hypotheses for Mr. L.

Diagnostic Hypotheses	Clinical Clues	Important Tests
Leading Hypothesis		
AAA	Orthostatic hypotension Pulsatile abdominal mass Decreased lower extremity pulses	Abdominal CT scan
Active Alternatives—Most Common		
Renal colic	Flank pain Radiation to groin Hematuria Costovertebral angle tenderness	Urinalysis Renal CT
Pancreatitis	Alcohol abuse Gallstones	Serum lipase
Diverticulitis	Left lower quadrant pain (usually) Diarrhea Fever	CT scan

Mr. L has no history of kidney stones or hematuria. He does not drink alcohol. On reexamination, orthostatic maneuvers reveal profound orthostatic hypotension. Supine BP and pulse were 110/65 mm Hg and 90 bpm. Upon standing his BP falls to 65/40 mm Hg and a pulse of 140 bpm. He remains afebrile. Again, you find that he lacks rebound or guarding and is not particularly tender in the LLQ. He has moderate flank and back tenderness to percussion. His abdominal aorta cannot be palpated due to his abdominal girth. Lower extremity pulses are intact. Plain abdominal radiographs do not demonstrate free air.

 Is the clinical information sufficient to make a diagnosis? If not, what other information do you need?

The most dramatic and important physical finding is the presence of profound orthostatic hypotension. It is critical to appreciate that his hypotension is clearly out of proportion to dehydration since he has only vomited once and his decreased oral intake only began 1 hour ago. As noted above *unexplained* hypotension is a pivotal finding suggesting either intra-abdominal hemorrhage or sepsis (Table 3-3). He has no fever or chills to suggest sepsis, but this is still possible. A serious consideration must be massive intra-abdominal hemorrhage, either within the GI tract or intraperitoneal. Large volume GI hemorrhage always exits the bowel quickly resulting in hematemesis, melena, or hematochezia and is rarely subtle. Therefore, you are more concerned about intraperitoneal hemorrhage. Causes of massive intraperitoneal hemorrhage include AAA rupture, splenic rupture, or rupture of an ectopic pregnancy. The patient's history is most suggestive of AAA rupture. You call for a stat vascular surgery consult.

 Orthostatic hypotension is always important. It significantly influences the differential diagnosis and the diagnostic and management decisions, and it may be marked despite a normal supine BP and pulse.

Leading Hypothesis: AAA

Textbook Presentation

Classically, patients are men with a history of smoking who have the triad of severe abdominal pain, a pulsatile abdominal mass, and hypotension.

Disease Highlights

A. Defined as an external diameter of the infrarenal abdominal aorta of ≥ 3 cm.

B. The highest prevalence of AAA is 5.9% in white male smokers between the ages of 50 and 79 years.

C. 10,000 deaths per year in United States

D. Risk factors

1. Smoking is the most significant risk factor (OR 5).

2. Men are affected 4 to 5 times more often than women.

3. Family history of AAA (OR 4.3)

4. Increased age

5. Hypertension (OR 1.2)

E. May present acutely with rupture and catastrophic consequences, occasionally chronically when expansion causes pain or a contained rupture, be discovered incidentally or with screening ultrasound.

1. Ruptured AAA

   a. Mortality with rupture is 70–90%.

   b. Misdiagnosis (most commonly renal colic) occurs in 16% of cases.

   c. Hypotension is a late finding, and palpable mass is often not present.

   d. Syncope may be present.

   e. Occasionally the rupture is contained and patients may have symptoms for months or longer (see below).

   f. Rupture into the duodenum is a rare complication, is more common in patients with prior AAA graft, and may result in GI bleeding over weeks.

2. Symptomatic, contained

   a. Rarely, patients present nonemergently with symptomatic contained rupture of the abdominal aorta. Symptoms are primarily secondary to retroperitoneal

hemorrhage and are occasionally present for weeks or even several years.

   b. Manifestations include

      (1) Abdominal pain 83%

      (2) Flank or back pain 61–66%

      (3) Syncope 26%

      (4) Abdominal mass on careful exam 52% (only 18% had abdominal mass noted on routine abdominal exam)

      (5) Hypotension or orthostasis 48%

      (6) Leukocytosis (> 11,000/mcL) 70%

      (7) Anemia (unusual)

3. Inflammatory AAA

   a. Comprise about 5–10% of AAAs and usually occurs at a slightly younger age.

   b. Distinguishing characteristic is marked inflammation of aortic adventitia.

   c. Back pain or abdominal pain is usual presentation (80% of patients); rupture is rarely presenting manifestation.

   d. Symptoms of inflammation (fever, weight loss) present in 20–50% of patients.

   e. Erythrocyte sedimentation rate is elevated in 40–90% of cases.

   f. CT or MRI reveal the aneurysm and marked thickening of the aortic wall. Periaortic fat stranding may be seen.

4. Rarely presents when intraluminal thrombus within the aneurysmal sac embolizes, leading to the blue toe syndrome

5. Asymptomatic AAA (discovered incidentally or on screening)

   a. The risk of rupture increases markedly as the diameter of the aneurysm increases. See Table 3-14.

Evidence-Based Diagnosis

A. Physical exam is *not* sufficiently sensitive to rule out AAA.

B. Bruits do not contribute to diagnosis.

C. Sensitivity of *focused* exam for *asymptomatic* AAA is poor overall (31–39%) and only 82% among patients with large AAA (≥ 5 cm). The sensitivity of the physical exam is less in obese patients (53% waist circumference > 39 inches vs 91% < 39 inches).

D. Sensitivity of abdominal exam in *symptomatic* AAA.

1. Abdominal pain, distention, and rupture all limit sensitivity.

Table 3-14. Annual rupture rate in AAA.

AAA Diameter (cm)	Rupture Risk (%)
3.0–3.9	0
4.0–4.9	1
5.0–5.9	1–11
6.0–6.9	10–22
>7.0	30–33

Data from Moll FL, Powell JT et al. Management of Abdominal Aortic Aneurysms Clinical Practice Guidelines of the European Society for Vascular Surgery. Eur J Vasc Endovasc Surg. 2011;41:S1–58.

2. Distention was reported in 52–100% in different series.

3. Palpable mass was found in 18%.

 A palpable mass is *unusual* in patients with a ruptured AAA.

E. Laboratory and radiologic tests

1. CT angiography is very accurate for ruptured AAA: sensitivity, 98.3%; specificity, 94.9%; LR+, 19.3; LR–, 0.02

2. Bedside emergency ultrasound has been demonstrated to be highly accurate: sensitivity, 96–100%; specificity, 98–100%.

3. For screening, ultrasound is preferred: sensitivity, 95%; specificity, 100%.

4. Preoperative evaluation prior to repair of *asymptomatic* AAA typically utilizes CT angiography.

Treatment

A. For ruptured AAA, proceed directly to the operating room.

B. Screening: See Chapter 2, Screening & Health Maintenance

C. Timing of elective surgery

1. Mortality with rupture exceeds 80%. Surgery is performed to minimize the risk of rupture.

2. The risk of rupture increases substantially with increasing AAA diameter (see above).

3. The standard recommendation is to electively repair AAAs ≥ 5.5 cm or those that are tender or have increased in size by ≥ 1 cm in 1 year.

4. Other risk factors for rupture include smoking (hazard ratio 2.02, 1.33–3.06) and female gender (HR 3.76, 2.58–5.47). Hypertension also increases the risk.

5. Some authorities recommend repair in women when the AAA reaches 5.2 cm.

D. Options include open surgical repair versus endovascular stent placement. Comparing stent to open repair:

1. 30-day mortality, length of hospital stay, and discharge to nursing home is lower with stent placement than open repair.

2. Minor revisions are required in 2–5% per year of patients with stent placements but the overall rate of all re-interventions for complications is lower in the stent placement group (21.2% vs 25.6%).

E. Surveillance of small AAA (4.0–5.4 cm)

1. The optimal frequency of follow-up ultrasonography has not been determined. A reasonable approach would be annual surveillance for aneurysms < 4.0 cm, every 6 months for aneurysms < 4.0–4.9 cm, and every 3 months for aneurysms 5.0–5.4 cm.

2. CT scan may be appropriate for patients with AAA of 5–5.4 cm. One study reported that 73% of patients found to have an AAA of 5–5.4 cm on ultrasound had an aneurysm that was ≥ 5.5 cm on CT.

F. Medical management

1. Smoking cessation and blood pressure control

2. AAAs are considered a coronary equivalent. Aspirin and statins are recommended.

MAKING A DIAGNOSIS

Further evaluation (eg, with CT) at this point depends on the index of suspicion. If AAA is very likely and the patient is unstable, many vascular surgeons proceed directly to the operating room without further studies in order to avoid the potential lethal delay of obtaining a CT scan. Bedside ultrasonography is a useful option if available. If AAA is less likely and the patient is stable, CT scanning is appropriate.

 Have you crossed a diagnostic threshold for the leading hypothesis, AAA? Have you ruled out the active alternatives? Do other tests need to be done to exclude the alternative diagnoses?

Alternative Diagnosis: Nephrolithiasis

Textbook Presentation

Patients typically experience rapid onset of excruciating back and flank pain, which may radiate to the abdomen or groin. The intensity of the pain is often dramatic as patients writhe and move about constantly (unlike peritonitis) in an unsuccessful attempt to get comfortable. The pain may be associated with nausea, vomiting, dysuria, or urinary frequency.

 Abdominal *tenderness* is unusual in patients with nephrolithiasis and should raise the possibility of other diagnoses.

Disease Highlights

A. Incidence: Symptomatic stones develop in 7–13% of people in the United States.

1. 35–50% recurrence at 5 years

2. Men affected 2–3 times more often than women

3. Positive family history increases the risk (relative risk 2.6)

B. Etiology

1. Calcium oxalate stones 75%

2. Calcium phosphate stones ($CaPO_4$) 5%

3. Uric acid stones 5–10%

4. Struvite stones ($MgNH_4PO_4$) 5–15%

5. Other: cystine and indinavir stones

C. Pathophysiology

1. Stones form when the concentration of salts (ie, calcium, oxalate, or uric acid) becomes supersaturated in the urine resulting in precipitation and crystallization.

2. Supersaturation is secondary to a combination of increased urinary salt excretion combined with inadequate diluting urinary volume. Numerous mechanisms can contribute to an increase in urinary mineral excretion including:

a. Calcium: idiopathic hypercalcuria, hypercalcemic disorders, primary hyperparathyroidism, immobilization, excessive sodium intake (which increases calcium excretion), systemic acidosis, and excessive vitamin D supplementation

b. Uric acid: Excessive dietary purines, myeloproliferative disorders, uricosuric agents (for the treatment of gout), and metabolic syndrome. Low urine pH also contributes to uric acid stone formation. Hyperuricosuria can lead to uric acid stones or calcium stones due to heterogeneous ossification.

    c. Oxalate: Increased excretion may be secondary to excessive oxalate intake (rhubarb, spinach, chocolate, nuts, vitamin C) and/or increased oxalate absorption.

      (1) Fat malabsorption increases oxalate absorption. The unabsorbed fat competes with oxalate to bind calcium leading to more intraluminal oxalate that is not bound to calcium. Unbound oxalate is absorbed and excreted in the urine.

      (2) Causes of fat malabsorption include short bowel syndrome, IBD, celiac sprue, and bariatric surgery.

  3. In some patients, a decrease in urinary stone inhibitors (urinary citrate) also contribute to stone formation.

  4. Infection with urea splitting organisms (ie, *Proteus*) plays a key role in the formation of struvite stones ($MgNH_4PO_4$).

  5. Renal colic develops when stones dislodge from the kidney and obstruct urinary flow.

D. Complications

  1. Ureteral obstruction

  2. Pyelonephritis

  3. Sepsis

  4. Renal failure is rare, occurring in patients with bilateral obstruction or obstruction of a solitary functioning kidney.

Evidence-Based Diagnosis

A. The evaluation is directed at establishing the diagnosis of nephrolithiasis *and* its underlying etiology so that measures to prevent its recurrence can be implemented.

B. Establishing the diagnosis

  1. Hematuria is present in 80% of patients; LR– is 0.57.

 The absence of hematuria does not rule out nephrolithiasis.

  2. Radiographs (kidneys, ureters, bladder) or ultrasound are not sufficiently sensitive to rule out nephrolithiasis (sensitivity 29–68% and 32–57%, respectively).

  3. Noncontrast renal CT is the test of choice.

    a. Sensitivity 95%; specificity 98%

    b. LR+, 48; LR–, 0.05

    c. Importantly, CT scan revealed alternative diagnoses in 33% of patients *clinically* suspected of nephrolithiasis.

  4. In pregnant women, ultrasound is the test of choice.

C. Evaluation of documented nephrolithiasis

  1. All patients should have a urinalysis and culture and basic serum chemistries, including several measurements of serum calcium. Urine culture, pH, and chemical analysis of any retrieved stones are also recommended.

  2. A more comprehensive evaluation, including several 24-hour urine specimens for analysis of calcium, oxalate, uric acid, sodium, creatinine and citrate as well as submission of retrieved stones for chemical analysis, is recommended for patients with recurrent stones. Some experts recommend this for patients with their first stone.

Treatment

A. Pain control

  1. NSAIDs

    a. Treat pain and diminish spasm

    b. Create less dependence than opioids

    c. To be avoided 3 days before lithotripsy due to antiplatelet effects

  2. Opioids

B. Hydration (oral if tolerated, otherwise IV)

C. Hospitalization indicated for uncontrolled pain, persistent nausea or vomiting, acute kidney injury or signs of infection.

D. Sepsis or acute kidney injury due to bilateral obstruction or unilateral obstruction in a solitary kidney

  1. Necessitate emergent drainage (via percutaneous nephrostomy tube or ureteral stent)

  2. For sepsis, broad-spectrum IV antibiotics to cover gram-negative organisms and enterococcus should also be administered.

E. Stone passage

  1. Nifedipine and tamsulosin have been demonstrated to significantly increase the likelihood of stone passage by 65%.

  2. Lithotripsy or ureteroscopy can be used to remove persistent ureteral stones.

F. Secondary prevention

  1. Patients with a single calcium stone:

    a. General measures include increasing fluid intake (≥ 2 L/d) (relative risk of recurrent stones 0.45, 0.24–0.84).

    b. Reducing phosphate-containing soft drinks may decrease recurrences (relative risk 0.83, 0.71–0.98).

  2. For patients with recurrent idiopathic calcium stones other options include:

    a. Thiazide diuretics decrease urinary calcium excretion (especially when combined with potassium supplementation) (relative risk 0.52, 0.39–0.69).

    b. Citrate supplementation is effective in patients with and without hypocitraturia (relative risk 0.25, 0.14–0.44).

    c. Allopurinol in patients with concomitant hyperuricemia or hyperuricosuria (relative risk 0.59, 0.42–0.84).

  3. More specific management (ie, dietary modification) is complex and depends on the underlying etiology of the patient's nephrolithiasis.

Alternative Diagnosis: Diverticulitis

Textbook Presentation

Patients typically complain of a constant gradually increasing LLQ abdominal pain, usually present for several days. Diarrhea or constipation and fever are often present. Guarding and rebound may be seen.

Disease Highlights

A. Diverticula are outpouchings of the colonic wall that may be asymptomatic (diverticulosis), become inflamed (diverticulitis), or hemorrhage.

B. Diverticulosis

  1. Develops in 5–10% of patients aged > 45 years, 50% in persons aged > 60 years, and 80% in those aged > 85 years.

2. Low-fiber diets are believed to cause diverticula by decreasing stool bulk, resulting in increased intraluminal pressure causing the mucosa and submucosa to herniate through weakness in the colonic wall where vessels penetrate creating diverticula.

C. Diverticulitis

1. Develops secondary to microscopic or frank perforation of diverticula.

2. 85–95% of diverticulitis occurs in sigmoid or descending colon

3. Mean age of onset is 63 years.

4. Complications of diverticulitis

   a. Abscess

   b. Peritonitis

   c. Sepsis

   d. Colonic obstruction

   e. Fistula formation (colovesicular fistula most common)

5. Simultaneous diverticular hemorrhage and *diverticulitis* are unusual; diverticular hemorrhage is discussed in Chapter 19, GI Bleeding.

Evidence-Based Diagnosis

A. LLQ tenderness increases the likelihood of diverticulitis (LR+, 3.4; LR–, 0.41).

B. Neither fever nor leukocytosis is very sensitive for diverticulitis or diverticular abscess.

1. In patients with uncomplicated diverticulitis, only 45% had temperature of $\geq$ 38.0°C or WBC > 11,000/mcL.

2. In patients with diverticular abscess, only 64% of patients had temperature of $\geq$ 38.0°C and 62% had WBC > 11,000/mcL.

C. Plain radiographs may demonstrate free air or obstruction.

D. CT scan is test of choice in men and non-pregnant women.

1. CT can confirm diverticulitis (diverticula with thickened bowel wall or pericolonic fat stranding); evaluate the extent, severity, and complications (abscess formation and perforation); and diagnose other conditions.

2. 93–97% sensitive

E. Colonoscopy

1. Colon cancer can be mistaken for diverticulitis on CT.

2. All patients with diverticulitis should have follow-up CT.

3. Colonoscopy should be delayed 4–6 weeks until there is resolution of acute inflammation.

Treatment

A. Outpatient management is appropriate for patients with a mild attack (ie, patients without marked fever or marked leukocytosis, pain manageable with oral analgesics, tolerating oral intake) and without significant comorbidities, immunocompromise, or advanced age.

1. Ciprofloxacin and metronidazole recommended for 7–10 days

2. Liquid diet

3. High-fiber diet after attack resolves

4. Follow-up colonoscopy (see above)

B. Moderate to severe attack (unable to tolerate oral intake, more severe pain) necessitates inpatient treatment.

1. Broad-spectrum IV antibiotics

2. No oral intake

3. CT-guided drainage for abscesses > 5 cm

4. Emergent surgery is recommended in patients with

   a. Frank peritonitis

   b. Uncontrolled sepsis

   c. Clinical deterioration despite medical management

   d. Obstruction or large abscesses that cannot be drained or are contaminated with frank fecal contents

5. The threshold for surgery should be lower in immunocompromised patients.

6. High-fiber diet once the attack has resolved

CASE RESOLUTION

The surgical resident evaluates the patient and agrees with your concern about an AAA. He orders a stat CT scan and contacts his attending. The attending immediately evaluates the patient and redirects the patient directly to the operating room bypassing the CT scan. Surgery reveals a leaking AAA that ruptures during surgery. The aorta is cross clamped, repaired, and the patient is stabilized.

REVIEW OF OTHER IMPORTANT DISEASES

Irritable Bowel Syndrome (IBS)

Textbook Presentation

Patients often complain of intermittent abdominal pain accompanied by diarrhea or constipation or both of *years'* duration. The diarrhea is often associated with cramps that are relieved by defecation. Pain cannot be explained by structural or biochemical abnormalities. Weight loss or anemia should alert the clinician to other possibilities.

New persistent *changes* in bowel habits (either diarrhea or constipation) should be thoroughly evaluated to exclude colon cancer, IBD, or other process. An assumption of IBS in such patients is inappropriate.

Disease Highlights

A. Affects 12% of adults, women 1.7 times more than men.

B. Etiology is a combination of altered motility, visceral hypersensitivity, autonomic dysfunction, and psychological factors.

C. Symptoms are often exacerbated by psychological or physical stressors.

D. Patients may have pain associated primarily with diarrhea (IBS-D) or constipation (IBS-C) or a mixed bowel pattern (IBS-M).

Evidence-Based Diagnosis

A. There are no known biochemical or structural markers for IBS.

B. A variety of symptoms are common in patients with IBS including lower abdominal pain, passage of mucous, feeling of incomplete evacuation, loose or frequent stools at onset of pain, and pain relieved by defecation. However, none of these are very predictive (LR+, 1.3–2.1 and LR–, 0.59–0.88).

C. Only abdominal pain is very sensitive (but required by the criteria).

D. Diarrhea pattern

1. One recent study suggested that patients with diarrhea-predominant IBS were more likely to have irregularly irregular diarrhea that fluctuated over days whereas patients with inflammatory diseases (IBD and celiac disease) were more likely to have persistent diarrhea that fluctuates over months.

2. Persistent diarrhea increased the likelihood of IBD (LR+ 4.2).

3. A more extensive workup may be indicated in patients with persistent, constant diarrhea.

E. The diagnosis is usually made by a combination of (1) a consistent history, (2) the absence of alarm features, and (3) a limited work-up to exclude other diseases.

1. Consistent history

   a. Although a variety of criteria have been developed (ie, Rome Criteria), a recent review by the American College of Gastroenterology suggested a consistent history was abdominal pain or discomfort that occurs in association with altered bowel habits for at least 3 months.

   b. Patients may also report a relief of pain with defecation.

2. Alarm symptoms (suggest alternative diagnosis and necessitate evaluation)

   a. Positive fecal occult blood test or rectal bleeding

   b. Anemia

   c. Weight loss > 10 lbs

   d. Fever

   e. Family history of colorectal cancer, IBD, or celiac disease

   f. Recent antibiotic use

3. Limited workup

   a. A CBC is appropriate to rule out anemia, which would suggest alternative diagnoses.

   b. Other diagnostic testing is not recommended for young patients without alarm features, with the exception of serologic testing for celiac sprue in patients with IBS-D.

      (1) Although recommended by the ACG, a recent study found the incidence of confirmed celiac disease in IBS-D patients (without alarm features) to be very low (0.41%) and not different from asymptomatic patients.

      (2) May best be reserved for the subset of IBS-D patients with other possible clues suggesting celiac disease (eg, anemia, autoimmune disease or family history)

   c. Lactose hydrogen breath testing can be considered if lactose intolerance remains a concern despite dietary lactose restriction.

   d. There is no evidence that routine flexible sigmoidoscopy or colonoscopy is necessary in young patients without alarm symptoms.

   e. Colonoscopy is recommended in patients with alarm symptoms and in those aged ≥ 50 years (if not already performed). Biopsy is also recommended in patients with IBS-D to rule out microscopic colitis.

f. The following should also be evaluated in patients with alarm symptoms:

   (1) Stool for occult blood

   (2) Thyroid-stimulating hormone levels

   (3) Basic chemistries

   (4) Stool for *Clostridium difficile* toxin and presence of ova and parasites

   (5) A variety of serum and fecal markers, including ASCA, pANCA, fecal calprotectin, and fecal lactoferrin, are useful in selected patients and can suggest bowel inflammation or IBD.

Treatment

A. Nonspecific management. A variety of treatments have been shown to be effective in IBS including:

1. Diets low in apples, cherries, nectarines, lactose, legumes, broccoli, cauliflower, Brussels sprouts and peas

2. Physical activity

3. Antispasmodics (including hyoscine and peppermint oil) help decrease abdominal pain.

4. Tricyclic antidepressants and selective serotonin reuptake inhibitors are effective. Psychological counseling may also be effective although the data are less robust.

5. Dietary fiber (psyllium) may be effective. Studies are conflicting.

B. Specific therapy is based on predominant syndrome.

1. Diarrhea-predominant IBS (IBS-D)

   a. Patients with IBS-D should have a trial of lactose-free diet. Such treatment in lactase-deficient individuals with IBS markedly reduces outpatient visits.

   b. Loperamide reduces diarrhea (but not abdominal pain or bloating).

   c. A single, short course of rifaximin, a nonabsorbed antibiotic is helpful. Doses have ranged from 400 mg to 550 mg twice daily for 10–14 days.

   d. Alosetron is a $5HT_3$-receptor antagonist whose use is restricted to prescribing program by US Food and Drug Administration. Expert consultation recommended.

   e. Probiotic treatment with *Bifidobacteria* may be useful.

2. Constipation predominant IBS (IBS-C)

   a. Lubiprostone

      (1) A selective C-2 chloride channel activator is more effective than placebo in women.

      (2) Women of childbearing years should have a negative pregnancy test before starting the medication and maintain contraception while taking lubiprostone.

      (3) Not yet recommended in men

Chronic Mesenteric Ischemia

Textbook Presentation

Patients with chronic mesenteric ischemia typically complain of recurrent postprandial abdominal pain (often in the first hour and diminishing 1–2 hours later), food fear, and weight loss. Patients often have a history of tobacco use (75%), peripheral vascular disease (55%), coronary artery disease (43%), or hypertension (37%).

Disease Highlights

A. Usually secondary to near obstructive atherosclerotic disease of the superior mesenteric artery or celiac artery or both.

B. Arterial stenosis results in an imbalance between intestinal oxygen supply and demand that is accentuated after eating leading to intestinal angina resulting in food fear and weight loss.

C. Two or more vessels (ie, superior mesenteric artery *and* celiac artery) are involved in 91% of affected patients.

Evidence-Based Diagnosis

A. Abdominal pain

1. Occurs in 94% and is postprandial in 88%.

2. It is typically epigastric or periumbilical.

3. Typically develops in the first hour after eating and diminishes 1–2 hours later.

B. Weight loss occurs in 78% of patients and is due to food aversion.

C. Diarrhea occurs in 36% of patients.

D. An epigastric bruit has been reported in 63% of patients (17–87%).

E. The abdomen is typically nontender even during a severe episode of pain.

F. Although stenoses are common (18% of population over age 65 years), symptomatic chronic ischemia is rare, and documented stenosis does *not* confirm the diagnosis of mesenteric ischemia. It is important to exclude more common disorders (ie, PUD and gallstone disease).

G. Duplex ultrasonography is very sensitive (> 90%) and can be used as the initial diagnostic tool. Normal results make the diagnosis very unlikely.

H. CT angiography and magnetic resonance angiography have also been used. Angiography should be considered if the results of noninvasive testing suggest vascular obstruction.

Treatment

Revascularization (surgical repair or angioplasty [with stent]) is the only treatment.

REFERENCES

Abbas S, Bisset IP, Parry BR. Oral water soluble contrast for the management of small bowel obstruction. Cochrane Database Syst Rev. 2007Jul 18;(3):CD004651.

American Society Gastroenterology Endoscopy Standards of Practice Committee. The role of endoscopy in the evaluation of suspected choledocholithiasis. Gastro Endo. 2010;71(1):1–9.

Andersson RE, Hugander AP, Ghazi SH et al. Diagnostic value of disease history, clinical presentation, and inflammatory parameters of appendicitis. World J Surg. 1999;23(2):133–40.

Andersson REB. Meta-analysis of the clinical and laboratory diagnosis of appendicitis. Br J Surg. 2004;91:28–37.

Biancari F, Poane R, Venermom M, D'Andrea V, Perala J. Diagnostic accuracy of computed tomography in patients with suspected abdominal aortic aneurysm rupture. Eur J Vasc Endovasc Surg. 2013;45(3):227–30.

Blankensteijn JD. A further meta-analysis of population-based screening for abdominal aortic aneurysm. J Vasc Surg. 2010;52:1103–8.

Bohner H, Yang Q, Franke C, Verreet PR, Ohmann C. Simple data from history and physical examination help to exclude bowel obstruction and to avoid radiographic studies in patients with acute abdominal pain. Eur J Surg. 1998;164: 777–84.

Brandt LJ, Chey WD. An Evidence-Based Systematic Review on the Management of Irritable Bowel Syndrome. Am J Gastro. 2009;104 Supplement 1:S1–36.

Cardall T, Glasser J, Guss DA. Clinical value of the total white blood cell count and temperature in the evaluation of patients with suspected appendicitis. Acad Emerg Med. 2004;11(10):1021–7.

Dholakia K, Pitchumoni CS, Agarwal N. How often are liver function tests normal in acute biliary pancreatitis? J Clin Gastroenterol. 2004;38(1):81–3.

Di Saverio S, Catena F, Ansaloni L, Gavioli M, Valentino M, Pinna AD. Water-soluble contrast medium (gastrografin) value in adhesive small intestine obstruction (ASIO): a prospective, randomized, controlled, clinical trial. World J Surg. 2008;32:2293–304.

Elmi A, Hedgire SS, Pargaonkar V, Cao K, McDermott S, Harisinghani M. Is early colonoscopy beneficial in patients with CT-diagnosed diverticulitis. AJR. 2013;200:1269–74.

Farid M, Fikry A, El Nakeeb A et al. Clinical impacts of oral gastrografin follow-through in adhesive small bowel obstruction (SBO). J Surg Res. 2009;162: 170–6.

Foo FJ, Hammond CJ, Goldstone AR et al. Agreement between computed tomography and ultrasound on abdominal aortic aneurysms and implications on clinical decisions. Eur J Vasc Endovasc Surg. 2011;42:608–14.

Ford AC, Talley NJ, Veldhuyzen van Zanten SJ, Vakil NB, Simel OL. Will the history and physical examination help establish that irritable bowel syndrome is causing this patient's lower gastrointestinal tract symptoms? JAMA. 2008;300(15):1793–805.

Frossard JL, Steer ML, Pastor CM. Acute pancreatitis. Lancet. 2008;371(9607): 143–52.

Gan SI, Romagnuolo J. Admission hematocrit: a simple, useful and early predictor of severe pancreatitis. Dig Dis Sci. 2004;49(11–12):1946–52.

Grootenboer N, van Sambeek MR, Arends LR Hendriks JM, Hunink MG, Bosch JL. Systematic review and meta-analysis of sex differences in outcome after intervention for abdominal aortic aneurysm. Br J Surg. 2010;97:1169–79.

Gurleyik G, Emir S, Kilicoglu G, Arman A, Saglam A. Computed tomography severity index, APACHE II score, and serum CRP concentration for predicting the severity of acute pancreatitis. JOP. 2005;6(6):562–7.

Ha M, MacDonald RD. Impact of CT scan in patients with first episode of suspected nephrolithiasis. J Emerg Med. 2004;27(3):225–31.

Hlibczuk V, Dattaro JA, Jin Z, Falzon L, Brown MD. Diagnostic accuracy of noncontrast computed tomography for appendicitis in adults: a systemic review. Ann Emerg Med. 2010;55(1):51–9.

Howell JM, Eddy OL Lukens TW, Thiessen ME, Weingart SD, Decker WW; American College of Emergency Physicians. Clinical policy: critical issues in the evaluation and management of emergency department patients with suspected appendicitis. Ann Emerg Med. 2010;55:71–116.

Huguier M, Barrier A Boelle PY, Houry S, Lacaine F. Ischemic colitis. Am J Surg. 2006;192(5):679–84.

Jacobs DO. Clinical practice. Diverticulitis. N Engl J Med. 2007;357(20):2057–66.

Jang TB, Schindler D, Kaji AH. Bedside ultrasonography for the detection of small bowel obstruction in the emergency department. Emerg Med J. 2011;28:676–8.

Hong JJ, Cohn SM Ekeh AP, Newman M, Salana M, Leblang SD; Miami Appendicitis Group. A prospective randomized study of clinical assessment versus computed tomography for the diagnosis of acute appendicitis. Surg Inf. 2003;4(3):231–9.

Krajewski S, Brown J Phang PT, Raval M, Brown CJ. Impact of computed tomography of the abdomen on clinical outcomes in patients with acute right lower quadrant pain: a meta-analysis. Can J Surg. 2011;54(1):43–53.

Kulvatunyou N, Joseph B, Gries L et al. A prospective cohort study of 200 acute care gallbladder surgeries: the same disease but a different approach. J Trauma Acute Care Surg. 2012;73(5):1039–45.

Lameris W, van Randen A, van Gulik TM et al. A clinical decision rule to establish the diagnosis of acute diverticulitis at the emergency department. Dis Colon Rectum. 2010;53(6):896–904.

Lederle FA, Simel DL. The rational clinical examination. Does this patient have abdominal aortic aneurysm? JAMA. 1999;281(1):77–82.

Lederle F, Etschells E. Update: abdominal aortic aneurysm. In: Simel DL, Rennie D, eds. *The Rational Clinical Examination: Evidence-Based Clinical Diagnosis.* New York, NY: McGraw-Hill; 2009.

Lee CC, Golub R, Singer AJ, Cantu R Jr,Levinson H. Routine versus selective abdominal computed tomography scan in the evaluation of right lower quadrant pain: a randomized controlled trial. Acad Emerg Med. 2007;14: 117–23.

Liu CL, Fan ST, Lo CM et al. Clinico-biochemical prediction of biliary cause of acute pancreatitis in the era of endoscopic ultrasonography. Aliment Pharmacol Ther. 2005;22(5):423–31.

Long SS, Long C, Lai H, Macura KJ. Imaging strategies for right lower quadrant pain in pregnancy. AJR. 2011;196:4–12.

Mayer EA. Clinical practice. Irritable bowel syndrome. N Engl J Med. 2008;358(16): 1692–9.

Moawa J, Gewertz BL. Chronic intestinal ischemia. Clinical presentation and diagnosis. Surg Clin N Am. 1977;77(2):357–69.

Park CJ, Jang MK, Shin WG et al. Can we predict the development of ischemic colitis among patients with lower abdominal pain? Dis Colon Rectum. 2007;50(2):232–8.

Petrov MS, Savides TJ. Systematic review of endoscopic ultrasonography versus endoscopic retrograde cholangiopancreatography for suspected choledocholithiasis. Br J Surg. 2009;96:967–74.

Pimentel M, Hwang L, Melmed GY et al. New clinical method for distinguishing D-IBS from other gastrointestinal conditions causing diarrhea: the LA/IBS diagnostic strategy. Dig Dis Sci. 2010;55:145–9.

Rao PM, Rhea JT Novelline RA, Mostafavi AA, McCabe CJ. Effect of computed tomography of the appendix on treatment of patients and use of hospital resources. N Engl J Med. 1998;338(3):141–6.

Schermerhorn M. A 66-year-old man with an abdominal aortic aneurysm. Review of screening and treatment. JAMA. 2009;302(18):2015–22.

Shea JA, Berlin JA, Escarce JJ et al. Revised estimates of diagnostic test sensitivity and specificity in suspected biliary tract disease. Arch Intern Med. 1994;154(22): 2573–81.

Snyder BK, Hayden SR. Accuracy of leukocyte count in the diagnosis of acute appendicitis. Ann Emerg Med. 1999;33(5):565–74.

Tenner S, Dubner H, Steinberg W. Predicting gallstone pancreatitis with laboratory parameters: a meta-analysis. Am J Gastroenterol. 1994;89(10):1863–6.

Trowbridge RL, Rutkowski NK, Shojania KG. Does this patient have acute cholecystitis? JAMA. 2003;289:80–6.

van Randen A, Bipat S Zwinderman AH, Ubbink DT, Stoker J, Boermeester MA. Acute appendicitis: meta-analysis of diagnostic performance of CT and graded compressions US related to prevalence of disease. Radiology. 2008;249(1):97–106.

Wagner JM, McKinney P, Carpenter JL. Does this patient have appendicitis? JAMA. 1996;276:1589–94.

Zakko SF, Afdhal NH. Clinical features and diagnosis of acute cholecystitis. In: UpToDate; 2007.

I have a patient with an acid-base abnormality. How do I determine the cause?

CHIEF COMPLAINT

PATIENT 1

Mr. L is a 42-year-old man with type 1 diabetes mellitus (DM) who complains of weakness, anorexia, abdominal pain, and vomiting. Laboratory studies demonstrate a HCO_3^- of 6 mEq/L.

His very low HCO_3^- suggests a significant acid-base abnormality. In addition to evaluating his abdominal pain, exploring his acid-base disorder is critical.

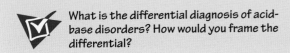

What is the differential diagnosis of acid-base disorders? How would you frame the differential?

CONSTRUCTING A DIFFERENTIAL DIAGNOSIS

The differential diagnosis of acid-base disorders is extensive (Table 4-1) but can be easily organized into 4 distinct subsets by first determining whether the *primary* disorder is a (1) metabolic acidosis, (2) metabolic alkalosis, (3) respiratory acidosis, or (4) respiratory alkalosis. The key pivotal feature that allows the clinician to narrow the differential to 1 of these subsets is to *first* evaluate the pH and *then* the HCO_3^- and $PaCO_2$.

Step 1: Determine Whether the Primary Disorder is an Acidosis or Alkalosis by Reviewing the pH.

A. pH < 7.4 indicates the *primary* disorder is an acidosis.

B. pH > 7.4 indicates the *primary* disorder is an alkalosis.

Step 2: Determine Whether the Primary Acidosis or Alkalosis is Metabolic or Respiratory by Reviewing the HCO_3^- and $PaCO_2$

A. Recall that $CO_2 + H_2O \Leftrightarrow H_2CO_3 \Leftrightarrow HCO_3^- + H^+$; therefore

B. $PaCO_2$ changes drive pH as follows:
   1. Increased $PaCO_2$ drives reaction to right: This increases H^+ which lowers pH, resulting in a respiratory acidosis.
   2. Decreased $PaCO_2$ drives reaction to left: This decreases H^+ which raises pH, resulting in a respiratory alkalosis.

C. HCO_3^- changes drive pH as follows:
   1. Increase HCO_3^- drives the reaction to left: This consumes H^+ which raises the pH, resulting in a metabolic alkalosis.
   2. Decreased HCO_3^- drives the reaction to right: This increases H^+ which lowers the pH, resulting in a metabolic acidosis. This occurs in 2 situations:
      a. Processes that produce H^+ ion (and consume HCO_3^-) (ie, ketoacidosis, lactic acidosis)
      b. Processes that lose HCO_3^- (ie, diarrhea)

D. For acidosis (pH < 7.4)
   1. $HCO_3^- < 24$ mEq/L: The primary disorder is a metabolic acidosis
   2. $PaCO_2 > 40$ mm Hg: The primary disorder is a respiratory acidosis

E. For alkalosis (pH > 7.4)
   1. $HCO_3^- > 24$ mEq/L: The primary disorder is a metabolic alkalosis
   2. $PaCO_2 < 40$ mm Hg: The primary disorder is a respiratory alkalosis

The differential diagnosis for metabolic acidosis is extensive but can be narrowed based on whether the anion gap is normal or elevated. The anion gap is an estimate of the unmeasured anions. Metabolic acidoses may be caused by processes that either produce acid (ie, ketoacids, lactic acid, sulfates, phosphates, or other organic acids), *or* by processes that lose HCO_3^- in the urine or stool (ie, diarrhea). Processes that produce acid also produce their associated unmeasured anions, resulting in an increased anion gap. On the other hand, processes that lose HCO_3^- do not generate unmeasured anions and the anion gap remains normal.

Step 3: Limit the Differential Diagnoses of Metabolic Acidosis by Calculating the Anion Gap

A. Anion gap = $Na^+ - (HCO_3^- + Cl^-)$

B. 12 ± 4 is often cited as an ideal cutoff, although in some institutions, a normal anion gap is only 7–9 mEq/L.

C. The normal anion gap is affected by the serum albumin level.
   1. Albumin is negatively charged so that lower serum albumin levels are associated with a lower anion gap.
   2. The normal anion gap is 2.5 mEq/L lower, for every 1 g/dL drop in the serum albumin (below 4.4 g/dL).
   3. The reference range at the institution performing the tests should be used.

D. An increased anion gap suggests that an anion gap metabolic acidosis is present.

Table 4-1. Differential diagnosis of primary acid-base disorders.

ACIDOSES pH < 7.4		
Metabolic Acidoses $HCO_3^- < 24$ mEq/L		**Respiratory Acidoses** $PaCO_2 > 40$ mm Hg
Anion gap	**Nonanion gap**	Lung diseases (most common)
Ketoacidoses	Diarrhea	COPD
DKA	RTA	Asthma
Alcoholic	Carbonic anhydrase inhibitors	Pulmonary edema
Starvation	Dilutional[1]	Pneumonia
	Early renal failure	
Lactic acidosis		Pleural disease
Hypoxia		Effusions
Shock		Pneumothorax
Septic		Neuromuscular disease
Hypovolemic		Brain: Stroke, intoxication, sleep apnea
Cardiogenic		Spinal cord: trauma, ALS, polio
Anaphylactic		Nerve: Guillain-Barre syndrome
CO or cyanide poisoning		Neuromuscular junction: Myasthenia gravis
Regional obstruction to blood flow		Chest wall: flail chest, muscular dystrophy
Seizures		
Uremia		
Toxins and miscellaneous		
Salicylate[2]		
Methanol[3]		
Ethylene glycol		
Rhabdomyolysis		
D-Lactic acidosis		

ALKALOSES pH > 7.4	
Metabolic Alkaloses $HCO_3^- > 24$ mEq/L	**Respiratory Alkaloses** $PaCO_2 < 40$ mm Hg
Vomiting or NG drainage	Hypoxemia
Diuretics	Pulmonary disorders
Hypokalemia	Pneumonia
Increased mineralocorticoid activity	Asthma
Primary hyperaldosteronism	Pulmonary edema
Hypercortisolism	Pulmonary embolism
Excessive licorice ingestion	Interstitial lung disease
	Mechanical ventilation
	Extrapulmonary disorders
	Anxiety
	Pain
	Fever
	Pregnancy
	CNS insult
	Drugs[4]
	Cirrhosis

[1]Following very large volume saline administration.
[2]Salicylate intoxication typically causes a primary respiratory alkalosis (due to CNS stimulation of the respiratory center) *and* a primary anion gap metabolic acidosis (with accumulation of lactate and ketones).
[3]Methanol and ethylene glycol ingestion may occur after ingestion of antifreeze, de-icing solutions, and other organic solvents
[4]Drugs include salicylates, nicotine, and catecholamines.
ALS, amyotrophic lateral sclerosis; CNS, central nervous system; CO, carbon monoxide; COPD, chronic obstructive pulmonary disease; DKA, diabetes ketoacidosis; NG, nasogastric; RTA, renal tubular acidosis.

Step 4: Explore the Differential Diagnoses of the Primary Disorder

After selecting the appropriate subset of hypotheses for the primary disorder, review the limited differential diagnoses (Table 4-1) and explore the demographics, risk factors, associated symptoms and signs of those diseases. This information allows the clinician to rank the differential diagnosis for the primary acid-base disorder and then determine the appropriate testing strategy.

Step 5: Diagnose Primary Disorder

Synthesize the clinical and laboratory information to arrive at a diagnosis of the primary acid-base disorder.

Step 6: Check for Additional Disorders

Step 6A: Calculate Anion Gap (Even in Patients Without Acidosis) to Uncover Unexpected Anion Gap Metabolic Acidosis

 Always check the anion gap. An elevated gap suggests an anion gap metabolic acidosis even when the HCO_3^- is above normal.

Step 6B: Calculate Whether Compensation Is Appropriate

A. The acid-base system attempts to maintain homeostasis. Alterations in 1 system (respiratory or metabolic) trigger compensatory changes in the other system to minimize the impact on pH.

B. Formulas predict the expected change in $PaCO_2$ to compensate for metabolic processes and the expected change in HCO_3^- to compensate for respiratory processes (Table 4-2).

C. Compensation that is greater or less than expected suggests that an *additional* acid-base abnormality is present, not just compensation.

D. If an additional process is implicated, the differential diagnosis for that additional disorder should be explored.

Table 4-2. Compensation in acid-base disorders.[1,2]

Primary Disorder	Duration	Expected Compensation
Metabolic acidosis	Acute/chronic	$PaCO_2$ ↓ 1.2 mm Hg per 1 mEq/L ↓ HCO_3^- (To a minimum $PaCO_2$ of 10-15 mm Hg)
Metabolic alkalosis	Acute/chronic	$PaCO_2$ ↑ 0.7 mm Hg per 1 mEq/L ↑ HCO_3^-
Respiratory acidosis	Acute	HCO_3^- ↑ 1 mEq/L per 10 mm Hg ↑ $PaCO_2$
	Chronic	HCO_3^- ↑ 4.0 mEq/L per 10 mm Hg ↑ $PaCO_2$
Respiratory alkalosis	Acute	HCO_3^- ↓ 2 mEq/L per 10 mm Hg ↓ $PaCO_2$
	Chronic	HCO_3^- ↓ 4 mEq/L per 10 mm Hg ↓ $PaCO_2$

[1]Metabolic compensation is slower than respiratory compensation and becomes more complete with time.
[2]Normal baseline is assumed to be $PaCO_2$ 40 mm Hg, HCO_3^- 24 mEq/L.
Reproduced with permission from Rose BD. Clinical Physiology of Acid-Base and Electrolyte Disorders. McGraw-Hill, 2001.

Step 7: Reach Final Diagnosis

Figure 4-1 outlines the stepwise approach to acid-base disorders.

 Mr. L reports that he has had diabetes since he was 10 years old. His diabetes has been complicated by peripheral vascular disease requiring a below the knee amputation and laser surgeries for retinopathy. Two days ago, he began experiencing nausea and some vomiting. He continued to take his insulin. Physical exam reveals supine BP of 90/50 mm Hg and pulse of 100 bpm. Upon standing, his vital signs are BP, 60/30 mm Hg; pulse, 150 bpm; RR, 24 breaths per minute; and temperature, 37.0°C. Retinal exam reveals dot-blot hemorrhages and multiple laser scars. Lungs are clear to percussion and auscultation. Cardiac exam reveals a regular rate and rhythm with a grade I/VI systolic murmur at the upper left sternal border. Abdominal exam is soft and nontender. Stool is guaiac-negative. Lab studies reveal Na^+, 138 mEq/L; K^+, 6.2 mEq/L; HCO_3^-, 6 mEq/L; Cl^-, 100 mEq/L; BUN, 40 mg/dL; creatinine, 1.8 mg/dL; glucose, 389 mg/dL; WBC, 10,500/mcL; HCT, 42%; ALT (SGPT), AST (SGOT), and lipase are normal.

 At this point what is the leading hypothesis, what are the active alternatives, and is there a must not miss diagnosis? Given this differential diagnosis, what tests should be ordered?

RANKING THE DIFFERENTIAL DIAGNOSIS

Step 1: Determine Whether the Primary Disorder Is an Acidosis or Alkalosis by Reviewing the pH

Although an arterial pH has not yet been obtained, the patient's very low HCO_3^- strongly suggests a metabolic acidosis. Commonly, sick patients are discovered to have a metabolic acidosis when a basic metabolic panel reveals a very low serum HCO_3^-. Although compensation for a respiratory alkalosis may result in a slightly low HCO_3^-, a HCO_3^- in this range is almost never seen unless there is in fact a primary metabolic acidosis. Nonetheless, an arterial blood gas (ABG) measurement can document the acidosis and evaluate respiratory compensation.

 ABG: pH of 7.15, PaO_2 of 80 mm Hg, and $PaCO_2$ of 20 mm Hg.

The low pH confirms that the primary disorder is an acidosis.

Step 2: Determine Whether the Primary Acidosis or Alkalosis Is Metabolic or Respiratory by Reviewing the HCO_3^- and $PaCO_2$

 $HCO_3^- = 6$ mEq/L and $PaCO_2 = 20$ mm Hg.

Both the HCO_3^- and $PaCO_2$ are low. Since only a low HCO_3^- would create an acidosis the primary disorder is a metabolic acidosis. (A low $PaCO_2$ drives the pH up [see above].)

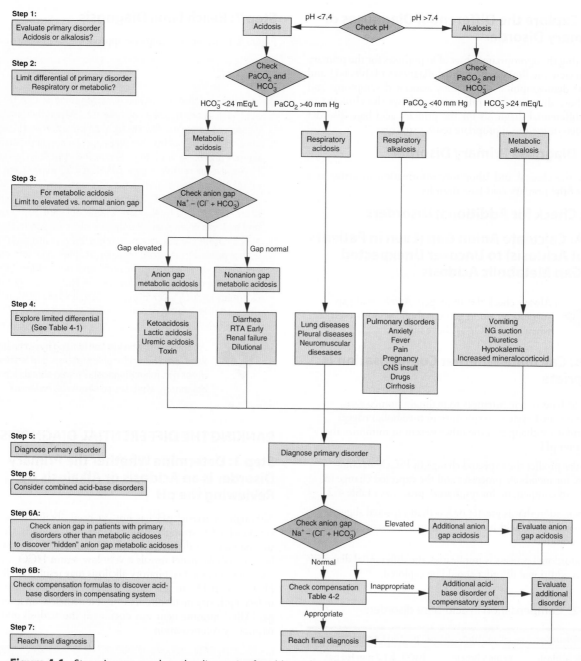

Figure 4-1. Stepwise approach to the diagnosis of acid-base disorders.

Step 3: For Patients With Metabolic Acidoses, Limit the Differential Diagnoses by Calculating the Anion Gap

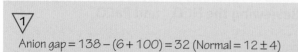

Anion gap = $138 - (6 + 100) = 32$ (Normal = 12 ± 4)

Clearly, the primary disorder is an anion gap metabolic acidosis. By referring to Table 4-1, the differential diagnosis can be narrowed to the remaining possibilities of diabetic ketoacidosis (DKA), other ketoacidosis, lactic acidosis, uremia, or toxin.

Step 4: Explore the Differential Diagnoses of the Primary Disorder

The history of childhood-onset DM strongly suggests insulin-dependent DM. This form of DM is associated with total or near total insulin deficiency increasing the risk of DKA. This is the leading hypothesis. Active alternative hypotheses include other ketoacidoses (starvation, alcohol) and uremia from renal failure (potentially secondary to long-standing diabetes). Finally, lactic acidosis (from hypoxemia or shock) is a "must not miss diagnosis" that should always be considered in sick patients with metabolic acidosis. Table 4-3 ranks the differential diagnoses considering the available demographic information, risk factors, and symptoms and signs.

Table 4-3. Diagnostic hypotheses for Mr. L.

Diagnostic Hypothesis	Demographics, Risk Factors, Symptoms and Signs	Important Tests
Leading Hypothesis		
Diabetic ketoacidosis	History of insulin-dependent diabetes mellitus Noncompliance with insulin Precipitating illness (eg, infection or stress)	Increased anion gap Increased serum or urine ketones Tests to identify precipitant (urinalysis, chest radiograph, ECG, lipase, abdominal imaging as indicated)
Active Alternatives—Most Common		
Uremic acidosis	Prior renal disease, hypertension, diabetes Dark urine Oliguria	Elevated BUN, creatinine, and anion gap Elevated FE_{Na} Urinalysis Renal ultrasound
Starvation ketoacidosis	A history of poor caloric intake	Urine ketones
Alcoholic ketoacidosis	Significant history of alcohol abuse and poor dietary intake of other calories	Urine ketones Lactate level
Active Alternatives—Must Not Miss		
Lactic acidosis from hypoxemia or shock	Shock (cardiogenic, hypovolemic or septic) Hypoxemia Fever Rigors Urinary frequency Dysuria Cough Diarrhea Oliguria Abdominal pain Hypotension Tachycardia Bounding pulses	Lactate level, anion gap, SaO_2, tests for sepsis (CBC, urinalysis, chest radiograph [imaging as indicated], blood cultures), ECG

ABG, arterial blood gas; BUN, blood urea nitrogen; ECG, electrocardiogram; FE_{Na}, fractional excretion of sodium; WBC, white blood cell.

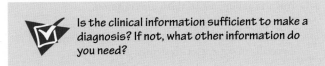

Is the clinical information sufficient to make a diagnosis? If not, what other information do you need?

Leading Hypothesis: DKA

Textbook Presentation

DKA often begins with an acute illness (ie, pneumonia, urinary tract infection, myocardial infarction [MI]) in a patient with type 1 DM. Patients often complain of symptoms related to hyperglycemia (polyuria, polydipsia, and polyphagia) and to the precipitating illness (eg, fever, cough, dysuria, chest pain). Nonspecific complaints are common (nausea, vomiting, abdominal pain, and weakness). Patients are profoundly dehydrated and exhibit orthostatic changes or frank hypotension. Confusion, lethargy, and coma may occur secondary to dehydration, hyperglycemia, acidosis, or the underlying precipitating event.

Disease Highlights

A. Occurs primarily in patients with complete or near complete insulin deficiency

1. Type 1 autoimmune insulin-dependent DM

2. Type 2 DM *can* cause DKA

   a. Studies report type 2 DM in 12–47% of diabetic patients with DKA

   b. Type 2 DM is more frequently found in African Americans and Hispanics presenting with DKA than non-Hispanic whites. (Up to 47% of Hispanic diabetics had type 2 DM.)

   c. Many such patients can eventually be treated with oral hypoglycemics without insulin after a short period of insulin therapy.

3. Diabetes secondary to severe chronic pancreatitis and near complete islet cell obliteration

B. Incidence is 4.6–8.0 cases/1000 person years in patients with DM

C. Precipitated by low insulin levels or illnesses that increase hormones counterregulatory to insulin (cortisol, epinephrine, glucagon, and growth hormone), or both.

1. The precipitant is the most frequent cause of mortality in DKA.

2. Most common precipitants

   a. Infection (urinary tract infections and pneumonia are most common). Patients may be afebrile.

   b. Discontinuation of insulin or oral hypoglycemics

   c. New-onset type 1 DM

3. Other precipitants

   a. Other infections

   b. MI

   c. Cerebrovascular accident

   d. Acute pancreatitis

   e. Pulmonary embolism

   f. Gastrointestinal hemorrhage

   g. Severe emotional stress

   h. Drugs (eg, corticosteroids, thiazides, cocaine, antipsychotics)

D. Pathogenesis: The *marked* decrease in insulin levels together with an increase in counterregulatory hormones lead to the following events:

1. Hyperglycemia: Caused by

   a. Reduced cellular uptake of glucose

   b. Increased hepatic glycogenolysis and gluconeogenesis

   c. Glucosuria helps prevent extreme hyperglycemia (> 500–600 mg/dL) but more extreme hyperglycemia occurs if urinary output falls.

2. Ketoacidosis

   a. Marked insulin deficiency increases glucagon which in turn increases acetyl CoA production within liver.

   b. Massive production of acetyl CoA overwhelms Krebs cycle resulting in ketone production and ketonemia (primarily beta hydroxybutyric acid and to a lesser extent acetoacetic acid).

   c. Ketonemia leads to anion gap metabolic acidosis.

3. Volume depletion: Ketonemia and hyperglycemia cause an osmotic diuresis, which results in profound dehydration and typical fluid losses of 3–6 L.

4. Potassium loss

   a. The osmotic diuresis also causes significant potassium losses.

   b. Dehydration-induced hyperaldosteronism aggravates potassium loss.

   c. Typical potassium deficit is 3–5 mEq/kg body weight.

5. Hyperkalemia

   a. Despite the total body potassium deficit, *hyper*kalemia is frequent.

   b. The etiology is multifactorial.

      (1) Insulin normally drives glucose and potassium into the cells. Insulin *deficiency* decreases cellular uptake and causes hyperkalemia.

      (2) Plasma hypertonicity drives water and potassium out of the cells and into the intravascular compartment accentuating the hyperkalemia.

6. Hyponatremia

   a. Despite a free water deficit due to osmotic diuresis, many patients with DKA have hyponatremia.

   b. Hyperglycemia leads to an osmotic shift of water from the intracellular space to the extracellular space, diluting sodium frequently causing hyponatremia.

   c. The elevated serum osmolality stimulates antidiuretic hormone (ADH) release further accentuating the hyponatremia.

   d. However, the patient's sodium concentration may be low, normal, or even high depending on the balance of the above factors (which act to lower serum sodium) with the free water loss from osmotic diuresis (which acts to raise serum sodium).

   e. Correction factors help predict the serum sodium concentration after the hyperglycemia is treated which shifts the intravascular water back to the intracellular space.

   f. Experiments suggest that the sodium concentration will increase by 2.4 mEq/L for every 100 mg/dL that the glucose falls with treatment. (See Pseudohyponatremia in Chapter 24.)

E. Mortality rate of DKA is 5–15%. Risk factors for death include:

1. Severe coexistent disease (adjusted OR 16.3)

2. pH < 7.0 at presentation (adjusted OR 8.7)

3. > 50 units of insulin required in first 12 hours (adjusted OR 7.9)

4. Glucose > 300 mg/dL after 12 hours (adjusted OR 8.3)

5. Depressed mental status after 24 hours (adjusted OR 8.6)

6. Fever (axillary temperature ≥ 38.0°C) after 24 hours (adjusted OR 5.8)

7. Increasing age

   a. Mortality rate < 1.25% in persons younger than 55 years

   b. Mortality rate 11.8% in persons older than 55 years

Evidence-Based Diagnosis

A. Diagnostic criteria established by the American Diabetes Association (ADA)

1. Glucose > 250 mg/dL

2. pH ≤ 7.3

3. HCO_3^- ≤ 18 mEq/L

4. Positive serum ketones

5. Anion gap > 10 mEq/L

B. Signs and symptoms

1. Polyuria and increased thirst are common.

2. Lethargy and obtundation may be seen in patients with markedly increased effective osmolality (> 320 mOsm/L), especially in patients with significant acidemia.

   a. Effective osmolality can be calculated:

      (1) $(2 \times Na^+) + Glucose/18$

      (2) eg, Na^+ of 140 mEq/L and glucose of 720 mg/dL = osmolality of 320 mOsm/L

   b. Consider neurologic insult (eg, cerebrovascular accident, drug intoxication) if neurologic changes are present in patients with a serum osmolality < 320 mOsm/L or if the neurologic abnormalities fail to resolve with therapy.

3. Abdominal pain

   a. Present in 50–75% of DKA cases

   b. May be secondary to the DKA or another process precipitating DKA (ie, appendicitis, pancreatitis, cholecystitis, abscess)

   c. Abdominal pain is increasingly common with increasing severity of DKA (Table 4-4).

Table 4-4. Frequency and etiology of abdominal pain in patients with DKA.

Serum HCO₃⁻	Frequency of Abdominal Pain	Patients with DKA as Etiology of Pain	Patients with Other Etiology of Pain
0–10 mEq/L	25–75%	70%	30%
> 10 mEq/L	12%	16%	84%

DKA, diabetic ketoacidosis.

 Always search for the etiology of abdominal pain in patients with DKA, especially if it occurs in patients with mild acidosis (HCO₃⁻ > 10 mEq/L), persists after resolution of the acidosis, or patients are older than 40 years.

    4. Nausea and vomiting are common and nonspecific.

C. Hyperglycemia
    1. Glucose level is variable.
    2. 15% of patients with DKA have glucose levels < 350 mg/dL (particularly in pregnancy, in patients with poor oral intake, or those given insulin in route to the hospital).
    3. Glucose > 250 mg/dL has poor specificity for DKA (11%).

D. Ketones
    1. 3 ketones: beta hydroxybutyrate, acetoacetate, acetone
    2. Standard ketone test uses the nitroprusside reaction, which detects acetoacetate but is insensitive for beta hydroxybutyrate. In severe DKA, beta hydroxybutyrate is the prominent ketone, and the nitroprusside test may be falsely negative. In addition, captopril causes a false-positive nitroprusside reaction.
    3. Beta hydroxybutyrate can be measured directly and rapidly. It is highly accurate for diagnosis of DKA: 98% sensitive, 79–85% specific, LR+ 6.5, LR– 0.02 (cutoff > 1.5 mmol/L).
    4. Urine ketones are sensitive for DKA (98%) but not specific (35–69%). Blood measurements are preferred.

E. Anion gap
    1. Anion gap is elevated in most patients with DKA (even when nitroprusside reaction is negative).
    2. In patients evaluated in the emergency department with glucose > 250 mg/dL, the anion gap is 84–90% sensitive and 85–99% specific; LR+, 6–84; LR–, 0.11–0.16.
    3. If anion gap is elevated and ketones are negative, beta hydroxybutyrate measurements should be measured. If beta hydroxybutyrate measurements are not available (or negative), lactic acid should be measured to rule out lactic acidosis.

F. Nonspecific findings
    1. Amylase: Nonspecific elevations in amylase are common.
    2. Leukocytosis
      a. Mild leukocytosis (10,000–15,000 cells/mcL) is common and may occur secondary to stress or infection.
      b. One study documented higher WBCs in DKA patients with major infection than in patients without infection (17,900/mcL vs 13,700/mcL).
      c. Band counts were also higher in patients with infection (23% vs 6%).

Treatment

A. Treatment of DKA must include the following:
    1. Initial evaluation and frequent monitoring
    2. Detection and therapy of the underlying precipitant

 The most common cause of death in patients with DKA is the underlying precipitant. It must be discovered and treated.

    3. Fluid resuscitation
    4. Insulin
    5. Potassium replacement

B. Initial evaluation and monitoring
    1. Check electrolytes, glucose, serum ketones, serum lactate, ABG, anion gap, plasma osmolality, blood urea nitrogen (BUN), and creatinine.
    2. Serum creatinine may be artificially elevated due to interference of assay by ketones.
    3. The serum glucose should be checked hourly and the electrolytes should be measured frequently (every 2–4 hours) and the anion gap calculated.

C. Detection and therapy of the underlying precipitant
    1. Urinalysis and urine culture, chest radiograph, CBC with differential, ECG and troponin levels are appropriate.
    2. Beta-HCG should be measured in women of childbearing age.
    3. Other tests as clinically indicated (blood cultures, lipase, etc.)

D. Fluid resuscitation
    1. Evaluate dehydration: Check BP, orthostatic BP and pulse, monitor hourly urinary output
    2. IV normal saline 0.5–1.5 L bolus initially.
      a. Larger volumes (1–1.5 L) are useful for patients with significant hypotension.
      b. Smaller volumes (500 mL) may allow for more rapid correction of acidosis in patients without marked volume depletion.
    3. Reevaluate after each liter by rechecking BP, orthostatic BP and pulse, urinary output, cardiac and pulmonary exams. Repeat boluses until hypotension and oliguria resolve.
    4. Normal saline should be switched to 0.45% normal saline when intravascular volume improves in patients with normal or elevated *corrected* serum sodium to restore the free water deficit. (Continue 0.9% saline if the corrected serum sodium concentration is low.)

E. Insulin
    1. The ADA recommends an IV bolus of regular insulin (0.1 units/kg) followed by IV regular insulin at 0.1 units/kg/h. Alternatively, the bolus may be omitted and the insulin initiated at 0.14 units/kg/h. If glucose fails to fall by ≥ 10% in first hour, adjust insulin therapy.
    2. Marked hypokalemia (< 3.3 mEq/L) should be excluded *before* insulin therapy is administered (see below).
    3. Administer in monitored setting.
    4. Monitor glucose levels hourly: Target reduction 75–90 mg/dL/h and adjust insulin dose accordingly.
    5. The ADA recommends continued IV insulin until glucose < 200 mg/dL and 2 of the following criteria are met: anion gap ≤ 12, serum HCO₃⁻ is ≥ 15 mEq/L, and the venous pH > 7.3.
      a. Premature discontinuation of IV insulin may result in rebound ketoacidosis.

b. If patient's glucose normalizes (< 200 mmol/d) before the anion gap normalizes and before the HCO_3^- is ≥ 18 mEq/L, reduce the insulin infusion and add glucose (D5W) to the IV to prevent hypoglycemia.

c. Patients should receive their first dose of SQ insulin 1–2 hours before IV insulin is discontinued in order to prevent an insulin free window and recurrent ketoacidosis.

 In DKA, it is important to continue IV insulin until the anion gap returns to normal. Administer glucose as necessary to prevent hypoglycemia.

F. Potassium replacement

1. Insulin shifts potassium back into the intracellular compartment. Fluid resuscitation and correction of the acidosis further lower the serum potassium concentration.

2. Despite hyperkalemia on presentation, profound and potentially life-threatening *hypokalemia* is a common *complication of therapy* and often develops within the first few hours.

3. Patients with normal or near normal serum potassium concentrations on admission should have cardiac monitoring due to the risk of arrhythmias.

4. Potassium levels should be monitored hourly, and replacement should be initiated when urinary output resumes and potassium is < 5.0–5.2 mEq/L.

5. Potassium therapy should be initiated immediately in patients with hypokalemia. In addition, insulin therapy should be delayed until the serum potassium > 3.3 mEq/L.

G. HCO_3^- therapy

1. Use is controversial; if used, monitor patient for hypokalemia.

2. HCO_3^- has not been shown to improve outcomes in patients with a serum pH > 6.9. It may also paradoxically lower CNS pH.

3. The ADA recommends HCO_3^- therapy in patients with a pH < 6.9.

H. Phosphate therapy

1. *Dramatic* falls in serum phosphate are common during treatment.

2. Replacement should be considered in patients with marked hypophosphatemia (< 1.0 mg/dL) or with respiratory depression, cardiac dysfunction, or anemia.

 Careful, frequent observation and evaluation of patients with DKA is critical.

MAKING A DIAGNOSIS

 Have you crossed a diagnostic threshold for the leading hypothesis, DKA? Have you ruled out the active alternatives uremia, starvation ketosis, alcoholic ketoacidosis, or lactic acidosis? Do other tests need to be done to exclude the alternative diagnoses?

Alternative Diagnosis: Uremic Acidosis

Textbook Presentation

Typically, patients with chronic kidney disease have low HCO_3^- levels, high creatinine levels (often > 4–5 mg/dL), and elevated BUN and phosphate levels. Patients often complain of a variety of constitutional symptoms secondary to their kidney disease, including fatigue, nausea, vomiting, anorexia, and pruritus.

Disease Highlights

A. Pathophysiology

1. Each day, ingested nonvolatile acids neutralize HCO_3^-.

2. In health, the kidneys regenerate the HCO_3^- and maintain the acid-base equilibrium.

3. Renal impairment results in failed HCO_3^- regeneration and a metabolic acidosis.

B. Acidosis in patients with kidney disease may be of the anion gap type or non–anion gap type.

1. In early kidney disease, ammonia-genesis is impaired, resulting in reduced acid secretion and a non–anion gap metabolic acidosis.

2. In more advanced chronic kidney disease, the kidney remains unable to excrete the daily acid load and also becomes unable to excrete anions such as sulfates, phosphates, and urate. Therefore, an anion gap acidosis develops. HCO_3^- levels stabilize between 12 mEq/L and 20 mEq/L.

C. The acidosis has several adverse effects.

1. Increased calcium loss from bone

2. Increased skeletal muscle breakdown

Treatment

A. $NaHCO_3^-$ replacement

B. Hemodialysis

Alternative Diagnosis: Starvation Ketosis

Typically, starvation ketosis occurs in patients with diminished carbohydrate intake. Ketosis is usually mild ($HCO_3^- ≥ 14$ mEq/L) and serum glucose is usually normal. Serum pH is usually normal.

Alternative Diagnosis: Alcoholic Ketoacidosis

Alcoholic ketoacidosis usually occurs in advanced alcoholism when the majority of calories come from alcohol. Ketoacidosis develops due to the combined effects of inadequate carbohydrate intake, ethanol conversion to acetic acid and stimulated lipolysis. Ketoacidosis may be precipitated by decreased intake, pancreatitis, gastrointestinal bleeding, or infection and may be profound. The plasma glucose level is typically normal to low. (Significant elevations suggest concomitant DKA.) It is important to consider other causes of metabolic acidosis in alcoholics with acidosis. First, patients with alcoholic ketoacidosis often have concomitant lactic acidosis. Shock and hypoxia should be carefully considered. Lactic acidosis may also occur due to an increase in NADH levels and can be particularly severe in patients with thiamine deficiency. Second, toxic ingestions (methanol, ethylene glycol, or salicylate) should also be considered, especially in patients with a large osmolar gap. (The osmolar gap = measured serum osmolality − calculated serum osmolality. The calculated osmolality = (2 × Na$^+$) + Glucose (mg/dL)/18 + BUN (mg/dL)/2.8 + ETOH (mg/dL)/3.7. A normal osmolar gap < 10 mosm/kg.) The treatment for alcoholic ketoacidosis should include IV thiamine prior to IV glucose to avoid precipitating Wernicke encephalopathy or Korsakoff syndrome.

Mr. L's serum ketones are large. He denies any history of heavy alcohol use or abuse. The serum lactate level is 1 mEq/L (normal 0.5–1.5 mEq/L).

Step 5: Diagnose Primary Disorder

The high serum ketones confirm ketoacidosis as the primary metabolic disturbance and the high glucose and diabetic history clearly suggest DKA as the cause of the primary acid base abnormality. The high glucose and profound acidosis are not consistent with starvation ketoacidosis and the absence of a significant alcohol history argues against alcoholic ketoacidosis. The normal lactate effectively rules out lactic acidosis, and uremic acidosis is very unlikely with mild renal insufficiency (Creatinine = 1.8).

Step 6: Check for Additional Disorders

Step 6A: Check Anion Gap

Already completed (see above)

Step 6B: Calculate Whether Compensation Is Appropriate

As shown in Table 4-2 the expected drop in $PaCO_2$ to compensate for a metabolic acidosis is 1.2 mm Hg per 1 mEq/L fall in HCO_3^-. The patient's HCO_3^- is 6 mEq/L (normal is 24 mEq/L), which is an 18 mEq/L decrement. The $PaCO_2$ should fall by $1.2 \times 18 = 21.6$ mm Hg. Since the normal $PaCO_2$ is approximately 40 mm Hg, the $PaCO_2$ would be expected to be approximately $40 - 21.6 \approx 18$. The actual $PaCO_2$ (20 mm Hg) is close to this predicted value suggesting that respiratory compensation is indeed appropriate.

Step 7: Reach Final Diagnosis

Therefore, Mr. L is suffering from an anion gap metabolic acidosis secondary to DKA with appropriate respiratory compensation.

CASE RESOLUTION

Evaluation and treatment identifies the precipitant of DKA and treats the acidosis, hyperglycemia, and profound dehydration.

Mr. L confirms he has been taking his insulin. He reports no fever, rigors, dysuria, cough, shortness of breath, diarrhea, or abdominal pain. Urinalysis, chest radiograph, and lipase were sent to search for the precipitating event. All of the results were normal. An ECG revealed T wave inversion in leads V1–V4, suggesting anterior myocardial ischemia. Troponin T levels were elevated consistent with an acute MI (believed to be the precipitant of his DKA). He was transferred to the ICU for monitoring. He received fluid resuscitation, IV insulin until his ketoacidosis resolved, and supplemental potassium (when his potassium fell below 5.3 mEq/L). His MI was treated with beta-blockers and aspirin. Subsequent cardiac catheterization revealed triple vessel disease. After stabilization, he underwent coronary artery bypass grafting and did well.

CHIEF COMPLAINT

PATIENT 2

Ms. S is a 32-year-old woman who complains of nausea and vomiting. She reports that she felt well until 5 days ago when she noticed urinary frequency and burning on urination. She increased her intake of fluids and cranberry juice but noticed some increasing right back pain 2 days ago. Yesterday, she felt warm and noticed that she had a fever of 38.8°C and teeth-chattering chills. Subsequently, she has been unable to keep down any food or liquids and has persistent nausea and vomiting. She feels weak and dizzy. Physical exam: supine BP, 95/62 mm Hg; pulse, 120 bpm; temperature, 38.9°C; RR, 24 breaths per minute. On standing, her BP falls to 72/40 mm Hg with a pulse of 145 bpm. Cardiac and pulmonary exam are notable only for the tachycardia. She has 2+ right costovertebral angle tenderness. Abdominal exam is soft without rebound, guarding, or focal tenderness. Initial laboratory results include Na^+, 138 mEq/L; K^+, 5.4 mEq/L; HCO_3^-, 14 mEq/L; Cl^-, 102 mEq/L; BUN, 30 mg/dL; creatinine, 1.2 mg/dL; glucose, 90 mg/dL.

The list of symptoms and signs can be grouped together to make evaluation more organized: (1) dysuria, urinary frequency, flank pain, fever, and chills, (2) nausea and vomiting, (3) hypotension and tachycardia, and (4) low serum HCO_3^-. In addition to investigating the probable urinary tract infection, it is critical to determine the nature of the acid-base abnormality.

At this point, what is the leading hypothesis, what are the active alternatives, and is there a must not miss diagnosis? Given this differential diagnosis, what tests should be ordered?

RANKING THE DIFFERENTIAL DIAGNOSIS

Step 1: Determine Whether the Primary Disorder Is an Acidosis or Alkalosis by Reviewing the pH

Similar to the first case, Ms. S has a low serum HCO_3^- suggesting a metabolic acidosis. On the other hand, it is conceivable (but unlikely), that the low serum HCO_3^- could occur in compensation for a profound respiratory alkalosis. An ABG can determine the primary disorder, limit the differential diagnosis of the primary disorder, and access compensation.

An ABG reveals a pH of 7.29, $PaCO_2$ of 30 mm Hg, PaO_2 of 90 mm Hg.

The low pH on the ABG confirms the primary process is an acidosis.

Step 2: Determine Whether the Primary Acidosis or Alkalosis is Metabolic or Respiratory by Reviewing the HCO_3^- and $PaCO_2$

Ms. S's serum HCO_3^- is 14 mEq/L, her $PaCO_2$ is 30 mm Hg. Both are quite low but only the low HCO_3^- would create an acidosis. (A low $PaCO_2$ would drive the pH up and cause an alkalosis.) Since her pH is low and the HCO_3^- is low the primary process is a metabolic acidosis.

Step 3: Limit the Differential Diagnoses of Metabolic Acidosis by Calculating the Anion Gap

The next step in the differential diagnosis is to calculate the anion gap. Her anion gap = 138 − (102 + 14) = 22.

Clearly, Ms. S is suffering from an anion gap metabolic acidosis. This is alarming because metabolic acidosis in the face of infection suggests lactic acidosis due to severe sepsis.

Step 4: Explore the Differential Diagnoses of the Primary Disorder

The leading and must not miss hypothesis would clearly be lactic acidosis, especially given the patient's hypotension. If confirmed, the cause of the lactic acidosis must be determined (which would most likely be sepsis for Ms. S) and then treated. Although unlikely, alternative causes of an anion gap metabolic acidosis (Table 4-1) that would be reasonable to consider include alcoholic ketoacidosis and toxin-related acidosis (including salicylates). The normal glucose and lack of history of diabetes rules out DKA, and the severity of acidosis is not consistent with starvation ketoacidosis. The normal creatinine rules out uremic acidosis. The differential diagnosis for Ms. S is listed in Table 4-5.

The patient denies any history of alcohol use, moonshine or antifreeze ingestion, or unusual salicylate use. Further lab studies include WBC, 18,500 cells/mcL with 62% granulocytes and 30% bands. Urinalysis reveals > 20 WBC/hpf.

Ms. S's history does not suggest toxic ingestions and her history of fever, dysuria, and flank pain as well as leukocytosis and pyuria clearly suggest urinary tract infection and pyelonephritis. Her teeth-chattering chills suggest bacteremia, which combined with her hypotension suggests severe sepsis. Septic shock can cause lactic acid production and thereby generate an anion gap metabolic acidosis.

Is the clinical information sufficient to make a diagnosis? If not, what other information do you need?

Leading Hypothesis: Lactic Acidosis

Textbook Presentation

The presentation of lactic acidosis depends on the underlying etiology. The most common causes are hypoxemia, septic shock, cardiogenic shock, or hypovolemic shock. Patients with shock usually have hypotension and tachycardia and often have impaired mentation and decreased urinary output. Patients with *septic* shock typically have fever and tachypnea. While patients with cardiogenic or hemorrhagic shock often have cold extremities, patients with septic shock often have warm extremities and bounding pulses after fluid resuscitation. (Pulses are bounding due to a widened pulse pressure.) See Chapter 25 for a review of sepsis.

Table 4-5. Diagnostic hypotheses for Ms. S.

Diagnostic Hypothesis	Demographics, Risk Factors, Symptoms and Signs	Important Tests
Leading Hypothesis		
Lactic acidosis		
Cardiogenic shock	History of CAD, HF, S_3 gallop, JVD, cold extremities, hypotension	ECG, troponin, echocardiogram
Hypovolemic shock	History of hemorrhage, dehydration, abdominal pain, tachycardia, hypotension, orthostatic hypotension	CBC, abdominal imaging if indicated
Septic	Fever	CBC with left shift
	Shaking chills	Blood cultures
	Localized symptoms and signs of infection (eg, cough, dysuria, skin redness)	Urinalysis
	Hypotension, tachycardia, bounding pulses	Chest radiograph
Active Alternatives—Most Common		
Alcoholic ketoacidosis	Significant history of alcohol abuse and poor dietary intake of other calories	Urine ketones
		Lactate level
Toxins Methanol Ethylene glycol Salicylate	History of alcoholism, "moonshine" or antifreeze ingestion, or salicylate use	Serum levels of salicylate, methanol, ethylene glycol and serum osmolality[1]

[1]Consider toxic ingestion in patients with an increased osmolar gap > 10 mosm/dL.
ABG, arterial blood gas; CAD, coronary artery disease; CBC, complete blood cell; ECG, electrocardiogram; HF, heart failure; JVD, jugular venous distention.

Table 4-6. Differential diagnosis of lactic acidosis.

Pathophysiology of Disorder	Examples
Common Causes	
Hypoxemia	Lung disease (eg, pneumonia, COPD, pulmonary embolism), HF
Shock (inadequate tissue perfusion; demand > supply)	Cardiogenic shock
	Hypovolemic shock
	Septic shock
Less Common Causes	
Regional blood flow obstruction	Mesenteric ischemia
Low environmental oxygen	High altitude
Severe anemia	
Low oxygen saturation (SaO_2) (despite normal PaO_2)	Carbon monoxide poisoning
	Methemoglobinemia
Cellular inability to utilize oxygen	Cyanide poisoning[1]
Increased demand	Intense anaerobic activity, seizures

[1]Most commonly seen in fire victims, industrial exposures (ie, electroplating jewelry) and certain medications (amygdalin and sodium nitroprusside).
COPD, chronic obstructive pulmonary disease; HF, heart failure.

Disease Highlights

A. Lactic acidosis develops when oxygen delivery to the cells is inadequate. This results in anaerobic metabolism and the production of lactic acid. Therefore, the differential diagnosis can be remembered by tracing the pathway of oxygen from the environment through the blood to the cells and mitochondria. Any disease that interferes with oxygen delivery can cause lactic acidosis (Table 4-6).

   1. Low oxygen carrying capacity

      a. Hypoxemia (from pulmonary or cardiac disease)

      b. Severe anemia

      c. Carbon monoxide poisoning (interferes with oxygen binding)

      d. Methemoglobinemia

   2. Inadequate tissue perfusion; causes include

      a. Hypovolemic shock

      b. Cardiogenic shock

      c. Septic shock

      d. Regional obstruction to blood flow (eg, ischemic bowel or gangrene)

   3. Inadequate cellular utilization of oxygen (cyanide poisoning)

   4. Occasionally, lactic acidosis develops secondary to unusually high demand exceeding oxygen supply (eg, intense exercise, seizures).

B. Lactate elevation is associated with a substantially increased mortality. The mortality rate of patients with shock and lactic acidosis is 70% compared with 25–35% in patients with shock without lactic acidosis.

Evidence-Based Diagnosis

A. Serum lactate levels are more sensitive and specific than an increase in the anion gap.

B. An elevated anion gap is 44–67% sensitive.

C. An elevated anion gap may suggest lactic acidosis, but a normal anion gap does not exclude lactic acidosis.

 The serum lactate level should be measured in critically ill patients in whom shock is suspected regardless of the anion gap.

Treatment

Treatment of lactic acidosis should target the underlying condition. A variety of buffering agents (ie, $NaHCO_3^-$) have been tried and failed to demonstrate improved hemodynamics or survival.

MAKING A DIAGNOSIS

 Have you crossed a diagnostic threshold for the leading hypothesis, lactic acidosis? Do other tests need to be done to exclude the alternative diagnoses?

 Serum lactate level of 8 mEq/L (nl 0.5–1.5 mEq/L) confirms lactic acidosis. Blood cultures and urine cultures grew *Escherichia coli*.

Step 5: Diagnose Primary Disorder

The serum lactate confirms an anion gap metabolic acidosis due to lactic acidosis as the primary acid-base disorder. The clinical scenario and positive cultures strongly suggest that the diagnosis is lactic acidosis secondary to sepsis. Other tests are not necessary to confirm the diagnosis.

Step 6: Check for Additional Disorders

Step 6A: Check Anion Gap
Already completed (see above).

Step 6B: Calculate Whether Compensation is Appropriate

In a metabolic acidosis, the $PaCO_2$ is expected to fall by 1.2 mm Hg per 1 mEq/L fall in HCO_3^- (see Table 4-1). The patient's HCO_3^- is 14 mEq/L (10 mEq/L below normal). The $PaCO_2$ should fall by $1.2 \times 10 = 12$. Since normal $PaCO_2$ is approximately 40 mm Hg, we would expect the $PaCO_2$ to be approximately 28 mm Hg ($40 - 12 = 28$ mm Hg). The actual $PaCO_2$ is 30 mm Hg, quite close to the prediction. This suggests that respiratory compensation is appropriate.

Step 7: Reach Final Diagnosis

In summary, Ms. S is suffering from a lactic acidosis with appropriate respiratory compensation.

CASE RESOLUTION

 Ms. S was treated with broad-spectrum antibiotics and IV fluid resuscitation. After initial stabilization, hypotension recurred and urinary output dropped. She was transferred to the ICU. Four hours later her oxygenation deteriorated and a chest film revealed a diffuse infiltrate consistent with acute respiratory distress syndrome. She was intubated and given IV fluids, norepinephrine, antibiotics, mechanical ventilation, and activated protein C. Over the next 24 hours, her BP stabilized and her anion gap lactic acidosis resolved. Seventy-two hours later she was extubated. She eventually made a full recovery.

CHIEF COMPLAINT

PATIENT

Mr. R is a 55-year-old man with chronic obstructive pulmonary disease (COPD) with a chief complaint of dyspnea. He reports that symptoms began 5 days ago with a cough productive of green sputum. The cough worsened, and 4 days ago he had a low-grade fever of 37.2°C. He noticed increasing shortness of breath 3 days ago. He reports that previously he was able to walk about 25 feet before becoming short of breath but now he is short of breath at rest. Last night his fever reached 38.8°C, and today his dyspnea intensified. He is unable to complete a sentence without pausing to take a breath. On physical exam he appears older than his stated age. He is gaunt, sitting upright, breathing through pursed lips, and in obvious distress. Vital signs are temperature, 38.9°C; RR, 28 breaths per minute; BP, 110/70 mm Hg; pulse, 110 bpm. His pulsus paradox is 20 mm Hg. Lung exam reveals significant use of accessory muscles and markedly decreased breath sounds. Cardiac exam is notable only for diminished heart sounds.

Your resident is concerned about the adequacy of Mr. R.'s ventilation and suggests checking his pulse oxymetry. You remind him that a pulse oximeter will not address the adequacy of the patient's ventilation nor will it determine whether respiratory failure is present.

An ABG reveals a pH of 7.22, PaCO$_2$ of 70 mm Hg, and PaO$_2$ of 55 mm Hg.

Always check an ABG when the adequacy of a patient's ventilation is a concern. Patients with adequate oxygenation may still be in respiratory failure.

Clearly Mr. R has several problems that are easily identified, including (1) fever, cough, and history of COPD, (2) respiratory distress, and (3) acidosis. All of these problems are obviously potentially life threatening. Furthermore, a thorough evaluation of the acidosis may shed light on the status of the other problems.

At this point, what is the leading hypothesis, what are the active alternatives, and is there a must not miss diagnosis? Given this differential diagnosis, what tests should be ordered?

RANKING THE DIFFERENTIAL DIAGNOSIS

Step 1: Determine Whether the Primary Disorder is an Acidosis or Alkalosis by Reviewing the pH

The low pH confirms the primary disorder is an acidosis.

Step 2: Determine Whether the Primary Acidosis or Alkalosis is Metabolic or Respiratory by Reviewing the HCO$_3^-$ and PaCO$_2$

Na$^+$, 138 mEq/L; K$^+$, 5.1 mEq/L; HCO$_3^-$, 27 mEq/L; Cl$^-$, 102 mEq/L; BUN, 30 mg/dL; creatinine, 1.2 mg/dL.

The PaCO$_2$ and HCO$_3^-$ are both elevated. An elevated PaCO$_2$ would lower pH and cause an acidemia (whereas an elevated HCO$_3^-$ would cause alkalemia). Since the patient is acidemic, the primary process is a respiratory acidosis.

Step 3: Explore the Differential Diagnoses of the Primary Disorder

Respiratory acidosis may be caused by lung diseases, pleural diseases, or a variety of neuromuscular diseases (see Table 4-1). His prior history of COPD and acute pulmonary complaints of cough and fever clearly suggest that his respiratory acidosis is due to a pulmonary process. Specifically, Mr. R's history of very poor exercise tolerance at *baseline* suggests severe COPD. Such severe COPD could result in chronic carbon dioxide retention and chronic respiratory acidosis. A "must not miss" possibility is that his acute respiratory infection has precipitated *acute* respiratory failure (and acute respiratory acidosis). This is suggested by his worsening symptoms, respiratory distress, upright posture, pursed lip breathing, pulsus paradox, and decreased breath sounds. *It is critical to distinguish acute respiratory acidosis from chronic respiratory acidosis* because the former is more likely to progress rapidly to *complete* respiratory failure and respiratory arrest. Therefore, acute respiratory acidosis is both the leading hypothesis and the "must not miss" diagnosis. Table 4-7 ranks the differential diagnosis considering the available demographic information, risk factors, and symptoms and signs.

Patients with a history of asthma or COPD should be asked about a prior history of intubation or ICU admission. Such patients are at greater risk for respiratory failure.

Is the clinical information sufficient to make a diagnosis? If not, what other information do you need?

Table 4-7. Diagnostic hypotheses for Mr. R.

Diagnostic Hypothesis	Demographics, Risk Factors, Symptoms and Signs	Important Tests
Leading Hypothesis		
Acute respiratory acidosis (from lung disease [eg, COPD, pneumonia])	Severe underlying lung disease Worsening symptoms Respiratory distress Pulsus paradox Decreased breath sounds Prior history of intubation or ICU admission	Decreased pH Elevated PCO$_2$ Near *normal* HCO$_3^-$
Active Alternatives—Most Common		
Chronic respiratory acidosis (from lung disease [eg, COPD, pneumonia])	Severe underlying lung disease Decreased breath sounds	Decreased pH Elevated PaCO$_2$ *Elevated* HCO$_3^-$

COPD, chronic obstructive pulmonary disease.

Leading Hypothesis: Respiratory Acidosis

Textbook Presentation

The presentation of respiratory acidosis depends primarily on the underlying cause. The most common causes are severe underlying lung disease (eg, COPD, pneumonia, or pulmonary edema). Such patients are typically in extreme respiratory distress.

Disease Highlights

A. Insufficient ventilation results in increasing levels of $PaCO_2$. This in turn lowers arterial pH. Compensation occurs over several days, with increased renal HCO_3^- regeneration.

B. Ventilation is assessed by measuring the arterial $PaCO_2$ and pH. Significant hypoventilation and acidosis may occur *without* significant hypoxia.

C. Etiology: Although most commonly due to lung disease, respiratory acidosis may result from any disease affecting ventilation—from the brain to the alveoli. (See differential diagnosis of acid-base disorders in Table 4-1.)

D. Manifestations are primarily CNS.

1. Severity depends on acuity. Patients with chronic hypercapnia have markedly fewer CNS effects than patients with acute hypercapnia.

2. Anxiety, irritability, confusion, and lethargy

3. Headache may be prominent in the morning due to the worsening hypoventilation that occurs with sleep.

4. Stupor and coma may occur when the $PaCO_2 > 70-100$ mm Hg.

5. Tremor, asterixis, slurred speech, and papilledema may be seen.

Evidence-Based Diagnosis

A. Typically characterized by $PaCO_2 > 43$ mm Hg.

1. Occasionally, a normal $PaCO_2$ suggests respiratory failure.

   a. For example, during asthma attacks, patients typically hyperventilate and present with a $PaCO_2$ *below* normal. A *normal* $PaCO_2$ in such a patient may reflect respiratory fatigue and herald the development of frank respiratory failure.

   b. Patients with primary metabolic acidoses typically hyperventilate to compensate, lowering the $PaCO_2$ below normal.

      (1) A $PaCO_2$ of ≥ 40 mm Hg is inappropriate in such cases and represents a respiratory acidosis.

      (2) Inability to compensate for a metabolic acidosis (hyperventilate) is associated with an increased risk of respiratory failure and the subsequent need for mechanical ventilation.

2. The alveolar-arterial oxygen gradient (PaO_2-PaO_2) can help distinguish hypercapnia due to pulmonary disease from hypercapnia due to CNS disease (central hypoventilation).

   a. This gradient compares the *calculated alveolar* partial pressure of oxygen (PaO_2) with the *measured arterial* partial pressure of oxygen (PaO_2).

      (1) In the absence of lung disease, there is little difference between the alveolar and arterial O_2.

      (2) A normal A-a gradient is around 10 mm Hg.

   b. Therefore, the A-a gradient is usually normal in hypoventilation due to CNS disease but increased in pulmonary disease.

c. The PaO_2 is measured in an ABG whereas the PaO_2 is calculated from the following formula:

$$PaO_2 = FIO_2 (pAtm - pH_2O) - PaCO_2/R.$$

(FIO$_2$ is the fraction of inspired oxygen: 0.21 for patients not on supplemental oxygen. pAtm = 760 at sea level, the partial pressure of H_2O = 47 and $PaCO_2$ is the arterial PCO_2 measured in the blood gas. R refers to the respiratory quotient and is often estimated at 0.8.)

B. Pulsus paradox

1. Defined as > 10 mm Hg drop in systolic BP during inspiration

2. May be seen in patients using unusually strong inspiratory effort due to asthma, COPD, or other respiratory diseases

3. When elevated in patients with asthma, it is highly specific for a severe attack but has poor sensitivity (Table 4-8).

4. When pulsus paradox is marked, there is a high LR of severe disease.

Treatment

A. Treat underlying disease process (ie, bronchodilators for asthma, naloxone for opioid overdose).

B. Supplemental oxygen should be given as necessary to prevent hypoxemia.

Supplemental oxygen occasionally worsens hypercapnia in some patients with severe COPD, asthma, and sleep apnea but should never be withheld from hypoxic patients.

C. Avoid hypokalemia and dehydration that may worsen metabolic alkalosis, raise the serum pH, and inadvertently further suppress ventilation.

D. Mechanical ventilation with either intubation or biphasic positive airway pressure (BiPAP) is lifesaving in some patients.

1. Institution of mechanical ventilation is considered when pH < 7.1–7.25 or $PaCO_2 > 80-90$ mm Hg.

2. In general, patients with acute hypoventilation require mechanical ventilation with milder hypercapnia than patients with chronic hypoventilation.

Step 4: Diagnose Primary Disorder

The patient's clinical picture and ABG clearly suggest the primary disorder is a respiratory acidosis.

Step 5: Check for Additional Disorders

Step 5A: Calculate Anion Gap (Even in Patients Without Acidosis) to Uncover Unexpected Anion Gap Metabolic Acidosis

Another "must not miss" diagnosis for Mr. R would be sepsis. His symptoms of fever and cough suggest the possibility of pneumonia, which can be complicated by sepsis resulting in an anion gap

Table 4-8. Pulsus paradox in severe asthma.

	Sensitivity %	Specificity %	LR+	LR−
Pulsus > 10 mm Hg	53-68	69-92	2.7	0.5
Pulsus > 20 mm Hg	19-39	92-100	8.2	0.8
Pulsus > 25 mm Hg	16	99	22.6	0.8

metabolic lactic acidosis. Although his elevated HCO_3^- does not immediately suggest a metabolic acidosis from sepsis, the HCO_3^- may *not* be low if there is also a superimposed metabolic alkalosis generating HCO_3^-. These hidden acidoses can be discovered by evaluating the anion gap (which is usually elevated due the accumulation of lactate) or by measuring the serum lactate level.

The anion gap = 138 − (102 + 27) = 9, and the serum lactate level is 0.8 mEq/L (normal 0.5–1.5 mEq/L).

Mr. R has a normal anion gap and normal lactate level, ruling out a coexistent hidden anion gap metabolic acidosis from sepsis.

Step 5B: Calculate Whether Compensation Is Appropriate

In this case, it is critical to determine whether the $PaCO_2$ is chronically elevated or whether this represents an acute decompensation. Acute respiratory acidosis can be distinguished from chronic respiratory acidosis by evaluating the degree of metabolic compensation (provided there are no other acidoses also effecting HCO_3^-). Because metabolic compensation takes time, chronic respiratory acidoses are associated with more complete compensation than acute respiratory acidoses. Table 4-2 shows the formulas that can be used to calculate the HCO_3^- levels. In acute respiratory acidosis, the HCO_3^- increases by only 1 mEq/L for every 10 mm Hg increase in $PaCO_2$ whereas in chronic respiratory acidosis, the HCO_3^- increases by 4 mEq/L for every 10 mm Hg increase in $PaCO_2$. In Mr. R's case, the $PaCO_2$ is 70 mm Hg, up by 30 mm Hg (from a normal of 40 mm Hg), so *if this were an acute respiratory acidosis,* the HCO_3^- level would be expected to increase by only 3 mEq/L (from a normal of 24 mEq/L to 27 mEq/L). If, on the other hand, this is a chronic respiratory acidosis, an increase of 4 mEq/L of HCO_3^- per 10 mm Hg increase in $PaCO_2$ would be expected. For a 30 mm Hg increase in $PaCO_2$, the predicted increase in HCO_3^- would be 3 × 4 = 12 mEq.

Mr. R's laboratory results reveal a HCO_3^- of 27 mEq/L, an increase of only 3 mEq/L from a normal baseline of 24 mEq/L. Other initial laboratory test results include WBC, 16,500/mcL with 62% granulocytes and 10% bands. Chest radiograph reveals hyperinflated lung fields and a left lower lobe infiltrate.

Step 6: Reach Final Diagnosis

The tiny metabolic compensation suggests that Mr. R is suffering from an acute respiratory acidosis with metabolic compensation. There is no evidence of a hidden anion gap acidosis. Therefore, Mr. R has an acute respiratory acidosis caused by pneumonia and COPD. He is at significant risk for complete respiratory failure and he is transferred him to the ICU.

It is vital to distinguish acute from chronic respiratory acidoses.

CASE RESOLUTION

In the ICU, Mr. R is placed on ventilatory support with BiPAP and antibiotics. Over the next 5 days, his pneumonia improves. On day 8, BiPAP is discontinued and he is sent to the medical floors.

REVIEW OF OTHER IMPORTANT DISEASES

Renal Tubular Acidosis (RTA)

Textbook Presentation

Although there are a variety of RTAs, the most common type in adults is type IV RTA, caused most commonly by long-standing diabetes. Laboratory abnormalities include mild renal insufficiency, a mild non-anion gap acidosis ($HCO_3^- \approx 17$ mEq/L) and hyperkalemia. Only the highlights of type IV RTA will be reviewed here.

Disease Highlights

A. Patients with type IV RTA have hypoaldosteronism.

B. Hypoaldosteronism decreases potassium and H^+ excretion resulting in hyperkalemia and acidosis.

C. The hyperkalemia also interferes with ammonia production (the major renal buffer) and further impairs acid secretion. The inability to excrete the daily acid load causes a non–anion gap acidosis.

D. In patients with diabetes mellitus, type IV RTA is also associated with low renin levels.

E. Etiologies of type IV RTA are numerous.

  1. Diabetes with mild renal impairment is the most common.

  2. Other causes include

    a. Drugs (NSAIDs, ACE inhibitors, potassium sparing diuretics, trimethoprim, heparin, and cyclosporine)

    b. Addison disease

    c. Systemic lupus erythematosus

    d. AIDS nephropathy

    e. Chronic interstitial renal disease

Treatment

Dietary potassium restriction, loop diuretics, and fludrocortisone are useful.

D-Lactic Acidosis

D-lactic acidosis is a rare disorder seen in some patients with jejunoileal bypass or short bowel. The bypass or short bowel results in carbohydrate malabsorption and delivery of this carbohydrate to the colon where colonic bacteria metabolize it into D-lactic acid, which is absorbed. (Endogenous lactate is L-lactic acid.) Presenting manifestations include encephalopathy and metabolic acidosis after carbohydrate ingestion. Patients may appear intoxicated and show the following symptoms and signs: altered mental status ranging from drowsiness to coma (100%), slurred speech (65%), ataxia (45%), and disorientation (21%) that may follow large carbohydrate meals. Attacks last from hours to days. It is unclear if the neurologic symptoms are secondary to the D-lactic acid or other absorbed toxins. Laboratory tests may reveal an anion gap acidosis. However, the anion gap may be smaller than expected because

D-lactate is not reabsorbed by the kidney (unlike L-lactate) and is excreted. Lactate measurements may be falsely negative since standard lactate tests measure L-lactate rather than D-lactate. Special assays must be requested to measure D-lactate.

Metabolic Alkalosis

Textbook Presentation

The most common clinical situations that give rise to metabolic alkalosis are recurrent vomiting or diuretic treatment. The metabolic alkalosis per se is usually asymptomatic. Muscle cramping due to coexistent hypokalemia may be seen.

Disease Highlights

A. Metabolic alkalosis develops only when there is *both* a source of additional HCO_3^- *and* a renal stimulus that limits its excretion.

1. *Increased HCO_3^- production* develops when H+ is (1) lost from the gastrointestinal tract (ie, due to vomiting) or (2) lost from the genitourinary tract (ie, due to hyperaldosteronism) or (3) during administration of HCO_3^-. Volume contraction around a constant amount of HCO_3^- also serves to increase the HCO_3^-.

2. *Decreased HCO_3^- excretion* is most commonly caused by decreased renal perfusion. This occurs when the *effective circulating volume* is reduced.

   a. Examples include dehydration or other pathologic states associated with decreased renal perfusion (ie, heart failure [HF], nephrotic syndrome).

   b. The mechanisms that interfere with HCO_3^- excretion are complex but include enhanced renal HCO_3^- reabsorption and decreased renal HCO_3^- secretion.

      (1) Decreased effective circulating volume promotes avid Na^+ absorption in the proximal tubule, which in turn facilitates HCO_3^- reclamation (Figure 4-2).

      (2) Decreased effective circulating volume and Cl^-depletion also decrease HCO_3^- *secretion* by the collecting cells, which compounds the metabolic alkalosis. This develops because HCO_3^- secretion occurs in exchange with Cl^- reabsorption in the distal tubules (Figure 4-3). This requires Cl^-

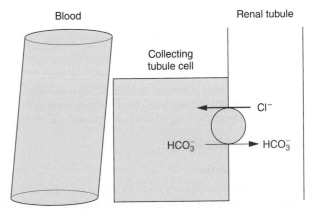

Figure 4-3. Chloride depletion interferes with HCO_3^- secretion. Distal HCO_3^- secretion is facilitated by Cl^- delivery. Hypovolemia increases proximal NaCl reabsorption, limiting distal chloride delivery, in turn interfering with HCO_3^- secretion.

delivery to the collecting tubules, which decreases both due to enhanced proximal Cl^- reabsorption and gastrointestinal or diuretic Cl^- losses.

      (3) Decreased effective circulating volume results in secondary hyperaldosteronism which activates H^+ secretion by the collecting tubule cells and production of HCO_3^- which is reabsorbed into the blood.

      (4) Low tubular Cl^- also draws chloride into the tubular cells (from the plasma) and promotes HCO_3^- reabsorption.

      (5) Hypokalemia is an important mechanism that promotes HCO_3^- reabsorption. In the collecting tubule, it stimulates potassium reabsorption in exchange for H^+ secretion. HCO_3^- is produced and reabsorbed into the blood.

B. Pathologic states associated with metabolic alkalosis (Table 4-1)

1. Vomiting or nasogastric drainage. Pathophysiology:

   a. Gastric acid production (and secretion) is matched by HCO_3^- production. The H^+ ion enters the gastric lumen, whereas the HCO_3^- enters the bloodstream.

   b. Dehydration decreases renal HCO_3^- excretion (see above).

2. Dehydration or other causes of reduced glomerular filtration rate (GFR) (ie, HF, nephrotic syndrome)

3. Diuretics

4. Hypokalemia

5. Hyperaldosteronism

   a. Adrenal adenoma

   b. Licorice ingestion or chewing tobacco (Normally, a renal enzyme converts cortisol to cortisone in order to prevent cortisol from exerting a significant mineralocorticoid effect. Licorice contains the steroid glycyrrhetinic acid which blocks this enzyme resulting in a heightened mineralocorticoid effect from endogenous cortisol.)

6. Bartter or Gitelman syndromes

7. Respiratory acidosis also promotes a compensatory metabolic alkalosis. Occasionally, rapid resolution of the respiratory failure will correct the hypercapnia, resulting in a transient inappropriate metabolic alkalosis (posthypercapnic metabolic alkalosis).

8. Milk-alkali syndrome

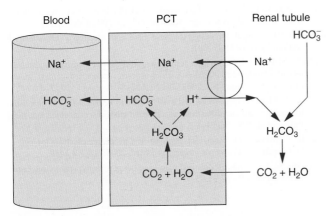

Figure 4-2. Reabsorption of HCO_3^- in hypovolemia. Hypovolemia increases reabsorption of sodium in exchange for hydrogen ion at the proximal convoluted tubule (PCT). The hydrogen ion reacts with HCO_3^- eventually forming CO_2 which crosses the cell membrane. HCO_3^- is then regenerated and delivered to the bloodstream.

Treatment

A. Volume resuscitation with NaCl in patients with true volume depletion usually results in resolution.

B. Replete potassium deficiency.

C. Carbonic anhydrase inhibitors and low bicarbonate dialysis can be used in severe cases, particularly in patients with HF (and ineffective circulating volume) who cannot tolerate NaCl.

Respiratory Alkalosis

Textbook Presentation

The presentation of respiratory alkalosis depends on the underlying disorder. Most causes are associated with tachypnea, which can be dramatic or subtle.

Disease Highlights

A. Hyperventilation induces hypocapnia causing respiratory alkalosis.

B. The most common causes are pulmonary diseases, cirrhosis, fever, pain, or anxiety (Table 4-1).

C. Hypocapnia acutely reduces CNS blood flow.

D. Symptoms include paresthesias (particularly perioral), vertigo, dizziness, anxiety, hallucinations, myalgias, and symptoms reflective of the underlying disorder.

E. Adverse effects include hypokalemia, hypocalcemia, lung injury, seizures, angina, and arrhythmias.

Treatment

Therapy is directed at the underlying disorder.

Mixed Disorders and the "Delta-Delta Gap"

A. Occasionally, 2 distinct metabolic processes will be present in the same patient (eg, 2 distinct acidoses, 1 anion gap and 1 non-anion gap). Alternatively, a patient may have both a metabolic alkalosis and metabolic acidosis (eg, metabolic alkalosis develops in a patient with vomiting and dehydration; if these symptoms are prolonged sufficiently, severe dehydration, hypovolemic shock, and lactic acidosis also develop).

B. These multiple metabolic processes can be difficult to tease out.

C. One approach to this problem is to evaluate the delta-delta gap. Here the absolute rise in the anion gap (ΔAG, the first delta) is compared with the absolute fall in HCO_3^- (ΔHCO_3^-, the second delta[1]).

  1. In simple anion gap acidoses, the deltas are similar.

  2. On the other hand, in a patient with both an anion gap and non-anion gap acidoses, the fall in HCO_3^- will be greater than the rise in the anion gap.

  3. In patients with an anion gap acidosis *and* a metabolic alkalosis, the fall in HCO_3^- will be antagonized by the

[1]ΔAG = Patients anion gap – normal anion gap; ΔHCO_3^- = 24 – patients' HCO_3^-

concomitant metabolic alkalosis whereas the anions will still accumulate. Therefore, the fall in HCO_3^- is less than the increase in the anion gap.

D. While occasionally useful, there are several limitations to applying the delta-delta gap.

  1. The normal anion gap varies from institution to institution and with the patient's serum albumin.

  2. Even in simple anion gap acidosis, bone buffering of acid and renal excretion of anions complicate the delta-delta gap and make it difficult to interpret.

E. In simple anion gap acidosis (without concomitant metabolic alkalosis or non-anion gap acidosis) the typical $\Delta AG/\Delta HCO_3^-$ is 1.6:1 in lactic acidosis and 1:1 in ketoacidosis.

REFERENCES

Bates DW, Cook EF, Goldman L, Lee TH. Predicting bacteremia in hospitalized patients. A prospectively validated model. Ann Intern Med. 1990;113(7):495–500.

Drage LA. Life-threatening rashes: dermatologic signs of four infectious diseases. Mayo Clin Proc. 1999;74(1):68–72.

Fall PJ, Szerlip HM. Lactic acidosis: from sour milk to septic shock. J Intensive Care Med. 2005;20(5):255–71.

Figge J, Jabor A, Kazda A, Fencl V. Anion gap and hypoalbuminemia. Crit Care Med. 1998;26(11):1807–10.

Howell MD, Donnino MW, Talmor D, Clardy P, Ngo L, Shapiro NI. Performance of severity of illness scoring systems in emergency department patients with infection. Acad Emerg Med. 2007;14(8):709–14.

Jaimes F, Arango C, Ruiz G et al. Predicting bacteremia at the bedside. Clin Infect Dis. 2004;38(3):357–62.

Kitabchi AE, Umpierrez GE, Murphy MB, Kreisberg RA. Hyperglycemic crises in adult patients with diabetes: a consensus statement from the American Diabetes Association. Diabetes Care. 2006;29(12):2739–48.

Leibovici L, Cohen O, Wysenbeek AJ. Occult bacterial infection in adults with unexplained fever. Validation of a diagnostic index. Arch Intern Med. 1990;150(6):1270–2.

Leibovici L, Greenshtain S, Cohen O, Mor F, Wysenbeek AJ. Bacteremia in febrile patients. A clinical model for diagnosis. Arch Intern Med. 1991;151(9):1801–6.

Levraut J, Bounatirou T, Ichai C et al. Reliability of anion gap as an indicator of blood lactate in critically ill patients. Intensive Care Med. 1997;23(4):417–22.

Mellors JW, Horwitz RI, Harvey MR, Horwitz SM. A simple index to identify occult bacterial infection in adults with acute unexplained fever. Arch Intern Med. 1987;147(4):666–71.

Naunheim R, Jang TJ, Banet G, Richmond A, McGill J. Point-of-care test identifies diabetic ketoacidosis at triage. Acad Emerg Med. 2006;13(6):683–5.

Rose BD PT. Clinical Physiology of Acid Base and Electrolyte Disorders.5th edition. McGraw Hill; 2001.

Safdar N, Maki DG. Inflammation at the insertion site is not predictive of catheter-related bloodstream infection with short-term, noncuffed central venous catheters. Crit Care Med. 2002;30(12):2632–5.

Slovis CM, Mork VG, Slovis RJ, Bain RP. Diabetic ketoacidosis and infection: leukocyte count and differential as early predictors of serious infection. Am J Emerg Med. 1987;5(1):1–5.

Tokuda Y, Miyasato H, Stein GH, Kishaba T. The degree of chills for risk of bacteremia in acute febrile illness. Am J Med. 2005;118(12):1417.

Umpierrez G, Freire AX. Abdominal pain in patients with hyperglycemic crises. J Crit Care. 2002;17(1):63–7.

I have patients with AIDS-related complaints.

I have a healthy patient without HIV risk factors who asks about HIV screening. How do I diagnose or exclude HIV infection?

CHIEF COMPLAINT

PATIENT 1

Mr. A asks his new primary care physician whether he should get an HIV test. He states that he has "absolutely no risk factors for HIV." He is a very healthy 21-year-old African American man who has been in a monogamous relationship with his current girlfriend for 2 years. The girlfriend was tested for HIV 6 months ago when a Board of Health nurse notified her that she might have been exposed to HIV, and retested 3 months ago. Both HIV tests were negative, effectively ruling out HIV infection.

Mr. A first became sexually active at age 15. Over the last 6 years, he has had only 4 female partners, although with a bit of overlap between the relationships (he had 2 simultaneous partners for about a year). He has never had sex with a male. He used condoms "pretty consistently." He had *Chlamydia trachomatis* urethritis 3 years ago, but no other sexually transmitted infections (STIs). He has never used injection drugs although he smokes marijuana once or twice a week. He stopped drinking excessively when he met his current girlfriend. He does not recall an episode of mononucleosis-like illness with fever and lymph node enlargement. His past medical history, review of systems, and physical exam are otherwise unremarkable.

 Is the clinical information sufficient to make a diagnosis? If not, what other information do you need?

Leading Hypothesis: Universal Screening for HIV Infection

Textbook Presentation

Chronic HIV infection may present in a myriad of ways. Many patients are entirely asymptomatic in spite of long-standing HIV infection and advanced immune deficiency as demonstrated by an absolute CD4 T lymphocyte (CD4TL) count below 200 cells/mcL (immunologic AIDS). Some patients may have symptoms that are often seen with HIV but are nonspecific, such as chronic diarrhea or nonspecific skin findings (seborrheic dermatitis, multiple molluscum contagiosum, poorly responsive psoriasis and prurigo nodularis). Other patients have conditions that are strongly associated with HIV infection but are also encountered in non–HIV-infected persons, such as tuberculosis (TB), idiopathic thrombocytopenic purpura,

nephropathy, cardiomyopathy, herpes zoster, and non-Hodgkin lymphoma. Unfortunately, too many patients are discovered to have HIV only when they are admitted to the hospital with a life-threatening AIDS-defining condition, such as *Pneumocystis jirovecii* pneumonia (PCP), *Cryptococcus* meningitis, central nervous system (CNS) toxoplasmosis, or primary brain lymphoma.

Disease Highlights

A. Prevalence and incidence of HIV in the United States

1. The Centers for Disease Control and Prevention (CDC) publishes yearly detailed data describing the HIV epidemic in the United States.

   a. 1,144,500 adolescents and adults lived with HIV (2010).

   b. 15.8% were not aware of their infection.

   c. Over the past decade, the prevalence of HIV has increased because HIV-infected people live much longer.

   d. The number of new infections has remained relatively stable at about 50,000 per year.

2. Sex ratio, risk factors, race, and ethnicity

   a. The sex ratio of new HIV infections is nearly 4 males to 1 female.

   b. Men who have sex with men (MSMs) are disproportionately infected. In 2011, MSMs accounted for 62% of new infections, heterosexual women 18%, heterosexual men 10%, and injection drug users 8%.

   c. African Americans are disproportionately affected. In 2011, African American men accounted for 46% of new infections, whites 28%, Hispanics 22%, and Asians 2%.

3. Transmission

   a. Common modes of transmission include male-to-male sexual transmission, heterosexual transmission, and drug paraphernalia sharing among injection drug users. Mother-to-child transmission has become uncommon in the United States but remains common elsewhere.

   b. The higher the viral load, the greater the risk of transmission.

      (1) The viral load is high in both acute HIV infection and advanced AIDS.

         (a) Coinfections (such as TB or syphilis) increase the viral load.

         (b) Effective antiretroviral therapy (ART) results in a very low viral load, decreasing the risk of transmission by about 95%.

c. Sexual practices and sexually transmitted infections (STIs)

   (1) The highest risk of sexual transmission is among persons with unprotected receptive anal intercourse, sex-for-hire workers, sexual contacts of sex-for-hire workers, and individuals with multiple sexual partners.

   (2) The presence of genital inflammation or breakdown of genital mucosa increases the risk of transmission. Receptive anal intercourse is frequently associated with trauma as well as an increased risk of STIs.

   (3) STIs, whether they cause genital ulceration or not, significantly increase the risk or either transmitting or acquiring HIV.

   (4) Risk is greater for persons with simultaneous rather than consecutive partners.

   (5) During heterosexual intercourse, man-to-woman transmission is significantly more likely than woman-to-man transmission.

   (6) Circumcised males are 65% less likely to acquire HIV through heterosexual intercourse.

   (7) The consistent use of barrier methods (either male or female condoms) is about 95% effective in preventing HIV sexual transmission, but adherence is poor in many high-risk situations.

d. Transmission through blood transfusion has been nearly eliminated by blood product screening. The risk associated with blood transfusion in the United States is estimated at less than 1 in 1,800,000 units.

e. Mother-to-child transmission is common without ART prophylaxis. Effective therapy markedly reduces this risk (see below).

B. HIV and its target, the CD4 T Lymphocyte (CD4TL)

  1. The HIV surface protein GP 120 binds first to the CD4 T receptor (main HIV receptor), then to 1 of 2 chemokine coreceptors (CCR5 or CXCR4) on CD4 T helper lymphocytes (CD4TL). Other cells are infected (eg, macrophages, dentritic cells, stem cells), but the main target is the CD4TL.

  2. HIV replicates mostly in activated CD4TL: 99% of HIV detected in the blood comes from recently infected, activated CD4TL.

  3. In acute HIV infection, there is a very rapid decrease in the number of CD4TL in the gut-associated lymphoid tissues but only a moderate and partially reversible decrease in the blood CD4TL.

  4. In chronic HIV infection, the absolute CD4TL count decreases slowly in the blood. About 2 billion CD4TL are destroyed and replaced every day. Both HIV-infected and non-infected CD4+TL (innocent bystanders) are destroyed.

  5. In most infected individuals, the high rate of CD4TL death results in a progressive fall in the blood CD4TL.

  6. When the absolute CD4TL count falls below 200 cells/mcL, the patient is susceptible to both opportunistic infections (OIs) and AIDS-defining malignancy. The lower the CD4TL count, the greater the risk of any OI and the greater the spectrum of OIs seen.

  7. About 5% of patients have stable CD4TL over many years ("long-term non-progressors"). Rarely, the viral load is also undetectable ("elite controller").

8. Accelerated evolution of HIV and quasi-species

   a. HIV mutates rapidly due to a high rate of mutations introduced by an error-prone reverse transcriptase and a very high replication rate (10 billion new HIV virions per day). This allows for the rapid development of genetic variants (quasi species), which may escape immune responses and be resistant to antiretroviral agents.

   b. Effective therapy requires complete suppression of viral replication to prevent the production of mutations associated with drug resistance (see below).

C. Staging

  1. Stages of HIV infection include viral transmission, primary infection, seroconversion, clinically latent period, early symptomatic HIV infection, and AIDS.

   a. Primary HIV infection

    (1) Up to 70% of patients experience a "mononucleosis syndrome" with fever, rash, sore throat, oral aphthous ulcers, diarrhea, lymphadenopathy, arthralgia, headache, and flu-like symptoms.

 Acute HIV infection needs to be considered when a patient with a mononucleosis syndrome has no evidence of infection by either the Epstein-Barr virus (negative heterophile antibody and negative Epstein-Barr virus viral capsid antibody IgM) or the cytomegalovirus (negative CMV IgM). Diagnosis of acute HIV requires a high index of suspicion.

    (2) In primary HIV infection, the viral load is > 10,000 and usually > 50,000/mcL.

   b. Seroconversion

    (1) Seroconversion rapidly causes a fall in HIV viral load (due to both humoral and cellular immune responses).

    (2) After about 6 months, the viral load is set at a level that remains stable in any specific patient (the viral load "set point") but varies from patient to patient.

    (3) In the absence of ART, the set point predicts the rate of disease progression (higher viral loads are associated with more rapid declines in CD4TL counts).

   c. Clinically latent period

    (1) Following primary infection, viral replication continues primarily within activated CD4TL cells, with progressive destruction of the CD4TL cell pool.

    (2) Persistent generalized lymphadenopathy is often seen.

    (3) Progression to an AIDS-defining illness is more common in patients with higher viral loads and lower CD4TL counts.

    (4) Progressive depletion of CD4TL renders patients increasingly susceptible to OIs and malignancies: predominantly T-cell immunodeficiency.

   d. Early symptomatic HIV infection: At relatively high CD4TL counts (200–350 cells/mcL) HIV infection is associated with an increased risk of infections by virulent pathogens, especially pneumococcal pneumonia and TB.

e. AIDS

(1) Advanced HIV disease is accompanied by severe CD4TL depletion (below 200 cells/mcL) and infection with less virulent, opportunistic pathogens.

(2) Specific opportunistic pathogens are mostly encountered when the CD4TL count falls below a critical level.

(a) CD4TL count is < 200 cells/mcL: PCP

(b) CD4TL count is < 100 cells/mcL: *Toxoplasma gondii* brain abscesses, *Candida* esophagitis, *Cryptococcus neoformans* meningitis, disseminated histoplasmosis, and meningeal coccidioidomycosis

(c) CD4TL count is < 50 cells/mcL: Cytomegalovirus (CMV) retinitis and disseminated MAI or MAC (*Mycobacterium avium/intracellulare* or *M avium* complex)

(3) AIDS diagnostic criteria

(a) CD4TL count < 200 cells/mcL (immunologic AIDS)

(b) AIDS indicator conditions (clinical AIDS):

(i) AIDS defining malignancies: primary CNS lymphoma, non-Hodgkin lymphoma, Kaposi sarcoma, and invasive cervical cancer

(ii) OIs: *P jirovecii*, TB, *M avium*, recurrent bacterial pneumonia, esophageal candidiasis, cryptococcosis, progressive multifocal leukoencephalopathy (PML), toxoplasmosis, cryptosporidiosis

(iii) Other conditions: HIV-associated dementia, wasting syndrome ("slim disease")

(c) Advanced HIV infection defined as CD4TL count < 50 cells/mcL

Evidence-Based Diagnosis

Similar to any other diagnosis, the positive predictive value is determined by 3 features: the pretest probability of disease, the sensitivity of the test, and the specificity of the test. Each feature must be carefully evaluated to properly interpret HIV results.

A. Estimating pretest probability of HIV infection

1. Risk factors include MSM, injection drug use, and multiple sexual partners.

2. The prevalence of HIV varies from 0.3% in the general US population to > 50% in very high-risk groups.

B. Sensitivity and specificity of tests for HIV

1. The diagnosis of chronic HIV infection involves the detection of antibody in a 2-step process: initial screening with HIV-1 enzyme immunoassay (EIA) and confirmatory positive HIV-1 Western blot to confirm a repeatedly positive EIA.

2. HIV EIA testing

a. HIV-1 EIA detects antibody to HIV-1 antigens (> 98% of HIV infections in the United States are HIV 1 of the main group M, subtype, or clade B).

b. Sensitivity > 99%, specificity 98–99%

c. False-positive results may be seen in a variety of circumstances: recent influenza or hepatitis B immunization, DNA virus infections, increasing parity, positive rapid plasma reagin (RPR), improper heating, clerical error, HIV vaccine, and cross reacting antibody.

d. Confirmatory testing with a positive HIV-1 Western blot is required before the diagnosis of HIV infection can be made.

e. False-negative EIA tests. Etiologies include

(1) Recent HIV infection prior to development of antibodies (window period). With the newer EIA tests, seroconversion occurs within 10 days to 6 weeks in most patients, and virtually all patients seroconvert within 3 months.

(2) Rare causes of false-negative results include advanced AIDS with sero-reversion (rare), immunosuppressive therapy, malignancy, bone marrow transplant, B-lymphocyte dysfunction, replacement transfusion, hypogammaglobulinemia, and rare HIV types.

3. HIV-1 Western blot

a. Detects antibody to multiple HIV antigens that are separated by electrophoresis.

b. Positive results require at least 2 of 3 specific bands: gp160/120, gp41, and p24. With such criterion, HIV-1 Western blot can still very rarely be falsely positive.

c. Negative HIV-Western blot results require the absence of any visible bands. False-negative HIV-1 Western blot (in the presence of a positive HIV EIA) occur in the window period.

d. Indeterminate HIV-Western blot results

(1) Indeterminate HIV-1 Western blot are common in noninfected patients (10–15%) in whom they usually show an isolated p24 or an isolated p17.

(2) May represent either early HIV infection (during the window period) or more often lack of HIV infection (cross-reacting antibodies). Infected patients in the window period have a high viral load.

(3) HIV-1 immunofluorescent antibody test is used to help decide whether a patient with a positive EIA and indeterminate Western blot has HIV or not.

(4) Patients with persistent, stable, indeterminate Western blot who have no new bands over 6 months are not infected with HIV 1.

4. Combination HIV-1 EIA and HIV-1 Western blot testing

a. Combination strategy uses initial testing with HIV-1 EIA or HIV-1 and HIV-2 EIA.

(1) Patients with negative HIV EIA are not tested further; they do not have chronic HIV, although recent HIV infection is possible.

(2) Positive HIV EIA must be **confirmed** by a second test.

b. Subsequent positive HIV-1 Western blot result confirms HIV infection.

c. Subsequent negative HIV-1 Western blot result rules out chronic HIV-1 infection although recent infection is still possible. HIV-2 infection is seen very rarely in the United States, usually in immigrants from West or Central Africa, or their sex partners.

d. The combined HIV EIA and HIV-1 Western blot strategy further decreases the risk of false-positive results.

e. False-negative results may still occur in patients who are tested following recent infection.

f. Sensitivity, 99%; specificity, > 99%

g. False-positive combined HIV-1 EIA and HIV-1 Western blot are very rare but should still be considered in very low prevalence populations (blood donors or pregnant women) or when an undetectable viral load makes untreated HIV infection unlikely. Only untreated "elite controllers" have undetectable HIV viral load.

C. Diagnosing primary HIV infection

1. Standard HIV EIA and HIV Western blot require an antibody response and are negative in the "window period" during the first weeks after HIV infection.

2. Later, HIV EIA becomes positive but HIV-1 Western blot may be indeterminate.

3. Finally both HIV EIA and HIV-1 Western blot are positive, confirming HIV infection.

4. In primary HIV infection, the HIV viral load is > 10,000 and usually > 50,000/mcL.

5. An HIV viral load can be used and is diagnostic in this situation if the viral load is higher than 10,000 copies/mcL.

6. Diagnosis of acute HIV requires a high index of suspicion.

Treatment

A. Prevention

1. As noted above, barrier methods are about 95% effective in preventing HIV sexual transmission, but adherence is poor in many high-risk situations.

2. Blood product screening has virtually eliminated transfusion-associated HIV transmission in the United States.

3. Effective ART results in a very low viral load, decreasing the risk of transmission by about 95%. The "treatment as prevention" strategy aims to identify HIV infection early and initiate effective therapy, which is highly successful in reducing the spread of HIV.

4. Preexposure prophylaxis

a. A highly effective strategy of treating a seronegative person with 2 antiretroviral drugs (tenofovir and emtricitabine) to prevent HIV infection.

b. Offered to HIV sero-discordant couples and high-risk individuals

c. The cost of the combination is usually covered by healthcare plans.

5. Needle-exchange programs are very useful in preventing the spread of HIV in injection drug users.

6. Mother-to-child transmission

a. Most of the transmission occurs at term (intrapartum) and with breastfeeding, but there is a significant risk from 28 weeks of pregnancy.

b. HIV-infected pregnant women are treated with ART so the viral load is undetectable at least from 28 weeks of pregnancy to the time of delivery.

c. Postpartum, mothers are told not to breastfeed, and the neonates receive postexposure ART prophylaxis.

d. Women who do not reach a low viral load at term (viral load > 1000 copies/mL) are candidates for an elective cesarean section to decrease the risk of mother-to-child transmission.

e. This strategy has reduced mother-to-child transmission by more than 90% in the United States.

B. Universal screening

1. Universal screening is now recommended by the CDC and USPSTF.

2. More than 1 million people live with HIV in the United States, and more than 15% of seropositive persons are unaware of their infection contributing to further spread of HIV.

3. As noted above, in the absence of screening, many patients may present with advanced immune deficiency and OIs.

a. Such patients are often very ill and severely immunocompromised and are at high risk for poor outcome.

b. Even if they do well on ART, most only partially recover their immune function.

4. Selective high-risk screening is often inefficient

a. Although most HIV-infected patients have increased risk factors, clinicians do not consistently inquire about risk factors and do not always screen patients who have another STI or blood-borne infection ("missed opportunities" for HIV testing).

b. Patients may not report risk factors accurately, especially if they fear the clinician may be judgmental.

c. Not all HIV-infected patients have identifiable risk factors, especially if HIV prevalence is higher in the general population.

d. Therefore, selective HIV screening of high-risk individuals is very inefficient.

C. Treatment

1. The First Encounter: the role of the primary care physician

a. The first encounter is essential in establishing a good clinician/patient relationship.

b. Patients who have just found out they have HIV tend to be distraught and confused even if they are not totally surprised by the diagnosis.

c. Often patients do not believe that the diagnosis is correct (HIV denial).

d. Patients may believe wrongly that their life is over because they perceive that they will die soon, they will be unable to live a productive and fulfilling life, they will face severe drug adverse effects, or they might infect their household contacts. Such misconceptions also enhance the stigma associated with HIV.

e. The primary care physician should take the required time necessary to reassure the patient that HIV can be managed well on a simple ART regimen with acceptable side effects in most people, and clarify the diagnosis, transmission, and natural history.

f. Providing ample time to answer questions and deal with anxiety, depression, addiction, housing issues, healthcare insurance coverage, partner notification is important.

g. Referral to an infectious disease specialist (or internist with specialized HIV practice) is required, but the primary care physician should strongly consider continuing to provide primary care.

2. HIV specialist

a. The HIV specialist does not work alone, but usually depends on nurses, social workers, case managers, HIV support groups, AIDS legal support group, addiction specialists, and psychiatrists to ensure effective HIV care and maximize adherence to ART.

b. HIV-infected patients who are adherent to ART are highly likely to do well over many years.

c. HIV-infected patients who do not take their ART as prescribed progress to AIDS and their virus may acquire resistance mutations to multiple agents.

3. Laboratory testing

a. Assess current immune competence: absolute CD4TL count and CD4/CD3 percentage

b. Test the HIV isolate: baseline HIV viral load and HIV genotype to look for transmitted resistance-associated mutations before any ART is introduced.

c. Test for coinfections common in HIV-positive populations.

   (1) RPR and if positive fluorescent treponemal antibody (FTA) to screen for syphilis

   (2) Test for hepatitis B (HBs Ag, HBs Ab) and C (HCV Ab, HCV viral load)

   (3) *T gondii* IgG

   (4) Latent TB infection: either purified protein derivative (PPD) (not very specific because it may be positive with exposure to non-TB mycobacteria or prior BCG) or interferon gamma release assay (which is much more specific for latent TB infection but may still be positive with exposure to *Mycobacterium kansasii* and *Mycobacterium marinum*).

   (5) In women, urinary or cervical nucleic acid amplification test detects *C trachomatis* and *Neisseria gonorrhoeae* infection, and any abnormal Papanicolaou smear suggests infection with one of the human papillomaviruses (HPV). HPV polymerase chain reaction (PCR) detects HPV serotypes most likely to cause cervical cancer (including HPV 16 and 18).

   (6) In men, urinary nucleic acid amplification test detects *C trachomatis* and *N gonorrhoeae* infection. In MSMs, anal Papanicolaou screening should be considered: men with abnormal anal Papanicolaou smear should be referred to specialists for "high-resolution anoscopy" to look for anal cancer.

4. Baseline labs: CBC, comprehensive metabolic panel, lipid panel, glucose-6-phosphate dehydrogenase (G6PD) level (in case either dapsone or primaquine are required to prevent or treat *Pneumocystis* infection)

5. Immunizations

a. All killed vaccines are safe in HIV.

b. In general live vaccines are not recommended, with the exception of MMR and chickenpox vaccines in patients who have a CD4TL count > 200 cells/mcL.

c. The response to vaccines often is suboptimal unless the CD4TL count is > 200 cells/mcL.

d. Since ART often leads to significant immune reconstitution, delaying or repeating immunizations may be very useful.

e. To decrease the high risk of invasive pneumococcal infection, conjugate pneumococcal vaccine (Prevnar-13) should be given first, followed by the polysaccharide pneumococcal vaccine (Pneumovax-23) > 2 months later, with a booster every 5 years.

f. Influenza causes severe morbidity and mortality, including in HIV and AIDS. Influenza vaccine should be administered yearly.

g. Tetanus, diphtheria, and acellular pertussis vaccine is recommended once, then tetanus-diphtheria vaccine every 10 years.

h. Hepatitis B vaccine is recommended in all HIV-infected persons. In nonresponders, the hepatitis B may have to be repeated with a double dosage.

i. Hepatitis A vaccine is recommended in many higher risk patients (including travelers, MSMs, patients with any chronic liver disease).

j. For efficiency, most HIV-infected patients are immunized with the combined hepatitis A and B vaccine series.

6. ART

a. ART has revolutionized HIV care. AIDS defining illnesses, mortality, and hospitalizations have decreased 60–80% since the introduction of ART.

b. Effective therapy requires complete suppression of viral replication to prevent the production of mutations associated with drug resistance.

c. The cornerstone of therapy is the *simultaneous* and *uninterrupted* use of at least 3 antiretroviral drugs to which the virus is susceptible.

d. Complete suppression is realistic in most patients and prevents the worsening of immune deficiency, results in partial immune reconstitution, and prevents the emergence of drug-resistance associated mutations.

e. Lifetime ART is necessary to prevent viral rebound due to non-replicating, latent HIV in the reservoirs (including macrophages, resting CD4TL, memory cells, and stem cells).

f. Even in patients with such "undetectable viral load," there is a "residual HIV viremia" (1–19 copies/mL), which can be assessed with advanced research techniques. When ART is interrupted, the residual viremia reinfects activated CD4TL leading to a quick relapse: HIV is not curable with ART.

g. Indications for ART

   (1) All HIV-infected patients benefit from ART, regardless of the presence of symptoms, CD4TL count, and viral load.

      (a) The lower the CD4TL count is, the greater the benefit and the stronger the evidence of benefit.

      (b) Asymptomatic patients with immunologic AIDS (CD4TL count < 200/mcL) who are at high risk of mortality associated with OIs and AIDS-defining malignancy benefit greatly from ART.

      (c) Asymptomatic patients with CD4TL count between 200/mcL and 500/mcL who receive ART have well-documented decreases in mortality and morbidity due to a decrease in immune activation, non–AIDS-related malignancy, and cardiovascular morbidity.

      (d) Asymptomatic patients with CD4TL count above 500/mcL also benefit but the evidence is still limited.

   (2) HIV-infected pregnant women must be treated to prevent mother-to-child transmission.

   (3) Symptomatic patients with life-threatening or serious HIV-associated conditions (such as nephropathy, cardiomyopathy, idiopathic thrombocytopenic purpura, thrombotic thrombocytopenic purpura) benefit from ART.

   (4) Early ART is recommended in acute HIV infection to prevent rapid immune destruction and seeding of HIV reservoirs.

h. Antiretroviral agents

  (1) Antiretroviral drugs belong to 5 classes.

   (a) Nucleoside reverse transcriptase inhibitors (NRTIs) block reverse transcription of viral RNA into DNA by incorporation in the elongating chain (chain terminators).

   (b) Nonnucleoside reverse transcriptase inhibitors (NNRTIs) block reverse transcription of viral RNA into DNA by binding to the "NNRTI pocket" in the p66 subunit.

   (c) Integrase inhibitors prevent the integration of HIV DNA into the cellular DNA.

   (d) Protease inhibitors inhibit the HIV protease, resulting in lack of cleavage of a viral polyprotein precursor.

   (e) Entry inhibitors (CCR5 receptor inhibitors and fusion inhibitors)

    (i) Prevent HIV cell entry by either blocking the CCR5 chemokine receptor (a co-receptor for HIV surface protein), or by blocking the fusion of the HIV membrane with the cell membrane (fusion inhibitor).

    (ii) CCR5 receptor inhibitors are effective only if HIV is exclusively CCR5-tropic, and does not use CXCR4 at all.

    (iii) The co-receptor tropism assay detects whether HIV is CCR5-tropic, CXCR4-tropic or dual-tropic.

   (f) Adherence

    (i) Patient adherence is key.

    (ii) Adherence of 90–95% is required to maintain viral control and prevent resistance.

    (iii) High adherence has been shown to decrease morbidity and mortality.

    (iv) Moderately poor adherence (50–90%) has still some clinical benefits but promotes viral resistance, leading to eventual failure of therapy.

    (v) Very poor adherence does not select for resistance but has no clinical benefits.

    (vi) Predictors of poor adherence include substance abuse, mental illness, lack of access to medical care or medications, lack of patient education, and poor trust between patient and physician.

i. Guidelines recommend monitoring CD4TL count and viral load every 3 months.

j. Goal of therapy: undetectable viral load (< 20/mcL) by 4–6 months.

k. Failure to achieve viral suppression usually is secondary to patient nonadherence, HIV drug resistance, or both. Occasionally other factors are involved: malabsorption, drug interactions, selection of a suboptimal regimen with lower potency, greater volume of distribution in late pregnancy.

l. Testing for viral resistance

  (1) Performed at baseline to detect transmitted resistance and whenever the patient does not achieve or maintain an undetectable viral load while taking ART.

  (2) Both genotype and phenotype are available, but the genotype is preferred because it provides faster results, costs less, and is as clinically useful as the phenotype.

  (3) Decisions are complex and require expert guidance. Database of resistance-associated mutations are available to help decision-making.

m. Primary and secondary prophylaxis of OIs

  (1) Primary prophylaxis prevents the *initial* OI.

  (2) Secondary prophylaxis prevents *subsequent symptomatic* episodes after the initial OI (may not eradicate the infection but can prevent illness).

  (3) Primary OI prophylaxis

   (a) The CD4TL cell count is the best predictor of susceptibility to OIs.

   (b) ART raises CD4TL count in most but not all patients, and markedly decreases the risk of OIs.

   (c) Susceptibility is determined by the *current* CD4TL count rather than the nadir CD4TL count.

    (i) CD4TL < 200/mcL: *Pneumocystis* prophylaxis recommended

    (ii) CD4TL < 100/mcL: Toxoplasmosis prophylaxis recommended if the serology is positive

    (iii) CD4TL < 50/mcL: MAI prophylaxis recommended

    (iv) Isoniazid therapy for latent TB infection is recommended if PPD causes > 5mm of induration or the interferon gamma release assay is positive.

   (d) Primary or secondary OI prophylaxis may be stopped in patients in whom ART restores the CD4TL count above the level recommended for primary prophylaxis.

n. Major socioeconomic barriers to diagnosis and treatment

  (1) Lack of timely access to high quality healthcare

  (2) Only partial drug cost coverage

  (3) Poor support for treatment of drug addiction and psychiatric conditions

  (4) Entrenched homelessness

  (5) Poor care of some patients in jail.

  (6) HIV-associated stigma remains an issue although significant progress has been achieved.

MAKING A DIAGNOSIS

As noted above, 3 factors determine the positive predictive value of the test: the pretest probability, the sensitivity, and the specificity. Mr. A is asymptomatic and denies high-risk behaviors. However he may not truly be at a low-risk of HIV, since he had a prior STI and did not *always* use a condom with his four life partners. His history of alcohol binges may also point to forgotten prior high-risk behaviors. The history of simultaneous sexual partners is also a risk factor. His pretest probability of HIV infection is therefore significantly higher than he believes.

An HIV EIA is repeatedly positive and HIV-1 Western blot is also positive, with multiple bands present. Because of the excellent specificity of the 2-step HIV EIA and HIV-1 Western blot test, (99%, 99.8%) his posttest probability of HIV infection is > 99%. The CD4TL count is 150 cells/ mcL (immunologic AIDS) and the HIV viral load is 80,000 copies/mcL (quite high). *Toxoplasma* antibody is negative. PPD is negative.

 Have you crossed a diagnostic threshold for the leading hypothesis, HIV? Do other tests need to be done to exclude the alternative diagnoses?

CASE RESOLUTION

Mr. A is HIV infected and his CD4TL count is diagnostic of immunologic AIDS. At this point, primary prophylaxis with trimethoprim-sulfamethoxazole (TMP-SMX) is indicated to prevent PCP because the CD4TL count is < 200/ mcL. However, MAI prophylaxis is not necessary because the CD4TL L count is > 50/ mcL. He does not need prophylaxis for toxoplasmosis either because he is seronegative for *T gondii*.

The patient should undergo blood testing for CBC with platelets, comprehensive metabolic panel, lipid panel, HBsAg, HBsAb, HCV Ab, G6PD level, interferon gamma release assay (since PPD often is negative at low CD4TL counts), and RPR. Urine nucleic acid amplification test for *Chlamydia* and *N gonorrhoeae* is recommended. He should receive the influenza vaccine, the tetanus-diphtheria-acellular pertussis vaccine, and the conjugated 13-valent pneumococcal vaccine. Two months later he can receive the polysaccharide pneumococcal vaccine. Hepatitis B and hepatitis A combined vaccine series should be started if he is not immune, but it is reasonable to wait for some level of immune reconstitution to improve immunogenicity.

He is in a monogamous sexual relationship with a probably HIV seronegative, uninfected female partner. To decrease her risk of acquiring HIV, they should use barrier precautions (male or female condom are 95% effective), and he should be started on ART to lower his HIV viral load to below the level of detection (treatment as prevention is also 95% effective). These combined interventions would decrease the risk of transmission of HIV to well below 1% ($5 . 10^{-2} \times 5. 10^{-2} = 2.5 \ 10^{-3}$). However, if their use of barrier precautions is inconsistent or the couple wishes to have a baby, preexposure prophylaxis (tenofovir and emtricitabine combination) administered to the partner is also a reasonable option.

I have an HIV-positive patient who complains of headache. How do I determine the cause?

CHIEF COMPLAINT

PATIENT 2

Mr. S is a 46-year-old man with AIDS and a CD4TL of 80/mcL. He arrives at the hospital complaining of having a headache for the last 2 weeks and low-grade fever for 5 days. He denies confusion, focal weakness, or seizures. He is febrile (temperature is 38.8°C). His neck is supple. The neurologic exam is nonfocal.

 What is the differential diagnosis of headache in HIV-positive patients? How would you frame the differential?

CONSTRUCTING A DIFFERENTIAL DIAGNOSIS

Three pivotal considerations help frame the differential diagnosis in HIV-infected persons with neurologic complaints: (1) the acuity of the symptoms, (2) the degree of immunosuppression (CD4TL), and (3) whether a mass lesion is seen on neuroimaging.

The first pivotal step in evaluating the HIV-positive patient with headache is to determine the **acuity** of the presentation. Most OIs have a subacute onset. In HIV-infected patients with an acute onset of headache and fever (< 3 days), virulent pathogens, including bacterial meningitis, herpes simplex virus type 1 encephalitis and West Nile virus encephalitis, must be considered.

The second pivotal issue is to assess the **degree of immunosuppression**. HIV-positive patients with intact immunity and CD4TL > 200/mcL are at markedly diminished risk for OIs. The differential diagnosis of such headaches is similar to patients without HIV infection. These disorders are covered in Chapter 20, Headache. However, as the immunosuppression worsens and the CD4TL falls < 200/mcL, the differential diagnosis broadens to include OIs and primary CNS lymphoma (PCL).

The third pivotal issue is to determine whether the patient has a **mass lesion.** The most common diagnoses in HIV-infected patients with low CD4TL and CNS mass lesions are toxoplasmosis, progressive multifocal leukoencephalopathy (PML), and PCL, whereas the most common diagnosis in such patients without a mass lesion is cryptococcal meningitis. CNS imaging and lumbar puncture (LP) are frequently required. In clinical practice, a CT scan is usually performed prior to LP because it rapidly rules out a large mass lesion that may cause post LP herniation. Platelet count, prothrombin time and partial thromboplastin time should be checked to ensure the patient is not at an increased risk for developing a spinal epidural hemorrhage. An MRI is often performed subsequently due to its substantially increased sensitivity for several diagnoses. A diagnostic algorithm for the evaluation of headache in HIV-positive patients is summarized in Figure 5-1 and Figure 5-2.

Differential Diagnosis of Headache in Patient With HIV

A. Meningoencephalitis
  1. Cryptococcal meningitis
  2. HIV encephalopathy
  3. TB meningoencephalitis
  4. Neurosyphilis
  5. Coccidioidomycosis (in southwestern United States)

B. Mass lesions
  1. Toxoplasmosis
  2. PML
  3. PCL

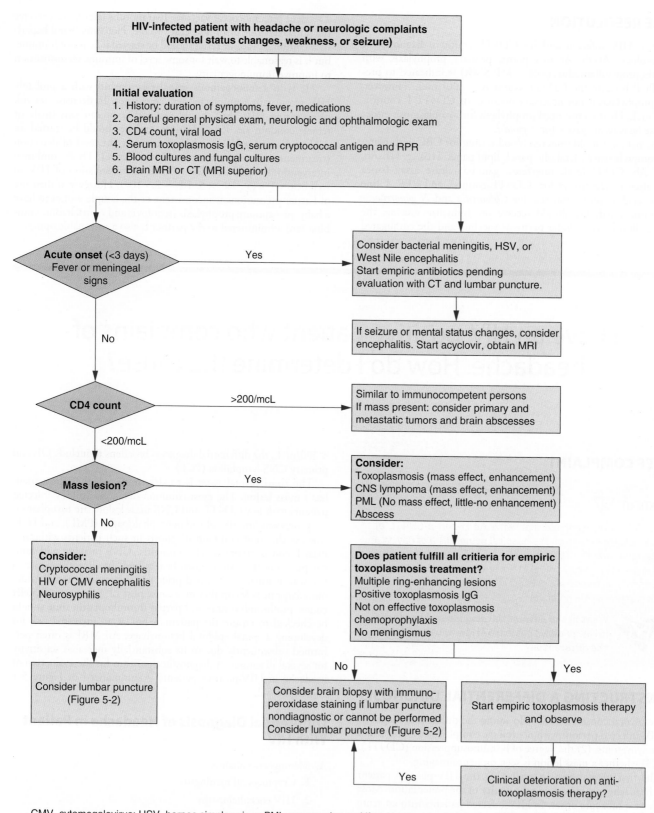

CMV, cytomegalovirus; HSV, herpes simplex virus; PML, progressive multifocal leukoencephalopathy; RPR, rapid plasma reagin.

Figure 5-1. Diagnostic approach: headache in HIV-positive patients.

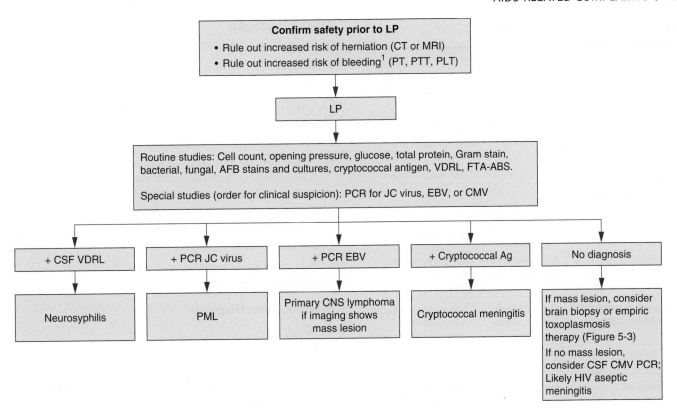

Confirm safety prior to LP
- Rule out increased risk of herniation (CT or MRI)
- Rule out increased risk of bleeding[1] (PT, PTT, PLT)

LP

Routine studies: Cell count, opening pressure, glucose, total protein, Gram stain, bacterial, fungal, AFB stains and cultures, cryptococcal antigen, VDRL, FTA-ABS.

Special studies (order for clinical suspicion): PCR for JC virus, EBV, or CMV

+ CSF VDRL	+ PCR JC virus	+ PCR EBV	+ Cryptococcal Ag	No diagnosis
Neurosyphilis	PML	Primary CNS lymphoma if imaging shows mass lesion	Cryptococcal meningitis	If mass lesion, consider brain biopsy or empiric toxoplasmosis therapy (Figure 5-3) If no mass lesion, consider CSF CMV PCR; Likely HIV aseptic meningitis

[1]Bleeding at the LP site can lead to a spinal epidural hemorrhage, cord compression, and paralysis.

AFB, acid-fast bacilli; CMV, cytomegalovirus; CSF, cerebrospinal fluid; EBV, Epstein-Barr virus; FTA-ABS, fluorescent treponemal antibody absorbption; LP, lumbar puncture; PCR, polymerase chain reaction; PLT, platelet; PML, progressive multifocal leukoencephalopathy; PT, prothrombin time; PTT, partial thromboplastin time; VDRL, Venereal Disease Research Laboratory.

Figure 5-2. Evaluation of headache in HIV-positive patients: lumbar puncture.

Mr. S reports that his headache began 14 days ago. The headache is described as frontal, unrelenting, and pounding. He complains of subjective fevers, sweats, and chills. He admits to mild photophobia. Persistent vomiting has also developed over the last 6 days. He denies any history of confusion or seizures.

Past medical history is remarkable for a long history of injection drug use. His last reported use was 2 years ago. HIV was diagnosed 9 years ago. He has not been adherent with ART or PCP prophylaxis with daily TMP-SMX. He takes no medications.

 At this point, what is the leading hypothesis, what are the active alternatives, and is there a must not miss diagnosis? Given this differential diagnosis, what tests should be ordered?

RANKING THE DIFFERENTIAL DIAGNOSIS

The first pivotal consideration is that Mr. S has had a headache for 2 weeks (subacute). This suggests a relatively less virulent OI rather than a virulent bacterial meningitis or herpes simplex virus type 1 encephalitis. Second, his prior CD4TL indicates profound immunosuppression. Therefore, he is at risk for all the serious OIs listed above. The third pivotal issue is whether there is a mass lesion. Ultimately, this will be confirmed or excluded on neuroimaging, but his photophobia suggests some form of meningoencephalitis. Cryptococcal meningitis is the most common meningitis seen in AIDS and is the leading hypothesis. Less common causes of meningoencephalitis include CMV, neurosyphilis, and tuberculous meningitis. Coccidioidomycosis is uncommon except in the southwestern United States. HIV meningitis may present with headache. Should neuroimaging confirm a mass lesion, common causes include toxoplasmosis, PML, and PCL. Since Mr. S has not taken TMP-SMX prophylaxis, he is at increased risk for toxoplasmosis, the most common CNS mass lesion in AIDS patients. Table 5-1 lists the differential diagnoses.

Physical exam reveals a thin man in moderate distress. Vital signs: temperature, 35.9°C; BP, 154/100 mm Hg; pulse, 66 bpm; RR, 20 breaths per minute. HEENT: disks sharp, neck supple. Kernig and Brudzinski signs are negative. Cardiac, pulmonary, and abdominal exams are within normal limits. Neurologic exam: alert and oriented; cranial nerves intact; motor, sensory, and cerebellar functions were normal.

A CT scan (with contrast) is reported as normal. No mass lesions or evidence of sinusitis are seen.

Table 5-1. Diagnostic hypotheses for Mr. S.

Diagnostic Hypotheses	Demographics, Risk Factors, Symptoms and Signs	Important Tests
Leading Hypothesis		
Cryptococcal meningitis	Headache, mental status changes	CD4 < 100/mcL
		Serum and CSF cryptococcal antigen
		CSF fungal culture
Active Alternatives		
Mass lesions Toxoplasmosis	Headache, focal findings, mental status changes Not receiving TMP-SMX prophylaxis	Toxoplasma IgG + MRI: multiple or single ring-enhancing lesions, mass effect and edema
Progressive multifocal leukoencephalopathy	Headache, focal findings, mental status changes	MRI single or multiple white matter nonenhancing lesions without mass effect. CSF + PCR JC virus
Primary CNS lymphoma	Focal findings, mental status changes	MRI single or multiple irregular enhancing lesions with mass effect CSF PCR + EBV
Meningoencephalitis CMV encephalitis	Headache, mental status changes	MRI normal or periventricular symmetric enhancement CSF PCR CMV +
Neurosyphilis	History of chancre, rash	Serum RPR, FTA-ABS; CSF VDRL, FTA-ABS, CSF pleocytosis

CMV, cytomegalovirus; CNS, central nervous system; CSF, cerebrospinal fluid; EBV, Epstein-Barr virus; FTA-ABS, fluorescent treponemal antibody-absorption; PCR, polymerase chain reaction; RPR, rapid plasma reagin; TMP-SMX, trimethoprim-sulfamethoxazole; VDRL, Venereal Disease Research Laboratory.

The normal CT scan markedly diminishes the likelihood of the diseases associated with mass lesion and increases the likelihood of one of the remaining causes of meningitis (*Cryptococcus,* CMV, neurosyphilis, TB); *Cryptococcus* is the most common. A brain MRI is more sensitive for mass lesions and should be performed.

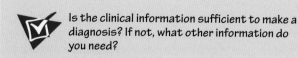

Is the clinical information sufficient to make a diagnosis? If not, what other information do you need?

Leading Hypothesis: Cryptococcal Meningoencephalitis

Textbook Presentation

Patients typically have a subacute headache, malaise, and fever that develop over days to weeks. Mental status changes may be seen. Importantly, meningismus is often absent due to the host's inability to mount an inflammatory reaction.

Disease Highlights

A. Most common cause of meningoencephalitis in AIDS

B. Encapsulated fungus acquired via inhalation

C. Meningitis due to dissemination of primary infection

D. Usually in patients with CD4TL < 100/mcL

E. Subacute onset over 2–4 weeks

F. CNS inflammation typically minimal

G. 70% of patients have increased intracranial pressure (ICP): > 20 cm H_2O in lateral decubitus position

   1. Elevated ICP associated with increased risk of death

   2. Patients with elevated ICP have worse symptoms (headaches, clouded sensorium).

H. Mortality 6–12%

I. Pulmonary involvement reported in 6–23% of patients with cryptococcal meningitis

Evidence-Based Diagnosis

A. History

   1. Fever: 65–95%

   2. Headache: 73–100%

   3. Median duration of symptoms: 31 days (1–120 days)

B. Physical exam

   1. Stiff neck: 22–27%

   2. Photophobia: 18–22%

   3. Mental status changes: 22%

   4. Focal neurologic signs or seizures: 10%

   5. No CNS signs or symptoms: 14%

Cryptococcal meningitis in AIDS patients is often indolent. Only a small percentage of patients exhibit meningismus or photophobia. Some patients have only fever and malaise. A supple neck does not rule out the diagnosis, and a high index of suspicion is required.

C. Laboratory findings

   1. Blood tests

     a. Blood cultures positive in 15–35%

     b. Serum cryptococcal antigen

       (1) 95–100% sensitive, 96% specific

       (2) LR+ 24, LR– 0.05

       (3) Negative serum cryptococcal antigen makes cryptococcal meningitis unlikely.

       (4) A positive serum cryptococcal antigen may precede clinical cryptococcal meningitis.

   2. LP

     a. Neuroimaging required before LP to rule out mass effect. Mass lesions are often due to concomitant toxoplasmosis or lymphoma and only rarely due to cryptococcoma.

     b. A platelet count, prothrombin time, and partial thromboplastin time are performed before LP to rule out a bleeding diathesis, with its risk of spinal epidural hematoma.

     c. LP is required in patients with suspected cryptococcal meningoencephalitis regardless of serum cryptococcal antigen results.

       (1) In patients with positive serum cryptococcal antigen, LP is necessary to confirm cryptococcal

meningitis, measure opening pressure, manage high ICP, and exclude other diagnoses.

   (2) In patients with negative serum cryptococcal antigen, LP is necessary to evaluate other diagnoses.

d. *Routine* cerebrospinal fluid (CSF) findings are often normal or minimally abnormal in patients with cryptococcal meningitis.

   (1) Normal glucose, protein, and WBC: 19–30%

   (2) Glucose < 50 mg/dL: 64%

   (3) Protein > 40 mg/dL: 64%

   (4) CSF WBCs > 5/mcL: 35%

   (5) Increased opening pressure: 50–75%

Routine CSF findings in patients with cryptococcal meningitis may be *normal*. Specific studies (fungal culture, cryptococcal antigen) must be obtained.

e. Special CSF studies

   (1) CSF cryptococcal antigen: 91–100% sensitive, 93–98% specific

   (2) CSF fungal culture: 95–100% sensitive, 100% specific

Treatment

A. Mortality is increased in patients with abnormal mental status and in patients with a marked elevated CSF cryptococcal antigen (> 1:1024). Low glycorrhachia and normal CSF cell counts also predict poor outcomes.

B. Induction therapy for 2 weeks should include lipsosomal amphotericin B with flucytosine. Flucytosine must be dose-adjusted in patients with renal insufficiency.

C. *After* induction therapy with amphotericin and flucytosine, fluconazole (400 mg/day) can be substituted in patients with clinical improvement for an additional 8–10 weeks or until CSF cultures are sterile.

D. Maintenance therapy should then be continued (fluconazole 200 mg/day) for a minimum of 1 year. Usually fluconazole is then stopped in patients with an excellent response to ART and CD4TL > 100/mcL.

E. In patients with high ICP, serial LPs are recommended to lower opening pressure to < 20 cm H_2O or by 50%; patients with hydrocephalus benefit from ventricular shunts.

MAKING A DIAGNOSIS

Blood cultures and serum cryptococcal antigen are ordered. A toxicology screen is positive for opioids and cocaine. CBC reveals a WBC of 3700/mcL (8% lymphocytes) a HCT of 36.6 and platelet count of 240,000/mcL. Prothrombin time and partial thromboplastin time are normal. Serum RPR and FTA-ABS are negative.

An LP is performed and reveals opening pressure of 30 cm H_2O, glucose 26 mg/dL (versus serum of 127 mg/dL); and protein, 68 mg/dL (normal 15–45 mg/dL). CSF shows 20 WBC/mcL and CSF Gram stain reveals numerous yeast forms.

Have you crossed a diagnostic threshold for the leading hypothesis, cryptococcal meningitis? Have you ruled out the active alternatives? Do other tests need to be done to exclude the alternative diagnoses?

The CSF findings strongly suggest cryptococcal meningitis. Positive cryptococcal antigen or culture will confirm the diagnosis. However, patients with AIDS may have more than 1 simultaneous infection and you review other diagnoses on the differential. There is no travel history to Arizona or the southwestern United States that would increase the probability of coccidioidomycosis. Neurosyphilis is unlikely with the negative VDRL and FTA absorbed (FTA-ABS). An MRI is more sensitive in the detection of CNS mass lesions than a contrast CT and is indicated to confidently exclude alternative diagnoses associated with masses. In addition, CMV encephalitis has not been excluded.

Alternative Diagnosis: Toxoplasmosis Encephalitis

Textbook Presentation

Toxoplasmosis encephalitis in AIDS patients typically presents subacutely over 1–2 weeks, although acute presentations with confusion or seizures may be seen. Focal neurologic manifestations are common. Confusion and mental status changes may dominate the clinical picture.

Disease Highlights

A. Most common CNS mass lesion in AIDS patients

B. 15% of US population seropositive for toxoplasmosis

C. Toxoplasmosis encephalitis develops secondary to reactivation of latent toxoplasmosis; therefore, most patients have positive IgG titers (see later discussion).

D. CD4TL < 100/mcL in 80% of patients

E. Probability of developing toxoplasmosis encephalitis is 30% in AIDS patients with CD4TL counts < 100/mcL and positive toxoplasmosis serology (if not receiving prophylaxis).

F. ART has decreased the incidence of toxoplasmosis encephalitis.

G. May be the initial manifestation or subsequent manifestation of HIV infection

H. 27% mortality despite treatment

I. Other concurrent CNS infections common

Evidence-Based Diagnosis

A. History

   1. Headache (often frontal and bilateral): 49–73%

   2. Seizures: 15–31%

   3. Hallucinations: 8%

   4. Fever: 4–68%

B. Physical exam

   1. Focal findings (weakness, abnormal gait, or other): 73–88%

   2. Mental status changes: 50–67%

   3. Mental status changes dominating clinical picture: 40%

   4. Cognitive impairment (with normal arousal): 66%

   5. Stiff neck: 0%

Meningismus is distinctly uncommon in cerebral toxoplasmosis and suggests an alternate or additional disease process.

C. Laboratory findings

1. Serology

   a. Toxoplasma IgG: ≈ 97% sensitive but does not confirm active CNS toxoplasmosis

   b. Toxoplasma IgM: insensitive (15%) because disease is usually secondary to reactivation.

   c. Cerebral toxoplasmosis is unlikely in patients with negative *Toxoplasma* IgG.

   d. Probability of toxoplasmosis encephalitis in seropositive patients with mass effect is markedly reduced (from 87% to 59%) in patients receiving TMP-SMX prophylaxis.

2. CSF analysis

   a. Standard CSF analysis may be normal or nonspecifically elevated.

   b. Percentage of patients with abnormal findings

      (1) WBC > 5 cells/mcL: 50%

      (2) Protein > 40 mg/dL: 81%

      (3) Low glucose: 14%

      (4) CSF *Toxoplasma* IgG: 33–69%

   c. CSF PCR insensitive for CNS toxoplasmosis but highly specific

      (1) 54% sensitive, 99% specific

      (2) LR+ 54, LR– 0.46

3. Neuroimaging

   a. MRI is test of choice.

      (1) Superior to contrast CT, affecting course in 40% of patients

      (2) 1 or more ring-enhancing lesions with mass effect and edema

      (3) Lesions may be located in basal ganglia, thalamus, and cortex.

      (4) Single lesion in 14% of patients

      (5) Single lesions make toxoplasmosis less likely and increase likelihood of PCL.

   b. CT scan with contrast is abnormal in 87–96%.

      (1) Single ring-enhancing lesion: 35%

      (2) ≥ 2 ring-enhancing lesions: 62%

      (3) Hypodense lesions: 13%

      (4) Moderate to severe cerebral edema: 48%

      (5) 75% of lesions located in cerebral hemispheres

      (6) MRI recommended in patients with normal contrast CT scan or a single enhancing lesion

   c. Single photon emission CT (SPECT) thallium 201 imaging usually reveals decreased isotope activity in patients with *Toxoplasma* encephalitis versus increased uptake in patients with PCL. This distinction is less reliable in patients receiving ART. 50% of patients with *Toxoplasma* encephalitis taking ART show increased uptake.

4. Brain biopsy

   a. Brain biopsy not done routinely due to complications and imperfect sensitivity.

   b. Toxoplasmosis is usually diagnosed presumptively and empiric treatment started in patients who fulfill diagnostic criteria (see below).

   c. When positive, it is the only method that confirms cerebral toxoplasmosis with certainty.

      (1) False-negative results can occur due to sampling error.

      (2) Can diagnose concomitant infection

   d. Sensitivity of standard hematoxylin and eosin staining only 50–66%. Immunoperoxidase staining improves sensitivity.

   e. Brain biopsy associated with 0.5–3.1% mortality and 10–40% morbidity.

   f. Biopsy reserved for atypical cases (ie, negative serology or nonresponders within 7–10 days).

5. **Presumptive diagnosis:** Toxoplasmosis probable and treatment instituted in patients with all of the following criteria:

   a. Multiple mass lesions

   b. CD4TL < 100/mcL

   c. Positive *Toxoplasma* serology

   d. Not already receiving toxoplasmosis prophylaxis (Figure 5-3).

Treatment

A. Pyrimethamine plus sulfadiazine or pyrimethamine plus clindamycin.

B. Folinic acid also administered to patients taking pyrimethamine.

C. TMP-SMX is an alternative therapy.

D. Clinical improvement is seen in > 90% of responders within first 2 weeks of drug therapy.

E. Radiologic improvement occurs in most patients within 3 weeks of treatment.

F. After induction therapy, suppressive therapy with lower doses is used. Suppressive therapy can be safely discontinued in asymptomatic patients in whom ART has restored CD4TL to > 200/mcL for ≥ 6 months. An MRI prior to discontinuation of suppressive therapy may be appropriate.

G. Corticosteroids are indicated for patients with cerebral edema *and* midline shift, or clinical deterioration within first 48 hours of therapy. Corticosteroids complicate interpretation of response to therapy since they reduce edema and the size of PCL lesions.

H. Prevention: HIV-positive patients with CD4TL < 200/mcL and positive *Toxoplasma* IgG should receive TMP-SMX as primary prophylaxis.

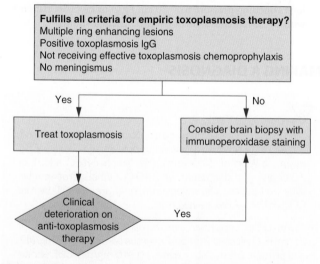

Figure 5-3. Empiric therapy for CNS toxoplasmosis in AIDS patients.

Alternative Diagnosis: Progressive Multifocal Leukoencephalopathy

Textbook Presentation

PML typically presents with progressive neurologic deficits, in particular weakness or gait disorders, over weeks to months. PML may also be present with visual problems, headache, alterations in mental status, or dementia with focal signs.

Disease Highlights

A. Etiologic agent is JC virus, a polyomavirus (not to be confused with Creutzfeldt-Jakob disease, a prion related illness).

B. Primary JC virus infection is common and asymptomatic; 80–90% of general population has antibodies to JC virus.

C. PML develops when profound immunosuppression allows latent JC virus in reticuloendothelial system and kidney to gain access to CNS and replicate.

D. Subsequent infection and lysis of the myelin-producing oligodendroglial cells results in PML. Astrocytes may be infected.

E. Pathogenesis may involve HIV-associated immunosuppression and a direct synergistic effect of HIV and JC virus.

F. Multifocal or unifocal white matter lesions are seen.

G. Mean CD4 TL count 84–104/mcL: 25% of patients have CD4TL count > 200/mcL.

H. PML occurs in 1–5% of AIDS patients.

Evidence-Based Diagnosis

A. History and physical exam
   1. Limb weakness: 50–70%
   2. Gait disorder: 26–64%
   3. Speech disorder: 31–51%
   4. Visual impairment (hemianopsia): 21–50%
   5. Seizures: 5–23%
   6. Headaches: 23%
   7. Cognitive abnormalities/mental status changes: 25–65%
   8. Cranial nerve palsies: 31%

B. Laboratory findings
   1. Serum antibodies to JC virus are not useful due to high prevalence of infection.
   2. CSF
      a. Routine studies may be normal or nonspecifically elevated.
      b. CSF PCR for JC virus DNA:
         (1) 80% sensitive, 98% specific
         (2) LR+ (average), 40; LR–, 0.20
         (3) Certain types of assays (repeat analysis) increase sensitivity to 90%.
         (4) Sensitivity is diminished in patients receiving ART.
   3. CNS imaging
      a. Typically shows extensive multifocal patchy white matter demyelination with sparing of the cortical gray matter
      b. MRI is more sensitive than CT scanning (CT 63% sensitive).
      c. Lesions hypodense on CT scanning, low intensity on T1-weighted MRI, hyperintense on T2-weighted MRI
      d. On imaging, lesions are restricted to the subcortical white matter, respecting the gray-white junction of the cerebrum.

   e. There is overlap in the MRI features of toxoplasmosis, primary CNS lymphoma, and PML. However certain features *suggest* PML:
      (1) Lack of enhancement
      (2) Lack of mass effect
      (3) Less well-circumscribed lesions
   f. MRI typically shows scalloping at gray-white matter interface.
   g. CT scanning typically demonstrates white matter hypodense lesions.
   h. Brain biopsy: 100% specific but sensitivities only 64% to 96% due to sampling error

 MRI is markedly superior to CT for diagnosis of PML

Treatment

A. ART associated with improvement or cure in some patients.
   1. Survival pre-ART averaged 4–6 months. Survival has improved to 50% since the introduction of ART.
   2. 80% of survivors have severe residual neurologic deficits
   3. Some patients receiving ART develop **immune reconstitution inflammatory syndrome** (IRIS) with worsening of symptoms and enhancement around the PML plaques on MRI.

B. Initiation of ART occasionally results in PML in previously asymptomatic patients due to increased inflammation associated with IRIS (**unmasking IRIS**).

Alternative Diagnosis: Primary CNS Lymphoma

Textbook Presentation

Typically, PCL develops in patients with advanced AIDS. While focal complaints (ie, weakness) may develop in some patients, altered mental status or seizures may be presenting complaints in many patients.

Disease Highlights

A. Biologically distinct from PCL in other immunocompromised states

B. Diffuse, high-grade, B cell, non-Hodgkin lymphoma arising and confined to the CNS (ie, not due to CNS involvement by *systemic* lymphoma)

C. CD4TL usually < 50/mcL

D. Consistently associated with Epstein-Barr virus in the tumor

E. Pathogenesis likely involves activation of latent Epstein-Barr virus genes due to immunodeficiency. The relative immunologic sanctuary of the CNS from immune surveillance may facilitate growth of these tumors at this location.

F. Rapidly progressive with a short interval from symptoms to diagnosis (1.8 months)

G. Median survival without treatment ≈1 month

H. Supratentorial location 3× more common than infratentorial

I. The most common cause of death in patients with PCL is *another* OI.

J. The incidence of PCL between 1995 and 2000 declined markedly (≈ 90%) because of the introduction of ART.

Evidence-Based Diagnosis

A. History and physical exam
   1. B symptoms (weight loss > 10%, unexplained temperatures > 38.0°C, drenching sweats): 80%

2. Focal neurologic deficits: 51%

3. Mental status changes: 53%

4. Seizures: 27%

5. Isolated headache 3%

B. Laboratory findings

1. CSF Epstein-Barr virus PCR:

   a. 87% sensitive, 98% specific

   b. LR+, 43; LR–, 0.13

2. Positive CSF cytology only 15–23% sensitive. Special studies are required to distinguish monoclonal proliferations from reactive T cell populations.

C. Radiologic studies

1. CT scanning

   a. 90% sensitive

   b. Usually reveals contrast enhancement (90%)

   c. 48% single lesion, 52% multiple lesions

   d. Usually associated with mass effect (similar to toxoplasmosis but not seen in PML)

2. MRI more sensitive than CT scanning

3. SPECT thallium imaging

   e. PCL usually demonstrates early uptake and retention (compared with decreased uptake in necrotic centers of toxoplasmosis).

   (1) 86–100% sensitive, 77–100% specific (higher specificity if retention index measured).

   (2) Increased uptake is noted in 15% of patients with toxoplasmosis encephalitis not receiving ART but up to 50% of patients with toxoplasmosis encephalitis receiving ART, making this test less useful in patients receiving ART.

D. Biopsy

1. Positive CSF Epstein-Barr virus PCR may make biopsy unnecessary.

2. Biopsy is useful when CSF Epstein-Barr virus PCR is negative.

3. Lympholytic effect of corticosteroids may render biopsy nondiagnostic.

 Corticosteroids should not be administered before brain biopsy in patients with suspected PCL unless the patient is at an increased risk for herniation.

Treatment

A. Prognosis is grave with or without therapy.

B. Chemotherapy, whole brain radiotherapy, and corticosteroids have been used. Chemotherapy modestly prolongs survival (median survival 7 months).

C. Surgical resection does not improve prognosis due to multifocal nature of disease.

CASE RESOLUTION

 Mr. S's LP reveals that cryptococcal antigen is positive at a titer of 1:512. Blood and CSF cultures are positive for *C neoformans*. An MRI confirmed the absence of a CNS mass. Subsequent CSF acid-fast bacilli (AFB) cultures and VDRL were negative.

Mr. S's CSF culture confirms cryptococcal meningitis. The subacute course and lack of meningeal findings are common features of this disease. CSF analysis did not suggest concomitant mycobacterial infection or neurosyphilis, and the MRI did not suggest toxoplasmosis, PML, or PCL.

 Mr. S was treated and showed gradual improvement. After 2 weeks of therapy, he was discharged to follow-up with the infectious disease clinic.

REVIEW OF OTHER IMPORTANT DISEASES

HIV Encephalopathy (HIV-Associated Dementia)

Textbook Presentation

Patients typically have advanced AIDS with a slowly progressive dementia eventually accompanied by motor symptoms.

Disease Highlights

A. Subcortical dementia characterized by cognitive, behavioral, and psychomotor slowing.

B. Prevalence of 15–20% in patients with AIDS prior to introduction of ART.

C. 40–50% decrease in incidence since the introduction of ART. However, prevalence is rising due to increasing survival.

D. Severe form of encephalopathy effectively eliminated by ART

E. Milder deficits still common

F. Principal target is perivascular CNS macrophages. Astrocytes may also become infected.

G. HIV encephalopathy develops late with CD4TL typically < 200/mcL.

H. Twofold increased risk in patients aged ≥ 50 years.

I. Neurotoxicity of HIV may be synergistic with that of cocaine or methamphetamine.

Evidence-Based Diagnosis

A. History and physical exam

1. Memory complaints: 70%

2. Cognitive slowing: 25–30%

3. Gait difficulty: 45%

4. Behavioral changes: 10–20%

5. Seizures: 5–10%

6. Focal findings uncommon

B. Laboratory findings

1. MRI: T2 images with hyperintensities in the deep white matter and basal ganglia without contrast enhancement and/or atrophy; the distribution of lesions is symmetric in contrast to PML lesions.

2. CSF

   a. Useful to rule out other infections

   b. Mild CSF leukocytosis and protein elevations seen

   c. CSF HIV RNA levels do not correlate with HIV encephalopathy.

   d. Cannot diagnose HIV encephalopathy with certainty

3. Neuropsychological testing is useful in evaluating the severity and response to ART.

 HIV encephalopathy is a diagnosis of exclusion. Diagnostic evaluations serve to exclude other OIs, malignancy, or substance abuse.

Treatment

A. Most patients treated with ART remain stable or show partial reversal of neurologic deficits. Early therapy is therefore important.

B. Elevated levels of CSF beta-microgbulin (suggesting ongoing inflammation) predicted better neurologic recovery with ART.

Neurosyphilis in HIV-Positive Patients

Textbook Presentation

Patients with neurosyphilis may be asymptomatic or have meningitis, stroke-like symptoms, visual or hearing loss, or other focal deficits due to CNS gummas.

Disease Highlights

A. Caused by spirochete *Treponema pallidum*

B. High-risk groups: MSMs, injection drug users, and patrons of paid sex workers

C. Association of HIV and syphilis infection
   1. Studies document 25–70% HIV coinfection rate in patients with syphilis.

 HIV infection in patients with syphilis is common.

   2. Neurosyphilis in HIV-infected less frequent (1%)

D. Syphilis commonly infects the CNS early in the course of disease in both HIV-infected and non–HIV-infected persons (25–33%).

E. The CNS infection is more often progressive in HIV-infected persons, increasing the need for detection in this group.

F. Infections develop in characteristic stages.
   1. Primary infection
      a. Characterized by chancre: a 0.5- to 2-cm painless, indurated, well-circumscribed ulcerated papule at the site of primary inoculation approximately 2–3 weeks after contact
      b. Multiple chancres seen in HIV-infected patients
      c. Lesion resolves with *or* without therapy.
   2. Secondary stage
      a. Symptoms include macular or maculopapular rash involving the palms and soles in 70%, fever, myalgias and lymphadenopathy; oral mucosal patches, perineal condyloma lata (often exuberant in HIV/AIDS).
      b. Develops within weeks to months of primary infection
      c. Symptoms of secondary syphilis may or may not be seen.
      d. Secondary syphilis and chancres may coexist in HIV-infected patients.
   3. Latent syphilis: 60–70% of untreated patients have no disease progression.
   4. Late or tertiary stage
      a. Develops in one-third of untreated patients
      b. Gummas (granulomas with caseating necrosis) affect involved organs and usually develop over 4–10 years but may develop within months in HIV-infected patients.
      c. Protean manifestations including cardiac (aortic root and coronary artery involvement), eyes, skin, and CNS

5. Neurosyphilis
   a. May be asymptomatic or symptomatic
   b. Neurosyphilis can develop early (< 1 year) or late after syphilis infection in HIV-infected patients.
      (1) Typical early symptoms include cranial nerve palsies, meningitis or meningovascular symptoms (strokes secondary to arteritis). One report found visual symptoms in 51%; headache in 32%; and gait difficulty, hearing loss, meningismus, or altered mental status in < 5%.
      (2) Early neurosyphilis develops in 1.7% of HIV-infected MSMs who acquire syphilis.
      (3) Typical late symptoms include tabes dorsalis, general paresis (dementia associated with psychotic features) and almost any focal finding.
      (4) May present with visual loss secondary to ophthalmic involvement (anterior uveitis, pan uveitis, optic atrophy) or neurosensory hearing loss.

Evidence-Based Diagnosis

A. Primary syphilis
   1. Dark field exam of chancre is the test of choice but availability is limited.
   2. Direct fluorescent antibody may be available.

B. Secondary syphilis
   1. Nonspecific treponemal tests of serum (RPR) is highly sensitive for secondary syphilis.
   2. Confirmation with FTA-ABS is required to prove diagnosis.

C. Tertiary syphilis
   1. RPR is positive in two-thirds of patients: confirmation by FTA-ABS is required.
   2. FTA-ABS is 100% sensitive.
   3. False-negative results occur rarely.

D. Neurosyphilis
   1. Approximately half of men with neurosyphilis have no other history or evidence of syphilis.

 Consider neurosyphilis in HIV-infected patients with new visual symptoms or headache.

   2. CD4TL count: 25–882/mcL; mean CD4TL count: 217–312/mcL
   3. Estimating test accuracy is difficult due to the lack of a gold standard.
   4. Commonly used criteria include *either* positive CSF VDRL *or* positive *serum* serology for syphilis *and* CSF pleocytosis.
      a. CSF VDRL is highly specific but sensitivity is only ≈ 50%.
      b. CSF pleocytosis is more sensitive but less specific due to other infections that increase CSF WBCs (including HIV and other OIs).
      c. Reverse transcriptase PCR testing of CSF for *T pallidum* has limited sensitivity.
      d. CSF FTA-ABS is highly sensitive but less specific: a negative CSF FTA-ABS makes neurosyphilis unlikely.
   5. Perform LP to look for neurosyphilis in any HIV patient with syphilis and either:
      a. Neurologic symptoms of any type, including meningitis, stroke-like syndrome, visual loss, hearing loss, dementia, or other focal deficit

b. Persistent signs of infection despite treatment: failure of RPR to fall fourfold with treatment

c. Serum RPR titer ≥ 1:32

(1) Increases the likelihood of neurosyphilis in HIV-infected persons with syphilis

(2) 76–96% sensitive, 59% specific

d. CD4TL count ≤ 350/mcL

(1) Increases the likelihood of neurosyphilis in HIV-infected persons with syphilis

(2) 69% sensitive, 53% specific

e. HIV-infected patients with late latent syphilis (> 1 year) or of unknown duration

Treatment

A. Primary and secondary syphilis

1. Single-dose benzathine penicillin IM

2. Penicillin allergy: doxycycline

3. Follow RPR every 3 months for 1 year to document 4 × fall in titer.

B. Latent syphilis

1. If duration is unknown, LP is recommended to rule out neurosyphilis.

2. If LP is negative, administer IM benzathine penicillin every week for 3 weeks.

3. Follow RPR every 6 months for 2 years to document 4 × fall in titer.

C. Neurosyphilis

1. IV penicillin for 10–14 days

2. Penicillin allergy: high-dose ceftriaxone, oral doxycycline, or desensitization to penicillin followed by IV penicillin for 10–14 days. The latter strategy is the most effective.

A summary of the clinical and radiologic features, CD4TL count, and tests of choice of the common CNS disorders in AIDS patients is presented in Table 5-2.

I have an HIV-positive patient with a cough and fever. How do I determine the cause?

CHIEF COMPLAINT

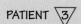

PATIENT 3

Mr. L is a 35-year-old man who is HIV-positive. His chief complaints are cough and fever lasting for 4 days.

What is the differential diagnosis of cough and fever in HIV-positive patients? How would you frame the differential?

CONSTRUCTING A DIFFERENTIAL DIAGNOSIS

The most common pneumonias in HIV-infected patients are bacterial pneumonia, PCP, and pulmonary tuberculosis (PTB). Taken together, they account for 91% of pulmonary infections in HIV-positive patients. Three pivotal features aid in the diagnosis of these common pneumonias in HIV-infected persons. First, the CD4TL count gauges the level of immunocompromise. Virulent infections, such as TB or bacterial pneumonia, may occur in patients with *any* CD4TL count. On the other hand, less virulent infections, such as PCP, are seen almost exclusively in patients with CD4TL < 200/mcL. Infections by nontuberculous mycobacteria, fungi, and CMV usually occur in patients with CD4TL < 100/mcL.

The second pivotal feature is that certain diseases present acutely (bacterial pneumonia), but other diseases present subacutely or chronically (PTB or PCP).

The final pivotal feature that aids in the diagnosis of these complaints is the pattern on chest radiograph. Lobar infiltrates suggest bacterial pneumonia, whereas diffuse or interstitial infiltrates are seen in PCP, CMV, and fungal pneumonia. Patterns that suggest PTB include apical or cavitary infiltrates, hilar lymphadenopathy, or nodular infiltrates. The chest radiographic pattern in PTB varies depending on the patient's degree of immunosuppression. Table 5-3 and Figure 5-4 summarize the typical CD4TL count, acuity, and chest radiographic pattern and approach to pulmonary infection in HIV-positive patients.

Tumors may also cause pulmonary complaints. Not surprisingly, aggressive neoplasms, such as lung cancer, may occur at any CD4TL count, whereas pulmonary lymphoma usually develops in patients with CD4TL counts < 500/mcL, and Kaposi sarcoma usually develops in patients with CD4TL < 200/mcL.

As noted above, the most common pneumonias in HIV-infected patients are bacterial pneumonia, PCP and PTB. PCP is reviewed in Chapter 10 and will be mentioned here only briefly. The remainder of this section will focus on bacterial pneumonia, PTB and nontuberculous mycobacterial infection in HIV-infected patients.

Differential Diagnosis of Pulmonary Processes in Patients With HIV

A. CD4TL count > 500/mcL

1. Bacterial pneumonia

2. TB

3. Lung cancer

B. CD4TL count 200–499/mcL: all of the above plus lymphoma

C. CD4TL count 100–199/mcL: all of the above plus PCP

Table 5-2. Summary of findings in CNS disorders in AIDS patients.

Disease	Common Clinical Features	Radiologic Features	Test of Choice
Mass Lesions			
Toxoplasmosis	Headache Focal findings Mental status changes Onset days CD4 < 100/mcL	MRI multiple ring enhancing lesions in most patients	Serum toxoplasma IgG almost always positive MRI
PML	Headache Focal findings Mental status changes Onset weeks-months CD4 average 100/mcL (may be > 200/mcL)	MRI single or multiple, asymmetric white matter lesions No mass effect or enhancement	CSF PCR JC virus If negative, consider brain biopsy MRI
Primary CNS lymphoma	Headache Focal findings Mental status changes Onset days-weeks CD4 < 50/mcL	MRI or CT => single (50%) or multiple (50%) irregular enhancing lesions; Lesions may be large (> 4 cm)	CSF PCR EBV If negative, perform brain biopsy MRI
Non-Mass Lesions			
Cryptococcal meningitis	Headache Mental status changes CD4 < 100/mcL	Mass lesions rare	Serum or CSF cryptococcal antigen CSF fungal culture
HIV encephalopathy	Dementia, ataxia, tremor CD4 < 200/mcL	MRI may show atrophy and/or hyperintensities in the deep white matter and basal ganglia without contrast enhancement	Diagnosis of exclusion Imaging may be very suggestive
CMV encephalitis	Mental status changes Headache Focal findings CD4 < 50/mcL	MRI may show periventricular enhancement, ventricular enlargement, or be normal	CSF CMV PCR
TB meningitis	Mental status changes Cranial nerve palsies Any CD4 count	MRI demonstrates meningeal enhancement, occasional mass, or may be normal	CSF AFB stain, large volume CSF for culture
Neurosyphilis	Visual symptoms, headache, cranial neuropathy, CVA, dementia Any CD4 count	May demonstrate CVA, rarely mass lesion	Serum RPR, Serum FTA-ABS CSF RPR, CSF FTA-ABS

AFB, acid-fast bacilli; CMV, cytomegalovirus; CNS, central nervous system; CSF, cerebrospinal fluid; CVA, cerebrovascular accident; EBV, Epstein-Barr virus; FTA-ABS, fluorescent treponemal antibody- absorbed; PCR, polymerase chain reaction; PML, progressive multifocal leukoencephalopathy; RPR, rapid plasma reagin; TB, tuberculosis.

D. CD4TL count < 100/mcL: all of the above plus the following:

1. Fungal infections uncommon (cryptococcosis, aspergillosis, histoplasmosis, blastomycosis, coccidioidomycosis)

2. CMV: commonly found in bronchoalveolar lavage (BAL) culture, but usually reflects asymptomatic reactivation; CMV rarely is responsible for pneumonia in AIDS.

3. Nontuberculous mycobacteria, especially MAI and *M kansasii*

4. Kaposi sarcoma

Mr. L reports that he was feeling well until 4 days ago when sudden-onset fever of 38.8°C, cough productive of green sputum, and right-sided chest pain with inspiration developed. He feels moderately short of breath with exertion. Medical history is remarkable for sexually acquired HIV infection diagnosed 2 years ago. His last CD4 T cell count 1 month ago was 400/mcL. At that time, his viral load was undetectable. He is compliant with ART.

Table 5-3. Summary of findings in pulmonary infection in HIV-positive patients.

Variable	Tuberculosis	Bacterial Pneumonia	PCP
Acuity	Subacute	Acute	Subacute
	Weeks to months	< 1 week	Weeks to months
CD4	Any count	Any count	< 200/mcL
Typical chest radiographic pattern	*CD4 > 200 /mcL:* Apical, cavitary or nodular lesions	Lobar consolidation	Bilateral perihilar diffuse symmetric interstitial pattern
	CD4 < 200 /mcL: Normal, or middle or lower lobe consolidation, miliary pattern, lymphadenopathy		
Risk factors	Foreign born or traveler to endemic area, recent exposure, prior positive PPD, injection drug use, prison	Injection drug use, Low CD4 count	Low CD4 count
Other clues	Pleural effusions may be seen		Elevated lactate dehydrogenase, more hypoxia than expected from chest radiographic findings
Diagnostic tests of choice	Sputum smear and culture. BAL if no productive cough; Biopsy if miliary TB	Sputum culture, Gram stain and blood culture	Sputum obtained by BAL[1]
			Silver stain, H&E, or DFA for PCP

[1]Most institutions lack the expertise to reliably detect PCP in expectorated sputum. BAL is usually required.
BAL, bronchoalveolar lavage; DFA, direct immunofluorescent assay; H&E, hematoxylin and eosin; PCP, *Pneumocystis jirovecii* pneumonia; PPD, purified protein derivative; TB tuberculosis.

At this point, what is the leading hypothesis, what are the active alternatives, and is there a must not miss diagnosis? Given this differential diagnosis, what tests should be ordered?

RANKING THE DIFFERENTIAL DIAGNOSIS

There are 2 key features to Mr. L's presentation. The first pivotal feature is that his CD4TL count is only moderately reduced. This makes a variety of OIs unlikely (PCP, MAI, CMV, and fungal infections). On the other hand, both PTB and bacterial pneumonia are sufficiently virulent to present in patients with normal or mildly impaired immune systems. The second pivotal feature is the rapid development of the pulmonary process, which strongly favors bacterial pneumonia over PTB. The differential diagnosis is summarized in Table 5-4.

Physical exam reveals the following: temperature, 38.6°C; BP, 120/75 mm Hg; pulse, 110 bpm; RR, 18 breaths per minute. Lung exam reveals crackles over the lower one-third of posterior right chest. Chest radiograph reveals a right lower lobe consolidation. No effusion is seen. WBC is 8000/mcL with 15% bands. Sputum Gram stain reveals numerous polymorphonuclear cells and gram-positive diplococci. The initial AFB smear is negative. Blood cultures are sent.

Is the clinical information sufficient to make a diagnosis? If not, what other information do you need?

Leading Hypothesis: Bacterial Pneumonia

Textbook Presentation

Typical onset is acute (< 1 week) with productive cough and fever. Patients may produce purulent sputum and complain of pleuritic chest pain. Presentation is similar to bacterial pneumonia in HIV-negative patients.

Disease Highlights

A. Bacterial infection is the most common cause of pneumonia associated with HIV and AIDS. HIV should therefore be considered in any patient with severe or recurrent community-acquired pneumonia.

B. Recurrent bacterial pneumonia (> 2 episodes within 1 year) is an AIDS-defining condition.

C. May occur at any time during course of HIV infection

D. Risk of bacterial pneumonia increases as CD4TL count falls. Injection drug use further increases the risk.

  1. CD4TL count

    a. Rate of bacterial pneumonia in HIV-negative patients: 0.9%/year

    b. Rate of bacterial pneumonia all HIV-positive patients: 5.5%/year

      (1) CD4TL > 500/mcL: 2.3%/year

      (2) CD4TL 200–500/mcL: 6.8%/year

      (3) CD4TL < 200/mcL: 10.8%/year

      (4) Two-thirds of cases in HIV-infected patients developed in those with CD4TL < 200/mcL.

  2. Injection drug use

    a. Pneumonia incidence in HIV-infected patients without injection drug use is 4.1%/year, compared with 11.1%/year in HIV-infected persons with injection drug use.

    b. Increased rate of septic emboli from infective endocarditis contributes to the increased risk of pneumonia.

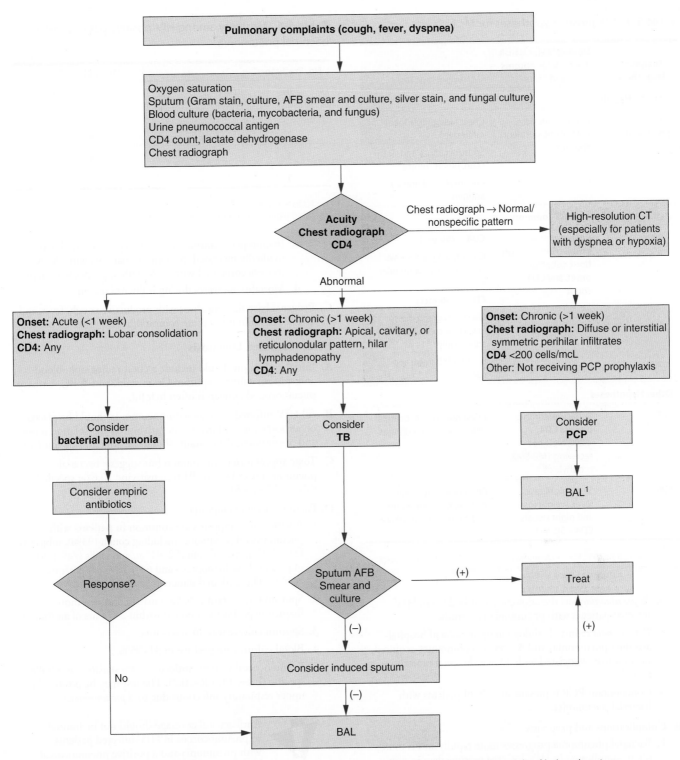

[1]BAL usually required for diagnosis of PCP except in few centers with unusual expertise in performing silver stain of induced sputums.

AFB, acid-fast bacilli; BAL, bronchoalveolar lavage; PCP, *Pneumocystis jiroveci* pneumonia; TB, tuberculosis.

Figure 5-4. Evaluation of pulmonary complaints in HIV-positive patients.

3. ART significantly reduces the risk of bacterial pneumonia (45%).

E. Etiology

1. *Streptococcus pneumoniae* is the most common cause of bacterial pneumonia. Other causes include *Haemophilus*

influenzae, Mycoplasma pneumoniae, Staphylococcus aureus, and *Pseudomonas aeruginosa.*

2. *S pneumoniae* is associated with higher WBC than *P aeruginosa* (12,400/mcL vs 5000/mcL) and higher average CD4TL count (106/mcL vs 19/mcL).

Table 5-4. Diagnostic hypotheses for Mr. L.

Diagnostic Hypotheses	Demographics, Risk Factors, Symptoms and Signs	Important Tests
Leading Hypothesis		
Bacterial pneumonia	Acute onset, any CD4 count, purulent sputum	Chest radiograph: lobar infiltrate(s)
		Sputum culture and Gram stain, blood culture
		Pneumococcal urinary antigen
Active Alternative—Most Common		
Tuberculosis	Recent exposure, positive PPD, foreign born, subacute onset, any CD4 count	**CD4 > 200/mcL:** Chest radiograph shows apical, cavitary or nodular lesion
		CD4 < 200/mcL: Chest radiograph shows lower lobe consolidation, adenopathy
		Sputum AFB smear and culture
Other Hypotheses		
PCP	Subacute/chronic process CD4 < 200/mcL, not receiving TMP-SMX prophylaxis	Chest radiograph: bilateral diffuse perihilar infiltrates
MAC	Systemic illness: fever, weight loss, and night sweats CD4 < 50/mcL	Chest radiograph: any pattern; AFB sputum smear and culture; blood culture

AFB, acid-fast bacillus; MAC, *Mycobacterium avium* complex; PCP, *Pneumocystis jirovecii* pneumonia; PPD, purified protein derivative; TMP-SMX, trimethoprim-sulfamethoxazole.

3. *M pneumoniae* was the etiologic agent in 21% of HIV-infected patients with pneumonia in 1 study.

4. *P aeruginosa* reported etiology in up to 38% of hospital-acquired pneumonias and 3–25% of community-acquired pneumonias; associated with 33% in-hospital mortality rate.

5. Concomitant PCP is present in 13% of patients with bacterial pneumonia.

F. Complications and prognosis

1. Bacterial pneumonia progresses more rapidly and is more often complicated in HIV-infected persons than in non-infected persons.

2. 30% of bacterial pneumonias associated with bacteremia; bacteremia is more common in *S pneumoniae* infections.

3. Among hospitalized patients, 9.3–27% overall mortality

   a. 6–13 × higher mortality than general US population (and 1.2–2.4 × higher than population > 65 years)

   b. 5 predictors of mortality include septic shock, CD4TL count < 100/mcL, significant pleural effusion (extending beyond costophrenic angle), cavities and multilobar infiltrates. Mortality is proportional to number of risk factors (Table 5-5).

Table 5-5. Mortality among HIV-positive patients with bacterial pneumonia.

No. Predictors[1]	Mortality (%)
0	1.3
1	7.5
2	8.7
3	34.5
4	42.8

[1]Predictors: septic shock, CD4 count < 100/mcL, significant pleural effusion (extending beyond costophrenic angle), cavities, and multilobar infiltrates.

   c. Inappropriate antimicrobial therapy associated with markedly increased mortality in patients with shock (85.7% compared with 25% with appropriate therapy).

   d. Mortality increases during influenza season.

G. Pyogenic bacterial bronchitis with productive cough, fever, and absence of infiltrates is more common in HIV-infected patients.

Evidence-Based Diagnosis

A. Initial evaluation should include a chest radiograph, blood and sputum cultures, sputum Gram stain, and WBC. Urinary pneumococcal antigen is often helpful.

B. All HIV-infected patients with pneumonia should be placed on airborne precautions in a negative-pressure isolation room, and 3 sputum acid-fast stains should be done to rule out PTB.

C. Toxic appearance is uncommon but suggests bacterial pneumonia over PCP or PTB (sensitivity, 10.6%; specificity, 97.8%; LR+, 4.8).

D. Pneumococcal pneumonia

1. A variety of symptoms are common in patients with pneumococcal pneumonia including cough (93%), subjective fever (90%), pleural pain (52–91%), and chills (74%). 51% of patients have hemoptysis and 63% have temperature > 38°C. The median duration of symptoms is 4 days.

2. Sputum Gram stain is 58% sensitive and was more frequently positive if collected within 24 hours of antibiotics.

3. Sputum culture was 56% sensitive.

4. Blood cultures are positive in 31–95%.

5. Pneumococcal urinary antigen: ≈79% sensitive and 94% specific (LR+, 13; LR–, 0.2). The test may be positive in upper respiratory infections due to *S pneumoniae*.

 Antibacterial coverage should not be limited to pneumococcus in HIV-infected patients with pneumonia and a positive pneumococcal urinary antigen.

E. *Legionella* pneumonia

1. One study reported that certain findings were more common in patients with *Legionella* pneumonia than *S pneumoniae*, including extra-respiratory symptoms (57% vs 24%), hyponatremia (57% vs 13%) and elevated creatine phosphokinase (57% vs 17%).

2. Respiratory failure was more common with *Legionella* than *S pneumoniae* (33% vs 2%).

F. *M pneumoniae* is usually diagnosed by IgM ELISA, four-fold change in IgG, or the presence of cold agglutination.

G. Chest radiograph

1. Standard imaging includes posteroanterior and lateral chest radiograph.

2. Chest radiograph typically demonstrates lobar or multifocal consolidation.

3. Lobar consolidation is not always seen but strongly suggests bacterial pneumonia over PCP or PTB (sensitivity, 54%; specificity, 90%; LR+, 5.6; LR–, 0.51).

4. Lobar infiltrates in patients with fever for less than 1 week strongly suggests bacterial pneumonia (sensitivity, 48%; specificity, 94%; LR+, 8.0; LR–, 0.55).

5. Chest radiographic patterns did not distinguish *S pneumoniae* from *P aeruginosa,* or *Legionella* infection.

6. One report found that 82% of HIV-infected persons with pulmonary complaints had abnormalities, including pleural effusions, cavities and abscess, on high-resolution CT scans that were not detected on chest radiograph.

 High-resolution CT scanning should be considered for HIV-infected patients who do not respond to therapy and for ill patients with respiratory symptoms or signs but an unexpectedly normal chest radiograph.

H. Bronchoscopy

1. Indicated in patients who do not respond to therapy or when concomitant infection is likely.

2. Sensitivity of BAL for bacterial pneumonia: 70%

Treatment

A. Prevention

1. TMP-SMX PCP prophylaxis in patients with a CD4TL count < 200/mcL also decreases the incidence of bacterial pneumonia by 67%.

2. Pneumococcal vaccines

   a. Two pneumococcal vaccines are recommended in HIV-infected persons: the conjugated pneumococcal vaccine (Prevnar-13) and the 23-valent polysaccharide pneumococcal vaccine. Both decreases pneumococcal disease significantly, but the combination is superior.

   b. The 23-valent polysaccharide pneumococcal vaccine covers 86% of serotypes but is not as immunogenic as the 13-valent conjugated pneumococcal vaccine.

   c. CDC recommends pneumococcal vaccine use as early as possible in HIV infection. Vaccination should be delayed 4 weeks in individuals initiating ART to allow for immune reconstitution. Usually, the conjugated pneumococcal vaccine is administered first and the polysaccharide vaccine 2 months later.

   d. A polysaccharide pneumococcal vaccine booster is recommended every 5 years. A booster may also be useful in patients whose initial CD4TL is < 200/mcL after significant immune reconstitution occurs (an increase of CD4TL > 100/mcL).

3. *Smoking cessation is strongly recommended.* HIV-infected persons die of tobacco-associated malignancy and chronic obstructive pulmonary disease at a much higher rate than the general population. Counseling patients again and again to stop smoking is essential.

4. Therapy for typical bacterial pneumonia is usually initiated empirically.

5. Antibiotics must cover frequent etiologies (*S pneumoniae, S aureus, H influenzae, M pneumoniae,* and *P aeruginosa*). Local resistance patterns should be considered.

6. There should be a low threshold for including anti-methicillin-resistant *S aureus* coverage particularly in patients with a history of injection drug use; patients receiving hemodialysis; MSMs; and patients with severe, presumably bacterial pneumonia during influenza season.

7. *Pseudomonas* coverage

   a. Should be considered when the CD4TL is low.

   b. Treated with an antipseudomonal beta-lactam antibiotic (piperacillin, ceftazidime, cefepime, meropenem)

   c. An aminoglycoside (usually tobramycin) may be added initially pending susceptibility data, but there is no benefit of continuing tobramycin if *Pseudomonas* is susceptible to the antipseudomonal beta-lactam.

8. Patients with uncomplicated pneumonia have a time course of clinical and radiologic response to therapy similar to non–HIV-infected persons.

MAKING A DIAGNOSIS

 Serial sputum samples are sent for AFB smear and culture. All AFB stains are negative.

 Have you crossed a diagnostic threshold for the leading hypothesis, bacterial pneumonia? Have you ruled out the active alternatives? Do other tests need to be done to exclude the alternative diagnoses?

A critical decision at this point in the evaluation of an HIV-infected patient with pulmonary complaints is whether the patient needs bronchoscopy with BAL to establish the etiologic agent. In HIV-positive patients with infiltrates, BAL is highly sensitive (86%). Transbronchial biopsy increases the sensitivity further to 96%. Due to the large number of potential pathogens, empiric treatment is often inappropriate *except* in the cases in which bacterial pneumonia is strongly suspected. Acute onset and focal infiltrates suggest bacterial pneumonia whereas subacute/chronic progression, diffuse infiltrates, and cavitary lesions suggest other etiologies. Bronchoscopy is often necessary in such cases unless sputum analysis is diagnostic (positive AFB or rarely positive silver stain). Figure 5-4 suggests one possible diagnostic algorithm. Mr. L' s acute illness, and focal findings on the chest radiograph strongly suggest bacterial pneumonia. You wonder if PTB would present similarly in an HIV-positive patient with this CD4TL count.

Alternative Diagnosis: Pulmonary TB in AIDS Patients[1]

Textbook Presentation

PTB typically presents subacutely with cough and fever that have gone on for over a week (and often much longer) and systemic symptoms of night sweats and weight loss are common. In patients with CD4TL > 200/mcL, the chest radiographic pattern is similar to non–HIV-infected patients—that is, with apical, cavitary, or nodular infiltrates. In patients with CD4TL < 200/mcL, the pattern on chest radiograph is often atypical: lower lobe infiltrates, miliary infiltrates

---

[1]TB in the non–HIV-infected patients is covered in Chapter 10, Cough, Fever, & Respiratory Infections.

and lymphadenopathy are more common. Extrapulmonary TB is also more common.

Disease Highlights

A. More worldwide cases of TB currently than at any time in human history

B. HIV-infected persons at highest risk for TB (170 times higher incidence).

    1. Risk increases further in patients from endemic areas and among injection drug users.

    2. 6000–9000 new cases in the United States each year

C. TB in turn increases both HIV replication and the risk of death.

D. Worldwide TB accounts for 30% of HIV-related deaths.

E. Epidemic in sub-Saharan Africa and parts of Asia

F. 50% of cases secondary to recent infection

G. TB may be the first manifestation of HIV infection and is an AIDS-defining illness.

 All patients with TB should be tested for HIV.

H. Clinical characteristics

    1. Early HIV infection: PTB is fairly typical.

    2. Advanced HIV infection

      a. Extrapulmonary TB more frequent

        (1) More common in the AIDS population (30%) than in patients without AIDS (15%)

        (2) Most common sites of extrapulmonary TB include blood, lymph nodes, bone marrow, genitourinary tract, CNS, and liver. 19% of patients had cervical or supraclavicular lymph node involvement.

        (3) Other syndromes seen in these patients include weight loss, fever of unknown origin, and TB meningitis.

      b. Chest radiographic pattern more frequently atypical (see below).

 Extrapulmonary TB is common in HIV-infected patients and extrapulmonary sites of infections may provide a target for procedures.

Evidence-Based Diagnosis

A. Prolonged fever (> 7 days) more common in HIV-infected persons with PTB than in PCP or bacterial pneumonia (sensitivity, 56%; specificity, 78%; LR+, 2.5; LR–, 0.57).

B. Weight loss also more common with PTB than with PCP or bacterial pneumonia (sensitivity, 66.7%; specificity, 68%; LR+, 2.08; LR–, 0.49).

C. Standard tests in patients with suspected PTB should include chest radiograph (with posteroanterior and lateral views), 3 sputum AFB stains and cultures, PPD or interferon gamma release assay, and blood and urine cultures.

D. Chest radiography

    1. Certain radiographic findings, including cavitary lesions, hilar lymphadenopathy, and nodular lesions, are infrequent but suggestive of PTB (Table 5-6).

    2. However, the radiographic manifestations of PTB vary with degree of immunosuppression (Table 5-7).

      a. Early HIV infection (CD4TL > 200/mcL): chest radiograph usually shows the typical reactivation

Table 5-6. Diagnostic accuracy of radiographic findings in HIV-infected patients for tuberculosis.

Radiographic Finding	Sensitivity	Specificity	LR+	LR–
Cavitary lesions	16.7%	98.4%	10.72	0.85
Hilar lymphadenopathy	11.1%	98.4%	7.15	0.90
Nodular lesions	25.0%	92.7%	3.45	0.81

Table 5-7. Frequency (%) of radiographic manifestations in HIV-infected patients with TB: Influence of CD4 count.

Radiographic Finding	CD4 Count (cells/mcL)		
	> 400	200–399	< 200
Cavitary lesions	63	44	29
Hilar lymphadenopathy	0	14	20
Pleural effusions	3	11	11
Miliary pattern	0	6	9

      pattern: upper lobe disease or apical segment of lower lobe with or without cavitation

      b. Advanced HIV infection (CD4TL count < 200/mcL):

        (1) Middle and lower lobe consolidation, lymph node enlargement, pleural effusions, and miliary patterns are more often seen.

        (2) Pleural involvement is more common.

          (a) Often accompanied by fever (85%), cough (77%), and chest pain (36%). Weight loss is common (74%).

          (b) Unilateral exudative effusion

          (c) Concomitant lower lobe parenchymal infiltrate present in 44–73%

    3. Cavitary lesions with night sweats or prolonged fever (> 7 days) is not sensitive for PTB but is virtually diagnostic (sensitivity, 8–11%; LR+, ∞).

    4. Hilar lymphadenopathy with weight loss or with prolonged cough (> 7 days) is not sensitive for TB but is highly suggestive (sensitivity, 8%; LR+, 8–∞).

 The chest radiograph in HIV-infected patients with PTB may be typical or atypical. PTB should be considered in patients with apical or cavitary disease, nodular infiltrates, or lymphadenopathy.

    5. Chest radiograph is normal in 10–21% of patients with PTB and advanced disease.

 PTB can be present despite a normal chest radiograph and should be considered in HIV-positive patients with CD4TL < 200/mcL and pulmonary symptoms.

E. PPD and interferon gamma release assay: sensitivity depends on the degree of immunosuppression.

    1. CD4TL > 300/mcL: PPD and interferon gamma release assay 90% sensitive

2. CD4TL < 100/mcL: PPD and interferon gamma release assay have different sensitivities

    a. PPD 0% sensitive.

    b. Interferon gamma release assay test interpretation is complex in patients CD4TL < 100/mcL. Most such patients have indeterminate results which are not diagnostic. However, a negative result makes the diagnosis of TB less likely.

F. Sputum analysis

  1. AFB smear results

    a. Poor sensitivity (29–60%) is often due to the patient's inability to produce adequate sputum. Sensitivity is 67% in patients able to produce adequate sputum.

    b. Specificity falls at lower CD4TL counts due to increasing incidence of MAI but remains remarkably high in this group (92%).

  2. AFB culture

    a. Sensitivity ranges from 43% to 100%. Sensitivity approaches 100% in patients able to produce adequate sputum.

    b. Induced sputum positive in 50% of patients with pleural TB without pulmonary infiltrates

G. *Mycobacterium tuberculosis* PCR testing of sputum

  1. Helps distinguish PTB from MAI, *M kansasii* or colonizing/contaminating nontuberculous mycobacteria (often *M gordonae*)

  2. Primarily used when AFB stains positive

  3. Particularly useful if suspicion of PTB is low

    a. Positive rapid tests help confirm PTB, negative tests make PTB less likely

    b. 95% sensitive and specific in this situation

  4. Also useful when clinical suspicion is high and smear negative

    a. Rapid tests reported 53% sensitive, 93% specific.

    b. Positive tests suggest PTB

    c. Cultures still required to test drug susceptibility

  5. A diagnostic algorithm is shown in Figure 5-5.

H. Blood culture for mycobacteria

  1. Blood cultures are positive in 26–42% of HIV-positive patients with TB.

  2. Sensitivity increases to 49% in patients with CD4TL < 100/mcL.

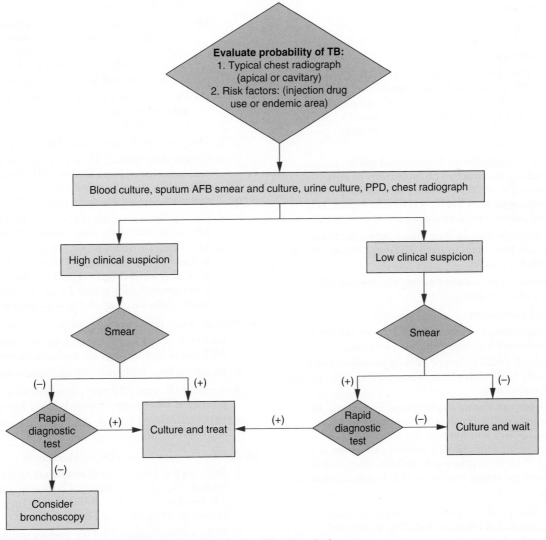

AFB, acid-fast bacillus; PPD, purified protein derivative; TB, tuberculosis.

Figure 5-5. Diagnosis of pulmonary tuberculosis: role of rapid diagnostic tests.

I. Bronchoscopy

1. Smear sensitivity: 50–57%; specificity: 99% in endemic area

2. Culture sensitivity: nearly 100%

3. Some studies report similar sensitivities to *induced* sputum.

4. Bronchoscopy associated with increased transmission of TB to medical personnel. Risk is minimal if bronchoscopy is performed in a pressure negative room.

5. Induced sputum is preferred.

6. If bronchoscopy is performed for suspected PTB, transbronchial biopsy is recommended to diagnose miliary TB.

J. Pleural evaluation

1. Pleural fluid smear is positive in 15%.

2. Culture of pleural fluid is positive in 33–90%.

3. Sputum smear or culture in patients with pleural TB is positive in 33–50%. Sputum may be positive in patients *without* parenchymal infiltrate.

4. Effusion is unilateral and exudative with lymphocyte predominance.

5. Pleural biopsy

   a. Positive smear: 44–69%

   b. Positive pathology (granuloma): 88%

Treatment

A. Chemoprophylaxis

1. Indicated for HIV-infected patients who have either a positive PPD (5 mm) or a positive interferon gamma release assay; also indicated for HIV-infected patients who have had a recent and significant exposure to persons with infectious PTB regardless of PPD/ interferon gamma release assay results.

2. A chest radiograph should be performed and the patient evaluated to rule out active TB (pulmonary or extra-pulmonary). In addition, even in patients with a normal chest radiograph but CD4TL < 200/mcL, sputum AFB stain and culture should be obtained.

3. Isoniazid prophylaxis for 9 months decreases the rate of progression from latent to active TB from 7.4% to 2.6% in HIV-infected patients.

4. Patients should be evaluated monthly to monitor adherence and side effects of therapy.

5. Isoniazid liver toxicity

   a. Transaminases are elevated in 10–20% of patients, but symptomatic hepatitis is much less common.

   b. Isoniazid should be stopped if transaminase elevation exceeds 5× the upper limit of normal, even if the patient is asymptomatic.

   c. Patients with alcohol abuse, chronic liver disease, or coinfection with hepatitis B or C virus should have monthly liver function tests to rule out isoniazid-induced hepatitis. All HIV-infected patients are at higher risk for hepatotoxicity (NASH, drug adverse effects) and should receive monthly liver function tests.

B. Active TB

1. Active TB is usually treated with rifampin, isoniazid, pyrazinamide, and ethambutol (RIPE). If the isolate is susceptible to rifampin and isoniazid, ethambutol is stopped. After 2 months of therapy, pyrazinamide is stopped. Rifampin and isoniazid are continued to complete 6 months of therapy.

2. Treating TB in HIV is complicated by clinically important drug interactions; consultation is recommended. Rifampin is rarely used in HIV patients because rifabutin interactions are easier to manage.

3. Directly observed therapy is recommended for all patients with active TB, including HIV-positive patients.

   a. Decreases relapse rate from 20% to 5%

   b. Decreases development of multi-drug resistant TB from 6% to 1%

4. Monthly follow-up sputum cultures are obtained: if the 2-month culture remains positive, treatment is extended from 6 to 9 months.

5. Multidrug resistance is a major health problem.

   a. Definitions

      (1) Drug-resistant TB is resistant to any of the first-line drugs (rifampin, isoniazid, pyrazinamide or ethambutol).

      (2) Streptomycin resistance is so common that streptomycin is no longer considered a first-line drug nor a very useful antituberculous drug.

      (3) Multi-drug resistant TB is defined as resistance to both rifampin and isoniazid.

      (4) Extensively drug resistant TB is defined as resistance to rifampin, isoniazid, fluoroquinolones (ciprofloxacin, moxifloxacin, levofloxacin) and 1 of the injectable second-line antituberculous drugs (capreomycin and specific aminoglycosides).

      (5) Drug-resistant TB is more common in HIV patients, but multi-drug resistant TB is uncommon in the United States.

   b. Drug-resistant TB arises in nonadherent patients.

   c. Suspect drug-resistant TB in patients with prior TB treatment, contact with known multi-drug resistant TB or immigrants from countries where multi-drug resistant or extensively drug resistant TB is prevalent.

   d. Case fatality rate is high in patients with multi-drug resistant or extensively drug resistant TB and HIV.

   e. Multi-drug resistant TB typically requires 5 to 6 drugs, including 3 drugs to which TB is susceptible. Expertise in treating multi-drug resistant TB is required. Therapy is recommended for at least 2 years. Surgical resection of localized disease is required in some patients.

C. Immune reconstitution inflammatory syndrome (IRIS)

1. Infiltrates worsen in 36% of patients upon institution of ART due to immunologically mediated reactions (ie IRIS).

2. Increasing fever, infiltrates, and adenopathy may be seen.

3. A second OI, poor adherence, drug resistance, or low potency of TB regimen needs to be excluded.

4. IRIS is usually self-limited with PTB, but more severe reactions benefit from corticosteroids.

D. Bacillus Calmette-Guérin (BCG) vaccination

1. BCG is a live-attenuated *Mycobacterium bovis* strain with limited efficacy: it may prevent TB meningitis and miliary TB, but does not prevent the more common presentations of primary or reactivation TB.

2. BCG is contraindicated in HIV-positive patients due to increased incidence of active infection or dissemination of the BCG strain.

CASE RESOLUTION

Mr. L's acute presentation and chest radiograph suggest bacterial pneumonia. PCP and MAC are unlikely given his relatively high CD4TL count. Similarly, TB would be unlikely with such an acute presentation. Furthermore, at this CD4TL level, TB would be expected to present more typically (ie, with upper lobe or apical segment of lower lobe disease). The LR of bacterial pneumonia given the acuity of symptoms and lobar infiltrate is 8.0. Therefore, empiric therapy for bacterial pneumonia would be appropriate. Bronchoscopy should be performed if Mr. L does not respond promptly to antibiotic therapy.

Mr. L is given ceftriaxone and azithromycin. Urinary antigen is positive for *S pneumoniae* and blood cultures return in 36 hours positive for *S pneumoniae*, sensitive to penicillin. Mr. L is treated with IV penicillin and improves over the next 3–4 days.

Table 5-8 summarizes the predictive value of clinical, radiologic, and combined findings for the diagnosis of bacterial pneumonia, PCP, and TB in HIV-infected patients.

REVIEW OF OTHER IMPORTANT DISEASES

Mycobacterium avium/intracellulare (MAI)

Textbook Presentation

MAI typically presents with constitutional symptoms, including fever, drenching sweats, and weight loss.

Disease Highlights

A. MAI (also known as MAC) refers to *M avium* and *M intracellulare*. *M avium* is by far the most common nontuberculous mycobacteria in AIDS patients.

B. *M avium* is acquired through inhalation or ingestion.

C. No human-to-human transmission

D. Infection is common in immunocompetent persons and pulmonary MAI disease may be progressive and require treatment.

E. Disseminated MAI infection
1. Usually occurs in patients with profound immunosuppression.
   a. CD4TL < 50/mcL in almost all disseminated MAI cases
   b. Mean CD4TL 7/mcL
2. Disseminated MAI involves the liver, spleen, gastrointestinal tract, lungs, and bone marrow.
   a. Cultures of blood, bone marrow, and urine may be positive.
   b. Predominantly pulmonary disease or gastrointestinal disease is seen uncommonly.
   c. Constitutional symptoms predominate.
3. MAI detection in sputum and stool often indicate colonization rather than disease.
4. Pulmonary disease occurs in < 5% of patients with disseminated disease. Nodules, infiltrates, lymphadenopathy, and cavities may be seen.

F. Marked decreased incidence of disseminated MAI since the introduction of ART.

Evidence-Based Diagnosis

A. Signs and symptoms
1. Fever: 18–87%
2. Night sweats: 78%
3. Cough: 78%
4. Diarrhea: 32–47%
5. Weight loss: 32–100%
6. Hepatosplenomegaly: 24%

B. Laboratory findings
1. Anemia: 85%
2. Increased alkaline phosphatase: 45–53%

C. Culture
1. Blood culture for AFB: 50–95% sensitive
2. Bone marrow culture: 82% sensitive

D. Sputum
1. Smears may be positive for AFB.
2. Rapid PCR testing can distinguish MAI from TB in patients with positive AFB smears.

E. Chest radiograph
1. Usually normal
2. May demonstrate patchy consolidation, nodules, or cavities

Treatment

A. Primary MAI prevention
1. Recommended for patients with CD4TL < 50/mcL. Options include azithromycin weekly or clarithromycin twice daily.
2. Therapy may be discontinued in patients responding to ART with CD4TL > 100/mcL for 3 months.

B. Treatment of MAI infection
1. Therapy usually includes clarithromycin and ethambutol, plus in sicker patients rifabutin. Drug interactions are complex and infectious disease consultation is mandatory.
2. Susceptibility testing to macrolides should be performed at baseline and whenever patients do not respond to the treatment regimen.
3. Therapy may be discontinued after 1 year in patients responding to ART with CD4TL > 100/mcL for more than 6 months.
4. Pulmonary infiltrates, hepatosplenomegaly, lymphadenopathy, or systemic symptoms may develop anew or worsen during institution of ART therapy (IRIS).

Kaposi Sarcoma

Textbook Presentation

The rash is usually seen in HIV-positive MSM who have nodular, nontender, pink to violaceous papules and nodules.

Disease Highlights

A. Human herpes virus 8 associated with HIV causes the angioproliferation seen in Kaposi sarcoma.

Table 5-8. The predictive value of clinical, radiologic, and combined findings for the diagnosis of bacterial pneumonia, Pneumocystis pneumonia, and tuberculosis in HIV-infected patients.

	Finding	LR+
Bacterial pneumonia		
Clinical findings	Toxic appearing	4.8
	Purulent sputum	1.9
Chest radiographic findings	Lobar infiltrate	5.6
Combined findings	Lobar infiltrate and cough ≤ 7 days	11.5
	Lobar infiltrate and pleuritic chest pain	10
Pneumocystis pneumonia		
Clinical findings	Clear sputum	2.3
	Dyspneic appearing	2.4
	Dyspnea on exertion	2.0
	Oral thrush	1.8
Chest radiographic findings	Diffuse infiltrate	2.3
	Interstitial infiltrate	4.3
Combined findings	Interstitial pattern and dyspnea on exertion	7.25
	Interstitial pattern and oral thrush	7.2
Tuberculosis		
Clinical findings	Fever > 1 week	2.5
	Weight loss	2.1
Chest radiographic findings	Cavitary lesion	10.7
	Hilar lymphadenopathy	7.2
	Nodular pattern	3.5
Combined findings	Cavitary and (night sweats or fever > 1 week)	∞
	Hilar lymphadenopathy and cough > 1 week	8

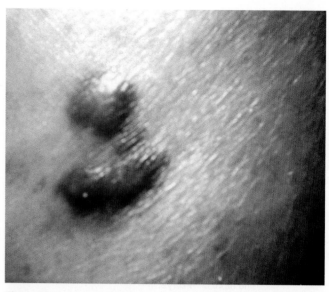

Figure 5-6. Kaposi sarcoma in an AIDS patient.

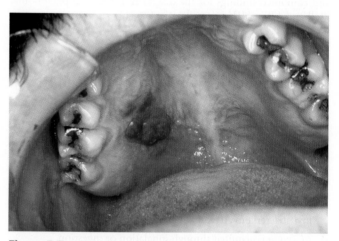

Figure 5-7. Involvement of oral cavity in AIDS patient with Kaposi sarcoma.

B. Most affected patients are MSMs. Individual lesions are pink, red, or purple, and nontender in most cases.

C. Lesions on the extremities, trunk, and face

D. With decreasing CD4TL, the number of lesions increases.

E. Skin involvement is almost always present in Kaposi sarcoma (Figure 5-6).

F. Extracutaneous involvement includes oral cavity (Figure 5-7), gastrointestinal tract, lymph nodes, and lungs.

G. Gastrointestinal involvement is common (40%) but usually asymptomatic. Occasionally, bleeding and perforation occur.

H. Pleuropulmonary involvement is common in advanced Kaposi sarcoma.

   1. Presentations of pulmonary Kaposi sarcoma include lung nodules, infiltrates, dyspnea, pleural effusions, and respiratory failure.

   2. Patient survival is shortened.

I. The incidence of Kaposi sarcoma has decreased dramatically, only in part due to the introduction of effective ART. A change in sexual behavior has also contributed to this decline.

Evidence-Based Diagnosis

A. Skin biopsy shows the typical angioproliferation with slit-like vascular spaces and spindle cells.

B. Immunohistochemistry can detect human herpes virus 8 in the endothelial cells.

C. Gastrointestinal Kaposi sarcoma: endoscopy is clinically suggestive, but the submucosal location of lesions makes tissue diagnosis difficult.

D. Pulmonary Kaposi sarcoma: high-resolution chest CT suggestive; bronchoscopy may show the lesions.

Treatment

Effective ART is highly effective in early Kaposi sarcoma, but chemotherapy is required in pulmonary involvement.

REFERENCES

Aberg JA, Gallant JE Ghanem KG, Emmanuel P Zingman BS, Horberg MA. Primary Care Guidelines for the Management of Persons Infected With HIV: 2013 Update by the HIV Medicine Association of the Infectious Diseases Society of America. Clin Infect Dis.2014;58(1):e1–34.

Achhra AC, Amin J, Law MG et al.Immunodeficiency and the risk of serious clinical endpoints in a well studied cohort of treated HIV-infected patients. AIDS.2010;24(12):1877–86.

Afessa B, Green B. Bacterial pneumonia in hospitalized patients with HIV infection: the Pulmonary Complications ICU Support and Prognostic Factors of Hospitalized Patients with HIV (PIP) Study. Chest.2000;117(4):1017–22.

Basso U, Brandes AA. Diagnostic advances and new trends for the treatment of primary central nervous system lymphoma. Eur J Can.2002;38(10):1298–312.

Berenguer J, Miralles P, Arrizabalaga J et al. Clinical course and prognostic factors of progressive multifocal leukoencephalopathy in patients treated with highly active antiretroviral therapy. Clin Infect Dis.2003;36(8):1047–52.

Boiselle PM, Tocino I, Hooley RJ et al.Chest radiograph interpretation of *Pneumocystis carinii* pneumonia, bacterial pneumonia, and pulmonary tuberculosis in HIV-positive patients: accuracy, distinguishing features, and mimics. J Thorac Imaging. 1997;12(1):47–53.

Chuck SL, Sande MA. Infections with *Cryptococcus neoformans* in the acquired immunodeficiency syndrome. N Engl J Med. 1989;321:794–9.

de Souza MC, Nitrini R. Effects of human immunodeficiency virus infection on the manifestations of neurosyphilis. Neurology.1997;49(3):893–4.

Eggers CH; German Neuro-AIDS Working Group. HIV-1 associated encephalopathy and myelopathy. J Neurol. 2002;249(8):1132–6.

Havlir DV, Barnes PF. Tuberculosis in patients with human immunodeficiency virus infection. N Engl J Med.1999;340(5):367–73.

Jones D, Havlir DV. Nontuberculous mycobacteria in the HIV infected patient. Clin Chest Med.2002;23(3):665–74.

Kovascs JA, Masur H. Prophylaxis against opportunistic infections in patients with human immunodeficiency virus infection. N Engl J Med.2000;342(19):1416–29.

Lin J, Nichol KL. Excess mortality due to pneumonia or influenza during influenza seasons among persons with acquired immunodeficiency syndrome. Arch Intern Med.2001;161(3):441–6.

Mamidi A, Desimone JA, Pomerantz RJ. Central nervous system infections in individuals with HIV-1 infection. J Neurovirology.2002;8(3):158–67.

McCutchan JA. Cytomegalovirus infections of the nervous system in patients with AIDS. Clin Infect Dis.1995;20(4):747–54.

Mellors JW, Munoz A, Giorgi JV et al.Plasma viral load and CD4+ lymphocytes as prognostic markers of HIV-1 infection. Ann Intern Med. 1997;126(12):946–54.

Panel on Antiretroviral Guidelines for Adults and Adolescents. Guidelines for the use of antiretroviral agents in HIV-1-infected adults and adolescents. Department of Health and Human Services. Last Updated on February 12, 2013. Accessed on December 24, 2013. Available at http://aidsinfo.nih.gov/ContentFiles/Adultand AdolescentGL.pdf.

Panel on Opportunistic Infections in HIV-Infected Adults and Adolescents. Guidelines for the prevention and treatment of opportunistic infections in HIV-infected adults and adolescents: recommendations from the Centers for Disease Control and Prevention, the National Institutes of Health, and the HIV Medicine Association of the Infectious Diseases Society of America. Last Updated on July 7 2013. Accessed on 12-24-2013. Available at http://aidsinfo.nih.gov/contentfiles/lvguidelines/adult_oi.pdf

Polsky B, Gold JW, Whimbey E et al.Bacterial pneumonia in patients with the acquired immunodeficiency syndrome. Ann Intern Med. 1986;104(1):38–41.

Raoof S, Rosen MJ, Khan FA. Role of bronchoscopy in AIDS. Clin Chest Med.1999;20(1):63–76.

Reichenberger F, Cathomas G, Weber R, Schoenenberger R, Tamm M. Recurrent fever and pulmonary infiltrates in an HIV-positive patient. Respiration.2001;68(5):548–54.

Shrosbree J, Campbell LJ, Ibrahim F et al.Late HIV diagnosis is a major risk factor for intensive care unit admission in HIV-positive patients: a single centre observational cohort study. BMC Infectious Diseases 2013;1323.

Skiest DJ, Crosby C. Survival is prolonged by highly active antiretroviral therapy in AIDS patients with primary central nervous system lymphoma. AIDS.2003;17(12):1787–93.

Zuger A, Louie E Holzman RS, Simberkoff MS, Rahal JJ. Cryptococcal disease in patients with the acquired immunodeficiency syndrome. Ann Intern Med.1986;104(2):234–40.

I have a patient with anemia. How do I determine the cause?

CHIEF COMPLAINT

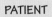

PATIENT ⟨1⟩

Mrs. A is a 48-year-old white woman who has had 2 months of fatigue due to anemia.

What is the differential diagnosis of anemia? How would you frame the differential?

CONSTRUCTING A DIFFERENTIAL DIAGNOSIS

Anemia can occur in isolation, or as a consequence of a process causing pancytopenia, the reduction of all 3 cell lines (white blood cells [WBCs], platelets, and red blood cells [RBCs]). This chapter focuses on the approach to isolated anemia, although a brief list of causes of pancytopenia appears in Figure 6-1. The first step in determining the cause of anemia is to identify the general mechanism of the anemia and organize the mechanisms using a pathophysiologic framework:

A. **Acute blood loss:** this is generally clinically obvious.

B. **Underproduction** of RBCs by the bone marrow; chronic blood loss is included in this category because it leads to iron deficiency, which ultimately results in underproduction.

C. Increased **destruction** of RBCs, called **hemolysis**.

Patients should always be assessed for signs and symptoms of acute blood loss.

A. Signs of acute blood loss
   1. Hypotension
   2. Tachycardia
   3. Large ecchymoses

B. Symptoms of acute blood loss
   1. Hematemesis
   2. Melena
   3. Rectal bleeding
   4. Hematuria
   5. Vaginal bleeding
   6. Hemoptysis

After excluding acute blood loss, the next pivotal step is to distinguish underproduction from hemolysis by checking the reticulocyte count:

A. Low or normal reticulocyte counts are seen in underproduction anemias.

B. High reticulocyte counts occur when the bone marrow is responding normally to blood loss; hemolysis; or replacement of iron, vitamin B_{12}, or folate.

C. Reticulocyte measures include:
   1. The **reticulocyte count:** the percentage of circulating RBCs that are reticulocytes (normally 0.5–1.5%).
   2. The **absolute reticulocyte count;** the number of reticulocytes actually circulating, normally 25,000–75,000/mcL (multiply the percentage of reticulocytes by the total number of RBCs).
   3. The **reticulocyte production index (RPI)**
      a. Corrects the reticulocyte count for the degree of anemia and for the prolonged peripheral maturation of reticulocytes that occurs in anemia.
         (1) Normally, the first 3–3.5 days of reticulocyte maturation occurs in the bone marrow and the last 24 hours in the peripheral blood.
         (2) When the bone marrow is stimulated, reticulocytes are released prematurely, leading to longer maturation times in the periphery, and larger numbers of reticulocytes present at any given time.
         (3) For a HCT of 25%, the peripheral blood maturation time is 2 days, and for a HCT of 15%, it is 2.5 days; the value of 2 is generally used in the RPI calculation.
      b. $RPI = \dfrac{\text{observed reticulocyte\%} \times (\text{Patient Hct}/45)}{\text{peripheral blood maturation time in days}}$
      c. The normal RPI is about 1.0. In the setting of anemia, values < 2.0 indicate underproduction; those > 2.0 indicate hemolysis or an adequate bone marrow response to acute blood loss or replacement of iron or vitamins.

The first steps in evaluating anemia are looking for acute blood loss and checking the RPI in patients who are not acutely bleeding.

After determining the general mechanism, the next step in diagnosing the cause of anemia is to determine the cause of the underproduction or increased destruction. Traditionally, the differential diagnosis for underproduction anemia is framed using the cell size. While this is a useful way to organize the differential, and may at times provide useful clues, it is important to keep in mind that the mean corpuscular volume (MCV) is not specific and should not be used to rule in or rule out a specific cause of anemia.

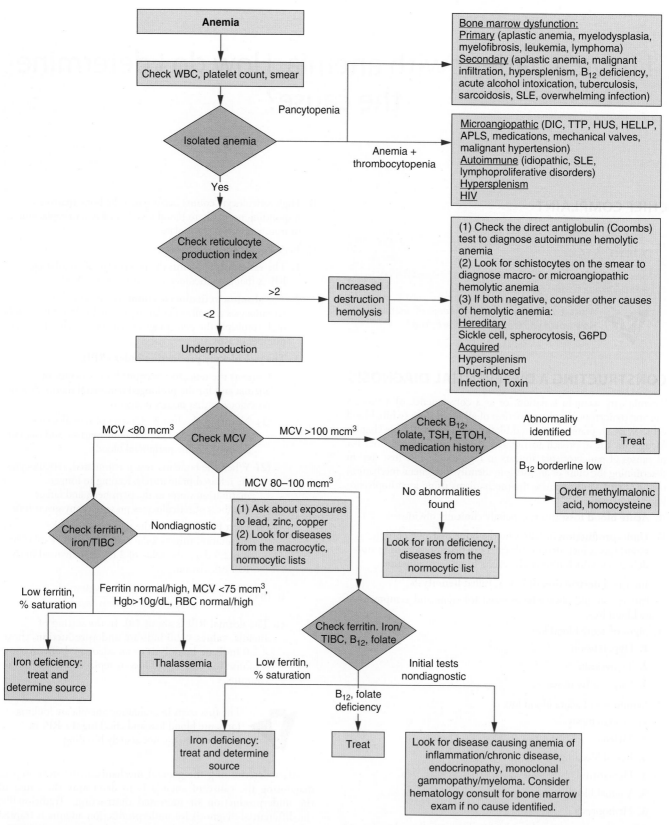

APLS, antiphospholipid syndrome; DIC, disseminated intravascular coagulation; ETOH, alcohol; G6PD, glucose-6-phosphate dehydrogenase; HELLP, hemolysis, elevated liver enzymes, and low platelet count; HUS, hemolytic uremic syndrome; MCV, mean corpuscular volume; SLE, systemic lupus erythematosus; TIBC, total iron-binding capacity; TTP, thrombotic thrombocytopenic purpura.

Figure 6-1. Diagnostic approach: anemia.

Use the MCV to organize your thinking, not to diagnose the cause of an anemia.

A. Microcytic anemias (MCV < 80 mcm³)

1. Iron deficiency

2. Thalassemia

3. Anemia of inflammation/chronic disease (more often normocytic)

4. Sideroblastic anemia (congenital, lead exposure, medications)—rare

5. Copper deficiency or zinc poisoning—rare

B. Macrocytic anemias (MCV > 100 mcm³)

1. Megaloblastic anemias (due to abnormalities in DNA synthesis; hypersegmented neutrophils also occur)

   a. Vitamin B$_{12}$ deficiency

   b. Folate deficiency

   c. Antimetabolite drugs, such as methotrexate or zidovudine

2. Nonmegaloblastic anemias (no hypersegmented neutrophils)

   a. Alcohol abuse

   b. Liver disease

   c. Hypothyroidism

   d. Myelodysplastic syndrome (often causes pancytopenia)

C. Normocytic anemias

1. Anemia of inflammation/chronic disease (chronic kidney disease, infection, inflammation, malignancy, aging)

2. Early iron deficiency

3. Bone marrow suppression

   a. Invasion by malignancy or granulomas

   b. Acquired pure red cell aplasia (parvovirus B19, HIV, medications [mycophenolate mofetil, trimethoprim-sulfamethoxazole, phenytoin, recombinant human erythropoietins], thymoma, other malignancies, immune disorders)

   c. Aplastic anemia (often causes pancytopenia)

4. Endocrine (hypopituitarism or hypothyroidism)

The framework for hemolytic anemias is pathophysiologic:

A. Hereditary

1. Enzyme defects, such as pyruvate kinase or glucose-6-phosphate dehydrogenase (G6PD) deficiency

2. Hemoglobinopathies, such as sickle cell anemia

3. RBC membrane abnormalities, such as spherocytosis

B. Acquired

1. Hypersplenism

2. Immune

   a. Autoimmune: warm IgG, cold IgM, cold IgG

   b. Drug induced: autoimmune or hapten

3. Mechanical

   a. Macroangiopathic (marching, prosthetic valves)

   b. Microangiopathic: disseminated intravascular coagulation (DIC), thrombotic thrombocytopenic purpura (TTP), and hemolytic uremic syndrome (HUS)

4. Infections, such as malaria

5. Toxins, such as snake venom and aniline dyes

Figure 6-1 outlines the approach to evaluating anemia, assuming acute bleeding has been excluded.

Mrs. A has a past medical history of obesity, reflux, depression, asthma, and osteoarthritis. She comes to your office complaining of feeling down, with progressive fatigue for the last 2 months. She has no chest pain, cough, fever, weight loss, or edema. Her only GI symptoms are poor appetite and her usual reflux symptoms; she has had no vomiting, melena, or rectal bleeding. She still has regular menses that are occasionally heavy. She brought in her medication bottles, which include ranitidine, sertraline, tramadol, cetirizine, and a fluticasone inhaler. Her physical exam shows a depressed affect, clear lungs, a normal cardiac exam, a nontender abdomen, guaiac-negative stool, no edema, and no pallor.

 How reliable is the history and physical for detecting anemia?

A. Symptoms in chronic anemia are due to decreased oxygen delivery to the tissues.

1. Fatigue is a common but not very specific symptom.

2. Dyspnea on exertion often occurs.

3. Exertional chest pain occurs most often in patients with underlying coronary artery disease or severe anemia or both.

4. Palpitations or tachycardia can occur.

5. Edema is sometimes seen.

   a. It is due to decreased renal blood flow leading to neurohormonal activation and salt and water retention, similar to that seen in heart failure.

   b. However, in contrast to the low cardiac output seen in patients with heart failure, the cardiac output in patients with anemia is high.

6. Mild anemia is often asymptomatic.

B. Symptoms of hypovolemia occur only in acute anemia caused by large volume blood loss.

C. Conjunctival rim pallor

1. Present when the anterior rim of the inferior palpebral conjunctiva is the same pale pink color as the deeper posterior aspect, rather than the normal bright red color of the anterior rim.

 2. The presence of conjunctival rim pallor strongly suggests the patient is anemic (LR+ 16.7).

3. However, the absence of pallor does not rule out anemia.

D. Palmar crease pallor has an LR+ of 7.9.

E. Pallor elsewhere (facial, nail bed) is not as useful, with LR+ < 5.

F. No physical sign rules out anemia.

G. The overall sensitivity and specificity of the physical exam for anemia is about 70%.

 Order a CBC if patients have symptoms that suggest anemia, even without physical exam signs, or if you observe conjunctival rim or palmar crease pallor.

Mrs. A's initial laboratory test results show a WBC of 7100/mcL, RBC of 2.6 million/mcL, Hgb of 6.7 g/dL, HCT of 23.3%, and MCV of 76 mcm³. Her platelet count is normal. A CBC 6 months ago showed an Hgb of 12 g/dL, HCT of 36%, and MCV of 82 mcm³.

At this point, what is the leading hypothesis, what are the active alternatives, and is there a must not miss diagnosis? Given this differential diagnosis, what tests should be ordered?

RANKING THE DIFFERENTIAL DIAGNOSIS

The first step is to determine the mechanism of Mrs. A's anemia. Mrs. A is not having any symptoms or signs of acute blood loss. She does have clinical findings suggestive of diseases associated with chronic blood loss: reflux possibly causing esophagitis and occasional menorrhagia. However, it is not possible to distinguish underproduction from hemolysis based on the history. Although the change in her CBC tells you a new process is going on, it also does not distinguish between these 2 mechanisms. The first pivotal point will be her reticulocyte count.

Always look at previous CBC results to see if the anemia is new, old, or progressive.

Mrs. A's reticulocyte count is 1.5%, which is an absolute reticulocyte count of 54,000/mcL, and an RPI of 0.39.

Now that you have found that Mrs. A has an underproduction anemia, what is the leading hypothesis, what are the active alternatives, and is there a must not miss diagnosis? Given this differential diagnosis, what tests should be ordered?

Mrs. A's MCV is 76 mcm³, so you should consider the differential diagnosis for microcytic anemia. However, it is important to keep in mind that the MCV is not specific and should not be used to rule in or rule out a specific cause of anemia.

A. In one study, normal MCVs were found in 50% of patients with abnormal serum vitamin B_{12}, folate, or iron studies.

  1. 5% of patients with iron deficiency had high MCVs

  2. 12% of patients with vitamin B_{12} or folate deficiency had low MCVs

B. What about the rest of the CBC? Do the other indices help?

  1. Other red cell indices (mean corpuscular hemoglobin [MCH] and mean corpuscular hemoglobin concentration [MCHC]) tend to trend with the MCV and are not particularly sensitive or specific.

  2. The red cell distribution width (RDW) is also not sensitive or specific in identifying the cause of an anemia.

Despite this caveat about the MCV, in a patient with a microcytic anemia and symptoms suggesting possible chronic blood loss, iron deficiency is by far the most likely cause, with a pretest probability of 80%. Therefore, the leading hypothesis for Mrs. A is iron deficiency anemia. Anemia of inflammation,

Table 6-1. Diagnostic hypotheses for Mrs. A.

Diagnostic Hypotheses	Demographics, Risk Factors, Symptoms and Signs	Important Tests
Leading Hypothesis		
Iron deficiency	Pica Blood loss (menorrhagia, melena, hematochezia, NSAID use)	Serum ferritin Transferrin saturation
Active Alternative---Most Common		
Anemia of chronic inflammation	History of renal or liver disease, inflammation, infection, malignancies	Iron, TIBC, ferritin, creatinine, transaminases, ESR, CRP
Other Hypotheses		
Thalassemia	Ethnic background	Hgb electrophoresis, DNA testing
Lead poisoning	Exposure to lead	Lead level
B_{12} deficiency	Diet Autoimmune diseases Neurologic symptoms	B_{12} level
Folate deficiency	Pregnancy Sickle cell anemia Alcohol abuse	Folate level

CRP, C-reactive protein; ESR, erythrocyte sedimentation rate; NSAID, nonsteroidal antiinflammatory drug; TIBC, total iron-binding capacity.

by virtue of being common, is the best active alternative; to make this diagnosis, keep in mind that the patient must have an inflammatory condition known to cause anemia. Sideroblastic anemia and lead exposure are other hypotheses. Thalassemia is excluded by the recently normal CBC. Because the MCV lacks specificity, the causes of normocytic and macrocytic anemia also need to be kept in mind as other hypotheses. Table 6-1 lists the differential diagnosis.

Leading Hypothesis: Iron Deficiency Anemia

Textbook Presentation

The most classic presentation would be a young, menstruating woman who has fatigue and a craving for ice. Typical presentations include fatigue, dyspnea, and sometimes edema.

Disease Highlights

A. The CBC varies with the degree of severity of the iron deficiency.

  1. In very early iron deficiency, the CBC is normal, although the ferritin is already decreasing.

  2. A mild anemia then develops, with an Hgb of 9–12 g/dL, and normal or slightly hypochromic RBCs.

  3. As the iron deficiency progresses, the Hgb continues to decrease, and hypochromia and microcytosis develop.

B. Causes of iron deficiency

1. Blood loss, most commonly menstrual or GI

2. Inadequate intake

   a. Males need 1 mg/day (need to consume 15 mg/day; absorption rate 6%).

   b. Females need 1.4 mg/day (need to consume 11 mg/day; absorption rate 12%).

   c. Iron is more bioavailable from meat than vegetables.

3. Malabsorption, seen in patients with gastrectomy, some bariatric surgery procedures, celiac sprue, or inflammatory bowel disease

4. Increased demand, seen with pregnancy, infancy, adolescence, erythropoietin therapy

Evidence-Based Diagnosis

A. Bone marrow exam for absence of iron stores is the gold standard.

B. The serum ferritin is the best serum test.

1. The LR+ for a decreased serum ferritin is very high, with reports ranging from LR+ of 51 for a ferritin < 15 ng/mL to a LR+ of 25.5 for a ferritin < 32 ng/mL.

2. Thus, a low ferritin rules in iron deficiency anemia.

3. In general populations, the LR– for a serum ferritin > 100 ng/mL is very low (0.08).

4. Thus, in general populations, a ferritin > 100 ng/mL greatly reduces the probability the patient has iron deficiency.

5. However, because ferritin is an acute phase reactant that increases in inflammatory states, interpreting it in the presence of such illnesses is difficult.

   a. There is a wide range of reported LRs, with many studies finding ferritin is *not* helpful in diagnosing iron deficiency in the presence of chronic illness.

   b. The level at which the serum ferritin suggests iron deficiency is probably much higher in patients with chronic illness, but the level may vary depending on the underlying illness.

   c. In chronic kidney disease, iron abnormalities are defined using the transferrin saturation (serum iron/total iron-binding capacity [Fe/TIBC]) and ferritin.

      (1) Absolute iron deficiency, due to dietary deficiency, poor absorption, GI or other bleeding: transferrin saturation < 20%, ferritin < 100 ng/mL

      (2) Functional iron deficiency, due to impaired iron transport to erythroblasts and inhibited intestinal absorption: transferrin saturation < 20%, ferritin ≥ 100 ng/mL

C. Other tests

1. The MCV, the transferrin saturation, red cell protoporphyrin, red cell ferritin, and RDW all are less sensitive and specific than ferritin.

2. The best of these is transferrin saturation ≤ 5%, with a LR+ of 10.46.

3. The reticulocyte-hemoglobin, measured by automated blood counters, is low in 80% of cases of iron deficiency anemia and normal in more than 80% of cases of anemia of chronic inflammation. It is also low in thalassemia trait. The normal range is 28–38 pg.

In patients without chronic inflammatory diseases, the serum ferritin is the best single test to diagnose iron deficiency anemia.

Treatment

A. Iron deficiency anemia is generally treated with oral iron replacement, with IV iron therapy reserved for patients who demonstrate malabsorption or who are unable to tolerate oral iron.

B. Transfusion is necessary only if the patient is hypotensive, orthostatic, or actively bleeding; or has angina, dizziness, syncope, or severe dyspnea or fatigue.

C. The best-absorbed oral iron is ferrous sulfate; the dose is 325 mg 3 times daily.

D. There are significant GI side effects, including nausea, abdominal pain, and constipation; these can be reduced by taking the iron with food, and slowly titrating the dose from 1 tablet daily to 3 tablets daily over 1–2 weeks.

E. There should be an increase in reticulocytes 7–10 days after starting therapy, and an increase in Hgb and HCT by 30 days; if there is no response, reconsider the diagnosis, keeping in mind that adherence with iron therapy is often low.

F. It is necessary to take iron for 6 months in order to replete iron stores.

MAKING A DIAGNOSIS

Since Mrs. A does not have any chronic, inflammatory diseases, the most useful test at this point is a serum ferritin. Serum iron and TIBC are often ordered simultaneously but are not necessary at this point.

You review the history, looking for symptoms of bleeding or chronic illness. She has no renal or liver disease and no symptoms of infection. Her ethnic background is Scandinavian, making thalassemia unlikely. You order a serum ferritin, which is 5 ng/mL.

CASE RESOLUTION

With a pretest probability of 80% and an LR+ of 51 for this level of ferritin, Mrs. A is clearly iron deficient. It is not necessary to test for any other causes of anemia, but it is necessary to determine why she is iron deficient.

Always look for a source of blood loss in iron deficiency anemia. Be alert for occult GI malignancies.

Iron deficiency is almost always due to chronic blood loss and rarely due to poor iron intake or malabsorption of iron; menstrual and GI blood loss are the most common sources. Because GI blood loss can be occult, many patients need GI evaluations.

A. Who needs a GI work-up? (also see Chapter 19, GI Bleeding)

1. All men, all women without menorrhagia, and women over age 50 even with menorrhagia.

2. Women under age 50 with menorrhagia do not need further GI evaluation, unless they have GI

symptoms or a family history of early colon cancer or adenomatous polyps.

3. Always ask carefully about minimal GI symptoms in young women, since celiac sprue often causes iron deficiency due to malabsorption, and the symptoms can easily be attributed to irritable bowel syndrome.

It is unclear from Mrs. A's history whether the menorrhagia is sufficient to cause this degree of iron deficiency anemia. In addition, she has upper GI symptoms of anorexia and reflux. Therefore, you order an EGD, which shows severe reflux esophagitis and also gastritis. Further history reveals she has been using several hundred milligrams of ibuprofen daily for several weeks because of a back strain. The severe esophagitis and gastritis are sufficient to explain her anemia. Although she has no lower GI symptoms or family history of colorectal cancer, the American Gastroenterological Association recommends performing a colonoscopy.

FOLLOW-UP OF MRS. A

Mrs. A stopped the ibuprofen, substituted a proton pump inhibitor for the H_2-blocker, and completed 6 months of iron therapy. She felt fine. A follow-up CBC showed an Hgb of 13 g/dL, an HCT of 39%, and a significantly elevated MCV of 122 mcm³.

At this point, what is the leading hypothesis, what are the active alternatives, and is there a must not miss diagnosis? Given this differential diagnosis, what tests should be ordered?

RANKING THE DIFFERENTIAL DIAGNOSIS

Although Mrs. A is not anemic now, she has a marked macrocytosis. The approach to isolated macrocytosis is the same as the approach to macrocytic anemia. The degree of macrocytosis is not a reliable predictor of the cause, but in general, the higher the MCV, the more likely the patient has a vitamin B_{12} or folate deficiency. The pretest probability of vitamin deficiency with an MCV of 115–129 mcm³ is 50%, and nearly all patients with an MCV > 130 mcm³ will have a vitamin deficiency.

B_{12} deficiency is seen more often than folate deficiency in otherwise healthy people, and so is the leading hypothesis, with folate deficiency being the active alternative. Use of antimetabolite drugs is excluded by history. Causes of nonmegaloblastic anemias need to be considered next. Hypothyroidism would be the most likely other hypothesis, with liver disease and alcohol abuse less likely based on her lack of a previous history of either. Hemolysis causing reticulocytosis is unlikely since she is not anemic. Table 6-2 lists the differential diagnosis.

Leading Hypothesis: B_{12} Deficiency

Textbook Presentation

The classic presentation is an elderly woman with marked anemia and neurologic symptoms such as paresthesias, sensory loss (especially vibration and position), and ataxia.

Table 6-2. Diagnostic hypotheses for Mrs. A's follow-up.

Diagnostic Hypotheses	Demographics, Risk Factors, Symptoms and Signs	Important Tests
Leading Hypothesis		
B_{12} deficiency	Vegan diet Other autoimmune diseases Elderly Neurologic symptoms	B_{12} level Homocysteine level Methylmalonic acid level (MMA)
Active Alternative---Most Common and Must Not Miss		
Folate deficiency	Alcohol abuse Starvation Pregnancy Sickle cell anemia	Serum folate level RBC folate level Homocysteine level
Other Hypothesis		
Hypothyroidism	Constipation Weight gain Fatigue Cold intolerance	TSH Free T4

Disease Highlights

A. It takes years to develop this deficiency because of extensive stores of vitamin B_{12} in the liver.

B. Anemia and macrocytosis are not always present.

1. In 1 study, 28% of patients with neurologic symptoms due to B_{12} deficiency had no anemia or macrocytosis; another study found that up to 84% of patients with B_{12} deficiency may be missed if B_{12} levels are checked only in patients with macrocytosis.

2. In another study, the following clinical characteristics were found in patients with B_{12} deficiency:

   a. 33% white, 41% black, 25% Latino

   b. 28% were not anemic

   c. 17% had a normal MCV

   d. 17% had leukopenia, 35% thrombocytopenia, 12.5% pancytopenia

   e. 36% had neuropsychiatric symptoms

      (1) Paresthesias occur initially, followed by ataxia with loss of vibration and position sense.

      (2) Neuropsychiatric symptoms can progress to severe weakness, spasticity, clonus, paraplegia, fecal and urinary incontinence.

      (3) Delirium and dementia can occur.

      (4) The severity of the anemia is inversely correlated with the degree of neurologic dysfunction.

 The CBC can be normal in B_{12} deficiency.

C. Intramedullary hemolysis can occur, leading to an increased lactate dehydrogenase (LD) and decreased haptoglobin.

D. B_{12} absorption requires normal gastric and intestinal function.

1. Dietary B_{12} is protein bound and is released by acid peptic digestion in the stomach.

2. Although intrinsic factor is made by the parietal cells of the gastric body and fundus, it does not bind to B_{12} until both reach the jejunum.

3. The B_{12}-intrinsic factor complex binds to receptors in the terminal ileum, where B_{12} is absorbed.

E. The most common causes of B_{12} deficiency are food cobalamin malabsorption, lack of intrinsic factor, and dietary deficiency; other causes of malabsorption are less common.

1. Dietary deficiency is rare unless the patient follows a vegan diet.

2. Food cobalamin malabsorption occurs when B_{12} is not released from food proteins due to impaired acid peptic digestion.

   a. The B_{12} deficiency in this condition is often subclinical and effects up to 20% of older adults.

   b. It is caused by atrophic gastritis and achlorhydria, which can be seen with chronic *Helicobacter pylori* infection, gastric surgery, and long-term use of acid suppressing drugs.

3. Lack of intrinsic factor is caused by gastrectomy (all patients with total gastrectomy and 5% of patients with partial gastrectomy will become B_{12} deficient) or pernicious anemia.

   a. Pernicious anemia is an immunologically mediated gastric atrophy leading to loss of parietal cells and a marked reduction in secretion of intrinsic factor.

   b. It is uncommon before age 30 and most often seen in patients over age 50, with a median age at diagnosis of 70–80 years.

   c. 25% of patients have a family history of pernicious anemia and 10% have autoimmune thyroid disease.

4. B_{12} deficiency can also be caused by malabsorption in the terminal ileum due to

   a. Ileal resection or bypass

   b. Tropical sprue

   c. Crohn disease

5. Blind loop syndrome can cause B_{12} deficiency due to utilization of B_{12} by the bacteria.

6. Sometimes drugs interfere with B_{12} absorption, most notably metformin, colchicine, ethanol, and neomycin.

7. Malabsorption may rarely be due to congenital disorders, such as transcobalamin II deficiency.

Evidence-Based Diagnosis

A. Determining whether a patient is B_{12} deficient is more complicated than it seems.

1. B_{12} levels can be falsely low in folate deficiency, pregnancy, and oral contraceptive use.

2. B_{12} levels can be falsely normal in myeloproliferative disorders, liver disease, and bacterial overgrowth syndromes.

3. The sensitivity of a B_{12} level < 200 pg/mL for proven clinical B_{12} deficiency is 65–95%; the specificity is 60–80%.

B. B_{12} is a cofactor in the conversion of homocysteine to methionine, and of methmalonyl CoA (MMA) to succinyl CoA.

1. Consequently, in B_{12} deficiency, the levels of homocysteine and MMA increase.

2. Therefore, another way to diagnosis B_{12} deficiency is to measure homocysteine and MMA levels.

   a. In addition to B_{12} deficiency, MMA can be elevated in chronic kidney disease and hypovolemia.

   b. Homocysteine can be elevated in folate or pyridoxine deficiency, chronic kidney disease, hypovolemia, and hypothyroidism.

   c. The sensitivity of MMA > 400 nmol/L for the diagnosis of B_{12} deficiency is 98%; modest elevations in the 300–700 nmol/L range can be seen in chronic kidney disease. MMA > 1000 nmol/L is highly specific for B_{12} deficiency.

   d. The sensitivity of homocysteine ranges from 85% to 96%; an elevated homocysteine is less specific than an elevated MMA.

C. Response to therapy is another way to establish the presence of B_{12} deficiency.

1. MMA and homocysteine normalize 7–14 days after the start of replacement therapy.

2. The reticulocyte count increases in 7–10 days, and the hemoglobin increases in 30 days.

D. An algorithm for diagnosing B_{12} deficiency in patients with macrocytic anemia

1. B_{12} level < 100 pg/mL: deficiency present

2. B_{12} level 100–350 pg/mL: check MMA and homocysteine levels

   a. If both normal, deficiency unlikely

   b. If both elevated, deficiency present

   c. If MMA alone elevated, deficiency present

   d. If homocysteine alone elevated, possible deficiency

3. B_{12} > 350 pg/mL: deficiency unlikely

Very low or very high B_{12} levels are usually diagnostic.

Patients with neurologic symptoms consistent with B_{12} deficiency should have MMA and homocysteine levels checked if the B_{12} level is normal.

Treatment

A. IM cobalamin, 1000 mcg weekly for 6–8 weeks, and then monthly for life

B. Can also use oral cobalamin, 1000–2000 mcg daily

1. Oral cobalamin is absorbed by a second, nonintrinsic factor dependent mechanism that is relatively inefficient.

2. Compliance can be a problem.

3. Patients with dietary deficiency and food cobalamin malabsorption can be treated with lower doses of oral B_{12}.

4. Randomized trials have shown that oral and intramuscular replacement are equally effective, even in patients with pernicious anemia or gastrectomies.

C. Sublingual and intranasal formulations are available but have not been extensively studied.

MAKING A DIAGNOSIS

Mrs. A's B_{12} level is 21 pg/mL, with a serum folate of 8.0 ng/mL.

Have you crossed a diagnostic threshold for the leading hypothesis, B_{12} deficiency? Have you ruled out the active alternatives? Do other tests need to be done to exclude the alternative diagnoses?

Alternative Diagnosis: Folate Deficiency

Textbook Presentation

The classic presentation is an alcoholic patient with malnutrition and anemia.

Disease Highlights

A. Anemia and macrocytosis are the most common manifestations; neurologic symptoms do not occur.

B. Most often caused by inadequate intake (especially in alcoholic patients) or increased demand due to pregnancy, chronic hemolysis, leukemia.

C. Since absorption occurs in the jejunum, malabsorption is rare in the absence of short bowel syndrome or bacterial overgrowth syndromes.

D. Some drugs can cause folate deficiency, including methotrexate, phenytoin, sulfasalazine, and alcohol.

E. Along with B_{12}, folate is a cofactor for the conversion of homocysteine to methionine, so homocysteine levels increase in folate deficiency.

Evidence-Based Diagnosis

A. The sensitivity and specificity of serum folate measurements for the diagnosis of folate deficiency are not clear.

B. Levels can decrease within a few days of dietary folate restriction, or with alcohol use, even though tissue stores can be normal; levels increase with feeding.

C. RBC folate, which reflects folate status over the previous 3 months, correlates more strongly with megaloblastic changes than does serum folate; however, the sensitivity and specificity of RBC folate for the diagnosis of true deficiency are both low (about 70% each).

D. Elevated homocysteine is about 80% sensitive for the diagnosis of folate deficiency; the specificity is unknown.

E. A positive response to therapy is diagnostic.

F. A patient with a normal serum folate, normal RBC folate, and no response to folate replacement does not have folate deficiency.

Treatment

A. In patients with an acute deficiency, treat with 1 mg of folic acid daily for 1–4 months, or until there is complete hematologic recovery.

   1. Never treat folate deficiency without determining whether the patient is B_{12} deficient.

   2. Folate replacement can correct hematologic abnormalities while worsening the neurologic symptoms specific to B_{12} deficiency.

B. Patients with long-term increased demand, such as those with sickle cell anemia, should take 1 mg of folic acid daily indefinitely.

C. Women who are trying to conceive should take 800 mcg/day of a prenatal vitamin (contains 1 mg folic acid); pregnant women should take a prenatal vitamin.

Always check for B_{12} deficiency in a patient with folate deficiency.

CASE RESOLUTION

Mrs. A's B_{12} level is diagnostic of B_{12} deficiency. She has no conditions associated with folate deficiency, so even though the test characteristics of the serum folate are unclear, in this case the normal level is sufficient to rule out folate deficiency.

The next step is to determine the cause of the B_{12} deficiency.

A. Test for pernicious anemia by sending anti-intrinsic factor and anti-parietal cell antibodies.

   1. Anti-intrinsic factor antibodies have a sensitivity of 50% and specificity of 100% for the diagnosis of pernicious anemia.

   2. Anti-parietal cell antibodies have a sensitivity of 80% and specificity of 50–100%.

B. Review history for other symptoms of malabsorption suggesting small bowel disease.

C. Assess for vegan diet

D. In older patients without other symptoms, negative antibodies, and adequate intake, consider food-cobalamin malabsorption.

It is not always possible to determine the site of malabsorption, and it is acceptable to treat such patients empirically with B_{12} replacement.

CHIEF COMPLAINT

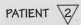

Mrs. L is a 70-year-old woman with a history of squamous cell carcinoma of the larynx, successfully treated with surgery and radiation therapy 10 years ago. She has a tracheostomy and a jejunostomy tube. One week ago, she fell and fractured her right humeral head. On routine preoperative laboratory tests, her CBC was unexpectedly abnormal: WBC 11,100/mcL (65% polymorphonuclear leukocytes, 12% bands, 4% monocytes, 19% lymphocytes), Hgb 8.7 g/dL, HCT 26.3%, MCV 85 mcm³; the platelet count is normal. One month ago, her Hgb was 12.0 g/dL, with a normal WBC.

At this point, what is the leading hypothesis, what are the active alternatives, and is there a must not miss diagnosis? Given this differential diagnosis, what tests should be ordered?

RANKING THE DIFFERENTIAL DIAGNOSIS

The relatively acute drop in HCT is a pivotal point that suggests either bleeding or hemolysis; these are also the "must not miss" diagnoses. The usual causes of normocytic anemia need to be considered next. Anemia of inflammation/chronic disease is a common cause of normocytic anemia, with bone marrow infiltration and RBC aplasia being less common. You would also include causes of microcytic and macrocytic anemia in your list of other hypotheses. Anemia is common in elderly patients, occurring in 10% of community dwelling older adults. In one study of patients over 65 referred to a hematology clinic for evaluation of anemia, 25% had iron deficiency, 10% anemia of inflammation, 7.5% hematologic malignancies (including myelodysplastic syndrome), 4.6% thalassemia, 3.4% chronic kidney disease, and 5.7% miscellaneous causes (including hypothyroidism, B_{12} deficiency, hemolysis, alcohol, medication). A specific cause could not be identified in 44% of the patients. However, since her anemia is acute, it is unlikely to be related solely to her age. Table 6-3 lists the differential diagnosis.

She has felt feverish, with a cough productive of brown sputum. She has had no nausea or vomiting, no melena, and no hematochezia. She has been postmenopausal for a long time and has had no vaginal bleeding. The orthopedic surgeon confirms it is unlikely that she has significant bleeding at the fracture site. Her rectal exam shows brown, hemoccult-negative stool. Her chest radiograph shows a new left lower lobe pneumonia.

Is the clinical information sufficient to make a diagnosis? If not, what other information do you need?

There are no symptoms or signs suggesting that she is having an active, acute episode of bleeding. The next step is to look for hemolysis and occult, subacute bleeding.

Table 6-3. Diagnostic hypotheses for Mrs. L.

Diagnostic Hypotheses	Demographics, Risk Factors, Symptoms and Signs	Important Tests
Leading Hypothesis		
Acute bleeding	Melena Hematochezia Hematemesis Menorrhagia	History Rectal exam for gross blood or positive guaiac test
Hemolysis	Fatigue	Reticulocyte count Haptoglobin Direct antiglobulin (Coombs) test Smear for schistocytes
Active Alternative---Must Not Miss		
Iron deficiency	Aspirin or NSAID use GI bleeding Pica Menorrhagia	Ferritin
Active Alternative---Most Common		
Anemia of inflammation	Acute infection Acute kidney injury Chronic inflammatory diseases	Fe/TIBC Ferritin Bone marrow
Other Alternatives		
Marrow infiltration	Pancytopenia Bleeding Malaise	Bone marrow
RBC aplasia	Drug exposure Viral symptoms	History Bone marrow Parvo IgM
Folate deficiency	Diet Alcohol abuse Pregnancy Sickle cell anemia	Serum or RBC folate Bone marrow
B_{12} deficiency	Vegan diet Other autoimmune diseases Elderly Neurologic symptoms	B_{12} level Homocysteine level Methylmalonic acid level (MMA)
Hypothyroidism	Constipation Weight gain Fatigue Cold intolerance	TSH Free T4

Fe/TIBC, serum iron/total iron-binding capacity.

MAKING A DIAGNOSIS

Further laboratory testing shows a reticulocyte count of 1.4% (RPI = 0.8). Her serum ferritin is 200 ng/mL. TSH, B_{12}, and folate levels are all normal.

Have you crossed a diagnostic threshold for the leading hypotheses, iron deficiency and hemolysis? Have you ruled out the active alternatives? Do other tests need to be done to exclude the alternative diagnoses?

The low RPI points toward an underproduction anemia, not hemolysis. The elevated serum ferritin substantially reduces the likelihood that she is iron deficient, especially since she has no history of chronic inflammatory diseases. She does not have hypothyroidism, B_{12} deficiency, or folate deficiency. She does not have pancytopenia, so bone marrow infiltration is unlikely.

Alternative Diagnosis: Anemia of Inflammation

Textbook Presentation

Because there is such a broad spectrum of underlying causes, there is no classic presentation of anemia of inflammation. It is most often discovered on a routine CBC that shows a normochromic, normocytic anemia, with a Hgb in the range of 8.5–9.5 g/dL.

Disease Highlights

A. Occurs in patients with acute or chronic immune activation

B. Cytokines (interferons, interleukins, tumor necrosis factor) induce *changes in iron homeostasis.*

  1. Dysregulation of iron homeostasis

    a. Increased uptake and retention of iron in reticuloendothelial system cells

    b. Limited availability of iron for erythropoiesis

  2. Impaired proliferation and differentiation of erythroid progenitor cells

  3. Blunted erythropoietin response

    a. Production of erythropoietin inadequate for degree of anemia

    b. Progenitor cells do not respond normally

  4. Increased erythrophagocytosis leads to decreased RBC half-life

C. Underlying causes of anemia of inflammation include

  1. Chronic kidney disease

    a. In patients with end-stage renal disease who undergo dialysis, the anemia is due to lack of erythropoietin and marked inflammation.

    b. In patients with lesser degrees of chronic kidney disease, the anemia is caused primarily by lack of erythropoietin and anti-proliferative effects of uremic toxins.

  2. Autoimmune diseases, such as systemic lupus erythematosus, rheumatoid arthritis, vasculitis, sarcoidosis, and inflammatory bowel disease

3. Acute infections caused by viruses, bacteria, fungi, or parasites

  a. Can occur within 24–48 hours in acute bacterial infections, with Hgb usually in the 10–12 g/dL range

  b. Occurs in as many as 90% of ICU patients, accompanied by inappropriately mild elevations of serum erythropoietin levels and blunted bone marrow response to endogenous erythropoietin

4. Chronic infections caused by viruses, bacteria, fungi, or parasites

5. Cancer, either hematologic or solid tumor

D. Noninflammatory chronic anemias also occur.

  1. Endocrinopathies, such as Addison disease, thyroid disease, panhypopituitarism can lead to mild chronic anemia.

  2. Liver disease can cause anemia.

Evidence-Based Diagnosis

A. There is no 1 test that proves or disproves a patient's anemia is from anemia of inflammation.

B. Instead, there are several diagnostic tests that can possibly be done, sometimes simultaneously and sometimes sequentially.

An Hgb of < 8 g/dL suggests there is a second cause for the anemia, beyond the anemia of inflammation.

1. Even in the presence of a disease known to cause anemia, it is important to rule out iron, B_{12}, and folate deficiencies.

2. As discussed above, it can be difficult to interpret iron studies in the presence of inflammatory diseases; however, the typical pattern in anemia of inflammation is a low serum iron, low TIBC, normal percent saturation, and elevated serum ferritin.

3. Erythropoietin levels will be low in chronic kidney disease and not appropriately elevated for the degree of anemia in inflammatory conditions; interpretation is difficult and measurement of the erythropoietin level is generally not useful diagnostically.

4. C-reactive protein is often elevated in patients with anemia of inflammation.

5. Pancytopenia suggests there is bone marrow infiltration or a disease that suppresses production of all cell lines.

When you see pancytopenia, think about bone marrow infiltration, B_{12} deficiency, viral infection, drug toxicity, hypersplenism, overwhelming infection, systemic lupus erythematosus, or acute alcohol intoxication.

6. Bone marrow examination is necessary to establish the diagnosis when pancytopenia is present, serum tests are not diagnostic, the anemia progresses, or there is not an appropriate response to empiric therapy.

Treatment

A. Treat the underlying chronic disease, if possible.

B. Indications for erythropoietin therapy and appropriate target Hgb levels are evolving; iron should be given to all patients being treated with erythropoietin.

CASE RESOLUTION

Mrs. L has normal liver function tests and a normal creatinine. Her iron studies show a serum iron of 25 mcg/dL, with a TIBC of 140 mcg/dL (% saturation = 18%).

Mrs. L has a very low RPI, ruling out hemolysis. She has no signs of bleeding, and iron studies are consistent with an anemia of inflammation. In addition, she has no pancytopenia to suggest bone marrow infiltration or diffuse marrow suppression, and no evidence of vitamin deficiency. She has a disease (acute bacterial pneumonia) known to be associated with acute anemia of inflammation. Thus, the diagnosis is acute anemia of inflammation. Her pneumonia is treated with oral antibiotics, and her CBC returns back to her baseline when checked 6 weeks later.

CHIEF COMPLAINT

PATIENT 3

Mr. J is a 77-year-old African American man with a history of an aortic valve replacement about 2 years ago. He brought in results of tests done at another hospital: Hgb, 9.0 g/dL; HCT, 27.4%; MCV, 90 mcm³; reticulocyte count, 7%; serum ferritin, 110 ng/mL; B_{12}, 416 pg/mL; folate 20.0 ng/mL. The RPI is 2.1.

At this point, what is the leading hypothesis, what are the active alternatives, and is there a must not miss diagnosis? Given this differential diagnosis, what tests should be ordered?

RANKING THE DIFFERENTIAL DIAGNOSIS

The leading hypothesis is hemolysis, with the pivotal point being the elevated reticulocyte count and RPI. Considering the normal ferritin and vitamin levels, the pretest probability of hemolysis is high. The only potential active alternative would be active bleeding, since an elevated reticulocyte count also occurs then; however, that would be clinically obvious. All other causes of anemia are alternative diagnoses to be considered only if the diagnosis of hemolysis is not supported by further testing. Table 6-4 lists the differential diagnosis.

Mr. J has no history of hematemesis, melena, hematochezia, or abdominal pain. His abdominal exam is normal, and rectal exam shows brown, hemoccult-negative stool.

Is the clinical information sufficient to make a diagnosis? If not, what other information do you need?

Leading Hypothesis: Hemolysis

Textbook Presentation

The presentation of hemolysis depends on the cause. Patients can be asymptomatic or critically ill.

Table 6-4. Diagnostic hypotheses for Mr. J.

Diagnostic Hypotheses	Demographics, Risk Factors, Symptoms and Signs	Important Tests
Leading Hypothesis		
Hemolysis	Mechanical valve Known hereditary condition Family history of anemia	Reticulocyte count Haptoglobin Indirect bilirubin Lactate dehydrogenase Examination of peripheral smear
	Sepsis Fever	Direct antiglobulin (Coombs) test
Active Alternative---Must Not Miss		
Active bleeding	Hematemesis Melena Hematochezia Vaginal bleeding Abdominal pain	

Disease Highlights

A. In macroangiopathic and microangiopathic hemolytic anemia and some complement-induced lysis, RBCs are destroyed in the **intravascular space**.
   1. Completely destroyed cells release free Hgb into the plasma, which then binds to **haptoglobin,** reducing the plasma haptoglobin level.
   2. Some Hgb is lysed intravascularly and then is filtered by the glomerulus, causing **hemoglobinuria.**
   3. Some filtered Hgb is taken up by renal tubular cells, stored as hemosiderin; **hemosiderinuria** occurs about a week later, when the tubular cells are sloughed into the urine.
   4. Damaged but incompletely hemolyzed cells are destroyed in the spleen.

B. Deformed RBCs and those coated with complement are usually destroyed in the **extravascular space,** in the liver or spleen.
   1. Most of the Hgb is degraded into biliverdin, iron, and carbon monoxide.
   2. Biliverdin is converted to **unconjugated bilirubin** and released into the plasma, increasing the unconjugated bilirubin level.

3. Some free Hgb is released, which then binds to **haptoglobin,** again reducing the plasma haptoglobin level.

Evidence-Based Diagnosis

A. The reticulocyte count is usually at least 4–5%; in 1 study of autoimmune hemolytic anemia, the median was 9%.

B. The serum haptoglobin should be < 25 mg/dL.

1. Sensitivity = 83%, specificity = 96% for hemolysis; LR+ = 21, LR– = 0.18

2. Haptoglobin is an acute phase reactant.

C. The LD is often increased.

1. Finding an increased LD *and* a decreased haptoglobin is 90% specific for the diagnosis of hemolysis.

2. Finding a normal LD *and* a normal serum haptoglobin (> 25 mg/dL) is 92% sensitive for the absence of hemolysis.

D. The unconjugated bilirubin may be increased.

E. Plasma and urine Hgb should be elevated if the hemolysis is intravascular.

Treatment

Treatment depends on the underlying cause. In an autoimmune condition, immunosuppressive therapy, especially prednisone, is used. If hemolysis is associated with TTP and HUS, the treatment is plasmapheresis and immunosuppressive therapy.

MAKING A DIAGNOSIS

Mr. J's serum haptoglobin is < 20 mg/dL, his serum bilirubin is normal, and his LD is elevated at 359 units/L.

 Have you crossed a diagnostic threshold for the leading hypothesis, hemolysis? Have you ruled out the active alternatives? Do other tests need to be done to exclude the alternative diagnoses?

The combination of the high pretest probability and the large LR+ for this level of haptoglobin confirms the diagnosis of hemolysis. Active bleeding has been ruled out by history and physical exam. At this point, any further testing should be aimed at determining the cause of the hemolysis.

A. The direct antiglobulin test (DAT), also known as the Coombs test, should be done in all patients to distinguish immune-mediated from non–immune-mediated hemolytic anemia.

1. Detects antibody or complement on the surface of the RBC

   a. The DAT is positive for IgG in patients with warm autoimmune hemolytic anemia.

   b. The DAT is positive for complement in patients with cold autoimmune hemolytic anemia.

   c. It is also positive in paroxysmal cold hemoglobinuria, transfusion-related hemolytic anemia, and some drug-induced hemolytic anemias.

2. The indirect Coombs test detects antibodies to RBC antigens in the patient's serum and is sometimes positive in drug-induced hemolytic anemias.

B. The smear should be examined for schistocytes, seen in macroangiopathic and microangiopathic hemolytic anemias.

1. Concomitant thrombocytopenia and coagulopathy are seen in DIC.

2. Concomitant thrombocytopenia, chronic kidney disease, or neurologic symptoms are seen in TTP and HUS.

C. Look for other causes of hemolytic anemia through history and physical exam and test selectively.

1. Does the patient have a mechanical valve?

2. Has the patient traveled to an area where malaria is endemic?

3. Has the patient been exposed to a toxin?

4. Does the patient have splenomegaly on exam or ultrasound?

5. Is there an undiagnosed hereditary cause (especially G6PD deficiency)?

CASE RESOLUTION

His WBC and platelet count as well as his renal function are all normal; the Coombs test is negative. He does have a few schistocytes on his peripheral smear. He has hemolysis due to his mechanical valve. Since he is asymptomatic, it is not necessary to consider removal of the valve.

REVIEW OF OTHER IMPORTANT DISEASES

Sickle Cell Anemia

Textbook Presentation

Sickle cell anemia is often identified at birth through screening. Adult patients generally seek medical attention for pain or some of the complications (see below). Occasionally, patients have very mild disease, and sickle cell is diagnosed late in life when evidence of a specific complication, such as sickle cell retinopathy, is identified.

Disease Highlights

A. Epidemiology

1. There are 5 haplotypes, 4 African and 1 Asian [Arab-Indian].

2. Common genotypes include

   a. Sickle cell anemia (homozygous HbS gene)

   b. SC disease (HbS + HbC genes)

   c. HbS-beta-thalassemia (HbS + beta^0 or beta$^+$ thalassemia gene)

   d. HbSO Arabia (HbS + HbO Arabia genes)

   e. HbSD Los Angeles [Punjab] (HbS + HbD genes)

3. In non-Hispanic white births, the gene frequency for sickle cell or thalassemia is 0.17%.

4. In African Americans, the gene frequency of Hgb S is 4%, of Hgb C is 1.5%, and of beta-thalassemia is 4%; the incidence of sickle cell anemia is about 1 in 600, with the incidence of all sickle cell disease genotypes approaching 1 in 300.

B. Pathophysiology (Figure 6-2) of sickle cell disease

1. Vaso-occlusion with ischemia-reperfusion injury

   a. Vascular obstruction is caused by precapillary obstruction by sickled cells and inflammatory triggers.

   b. Episodic microvascular occlusion and ischemia is followed by restoration of blood flow, leading to further injury during reperfusion as oxidases, cytokines, and other inflammatory mediators are activated.

2. Hemolysis

   a. Contributes to progressive vasculopathy

   b. Patients with high hemolytic rates are more anemic and have more cholelithiasis, leg ulcerations, priapism, and pulmonary hypertension than patients with lower hemolytic rates.

   c. Patients with lower hemolytic rates tend to have more episodes of acute pain and possibly acute chest syndrome.

C. Prognosis

1. Median age at death is 42 for men and 48 for women.

2. Genetic factors can affect prognosis.

   a. Higher levels of fetal hemoglobin are associated with increased life expectancy, fewer acute pain episodes, and fewer leg ulcers; levels range from 1% to 30%.

   b. Coexistent alpha-thalassemia (30% of patients of African origin, 50% of patients of Arabian or Indian origin) leads to decreased rates of hemolysis and increased hemoglobin levels; pain frequency is not reduced, but the rates of stroke, gallstones, leg ulcers, and priapism are lower.

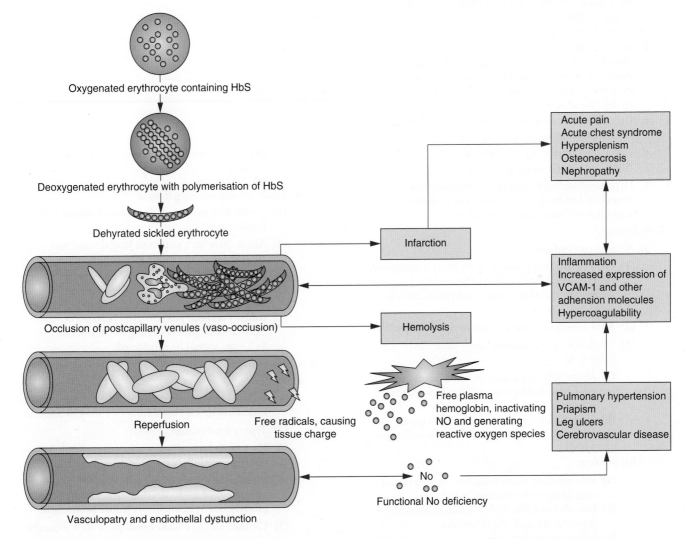

HbS, sickle hemoglobin; NO, nitric oxide; VCAM, vascular cell adhesion molecule.

Figure 6-2. Pathophysiology of sickle cell disease. The roles of HbS polymerization, hyperviscosity, vaso-occlusion, hemolysis, and endothelial dysfunction are shown. Deoxygenation causes HbS to polymerize, leading to sickled erythrocytes. Vaso-occlusion results from the interaction of sickled erythrocytes with leukocytes and the vascular endothelium. Vaso-occlusion then leads to infarction, hemolysis, and inflammation; inflammation enhances the expression of adhesion molecules, further increasing the tendency of sickled erythrocytes to adhere to the vascular endothelium to worsen vaso-occlusion. Reperfusion of the ischemic tissue generates free radicals and oxidative damage. The damage erythrocytes release free hemoglobin into the plasma, which strongly bind to nitric oxide, causing functional nitric oxide deficiency and contributing to the development of vasculopathy. Reproduced, with permission, from Rees DC, Williams TN, Gladwin MT. Sickle-cell disease. Lancet. 2010;376:2018–31.

D. Sickle cell trait

   1. 8% of African Americans have sickle cell trait

   2. Patients with sickle cell trait are not anemic, do not have pain crises, and do not have increased mortality rates.

   3. Most cannot concentrate urine normally, but this is clinically important only if hydration is inadequate.

   4. Benign, self-limited hematuria due to papillary necrosis is common; however, renal medullary cancer, stones, glomerulonephritis, and infection should be ruled out.

   5. There is no need to routinely screen for sickle cell trait prior to surgery.

   6. Patients with sickle cell trait have a 2-fold increased risk for venous thromboembolism.

E. Clinical manifestations of sickle cell anemia

   1. Hematologic

   a. HCT usually 20–30%, with reticulocyte count of 3–15%; patients with HbSC disease and HbS-beta+-thalassemia tend to be less anemic.

   b. Hemoglobin levels decrease slightly during acute pain episodes and episodes of acute chest syndrome; acute, marked decreases can occur due to transient aplasia from parvovirus B19 infections or sudden sequestration by the liver or spleen.

   c. Unconjugated hyperbilirubinemia, elevated LD, and low haptoglobin are present.

   d. Hgb F level usually slightly elevated.

   e. WBC and platelet count usually elevated.

   f. Hypercoagulability occurs due to high levels of thrombin, low levels of protein C and S, abnormal activation of fibrinolysis and platelets

   2. Pulmonary

   a. Acute chest syndrome

   (1) Defined as a new pulmonary infiltrate accompanied by fever and a combination of respiratory symptoms, including cough, tachypnea, and chest pain.

   (2) Most common cause of death in sickle cell patients

   (3) Clinical manifestations in adults shown in Table 6-5.

   (a) About 50% of patients in whom acute chest syndrome develops are admitted for another reason.

   (b) Over 80% have concomitant pain crises.

   (c) Up to 13% require mechanical ventilation; 3% die.

   (4) Etiology

   (a) Fat embolism (from infarction of long bones), with or without infection in 12%

   (b) Infection in 27%, with 8% due to bacteria, 5% mycoplasma, and 9% chlamydia

   (c) Infarction in about 10%

   (d) Hypoventilation and atelectasis due to pain and analgesia may play a role, as might fluid overload

   (e) Unknown in about 50% of patients

   (5) General principles of management

   (a) Supplemental oxygen

   (b) Empiric treatment with broad-spectrum antibiotics

   (c) Incentive spirometry (can be preventive)

Table 6-5. Clinical manifestations of acute chest syndrome in adults.

Symptom or Sign	Frequency (%)
Fever	70
Cough	54
Chest pain	55
Tachypnea	39
Shortness of breath	58
Limb pain	59
Abdominal pain	29
Rib or sternal pain	30
Respiratory rate > 30 breaths per minute	38
Crackles	81
Wheezing	16
Effusion	27
Mean temperature:	38.8°C

   (d) Bronchodilators for patients with reactive airways

   (e) Transfusion

   b. Sickle cell chronic lung disease

   (1) 35–60% of patients with sickle cell disease have reactive airways.

   (2) About 20% have restrictive lung disease, and another 20% have mixed obstructive/restrictive abnormalities.

   (3) Up to 30% have pulmonary hypertension, with a very high risk of death compared to patients without pulmonary hypertension. Echocardiographic screening of adults every 1–3 years should be considered.

   3. Genitourinary

   a. Renal

   (1) Inability to concentrate urine (hyposthenuria), with maximum urinary osmolality of 400–450 mOsm/kg

   (2) Type 4 renal tubular acidosis

   (3) Hematuria is usually secondary to papillary necrosis, but renal medullary carcinoma has been reported.

   (4) Microalbuminuria is common in childhood, with up to 20% of adults developing nephrotic range proteinuria; ACE inhibitors reduce proteinuria.

   (5) Chronic kidney disease develops in 30% of adults.

   b. Priapism

   (1) 30–40% of adult males with sickle cell disease report at least 1 episode.

   (2) Bimodal peak incidences in ages 5–13 and 21–29.

   (3) 75% of episodes occur during sleep; the mean duration is 125 minutes.

   (4) Treatment approaches include hydration, analgesia, transfusion, and injection of alpha-adrenergic drugs.

4. Neurologic
   a. Highest incidence of first infarction is between the ages of 2 and 5, followed by another peak in incidence between the ages of 35 and 45.
   b. Hemorrhagic stroke can also occur.
   c. Recurrent infarction occurs in 67% of patients.
   d. Silent infarction is common (seen in 18–23% of patients by age 14); cognitive deficits also common.
   e. Patients over 2 years of age should undergo annual transcranial Doppler screening to assess stroke risk.
      (1) Patients with elevated transcranial Doppler velocities (> 200 cm/s) are at high risk.
      (2) Regular transfusions to keep the HbS level below 30% reduces the risk of stroke in such patients by 90% (10% stroke rate in control group, 1% in treatment group, number needed to treat (NNT) = 11).
5. Musculoskeletal
   a. Bones and joints often the sites of vaso-occlusive episodes.
   b. Avascular necrosis of hips, shoulders, ankles, and spine can cause chronic pain.
      (1) Often best detected by MRI
      (2) May require joint replacement
6. Other
   a. Retinopathy
      (1) More common in patients with Hgb SC disease than with sickle cell (SS) disease
      (2) Treated with photocoagulation
   b. Leg ulcers
      (1) Present in about 20% of patients
      (2) Most commonly over the medial or lateral malleoli
   c. Cholelithiasis: nearly universal due to chronic hemolysis
   d. Splenic sequestration and autosplenectomy: seen in children; leads to increased risk of infection with encapsulated organisms and the need for antibiotic prophylaxis
   e. Liver disease: multifactorial, due to causes such as iron overload or viral hepatitis

Evidence-Based Diagnosis

A. Newborn screening
   1. Universal screening identifies many more patients than screening targeted at high-risk groups.
   2. Homozygotes have an FS pattern on electrophoresis, which is predominantly Hgb F, with some Hgb S, and no Hgb A.
   3. The FS pattern in not specific for sickle cell disease, and the diagnosis should be confirmed through family studies, DNA based testing, or repeat Hgb electrophoresis at 3–4 months of age.
B. Testing in older children and adults
   1. Cellulose acetate electrophoresis separates Hgb S from other variants; however, S, G, and D all have the same electrophoretic mobility.
   2. Only Hgb S will precipitate in a solubility test such as the Sickledex.

Treatment

A. General principles
   1. All pediatric patients should receive prophylactic penicillin to prevent streptococcal sepsis.

2. Indications for transfusion (preoperative transfusions and those for stroke prevention are evidence based; other indications are based on expert opinion or clinical practice)
   a. Acute transfusions: acute exacerbation of anemia, acute chest syndrome, acute stroke, multiorgan failure, preoperative management
   b. Chronic regular transfusions: primary and secondary stroke prevention, recurrent acute chest syndrome despite hydroxyurea therapy, progressive organ failure
   c. Patients should be monitored for iron overload and treated as needed.
3. Hydroxyurea
   a. In patients with moderate to severe sickle cell disease, hydroxyurea therapy reduced the rate of pain crises and development of acute chest syndrome by about 50%.
   b. Hydroxyurea use is associated with a lower mortality rate.
4. Stem cell transplant is an experimental therapy.
B. Management of vaso-occlusive crises
   1. The general approach should be similar to that used in patients with other causes of severe pain, such as cancer.
      a. Analgesics should be dosed regularly, rather than as needed.
      b. Patient-controlled analgesia can also be used.
      c. Remember that patients who use opioids long-term become tolerant and often require high doses for acute pain.
      d. Adding NSAIDs or tricyclic antidepressants to opioids is sometimes beneficial.
      e. Patients often need a long-acting opioid for baseline analgesia, combined with a short-acting opioid for breakthrough pain.
      f. A multidisciplinary approach to pain management involving nurses and social workers may help optimize pain management.
   2. Oral hydration is preferable to IV hydration.
   3. Oxygen is indicated only if the patient is hypoxemic.

Beta-Thalassemia

Textbook Presentation

Beta-thalassemia major (homozygotes) presents in infancy with multiple severe abnormalities. Heterozygotes are usually asymptomatic.

Disease Highlights

A. Impaired production of beta globin chains.
B. Common in patients of Mediterranean origin.
C. Beta-thalassemia minor: heterozygotes with 1 normal beta globin allele and 1 beta thalassemic allele.
D. Anemia is generally mild (HCT > 30%), and microcytosis is severe (MCV < 75 mcm^3).
E. In pregnancy, anemia can be more severe than usual.
F. Splenomegaly is asymptomatic in 15–20% of patients.

Evidence-Based Diagnosis

A. Iron studies should be normal; RDW usually normal; target cells abundant; RBCs may be normal or high.
B. On Hgb electrophoresis, the Hgb A$_2$ can be elevated, but a normal A$_2$ does not rule out beta-thalassemia minor.

Treatment of Beta-Thalassemia Minor

None.

Alpha-Thalassemia

Textbook Presentation

Loss of 3 or 4 alpha globin genes causes severe disease that presents at birth or is fatal in utero. Patients with loss of 1 or 2 genes are usually asymptomatic.

Disease Highlights

A. Impaired production of alpha globin chains.

B. Common in patients of African or Asian origin.

C. Alpha-thalassemia-2 trait: loss of 1 alpha globin gene; CBC normal.

D. Alpha-thalassemia-1 trait (alpha-thalassemia minor): loss of 2 alpha globin genes; mild microcytic anemia with target cells and normal Hgb electrophoresis.

Evidence-Based Diagnosis

Alpha-thalassemia is diagnosed by polymerase chain reaction genetic analysis.

Treatment of Alpha-Thalassemia Trait

None.

REFERENCES

Artz A, Thirman MJ. Unexplained anemia predominates despite an intensive evaluation in a racially diverse cohort of older adults from a referral anemia clinic. J Gerontol A Biol Sci Med Sci. 2011:1–8.

Anand IS, Chandrashekhar Y, Ferrari R, Poole-Wilson PA , Harris PC . Pathogenesis of oedema in chronic severe anaemia: studies of body water and sodium, renal function, haemodynamic variables, and plasma hormones. Br Heart J. 1993;70:357–62.

Charache S, Terrin ML, Moore RD et al. Effect of hydroxyurea on the frequency of painful crises in sickle cell anemia. N Engl J Med. 1995;332:1317–22.

Guyatt GH, Oxman AD, Ali M et al. Laboratory diagnosis of iron deficiency anemia: an overview. J Gen Intern Med. 1992;7(2):145–53.

Lindenbaum J, Healton E, Savage D et al. Neuropsychiatric disorders caused by cobalamin deficiency in the absence of anemia or macrocytosis. N Engl J Med. 1988;318:1720–8.

Marchand A, Galen R, Van Lente F . The predictive value of serum haptoglobin in hemolytic disease. JAMA. 1980;243:1909–11.

Rees DC, Williams TN, Gladwin MT. Sickle-cell disease. Lancet. 2010;376: 2018–31.

Snow C. Laboratory diagnosis of vitamin B12 and folate deficiency. Arch Intern Med. 1999;159:1289–98.

Stabler DP. Vitamin B12 deficiency. N Engl J Med. 2013;368:149–60.

Steinberg MH. In the clinic: Sickle cell disease. Ann Intern Med. 2011 Sep 6;155(5): ITC31-15.

Steinberg M, Barton F, Castro O. Effect of hydroxyurea on mortality and morbidity in adult sickle cell anemia. JAMA. 2003;289:1645–51.

Vichinsky EP, Neumayr LD, Earles AN et al. Causes and outcomes of the acute chest syndrome in sickle cell disease. N Engl J Med. 2000;342:1855–65.

Weiss G, Goodnough LT. Anemia of chronic disease. N Engl J Med. 2005;352: 1011–23.

I have a patient with low back pain. How do I determine the cause?

CHIEF COMPLAINT

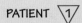

PATIENT

Mr. Y is a 30-year-old man with low back pain that has lasted for 6 days.

What is the differential diagnosis of low back pain? How would you frame the differential?

CONSTRUCTING A DIFFERENTIAL DIAGNOSIS

Most low back pain is caused by conditions that are troublesome but not progressive or life-threatening. The primary task when evaluating patients with low back pain is to identify those who have a serious cause of back pain that requires specific, and sometimes rapid, diagnosis and treatment. In practice, this means distinguishing *serious* back pain (pain due to a systemic or visceral disease or pain with significant neurologic symptoms or signs) from *nonspecific* back pain related to the musculoskeletal structures of the back, called mechanical back pain. The framework for the differential diagnosis reflects this task.

A. Back pain due to disorders of the **musculoskeletal** structures

1. Nonspecific (mechanical) back pain: no definite relationship between anatomic abnormalities seen on imaging and symptoms

2. Specific musculoskeletal back pain: clear relationship between anatomic abnormalities and symptoms

   a. Lumbar radiculopathy due to herniated disk, osteophyte, facet hypertrophy, or neuroforaminal narrowing

   b. Spinal stenosis

   c. Cauda equina syndrome

B. Back pain due to **systemic disease** affecting the spine

1. Serious and emergent (requires specific and often rapid treatment)

   a. Neoplasia

   (1) Multiple myeloma, metastatic carcinoma, lymphoma, leukemia

   (2) Spinal cord tumors, primary vertebral tumors

   b. Infection

   (1) Osteomyelitis

   (2) Septic diskitis

   (3) Paraspinal abscess

   (4) Epidural abscess

2. Serious but nonemergent (requires specific treatment but not urgently)

   a. Osteoporotic compression fracture

   b. Inflammatory arthritis

   (1) Ankylosing spondylitis

   (2) Psoriatic arthritis

   (3) Reactive arthritis

   (4) Inflammatory bowel disease–associated arthritis

C. Back pain due to **visceral disease** (serious, requires specific and rapid diagnosis and treatment)

1. Retroperitoneal

   a. Aortic aneurysm

   b. Retroperitoneal adenopathy or mass

2. Pelvic

   a. Prostatitis

   b. Endometriosis

   c. Pelvic inflammatory disease

3. Renal

   a. Nephrolithiasis

   b. Pyelonephritis

   c. Perinephric abscess

4. GI

   a. Pancreatitis

   b. Cholecystitis

   c. Penetrating ulcer

Figure 7-1 reorganizes the differential diagnosis using pivotal points and outlines the diagnostic approach to low back pain. In every patient with back pain, it is essential to systematically ask about and look for the clinical clues and pivotal points associated with serious causes of back pain (Table 7-1). In patients with positive findings, the initial patient-specific differential is quickly limited to serious systemic causes of back pain or specific musculoskeletal back pain. Likelihood ratios (LRs) for these findings, when available, will be discussed later in the chapter. It is also essential to understand the clinical neuroanatomy of the lower extremity to properly examine patients with low back pain (Figures 7-2 and 7-3).

Mr. Y felt well until 1 week ago, when he helped his girlfriend move into her third floor apartment. Although he felt fine while helping her, the next day he woke up with

(continued)

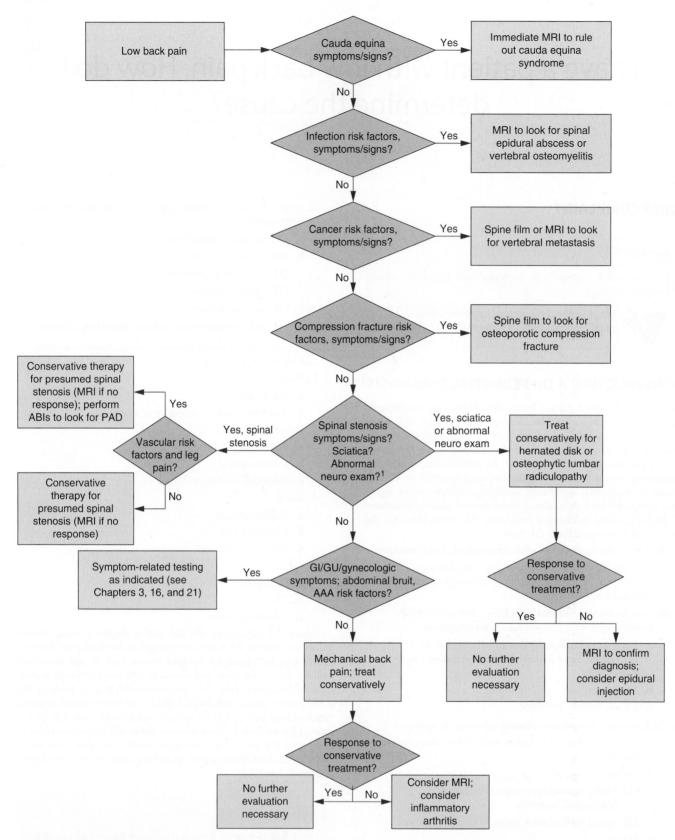

[1]Abnormal neurologic exam means abnormalities consistent with lumbar radiculopathy. Finding any other abnormalities requires consideration of other neurologic causes.

AAA, abdominal aortic aneurysm; ABIs, ankle-brachial index; GI, gastrointestinal; GU, genitourinary; MRI, magnetic resonance imaging; PAD, peripheral arterial disease.

Figure 7-1. Diagnostic approach: low back pain.

Table 7-1. Pivotal points and clinical clues in the diagnosis of low back pain.

Diagnosis	Pivotal Points/Clinical Clues
Cauda equina syndrome	Urinary retention Saddle anesthesia Bilateral leg weakness Bilateral sciatica
Infection	Fever Recent skin or urinary tract infection Immunosuppression Injection drug use
Malignancy	Cancer history, especially active cancer Unexplained weight loss Age over 50 Duration > 1 month
Compression fracture	Age over 70 Female sex Corticosteroid use History of osteoporosis Trauma
Lumbar radiculopathy	Sciatica Abnormal neurologic exam

diffuse pain across his lower back and buttocks. He spent that day lying on the floor, with some improvement. Ibuprofen has helped somewhat. He feels better when he is in bed and had transiently worse pain after doing his usual weight lifting at the gym.

 At this point, what is the leading hypothesis, what are the active alternatives, and is there a must not miss diagnosis? Given this differential diagnosis, what tests should be ordered?

RANKING THE DIFFERENTIAL DIAGNOSIS

Mr. Y's history of a specific precipitant and diffuse back pain is consistent with nonspecific mechanical back pain, which is the cause of 97% of the back pain seen in a primary care practice. History and physical exam should focus on looking for neurologic signs and symptoms that would suggest a specific musculoskeletal cause, such as a herniated disk, and for signs and symptoms that would suggest the presence of a systemic disease. Signs and symptoms of neurologic or systemic disease are pivotal points in the assessment of back pain. It is necessary to further explore the differential by looking for findings listed in Tables 7-1 and 7-2. Table 7-2 lists the differential diagnosis.

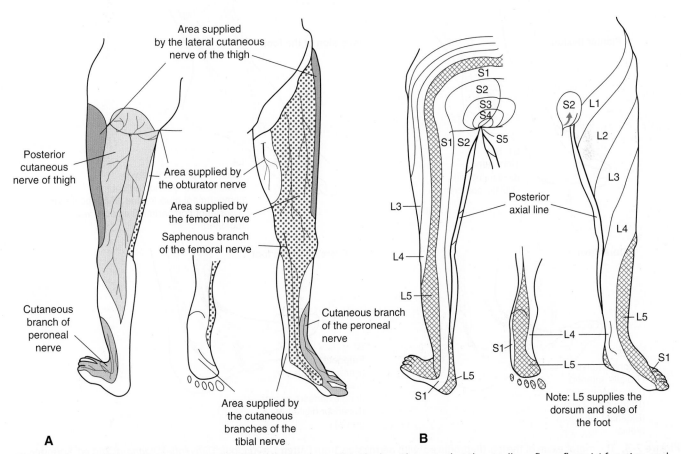

Figure 7-2. Distribution of cutaneous nerves (A) and nerve roots (B) in the leg. Also note that the patellar reflex reflects L4 function, and the Achilles reflex reflects S1 function. (Reproduced, with permission, from Patten J. *Neurologic Differential Diagnosis,* 2nd ed. Springer, 1996.)

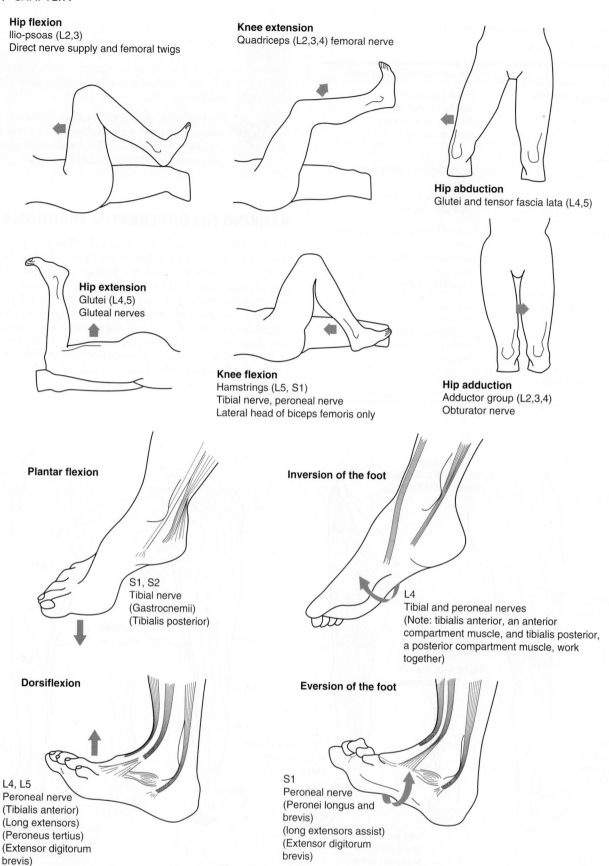

Hip flexion
Ilio-psoas (L2,3)
Direct nerve supply and femoral twigs

Knee extension
Quadriceps (L2,3,4) femoral nerve

Hip abduction
Glutei and tensor fascia lata (L4,5)

Hip extension
Glutei (L4,5)
Gluteal nerves

Knee flexion
Hamstrings (L5, S1)
Tibial nerve, peroneal nerve
Lateral head of biceps femoris only

Hip adduction
Adductor group (L2,3,4)
Obturator nerve

Plantar flexion
S1, S2
Tibial nerve
(Gastrocnemii)
(Tibialis posterior)

Inversion of the foot
L4
Tibial and peroneal nerves
(Note: tibialis anterior, an anterior compartment muscle, and tibialis posterior, a posterior compartment muscle, work together)

Dorsiflexion
L4, L5
Peroneal nerve
(Tibialis anterior)
(Long extensors)
(Peroneus tertius)
(Extensor digitorum brevis)

Eversion of the foot
S1
Peroneal nerve
(Peronei longus and brevis)
(long extensors assist)
(Extensor digitorum brevis)

Figure 7-3. The motor exam of the leg. (Reproduced, with permission, from Patten J. *Neurologic Differential Diagnosis,* 2nd ed. Springer, 1996.)

Table 7-2. Diagnostic hypotheses for Mr. Y.

Diagnostic Hypotheses	Demographics, Risk Factors, Symptoms and Signs	Important Tests
Leading Hypothesis		
Mechanical back pain	Absence of symptoms listed below	Resolution within 4–6 weeks
Active Alternative—Most Common		
Herniated disk	Sciatica Abnormal neurologic exam, especially in L5–S1 distribution	CT or MRI
Active Alternative—Must Not Miss		
Malignancy	Duration of pain > 1 month Age > 50 Previous cancer history Unexplained weight loss (> 10 lbs over 6 months)	Spine radiograph MRI
Infection	Fever Chills Recent skin or urinary infection Immunosuppression Injection drug use	MRI
Cauda equina syndrome	Urinary retention Saddle anesthesia Bilateral sciatica Leg weakness Decreased anal sphincter tone	MRI
Other Hypotheses		
Compression fracture	Age > 70 Female sex Significant trauma History of osteoporosis Corticosteroid use	Spine radiograph MRI

 The clinical clues (sometimes called "red flags") listed in Table 7-1 should be assessed in all patients with back pain.

Mr. Y has no history of other illnesses. He has had no trauma, weight loss, fever, chills, or recent infections. He takes no medications and does not smoke, drink, or use injection drugs. The back pain does not radiate to his legs. On physical exam, he has mild tenderness across his lower back; lower extremity strength, sensation, and reflexes are normal. Straight leg raise test is negative.

 Is the clinical information sufficient to make a diagnosis? If not, what other information do you need?

The exploration does not undercover new findings suggestive of specific or serious causes of back pain, limiting the differential at this point to nonspecific, mechanical low back pain.

Leading Hypothesis: Mechanical Low Back Pain

Textbook Presentation

The classic presentation is nonradiating pain and stiffness in the lower back, often precipitated by heavy lifting.

Disease Highlights

A. Can also have pain and stiffness in the buttocks and hips

B. Often occurs hours to days after a new or unusual exertion and improves when the patient is supine, but patients do not always identify a specific precipitant

C. Can rarely make a specific anatomic diagnosis

D. New neurologic abnormalities on history or physical exam should prompt investigation of another diagnosis.

E. Lifetime prevalence of mechanical low back pain is 84%.

F. Prognosis

1. 75–90% of patients improve within 1 month; of the subset with pain at 3 months, only 40% recover by 12 months.

2. 25–50% of patients have additional episodes over the next year

3. Risk factors for persistent low back pain, which occurs in 10–15% of patients, include

a. Maladaptive pain coping behaviors

b. High level of baseline functional impairment

c. Low general health status

d. Presence of psychiatric comorbidities

e. Presence of "nonorganic signs" (signs suggesting a strong psychological component to pain, such as superficial or nonanatomic tenderness, overreaction, nonreproducibility with distraction, nonanatomic weakness or sensory changes)

Evidence-Based Diagnosis

A. The absence of all red flags is 99% predictive of a nonserious etiology of low back pain.

B. Many *asymptomatic* patients will have anatomic abnormalities on imaging studies.

1. 20% of patients aged 14–25 have degenerative disks on plain radiographs.

2. 20–75% of patients younger than 50 years have herniated disks on MRI.

3. 40–80% of patients have bulging disks on MRI.

4. Over 90% of patients older than age 50 have degenerative disks on MRI.

5. Up to 20% of patients over age 50 have spinal stenosis.

C. Even in symptomatic patients, anatomic abnormalities are not necessarily causative, and identifying them does not influence initial treatment decisions.

D. A specific pathoanatomic diagnosis cannot be made in 85% of patients with isolated low back pain.

E. Imaging does not improve clinical outcomes such as pain or functional status, especially in patients with acute (< 4 weeks) or subacute (4–12 weeks) pain.

 Patients who have none of the clinical clues should not have any diagnostic imaging performed. If done, diagnostic imaging will often find clinically unimportant abnormalities.

Treatment

A. Acute low back pain

1. Randomized controlled trials have shown that acetaminophen, nonsteroidal antiinflammatory drugs (NSAIDs), and skeletal muscle relaxants are effective in relieving acute low back pain.

2. There is little data regarding the effects of opioids and tramadol in acute low back pain, but they are sometimes used in patients whose pain is not controlled with acetaminophen, NSAIDS, and muscle relaxants.

3. Specific back exercises do not help acute low back pain but do help prevent recurrent back pain.

4. Heat and spinal manipulation have been shown to reduce acute low back pain.

5. The best approach is acetaminophen or NSAIDs and heat during the acute phase and activity as tolerated until the pain resolves, followed by specific daily back exercises.

 Bed rest does not help acute pain and may prolong the duration of pain. Activity will not worsen the injury, and patients should be as active as is tolerated.

B. Subacute or chronic low back pain

1. Tricyclic antidepressants, tramadol, opioids, gabapentin, and benzodiazepines have all been shown to be effective in treating chronic low back pain; the best evidence is for tricyclic antidepressants.

2. There is good evidence that cognitive-behavioral therapy, exercise, spinal manipulation, and interdisciplinary rehabilitation are effective for chronic low back pain.

3. There is fair evidence that acupuncture, massage, and some yoga techniques are effective.

4. Facet and epidural injection has not been shown to be beneficial; local trigger point injection might be helpful.

MAKING A DIAGNOSIS

Considering Mr. Y's history and physical exam, there is no need to consider other diagnoses at this point. Should he not respond to conservative therapy, the alternative diagnoses would need to be reconsidered.

CASE RESOLUTION

You reassure Mr. Y that his pain will resolve within another 2–3 weeks. You recommend that he use ibuprofen as needed and be as active as possible within the limits of the pain. Rather than weight lifting, you suggest swimming or walking for exercise until his pain resolves. You also provide a handout on proper lifting techniques and back exercises, to be started after the pain resolves. He cancels a follow up appointment 1 month later, leaving a message that his pain is gone and he has resumed all of his usual activities.

CHIEF COMPLAINT

 PATIENT 2

Mrs. H, a 47-year-old woman, was well until 2 days ago, when she started having low back pain after working in her garden and pulling weeds for several hours. The pain is a constant, dull ache that radiates to her right buttock and hip. Yesterday, after sitting in a movie, the pain began radiating to the back of the right knee. She has taken some acetaminophen and ibuprofen without much relief. Her past medical history is unremarkable, and she takes no medicines. She has no constitutional, bowel, or bladder symptoms.

 At this point, what is the leading hypothesis, what are the active alternatives, and is there a must not miss diagnosis? Given this differential diagnosis, what tests should be ordered?

RANKING THE DIFFERENTIAL DIAGNOSIS

Similar to the patient discussed in the first case, Mrs. H's low back pain developed after an unusual exertion, and she has no systemic symptoms. However, her pain is worsened by sitting and radiates down the back of her leg (a pain distribution that suggests radicular pain in the L5–S1 distribution, often called sciatica). Both of these pivotal features increase the probability that she has a herniated disk. She has no findings that suggest a systemic cause of her back pain, so the initial differential is limited. Table 7-3 lists the differential diagnosis.

Table 7-3. Diagnostic hypotheses for Mrs. H.

Diagnostic Hypotheses	Demographics, Risk Factors, Symptoms and Signs	Important Tests
Leading Hypothesis		
Herniated lumbar disk	Sciatica Neurologic signs and symptoms, especially in L5–S1 distribution Positive straight leg raise	CT or MRI
Active Alternative—Most Common		
Nonspecific mechanical back pain	No neurologic or systemic symptoms	Resolution of pain

On physical exam, Mrs. H is clearly uncomfortable. She has no back tenderness and has full range of motion of both hips. When her right leg is raised to about 60 degrees, pain shoots down the leg. When her left leg is raised, she has pain in her lower back. Her strength and sensation are normal, but the right ankle reflex is absent.

 Is the clinical information sufficient to make a diagnosis? If not, what other information do you need?

Leading Hypothesis: Lumbar Radiculopathy due to a Herniated Disk

Textbook Presentation

The classic presentation is moderate to severe pain radiating from the back down the buttock and leg, usually to the foot or ankle, with associated numbness or paresthesias. This type of pain is called sciatica, and it is classically precipitated by a sudden increase in pressure on the disk, such as after coughing or lifting.

Disease Highlights

A. Disk disease is frequently asymptomatic.

B. 98% of clinically important disk herniations occur at L4–L5 and L5–S1, so pain and paresthesias are most often seen in the distributions of these nerves (Figures 7–2 and 7–3).

   1. Radicular pain is often described as sharp, shooting or burning but can also be described as throbbing, tingling, or dull.

   2. Neurologic abnormalities such as paresthesias/sensory loss and motor weakness are found variably and can occur in the absence of pain. Table 7-4 describes the typical findings.

C. Myofascial pain syndromes and hip and knee pathology can be difficult to distinguish from radiculopathy; many patients have both radiculopathy *and* other musculoskeletal conditions.

D. Coughing, sneezing, or prolonged sitting can aggravate radicular pain from a herniated disk.

E. 50% of patients recover in 2 weeks and 70% in 6 weeks.

F. Risk factors for herniated disks include sedentary activities, especially driving, chronic cough, lack of physical exercise, and possibly pregnancy. Jobs involving lifting and pulling have not been associated with increased risk.

G. There are no bowel or bladder symptoms with unilateral disk herniations.

H. Large midline herniations can cause the **cauda equina syndrome.**

   1. Cauda equina syndrome is a rare condition caused by tumor or massive midline disk herniations.

   2. It is characterized by the following:

   a. Urinary retention [CE1](sensitivity 90%, specificity 95%; LR+ = 18, LR– = 0.1)

   b. Urinary incontinence

   c. Decreased anal sphincter tone (80% of patients)

   d. Sensory loss in a saddle distribution (75% of patients)

   e. Bilateral sciatica

   f. Leg weakness

   g. The combination of measured urinary retention > 500 mL, and at least 2 of 3 typical symptoms (bilateral sciatica, subjective urinary retention, and rectal incontinence) is highly predictive of cauda equina syndrome on MRI.

 Suspected cauda equina syndrome is a medical emergency that requires immediate imaging and decompression.

Evidence-Based Diagnosis

A. History and physical exam (Table 7-5)

   1. Sciatica has an LR+ of 7.9 for the diagnosis of L4–5 or L5–S1 herniated disk.

   2. Straight leg test is performed by holding the heel in 1 hand and slowly raising the leg, keeping the knee extended.

   a. A positive test reproduces the patient's sciatica when the leg is elevated between 30 and 60 degrees.

   b. The patient should describe the pain induced by the maneuver as shooting down the leg not just a pulling sensation in the hamstring muscle.

Table 7-4. Typical abnormalities in lumbosacral radiculopathies.

Nerve Root	Distribution of Pain	Paresthesias/ Sensory changes	Motor weakness	Absent Reflexes
L4	Medial thigh	Medial lower leg	Knee extension, hip adduction	Knee
L5	Lateral thigh, lateral lower leg, dorsum of foot	Lateral thigh, lateral lower leg, dorsum of foot	Ankle dorsiflexion, foot eversion + inversion, hip abduction	
S1	Posterior thigh, calf, heel	Sole, lateral foot + ankle, fourth + fifth toes	Foot plantar flexion, knee flexion, hip extension	Ankle

Table 7-5. Physical exam findings for the diagnosis of disk herniation.

Finding	Sensitivity	Specificity	LR+	LR–
Sciatica	95%	88%	7.9	0.06
Positive crossed straight leg raise	25%	90%	2.5	0.83
Positive ipsilateral straight leg raise	85–91%	26–50%	1.2–1.8	0.18–0.3
Great toe extensor weakness	50%	70%	1.7	0.71
Impaired ankle reflex	50%	60%	1.3	0.83
Ankle dorsiflexion weakness	35%	70%	1.2	0.93
Ankle plantar flexion weakness	6%	95%	1.2	0.99

3. Crossed straight leg test is performed by lifting the contralateral leg; a positive test reproduces the sciatica in the affected leg.

 A straight leg raise test that elicits just back pain is negative.

4. Combinations of abnormal findings (eg, positive straight leg raise and neurologic abnormalities such as absent ankle reflex, impaired plantar flexion or dorsiflexion, impaired sensation in L5–S1 distribution) are presumably more specific than isolated findings.

B. Imaging

1. Plain radiographs do not image the disks and are useless for diagnosing herniations.

2. CT and MRI scans have similar test characteristics for diagnosing herniated disks.

   a. CT: sensitivity, 62–90%; specificity, 70–87%; LR+, 2.1–6.9; LR–, 0.11–0.54

   b. MRI: sensitivity, 60–100%; specificity, 43–97%; LR+, 1.1–33; LR–, 0–0.93

C. Electromyography (EMG)

1. Primarily used to confirm lumbosacral radiculopathy and exclude other peripheral nerve abnormalities, particularly when physical exam abnormalities do not correlate with imaging abnormalities

2. Also used to determine the severity and chronicity of a radiculopathy, and the functional significance of an imaging abnormality

3. Most useful for subacute abnormalities (3 weeks to 3 months after onset of symptoms)

4. Data regarding sensitivity and specificity are flawed but estimates are 71–100% sensitivity and 38–88% specificity.

Treatment

A. In the absence of cauda equina syndrome or progressive neurologic dysfunction, conservative therapy should be tried for 4–6 weeks.

1. NSAIDs are the first choice.

2. Tramadol or opioids are often necessary.

3. Short courses of oral corticosteroids may be helpful for acute, severe pain.

4. Bed rest does not accelerate recovery.

5. Epidural corticosteroid injections may provide temporary pain relief.

B. Surgery

1. Indications include

   a. Impairment of bowel and bladder function (cauda equina syndrome)

   b. Gross motor weakness

   c. Progressive neurologic symptoms or signs

2. Surgery should not be done for painless herniations or when the herniation is at a different level than the symptoms.

3. In the absence of progressive neurologic symptoms, surgery is elective; patients with disk herniations and radicular pain generally recover with or without surgery.

a. Recent randomized trials of surgery versus conservative therapy for symptomatic L4–5 or L5–S1 herniated disks found short-term benefits for surgery.

   (1) Patients who received surgery had better pain and function scores at 12 weeks, but both groups had identical scores at 52 weeks.

   (2) The median time to recovery was 4 weeks for the surgery group and 12 weeks for the conservative therapy group.

b. Patient preference should drive decision making with regard to surgery.

MAKING A DIAGNOSIS

Mrs. H has sciatica, a positive straight leg raise test, and an absent ankle reflex, a combination that strongly suggests nerve root impingement at L5–S1. One option at this point would be to order an MRI or CT scan to confirm a herniated disk. However, there are 2 questions to consider before ordering a scan:

 1. Will the scan be diagnostic? Remember that a significant percentage of asymptomatic people have herniated disks on CT or MRI.

 2. If the scan is diagnostic, will the finding change the initial management of the patient? Conservative therapy, similar to that for nonspecific back pain, is indicated initially unless the patient has cauda equina syndrome or other rapidly progressive neurologic impairment.

 The abnormality on imaging studies must correlate with the findings on history and physical exam; in other words, the herniation must affect the nerve associated with the dermatome that matches the symptoms.

CASE RESOLUTION

You decide not to order any imaging studies initially and prescribe ibuprofen (800 mg 3 times daily) and activity as tolerated. Mrs. H calls the next day, reporting that she was unable to sleep because of the pain. You then prescribe acetaminophen with codeine, which provides good pain relief. Two weeks later, she is rarely using the codeine, and is only using ibuprofen 1 to 2 times a day. Two months later, she is pain free and back to her usual activities, although her ankle reflex is still absent—a common and not significant finding. She is fine until about a year later, when identical pain develops after a bad bronchitis. Her pain resolves with a few days of acetaminophen with codeine.

CHIEF COMPLAINT

PATIENT

Mrs. P is a 75-year-old white woman who was well until 2 days ago when pain developed in the center of her lower back. The pain is constant and becoming more severe. There is no position or movement that changes the pain, and it is not relieved with acetaminophen or ibuprofen. It sometimes radiates in a belt like fashion across her lower back, extending around to the abdomen. She has no fever or weight loss. Her past medical history is notable for a radial fracture after falling off her bicycle 15 years ago, and breast cancer 2 years ago, treated with lumpectomy and radiation therapy. She currently takes only 1 medication, letrozole. Her last mammogram was normal 6 months ago.

 At this point, what is the leading hypothesis, what are the active alternatives, and is there a must not miss diagnosis? Given this differential diagnosis, what tests should be ordered?

RANKING THE DIFFERENTIAL DIAGNOSIS

Mrs. P has several pivotal clinical findings that suggest her back pain could be due to a more serious, systemic disease rather than being nonspecific, mechanical back pain. First, she is older and has a history of cancer; both findings are associated with malignancy as a cause of back pain. Second, her age, race, and history of a previous fracture are established risk factors for osteoporosis. In addition, 5–15% of patients using aromatase inhibitors such as letrozole have increased bone loss or fractures. Metastatic breast cancer is more emergent than vertebral compression fracture and is therefore both the leading and must not miss hypothesis. Table 7-6 lists the differential diagnosis.

Table 7-6. Diagnostic hypotheses for Mrs. P.

Diagnostic Hypotheses	Demographics, Risk Factors, Symptoms and Signs	Important Tests
Leading Hypothesis		
Metastatic breast cancer	Duration of pain > 1 month Age > 50 Previous cancer history Unexplained weight loss (> 10 lbs over 6 months)	Spine radiograph MRI
Active Alternative		
Osteoporotic compression fracture	Age > 70 Female sex Significant trauma History of osteoporosis Corticosteroid use Prior fracture	Spine radiograph MRI

On physical exam, she is in obvious pain. She is 5 ft 2 in and weighs 115 lbs. There is diffuse tenderness across her lower back, with no point tenderness of the vertebrae. There is no rash as would be seen in herpes zoster, and abdominal exam is normal. Her reflexes, strength, and sensation are all normal, and straight leg raise is negative.

Is the clinical information sufficient to make a diagnosis? If not, what other information do you need?

Leading Hypothesis: Back Pain Due to Metastatic Cancer

Textbook Presentation

The classic presentation is the development of constant, dull back pain that is not relieved by rest and is worse at night in a patient with a known malignancy.

Disease Highlights

A. Bone metastases can be limited to the vertebral body or extend into the epidural space, causing cord compression.

B. Pain can precede cord compression by weeks or even months, but compression progresses rapidly once it starts.

> Cancer + back pain + neurologic abnormalities = an emergency.

C. Malignancy causes < 1% of back pain in general but is the cause in most patients with active cancer who have back pain.

D. Most common sources are breast, lung, or prostate cancer.
   1. Renal and thyroid cancers also commonly metastasize to bone.
   2. Myeloma and lymphoma frequently involve the spine.

E. In most cases of cancer metastasis, the thoracic vertebrae are affected, while metastasis of prostate cancer most often affects the lumbar vertebrae.

F. Blastic lesions are seen with prostate cancer, small cell lung cancer, Hodgkin lymphoma.

G. Lytic lesions are seen with renal cell, myeloma, non-Hodgkin lymphoma, melanoma, non–small cell lung cancer, thyroid cancer.

H. Mixed blastic and lytic lesions are seen with breast cancer and GI cancers.

Evidence-Based Diagnosis

A. History and physical exam
   1. Previous history of cancer has an LR+ of 14.7 for the diagnosis of vertebral metastasis as a cause of back pain.
   2. Table 7-7 lists the historical and physical exam findings associated with low back pain due to cancer.

 Cancer is not likely to be the cause of back pain if the patient is younger than 50 years, has no history of cancer, has not experienced unexplained weight loss, and has not failed conservative therapy.

Table 7-7. History and physical exam findings in the diagnosis of cancer as a cause of low back pain.

Finding	Sensitivity	Specificity	LR+	LR−
Previous history of cancer	31%	98%	14.7	0.7
Failure to improve after 1 month of therapy	31%	90%	3.0	0.77
Age > 50	77%	71%	2.7	0.32
Unexplained weight loss	15%	94%	2.7	0.9
Duration of pain > 1 month	50%	81%	2.6	0.62
No relief with bed rest	90%	46%	1.7	0.21
Any of the following: age > 50, history of cancer, unexplained weight loss, or failure of conservative therapy	100%	60%	2.5	0.0

B. Imaging
1. Plain radiographs
   a. Lytic lesions are not visible until about 50% of trabecular bone is lost.
   b. Blastic lesions can be seen earlier on radiographs than lytic lesions.
   c. Sensitivity, 60%; specificity, 96–99.5%
   d. LR+, 12–120; LR−, 0.4–0.42
2. CT scan: Sensitivity and specificity for diagnosing metastatic lesions are unknown.
3. MRI
   a. Sensitivity, 83–93%; specificity, 90–97%
   b. LR+, 8.3–31; LR−, 0.07–0.19
4. Bone scan
   a. Sensitivity, 74–98%; specificity, 64–81%
   b. LR+, 3.9-10; LR−, 0.1–0.32
   c. Better for blastic lesions than lytic lesions; myeloma, in particular, can be missed on bone scan.

MRI scan is the best test for diagnosing or ruling out cancer as a cause of back pain and for determining whether there is cord compression.

C. Laboratory tests: the erythrocyte sedimentation rate (ESR) is sometimes helpful.
1. ≥ 20 mm/h: sensitivity, 78%; specificity, 67%; LR+, 2.4
2. ≥ 50 mm/h: sensitivity, 56%; specificity, 97%; LR+, 19.2
3. ≥ 100 mm/h: sensitivity, 22%; specificity, 99.4%; LR+, 55.5

Treatment

A. Surgery, radiation therapy, and chemotherapy
B. Choice of therapy depends on the type of cancer and the extent of the lesion.

MAKING A DIAGNOSIS

Since Mrs. P has no neurologic abnormalities, and plain radiographs are relatively quick to perform, it is reasonable to start with lumbar spine films. However, because of the suboptimal LR− of about 0.4, it will be necessary to perform additional imaging if the plain radiographs are normal.

The lumbar spine films show a vertebral compression fracture at L1, which is new when compared with films done several months ago.

Have you crossed a diagnostic threshold for the leading hypothesis, metastatic cancer? Have you ruled out the active alternatives? Do other tests need to be done to exclude the alternative diagnoses?

Alternative Diagnosis: Osteoporotic Compression Fracture

Textbook Presentation

The classic presentation is acute, severe pain that develops in an older woman and radiates around the flank to the abdomen, occurring either spontaneously or brought on by trivial activity such as minor lifting, bending, or jarring.

Disease Highlights

A. Fractures are usually in the mid to lower thoracic or lumbar region.
B. Fractures at T4 or higher are more often due to malignancy than osteoporosis.
C. Pain is often increased by slight movements, such as turning over in bed.
D. Can also be asymptomatic
E. Pain usually improves within 1 week and resolves by 4–6 weeks, but some patients have more chronic pain.
F. Osteoporosis is most commonly primary, related to menopause and aging.
G. Can occur as a complication of a variety of diseases and medications.
   1. Most common diseases include hyperthyroidism, primary hyperparathyroidism, vitamin D deficiency, hypogonadism, and malabsorption.
   2. Medications that can lead to osteoporosis include corticosteroids (most common), anticonvulsants, aromatase inhibitors, and long-term heparin therapy.
H. Risk factors for osteoporosis include
   1. Age
      a. Strongest risk factor
      b. Relative risk of almost 10 for women aged 70–74 (compared with women under 65), increasing to a relative risk of 22.5 for women over 80
   2. Personal history of rib, spine, wrist, or hip fracture
   3. Current smoking
   4. White, Hispanic, or Asian ethnicity
   5. Weight < 132 lbs
   6. Family history of osteoporosis

I. Risk of developing osteoporosis is decreased in women who are obese, are of African American descent, and use estrogen after menopause.

J. Over 15 years, the absolute risk of vertebral fracture is about 10% for women with T scores of 0 to −1.0 and about 30% for women with T scores of − 2.5 or worse; the T score is defined as the number of standard deviations different the current bone density is compared to a young adult reference population.

K. Women with a prevalent vertebral fracture and a T score > −1.0 have the same absolute risk of subsequent fracture (~25%) as women without prevalent fractures and T scores ≤ −2.5.

L. The FRAX score, used to estimate the 10-year probability of a hip fracture or a major osteoporotic fracture, is available at http://www.shef.ac.uk/FRAX/

Evidence-Based Diagnosis

A. History and physical exam

1. Not well studied
2. Age > 70 has LR+ of 5.5

3. History of corticosteroid use has LR+ of 12.0 for diagnosis of osteoporotic compression fracture as a cause of back pain
4. Patients with at least 3 typical risk factors (female sex, age over 70, trauma, and use of corticosteroids) have a very high likelihood of having an osteoporotic compression fracture.

B. Imaging

1. MRI is thought to be more sensitive and specific than radiographs, but data are not available; most compression fractures are diagnosed with radiographs, unless there is a concern for malignancy.
2. MRI scan can distinguish between benign and malignant osteoporotic compression fractures, with sensitivity of 88.5–100% and specificity of 89.5–93% (LR+ = 8–14, LR− = 0–0.12).
3. Bone scan can be useful for determining acuity.

 MRI scan is the best way to distinguish malignant from benign osteoporotic compression fractures.

Treatment

A. Osteoporosis

1. Total calcium intake (dietary plus supplementation, if necessary) should be 1200–1500 mg daily; total vitamin D intake should be 700–800 international units daily. Excessive supplementation may be harmful.
2. Bisphosphonates both increase bone density and reduce risk of subsequent spine and hip fractures.
   a. Alendronate and risedronate are given orally once per week.

b. Ibandronate is given orally once per month.

c. Zoledronic acid is given intravenously once per year.

3. Raloxifene reduces risk of spine fractures but not hip fractures.
   a. It also reduces the risk of estrogen receptor–positive breast cancer (relative risk = 0.56).
   b. It increases the risk of venous thromboembolism (relative risk about 3).
4. Parathyroid hormone (teriparatide) increases bone density and prevents fractures at the spine and the hip.
5. Estrogen can prevent fractures but is no longer recommended for long-term therapy due to such adverse events as the following:
   a. Deep venous thrombosis
   b. Pulmonary embolism
   c. Breast cancer
   d. Myocardial infarction
   e. Cerebrovascular accidents
6. Calcitonin does not significantly increase bone density or prevent fractures.

B. Compression fractures

1. Calcitonin may reduce the pain from an acute vertebral compression fracture.
2. Vertebroplasty (percutaneous injection of bone cement under fluoroscopic guidance into a collapsed vertebra) and kyphoplasty, (introduction of bone cement and inflatable bone tamps into the fractured vertebral body) have *not* been shown to reduce pain in well-done randomized controlled trials using sham procedures in the control groups.

CASE RESOLUTION

Mrs. P undergoes an MRI scan, which confirms the diagnosis of osteoporotic compression fracture. She is treated with opioids, and her pain resolves over 3–4 weeks. Her bone density results show a spine T score of −2.1, and a hip T score of −2.6. Her osteoporosis is probably largely primary osteoporosis, perhaps worsened by exposure to an aromatase inhibitor. Treatment is started.

Regardless of Mrs. P's bone density results, the presence of a vertebral compression fracture mandates treatment for osteoporosis. Reviewing her history, she had several risk factors for osteoporosis, including her age, weight, and history of a wrist fracture.

CHIEF COMPLAINT

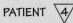
PATIENT

Mr. F is a 65-year-old man with type 2 diabetes, hypertension, and osteoarthritis who comes into your office

complaining of several months of low back pain. Sometimes the pain is limited to his back, but it sometimes radiates to his buttocks, hips, thighs and calves when he walks. Although generally achy in character, he sometimes feels

(continued)

numbness in both thighs. The pain gets better when he sits down, although he finds it also goes away while he is grocery shopping if he bends a bit to push the cart. He does not have pain while in bed, and he has more pain standing than sitting. Over-the-counter ibuprofen helps somewhat, but he feels quite limited in his activity. He has no fever, history of instrumentation, or injection drug use.

 At this point, what is the leading hypothesis, what are the active alternatives, and is there a must not miss diagnosis?

RANKING THE DIFFERENTIAL DIAGNOSIS

The differential for back pain in a man this age is broad. He does not have pivotal systemic symptoms suggesting that infection should be included in the initial differential diagnosis. Exploring his history, there are 2 historical findings strongly suggesting spinal stenosis: the sensation of numbness with exertion (neurogenic or "pseudoclaudication"), and the improvement in the pain when he bends forward to push a grocery cart. Although he does not have the unremitting pain characteristic of metastatic cancer, that is still a possibility because of his age. Another pivotal clue is that he has risk factors for vascular disease, and so peripheral arterial disease (PAD) must be considered. Mechanical low back pain, although common, is very unlikely given the pivotal clue of neurologic symptoms (thigh numbness). Disk herniation is a final possibility, although it would have to be a central herniation to explain the bilateral symptoms. Table 7-8 lists the differential diagnosis.

Table 7-8. Diagnostic hypotheses for Mr. F.

Diagnostic Hypotheses	Demographics, Risk Factors, Symptoms and Signs	Important Tests
Leading Hypothesis		
Spinal stenosis	Wide-based gait Neurogenic claudication Age > 65 Improvement with sitting/bending forward	MRI
Active Alternative—Must Not Miss		
Metastatic cancer	Duration of pain > 1 month Age > 50 Previous cancer history Unexplained weight loss (> 10 lbs over 6 months)	Spine radiograph MRI
Peripheral arterial disease	Vascular risk factors; leg pain with walking	ABIs
Active Alternative—Most Common		
Mechanical back pain	No neurologic or systemic symptoms	Resolution of pain
Central disk herniation	Bilateral radicular pain	MRI

Mr. F's past medical history is notable for hypertension, type 2 diabetes, and osteoarthritis of his knees. He quit smoking 10 years ago, having smoked 1 pack per day for 30 years. His medications include lisinopril, glipizide, atorvastatin, aspirin, and acetaminophen or ibuprofen. He has no history of cancer, and his prostate-specific antigen (PSA) was 0.9 ng/mL 1 month ago. He has no back or hip tenderness. Straight leg raise test is negative bilaterally; reflexes are symmetric; strength is normal; and sensation is normal, except for decreased vibratory sense in his feet. Dorsalis pedis and posterior tibialis pulses are easily palpable. His gait is normal.

 Is the clinical information sufficient to make a diagnosis? If not, what other information do you need?

Leading Hypothesis: Spinal Stenosis

Textbook Presentation

The classic presentation is somewhat vague, but persistent back and leg discomfort brought on by walking or standing that is relieved by sitting or bending forward is typically seen.

Disease Highlights

A. The clinical syndrome of lumbar spinal stenosis consists of characteristic symptoms **and** radiographic abnormalities.

    1. Neurogenic claudication, a variable pain or discomfort with walking or prolonged standing that radiates into the buttocks, thighs, or lower legs, is the most common symptom.

    2. Radicular or polyradicular pain can occur and is not as related to position as neurogenic claudication.

    3. Descriptions of pain from spinal stenosis differ qualitatively from textbook descriptions of vascular claudication (Table 7-9).

B. Neurologic symptoms and signs are variable.

C. Stenosis is seen most often in the lumbar spine, sometimes in the cervical spine, and rarely in the thoracic spine.

D. Spinal stenosis is due to hypertrophic degenerative processes

Table 7-9. Findings that differentiate vascular from neurogenic claudication.

Vascular	Neurogenic
Fixed walking distance before onset of symptoms	Variable walking distance before onset of symptoms
Improved by standing still	Improved by sitting or bending forward
Worsened by walking	Worsened by walking or standing
Painful to walk uphill	Can be painless to walk uphill due to tendency to bend forward
Absent pulses	Present pulses
Skin shiny with loss of hair	Skin appears normal

and degenerative spondylolisthesis compressing the spinal cord, cauda equina, individual nerve roots, and the arterioles and capillaries supplying the cauda equina and nerve roots.

E. Pain is worsened by extension and relieved by flexion.

F. Patients with central stenosis generally have bilateral, non-dermatomal pain involving the buttocks and posterior thighs.

G. Patients with lateral stenosis generally have pain in a dermatomal distribution.

H. Repeating the physical exam after rapid walking might demonstrate subtle abnormalities.

I. About 50% of patients have stable symptoms; when worsening occurs, it is gradual.

  1. Lumbar spinal stenosis does not progress to paralysis and should be managed based on severity of symptoms.

  2. Progression of cervical and thoracic stenoses can cause myelopathy and paralysis and requires surgery more often than lumbar spinal stenosis.

Evidence-Based Diagnosis

A. History and physical exam

  1. Wide-based gait has an LR+ of 13 for the diagnosis of spinal stenosis.

  2. Table 7-10 outlines the historical and physical exam findings associated with the diagnosis of spinal stenosis.

B. Imaging

  1. Plain radiographs are not necessary: they do not change management, or provide the degree of anatomic detail necessary to guide interventional treatment (such as epidural injection or surgery).

Table 7-10. History and physical exam findings in the diagnosis of spinal stenosis.

Finding	Sensitivity	Specificity	LR+	LR−
History				
No pain when seated	47%	94%	7.4	0.57
Burning sensation around buttocks	6%	99%	7.2	0.95
Improvement with bending forward	52%	92%	6.4	0.52
Bilateral buttock or leg pain	51%	92%	6.3	0.54
Neurogenic claudication	82%	78%	3.7	0.23
Symptoms improve when seated	51%	84%	3.3	0.58
Age > 65	77%	69%	2.5	0.34
Physical Exam				
Wide-based gait	42%	97%	13	0.6
Abnormal Romberg sign[1]	40%	91%	4.2	0.67
Vibration deficit	53%	81%	2.8	0.57

[1] Defined as compensatory movements required to maintain balance within 10 seconds of standing with feet together and eyes closed.

2. Noninfused CT and noninfused MRI have similar test characteristics.

  a. CT scan: sensitivity, 90%; specificity, 80–96%; LR+, 4.5–22; LR−, 0.10–0.12

  b. MRI: sensitivity, 90%; specificity, 72–99%; LR+, 3.2–90; LR−, 0.10–0.14

  c. Up to 21% of asymptomatic patients over age 65 have spinal stenosis on MRI.

3. Patients with typical symptoms who respond to conservative therapy can be managed without imaging.

> CT and MRI scans can rule out spinal stenosis but cannot necessarily determine whether visualized stenosis is causing the patient's symptoms.

Treatment

A. Evidence to guide treatment decisions is minimal.

B. Nonoperative treatment is variably successful. 15–70% of patients stabilize or improve.

  1. Medications used for pain relief include NSAIDs, tricyclic antidepressants, gabapentin, pregabalin, tramadol, and sometimes opioids.

  2. Physical therapy improves stamina and muscle strength in the legs and trunk; exercises performed with lumbar flexion, such as cycling, may be better tolerated than walking.

  3. Epidural corticosteroid injection helps some patients, especially those with radicular pain.

C. Surgery

  1. Primary indication is increasing pain that is not responsive to conservative measures.

  2. Observational data show the following:

  a. More effective in reducing leg pain than back pain

  b. Reported improvement rates range between 64% and 91%.

  c. Reoperation rates range from 6% to 23%.

  d. Predictors of a positive response to surgery include male gender, younger age, better walking ability, better self-rated health, less comorbidity, and more pronounced canal stenosis.

  3. A recent trial with both a randomized and observation cohort showed the following:

  a. In the intention to treat analysis of the randomized cohort, patients randomized to surgery reported better scores on 1 measure of bodily pain at 2 years than did those randomized to conservative therapy.

  b. In the analysis of the observational cohort, patients who chose surgery reported better pain and function scores than those who chose conservative therapy.

MAKING A DIAGNOSIS

Mr. F's history remains suggestive of spinal stenosis; his physical exam neither rules in nor rules out the diagnosis. You prescribe acetaminophen and gabapentin, refer him to

(continued)

physical therapy, and plan to order an MRI if he does not respond to conservative treatment.

Have you crossed a diagnostic threshold for the leading hypothesis, spinal stenosis? Have you ruled out the active alternative, PAD? Do other tests need to be done to exclude the alternative diagnoses?

Alternative Diagnosis: Peripheral Arterial Disease (PAD)

Textbook Presentation

Classic claudication is defined as reproducible, exercise-induced calf pain that requires stopping and is relieved with < 10 minutes of rest. Critical limb ischemia classically presents with pain in the feet at rest that may be relieved by placing the feet in a dependent position.

Disease Highlights

A. In a study of outpatients over the age of 70, or aged 50–69 with a history of smoking or diabetes, the prevalence of PAD was 29%.

  1. Only 11% of the patients with PAD had classic claudication.

  2. 47% of patients had atypical symptoms (exertional leg pain that was not in the calf or was not relieved by rest), and 42% had no leg pain.

B. Critical limb ischemia is the presenting manifestation in 1–2% of patients.

C. Risk factors include

  1. Smoking (relative risk of PAD increases by 1.4 for every 10 cigarettes smoked/day)

  2. Hypertension (risk of PAD increases by 1.5 for mild and 2.2 for moderate hypertension)

  3. Diabetes (risk of PAD increases by 2.6)

  4. Hyperlipidemia (risk of PAD increases by 1.2 for each 40 mg/dL increase in cholesterol)

D. Patients with PAD have a high prevalence of coronary artery disease and cerebrovascular disease with an annual rate of cardiovascular events of 5–7%.

E. PAD is associated with a progressive decline in walking endurance and an increased rate of depression.

F. Pretest probabilities of PAD in patients with a variety of risk factors are shown in Table 7-11.

Evidence-Based Diagnosis

A. History

  1. The presence of classic claudication has an LR+ = 3.30.

  2. The absence of classic claudication has an LR– = 0.89.

B. Physical exam

  1. Skin changes

    a. In symptomatic patients, skin being cooler to the touch and the presence of a foot ulcer in the affected leg both have a LR+ = 5.9 and a LR– of about 1.0.

    b. Skin changes (atrophic or cool skin, blue/purple skin, absence of lower limb hair) are not useful in assessing for PAD in asymptomatic patients.

Table 7-11. Pretest probabilities of PAD.

	Patients with Leg Complaints	Asymptomatic Patients
Age 60–80	15%	
Age 60–69		5%
Age 70–79		12%
Stroke	26%	15%
Ischemic heart disease	19%	13%
Diabetes	18%	11%
Hypercholesterolemia	15%	6%
Hypertension	12%	7%
Male sex	12%	5%
Smoking (current or quit in last 5 years)	11%	7%

PAD, peripheral arterial disease.

  2. Bruits

    a. In symptomatic patients the presence of an iliac, femoral, or popliteal bruit has a LR+ = 5.6; the absence of a bruit in **all** 3 locations has a LR– = 0.39.

    b. In asymptomatic patients, the finding of a femoral bruit has a LR+ = 4.8; the absence of a femoral bruit does not change the probability of PAD.

  3. Pulses

     a. An abnormal femoral pulse has a LR+ = 7.2; an abnormal posterior tibial pulse has an LR+ = 8.10.

    b. An abnormal dorsalis pedis pulse does not substantially increase the probability of PAD (LR+ = 1.9); the dorsalis pedis pulse is not palpable in 8.1% of normal individuals.

    c. The absence of an abnormality in any pulse has a wide range of negative LRs (0.38–0.87).

  4. Capillary refill time

    a. Apply firm pressure to the plantar aspect of the great toe for 5 seconds; after releasing the toe, normal color should return in ≤ 5 seconds.

    b. Neither sensitive nor specific for diagnosing PAD

 *Lack of typical symptoms and physical findings does **not** lower the likelihood of PAD.*

C. Ankle-brachial index (ABI)

  1. Systolic pressures are measured in the arms and at the ankles. The formula for the ABI is: Highest ankle pressure (mm Hg)/Highest arm pressure (mm Hg)

  2. Using a cutoff of 0.90 or less to define abnormal, the sensitivity is 95% and specificity 99% for the diagnosis of PAD (LR+ = 95, LR– = 0.05)

  3. An ABI of 0.71–0.9 = mild PAD; 0.41–0.70 = moderate PAD; 0.00–0.40 = severe PAD

Treatment

A. Risk factor modification: smoking cessation, control of hypertension and diabetes, reduction of LDL to < 100 mg/dL

B. Antiplatelet therapy with aspirin or clopidogrel reduces myocardial infarction, stroke, and death from vascular causes; there is no additional benefit with combination therapy.

C. Cilostazol 100 mg twice daily increases walking distance by 50% after 3–6 months of use; pentoxifylline has no effect on walking distance.

D. Ramipril increases mean pain free walking time by over 200 yards in patients with uncomplicated, stable claudication not already taking an angiotensin-converting enzyme inhibitor or angiotensin receptor blocker.

E. Exercise, especially a supervised exercise program, can increase walking by up to 150% over 3–12 months.

F. Revascularization, either surgical or percutaneous transluminal angioplasty, is indicated for the following:

    1. Critical limb ischemia

    2. Claudication unresponsive to exercise and pharmacologic therapy that limits patients' lifestyle or ability to work

CASE RESOLUTION

Mr. F's pretest probability of PAD is at least 18%. You order ABIs, which show mild PAD (bilateral indices of 0.89). After attending physical therapy for presumed spinal stenosis for 8 weeks, he reports some improvement in his exercise tolerance, although he still has daily pain. He has not had sufficient relief from a variety of analgesics. An MRI scan shows moderate central canal stenosis and neuroforaminal narrowing at L3, L4, and L5. An epidural corticosteroid injection provides more pain relief, and he is able to continue a walking program.

REVIEW OF OTHER IMPORTANT DISEASES

Spinal Epidural Abscess

Textbook Presentation

The classic presentation is a patient with a history of diabetes or injection drug use who has fever and back pain, followed by neurologic symptoms (eg, motor weakness, sensory changes, and bowel or bladder dysfunction).

Disease Highlights

A. Pathogenesis

    1. Most patients have 1 or more predisposing conditions.

        a. Underlying disease (diabetes mellitus, alcoholism, HIV)

        b. Spinal abnormality or intervention (degenerative joint disease, trauma, surgery, drug injection)

        c. Potential local or systemic source of infection (skin or soft tissue infection, endocarditis, osteomyelitis, urinary tract infection, injection drug use, epidural anesthesia, indwelling vascular access)

    2. Infection occurs by contiguous spread in 33% of cases and by hematogenous spread in 50%.

    3. *Staphylococcus aureus* is the organism in 66% of cases.

        a. Other organisms include *Staphylococcus epidermidis, Escherichia coli, Pseudomonas aeruginosa.*

        b. Anaerobes, mycobacteria, fungi, and parasites are occasionally found.

B. Clinical manifestations

    1. Back pain in 75% of patients

    2. Fever in about 50% of patients

    3. Neurologic deficits are found in about 33% of patients.

    4. More common in posterior than anterior epidural space, and more common in the thoracolumbar than cervical areas.

    5. Generally extend over 3–5 vertebrae

C. Staging

    1. Stage 1: back pain at the level of the affected spine

    2. Stage 2: nerve root pain radiating from the involved spinal area

    3. Stage 3: motor weakness, sensory deficit, bladder/bowel dysfunction

    4. Stage 4: paralysis

    5. Rate of progression from 1 stage to another is highly variable.

    6. The most important predictor of the final neurologic outcome is the neurologic status before surgery, with the postoperative neurologic status being as good as or better than the preoperative status.

Evidence-Based Diagnosis

A. ESR and C-reactive protein are usually elevated.

B. Leukocytosis is present in about 66% of patients.

C. Bacteremia is present in 60% of patients.

D. MRI is best imaging study, with a sensitivity of > 90%.

Treatment

A. Emergent surgical decompression and drainage

B. Antibiotics

Vertebral Osteomyelitis

Textbook Presentation

The classic presentation is unremitting back pain often, but not always, with fever.

Disease Highlights

A. Pathogenesis

    1. Most commonly from hematogenous spread

        a. Urinary tract, skin, soft tissue, vascular access site, endocarditis, septic arthritis most commonly found sources, with endocarditis found in one-third of patients with vertebral osteomyelitis

        b. Patients usually have underlying chronic illnesses or injection drug use

    2. Can also occur due to contiguous spread from an adjacent soft tissue infection or direct infection from trauma or surgery.

    3. Generally causes bony destruction of 2 adjacent vertebral bodies and collapse of the intervertebral space.

        a. Found in the lumbar spine in 58% of cases, thoracic spine in 30%, and cervical spine in 11%

        b. Complicated by epidural abscess in 17% of cases, by paravertebral abscess in 26%, and disk space abscess in 5%

B. Microbiology

1. *S aureus* in over 50% of patients

2. Group B and G hemolytic streptococcus, especially in diabetic patients

3. Enteric gram-negative bacilli, especially after urinary tract instrumentation

4. Coagulase-negative staphylococci sometimes causative

Evidence-Based Diagnosis

A. History and physical exam

1. Back pain reported in 86% of patients

2. Spinal tenderness: sensitivity, 86%; specificity, 60%; LR+, 2.1; LR–, 0.23

3. Fever: sensitivity, 52%; specificity, 98%; LR+, 26; LR– 0.49

B. Laboratory tests

1. Leukocytosis: sensitivity, 43%; specificity, 94%; LR+, 7.2; LR– 0.6

2. ESR: sensitivity and specificity unknown, but nearly all patients in reported case series have an elevated ESR, often over 100 mm/h

3. C-reactive protein also elevated in nearly all patients, and may be a better marker of response to therapy.

4. Blood cultures are positive in about 58% of patients (range in studies 30–78%).

5. Culture of a biopsy specimen is positive in about 77% of patients (range in studies 47–100%).

C. Imaging

1. Radiographs: sensitivity, 82%; specificity, 57%; LR+, 1.9; LR–, 0.32

2. MRI: sensitivity, 96%; specificity, 92%; LR+, 12; LR–, 0.04

3. Bone scan: sensitivity, 90%; specificity, 78%; LR+, 4.1; LR–, 0.13

Treatment

A. Antibiotics for at least 4–6 weeks

B. Surgery is necessary only if neurologic symptoms suggest onset of vertebral collapse causing cord compression or development of spinal epidural abscess; surgery is always necessary for osteomyelitis associated with a spinal implant.

 Endocarditis should be considered in patients with either vertebral osteomyelitis or a spinal epidural abscess.

REFERENCES

Balague F, Mannion A, Pellise F, Cedraschi C. Non-specific low back pain. Lancet. 2012;379:482–91.

Chou R, Qaseem A, Snow V et al; Clinical Efficacy Assessment Subcommittee of the American College of Physicians; American College of Physicians; American Pain Society Low Back Pain Guidelines Panel. Diagnosis and treatment of low back pain: a joint clinical practice guideline from the American College of Physicians, and the American Pain Society. Ann Intern Med. 2007;147:478–91.

Chou R, Qaseem A, Owens DK, Shekelle P; Clinical Guidelines Committee of the American College of Physicians. Diagnostic imaging for low back pain: advice for high-value health care from the American College of Physicians. Ann Intern Med. 2011;154:181–9.

Chou R, Shekelle P. Will this patient develop persistent disabling low back pain? JAMA. 2010;303:1295–1302.

Dauouich RO. Spinal epidural abscess. N Engl J Med. 2006;355:2012–20.

Domen PM, Hofman PA, van Santbrink H, Weber WE. Predictive value of clinical characteristics in patients with suspected cauda equina syndrome. Eur J Neurol. 2009;16:416–9.

Katz JN, Harris MB. Lumbar spinal stenosis. N Engl J Med. 2008;358:818–25.

Khan NA, Rahim SA, Anand SS, Simel DL, Panju A. Does the clinical examination predict lower extremity peripheral arterial disease? JAMA. 2006;295:536–46.

Lurie JD. What diagnostic tests are useful for low back pain? Best Pract Res Clin Rheumatol. 2005;19:557–75.

Sandoval AEG. Electrodiagnostics for low back pain. Phys Med Rehabil Clin N Am. 2010;4:767–76.

Suri P, Rainville J, Kalichman L, Katz JN. Does this older adult with lower extremity pain have the clinical syndrome of lumbar spinal stenosis? JAMA. 2010;304:2628–36.

Tarulli AW, Raynor EM. Lumbosacral radiculopathy. Neurol Clin. 2007;25:387–405.

Watson J. Office evaluation of spine and limb pain: spondylotic radiculopathy and other nonstructural mimickers. Semin Neurol. 2011;31:85–101.

White C. Intermittent claudication. N Engl J Med. 2007;356:1241–50.

Zimmerli W. Vertebral osteomyelitis. N Engl J Med. 2010;362:1022–9.

8

I have a patient with a bleeding disorder. How do I determine the cause?

CHIEF COMPLAINT

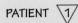

PATIENT 1

Ms. A is a 24-year-old woman who comes to see you because her gums are bleeding when she brushes her teeth.

What is the differential diagnosis of bleeding? How would you frame the differential?

CONSTRUCTING A DIFFERENTIAL DIAGNOSIS

The framework for bleeding distinguishes between structural causes (ie, an injury to the tissue or organ), platelet-related causes, and clotting factor–related causes. Bleeding due to platelet abnormalities, whether due to reduced number or abnormal function of platelets, is usually small vessel bleeding, and produces such findings as petechiae, bruising, gum bleeding, or nosebleeds. The bleeding occurs immediately upon the injury that induces it. Platelet-related bleeding is generally not quantitatively significant (ie, platelet-related bleeding tends not to cause serious blood loss requiring red cell transfusions). Nonetheless, platelet-related bleeding can still be clinically important if a patient bleeds a small amount into the brain (unusual unless the platelet count is < 10,000/mcL) or induces an abdominal hematoma from vigorous coughing, for example. By contrast, bleeding due to coagulation factor deficiencies or inhibitors tends to be delayed; that is, a platelet plug slows or stops the bleeding immediately after an injury, but the platelet plug is then not bolstered by the stable fibrin clot that is meant to definitively stop the bleeding. Bleeding due to coagulation factor abnormalities is more likely to be quantitatively significant, generally occurring in joints, the gastrointestinal tract, brain, retroperitoneum, or at sites of recent injury or medical or surgical intervention.

A. Structural causes

  1. Tissue injury from trauma
  2. Abnormality of the tissue such that minor trauma causes bleeding, such as a toothbrush causing gum bleeding from inflammatory gingival disease

B. Bleeding due to platelet disorders

  1. Disorders of platelet number (thrombocytopenia)
     a. Decreased production of platelets
        (1) Medications (examples include valproic acid, linezolid, thiazide diuretics, gold compounds, antineoplastic chemotherapy drugs)

        (2) Bone marrow replacement by malignancy, fibrosis, granulomas
        (3) Bone marrow aplasia
        (4) Alcohol
        (5) B_{12} deficiency
     b. Increased loss or consumption of platelets
        (1) Splenic sequestration
        (2) Autoimmune thrombocytopenia
           (a) Idiopathic (also called idiopathic thrombocytopenic purpura [ITP])
           (b) HIV
           (c) Systemic lupus erythematosus (SLE)
           (d) Lymphoproliferative disorders
           (e) Medications (examples include heparin, phenytoin, carbamazepine, sulfonamides, quinine, antiplatelet drugs used for coronary syndromes such as abciximab or tirofiban)
        (3) Disseminated intravascular coagulation (DIC)
        (4) Thrombotic thrombocytopenic purpura (TTP)
        (5) Sepsis
  2. Disorders of platelet function
     a. Congenital
        (1) von Willebrand disease
        (2) Other rare genetic abnormalities
     b. Acquired
        (1) Medications, such as aspirin, nonsteroidal antiinflammatory drugs (NSAIDs)
        (2) Myeloproliferative disorders, such as essential thrombocythemia, polycythemia vera
        (3) Coating of platelets by abnormal proteins, such as in multiple myeloma and, occasionally, immune thrombocytopenia
        (4) Uremia

C. Bleeding due to clotting factor abnormalities
  1. Congenital
     a. Hemophilia A (the most common)
     b. Other clotting factor deficiencies
  2. Acquired
     a. Deficiency of a factor or factors
        (1) Liver disease
        (2) Vitamin K deficiency (nutritional or due to warfarin therapy)

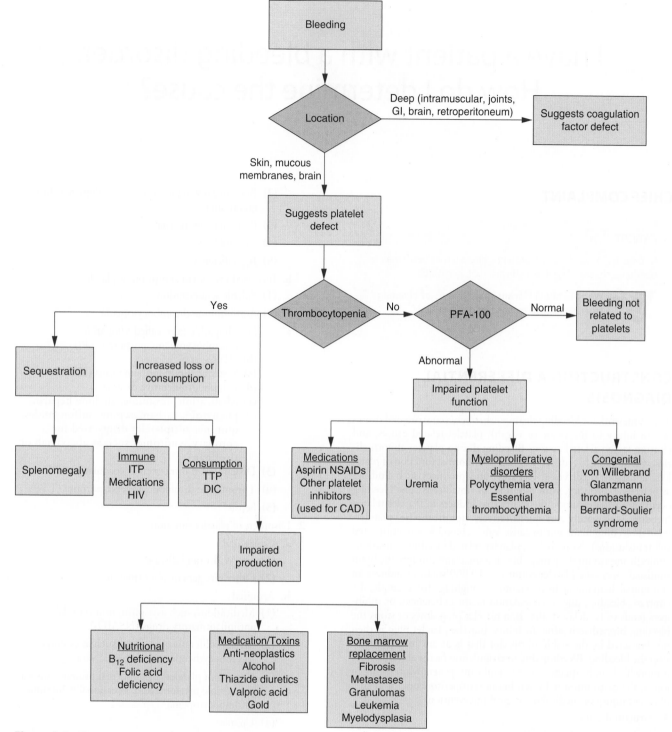

Figure 8-1. Diagnostic approach to the bleeding patient.

(3) Abnormal adsorption of a factor, eg, factor X adsorption to amyloid fibrils

(4) Consumption of factors, eg, DIC

(5) Dilution of factors, eg, massive transfusion

b. Acquired inhibitor to clotting factor or factors

Figure 8-1 shows the diagnostic approach to bleeding disorders.

About 2 weeks ago, Ms. A noticed bleeding from her gums while she was brushing her teeth. The bleeding lasts only briefly, and she does not consider it to be a large amount

(continued)

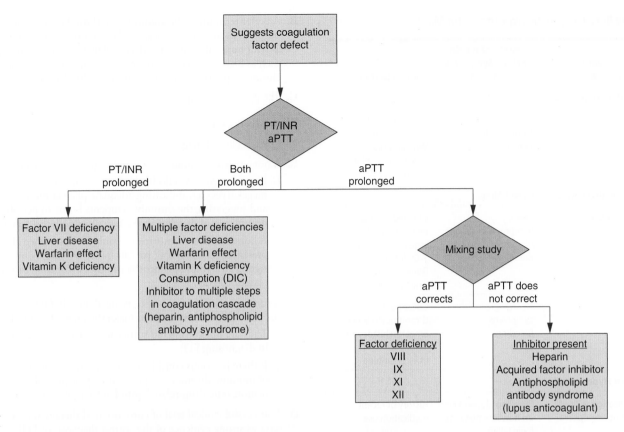

aPTT, activated partial thromboplastin time; CAD, coronary artery disease; DIC, disseminated intravascular coagulation; GI, gastrointestinal; INR, international normalized ratio; ITP, idiopathic thrombocytopenia purpura; NSAIDs, nonsteroidal antiinflammatory drugs; PT, prothrombin time; TTP, thrombotic thrombocytopenic purpura.

Figure 8-1. *(Continued)*

of blood. Her gums do not hurt, and she is timely with her dental care. At her last cleaning a month ago, she was told all was well. She has also noted some tiny red dots on her ankles in the past week—they are not raised and do not itch or hurt. She notes that her last menstrual period was somewhat heavier than usual, and she has had an intermittent headache over the last 2 days, partially relieved by acetaminophen. Otherwise, she has taken no medications. On examination, she looks well and has normal vital signs. Her oral examination shows evidence of recent gingival bleeding, and there are a few palatal petechiae. She also has petechiae on her antecubital fossae and ankles. There is no lymphadenopathy. Chest and abdominal examinations are normal, with no splenomegaly noted.

 At this point, what is the leading hypothesis, what are the active alternatives, and is there a must not miss diagnosis? Given this differential diagnosis, what tests should be ordered?

RANKING THE DIFFERENTIAL DIAGNOSIS

There are several pivotal points in Ms. A's presentation that suggest her bleeding is due to a platelet disorder: the bleeding occurs immediately after the trauma of tooth brushing, she has petechiae on her skin, and the bleeding is small volume.

The second pivotal point is that her history further suggests that her platelet disorder is acquired. If she had a congenital platelet disorder, such as von Willebrand disease, she might have had life-long heavy menses and other manifestations of bleeding. In this case, her symptoms just began 2 weeks ago. A platelet count will confirm that her bleeding is related to thrombocytopenia, rather than platelet dysfunction, which is less commonly seen. (When platelet dysfunction is suspected, a test such as the PFA-100 assay should be ordered. This test is a reproducible screening tool for platelet function abnormalities. It measures the time to formation of a platelet plug in response to collagen along with adenosine diphosphate [ADP] or epinephrine.) The most common cause of thrombocytopenia in a young woman with no signs of systemic illness is idiopathic autoimmune thrombocytopenia. Although Ms. A's headache is mild and she looks well, TTP can present with headache and thrombocytopenia and also tends to occur in young women. Finally, it is critical to remember that the platelets are only 1 of the cell lines affected by bone marrow disorders, and that a serious bone marrow condition (eg, leukemia) might first manifest as thrombocytopenia. A key step, then, is to decide if the thrombocytopenia is isolated or part of a pancytopenia picture, such as one might encounter with acute leukemia.

Table 8-1 lists the differential diagnosis.

Table 8-1. Diagnostic hypotheses for Ms. A

Diagnostic Hypotheses	Demographics, Risk Factors, Symptoms and Signs	Important Tests
Leading Hypothesis		
ITP	Young woman Gum bleeding Petechiae	CBC: isolated low platelets, normal WBC and Hb Smear: Large platelet forms
Active Alternative—Must Not Miss		
Acute leukemia	Fever, Symptoms and signs of anemia Bleeding	CBC: reduced or increased WBC Smear: immature WBC forms Bone marrow examination
TTP	Neurologic symptoms Bleeding Fever	CBC: anemia, thrombocytopenia Smear: schistocytes Serum LD BUN, creatinine
Other Hypothesis		
Medication related thrombocytopenia	Bleeding, depending on how low platelets have fallen	History of recent medication use

BUN, blood urea nitrogen; CBC, complete blood cell; Hg, hemoglobin; ITP, idiopathic thrombocytopenia purpura; LD, lactate dehydrogenase; TTP, thrombotic thrombocytopenia purpura; WBC, white blood cell.

Ms. A's laboratory tests indicate a WBC of 5600/mcL, RBC of 3.9 million/mcL, Hgb of 11.2 g/dL, HCT of 33.5%, and platelet count 8,000/mcL. Examination of the peripheral blood smear shows markedly decreased platelets with some large platelet forms, and normal RBC and WBC morphology.

Is the clinical information sufficient to make a diagnosis? If not, what other information do you need?

Leading Hypothesis: ITP

Textbook Presentation

The classic presentation is a previously healthy person not exposed to medications that can cause thrombocytopenia in whom gum bleeding or petechiae are present. The platelet count is low, with large platelets seen on peripheral blood smear; other cell lines are normal. Physical exam, other than the minor bleeding, is normal.

Disease Highlights

A. ITP is an autoimmune disorder primarily of young women. This is the demographic group that commonly suffers from other autoimmune disorders.

B. A better term might be autoimmune thrombocytopenic purpura, as some cases are secondary to other conditions, such as lymphoproliferative disorders, collagen vascular disorders such as SLE, or infectious or inflammatory disorders such as chronic hepatitis, HIV infection, or Crohn disease.

C. The prevalence is approximately 100 cases per million persons.

Evidence-Based Diagnosis

A. ITP is a clinical diagnosis.

B. A bone marrow examination is not required for diagnosis.
1. If performed, it would likely show normal or increased megakaryocytes, indicating adequate platelet production and suggesting the thrombocytopenia is due to peripheral destruction of platelets in the reticuloendothelial system.
2. A bone marrow examination should be done when the presentation is atypical: patient has splenomegaly or significant lymphadenopathy or other cytopenias or the patient is older.

C. Serum antiplatelet antibody tests are about 50–60% sensitive, and not sufficiently specific to make the diagnosis of ITP.
1. They are not considered sufficiently reliable for general use in diagnosing ITP.
2. If there is serious consideration of a drug-induced cause of immune thrombocytopenia, it may be possible to demonstrate drug-related antiplatelet antibodies.

D. A successful clinical trial of corticosteroid therapy may also serve as strong evidence of the correct diagnosis of ITP.

E. Serologic studies to evaluate for lupus erythematosus or HIV infection would also be indicated if there is any clinical suspicion for their presence.

Treatment

A. Prednisone is the initial treatment for all patients.

B. Patients who do not respond to prednisone or whose thrombocytopenia recurs when the prednisone is stopped undergo splenectomy, which removes a site of antibody production as well as a site of reticuloendothelial system destruction of antibody-coated platelets.

C. In refractory cases, other immunosuppressants may be used, such as rituximab, azathioprine, or cyclophosphamide.

D. Thrombopoietin analogues such as romiplostim and eltrombopag have recently become available for treatment of refractory cases of ITP.

MAKING A DIAGNOSIS

Ms. A's WBC count and hemoglobin are normal, eliminating leukemia as a possible diagnosis. Her reticulocyte production index is low and there are no schistocytes seen on her blood smear, suggesting that she does not have a hemolytic anemia. Her neurologic exam is normal as is her serum creatinine.

Have you crossed a diagnostic threshold for the leading hypothesis, ITP? Have you ruled out the active alternatives? Do other tests need to be done to exclude the alternative diagnoses?

Alternative Diagnosis: TTP

Textbook Presentation

Patients with TTP appear systemically ill. The 5 classic manifestations are thrombocytopenia; microangiopathic hemolytic anemia; neurologic abnormalities such as confusion, headache, lethargy, or seizures; fever; and acute kidney injury.

Disease Highlights

A. Only 2 or 3 of the classic manifestations are present in many patients.

B. Thrombocytopenia and microangiopathic hemolytic anemia must be present to diagnose TTP, regardless of whether the other manifestations are present.

C. Neurologic abnormalities are present in about two-thirds of patients, acute kidney injury or renal failure in about half, and fever in about one-quarter.

D. Pathophysiology
   1. The ADAMTS13 enzyme is responsible for cleaving ultra-large von Willebrand factor multimers into smaller components.
   2. An anti-ADAMTS13 antibody inactivates the enzyme; the trigger for antibody formation is unknown.
   3. The lack of the enzyme leads to the ultra-large multimers causing platelet aggregation and clumping in the microcirculation, leading to thrombocytopenia.
   4. These clumps cause red blood cells passing over them to be physically damaged, leading to the characteristic finding on the blood smear of schistocytes, or fragmented red blood cells.

Evidence-Based Diagnosis

A. A serum test demonstrating reduced ADAMTS13 activity and a positive test for the anti-ADAMTS13 antibody reliably establish the diagnosis.

B. The diagnosis of TTP is made clinically, since the ADAMTS13 assay result may take several days to return, and the disease has critical morbidity and mortality if treatment is delayed.
   1. Any patient with thrombocytopenia (usually below 30,000/mcL) and evidence of microangiopathic hemolysis (schistocytes on peripheral blood smear, elevated serum lactate dehydrogenase (LD) level, reduced serum haptoglobin level) should raise concern about TTP.
   2. If neurologic signs or acute kidney injury is present, the diagnosis becomes even more likely.

 Think about TTP in patients with thrombocytopenia and signs of hemolytic anemia.

Treatment

A. Plasma exchange is the treatment of TTP. While it is complicated and expensive, it does not carry substantial medical risk.
   1. Large volumes of plasma are removed from the patient and fresh plasma reinfused.
   2. This removes the antibody to ADAMTS13, and provides plasma with a normal complement of the enzyme.
   3. It is possible to treat TTP with plasma infusion alone, but plasma exchange allows for infusion of much higher volumes of plasma.
   4. Plasma exchange is performed daily, typically for 7–14 days, while monitoring the platelet count and LD levels.
   5. Prior to the advent of plasma exchange, the mortality rate for TTP was about 90%. With plasma exchange, the survival rate is now about 90%.

B. Immunosuppressive drugs such as prednisone or rituximab are also used in an effort to reduce the production of the anti-ADAMTS13 antibody.

 It is essential to treat TTP as soon as it is suspected, even if the diagnosis is not absolutely firm.

CASE RESOLUTION

Ms. A's presentation does not meet criteria for TTP. She has no other symptoms or signs of bone marrow dysfunction, no history of recent medication use, and no underlying other conditions. Her bleeding is consistent with platelet-induced bleeding, and so the diagnosis of ITP appears firm.

Ms. A begins treatment with prednisone at a dose of 1 mg/kg orally daily. After 1 week, her platelet count rises to 40,000/mcL, and after 2 weeks, to 130,000/mcL. She then begins a prednisone taper over many weeks, and her platelet count remains above 100,000/mcL.

The goal of therapy in ITP is a safe platelet count, typically a count above 30,000/mcL, rather than a normal count. If it is not possible to taper prednisone off, or to a very low dose, while maintaining a safe platelet count, alternative therapies such as splenectomy or thrombopoietin analogues are indicated, since the long-term risks of corticosteroids (infections, osteoporosis, adrenal suppression, muscle weakness, electrolyte disturbances) should be avoided if possible.

CHIEF COMPLAINT

 PATIENT 2

Mr. J is a 62-year-old man who underwent a coronary bypass graft operation 1 week ago for severe coronary artery disease. He has remained in the hospital for management of a postoperative sternal wound infection, has been doing well, and is scheduled for discharge later in the day.

His past history is notable for an autoimmune hemolytic anemia several years ago, successfully treated with prednisone. He drank 6 beers per day for years, quitting about 6 months ago. The laboratory pages you to report that his platelet count is 56,000/mcL.

 At this point, what is the leading hypothesis, what are the active alternatives, and is there a must not miss diagnosis? Given this differential diagnosis, what tests should be ordered?

RANKING THE DIFFERENTIAL DIAGNOSIS

The most common causes of new thrombocytopenia in hospitalized patients are medications, heparin-induced thrombocytopenia (HIT), and sepsis. Therefore, the first steps in diagnosing thrombocytopenia in a hospitalized patient are to review previous platelet counts to determine whether the thrombocytopenia is new, review the medication list, and look for vital signs suggestive of sepsis. Because Mr. J has a history of autoimmune hemolytic anemia, it is also important to consider autoimmune thrombocytopenia as an accompanying autoimmune phenomenon (also called Evans syndrome, characterized by seeing spherocytes rather than schistocytes in the peripheral smear), although this would otherwise be uncommon in his age group. Finally, he could have cirrhosis due to his extensive alcohol intake over the years, with hypersplenism causing mild-to-moderate thrombocytopenia. Chronic autoimmune hemolytic anemia might also cause splenic enlargement. If hypersplenism is the cause, his platelet count at admission would probably have been somewhat low, typically between 40,000/mcL and 120,000/mcL. Table 8-2 lists the differential diagnosis.

Mr. J's vital signs are normal, and a recent nursing note reports that he finished his breakfast and looked fine. He is receiving antibiotics for the wound infection and subcutaneous heparin every 8 hours for prophylaxis against deep venous thrombosis. His last platelet count was 175,000/mcL 3 days ago. The rest of his CBC results from today include WBC 14,600/mcL and Hgb 11.8 g/dL, unchanged from previous Hgb levels. A chemistry profile, including liver enzymes and albumin, is normal.

Is the clinical information sufficient to make a diagnosis? If not, what other information do you need?

Table 8-2. Diagnostic hypotheses for Mr. J.

Diagnostic Hypotheses	Demographics, Risk Factors, Symptoms and Signs	Important Tests
Leading Hypothesis		
HIT	Heparin exposure Cold toe	Platelet count HIT ELISA assay
Active Alternative—Must Not Miss		
Autoimmune thrombocytopenia (idiopathic or secondary)	Gum bleeding Petechiae Known associated disease (SLE, HIV, autoimmune hemolytic anemia)	CBC: isolated low platelets, normal WBC and Hb Smear: Large platelet forms
Hypersplenism	Known cirrhosis Risk factors for liver disease	History Splenomegaly on exam or imaging
Sepsis	Fever Rigors Hypotension Tachycardia	CBC Blood cultures

CBC, complete blood cell; ELISA, enzyme-linked immunosorbent assay; Hg, hemoglobin; HIT, heparin-induced thrombocytopenia; SLE, systemic lupus erythematosus.

Mr. J's thrombocytopenia is new, and he is receiving heparin, a very common cause of medication-related thrombocytopenia. He is clinically stable, and so sepsis is not a serious consideration.

Leading Hypothesis: HIT

Textbook Presentation

The classic presentation of HIT is a hospitalized patient receiving heparin whose platelet count falls by more than 50% from baseline, though generally to a level still above 50,000/mcL. There may be associated thrombosis, more commonly venous (deep venous thrombosis, pulmonary embolism, venous limb gangrene) than arterial (cold digits or extremity). Skin necrosis at the site of heparin injections may also be seen.

Disease Highlights

A. Caused by the development of an antibody directed against a heparin-platelet factor 4 complex; the antibody occurs more commonly with unfractionated heparin than with low-molecular-weight heparin.

B. Develops in about 5% of patients who receive heparin.

C. Surgical patients are at higher risk.

D. HIT manifests between 5 and 10 days after starting any kind of heparin—full dose intravenous heparin, low-dose prophylactic heparin, or even just heparin flushes to maintain patency of indwelling intravascular catheters. Thrombocytopenia may develop earlier in patients with recent heparin exposure.

E. Thrombosis develops in about 50% of patients who have HIT, and the thrombosis may be evident at the same time as the platelet count drop. Thrombosis may be arterial (previously called the white clot syndrome), although it is more often venous.

F. The platelet count does not usually drop below 50,000/mcL in HIT; a lower platelet count suggests another etiology.

Evidence-Based Diagnosis

A. The most sensitive, readily available, screening test is an enzyme-linked immunosorbent assay (ELISA) assay for anti-PF4 antibody.

   1. It is nearly 100% sensitive, although specificity is between 75% and 85%. Thus, a negative test is very reassuring that HIT is not present, but false-positive tests are not uncommon.

   2. The serotonin-release assay is more specific but not readily available.

B. Because the poor specificity of the anti-PF4 assay leads to overdiagnosis of HIT, a pretest probability scoring system (the 4"T's") has been validated.

   1. **Thrombocytopenia**

      a. Fall of platelets by > 50% and nadir > 20,000/mcL = 2 points

      b. Fall of platelets by 30–50% or nadir 10–19,000/mcL = 1 point

      c. Fall by < 30% or nadir < 10,000/mcL = 0 points

   2. **Timing of platelet fall**

      a. Clear onset between days 5 and 10 after exposure, or < 1 day if prior heparin exposure within 30 days = 2 points

      b. Consistent with fall between 5 and 10 days, but some data missing, or fall > 10 days, or < 1 day if prior heparin exposure within 30–100 days = 1 point

      c. Fall at < 4 days and without recent exposure = 0 points

3. **T**hrombosis or other sequelae

   a. Confirmed new thrombosis, skin necrosis, or acute systemic reaction after IV unfractionated heparin bolus = 2 points

   b. Progressive or recurrent thrombosis, non-necrotizing skin lesions or suspected thrombosis that has not been proven = 1 point

   c. None of the above = 0 points.

4. **OT**her causes for thrombocytopenia present:

   a. None apparent = 2 points

   b. Possible = 1 point

   c. Definite = 0 points.

5. Test interpretation: 0–3 points: low probability; 4–5 points: intermediate probability; 6–8 points: high probability.

   a. In 1 large series of 111 patients with a low pretest probability of HIT using this scoring system, only 1 had clinically significant HIT antibodies (0.9%).

   b. In contrast, the overall rate of clinically significant HIT antibodies was 11.4% and 34% in those with intermediate and high scores, respectively.

6. An online calculator is available at http://www.qxmd.com/calculate-online/hematology/hit-heparin-induced-thrombocytopenia-probability

Treatment

A. Heparin must be discontinued whenever HIT is suspected, even when the anti-PF4 assay result is not yet available.

B. An alternative anticoagulant must be started to prevent HIT-associated thrombosis, regardless of whether the initial indication for anticoagulation is still present; generally, a direct thrombin inhibitor such as argatroban or lepirudin is used.

   1. Low-molecular-weight heparin may not be substituted: although the incidence of HIT with low-molecular-weight heparin is much lower than with unfractionated heparin, once HIT occurs, there is too much risk for cross-reactivity.

   2. Similarly, warfarin should not be used until the platelet count has recovered (this takes a few days) but can then be started while the direct thrombin inhibitor is being given.

   3. Anticoagulation should continue for 2–3 months.

C. Although not approved for this indication, fondaparinux, a factor X inhibitor, has sometimes been used as an alternative anticoagulant in patients with HIT.

D. Surprisingly, patients with a history of HIT may safely be reexposed to heparin if necessary after a year has passed and the antibody has presumably disappeared.

MAKING A DIAGNOSIS

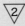

Before you have finished reviewing Mr. J's chart, the nurse pages you to report that he is complaining of severe pain in his right great toe. It is cool and dusky when you examine it.

 Have you crossed a diagnostic threshold for the leading hypothesis, HIT? Have you ruled out the active alternatives? Do other tests need to be done to exclude the alternative diagnoses?

The findings of a painful, cool, and dusky toe suggest arterial occlusion. While post cardiac surgery patients can have arterial emboli from a left ventricular clot or postoperative atrial fibrillation, the combination of new thrombocytopenia, heparin exposure, and thrombosis points toward HIT. Mr. J's "4T" score is 8, consistent with a high probability of HIT: 2 points for the degree of thrombocytopenia, 2 points for the time course, 2 points for the presence of new thrombosis, and 2 points for lack of other apparent causes of thrombocytopenia (despite his alcohol history, his liver tests are normal, making cirrhosis and hypersplenism unlikely, and ITP is not associated with thrombosis).

CASE RESOLUTION

You immediately stop all heparin exposure and start Mr. J on argatroban. His HIT ELISA assay is positive. His toe returns to normal, and his platelet count increases to 180,000/mcL within 4 days. He is receiving warfarin therapy when he is discharged.

CHIEF COMPLAINT

 PATIENT

Ms. W is a 56-year-old woman who comes to the office complaining of poor appetite for several weeks and black, tarry stools with generalized weakness for 1 day.

She has no prior history of bleeding, and her 3 prior obstetric deliveries were uncomplicated. Her past history is notable for cirrhosis due to chronic hepatitis C. Her medications include spironolactone and metoprolol; additionally, she has been taking ibuprofen for back pain.

On examination, she is pale. Her blood pressure is 110/80 mm Hg, pulse is 112 bpm, RR is 16 breaths per minute, temperature is 37.1°C. Her conjunctivae are pale, mucous membranes moist, lungs clear, heart regular rhythm with a systolic flow murmur at the left sternal border, liver minimally enlarged with a nodular edge, spleen palpable 3 cm below the left costal margin in the anterior axillary line, and she has no edema. Digital rectal examination discloses black stool that is Hemoccult-positive.

 At this point, what is the leading hypothesis, what are the active alternatives, and is there a must not miss diagnosis? Given this differential diagnosis, what tests should be ordered?

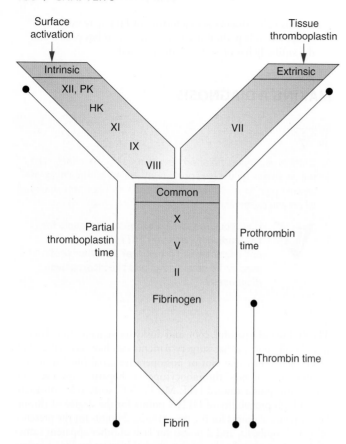

Surface activation

Tissue thromboplastin

Intrinsic

Extrinsic

XII, PK

HK

XI

IX

VIII

VII

Common

X

V

II

Fibrinogen

Partial thromboplastin time

Prothrombin time

Thrombin time

Fibrin

Figure 8-2. The coagulation cascade. Organization of the coagulation system based on current assays. The **intrinsic** coagulation system consists of the proteins factors XII, XI, IX, and VIII and prekallikrein (PK) and high molecular weight kininogen (HK). The **extrinsic** coagulation system consists of tissue factor (tissue thromboplastin) and factor VII. The **common pathway** of the coagulation system consists of factors X, V, and II, and fibrinogen (I). (Reproduced, with permission, from McPherson RA, Pincus MR, eds. *Henry's Clinical Diagnosis and Management by Laboratory Methods,* 22nd ed. Philadelphia, Elsevier Saunders, 2011, page 791.)

Table 8-3. Common factor deficiency patterns.

Clinical Setting	Factors Deficient	PT, aPTT Results
Liver disease	All but VIII[1]	Both prolonged
DIC	Fibrinogen, V, VIII, platelets	Both prolonged; thrombin time especially prolonged.
Vitamin K deficiency	II, VII, IX, X	PT and aPTT both prolonged, PT to greater extent
Warfarin effect	II, VII, IX, X	PT and aPTT both prolonged, PT to greater extent

[1] The only factor not produced by hepatocytes.
aPTT, activated partial thromboplastin time; DIC, disseminated intravascular coagulation; PT, prothrombin time.

Ms. W's presentation suggests that she is having an upper gastrointestinal (GI) bleed. In addition to the specific GI causes of upper GI bleeding discussed in Chapter 19, GI Bleeding, it is important to consider whether patients who are bleeding have an underlying platelet or coagulation disorder contributing to the bleeding. Ms. W does have cirrhosis with splenomegaly that could lead to thrombocytopenia due to splenic sequestration; however, the large volume of the bleeding may suggest a coagulation factor disorder.

The prothrombin time (PT) measures what is commonly called the extrinsic clotting pathway (Figure 8-2), wherein tissue factor from an injury activates factor VII, followed by activation of the coagulation cascade through the "common pathway" factors (factors V, X, II [prothrombin] and I [fibrinogen]). Because the source of tissue factor reagents used in the laboratory to trigger the cascade vary, the PT will vary among different laboratories when testing the same sample. To overcome this problem of PT results not being comparable from one lab to another, the international normalized ratio (INR) was developed, to standardize PT results based on a constant associated with each laboratory reagent. The INR, which is routinely reported along with the PT,

allows the clinician to feel confident that the data from different laboratories are comparable.

The activated partial thromboplastin time (aPTT) measures what is commonly called the intrinsic clotting pathway, starting with factor XII and working through factors XI, IX and VIII before entering the "common pathway."

In the evaluation of a prolonged clotting time, either PT or aPTT, one considers whether only 1 test is prolonged, and which factors contribute to each test. For example, an isolated prolonged PT suggests a deficiency of factor VII, since that is the only factor unique to the PT assay. An isolated prolonged aPTT raises concern about the 4 factors that are unique to the aPTT—factors, XII, XI, IX, and VIII. Prolongation of both the PT and aPTT raises concern either about the factors in the common pathway—I, II, V, and X—or a defect in multiple factors. Table 8-3 summarizes commonly seen patterns of factor deficiencies.

In clinical practice, prolongation of clotting times is most commonly acquired, either due to acquired deficiencies (eg, from malnutrition or liver disease) or acquired factor inhibitors. (While congenital factor deficiencies such as hemophilia certainly cause prolonged clotting times, these are far less commonly seen, and patients are well aware of them, making complex diagnostic evaluations unnecessary.) In order to distinguish between a factor deficiency and an inhibitor, it is often helpful to perform a mixing study, wherein one mixes 1:1 the patient's plasma and normal plasma, to see if the clotting time corrects. If it does correct, the normal plasma has provided the missing factor to the patient's plasma, indicating the abnormality is due to a factor deficiency. If it does not correct, the implication is that an inhibitor in the patient's plasma is inactivating the clotting factor(s) from the normal plasma. Such inhibitors may be exogenous, such as inadvertent heparin in the mixture; or endogenous, such as an acquired factor inhibitory antibody.

Based on the data we have so far, Ms. W's GI bleeding is most likely from the upper GI tract, probably induced by use of the NSAID ibuprofen. The severity of the bleeding may be exacerbated by a coagulopathy related to her cirrhosis. The history of poor appetite for a few weeks raises the consideration of vitamin K deficiency, and the presence of splenomegaly on examination suggests that thrombocytopenia due to splenic sequestration may also be contributing.

Table 8-4 lists the differential diagnosis.

Table 8-4. Diagnostic hypotheses for Ms. W.

Diagnostic Hypotheses	Demographics, Risk Factors, Symptoms and Signs	Important Tests
Leading Hypothesis		
Coagulopathy due to liver disease	History of hepatitis C or other chronic liver disease Signs of GI bleeding Jaundice, ascites	PT aPTT Platelet count LFTs
Active Alternatives—Must Not Miss		
Vitamin K deficiency	Lack of dietary vitamin K Recent use of antibiotics	Prolonged PT and aPTT, with PT disproportionately prolonged compared with aPTT
Acquired factor inhibitor	Older patient Abrupt onset of serious bleeding manifestations	Prolonged aPTT, as factor VIII most common example Failure to correct with mixing study Demonstrable factor VIII inhibitor
DIC	Inciting cause, such as sepsis, tissue injury, shock, obstetric crisis	Thrombocytopenia Prolongation of PT and aPTT Reduced fibrinogen Elevated D-dimer and fibrin degradation products
Other Hypothesis		
Hypersplenism	Splenomegaly on examination or radiographic study	Mild to moderate reductions in all cell lines

aPTT, activated partial thromboplastin time; DIC, disseminated intravascular coagulation; GI, gastrointestinal; LFTs, liver function tests; PT, prothrombin time.

A CBC shows WBC 9400/mcL, Hgb 7.8 g/dL, platelet count 76,000/mcL. A chemistry profile shows mild elevation of the transaminases but is otherwise normal. Her CBC 6 months ago showed an Hgb of 11.7 g/dL and platelet count of 80,000/mcL. Coagulation studies include a PT of 22 seconds (normal range 11–13 seconds), with an INR of 1.8 (normal 0.9–1.2). The aPTT is 39 seconds (normal 24–34 seconds).

Is the clinical information sufficient to make a diagnosis? If not, what other information do you need?

Ms. W has the stable, moderate thrombocytopenia generally seen in patients with portal hypertension and hypersplenism. Moderate thrombocytopenia such as this does not substantially increase the risk of bleeding, especially not the large volume GI

bleeding she is experiencing. The coagulation abnormalities she has can certainly contribute to large volume bleeding.

Leading Hypothesis: Liver Disease–Induced Coagulopathy

Textbook Presentation

The classic presentation of liver disease–induced coagulopathy is variable. Patients may be asymptomatic, only discovered to have a coagulopathy incidentally on coagulation laboratory studies. Spontaneous bleeding is uncommon, but anything that stresses the patient (such as an injury, an operative procedure, or perhaps drug-induced gastritis) may lead to more bleeding than one might normally anticipate with that event in someone without liver disease.

Disease Highlights

A. Patients with liver disease–induced coagulopathy typically have a disproportionately longer PT (and therefore higher INR) than aPTT.

B. The coagulopathy is caused by impaired production of clotting factors by the diseased liver; the clotting factor with the shortest half-life, namely factor VII, would be expected to be most prominently affected. Since the PT/INR is so sensitive to factor VII levels, that test is more notably abnormal.

C. Coagulopathy is seen primarily in patients with severe liver disease. The liver has considerable reserve, and only when the impairment is severe does one find significant coagulopathy.

Evidence-Based Diagnosis

A. In a patient with liver disease who is bleeding or in whom an invasive procedure is planned, the PT/INR and aPTT should be checked in order to screen for coagulation factor deficiencies.

   1. If the screening tests are prolonged, it may be worth checking the levels of factor VII, factor V, factor II, factor IX, and factor X as well as fibrinogen to help determine which replacement therapy is most appropriate.

   2. If factor VII is low but factor V normal, it suggests that vitamin K deficiency may be playing a role, whereas in severe liver impairment, both factors V and VII are reduced.

   3. Because all the clotting factors except factor VIII are produced in the hepatocytes, all of them except factor VIII may be low in severe liver disease. Factor VIII is typically normal or even elevated in liver disease, a finding that may distinguish liver disease from DIC, in which factor VIII is low.

B. Another finding that may contribute to bleeding risk in severe liver disease is excessive fibrinolysis, the cause of which is a complex interplay between the production of and hepatic clearance of fibrinolytic activators and inhibitors.

C. While it may seem paradoxical, there may also be increased risk of thrombosis in liver disease. Several findings may account for this: reduction of the vitamin K-dependent *anti*coagulant proteins, protein C and protein S; and increases in factor VIII and sometimes von Willebrand factor.

Treatment

A. Correct the coagulopathy using fresh frozen plasma to replete clotting factors. If the plasma fibrinogen level is particularly low (eg, < 100 mg/dL), infusion of cryoprecipitate may be helpful.

B. In severe cases, administration of recombinant activated factor VIIa may help stop the bleeding associated with liver disease; it is extremely expensive, however, and carries some risk of inducing thrombosis.

MAKING A DIAGNOSIS

An esophagogastroduodenoscopy (EGD) shows a duodenal ulcer consistent with NSAID use. Ms. W is treated with a proton pump inhibitor and fresh frozen plasma. Her PT and PTT normalize, and the bleeding stops.

Have you crossed a diagnostic threshold for the leading hypothesis, liver disease–induced coagulopathy? Have you ruled out the active alternatives? Do other tests need to be done to exclude the alternative diagnoses?

Alternative Diagnosis: Vitamin K Deficiency

Textbook Presentation

The usual presentation of vitamin K deficiency is a hospitalized patient who is found to have a prolonged PT/INR, rarely with bleeding manifestations.

Disease Highlights

A. The most common cause of vitamin K deficiency is inadequate oral intake.

B. Patients who have been hospitalized and need to start warfarin therapy may require smaller than expected doses to achieve therapeutic levels, because they may be unduly sensitive as a result of baseline vitamin K deficiency.

C. Vitamin K deficiency can also occur with the recent use of antibiotics that alter the gut flora's ability to convert vitamin K to an absorbable form.

Evidence-Based Diagnosis

A. As with liver disease, patients with vitamin K deficiency have PT/INR levels disproportionately longer than aPTT levels.

B. This is due to factor VII having the shortest half-life of the vitamin K–dependent factors (II, VII, IX, and X), thus making the factor VII–dependent PT/INR more sensitive to vitamin K alterations.

C. The aPTT will also go up eventually, as the levels of factors II, IX and X, with much longer half-lives, fall.

Treatment

A. Vitamin K repletion, either orally or parenterally, is the treatment of choice.
   1. If parenteral treatment is chosen, it should be administered subcutaneously or intravenously—not intramuscularly.
   2. Intramuscular injections should be avoided in patients with coagulopathies, in order to avoid the development of hematomas in muscles that can lead to neuropathy if a major nerve traverses the area.

B. Vitamin K administration takes 18–24 hours to have its effect, so if a patient with vitamin K deficiency is bleeding, fresh frozen plasma may be required.

Alternative Diagnosis: DIC

Textbook Presentation

Disseminated intravascular coagulation (DIC, also called consumptive coagulopathy) is a catastrophic activation of the coagulation system that classically presents as the abrupt onset of uncontrolled spontaneous diffuse bleeding from multiple sites (venipuncture sites, catheter sites, endotracheal tubes, recent surgical sites) in patients with severe illness such as shock states, major trauma, sepsis, obstetric emergencies, and advanced cancer.

Disease Highlights

A. The common denominator of conditions that cause DIC is tissue injury and activation of the clotting cascade via entry of procoagulants into the circulation.

B. A variety of conditions activate the clotting cascade.
   1. Trauma
   2. Advanced adenocarcinomas of any site, such as colon, pancreas, or lung.
   3. Obstetric crises such as amniotic fluid embolism or placental abruption.
   4. Acute promyelocytic leukemia, wherein the granules of the malignant promyelocytes activate the clotting system.

C. Although the classic presentation is major bleeding due to activation of the clotting cascade leading to secondary consumption of clotting factors, in some cases clotting manifestations may predominate.
   1. Patients with advanced cancer may have recurrent deep venous thrombosis or pulmonary embolism or arterial emboli in the extremities, without signs of bleeding.
   2. This is considered chronic DIC.

D. Renal, hepatic, and pulmonary dysfunction may accompany acute DIC.

Evidence-Based Diagnosis

A. In acute DIC, consumption of clotting factors is demonstrated by thrombocytopenia, prolongation of the PT/INR and aPTT, reduction of plasma fibrinogen level, and increases in D-dimer and fibrin degradation products (FDP).

B. The D-dimer and FDP reflect fibrinolytic activity acting upon fibrin formed during the clotting process.
   1. D-dimer is the product of lysis of cross-linked fibrin.
   2. FDP is the product of lysis of both fibrin and fibrinogen.
   3. Fibrinogen levels below 100 mg/dL may correlate with bleeding risk.

If DIC is suspected, testing should include platelet count, PT/INR, aPTT, fibrinogen, and D-dimer.

Treatment

A. Treat the underlying condition if possible.

B. Replete clotting factors that have been depleted, with platelet transfusions, fresh frozen plasma, and cryoprecipitate if fibrinogen is particularly low.

C. In rare instances, the use of low-dose heparin is considered. While it is logical to consider undertaking *anti*coagulation if the initiation of the process was coagulation, the additional bleeding risk is of great concern, and efforts are generally focused more on providing clotting factors while addressing the underlying cause.

CASE RESOLUTION

You instruct Ms. W to avoid all aspirin products and NSAIDs. She is seen by the dietician for review of vitamin K–rich foods. Her hemoglobin is stable at a follow up visit 2 weeks later.

REFERENCES

Bell WR, Braine HG, Ness PM, Kickler TS. Improved survival in thrombotic thrombocytopenic purpura-hemolytic uremic syndrome. Clinical experience in 108 patients. N Engl J Med. 1991 Aug 8;325(6):398–403.

Cuker A, Gimotty PA, Crowther MA, Warkentin TE. Predictive value of the 4Ts scoring system for heparin-induced thrombocytopenia: a systematic review and meta-analysis. Blood. 2012 Nov 15;120(20):4160–7.

George JN. Clinical practice. Thrombotic thrombocytopenic purpura. N Engl J Med. 2006 May 4;354(18):1927–35.

Greinacher A, Warkentin TE. Recognition, treatment, and prevention of heparin-induced thrombocytopenia: review and update. Thromb Res. 2006;118(2):165–76.

Levi M, Toh CH, Thachil J, Watson HG. Guidelines for the diagnosis and management of disseminated intravascular coagulation. British Committee for Standards in Haematology. Br J Haematol. 2009 Apr;145(1):24–33.

Linkins LA, Dans AL, Moores LK et al; American College of Chest Physicians. Treatment and prevention of heparin-induced thrombocytopenia: Antithrombotic Therapy and Prevention of Thrombosis, 9th ed: American College of Chest Physicians Evidence-Based Clinical Practice Guidelines. Chest. 2012 Feb;141(2 Suppl):e495S–530S.

Neunert C, Lim W, Crowther M, Cohen A, Solberg L Jr, Crowther MA; American Society of Hematology. The American Society of Hematology 2011 evidence-based practice guideline for immune thrombocytopenia. Blood. 2011 Apr 21;117(16):4190–207.

Sallah S, Wan JYU, Nguyen NP, Hanrahan LR, Sigounas G. Disseminated intravascular coagulation in solid tumors: clinical and pathologic study. Thromb Haemost. 2001 Sep;86(3):828–33.

Tripodi A, Mannucci PM. The coagulopathy of chronic liver disease. N Engl J Med. 2011 Jul 14;365(2):147–56.

I have a patient with chest pain. How do I determine the cause?

CHIEF COMPLAINT

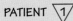

PATIENT ▽1

Mr. W is a 56-year-old man who comes to your office with chest pain.

 What is the differential diagnosis of chest pain? How would you frame the differential?

CONSTRUCTING A DIFFERENTIAL DIAGNOSIS

A patient with chest pain poses one of the most complicated diagnostic challenges. The differential diagnosis is extensive and includes diagnoses that can be imminently life-threatening. The initial pivotal points are the acuity of onset of the pain and the presence of vital sign abnormalities. Later in the evaluation, the presence of ECG or chest film abnormalities, symptoms consistent with aortic dissection, and the presence or absence of pleuritic pain (pain that worsens with inspiration) are important pivotal points. An algorithm to guide the consideration of the patient with chest pain is shown in Figure 9-1.

The differential diagnosis of chest pain is best remembered using an anatomic approach. Consideration needs to be given to the structures from the skin to the internal organs. The differential below is organized anatomically.

A. Skin: Herpes zoster

B. Breast
   1. Fibroadenomas
   2. Mastitis
   3. Gynecomastia

C. Musculoskeletal
   1. Costochondritis
   2. Precordial catch syndrome
   3. Pectoral muscle strain
   4. Rib fracture
   5. Cervical or thoracic spondylosis (C4–T6)
   6. Myositis

D. Esophageal
   1. Spasm
   2. Rupture
   3. Esophagitis
      a. Reflux
      b. Medication-related
   4. Neoplasm

E. Gastrointestinal (GI)
   1. Peptic ulcer disease
   2. Gallbladder disease
   3. Liver abscess
   4. Subdiaphragmatic abscess
   5. Pancreatitis

F. Pulmonary
   1. Pleura
      a. Pleural effusion
      b. Pneumonia
      c. Neoplasm
      d. Viral infections
      e. Pneumothorax
   2. Lung
      a. Neoplasm
      b. Pneumonia
   3. Pulmonary vasculature
      a. Pulmonary embolism
      b. Pulmonary hypertension

G. Cardiac
   1. Pericarditis
   2. Myocarditis
   3. Myocardial ischemia (stable angina, myocardial infarction, or unstable angina)

H. Vascular: Thoracic aortic aneurysm or aortic dissection

I. Mediastinal structures
   1. Lymphoma
   2. Thymoma

J. Psychiatric

▽1

Mr. W has a history of well-controlled hypertension and diabetes. He has been having symptoms for the last 4 months. He feels squeezing, substernal pressure while climbing stairs to the elevated train he rides to work. The pressure resolves after about 5 minutes of rest. He also occasionally feels the sensation during stressful periods at work. It is occasionally associated with mild nausea and jaw pain. Medications are metformin, aspirin, and enalapril.

(continued)

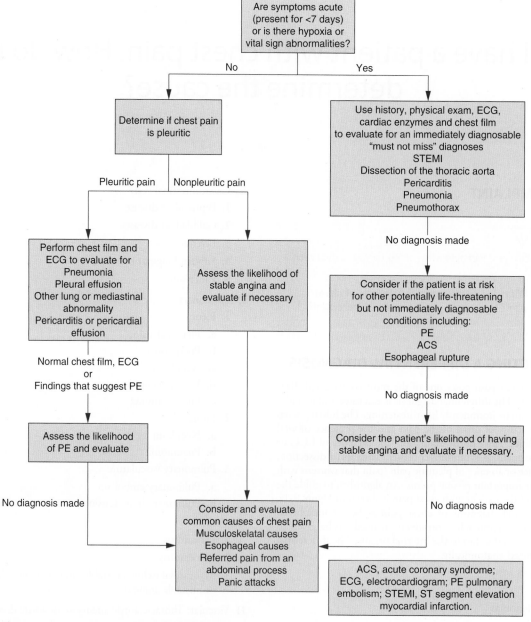

Figure 9-1. Evaluation of the patient with chest pain.

 At this point, what is the leading hypothesis, what are the active alternatives, and is there a must not miss diagnosis? Given this differential diagnosis, what tests should be ordered?

RANKING THE DIFFERENTIAL DIAGNOSIS

Mr. W is a middle-aged man with chronic, nonpleuritic chest pain and risk factors for coronary artery disease (CAD). His symptoms are consistent with stable angina. The pivotal points in this case are the chronicity, exertional nature, and substernal location of the pain. Given the seriousness and prevalence of CAD, it must lead the differential diagnosis. Gastroesophageal reflux disease (GERD) and musculoskeletal disorders are common causes of chest pain that can mimic angina (exacerbated by activity, sensation of pressure)

and thus should be considered. The chronicity of his symptoms argues against many other worrisome diagnoses (eg, pulmonary embolism [PE], pneumothorax, pericarditis, or aortic dissection). Pain from a mediastinal abnormality is possible. Table 9-1 lists the differential diagnosis.

 Physical exam is entirely unremarkable except for mild, stable, peripheral neuropathy presumably related to diabetes. The patient's ECG is remarkable only for evidence of left ventricular hypertrophy with strain.

 Is the clinical information sufficient to make a diagnosis? If not, what other information do you need?

Table 9-1. Diagnostic hypotheses for Mr. W.

Diagnostic Hypotheses	Demographics, Risk Factors, Symptoms and Signs	Important Tests
Leading Hypothesis		
Stable angina	Substernal chest pressure with exertion Risk factors for CAD	Exercise tolerance test Angiogram
Active Alternative—Most Common		
GERD	Symptoms of heartburn, chronic nature	EGD Esophageal pH monitoring
Active Alternative		
Musculoskeletal disorders	History of injury or specific musculoskeletal chest pain syndrome	Physical exam Response to treatment

CAD, coronary artery disease; EGD, esophagogastroduodenoscopy; GERD, gastroesophageal reflux disease.

Leading Hypothesis: Stable Angina

Textbook Presentation

Although atypical presentations are common, stable angina usually presents with symptoms of substernal chest discomfort precipitated by exertion. These symptoms resolve promptly with rest or nitroglycerin and do not change over the course of weeks. Affected patients usually have risk factors for CAD.

Disease Highlights

A. Stable angina is a chest pain syndrome caused by a mismatch between myocardial oxygen supply and demand.

 1. The mismatch is most often caused by coronary artery stenoses.

 2. It can also occur in the setting of normal or nearly normal coronary arteries and

 a. Anemia

 b. Tachycardia of any cause (atrial fibrillation, hyperthyroidism)

 c. Aortic stenosis

 d. Hypertrophic cardiomyopathy

 e. Heart failure (HF) (the result of high filling pressures)

 It is important to consider causes of angina other than CAD.

B. Stable angina is a common presentation for CAD.

C. Although exertional chest pain is the most common symptom of stable angina, other presentations are possible. Presentations may vary by what elicits the pain and what the symptoms are.

 1. Eliciting factors other than exercise

 a. Cold weather

 b. Extreme moods (anger, stress)

 c. Large meals

 2. Symptoms other than chest pain

 a. Dyspnea

 b. Nausea or indigestion

 c. Pain in areas other than the chest (eg, jaw, neck, teeth, back, abdomen)

 d. Palpitations

 e. Syncope

 f. Weakness and fatigue

D. The risk factors for CAD are important to elicit when the patient's history is suspicious. The traditional risk factors follow:

 1. Male sex

 2. Age > 55 years in men and > 65 years in women

 3. Tobacco use

 4. Diabetes

 5. Hypertension

 6. Family history of premature cardiovascular disease (younger than age 55 in men and younger than age 65 in women).

 7. Abnormal lipid profile

 a. Elevated low-density lipoprotein (LDL)

 b. Elevated triglycerides

 c. Elevated cholesterol/high-density lipoprotein (HDL) ratio (normal < 5:1, ideally < 3.5:1).

 d. Low HDL

E. Other risk factors

 1. Other vascular diseases (peripheral, cerebral)

 2. Hyperhomocysteinemia

 3. Elevated levels of inflammation (C-reactive protein)

 4. Chronic kidney disease

 5. Cocaine use should be asked about because, although it is not a risk factor for CAD, it can cause both angina and myocardial infarction (MI).

 Asking about the traditional cardiac risk factors should be a part of the history for any patient with chest pain.

F. Stable angina and CAD in women

 1. Although the pathophysiology of stable angina is the same in men and women, it raises some unique issues in women that deserve comment.

 2. Stable angina presents differently in women than in men.

 a. Because angina usually presents in women at an older age than in men, there are more comorbid diseases to confuse the presentation.

 b. Women describe their chest pain differently, using terms like "burning" and "tender" more frequently.

 3. There is good evidence that the diagnostic tests used for CAD, which are discussed later in this chapter, are less accurate in women than in men.

 4. Because there is a lower prevalence of disease among women,

 a. Physicians often do not consider the diagnosis.

 b. Lower pretest probability leads to worse positive predictive value of diagnostic tests (there are more false-positive results on noninvasive tests).

Evidence-Based Diagnosis

A. History

1. The first step in diagnosing CAD is taking an accurate history of the patient's chest pain.

2. There are reliable data on the prevalence of disease in patients with typical angina, atypical angina, nonanginal chest pain, and in patients who are asymptomatic. The answers to the following questions categorize the patient's chest pain:

   a. Is your chest discomfort substernal? ("Where is your pain?")

   b. Are your symptoms precipitated by exertion? ("Does your pain come on or get worse when you walk, walk fast, or climb stairs?")

   c. Does rest provide prompt relief of your symptoms (within 10 minutes)? ("Does your pain get better with rest?")

 Use the patient's own words when taking a history (eg, pressure, burning, aching, squeezing, piercing).

3. Patients who answer yes to all 3 questions are classified as having typical angina, 2 positive answers as atypical angina, and 1 positive as nonanginal chest pain. A patient who answers no to all questions is asymptomatic.

4. The prevalence of CAD in each group is shown in Table 9-2.

5. It is also useful to think of these data in terms of low-, intermediate-, and high-risk groups.

   a. Patients with a low pretest probability of CAD (< 15%) are all asymptomatic patients, men with nonanginal chest pain who are younger than 50 years and women with nonanginal chest pain who are younger than 60 years. Women under age 50 with atypical angina are also low risk.

   b. Patients with intermediate pretest probability (15–85%) are men over age 50 and women over age 60 with nonanginal chest pain, any man and any woman over age 50 with atypical angina as well as men under age 40 and women under age 60 with typical angina.

   c. Men older than 40 years and women older than 60 years with typical angina have a high (>85%) pretest probability.

6. It is important to recognize that comorbidities can markedly influence the probability of disease. As an example, the rate of CAD in a 55-year-old woman with atypical angina goes from about 32% with no risk factors to 47% with 1 risk factor (eg, diabetes, tobacco use, hypertension).

7. The remainder of the history should be aimed at collecting evidence that makes the diagnosis of CAD more likely, such as

   a. Cardiac risk factors

   b. Past history of cardiac disease

   c. Symptoms classic for other causes of chest pain

8. Factors that make the diagnosis of CAD less likely include

   a. Unremitting pain of prolonged duration

   b. Other explanations for the patient's symptoms

9. Initial tests that should be done at the initial presentation include

   a. Glucose and lipid profile to identify diseases that increase the likelihood of chest pain being ischemic in origin.

   b. Hgb and thyroid-stimulating hormone (TSH) to identify other diseases that may cause angina.

   c. Resting electrocardiogram (ECG), looking for evidence of previous infarction.

   d. Troponin, if recent anginal symptoms had been particularly severe or long lasting.

B. Exercise testing

1. Except in very rare cases, patients with symptoms of stable angina should have an exercise test.

2. The test is used for 2 purposes: to diagnose CAD and for risk stratification (determining whether patients should be treated with medication only, percutaneous coronary intervention (PCI), or bypass surgery.

3. Decisions about treatment are based on a number of factors, many coming from the results of exercise testing:

   a. The extent and severity of ischemia (most important)

   b. Other prognostic variables, such as aerobic ability, blood pressure and heart rate response to exercise, and inducible left ventricular dysfunction.

4. All exercise tests attempt to induce and detect myocardial ischemia.

   a. Myocardial ischemia may be induced by exercise, dobutamine, adenosine, or dipyridamole.

   b. Myocardial ischemia may be detected by ECG, echocardiogram, or nuclear imaging.

   c. The sensitivity of an exercise test will fall if the patient does not reach an adequate degree of exercise, as measured by the rate-pressure product.

Table 9-2. Prevalence of coronary artery disease (%).[1]

Age	Asymptomatic		Nonanginal Chest Pain		Atypical Angina		Typical Angina	
	Male	Female	Male	Female	Male	Female	Male	Female
30–39	1.9	0.3	5.2	0.8	21.8	4.2	69.7	25.8
40–49	5.5	1.0	14.1	2.8	46.1	13.3	87.3	55.2
50–59	9.7	3.2	21.5	8.4	58.9	32.4	92	79.4
60–69	12.3	7.5	28.1	18.6	67.1	54.4	94.3	90.6

[1]See text for definitions.
Data from Diamond GA, Forrester JS. Analysis of probability as an aid in the clinical diagnosis of coronary-artery disease. N Engl J Med. 1979;300:1350–8.

Table 9-3. Test characteristics of exercise tests.

Test	Sensitivity	Specificity	LR+	LR−
Exercise ECG > 1 mm depression	65–70%	70–75%	≈ 2.5	≈ .45
Exercise echocardiography	80–85%	80–85%	≈ 4.8	≈ 0.21
Dobutamine echocardiography	80–85%	85–90%	≈ 6.7	≈ 0.23
Exercise myocardial perfusion SPECT	85–90%	85–90%	≈ 6.9	≈ 0.15
Pharmacologic myocardial perfusion SPECT	80–90%	80–90%	≈ 7	≈ 0.18

SPECT, single photon emission computed tomography.

5. Exercise electrocardiography is the simplest and least expensive test.
   a. It requires a normal resting ECG.
   b. The sensitivity of the exercise stress test can be improved (at the cost of lower specificity) by reducing the degree of ST depression needed for a positive test.
6. The sensitivity, specificity, and LRs of some of the various tests are shown in Table 9-3. (It should be noted that the test characteristics of stress thallium and dobutamine echocardiography vary among healthcare centers.)
7. The decision whether to order a routine exercise test or one with imaging is difficult. In general, reasons to obtain imaging are
   a. Abnormal resting ECG
   b. Previous coronary artery bypass grafting (CABG) surgery or PCI
   c. A more sensitive test is required to rule out CAD, such as in patients with a high likelihood of CAD.

 Because of the relatively low sensitivity of ECG stress tests, these should only be used to exclude the diagnosis of CAD in low-risk patients.

8. Means of increasing coronary demand other than exercise (pharmacologic stress tests) are indicated for patients who are unable to exercise. They may also be more accurate in patients with a left bundle-branch block.
9. A patient with stable angina might not undergo an exercise test if he has a high likelihood of disease (a test therefore does not need to be done for diagnostic purposes) and would not benefit from determining the distribution or severity of the disease (usually because he would not, or could not, undergo revascularization).

C. Angiography
   1. The gold standard for diagnosing CAD.
   2. The indications for patients with stable angina to undergo angiography include
      a. Abnormal stress indicating substantial ischemia.
      b. Ischemia at a low workload on an exercise test.
      c. Diagnostic uncertainty after an exercise test.

3. Patients may undergo angiography without first having an exercise test in 2 circumstances when they will almost certainly require invasive therapy (PCI or CABG).
   a. When their symptoms are disabling despite therapy.
   b. When they have HF.

Treatment

A. The goal of treatment in patients with stable angina is to decrease symptoms and inhibit disease progression. Patients with stable angina have about a 3%/year risk of both MI and death.

B. Nonpharmacologic
   1. Smoking cessation
   2. Exercise (intensity guided by exercise testing)
   3. Low fat, low cholesterol diet

C. Pharmacologic
   1. Symptomatic treatment. It is important to recognize that patients often need a combination of medicines to control their symptoms.
      a. Decrease oxygen demand: beta-blocker or the calcium channel blockers verapamil or diltiazem
      b. Increase oxygen supply: long- and short-acting nitrates
      c. Ranolazine, a sodium channel blocker, is an effective antianginal, usually used in combination with a beta-blocker.
   2. Inhibit disease progression
      a. Aspirin
      b. Clopidogrel in patients who are intolerant of aspirin or who have had PCI.
      c. Risk factor modification
         (1) BP control in patients with hypertension.
         (2) High intensity HMG-CoA reductase inhibitor (statin) therapy.
         (3) Angiotensin-converting enzyme (ACE) inhibitor or angiotensin receptor blocker (ARB) in patients at the highest risk, such as those with diabetes or HF.
         (4) Glycemic control in patients with diabetes

D. Interventional therapy (either via PCI or bypass surgery) is the mainstay of treatment for the acute coronary syndromes discussed below. For stable angina, it plays a role in the care of patients with more advanced disease. An overview of the data is below.
   1. In low-risk patients (such as those with single vessel disease)
      a. There is no difference in mortality between medical management and PCI.
      b. Patients who undergo a PCI tend to have better control of their symptoms but undergo more procedures.
   2. In moderate-risk patients (such as those with multivessel disease but an otherwise normal heart)
      a. PCI and CABG are about equal in terms of mortality and both are superior to medical therapy.
      b. PCI leads to more procedures.
   3. In high-risk patients (such as those with disease of the left main coronary artery, 3 vessel disease, or 2 vessel disease involving the proximal left anterior descending artery)
      a. Bypass surgery has a survival benefit compared with medical therapy.
      b. For selected patients, PCI can have a similar outcome to surgery.
      c. Bypass surgery is superior in patients with diabetes.

A tentative diagnosis of stable angina from CAD is made. Laboratory data are notable for normal blood counts and chemistries. There is hypercholesterolemia (LDL, 136 mg/dL; HDL, 42 mg/dL). Mr. W is referred for an exercise tolerance test. Because of his abnormal resting ECG, an exercise myocardial perfusion SPECT was performed. Although chest pain developed during the test, his results were normal without evidence of myocardial ischemia.

Have you crossed a diagnostic threshold for the leading hypothesis, stable angina? Have you ruled out the active alternatives? Do other tests need to be done to exclude the alternative diagnoses?

MAKING A DIAGNOSIS

The results of the patient's exercise test are surprising. Stable angina remains high in the differential despite the normal stress test but alternative diagnoses must be considered. The intermittent nature of the pain and the lack of constitutional symptoms both make a mediastinal lesion unlikely. The absence of a recent injury, change in activity or reproducible pain on physical exam moves musculoskeletal pain down on the differential. GERD is a common cause of chest pain and should be considered.

Alternative Diagnosis: Gastroesophageal Reflux Disease (GERD)

Textbook Presentation

Heartburn (a burning, substernal, chest discomfort) is usually the presenting symptom in a patient with GERD. Other classic symptoms are regurgitation or dysphagia; chest pain is a common alternative presentation. Patients often report that their symptoms are worst at night and after large meals.

Although dysphagia is a common presentation of GERD, its presence raises the possibility of an obstructing lesion and thus mandates prompt evaluation, usually with upper endoscopy.

Disease Highlights

A. The symptoms of GERD are so well known that most patients diagnose themselves before visiting a physician.

B. GERD is a common cause of chest pain.

C. There are GI and non-GI complications of GERD.

  1. GI

    a. Esophagitis

    b. Stricture formation

    c. Barrett esophagus

    d. Esophageal adenocarcinoma

  2. Non-GI

    a. Chronic cough

    b. Hoarseness

    c. Worsening of asthma

D. Esophageal disorders, other than GERD, might also present as chest pain.

  1. Esophagitis or esophageal ulcer

    a. Odynophagia common

    b. Multiple causes include infection and pill esophagitis.

    c. Pill esophagitis is especially associated with certain medications:

      (1) Bisphosphonates

      (2) Tetracyclines

      (3) Antiinflammatories

      (4) Potassium chloride

  2. Esophageal cancer

    a. Often associated with dysphagia

    b. Smoking, alcohol use, and chronic reflux are risk factors.

  3. Esophageal rupture (Boerhaave syndrome). Often presents with acute pain after retching.

  4. Esophageal spasm and motility disorders. Often presents with intermittent chest pain and dysphagia.

Evidence-Based Diagnosis

A. GERD should be high in the differential diagnosis of chest pain when heartburn, regurgitation, or dysphagia is present or when other commonly associated symptoms or complications (eg, chronic cough and asthma) are present.

B. Identifying factors that exacerbate the symptoms of GERD is helpful both in diagnosis and management.

  1. Ingesting large (especially fatty) meals

  2. Lying down after a meal

  3. Using tobacco

  4. Eating any of the (delicious) foods that relax the lower esophageal sphincter

    a. Chocolate

    b. Alcohol

    c. Coffee

    d. Peppermint

C. Historical features help differentiate esophageal from cardiac chest pain.

  1. A small study analyzed the prevalence of several historical features in 100 patients in an emergency department with either esophageal or cardiac chest pain.

  2. The differences that reached statistical significance are listed in Table 9-4. Although the study was small, the data are instructive.

  3. From these data, it is clear that history cannot differentiate esophageal chest pain from pain due to cardiac ischemia. That said, pain that occurs with swallowing, is persistent, wakes the patient from sleep, is positional, and is associated with heartburn or regurgitation is more likely to be of esophageal origin.

  4. It is interesting that only 83% of patients with an esophageal cause of pain in this study had GI symptoms (ie, heartburn, regurgitation, dysphagia, or vomiting).

  5. Striking were some of the features not significantly different between the 2 groups:

    a. Radiation to the left arm

    b. Exacerbation with exercise

    c. Relief with nitroglycerin

  6. The effect of nitroglycerin in relieving chest pain has consistently been found to be useless in differentiating anginal chest pain from esophageal or other causes of chest pain.

 Response to nitroglycerin should not be used as a diagnostic test in the evaluation of chest pain.

Table 9-4. Prevalence of symptoms in patients with cardiac and esophageal chest pain.

Symptom	Prevalence (%)	
	Among patients with cardiac cause	Among patients with esophageal cause
Lateral radiation	69	11
More than 1 spontaneous episode per month	13	50
Pain persists as ache for several hours	25	78
Nighttime wakening caused by pain	25	61
Provoked by swallowing	6	39
Provoked by recumbency or stooping	19	61
Variable exercise tolerance	10	39
Pain starts after exercise completed	4	33
Pain relieved by antacid	10	44
Presence of heartburn	17	78
Presence of regurgitation	17	67
Presence of GI symptoms	46	83

D. Esophageal pH testing, the gold standard for the diagnosis of GERD, is seldom necessary.

E. The combination of a suspicious history and consistent endoscopic findings has a 97% specificity for GERD.

F. Suggestive symptoms and response to therapy is generally considered diagnostic.

G. Esophagogastroduodenoscopy (EGD) should be done when
1. Patients have symptoms of complicated disease
   a. Dysphagia
   b. Extra-esophageal symptoms
   c. Bleeding
   d. Weight loss
   e. Chest pain of unclear etiology
2. Patients are at risk for Barrett esophagus (long-standing symptoms of reflux).
3. Patients require long-term therapy.
4. Patients respond poorly to appropriate therapy.

H. Ambulatory pH monitoring is useful in 2 settings:
1. In patients with symptoms of GERD and a normal endoscopy.
2. To monitor therapy in refractory cases.

Treatment

A. Nonpharmacologic
1. Elevate the entire head of the bed; adding extra pillows may actually worsen reflux.
2. Avoid lying down for 3 hours after meals.
3. Stop smoking.
4. Stop ingesting foods and beverages that relax the lower esophageal sphincter or worsen symptoms of GERD.

B. Pharmacologic
1. Antacids
2. H_2-blockers
3. Proton-pump inhibitors
   a. First-line therapy in patients with reflux severe enough to prompt a physician visit.
   b. Many patients require long-term therapy.
4. Motility agents (such as metoclopramide) are useful in patients who need adjuvant therapy or who have significant symptoms of regurgitation.
5. Surgery
   a. Antireflux surgery currently has only a very small role.
   b. May be warranted in some patients with particularly severe disease.
   c. One randomized trial has suggested that patients treated with surgery had a higher mortality rate than those treated medically at a mean follow-up of about 11 years (number needed to harm [NNH] = 8.3).

Because GERD is a common cause of chest pain, if the suspicion of the disease is high, it is appropriate to prescribe an empiric course of proton-pump inhibitors after more ominous causes of chest pain have been ruled out.

CASE RESOLUTION

Prior to the stress test, Mr. W's probability of having CAD was at least 92% (see Table 9-2). It is important to understand why the exercise test was done in this case. The diagnosis of coronary disease was essentially made by the history and physical. The exercise test was meant to guide therapy. Considering a pretest probability of 92%, and a LR– of about 0.15 for the exercise test, the posttest probability is 60%. This is still well above the test threshold for a potentially fatal disease like CAD.

Despite the results of the stress test, stable angina was considered more likely than GERD. Mr. W was given aspirin and a beta-blocker and underwent an angiogram the week after the visit. He was found to have a 90% stenosis of the mid left anterior descending artery and underwent PCI with stent placement.

Before ordering an exercise test, ask yourself why you are doing it: Are you trying to diagnose CAD or determine the severity of the disease?

CHIEF COMPLAINT

PATIENT 2

Mrs. G is a 68-year-old woman with a history of hypertension who arrives at the emergency department by ambulance complaining of chest pain that began 6 hours ago. Two hours after eating, moderate (5/10) chest discomfort developed. She describes it as a burning sensation beginning in her mid chest and radiating to her back. She initially attributed the pain to heartburn and used antacids. Despite multiple doses over 3 hours, there was no relief. Over the last hour, the pain became very severe (10/10) with radiation to her back and arms. The pain is associated with diaphoresis and shortness of breath. The pain is not pleuritic.

 At this point, what is the leading hypothesis, what are the active alternatives, and is there a must not miss diagnosis? Given this differential diagnosis, what tests should be ordered?

RANKING THE DIFFERENTIAL DIAGNOSIS

Mrs. G is experiencing acute, severe, nonpleuritic chest pain. This presentation is associated with multiple "must not miss" diagnoses. The acuity of the pain is a pivotal point in this history. MI with and without ST elevations and unstable angina, as a group referred to as acute coronary syndromes, are the most common life-threatening causes of acute chest pain and need to be considered first. Aortic dissection also needs to be considered given the severity of the pain, the history of hypertension, and the radiation of the pain to the back. PE is another possible cause even though the chest pain is not pleuritic. Other alternative causes of this type of pain are esophageal spasm and pancreatitis (though it would be atypical for pancreatitis to begin so acutely). Table 9-5 lists the differential diagnosis.

2

The patient takes enalapril for hypertension. She lives alone, is sedentary, and smokes 1 pack of cigarettes each day. She has an 80 pack-year smoking history.

On physical exam, the patient is in moderate distress. She thinks that she is having a heart attack. Vital signs are temperature, 37.0°C; BP, 156/90 mm Hg in both arms; pulse, 100 bpm; RR, 22 breaths per minute. Head and neck exam, including jugular and carotid pulsations, are normal. The lung exam is clear. Heart exam is notable for a normal S_1 and S_2 and a soft, II/VI systolic ejection murmur. Abdominal exam is unremarkable with no tenderness, hepatosplenomegaly, or bruits.

 Is the clinical information sufficient to make a diagnosis? If not, what other information do you need?

Leading Hypothesis: Acute MI

Textbook Presentation

The classic presentation of an acute MI is crushing substernal chest pressure, diaphoresis, nausea, shortness of breath, and a feeling of impending doom in a middle-aged man with risk factors for CAD.

Table 9-5. Diagnostic hypotheses for Mrs. G.

Diagnostic Hypotheses	Demographics, Risk Factors, Symptoms and Signs	Important Tests
Leading Hypothesis		
Acute MI	Presence of cardiac risk factors Acute onset	ECG Cardiac enzymes (CK and troponin) Coronary angiography
Active Alternative—Must Not Miss		
Unstable angina	Presence of cardiac risk factors Ischemic symptoms that are new or increasing in frequency	ECG Cardiac enzymes (CK and troponin) Stress testing Coronary angiography
Thoracic aortic aneurysm dissection	Presence of hypertension Radiation of pain to back BP differential	Transesophageal echocardiography CT scan
Other Alternative		
Esophageal spasm	Recurrent chest pain, often with radiation to back	Esophageal manometry and exclusion of other causes

CK, creatine kinase, ECG electrocardiogram, MI, myocardial infarction.

Even more than other "textbook presentations," this description is often inaccurate because it does not take into account the frequency of MIs in women, younger and older patients, and the frequency of atypical presentations.

Disease Highlights

A. MI occurs when there is a prolonged failure to perfuse an area of myocardium leading to cell death.

B. Most commonly occurs when a coronary plaque ruptures causing thrombosis and subsequent blockage of a coronary artery.

C. The universal definition of MI describes 5 subtypes of MI based on their clinical presentation:

   1. Spontaneous MI due to a primary coronary event.

   2. MI secondary to ischemia due to either increased oxygen demand or decreased supply, eg, coronary artery spasm, anemia, or arrhythmias.

   3. Sudden unexpected cardiac death, including cardiac arrest, often with symptoms suggestive of myocardial ischemia.

   4. MI associated with PCI or stent thrombosis.

   5. MI associated with CABG.

D. Acute MIs are classified as either ST segment elevation MI (STEMI) or non–ST segment elevation MI (NSTEMI).

   1. ST elevations signify transmural ischemia or infarction.

   2. NSTEMI

      a. Are less severe, usually injuring only subendomyocardial tissue

      b. Have a higher subsequent risk for STEMI than for patients who have had a STEMI

Table 9-6. Criteria for diagnosing acute MI.

1. A rise and fall of cardiac biomarkers (preferably troponin) with at least 1 value above the 99th percentile of the URL along with 1 of the following:
   a. Symptoms of ischemia
   b. ECG changes consistent with new ischemia
   c. Development of pathologic Q waves
   d. Imaging evidence of new loss of viable myocardium or myocardial function.
2. Sudden cardiac death accompanied by ECG changes, angiographic findings, or autopsy findings supporting MI as the cause.
3. Elevation of cardiac biomarkers above 3 times the 99th percentile of the URL in the setting of PCI.
4. Elevation of cardiac biomarkers above 5 times the 99th percentile consistent with MI, angiographic evidence of MI, or imaging evidence of new loss of viable myocardium of myocardial function.
5. Pathologic evidence of an MI.

MI, myocardial infarction; PCI, percutaneous coronary intervention; URL, upper reference limit.

Table 9-7. Likelihood ratios of historical features and physical exam findings and the effect on posttest probability of acute MI.

Feature or Finding	LR+	Posttest Probability[1]
Radiation to both arms	9.7	63%
Radiation to right arm	7.3	56%
Third heart sound	3.2	36%
Hypotension	3.1	35%
Radiation to left arm	2.2	28%
Radiation to right shoulder	2.2	28%
Crackles	2.1	27%
Diaphoresis	2.0	26%
Nausea and vomiting	1.9	25%

[1]Assuming 15% pretest probability.

3. These 2 types of MI are managed differently. The discussion of STEMI is covered in this section while the management of NSTEMI is discussed in the next section on unstable angina.

Evidence-Based Diagnosis

A. The diagnostic criteria for acute MI have been clearly established. There are 5 criteria that vary somewhat, based partly on the subtype of MI. They are shown in Table 9-6.

B. Clinical findings suggestive of MI
   1. Pretest probability
      a. About 15% of patients who arrive at the emergency department complaining of chest pain are having an MI.
      b. About 33% of patients admitted to the hospital with suspicion of an MI are found to be having one.
      c. About 50% of patients admitted to the CCU with suspicion of an MI are found to be having one.
   2. Historical and physical exam features are never sufficient to diagnose an MI and only (nearly) exclude MI in the lowest risk patients. Test characteristics for some common signs and symptoms appear in Table 9-7.
   3. Types of chest pain that decrease the likelihood of MI include pleuritic pain, sharp or stabbing pain, or positional pain.

C. ECG findings suggestive of MI
   1. All guidelines recommend an ECG be performed within 10 minutes of a patient's arrival at a healthcare facility when an MI is suspected.

 Patients with chest pain should have an ECG within 10 minutes of arriving at a healthcare facility.

   2. Prevalence rates of MI among emergency department patients with chest pain and various ECG findings follow:
      a. New ST elevation of 1 mm: 80%
      b. New ST depression or T wave inversion: 20%
      c. No new changes in a patient with known CAD: 4%
      d. No new changes in a patient without known CAD: 2%
   3. Table 9-8 shows the test characteristics for ECG findings in patients with acute chest pain. (Because numbers vary from study to study, these likelihood ratios should be treated as estimates.)

 A patient with chest pain and ≥ 1-mm ST elevations in 2 contiguous leads or a new left bundle-branch block is having an acute MI and should receive immediate therapy.

D. Cardiac enzymes
   1. As is clear from the diagnostic criteria, abnormal levels of cardiac enzymes define the presence of MI.

Table 9-8. Test characteristics for ECG findings in patients with chest pain for the diagnosis of acute MI.[1]

ECG Finding	LR+	LR−
New ST elevation > 1 mm	5.7–53	
New Q wave	5.3–24.8	
Any ST elevation	11.2	
New Q or ST elevation	11	0.24
New conduction defect	6.3	
Any Q wave	3.9	
T wave peaking	3.1	
Any conduction defect	2.7	
Any ECG abnormality	1.3	0.04

[1]Data are unavailable when not given.
Adapted from Panju AA et al. The rational clinical examination. Is this patient having a myocardial infarction? JAMA. 1998;280:1256–63.

2. When an MI is suspected, creatine kinase MB subunit (CK-MB) and troponin should be ordered and processed immediately.

3. These tests are highly reliable in diagnosing MI. (Note that the definition of MI is based on enzyme results whenever they are available.)

   a. Troponin: sensitivity, 95%; specificity, 98%; LR+, 47; LR-, 0.3.

   b. Serial CK-MB: in the first 24 hours—sensitivity, 99%; specificity, 98%; LR+, 50; LR-, 0.1.

4. Troponin levels in patients with kidney disease

   a. Patients with kidney disease often have elevated troponin levels raising the risk of false-positive tests for MI.

   b. Patients with elevated troponin levels at baseline will still have a diagnostic rise and fall with MI.

   c. In patients with chronic kidney disease, higher baseline troponin levels are predictive of poor cardiovascular outcomes.

E. MI in women

   1. Presentation

      a. Acute MIs present differently in women than in men.

      b. Women often report prodromal symptoms such as fatigue, dyspnea, and insomnia.

      c. Women are more likely to present without chest pain than men (42% vs 30.7%). This difference becomes less pronounced as patients age (as both men and woman present more frequently without chest pain).

 Just under half of women suffering an MI have a chief complaint other than chest pain.

      d. Dyspnea, weakness, and fatigue are the other common presenting symptoms.

   2. Outcomes

      a. Women who suffer an MI are more likely to die. Recent data show an in-hospital mortality rate of 14.6% for women and 10.3% for men.

      b. The cause of this disparity is multifactorial but includes the fact that patients without chest pain receive delayed and less aggressive care.

      c. The mortality difference becomes less pronounced and eventually reverses as patients age.

F. Unrecognized MI

   1. Although the combination of symptoms, ECG findings, and enzymes make most MIs easy to diagnose, about 2% of patients with acute MI are not diagnosed and are discharged from the emergency department.

   2. Failure to recognize an MI results in worse outcomes for patients and serious medicolegal issues.

   3. MIs most commonly go unrecognized when they present in unusual ways or in people not expected to have MI.

   4. A patient with an MI or unstable angina who is mistakenly discharged is most likely to:

      a. Be a woman younger than age 55

      b. Be non-white

      c. Have a chief complaint of shortness of breath

      d. Have a nondiagnostic ECG

   5. The most common alternative presentations of MI are listed below. MI should at least be considered in patients being discharged from the emergency department with 1 of these diagnoses:

      a. HF

      b. Stable angina

      c. Arrhythmia

      d. Atypical location of pain

      e. Central nervous system manifestations (symptoms of cerebrovascular accident)

      f. Nervousness, mania, or psychosis

      g. Syncope

      h. Weakness

      i. Indigestion

 MI can present in many different ways. A high index of suspicion should always be present. Certain groups of patients (elderly, women, minorities, diabetics) are most likely to be misdiagnosed.

Treatment

A. Once an MI is diagnosed, therapy must be initiated immediately. The following applies to the treatment of STEMI:

   1. Medications

      a. Antiplatelet agents: aspirin, P2Y12 receptor blockers (eg, clopidogrel) and, in patients undergoing primary PCI, a glycoprotein IIb/IIIa inhibitor

      b. Beta-blockers

      c. Oxygen

      d. Nitroglycerin

      e. High intensity HMG-CoA reductase inhibitors (statins)

      f. Other therapy based on presentation

         (1) Opioids for patients in pain

         (2) Atropine for patients with pathologic bradycardia

         (3) Antiarrhythmic agents

B. Reperfusion with either systemic thrombolysis or primary PCI.

   1. Although not universally available, primary PCI is the preferred option.

   2. Primary PCI is associated with

      a. Lower mortality (even in patients who must be transferred—albeit quickly—to a hospital with the capability)

      b. Significantly lower risk of serious bleeding complication. Hemorrhagic stroke is not a potential complication as it is with systemic thrombolysis.

   3. The ability to do primary PCI depends on the presence of an interventional cardiology team who can rapidly (within 90 minutes) bring the patient to the catheterization laboratory.

   4. Primary PCI with stent placement is the most efficacious treatment.

   5. Both primary angioplasty and thrombolysis are most effective when completed within 12 hours of symptom onset.

C. Once the culprit vessel has been opened, various medications have been shown to improve survival after acute MI.

   1. Beta-blockers

   2. ACE inhibitors

3. Aspirin

4. P2Y12 receptor blockers (duration based on intervention and risk of bleeding)

5. HMG-CoA reductase inhibitors, dosed to achieve an LDL < 70 mg/dL.

6. Glycoprotein IIB/IIIA inhibitors are recommended for patients with MIs who undergo stenting.

D. An exercise test is also recommended within 3 weeks of an MI in patients not undergoing PCI or angiography for information on prognosis, functional capacity, and risk stratification.

Mrs. G's ECG shows ST depression in leads II, III, AVL, and V3–V6. The chest radiograph is normal.

Have you crossed a diagnostic threshold for the leading hypothesis, acute MI? Have you ruled out the active alternatives? Do other tests need to be done to exclude the alternative diagnoses?

MAKING A DIAGNOSIS

The ST depression is consistent with cardiac ischemia but is less specific than ST elevation and does not conclusively make the diagnosis of an acute MI; the diagnosis will be confirmed when cardiac enzyme levels are available. The abnormal ECG certainly makes the alternative diagnosis, unstable angina, quite likely if an MI is excluded. Aortic dissections can cause cardiac ischemia, so this too must remain in the differential.

Alternative Diagnosis: Unstable Angina

Textbook Presentation

New or worsening symptoms of CAD are the presenting symptoms of unstable angina. Unstable angina and an acute MI without ST elevation (NSTEMI) may be identical in their presentation, only differentiated by the presence or absence of myocardial enzyme elevation.

Disease Highlights

A. Unstable angina is defined as angina that is new, worsening in severity or frequency, or occurs at rest.

B. Pathophysiology
   1. Primarily caused by acute plaque rupture followed by platelet aggregation
      a. 67% of episodes occur in arteries with < 50% stenosis.
      b. 97% occur in arteries with < 75% stenosis.
   2. Caused less commonly by changes in oxygen demand or supply (eg, hyperthyroidism, anemia, high altitude)

C. The diagnosis of unstable angina can be difficult, often depending on a careful history to differentiate stable from unstable angina.

D. The clinician seeing a patient with unstable angina or a NSTEMI must
   1. Recognize that the patient has an acute coronary syndrome
   2. Institute care

3. Determine the patient's risk of progressing to an MI or death
4. Treat accordingly

E. Vasospastic angina
   1. Vasospastic angina (also called Prinzmetal or variant angina) is a phenomenon that presents in a similar way to unstable angina.
   2. Patients with vasospastic angina periodically have episodes of cardiac ischemia with ST elevation.
   3. The attacks
      a. Are often associated with chest pain or other ischemic symptoms
      b. Resolve spontaneously or with nitroglycerin
      c. May occur in normal or diseased coronary arteries
      d. Can result in MI or death (often secondary to arrhythmia)
      e. Often occur at the same time each day
   4. Vasospastic angina is usually diagnosed clinically but can also be diagnosed by inducing it with ergonovine infusion in the catheterization laboratory.
   5. Vasospastic angina is treated effectively with calcium channel blockers and nitrates.

Vasospastic angina should be considered in patients whose symptoms are consistent with cardiac ischemia and occur at about the same time each day. The diagnosis should also be considered when transient ST elevations develop.

Evidence-Based Diagnosis

A. Diagnosis
   1. There are 3 presentations of unstable angina:
      a. Rest angina
      b. New-onset (< 2 months) angina
      c. Increasing angina
   2. The American College of Cardiology and American Heart Association have endorsed a number of findings that increase the likelihood that a patient's symptoms represent an acute coronary syndrome. These include
      a. Chest or left arm pain that reproduces prior angina
      b. Known history of CAD
      c. Transient mitral regurgitation murmur
      d. Hypotension
      e. Diaphoresis
      f. Pulmonary edema
      g. Crackles

B. Risk stratification
   1. Appropriate risk stratification ensures that the patient is triaged to the proper location for care (ICU, inpatient ward, home) and receives the most beneficial therapy.
   2. Patients can be stratified by various validated scores. The TIMI score is probably most commonly used and is shown in Table 9-9.
   3. Other characteristics that portend high risk are
      a. Recurrent angina or ischemia at rest or with low-level activities despite intensive medical therapy
      b. Elevated cardiac biomarkers (troponin)
      c. Signs or symptoms of HF or new or worsening mitral regurgitation

Table 9-9 TIMI risk score for unstable angina/NSTEMI.

TIMI Score[1]	All cause mortality, new or recurrent MI, or severe or recurrent ischemia requiring urgent revascularization within 14 days
0–1	4.7
2	8.3
3	13.2
4	19.9
5	26.2
6–7	40.9

[1]Patients receive 1 point for each of the following variables: age ≥ 65, ≥ 3 cardiac risk factors, prior coronary stenosis of ≥ 50%, ST segment deviation on admission ECG, ≥ 2 anginal events in preceding 24 hours, use of aspirin in previous 7 days, elevated cardiac biomarkers.

MI, myocardial infarction; NSTEMI, non–ST segment elevation MI.

   d. High-risk findings from noninvasive testing

   e. Hemodynamic instability

   f. Sustained ventricular tachycardia

   g. PCI within 6 months

   h. Prior CABG

   i. Reduced left ventricular function

Treatment

A. The following treatments should be started as soon as unstable angina or a NSTEMI is suspected:

   1. Oxygen

   2. Antiplatelet agents aspirin and a P2Y12 receptor blocker

   3. Anticoagulation with enoxaparin, unfractionated heparin, or bivalirudin

   4. Beta-blockers

   5. Nitrates

   6. High doses of HMG-CoA reductase inhibitors are probably beneficial when given early in the course of the presentation.

B. Patients whose risk stratification identifies them as having a low risk of death or complications should undergo conservative management strategy.

   1. If the patient is stable (no ongoing ischemia, arrhythmias or decreased ejection fraction on echocardiogram), a stress test should be done to determine whether angiography is indicated.

   2. If the stress test finds the patient to be at low risk, the patient can be discharged with prescriptions for aspirin, clopidogrel, beta-blockers, and an HMG-CoA reductase inhibitor.

C. Patients found to be at higher risk benefit from an early invasive strategy. These patients undergo angiography to determine further management (PCI, CABG, or medical therapy for coronary disease).

Alternative Diagnosis: Aortic Dissection

Textbook Presentation

The textbook presentation of an aortic dissection is an older man with a history of hypertension and possibly atherosclerotic disease who complains of "tearing" chest or back pain. The pain might be associated with vascular complications such as syncope, stroke, cardiac ischemia, or HF secondary to acute aortic regurgitation. On physical exam, there is asymmetry in the upper extremity BPs, and the chest radiograph shows a widened mediastinum.

Disease Highlights

A. Dissection begins with a tear in the aortic intima allowing blood to dissect the aorta between the intima and media.

B. Risk factors

   1. Hypertension, present in 72% of patients

   2. Atherosclerosis, present in 31% of patients

   3. Known aortic aneurysm, present in 16% of patients

      a. Aortic aneurysms are usually detected while they are asymptomatic on a chest radiograph.

      b. They may also present with aortic regurgitation, pain, or through impingement on other structures such as the trachea, esophagus, or recurrent laryngeal nerve.

   4. Prior aortic dissection (6%)

   5. Diabetes (5%)

   6. Marfan syndrome (5%)

C. An additional risk factor for aortic dissection is cocaine use. This is associated with dissections in younger patients (mean age 41).

 In addition to MI, thoracic aortic dissection should be considered in the differential of a young hypertensive patient who has chest pain after using cocaine.

D. The symptoms of dissection include pain as well as symptoms of vascular complications of the dissection. The type of complication depends on what type of dissection occurs.

E. Type A dissections involve the ascending aorta with or without the descending aorta.

   1. Account for about 60% of dissections

   2. Carry a mortality of about 35%

   3. May be associated with

      a. Acute aortic insufficiency

      b. Myocardial ischemia due to coronary occlusion

      c. Neurologic deficits

      d. Cardiac tamponade due to hemopericardium

F. Type B dissections involve only the descending aorta and are associated with a mortality rate of about 15%.

Evidence-Based Diagnosis

A. The diagnosis of aortic dissection is notoriously difficult. There are no signs or symptoms that are consistently associated with very high or very low LRs.

B. A study of 464 patients with aortic dissection helps describe the common presenting signs and symptoms of people with this diagnosis.

   1. Demographics:

      a. Mean age ≈ 63 years

      b. Hypertension in about three-quarters

   2. The presenting signs and symptoms were notable for the infrequency of some classic findings.

      a. Pulse deficit was noted in only 15% of patients, syncope in 9%, cerebrovascular accident in 5%, and HF in 7%.

Table 9-10. Prevalence of various findings and symptoms in patients with thoracic aortic aneurysm dissection (type A).

Finding or Symptom	Prevalence
Severe or worst ever pain	90%
Abrupt onset pain	85%
Chest pain	79%
Sharp pain	62%
Widened mediastinum	63%
Tearing pain	51%
Back pain	47%
Nonspecific ST-segment or T-wave changes	43%
Normal mediastinum and aortic contour	17%
Normal chest film	11%

Data from Hagan PG et al. The International Registry of Acute Aortic Dissection (IRAD): new insights into an old disease. JAMA. 2000;283:897–903. Copyright © 2000. American Medical Association. All rights reserved.

    b. Some of the more common symptoms are shown in Table 9-10.

    c. Chest radiograph and ECG were found to be very insensitive diagnostic tools.

 The aorta is normal on the chest film in about 40% of patients with a dissection of the thoracic aorta.

C. Another study stratified patients by 3 independent predictors of aortic dissection: aortic type pain (pain of acute onset or tearing or ripping character), aortic or mediastinal widening on chest radiograph, and pulse or BP differentials.

    1. Low-risk patients had none of the characteristics.

        a. Only 7% of these patients had a dissection

        b. The test characteristics of these findings for excluding dissection were sensitivity, 96%; specificity, 48%; LR+, 1.85; LR–, 0.08.

    2. Intermediate-risk patients had only consistent pain or a consistent chest radiograph. Between 30% and 40% of these patients had a dissection.

    3. High-risk patients had pulse or both consistent pain and an abnormal chest film.

        a. > 84% of these patients had a dissection.

        b. The test characteristics of these findings for predicting dissection were sensitivity, 76%; specificity, 91%; LR+, 8.4; LR–, 0.26.

    4. The test characteristics for pulse or BP differentials in a patient in whom aortic dissection is suspected were sensitivity, 37%; specificity, 99%; LR+, 37; LR–, 0.64.

D. Summarizing the clinical diagnosis of aortic dissection

    1. Patients with dissections are likely to have a history of hypertension and experience severe, acute pain.

    2. Patients with chest pain are unlikely to have a dissection if they do not have any of the following:

        a. Acute or tearing or ripping pain

        b. Aortic or mediastinal widening

        c. Asymmetric pulse or BPs

E. The gold standard for diagnosis is angiography but most patients undergo noninvasive tests (CT or transesophageal echocardiography).

F. Both noninvasive tests have sensitivities and specificities above 95%.

G. Angiography is recommended to help guide therapy if there is evidence of organ ischemia.

Treatment

A. Because dissection is associated with extremely high mortality, the goal is to identify and repair the aneurysm prior to rupture.

B. Thoracic aortic dissection

    1. Dissection of the thoracic aorta is a medical emergency.

    2. Type A dissections generally are operated on immediately.

    3. Type B dissections usually are managed medically.

C. Thoracic aortic aneurysms (without dissection)

    1. When aneurysms are detected prior to rupture, the goal of therapy is to slow their growth and operate when the aneurysm reaches a certain size.

    2. Patients with aneurysms should have tight BP control.

    3. Patients should be closely monitored for increasing aneurysm size.

    4. Indications for surgery are based on the size of the aneurysm.

        a. 5.5 cm for ascending aneurysms

        b. 6.5 cm for descending aneurysms

        c. Rapid growth

CASE RESOLUTION

Mrs. G's initial troponin was elevated at 3.5 ng/mL with a CK of 750 units/L and positive MB fraction. The final diagnosis is NSTEMI. Following treatment in the emergency department with aspirin, clopidogrel, oxygen, beta-blockers, nitrates, and enoxaparin, she was taken directly to the cardiac catheterization laboratory. There she was found to have a left dominant system and an acute thrombosis of a branch of the left circumflex artery. This was opened with intracoronary thrombolysis and a stent was placed.

The patient's troponin and CK make the diagnosis of an acute MI. It should be realized that the presence of an MI does not rule out dissection of the thoracic aorta. Between 3% and 5% of patients with dissections have associated MIs. Even before the catheterization results, the subacute onset of the pain, the normal chest film, the lack of "tearing pain," and symmetric pulses made aortic dissection unlikely.

Four days after her MI, Mrs. G was discharged with prescriptions for the following medications:

1. Atorvastatin 80 mg
2. Lisinopril 20 mg
3. Metoprolol 100 mg
4. Aspirin 81 mg
5. Clopidogrel 75 mg

CHIEF COMPLAINT

PATIENT

Mr. H is a 31-year-old man, previously in excellent health, who arrives at the emergency department complaining of chest pain. He reports that the pain began 10 days earlier. It was initially mild but has become more severe. The pain is accompanied by mild cough and shortness of breath. Five days earlier, he came to the emergency department and was diagnosed with musculoskeletal chest pain; he was given non-steroidal antiinflammatory drugs (NSAIDs) and discharged.

Since then the pain has become more severe and has become pleuritic. He says it is located over the right lateral lower chest wall. His dyspnea is still only mild. He also has noted low-grade fevers with temperatures running about 38°C.

At this point, what is the leading hypothesis, what are the active alternatives, and is there a must not miss diagnosis? Given this differential diagnosis, what tests should be ordered?

RANKING THE DIFFERENTIAL DIAGNOSIS

This is a healthy young man with an acute illness. He reports pleuritic chest pain, cough, dyspnea, and fevers. The acuity of the symptoms as well as the pleuritic nature of the pain are pivotal points in this case. The first diagnoses to consider are infectious diseases that could cause pleuritic chest pain and fever. Pneumonia or pleural effusion could cause these symptoms, either individually or as part of the same process. (Pleural effusions will be discussed below while pneumonia will be discussed in Chapter 10.) Pericarditis can also cause pleuritic chest pain and can be associated with fevers. PE is a classic cause of pleuritic chest pain and shortness of breath and may be associated with fever (see Chapter 15). Intra-abdominal processes, such as subdiaphragmatic abscess should be kept in mind as causes of pleuritic chest pain. The combination of fever, dyspnea, and chest pain places pneumonia or pleural effusion at the top of the list. Table 9-11 lists the differential diagnosis.

During further history taking, Mr. H reports no radiation of the pain. He denies abdominal pain, nausea, vomiting, or change in appetite. Deep breathing and sudden movements tend to worsen the pain. There are no other palliative or provocative features.

On physical exam, Mr. H is a healthy appearing man who appears in mild distress. He moves gingerly because of the pain and he is dyspneic. He coughs occasionally during the history. This causes great pain. Vital signs are temperature, 38.9°C; BP, 130/84 mm Hg; pulse, 110 bpm; RR, 26 breaths per minute. Head and neck exam is normal; there is no jugular venous distention. Lung exam is notable for dullness to percussion and decreased breath sounds at the right base. There is an area of egophony just superior to the decreased breath sounds and normal breath sounds superior to this. The left chest is clear. Heart exam is normal as are the abdomen and extremities.

Is the clinical information sufficient to make a diagnosis? If not, what other information do you need?

Table 9-11. Diagnostic hypotheses for Mr. H.

Diagnostic Hypotheses	Demographics, Risk Factors, Symptoms and Signs	Important Tests
Leading Hypothesis		
Pleural effusion or pneumonia with pleural effusion	Cough and shortness of breath with physical exam findings for pleural effusion Fever	Chest radiograph Thoracentesis
Active Alternative		
Pericarditis	Pain relieved by leaning forward Friction rub ECG changes	ECG Echocardiogram
Active Alternative—Must Not Miss		
Pulmonary embolism	Risk factors Dyspnea Tachycardia Unilateral leg swelling	CT angiography Ventilation-perfusion scan D-dimer Pulmonary angiogram
Other Alternative		
Subdiaphragmatic abscess	Intra-abdominal process Fevers	Abdominal ultrasound CT

Leading Hypothesis: Pleural Effusion

Textbook Presentation

Small effusions are usually asymptomatic while large effusions reliably cause dyspnea with or without pleuritic chest pain. The presentation depends on the cause of the effusion. Parapneumonic effusions will be accompanied by the signs and symptoms of pneumonia while effusions related to neoplasm, HF, PE or rheumatologic disease will be accompanied by signs of those underlying diseases.

Disease Highlights

A. Pathophysiology of pleural effusions vary by etiology but may be due to 1 or any combination of the following:

   1. Increased capillary permeability

   2. Increased hydrostatic pressure

   3. Decreased oncotic pressure

   4. Increased negative intrapleural pressure

   5. Disruption of pulmonary lymphatics

B. The most common causes of pleural effusions with their approximate yearly incidence are listed in Table 9-12.

C. The most useful way of organizing the differential diagnosis is by whether the effusion is exudative or transudative.

   1. Exudative effusions are caused by increased capillary permeability or disruption of pulmonary lymphatics.

   2. Transudative effusions are caused by increased hydrostatic pressure, decreased oncotic pressure, or increased negative intrapleural pressure.

D. Table 9-13 lists some common transudative and exudative effusions.

Table 9-12. The incidences of several causes of pleural effusion.

Etiology	Incidence
Heart failure	500,000
Pneumonia	300,000
Malignancy	200,000
Pulmonary embolism	150,000
Viral disease	100,000
Coronary artery bypass surgery	60,000
Cirrhosis with ascites	50,000
Less common but prevalent causes, including uremia, tuberculosis, chylothorax, and rheumatologic disease (RA and SLE)	

Data from Light RW. Clinical practice. Pleural effusion. N Engl J Med. 2002;346:1971–1977. RA, rheumatoid arthritis; SLE, systemic lupus erythematosus.

Table 9-13. Common transudative and exudative effusions.

Transudative Effusions	Exudative Effusions
Heart failure	Parapneumonic effusions
Cirrhosis with ascites	Malignancy
Pulmonary embolism (1/4)	Pulmonary embolism (3/4)
Nephrotic syndrome	Viral infections
Severe hypoalbuminemia	Post CABG
	Subdiaghragmatic infections and inflammatory states
	Chylothorax, uremia, connective tissue diseases

CABG, coronary artery bypass grafting.

E. Exudative effusions commonly complicate the following diagnoses:

1. Pneumonia
   a. Any effusion associated with pneumonia, lung abscess, or bronchiectasis is considered a parapneumonic effusion.
   b. Empyemas are parapneumonic effusions that have become infected.
   c. Empyemas, and certain parapneumonic effusions called complicated parapneumonic effusions, are more likely to form fibrotic, pleural peels. The diagnostic criteria for these types of effusions are described in the evidence-based diagnosis section.
   d. Parapneumonic effusions accompany 40% of all pneumonias while empyemas are rare complications.
   e. Effusions are more likely to form and are more likely to become infected if the treatment of the underlying pneumonia is delayed.
   f. The bacteriology of parapneumonic effusions is shown in Table 9-14.

Table 9-14. Bacteriology of parapneumonic effusions.

Bacteria	Percentage of Pneumonias with Effusion	Percentage of Effusions that are Empyemas
Streptococcus pneumoniae	40–60	< 5
Anaerobes	35	90
Staphylococcus aureus	40	20
Haemophilus influenzae	50	20
Escherichia coli	~50	~99

2. Malignancy
   a. Cancers most commonly associated with effusions are
      (1) Lung
      (2) Breast
      (3) Lymphoma
      (4) Leukemia
      (5) Adenocarcinoma of unknown primary
   b. The effusion may occur as the presenting symptom of the cancer or occur in patients with a previously diagnosed malignancy.
   c. The presence of a malignant effusion is generally a very poor prognostic sign.
3. PE
   a. Effusions are present in 26–56% of patients with PE.
   b. Effusions accompany PE most commonly in patients with pleuritic pain or hemoptysis.
4. Viral infections
   a. Considered to be a common cause of effusions
   b. Difficult to diagnose; definitive diagnosis is rarely made
   c. Usually diagnosed in patients with febrile or nonfebrile illness with a transient effusion and negative evaluation for other causes.
   d. Other clues such as atypical lymphocytes, monocytosis, and leukopenia are helpful in diagnosing viral infection.

 A pleural effusion should only be diagnosed as viral in an appropriate clinical setting when more serious causes of effusion have been ruled out.

5. CABG
   a. Pleural effusions develop in up to 90% of patients immediately following CABG.
   b. Can be left sided or bilateral
   c. Usually resolve spontaneously
6. Other diseases that are not common causes of exudative pleural effusions include
   a. Uremia
   b. Tuberculosis (TB)
   c. Chylothorax
   d. Rheumatologic disease (eg, rheumatoid arthritis and systemic lupus erythematosus)

F. The most common causes of transudative effusions are

1. HF

   a. Effusions are accompanied by other findings of left HF.

   b. Effusions are usually bilateral; unilateral effusions can occur, but they are less common.

2. Cirrhosis with ascites

   a. About 6% of patients with ascites have pleural effusions.

   b. Effusion is thought to be secondary to ascites moving into the thorax via defects in the diaphragm.

   c. It is extremely rare to have pleural effusions on the basis of cirrhosis without ascites.

Evidence-Based Diagnosis

A. Detecting a pleural effusion

1. The test characteristics for dullness to chest percussion are not well defined. The best estimates are sensitivity, 77%; specificity, 92%; LR+, 7.7; LR–, 0.27.

2. There is often an area of egophony just superior to the effusion.

3. Once detected, a pleural effusion is confirmed on chest radiograph, ultrasound, or other form of chest imaging.

B. Determining the etiology of a pleural effusion

1. Any clinically significant effusion (> 1 cm on a chest film) should be sampled via thoracentesis.

2. The only exception to this is in the case of HF. If the clinical suspicion for HF as the sole cause of the effusion is high, the effusion can be observed while the patient is treated. If the effusion persists or the diagnosis becomes unclear, the effusion should then be sampled.

 Pleural effusions are abnormal; any new pleural effusion should be evaluated.

3. The first step in determining the cause of an effusion is to differentiate transudative from exudative effusions.

   a. Light criteria are the most widely used test for differentiating transudative from exudative effusions. By these criteria, an effusion is considered to be an exudate if any of the following are present:

      (1) Pleural fluid protein/serum protein > 0.5

      (2) Pleural fluid lactate dehydrogenase (LD)/serum LD > 0.6

      (3) Pleural fluid LD > two-thirds upper limit of normal for serum LD

   b. The test characteristics for Light criteria are

      (1) Sensitivity, 98%; specificity, 83%

      (2) LR+, 5.76; LR–, 0.02

   c. The most specific test for an exudative effusion is a difference between the serum albumin and pleural fluid albumin of < 1.2 g/dL (LR+ 10.88).

4. Once the diagnosis of a transudate or exudate is made, various other tests will help determine the exact diagnosis.

   a. Positive Gram stain or culture makes the diagnosis of an empyema.

   b. Fluid pH: A low pH (< 7.2) is commonly seen with

      (1) Empyemas

      (2) Malignant effusions

      (3) Esophageal rupture

   c. Cell count

      (1) Neutrophil count over 50% argues for an acute process

         (a) Parapneumonic effusion (sensitivity = 91%)

         (b) PE

      (2) High neutrophil count is rarely seen in other diseases, such as TB and malignancy.

      (3) Lymphocyte predominant exudative effusions are almost always caused by TB or malignancy (positive predictive value = 97%).

      (4) Pleural fluid eosinophilia is a nonspecific finding. It is seen frequently with inflammatory diseases, pneumococcal pneumonia, viral pleuritis, TB, and even repeated thoracentesis.

      (5) A low mesothelial cell count (< 5%) is highly suggestive of TB.

   d. Cytology

      (1) Highly specific for the diagnosis of cancer

      (2) Sensitivity is 70% at best, with significantly lower values for some cancers.

5. Other tests for certain diseases are done if the clinical suspicion is high.

   a. Tuberculous effusions

      (1) Usually suspected based on clinical presentation and pleural fluid lymphocytosis

      (2) The sensitivity of commonly used tests for the diagnosis of tuberculous pleurisy are

         (a) Pleural fluid culture, 42%

         (b) Pleural biopsy culture, 64%

         (c) Pleural biopsy histology (caseating granulomas), 70–80%

         (d) Histology and pleural tissue culture > 90%

         (e) Sputum culture, 20–50%

      (3) Two newer tests, pleural fluid adenosine deaminase and interferon-gamma, are proving useful in the diagnosis of tuberculous effusions. Test characteristics from recent meta-analyses are

         (a) Adenosine deaminase: sensitivity and specificity of 92.2%; LR+, 11.82; LR–, 0.08

         (b) Interferon-gamma: sensitivity, 89%; specificity, 97%; LR+, 23.45; LR–, 0.11

   b. Glucose levels < 60 mg/dL are seen in

      (1) Empyema

      (2) TB

      (3) Rheumatoid arthritis

      (4) Systemic lupus erythematosus

   c. Triglycerides are > 110 mg/dL in patients with chylothorax. The fluid is also a milky white.

   d. Thoracoscopy with pleural biopsy is necessary when there is a suspicion for malignancy and cytology is negative.

 Pleural fluid testing should always include LD, protein, albumin, pH, and cell count. Other tests, such as cytology, are often sent.

Treatment

A. Pleural effusions are managed by treating the underlying disease (eg, pneumonia, uremia, HF).

B. Specific treatment of the effusion is necessary in certain circumstances.

1. Complicated parapneumonic effusions

   a. Evacuation by chest tube drainage prevents pleural scarring and the development of restrictive pleural disease.

   b. Indications for chest tube placement are

   (1) Purulent fluid or positive Gram stain

   (2) pH < 7.2

   (3) LD > 1000 units/L

   (4) Glucose < 40 mg/dL

   (5) Small effusions that are close to the above 3 cutoffs can sometimes be carefully monitored.

2. Malignant pleural effusions

   a. Usually managed by treating the underlying disease and periodic therapeutic thoracentesis.

   b. If thoracentesis is required frequently and the patient's life expectancy is long, there are a number of options among which are

   (1) Pleurodesis, obliteration of the pleural space by the installation of a chemical irritant

   (2) Catheter drainage, in which a semi-permanent catheter is placed to allow constant drainage of the effusion.

3. Chylothorax

   a. Caused by nontraumatic (primarily lymphoma) or traumatic (usually surgical) disruption of the thoracic duct.

   b. In nontraumatic cases, the underlying disease is treated.

   c. In both nontraumatic and traumatic disease, the pleural space is evacuated with chest tube drainage.

   d. A diet of medium chain fatty acids or a trial of total parenteral nutrition is used to decrease flow through the thoracic duct.

   e. Pleurodesis and surgical management reserved for refractory cases.

MAKING A DIAGNOSIS

The patient's physical exam findings are consistent with a pleural effusion. A posteroanterior, lateral, and decubitus chest film were done that revealed an effusion. The effusion was aspirated and yielded pale, turbid fluid. The initial results are glucose, < 20 mg/dL; LD = 38,400 units/L; protein = 4.4 g/dL; fluid pH, 6.2; RBC, 3200/mcL; WBC, 144,000/mcL; Gram stain positive for gram-positive cocci in pairs and chains. Serum values at the time included total protein of 7.8 g/dL and LD 141 units/L.

Have you crossed a diagnostic threshold for the leading hypothesis, pleural effusion? Have you ruled out the active alternatives? Do other tests need to be done to exclude the alternative diagnoses?

Mr. H has a pleural effusion. Given the size of the effusion on the chest film, a thoracentesis was clearly indicated. The results of the aspirate are diagnostic. The fluid is an exudate and the low glucose, low pH, high WBC, and positive Gram stain make the diagnosis of an empyema.

It is worth noting that Mr. H's previous diagnosis of musculoskeletal chest pain was incorrect. A chest radiograph done on his previous visit to the emergency department may have made the correct diagnosis and treatment could, potentially, have prevented the development of an empyema. There are many indications for chest films, one is to diagnose a cause for chest pain.

A chest film should be performed in any patient with chest pain and no clear diagnosis.

Alternative Diagnoses: Acute Pericarditis

Textbook Presentation

Acute pericarditis typically presents in young adults, with 1 week of viral symptoms and chest pain that improves with leaning forward. Physical exam reveals a 3-part friction rub. ECG reveals ST elevations and PR depressions in all leads.

Disease Highlights

A. Differential diagnosis

1. Viral pericarditis is primarily caused by coxsackievirus, echovirus, and adenovirus.

2. Other infectious causes of pericarditis include TB (historically the most common) and HIV.

3. Pericarditis may occur after myocardial injury (post MI and postcardiac surgery).

4. Rheumatologic causes include systemic lupus erythematosus and rheumatoid arthritis.

5. Procainamide and hydralazine are among the drugs that can cause pericarditis.

6. Neoplastic causes

   a. Malignancy metastatic to the pericardium

   b. Pericarditis can also be caused by chest irradiation.

7. Uremia: approximately 50% of patients with uremia have pericardial effusions.

B. Although the differential diagnosis of pericarditis is long, 85–90% of cases are considered idiopathic or due to an undiagnosed virus.

Evidence-Based Diagnosis

A. Pericarditis is diagnosed when the characteristic pericardial friction is heard or when a patient with chest pain has characteristic ECG findings.

1. History

   a. Chest pain is almost always present.

   b. The pain is usually pleuritic.

   c. It classically radiates to the trapezius ridge.

   d. Pain improves with sitting and worsens with reclining.

2. Physical exam

    a. The pericardial friction rub is insensitive but nearly 100% specific; it is diagnostic of pericarditis.

b. The rub is usually triphasic.

  (1) Triphasic in 58% of cases

  (2) Biphasic in 24% of cases

  (3) Monophasic in 18% of cases

c. Pericarditis is usually complicated by a pericardial effusion. Although the physical exam is insensitive for effusions, it is good for detecting tamponade.

  (1) Sensitivity of jugular venous distention to detect tamponade is 100%.

  (2) Sensitivity of tachycardia to detect tamponade is 100%.

  (3) Pulsus paradoxus > 12 mm Hg

    (a) Sensitivity, 98%; specificity, 83%
    (b) LR+, 5.9; LR–, 0.03

d. Beck triad (hypotension, jugular venous distention, and the presence of muffled heart sounds) is seldom seen but is very specific for tamponade.

3. ECG

a. The ECG most commonly shows widespread ST elevations and PR depressions. This finding is highly specific but the sensitivity is only about 60%.

b. The differentiation of pericarditis from acute MI on ECG can be difficult. Some of the key differentiating factors are

  (1) ST elevation in pericarditis is usually diffuse while in MI it is usually localized.

  (2) ST elevations in MI are often associated with reciprocal changes.

  (3) PR depression is very uncommon in acute MI.

  (4) Q waves are not present with pericarditis.

Pericarditis can mimic MI. The presence of a rub and careful analysis of the ECG should enable their distinction.

4. Other diagnostic tests

a. An echocardiogram is always done when pericarditis has been diagnosed to evaluate the presence of a significant pericardial effusion and exclude the presence of tamponade.

b. Cardiac enzymes are frequently positive and are therefore not helpful for distinguishing the chest pain of pericarditis from that of cardiac ischemia.

B. Determining the etiology of pericarditis

1. Because most pericarditis is either idiopathic or viral, requiring only supportive care, extensive work-up is generally not indicated.

2. After a thorough history, most experts recommend only a few diagnostic tests.

a. Chest radiograph

b. Blood urea nitrogen and creatinine

c. Purified protein derivative, interferon-gamma release assays (Quantiferon)

d. Antinuclear antibodies

e. Blood cultures

3. More extensive evaluation is appropriate for patients with refractory or recurrent disease. Even the most invasive diagnostic studies, pericardiocentesis and pericardial biopsy, are generally not helpful. Their diagnostic yield is only about 20%.

Treatment

A. Because most patients have viral or idiopathic disease, the treatment of acute pericarditis is supportive.

1. NSAIDs are the treatment of choice, usually providing good pain relief.

2. The addition of colchicine may improve response to therapy and decrease rates of recurrent disease.

B. Prednisone is effective in patients with refractory disease but only after excluding the presence of diseases (such as TB) that could be worsened by corticosteroids.

C. Pericardiocentesis is required in patients with tamponade.

CASE RESOLUTION

Mr. H underwent chest tube drainage of the effusion. Because the effusion was loculated, 3 tubes were placed under thoracoscopic guidance. He was given a third-generation cephalosporin while sensitivities of his presumed pneumococcus were pending. He became afebrile after 2 days of antibiotics and chest tube drainage. The tube output declined over 5 days and the tubes were removed on day 6. Total output was about 3 L.

He was discharged with a prescription for 6 weeks of oral antibiotics.

Empyemas are a medical emergency. They are closed space infections that need to be drained in order to cure them and preserve future lung function. As soon as one is detected, steps should be taken to drain it.

REFERENCES

Abrams J. Clinical practice. Chronic stable angina. N Engl J Med. 2005; 352(24):2524–33.

Anderson JL, Adams CD, Antman EM et al. ACC/AHA 2007 guidelines for the management of patients with unstable angina/non ST-elevation myocardial Infarction. J Am Coll Cardiol. 2007;50(7):e1–157.

Antman EM, Anbe DT, Armstrong PW et al. ACC/AHA guidelines for the management of patients with ST-elevation myocardial infarction. J Am Coll Cardiol. 2004;44(3):E1–E211.

Canto JG, Rogers WJ, Goldberg RJ et al. Association of age and sex with myocardial infarction symptom presentation and in-hospital mortality. JAMA. 2012;307(8):813–22.

Goto M, Noguchi Y, Koyama H, Hira K, Shimbo T, Fukui T. Diagnostic value of adenosine deaminase in tuberculous pleural effusion: a meta-analysis. Ann Clin Biochem. 2003;40:374–81.

Jiang J, Shi HZ, Liang QL, Qin SM, Qin XJ. Diagnostic value of interferon-gamma in tuberculous pleurisy: a meta-analysis. Chest. 2007;131(4):1133–41.

Kimble LP, McGuire DB, Dunbar SB et al. Gender differences in pain characteristics of chronic stable angina and perceived physical limitation in patients with coronary artery disease. Pain. 2003;101:45–53.

Klompas M. Does this patient have an acute thoracic aortic dissection? JAMA. 2002;287(17):2262–72.

Light RW. Parapneumonic effusions and empyema. Clin Chest Med. 1985;6(1): 55–62.

McGee SR. Evidence-based physical diagnosis. Philadelphia, PA: Saunders; 2001.

Permanyer-Miralda G, Sagrista-Sauleda J, Soler-Soler J. Primary acute pericardial disease: a prospective series of 231 consecutive patients. Am J Cardiol. 1985;56(10):623–30.

Simel DL, Rennie D, eds. The Rational Clinical Examination: Evidence-Based Clinical Diagnosis. New York, NY: McGraw-Hill; 2010.

Spodick DH. Pericardial friction. Characteristics of pericardial rubs in fifty consecutive, prospectively studied patients. N Engl J Med. 1968;278(22):1204–7.

Thygesen K, Alpert JS, White HD. Universal definition of myocardial infarction. Circulation. 2007;116(22):2634–53.

von Kodolitsch Y, Schwartz AG, Nienaber CA. Clinical prediction of acute aortic dissection. Arch Intern Med. 2000;160(19):2977–82.

Williams SV, Fihn SD, Gibbons RJ. Guidelines for the management of patients with chronic stable angina: diagnosis and risk stratification. Ann Intern Med. 2001;135(7):530–47.

Wong CL, Holroyd-Leduc J, Straus SE. Original article: does this patient have a pleural effusion? In: Simel DL, Rennie D, eds. *The Rational Clinical Examination: Evidence-Based Clinical Diagnosis.* New York, NY: McGraw-Hill; 2010.

http://www.jamaevidence.com/content/3494687. Accessed 11/20/2013

Yeghiazarians Y, Braunstein JB, Askari A, Stone PH. Unstable angina pectoris. N Engl J Med. 2000;342(2):101–14.

I have a patient with acute respiratory complaints of cough and congestion. How do I determine the cause?

CHIEF COMPLAINT

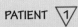

Ms. L is a 22-year-old woman who comes to your office in August complaining of cough and fever. She reports that she was in her usual state of health until 3 days ago when a cough developed. Two days ago, a low-grade fever (37.8°C) developed, which increased to 38.8°C yesterday. She reports that her sputum is yellow and that she has no chest pain or shortness of breath.

CONSTRUCTING A DIFFERENTIAL DIAGNOSIS

The causes of cough and congestion vary from trivial self-limited upper respiratory viral infections to serious, imminently life-threatening forms of pneumonia. The approach to such patients focuses on 2 pivotal questions. First, does the patient have symptoms, signs, or risk factors for pneumonia that warrant a chest radiograph or other evaluation? Second, in patients with pneumonia, is it simply a community-acquired pneumonia (CAP) or another type of pneumonia that requires alternative/additional treatment (such as *Pneumocystis jirovecii* pneumonia [PCP] or tuberculosis [TB])?

A variety of symptoms suggest pneumonia because they are unusual in upper respiratory tract infections or bronchitis. These include dyspnea, high fever (with the exception of influenza [see below]), altered mental status, hypoxia, hypotension, dullness to percussion, crackles, decreased breath sounds, bronchophony, or egophony. Any patient with such symptoms or signs requires a minimum evaluation with a chest radiograph to rule out pneumonia. A chest radiograph should also be strongly considered in patients at increased risk for poor outcomes, including immunocompromised patients; elderly patients; and those with heart failure (HF), chronic kidney disease, or chronic obstructive pulmonary disease (COPD) (in whom abnormal lung findings are also more difficult to appreciate). Figure 10-1 shows a diagnostic algorithm illustrating the initial approach to patients with cough and congestion.

In patients with pneumonia, the next pivotal step is to determine the likely etiologic pathogen(s), which will ensure patients receive appropriate therapy. Even in patients coming from the community, it is *not safe to assume that all have the typical CAP pathogens*. In many such patients, other types of pneumonia that require different/additional antimicrobial therapy will ultimately be diagnosed. A careful review of both the patient's risk factors and chest radiograph often provide critical clues that suggest additional microorganisms needing antibiotic coverage. Figure 10-2 illustrates the approach to patients with pneumonia. Pneumonia in patients with known immunocompromise will not be covered in this chapter (known HIV, transplant recipients, and patients with granulocytopenia).

Differential Diagnosis of Acute Cough and Congestion

A. Common cold

B. Sinusitis

C. Bronchitis

D. Influenza

E. Pneumonia
1. CAP
2. Aspiration pneumonia
3. TB
4. Opportunistic (eg, PCP)

On physical exam, Ms. L is in no acute distress. Vital signs are RR, 18 breaths per minute; BP, 110/72 mm Hg; pulse, 92 bpm; temperature, 38.6°C. Pharynx is unremarkable; lung exam reveals normal breath sounds without crackles, dullness, bronchophony, or egophony.

 At this point, what is the leading hypothesis, what are the active alternatives, and is there a must not miss diagnosis? Given this differential diagnosis, what tests should be ordered?

RANKING THE DIFFERENTIAL DIAGNOSIS

The differential diagnosis for Ms. L includes acute bronchitis, influenza, aspiration pneumonia, and CAP. Ms. L's high fever is a pivotal feature of this case. Acute bronchitis is *not* usually associated with significant fever (unless caused by influenza). Influenza can cause high fevers and chest symptoms but almost always occurs between December and May. Therefore, despite Ms. L's normal lung exam, the high fever raises the possibility of CAP and makes this the leading diagnosis. Table 10-1 lists the differential diagnosis.

 A high fever (temperature > 38°C) should raise the suspicion of pneumonia.

 Influenza occurs from December to May in the northern hemisphere; it is highly unlikely at other times.

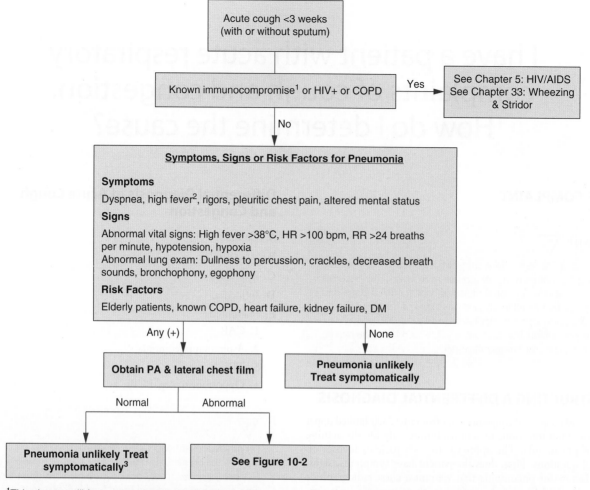

Figure 10-1. Initial approach to the patient with cough and congestion.

[1]This chapter will focus on patients without known immunocompromise. For patients known to be HIV+ see Chapter 5. See Chapter 33 for patients with underlying COPD. Readers are referred elsewhere for transplant recipients, granulocytopenia, or other immunosuppressive conditions.

[2]Febrile patients very likely to have influenza may not require a chest radiograph. That would include patients fulfilling all of the following criteria: influenza season, unvaccinated patient, maximum fever within the first 24 hours and without dyspnea or focal lung findings. Clinical judgment is required.

[3]A normal chest film does not completely rule out pneumonia. Patients in whom there is a high clinical suspicion (eg, those with focal crackles and fever) should be empirically treated for pneumonia with consideration for additional radiographic imaging (eg, follow-up chest film or CT scan. See Community-acquired pneumonia, Evidence-Based Diagnosis section.)

COPD, chronic obstructive pulmonary disease; DM, diabetes mellitus; PA, posterior-anterior

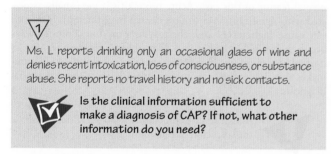

Ms. L reports drinking only an occasional glass of wine and denies recent intoxication, loss of consciousness, or substance abuse. She reports no travel history and no sick contacts.

Is the clinical information sufficient to make a diagnosis of CAP? If not, what other information do you need?

Leading Hypothesis: CAP

Textbook Presentation

Productive cough and fever are usually the presenting symptoms in patients with pneumonia. Symptoms may worsen over days or develop abruptly. Pleuritic chest pain, shortness of breath, chills, and rigors may also develop.

Disease Highlights

A. Most common cause of infectious death in the United States

B. *Streptococcus pneumoniae* is the most commonly identified pathogen in patients hospitalized for pneumonia whereas *Mycoplasma pneumoniae* is the most commonly identified pathogen in outpatients.

C. Other common pathogens include *Chlamydia, Haemophilus influenzae, Legionella,* and respiratory viruses (influenza, parainfluenza, respiratory syncytial virus, and adenovirus).

D. 3.4% of pneumonias are associated with underlying malignancy (postobstructive pneumonias)

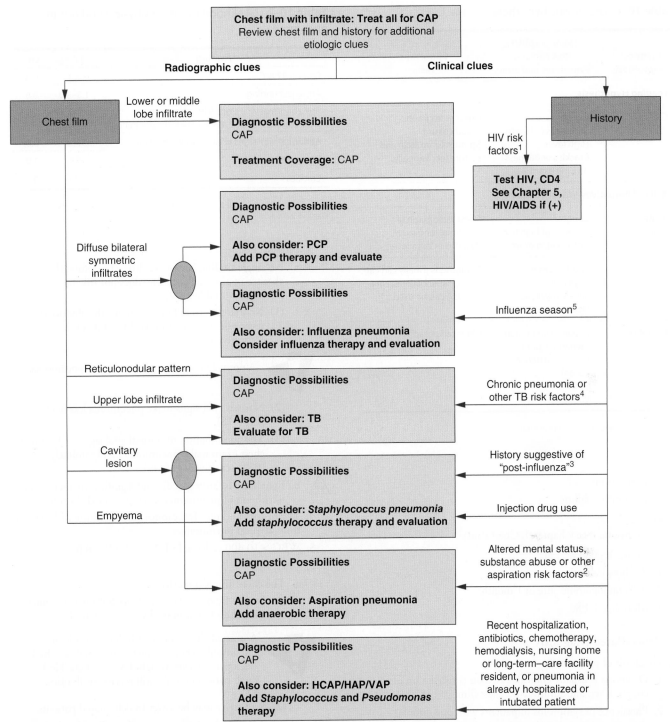

```
Chest film with infiltrate: Treat all for CAP
Review chest film and history for additional
            etiologic clues
```

Radiographic clues   Clinical clues

Chest film — Lower or middle lobe infiltrate →

Diagnostic Possibilities
CAP

Treatment Coverage: CAP

History

HIV risk factors[1]

**Test HIV, CD4
See Chapter 5,
HIV/AIDS if (+)**

Diffuse bilateral symmetric infiltrates →

Diagnostic Possibilities
CAP

**Also consider: PCP
Add PCP therapy and evaluate**

Diagnostic Possibilities
CAP

**Also consider: Influenza pneumonia
Consider influenza therapy and evaluation**

Influenza season[5]

Reticulonodular pattern →
Upper lobe infiltrate →

Diagnostic Possibilities
CAP

**Also consider: TB
Evaluate for TB**

Chronic pneumonia or other TB risk factors[4]

Cavitary lesion →
Empyema →

Diagnostic Possibilities
CAP

**Also consider: *Staphylococcus pneumonia*
Add *staphylococcus* therapy and evaluation**

History suggestive of "post-influenza"[3]

Injection drug use

Diagnostic Possibilities
CAP

**Also consider: Aspiration pneumonia
Add anaerobic therapy**

Altered mental status, substance abuse or other aspiration risk factors[2]

Diagnostic Possibilities
CAP

**Also consider: HCAP/HAP/VAP
Add *Staphylococcus* and *Pseudomonas* therapy**

Recent hospitalization, antibiotics, chemotherapy, hemodialysis, nursing home or long-term–care facility resident, or pneumonia in already hospitalized or intubated patient

[1]HIV clues include high-risk sexual behavior, injection drug use, blood product recipient (prior to blood screening), thrush, or Kaposi sarcoma.
[2]Aspiration risk factors include difficulty swallowing, sedation, alcohol or drug abuse, delirium or dementia, cerebrovascular accident, vomiting, endoscopy, bronchoscopy, nasogastric feeding.
[3]Post-influenza pneumonia clues include a patient with influenza who improves initially with resolution of fever and then worsens with recurrent fever.
[4]TB clues include (1) recent exposure to a patient with documented active TB, (2) history of a positive purified protein derivative, (3) fever or night sweats for ≥ 3 weeks, (4) > 10% weight loss.
[5]Influenza clues include influenza season (typically December-May in Northern Hemisphere), nonvaccinated patient against the current strain (vaccine nonrecipients, or poor strain-vaccine match). Other common symptoms include headache, sore throat, myalgias, and sudden onset of symptoms.
CAP, community-acquired pneumonia; HAP, hospital-acquired pneumonia; HCAP, healthcare-associated pneumonia; PCP, Pneumocystis jirovecii pneumonia; TB, tuberculosis; VAP, ventilator-associated pneumonia

Figure 10-2. Approach to patient with cough, congestion, and infiltrate on chest film.

Table 10-1. Diagnostic hypotheses for Ms. L.

Diagnostic Hypothesis	Demographics, Risk Factors, Symptoms and Signs	Important Tests
Leading Hypothesis		
CAP	Cough Shortness of breath High fever Crackles or dullness on lung exam	Chest radiograph Blood culture Sputum Gram stain and culture (occasionally)
Active Alternatives—Most Common		
Acute bronchitis	Cough Absence of high fever Normal lung exam	Chest radiograph (if abnormal lung exam, dyspnea or high fever)
Influenza	Sudden onset High fever Severe myalgias December to May	Diagnosis is usually clinical Direct immunofluorescence or ELISA can be used
Aspiration pneumonia	Impaired mentation (dementia, prior stroke, substance abuse) Seizure Vomiting	Chest radiograph

ELISA, enzyme-linked immunosorbent assay.

E. Complications
   1. Respiratory failure
   2. Death
   3. Empyema (See Chapter 9, Chest Pain)
F. Prognosis is good overall.
   1. 8% hospitalization rate
   2. 95% radiographic cure in 1 month
   3. Mortality 1.2%

Evidence-Based Diagnosis

A. Diagnosis of pneumonia
   1. Diagnosis is usually clinical, based on constellation of cough, fever, and infiltrate on chest film.
   2. Prevalence of symptoms in patients with pneumonia
      a. Cough, 96%
      b. Fever, 81% but 53% in the elderly

Elderly patients with pneumonia often *do not* have a fever. Clinicians should have a low threshold for obtaining a chest radiograph in elderly patients or in patients with COPD with cough or with mental status changes.

   c. Dyspnea, 46–66%
   d. Pleuritic chest pain, 37–50%
   e. Chills, 59%
   f. Headache, 58%

Table 10-2. Likelihood ratios for physical findings in pneumonia.

Finding	LR+	LR−
Fever > 37.8°C	4.4	0.8
Any chest finding	1.3–3.0	0.6
Any abnormal vital signs (HR > 100 bpm, temperature > 37.8°C, RR ≥ 30 breaths per minute)	1.2	0.18
Abnormal vital signs or abnormal lung exam	2.2	0.09[1]
Egophony	8.6	1.0
Crackles	2.7	0.9

[1]The negative LRs refer to the likelihood of pneumonia if both the vital signs and lung exam are normal.

3. Physical exam
   a. No single finding is very sensitive. Therefore, the absence of any single finding does not rule out pneumonia (Table 10-2).
      (1) Neither a normal lung exam nor the absence of fever rule out pneumonia (LR–, 0.6 and 0.8, respectively).

A normal lung exam *does not* rule out pneumonia.

      (2) Normal vital signs make pneumonia less likely (LR 0.18).
      (3) The combination of normal vital signs and normal chest exam make pneumonia highly unlikely (95% sensitive, LR 0.09).

   b. Egophony is fairly specific and significantly increases the likelihood of pneumonia when present (LR+ 8.6).
4. The history and physical cannot reliably distinguish typical from atypical pneumonias.
5. WBC > 10,400 cells/mcL: LR+, 3.7; LR–, 0.6
6. Chest film
   a. The chest film is imperfect.
      (1) Sensitivity 67–75%, specificity 85% when compared with chest CT scan or discharge diagnosis.

A normal chest radiograph does *not* rule out pneumonia when the pretest probability is high (ie, a patient with cough, fever, and crackles). Such patients should still receive antibiotics.

      (2) Sensitivity may be lower in dehydrated patients.
      (3) A single anterior-posterior chest film view has a lower sensitivity than posteroanterior and lateral (59% vs 90%) views.

Posteroanterior and lateral chest film views are superior to single anterior-posterior views and should be obtained when possible.

   b. 94% of infiltrates are in the lower and middle regions.

CAP rarely affects the upper lobes; consider TB or aspiration pneumonia when upper lobe involvement is seen.

   c. The chest radiograph cannot distinguish typical from atypical pneumonias.

Treatment

A. Prevention

1. Two vaccines are currently available to prevent invasive pneumococcal disease:

   a. An older 23-valent pneumococcal polysaccharide vaccine (PPSV 23) and a newer 13-valent pneumococcal conjugate vaccine (PCV 13)

   b. PCV 13 vaccine has fewer serotypes but generates an equivalent or larger immune response.

2. Vaccine recommendations (Advisory Committee on Immunization Practices [ACIP])

   a. All adults aged ≥ 65 years: A single dose of PPSV 23 regardless of previous history of pneumococcal vaccination

   b. Any adult who received PPSV prior to age 65 should receive a second dose at 65 or later once at least 5 years have passed since the first vaccination.

   c. The recommendations for immunocompromised adults and those with high risk conditions[1] are complex. Certain patients require PPSV 23 alone, some PCV 13 and PPSV 23, and others revaccination. Details can be found at the CDC Web site http://www.cdc.gov/mmwr/preview/mmwrhtml/mm6140a4.htm

B. Evaluation

1. Chest film is recommended in the evaluation of all patients with CAP.

2. Evaluate oxygenation in all patients (arterial blood gas [ABG] or SaO_2)

3. An ABG is required in patients with respiratory distress, particularly those with preexistent COPD.

 A normal SaO_2 on pulse oximetry does not exclude *hypercarbia* and respiratory failure. A blood gas to check $PaCO_2$ is required for patients with respiratory distress.

4. Determining the causative agent

   a. CAP is the most common pneumonia among outpatients with an infiltrate and fever.

   b. Nonetheless, clinicians should always consider other less common pneumonias including aspiration, TB, pneumocystis and HCAP (see Figure 10-2), which may warrant additional testing or therapy (see below for details).

      (1) A history of neurologic impairment or drug abuse increases the likelihood of aspiration pneumonia.

      (2) Chronic symptoms, upper lobe disease, or cavitary lesions increase the likelihood of TB.

      (3) HIV risk factors or bilateral fluffy infiltrates increase the likelihood of PCP.

      (4) Recent nursing home or institutional living or hospitalization warrants coverage for HCAP or hospital-acquired pneumonia.

   c. In the absence of clinical or radiographic clues that suggest other types of pneumonia, most patients are treated empirically, to cover the most common organisms responsible for CAP.

   d. However, a variety of tests, including sputum culture, sputum Gram stain, blood culture, and urinary antigen tests for pneumococcus and *Legionella,* can help determine the pathogen in CAP.

      (1) The yield of these tests in outpatients with CAP is low and routine testing is optional in outpatients.

      (2) Sputum cultures are often unreliable due to contamination by oral flora.

         (a) Normal flora should not be misinterpreted to mean no infection.

         (b) When positive, sputum cultures can help determine the resistance pattern.

      (3) Sputum Gram stains are also often unreliable due to poor quality, preparation, and interpretation.

         (a) Overall, only 14% of hospitalized patients had an adequate specimen with a dominant organism.

         (b) In patients with pneumococcal bacteremia, the Gram stain was positive in 63–80%.

      (4) Blood cultures are positive in 5–14% of patients.

      (5) Pneumococcal urinary antigen is 50–80% sensitive and 90% specific (false-positives may occur secondary to colonization).

      (6) *Legionella* urinary antigen is 70–90% sensitive and 99% specific.

      (7) The Infectious Diseases Society of America (IDSA) has published guidelines for more extensive testing on select inpatients (Table 10-3).

   e. Patients with severe pneumonia should have blood and sputum cultures, sputum Gram stain, and urinary tests for pneumococcal and *Legionella* antigen.

5. Patients with pleural effusions require diagnostic thoracentesis to rule out empyema or complicated parapneumonic effusions, which require chest tube drainage in addition to antibiotics (see Chapter 9, Chest Pain).

6. HIV testing is recommended for all adults aged 15–65 years who have CAP.

C. Determine the need for hospitalization

1. Indications for admission

   a. Hypoxia

   b. Shock

   c. Pleural effusion

   d. Multilobar infiltrates on chest film

   e. Failure of prior outpatient therapy

   f. Confusion

   g. Unable to tolerate oral intake

   h. Unreliable social situation

   i. Certain underlying diseases (sickle cell disease, immunocompromise, severe COPD or HF)

2. Prospective validated clinical tools can help determine the need for admission. The CURB-65 score is the most widely used, validated model that predicts mortality.

   a. Criteria are **c**onfusion (to person, place, or time), **u**remia (BUN > 20 mg/dL), **R**R ≥ 30 breaths per minute, systolic **B**P < 90 mm Hg or diastolic BP ≤ 60 mm Hg, age ≥ **65.**

   b. Scores of > 1 are associated with an increased mortality and the need for hospital admission.

[1]Chronic kidney disease, nephrotic syndrome, chronic HF, chronic liver disease, diabetes mellitus, functional or anatomic asplenia, hemoglobinopathy, congenital or acquired immunodeficiency, HIV, leukemia, lymphoma, generalized malignancy, iatrogenic immunosuppression, solid organ transplant, multiple myeloma, CSF leak, cochlear implant, alcoholism.

Table 10-3. IDSA guidelines for more extensive testing in persons with CAP.

Indication	Blood Culture	Sputum Culture	*Legionella* UAT	Pneumococcal UAT	Other
Intensive care unit admission	X	X	X	X	X[1]
Failure of outpatient antibiotic therapy		X	X	X	
Cavitary infiltrates	X	X			X[2]
Leukopenia	X			X	
Active alcohol abuse	X	X	X	X	
Chronic severe liver disease	X			X	
Severe obstructive/structural lung disease		X			
Asplenia (anatomic or functional)	X			X	
Recent travel (within past 2 weeks)			X		X[5]
Positive *Legionella* UAT result		X[3]	NA		
Positive pneumococcal UAT result	X	X		NA	
Pleural effusion	X	X	X	X	X[4]

NOTE. NA, not applicable; UAT, urinary antigen test.
[1]Endotracheal aspirate if intubated, possibly bronchoscopy or nonbronchoscopic bronchoalveolar lavage.
[2]Fungal and tuberculosis cultures.
[3]Special media for *Legionella*.
[4]Thoracentesis and pleural fluid cultures.
[5]Consider pathogens endemic to visited region(s).
CAP, community-acquired pneumonia; IDSA, Infectious Diseases Society of America; NA, not applicable; UAT, urinary antigen test. (Reproduced, with permission, from Mandell LA, Wunderink RG, Anzueto A et al. Infectious Diseases Society of America/American Thoracic Society consensus guidelines on the management of community-acquired pneumonia in adults. Clin Infect Dis. 2007;44 Suppl 2:S27–72.)

D. Determine the need for ICU admission: The IDSA and ATS have published guidelines on ICU admissions for patients with severe pneumonia. ICU admission is recommended for septic shock requiring vasopressors and those on mechanical ventilation as well as patients with ≥ 3 minor criteria (RR > 30 breaths per minute, PaO_2/FiO_2 ratio ≤ 250, multilobar infiltrates, confusion, BUN ≥ 20 mg/dL, WBC < 4000 cells/mL, platelet count < 100,000 cells/mL, temperature < 36°C, or hypotension requiring aggressive fluid resuscitation).

E. Antibiotics
1. Treatment must cover pyogenic (*S pneumoniae*) and atypical (*Mycoplasma* and *Chlamydia*) organisms.
2. Penicillin-resistant *S pneumoniae* (PRSP)
   a. Increasing resistance in United States
   b. Marked geographic variability in frequency of resistance but up to 65% in some areas
   c. PRSP often resistant to cephalosporins and macrolides but not quinolones with extended activity against *S pneumoniae*.
3. Empiric therapy (recommendations from the IDSA 2007)
   a. Outpatients
      (1) Previously healthy outpatients are usually treated with an advanced macrolide (azithromycin or clarithromycin) or doxycycline. (Macrolides are preferred.)
      (2) Certain patients require alternative therapy with either a respiratory quinolone (moxifloxacin, levofloxacin, or gemifloxacin) or combination therapy of a beta-lactam (amoxicillin or amoxicillin-clavulanate or

cefpodoxime) and macrolide. This includes patients with any of the following:
      (a) Comorbidities (heart, lung, liver, or kidney disease; diabetes mellitus; alcoholism; cancer; asplenia; immunosuppression)
      (b) Antibiotic use within the last 3 months
      (c) Exposure to children in day care centers (increasing the risk for *S pneumoniae* resistance)
      (d) Evidence of pneumococcal pneumonia (diplococci on Gram stain, positive pneumococcal urine antigen, positive sputum culture for pneumococcus, or sudden onset of high fever and rigors)
      (e) Areas with a rate of macrolide resistance > 25%
   b. Inpatients should be treated with respiratory fluoroquinolone (levofloxacin or moxifloxacin) or advanced macrolide with a beta-lactam (ceftriaxone, cefotaxime or ampicillin-sulbactam).

F. Consultation is recommended for patients admitted to the ICU for antibiotic choice and consideration of other interventions including drotrecogin alpha (activated protein C) and screening for adrenal insufficiency.

G. Follow-up chest film
1. 3.4% of pneumonias are associated with an underlying tumor (postobstructive pneumonia) that may be obscured by the infiltrate
2. Follow-up radiography can ensure pneumonia resolution and discover an underlying mass.
3. Particularly important in patients at increased risk for pneumonia, including patients over 50 or who are smokers.

4. Chest film resolution lags behind clinical resolution.

   a. By day 10, most patients have clinical resolution but only 31% had a normal chest radiograph and 68% of patients had a normal chest radiograph by day 28.

   b. Follow-up chest film should be performed promptly in any patient with clinical deterioration and after day 28 in patients at risk for malignancy.

MAKING A DIAGNOSIS

Ms. L does not have risk factors for aspiration pneumonia. Influenza is highly unlikely in August. The differential diagnosis is narrowed to CAP and acute bronchitis.

 Have you crossed a diagnostic threshold for the leading hypothesis, CAP? Have you ruled out the active alternatives? Do other tests need to be done to exclude the alternative diagnosis?

Alternative Diagnosis: Acute Bronchitis

Textbook Presentation

Acute bronchitis presents in the healthy adult primarily as a cough of 1–3 weeks duration. Myalgias and low-grade fevers may be seen. This is distinct from an acute exacerbation of COPD (see Chapter 33, Wheezing & Stridor).

Disease Highlights

A. Etiology
   1. Viruses
      a. Influenza
      b. Parainfluenza
      c. Respiratory syncytial virus
      d. Adenovirus
      e. Rhinovirus
      f. Coronavirus
   2. Bacterial
      a. Bacteria cause < 10% of cases
      b. Organisms include *Bordetella pertussis, Mycoplasma,* and *Chlamydia.*
   3. Noninfectious
      a. Asthma
      b. Pollution
      c. Tobacco
      d. Cannabis

B. Symptoms
   1. Initial phase: Cough and systemic symptoms secondary to infection are seen.
   2. Fever absent or low grade. Consider pneumonia in patients whose fever is high-grade (> 38°C) or persistent.
   3. Protracted phase
      a. 40–65% of patients without prior pulmonary disease show evidence of reactive airway disease during acute bronchitis.
      b. In 26% of patients, cough persists secondary to bronchial hyperresponsiveness and lasts ≥ 2–4 weeks.

Evidence-Based Diagnosis

A. Sputum may be clear or discolored. Discoloration arises from tracheobronchial epithelium cells and WBCs and is *not* diagnostic of bacterial infection.

 Purulent sputum is not an indication for antibiotic therapy in patients with acute bronchitis.

B. Chest film is not routine but should be obtained when pneumonia is being considered (see Figure 10-1); indications include
   1. Patients at risk for pneumonia: elderly patients and those with heart, lung, kidney disease or are immunocompromised
   2. Symptoms of dyspnea, high fever, rigors, pleuritic chest pain, or altered mental status
   3. Abnormal vital signs including high fever (temperature > 38°C), tachypnea (RR > 24 breaths per minute), tachycardia (HR > 100 bpm)
   4. Focal findings on lung exam or hypoxemia

C. Testing for influenza can be considered in febrile patients who present during influenza season within 48 hours of symptoms onset in whom antiviral therapy is being considered (see below).

Treatment

A. Antibiotics
   1. Antibiotics do not provide major clinical benefit and are *not* recommended for most patients with acute bronchitis. Antibiotics can be considered in high-risk patients (those with underlying heart, lung, kidney disease or immunosuppression) or when the clinical index of suspicion for CAP is high despite a normal chest film.
   2. Influenza treatment shortens the course of illness in patients with influenza treated within 48 hours of symptoms (see below) and can be considered in patients with bronchitis due to this pathogen.

B. Bronchodilators significantly reduce cough in patients with bronchial hyperreactivity, wheezing, or airflow obstruction at baseline.

C. Antitussives are useful symptomatic measures.

CASE RESOLUTION

At this point, obtaining a chest radiograph is critical. A CBC, sputum and blood cultures can be obtained but are not sensitive enough to rule out pneumonia.

 A chest film reveals a left lower-lobe infiltrate, confirming the diagnosis of pneumonia.

 25–50% of patients with pneumonia do not have crackles on auscultation. Chest film is required when pneumonia is suspected.

WBC is 10,200 cells/mcL with 67% neutrophils and 5% bands. Her SaO$_2$ is 96% on room air. An HIV test should be ordered, antibiotics must be chosen, and a decision must be made to admit or discharge Ms. L.

Ms. L's CURB-65 score is 0 and she has no indications for admission (see above under CAP treatment). She has no

(continued)

risk factors for aspiration, and her chest radiograph does not suggest TB or PCP. Her HIV test is negative. She is treated for CAP with azithromycin and instructed to call immediately if her fever increases or increasing shortness of breath or chest pain develop.

One week later, she reports feeling much better. A follow-up chest film 6 weeks later shows resolution of the pneumonia.

A follow-up chest radiograph is indicated in patients with pneumonia to exclude an underlying obstructing mass.

CHIEF COMPLAINT

PATIENT 2

Mr. P is a 32-year-old man with cough and progressive shortness of breath over the last 4 weeks. He complains of a persistent cough productive of purulent sputum and low-grade fever. His past medical history is unremarkable. Social history: Mr. P reports that he is homeless. He admits to drinking 1 pint of gin per day. He reports no history of recreational or injection drug use. He reports that he has rarely used paid sex workers. He has no history of sex with men. He denies using condoms.

On physical exam he appears disheveled and smells of alcohol and urine. Vital signs are pulse, 95 bpm; temperature, 37.0°C; RR, 20 breaths per minute; BP, 140/90 mm Hg. There is temporal wasting. Lung exam reveals diffuse fine crackles in the lower lung fields bilaterally. Cardiac exam is normal. His chest radiograph demonstrates bilateral lower lobe infiltrates. No cardiomegaly is seen. A CBC is normal. SaO$_2$ is 88%. His BUN is 18 mg/dL.

At this point, what is the leading hypothesis, what are the active alternatives, and is there a must not miss diagnosis? Given this differential diagnosis, what tests should be ordered?

RANKING THE DIFFERENTIAL DIAGNOSIS

The clinical findings of cough, shortness of breath, crackles on pulmonary exam, and infiltrates on chest film all suggest pneumonia. One pivotal feature of this case is the long duration of symptoms. CAP is possible but less likely with such protracted symptoms. More chronic processes such as aspiration pneumonia or TB should be considered. Another pivotal feature of Mr. P's case is his alcoholism. Alcoholism, substance abuse, and neurologic disorders are leading risk factors for aspiration, and his alcoholism makes aspiration pneumonia the leading diagnosis. The duration of his complaints and temporal wasting also raise the possibility of more chronic pneumonias caused by TB, fungi, or PCP. TB is more common in alcoholic patients and malnourished patients.

Given the public health risks, TB is a must not miss possibility. A third pivotal feature in this patient is his high-risk sexual behavior increasing his risk for HIV infection and PCP. PCP primarily affects HIV-infected patients. It is important to consider PCP even in patients without a history of *known* HIV infection because PCP can be the first sign of HIV infection. The sexual history makes PCP (or another HIV-related pneumonia) an active alternative diagnosis. Finally, uncomplicated influenza does not persist for 4 weeks, although a postinfluenza pneumonia could be considered in the proper season. Table 10-4 lists the differential diagnosis.

Is the clinical information sufficient to make a diagnosis? If not what other information do you need?

Leading Hypothesis: Aspiration Pneumonia

Textbook Presentation

Aspiration pneumonia typically develops in patients with impaired mentation (ie, the demented elderly patient or alcoholic). Classic symptoms include fever, cough, chest pain, and putrid sputum. The syndrome most commonly evolves over days to weeks rather than acutely.

Disease Highlights

A. There are 2 types of aspiration: Small volume aspiration, typically of oropharyngeal secretions, and large volume aspiration, typically of gastric contents.

1. Aspiration of colonized oropharyngeal secretions is common but may be complicated by pneumonia when the combination of a large bacterial load (due to poor dentition) and virulence overcome host defenses (particularly cough).

2. Gastric acid aspiration may result in chemical damage (aspiration *pneumonitis*), which may be accompanied by subsequent infection (aspiration *pneumonia*).

B. Risk factors for aspiration

1. Neurologic disease (dementia, cerebrovascular accident, seizures)

2. Sedation (illicit drug or alcohol overdose, general anesthesia)

Table 10-4. Diagnostic hypotheses for Mr. P.

Diagnostic Hypothesis	Demographics, Risk Factors, Symptoms and Signs	Important Tests
Leading Hypothesis		
Aspiration pneumonia	Impaired mentation (dementia, prior stroke, substance abuse) Seizure Vomiting	Chest radiograph
Active Alternatives—Most Common		
CAP	Cough Shortness of breath High fever Crackles or dullness on lung exam	Chest radiograph Blood culture Sputum culture and Gram stain (occasionally)
PCP	Injection drug use, men who have sex with men, engaging in sex with paid sex workers	HIV CD4 count Chest radiograph demonstrating diffuse bilateral infiltrates
Active Alternatives—Must Not Miss		
TB	Long duration of symptoms	Chest radiograph shows upper lobe, cavitary or reticulonodular disease
	Risk factors for TB (alcoholism, HIV infection, foreign-born persons, cancer, diabetes, homeless persons, end-stage renal disease, use of corticosteroids, incarceration)	Sputum for acid-fast stain and culture

CAP, community-acquired pneumonia; PCP, *Pneumocystis jiroveci* pneumonia; TB, tuberculosis.

3. Dysphagia (status post head and neck surgery)
4. Gastroesophageal reflux disease, vomiting
5. Endoscopy, tracheostomy, bronchoscopy, nasogastric feeding

C. Aspiration *pneumonitis*
 1. Aspirated contents with lower pHs and larger volumes lead to more damage
 2. Clinical syndrome
  a. Usually follows large volume aspiration (ie, during anesthesia)
  b. Cyanosis, shortness of breath, and pulmonary infiltrates develop within 2 hours.
  c. Fever is usually low grade.
  d. Sputum may be putrid.
  e. Outcome varies
   (1) Rapid recovery within 24–36 hours (62%), bacterial superinfection (26%), acute respiratory distress syndrome (12%)
   (2) Bacterial superinfection may lead to pneumonia, lung abscess, or empyema.

D. Aspiration *pneumonia* refers to infection due to aspirated organisms.
 1. Accounts for 5–15% of pneumonias
 2. Poor dentition increases the risk of aspiration pneumonia.
 3. Aspiration is usually not witnessed.
 4. Clinical features include cough, fever, sputum production, and shortness of breath, which may progress over days to weeks.
 5. Organisms
  a. Community-acquired aspiration pneumonia may be caused by anaerobes, aerobic streptococci, *S pneumoniae*, *Staphylococcus aureus*, and *H influenzae*.
  b. Hospital-acquired aspiration pneumonias may be caused by anaerobes, gram-negative organisms (including *Pseudomonas*), or *S aureus*.

Evidence-Based Diagnosis

A. Often presumptive based on aspiration risk factors, putrid sputum, and typical chest film. Many patients have periodontal disease.

B. Oropharyngeal motility studies can identify certain patients at risk, particularly those with neurologic impairment.

C. Rigors and acute onset suggest more virulent organisms (ie, *S pneumoniae* and *S aureus*).

D. Chest film
 1. Aspiration pneumonia classically involves the basal segment of lower lobes but can involve the posterior segments of the upper lobes if aspiration occurred while the patient was recumbent.
 2. Cavitation is more common in aspiration pneumonia than in CAP.

Treatment

A. Prevention
 1. Soft diets and feeding strategies can reduce subsequent aspiration.
 2. Tube feedings decrease the incidence of aspiration pneumonia in patients with dysphagia (54% vs 13% with oral feeding). However, despite tube feedings, patients can still aspirate from gastroesophageal reflux, vomiting, and aspiration of oropharyngeal contents.
 3. Several studies suggest that angiotensin-converting enzyme (ACE) inhibitors increase the cough reflex and decrease the rate of pneumonia in persons at-risk (NNT 9–19).
 4. Amantadine promotes dopamine release (which facilitates cough and decreases dysphagia). It also has been shown to decrease the rate of pneumonia in elderly patients with prior stroke (NNT 4.3).
 5. Oral hygiene decreases colonization and subsequent pneumonia.
 6. Postprandial semirecumbent positions decrease the rate of aspiration pneumonia compared with supine positions.

B. Supportive treatment
 1. Suction any material in airway.
 2. Intubation if necessary for ventilation, oxygenation, or to protect airway in patients with altered level of consciousness.

C. Aspiration *pneumonitis*

1. Antibiotics

   a. Often used initially due to the high frequency of subsequent superinfection.

   b. Can be discontinued if no infiltrates develop within 48–72 hours.

   c. Pneumonia is more likely in patients with gastric colonization (resulting from a H_2-blocker, proton pump inhibitor, or from bowel obstruction).

2. Corticosteroids are controversial.

D. Aspiration *pneumonia*: antibiotics are indicated.

1. Community-acquired aspiration: First-line options include clindamycin or amoxicillin/clavulanate or amoxicillin with metronidazole.

2. Hospital-acquired aspiration:

   a. Coverage requires addition of an antibiotic that is effective against gram-negative organisms and *S aureus*.

   b. Options include carbapenem or piperacillin-tazobactam.

MAKING A DIAGNOSIS

At this point, it is appropriate to order blood cultures, sputum cultures, and Gram stain. The patient's chest radiograph does not have any features that suggest TB (see below), which makes TB less likely. Nonetheless, purified protein derivative (PPD) placement or QuantiFERON testing and obtaining sputum for acid-fast bacillus (AFB) stain and culture would be reasonable. Finally, given the diffuse symmetric infiltrate on chest radiograph and his sexual history, PCP must be considered and testing for HIV is mandatory. Although the patient's CURB-65 score is 0, his hypoxia and lack of a reliable social structure make admission mandatory. Antibiotics that cover both CAP and aspiration pneumonia should be started.

Mr. P is admitted to an isolation bed on the general medical floor. He is empirically treated with clindamycin (for presumed aspiration pneumonia), azithromycin, and ceftriaxone. The PPD test is done and is negative. Blood cultures are negative and sputum cultures reveal normal flora.

 Have you crossed a diagnostic threshold for the leading hypothesis, aspiration pneumonia? Have you ruled out the active alternatives TB and PCP? Do other tests need to be done to exclude the alternative diagnosis?

Alternative Diagnosis: PCP

Textbook Presentation

Patients with PCP may have diagnosed or *undiagnosed* advanced HIV disease. Patients commonly complain of progressive shortness of breath and dry cough of 1–3 weeks duration.

 PCP is often the *presenting* manifestation of AIDS. Suspect PCP in patients with diffuse bilateral pneumonia, particularly of subacute onset.

Disease Highlights

A. PCP is caused by the fungal organism *P jirovecii* and typically presents as a diffuse bilateral pneumonia.

B. PCP occurs most commonly in patients with HIV disease and CD4 counts < 200 cells/mcL.

C. PCP is the most common cause of acute *diffuse* lung disease in immunocompromised patients and is the leading cause of AIDS-related death in HIV-infected patients.

D. PCP may also develop in patients undergoing organ transplantation or chemotherapy and in patients with idiopathic CD4 lymphocytopenia.

Evidence-Based Diagnosis

A. History

1. Patients may *or may not* already carry diagnosis of HIV or AIDS.

2. Fever is present in 79–100% of cases.

3. Cough is present in 95% of cases. It is usually (but not always) nonproductive.

4. Progressive dyspnea is present in 95% of cases.

B. Physical exam

1. Fever is present in 84%.

2. Tachypnea is present in 62%.

3. Chest auscultation is normal in 50% of cases.

C. Chest film

1. Usually shows diffuse symmetric bilateral alveolar or interstitial infiltrates (81–93% of cases)

2. In HIV-infected patients, interstitial infiltrates are present in 69% of patients and increase the likelihood of PCP (versus TB or bacterial pneumonia) (LR+ 4.25).

3. Isolated upper lobe disease may be seen in patients taking inhaled pentamidine as PCP prophylaxis.

4. Occasionally shows pneumothorax

5. Normal in 10–25% of cases

 PCP should be considered in dyspneic patients with HIV and CD4 counts < 200 cells/mcL even when the chest exam and chest radiograph are normal.

D. Specific diagnostic tests

1. Although the chest radiograph and lactate dehydrogenase (see below) can suggest PCP or make the diagnosis less likely, patients require specific tests to confirm or exclude PCP.

2. Clinical diagnosis (without confirmational staining of sputum or bronchoalveolar lavage [BAL]) is incorrect in 43% of patients.

3. Induced sputums are typically the first test used to diagnose PCP.

   a. 55–92% sensitive, 100% specific

   b. The addition of immunofluorescent monoclonal staining increases sensitivity.

4. BAL is used to diagnose PCP when sputum stains are negative.

   a. Diagnosis is based on staining the fluid obtained during BAL.

b. Silver, Giemsa or immunofluorescent staining using monoclonal antibodies have been used.

c. Sensitivity is 86–97%.

d. Sensitivity of BAL is lower (62%) after inhaled pentamidine prophylaxis. Transbronchial biopsy improves the diagnostic yield in these patients.

5. The most common diagnostic strategy is sputum analysis with silver stain and immunofluorescence. Positive results confirm PCP. Negative results should prompt BAL.

6. Other diagnostic tools being investigated include the study of sputum, blood, and nasal pharyngeal specimens with polymerase chain reaction (PCR) and a serum measurement of 1,3-beta-D-glucan (See below).

E. Nonspecific diagnostic tests

1. 1,3-beta-D-glucan

a. A cell wall component of pneumocystis and other fungi (*Candida, Aspergillus,* but not *Cryptococcus*)

b. Sensitivity 96%, specificity 84%, LR+ 6.0, LR– 0.05

c. May prove to be a useful serum tool to rule out PCP if negative, but given the low specificity other tests would be needed to confirm PCP if positive.

d. Also can be elevated in invasive candidiasis and aspergillosis

2. High-resolution chest CT scan

a. Patchy or nodular ground-glass appearance; ground glass most marked in perihilar regions. Cystic lesions may be seen.

b. 100% sensitive, 83–89% specific

c. LR+, 5.9; LR–, 0

3. Pulmonary function tests

a. Carbon monoxide diffusing capacity of the lungs (DLCO) is usually low in PCP and highly sensitive.

b. Likelihood of PCP is < 2% if DLCO is > 75% predicted.

Treatment

A. Antimicrobial therapy

1. Trimethoprim-sulfamethoxazole (TMP-SMX) is initial treatment of choice.

2. Side effects are common including rash, fever, GI symptoms, hepatitis, neutropenia and hyperkalemia. CBC, liver function tests (LFTs), and K+ should be monitored.

3. Antibiotic therapy may markedly *worsen* preexisting hypoxia. Many patients require concomitant corticosteroids to prevent acute respiratory distress syndrome (see below).

4. Alternatives are available for patients intolerant to TMP-SMX but some allergic patients may be desensitized.

5. Occasional resistance to TMP-SMX has been reported.

6. Other options reserved for patients with mild to moderate PCP infections include clindamycin plus primaquine, dapsone plus TMP or atovaquone.

B. Corticosteroids

1. Reduce mortality and respiratory failure in patients with severe PCP treated with TMP-SMX (relative risk for mortality 0.56)

2. Initiate at time of PCP therapy if room air PaO₂ < 70 mm Hg or the A-a gradient ≥ 35 mm Hg.

3. Should be added to patients who do not initially qualify for corticosteroid treatment but deteriorate while taking TMP/SMX.

4. Prednisone 40 mg twice daily for 5 days, then 40 mg daily for 5 days, then 20 mg daily for 11 days.

 Concomitant corticosteroid therapy is lifesaving in patients with PCP whose PaO₂ < 70 mm Hg.

C. Highly active antiretroviral therapy (HAART) should also be initiated within 2 weeks of treatment for PCP in HIV-infected patients (not already receiving HAART).

D. Prophylaxis

1. Indications (any of the following)

a. Prior PCP

b. CD4 counts < 200 cells/mcL

c. HIV-infected patients with unexplained persistent fevers or oral candidiasis for more than 2 weeks

2. TMP-SMX is superior to pentamidine and the drug of choice. In addition, it is effective prophylaxis against toxoplasmosis and some bacterial infections.

3. Significant adverse reactions are common with TMP-SMX. Rash, fever, neutropenia, and hypotension may necessitate discontinuation of TMP-SMX. Consultation with an infectious disease specialist is recommended.

4. Dapsone, pentamidine, and atovaquone are alternative therapies in patients intolerant of TMP-SMX. Some authorities recommend screening patients for glucose 6-phosphate dehydrogenase (G6PD) deficiency prior to instituting dapsone.

5. HAART can restore the CD4 count and allow for discontinuation of prophylaxis when CD4 count > 200 cells/mcL for approximately 3 months (unless PCP developed in patients with CD4 counts above 200 cells/mcL).

Alternative Diagnosis: TB

Textbook Presentation

TB pneumonia usually develops due to reactivation of latent mycobacteria residing in the upper lobes. Symptoms are chronic and include cough, fever, weight loss, and night sweats. By the time patients seek medical attention, they have often had these symptoms for weeks or months. The weight loss and duration of symptoms often suggest cancer.

Disease Highlights

A. Obligate aerobe has predilection for lung apices.

B. The organism is slow growing; the generation time is 20–24 hours, resulting in slow progression.

C. Common and serious

1. Infects 33% of the world's population

2. 8.7 million new cases per year (2011 data) and 1.4 million deaths (worldwide)

3. 95% of cases occur in developing countries.

D. Epidemiology

1. 7% of US population is PPD positive.

2. Foreign-born persons have the highest rate of TB (9.7 times higher than US-born persons) and account for 85% of multidrug resistant TB (MDR-TB) in the United States.

3. Asians, blacks, and Hispanics have higher rates of TB than whites (22.9, 8.3 and 7.4 times, respectively). Foreign-born persons account for a majority of TB cases in Asians and Hispanics but not blacks.

4. 67% of cases occur in the nonwhite population.

5. In the nonwhite population, the median age is 39. In whites, the median age is 62.

6. Reactivation TB accounts for 90% of TB in older patients and 67% of TB in younger patients.

7. High risk groups

   a. HIV

     (1) HIV-infected patients are at highest risk for TB (200 times increased incidence).

     (2) In 2011, HIV-infected persons accounted for 1.1 million TB cases worldwide (13% of the total).

     (3) TB may be the first manifestation of HIV.

 Patients with active or latent TB should be tested for HIV.

     (4) Extrapulmonary TB without pulmonary disease is more common in patients with AIDS (30%) than in those without AIDS (15%).

     (5) In early HIV infection, TB is fairly typical. However, in advanced HIV infection, pulmonary TB is much more often atypical.

   b. Alcoholics

   c. Other high-risk groups

     (1) Foreign-born persons

     (2) Immunosuppressed patients (including patients taking corticosteroids)

     (3) Patients with cancer, diabetes mellitus, end-stage renal disease, transplants, or malnutrition

     (4) PPD-positive patients

     (5) Patients with evidence of prior TB on chest film

     (6) Economically disadvantaged, inner city residents

     (7) Nursing home residents

     (8) Hispanics and African Americans

     (9) Drug-dependent persons, homeless persons, prison inmates

E. Pathophysiology

   1. Inhaled organism lands in the middle and lower lobes (due to increased ventilation).

   2. Multiplies over next 3 weeks, spreads to hilar nodes and often bloodstream.

   3. Organism reproduces preferentially in areas of high PaO_2 (lung apices, renal cortex, vertebrae).

   4. In 90% of patients, the immune system then contains the organism resulting in typical scarring (Ghon complex). However, the chest film can be normal.

   5. Above sequence usually asymptomatic.

   6. In some patients a few viable organisms remain. This is referred to as **latent TB infection** (LTBI). Latent TB can reactivate later **(reactivation TB).**

   7. The PPD is positive 6–8 weeks after the initial infection. These patients are resistant to subsequent *exogenous* infection (but not reactivation).

8. Primary TB

   a. In approximately 10% of patients (higher in immunocompromised patients and children), the initial infection is not controlled and causes primary TB.

   b. Primary TB accounts for 23–34% of adult cases.

   c. Fever is the most common symptom (70%) and usually occurs in isolation.

   d. Chest radiograph usually shows consolidation (50%).

     (1) Disease is usually unifocal (75%) but may be multifocal.

     (2) Usually involves lower and middle lobes (63% of cases).

     (3) Lymphadenopathy is seen in 10–67% of adults and is rarely the sole radiologic manifestation.

     (4) Pleural effusions, usually unilateral, develop in 24% and may occur with or without infiltrates.

     (5) Normal in 15% of patients with primary pulmonary TB

     (6) Other findings include miliary pattern 6%, cavitation 15%.

   e. Often occurs in those unable to mount a sensitized macrophage response.

   f. PPD may be negative in these patients.

   g. Most cases of primary TB resolve spontaneously without treatment.

   h. Pneumonia progresses without treatment in 10–15% of patients.

9. Reactivation TB

   a. 3–5% of patients with LTBI experience reactivation due to declining immune function.

   b. Reactivation TB results in 90% of adult non–AIDS-related TB.

   c. 71% of cases occur in foreign-born patients.

   d. Symptoms are usually insidious and include chronic cough, weight loss, night sweats, anorexia, and low- or high-grade fevers.

   e. Reactivation TB progresses unless patient is treated.

10. Pleural TB takes 2 forms: tuberculous empyema and tuberculous pleural effusions.

   a. Tuberculous empyema

     (1) Secondary to direct infection of pleural space (often from rupture of neighboring tuberculous cavity)

     (2) Rare

     (3) Pleural fluid characterized by pus and numerous TB organisms

   b. Tuberculous effusions

     (1) Tuberculous effusions result from a delayed hypersensitivity reaction to mycobacterial antigens in the pleural space.

     (2) Usually due to reactivation in adults (75%)

     (3) Typical features include acute high fever, cough (94%), and pleuritic chest pain (78%).

     (4) Chest radiograph shows unilateral effusion in 95% of cases. Parenchymal infiltrate is seen in 50% of cases.

     (5) Effusion is usually exudative (see below).

     (6) PPD is usually positive (69–93%).

11. Extrapulmonary TB may involve the spine, kidney, pericardium, and central nervous system.

Evidence-Based Diagnosis

A. A variety of risk factors, symptoms, and radiographic findings can suggest TB (Table 10-5). Sensitivity is likely to be overestimated because TB was not systematically evaluated in all patients.

1. Risk factors: The most important risk factors are immigrant from TB endemic areas (LR+ 4.1), history of positive PPD test (LR+ 3.8), or history of TB (LR+ 3.6)

2. Symptoms

   a. No symptom is terribly sensitive for TB. Weight loss and cough for > 2 weeks increase the likelihood of TB more significantly than night sweats or hemoptysis.

   b. Hemoptysis was neither sensitive nor specific for TB.

   c. Fever is present in only 55%.

   d. Other clues may include lack of systemic toxicity or failure to respond to antibacterial therapy.

 Patients with TB may complain primarily of weight loss or night sweats and have a normal lung exam. Fever and hemoptysis may be absent. Pulmonary TB still needs to be considered in such patients.

   e. Symptoms and risk factors for disease tend to vary between older patients who often have reactivation TB and younger patients in whom primary TB is more common. Compared with older patients, younger patients have a higher incidence of alcoholism (66% vs 37%). In addition, younger patients more frequently have fever (62% vs 31%), night sweats (48% vs 6%), and hemoptysis (40% vs 17%).

3. Radiography

   a. A normal chest film is very unlikely in patients with pulmonary TB (97% sensitive).

   b. Cavitary disease and apical disease markedly increase the likelihood of TB (LR+ 8.3 and 4.8, respectively).

   c. Most patients with TB have one of three radiographic patterns: apical, cavitary, or reticulonodular disease (LR+, 5.0; LR−, 0.16).

 TB should be considered in patients with apical, cavitary, or reticulonodular patterns on chest radiograph. TB is unlikely if none of these features are present.

   d. Calcification can be seen in *active* lesions. Demonstrating stability requires comparison of prior films.

   e. The chest radiograph in HIV-positive patients is often atypical (see Chapter 5, AIDS/HIV).

B. Clinical decision rules:

1. A variety of clinical decision rules can help determine the likelihood of TB in patients with pneumonia and the need for isolation on admission.

2. None have ideal sensitivity and specificity.

3. High sensitivity is preferred to ensure patients with TB are isolated and reduce the risk of nosocomial transmission of TB.

4. The clinical decision rules with the highest sensitivity (96–98% sensitive, 20–48% specific) categorized patients at high risk if they had *any* of the following risk factors:

   a. Immigrants from TB prevalent areas

   b. Positive TB history or history of positive PPD

   c. Homelessness, incarceration

   d. Weight loss

   e. Chest film with apical or cavitary infiltrates

C. PPD

1. Immune response to 0.1 mL intradermal PPD

2. Turns positive 4–7 weeks after primary infection

3. Test results are determined by measuring the maximal diameter of *induration* (not redness).

4. Maximal induration occurs 48–72 hours after injection.

5. The criteria for a positive reaction depend on the clinical situation.

   a. An induration of ≥ 5 mm is considered positive in HIV-infected persons, organ-transplant recipients, patients on immunosuppressive agents (including > 15 mg per day of prednisone or TNF-alpha antagonists), those with recent contact with active TB, or persons with radiographic findings consistent with prior TB.

   b. An induration of ≥ 10 mm is considered positive in recent immigrants (< 5 years) from high prevalence areas, injection drug users, persons with clinical conditions that place them at high risk (including end-stage renal disease, malnutrition; diabetes mellitus; lymphoma; leukemia; carcinoma of the lung, head, or neck; silicosis, gastrectomy; or jejunoileal bypass), residents and employees of nursing homes, prisons, or homeless shelters.

   c. An induration of ≥ 15 mm is considered positive in any person.

Table 10-5. Clinical and radiographic findings in TB.

Finding	Sensitivity%	Specificity%	LR+	LR−
Risk Factor				
Immigrant from TB area	37	91	4.1	0.69
History of PPD (+)	19	95	3.8	0.85
History of TB	29	92	3.6	0.77
Known TB exposure	11	95	2.2	0.94
Homeless	19	88	1.6	0.92
Prison	16	89	1.5	0.94
Symptoms				
Weight loss	52	80	2.6	0.60
Cough > 2 weeks	62	73	2.3	0.52
Night sweats	40	75	1.6	0.80
Hemoptysis	16	87	1.2	0.97
Fever	55	35	0.85	1.3
Radiographic Findings				
Cavitary infiltrate	25	97	8.3	0.77
Apical infiltrate	53	89	4.8	0.53
Either cavitary, apical, or reticulonodular disease	86	83	5.0	0.16

6. *Significant* reaction suggests prior infection, not necessarily active disease. Patients with positive tests who do not have active TB are classified as having LTBI.

7. Sensitivity (for active TB) 70–80%

    a. Primary TB: PPD is often negative.

    b. Reactivation TB: PPD is positive in 80% of cases.

    c. Tuberculous pleurisy: PPD is usually positive.

    d. AIDS patients with TB: PPD is positive in 50% of cases.

 A negative PPD does *not* rule out active TB.

8. Specificity is 98–99% but is lower in patients who received bacillus Calmette-Guérin (BCG) vaccination after infancy.

    a. BCG is a TB vaccine used in some countries to prevent TB.

    b. BCG has some similarities to PPD and may cause false-positive PPD reactions.

       (1) False-positive PPD reactions (≥ 10 mm) are rare in adults who received BCG in infancy (≈1%).

       (2) However, false-positives are more common in BCG recipients who were vaccinated ≥ 2 years of age (40%). False-positive PPDs remained common in this group even more than 10 years later (20%).

       (3) Interferon gamma assays are more accurate in patients previously vaccinated with BCG (see below).

9. Indications for single PPD test

    a. Clinical suspicion of active TB

    b. Immigrants from high-incidence areas (eg, Africa, Asia, Latin America)

    c. Status post exposure to TB

    d. Fibrotic lung lesion

10. Annual PPD

    a. Useful to determine whether patient has recently converted

    b. Recent converters are at higher risk for developing active TB.

    c. Conversion defined as *increase* in induration of ≥ 10 mm

    d. Therapy is indicated for patients who have recently converted due to high risk of developing active TB.

    e. Indications for annual PPD

       (1) HIV infection

       (2) Health care workers

       (3) Correctional facility workers

       (4) Residents in long-term–care facilities

       (5) Medical conditions that carry an increased risk of active TB (see above)

       (6) Homeless persons

11. Booster phenomenon

    a. In patients with latent TB, the PPD may revert to negative many years after infection.

    b. In such patients, the *initial* PPD may be negative but stimulate immune memory cells such that *subsequent* PPD tests may be positive.

    c. Subsequent positive tests may be *misinterpreted* as recent conversion.

    d. Misinterpretation can be avoided by performing the 2-step skin tests in patients scheduled for annual PPD.

    e. Patients with initial negative PPD are retested 1 week later.

       (1) Patient in whom the second PPD test is positive should be treated as though the first test was positive.

       (2) Patients in whom the second PPD test is negative are truly negative. Any future positive reactions in these patients should be considered recent conversions.

D. Interferon gamma assays

    1. Lymphocytes from patients with LTBI or active TB produce interferon gamma when exposed to TB antigens.

    2. Blood tests have been recently developed that expose the patient's lymphocytes to *highly* specific TB antigens (not shared with BCG or most nontuberculous mycobacteria) and measure the production of interferon gamma by the patient's lymphocytes.

    3. These tests are highly specific for *active* or *latent* TB infection.

    a. Prior BCG vaccination and infection with nontuberculous mycobacteria may cause false-positive PPD reactions but do not cause false-positive reactions with interferon gamma assays. A positive interferon gamma assay is much more accurate than a positive PPD in such patients (LR+ > 10 vs 1.9, respectively).

    b. A CDC report summarized the accuracy of these tests in patients who have not previously received BCG Table 10-6.

    4. Positive results confirm either active or latent TB.

    5. Positive results do not distinguish active TB from LTBI. In patients with pneumonia, a positive result could be due to active TB or latent TB in a patient with some other form of pneumonia (ie, streptococcal).

    6. Negative tests decrease the likelihood of TB infection but are not sufficiently sensitive to rule out active TB when the clinical suspicion is high (LR–, 0.13–0.25).

    7. In addition to the higher specificity and sensitivity of these assays over PPD, they have the added advantage of not requiring a return visit by the patient to have the PPD read, and do not require the expertise of an intradermal injection or reading.

    8. The CDC has recommended that interferon assays be used in prior recipients of BCG and in patients at low likelihood of returning for a second visit to have their PPD interpreted (eg, homeless persons).

Table 10-6. Characteristics of various TB tests in patients without prior BCG vaccination.

Test	Sensitivity	Specificity	LR+	LR–
QuantiFERON-TB Gold In-Tube	81–84%	99%	83	0.18
T-SPOT.TB	90–91%	88%	7.5	0.11
PPD	89–95%	85–86%	6.3	0.09

E. Diagnosis of active TB

1. AFB stain and culture

   a. Culture is the gold standard and is specific.

   b. Sensitivity depends on the number of specimens (Table 10-7).

   c. Microscopy

      (1) Patients with positive smears are more infectious than patients who are culture positive but have negative smears; 35% of family members of persons with positive smears are PPD positive compared with 9% of family members when patients are smear negative.

      (2) Sputum or other specimens may be stained with Ziehl-Neelsen or a fluorochrome dye.

      (3) Fluorochrome dyes are more sensitive

      (4) Ziehl-Neelsen and fluorochrome dyes are nonspecific staining both TB and atypical mycobacteria.

2. Specific nucleic acid amplification tests of sputum for TB RNA or DNA are specific for TB and can help distinguish TB from other mycobacteria.

   a. Unlike culture, rapidly available within 1–2 days

   b. More specific than AFB smears and helps distinguish TB from *Mycobacterium avium* complex (MAC) or commensual organisms that are also acid-fast positive.

   c. The CDC recommends nucleic acid amplification testing for all patients being evaluated for TB.

   d. Useful when AFB stains positive

      (1) Positive rapid tests help confirm TB, negative tests make TB less likely.

      (2) 95% sensitive and specific in this situation.

   e. Also useful if suspicion of TB is high and smear is negative

      (1) Rapid tests reported to be 50–80% sensitive, 93% specific.

      (2) Positive tests suggest TB.

      (3) Cultures are still required to test for drug susceptibility.

   f. Inhibitors of nucleic acid amplification present in 3–7% of sputum samples. Tests can detect inhibitors when suspected.

3. A diagnostic algorithm that incorporates sputum smear, nucleic acid amplification and culture for the diagnosis of TB is shown in Figure 10-3.

Table 10-7. Sensitivity of test according to the number of sputum specimens sent to the laboratory.

Number of Specimens	Sensitivity		
	Culture Alone	Sputum Stain Alone	Either positive
1	79%	58%	81%
2	96%	82%	97%
3	99%	93%	99%

Reprinted, with permission, from Scott B. Early identification and isolation of inpatients at high risk for tuberculosis. Arch Intern Med. 1994;154:326–30.

4. Bronchoalveolar lavage (BAL)

   a. Bronchoscopy with BAL can be used to diagnose TB and other conditions.

   b. Useful when clinical suspicion of TB is high, sputum AFB smears are negative, and patients are unable to produce sputum

   c. The diagnostic yield of BAL can be augmented by testing BAL specimens with nucleic acid amplification and having patients submit *post* bronchoscopy sputums for AFB (which are occasionally diagnostic in patients with both negative pre-endoscopy specimens and negative BAL specimens).

5. Tuberculous pleurisy with effusion

   a. Typical pleural fluid findings

      (1) Exudative effusion

      (2) Pleural fluid glucose variable

      (3) Pleural fluid pH always < 7.4

      (4) WBC 1000–6000 cells/mcL with neutrophilic predominance early and lymphocytic predominance later

      (5) Pleural fluid eosinophils > 10% suggests alternative diagnosis (unless prior thoracentesis).

   b. Sensitivity of tests for diagnosis of tuberculous pleurisy

      (1) Pleural fluid culture, < 30%

      (2) Pleural biopsy culture, 40–80%

      (3) Pleural biopsy histology (caseating granulomas), 50–97%

      (4) Histology and pleural tissue culture > 60–95%

      (5) Sputum culture, 20–50%

   c. Adenosine deaminase: Utility unclear due to different cut points and different isoenzymes.

   d. Pleural fluid interferon gamma 89% sensitive, 97% specific

Treatment

A. Isolation: see above

B. Principles of therapy

1. Multidrug resistance TB (MDR-TB) is a significant problem.

2. Precise drug recommendations evolve due to resistance.

3. Susceptibility testing is critical to ensure an appropriate regimen is used.

4. Direct observed therapy (DOT)

   a. Premature discontinuation and nonadherence promotes drug resistance and must be avoided.

   b. DOT refers to treatment protocols where public health officials directly observe patients swallow *each* dose of medication (administered 2–3 times/week).

   c. DOT is strongly recommended.

5. Due to the public health risks of MDR-TB, the responsibility for prescribing appropriate therapy and ensuring adherence rests on the public health program and clinician.

6. Effective regimens require at least 2 drugs to which the organism is susceptible.

7. Effective therapy takes many months.

8. To determine the duration of therapy, all patients should have monthly sputum smears analyzed for AFB stain and culture until 2 consecutive sputum cultures are negative.

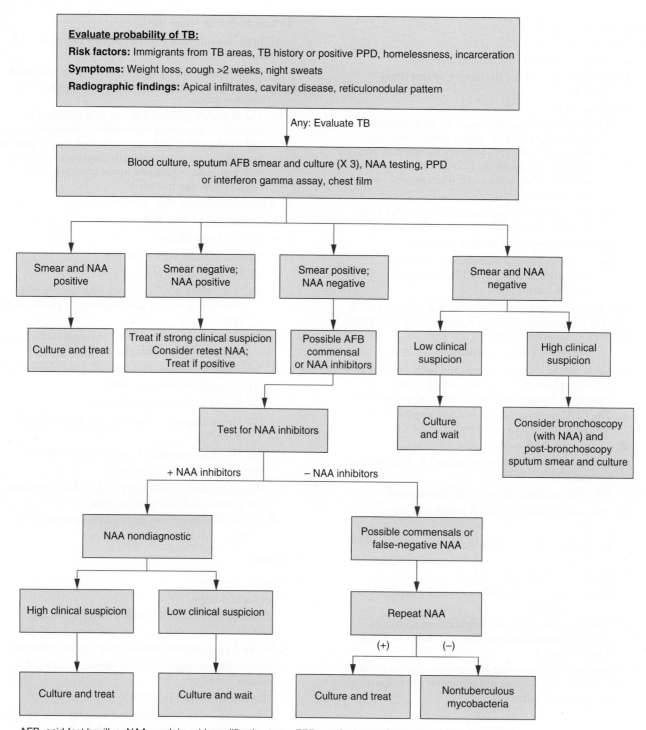

AFB, acid-fast bacillus; NAA, nucleic acid amplification tests; PPD, purified protein derivative; TB, tuberculosis.

Figure 10-3. Diagnostic approach: TB.

9. All patients should be seen monthly to assess symptoms, side effects, and adherence to therapy.

10. Infectious disease consultation is advised.

11. TB therapy in HIV-infected patients is complex due to innumerable drug interactions with HAART and the need for differing regimens depending on the degree of immunosuppression. Consultation is advised

C. Multidrug resistant TB (MDR-TB)

1. Defined as organisms that are resistant to isoniazid and rifampin

2. Accounts for 3.7% of new cases and 20% of previously treated cases worldwide.

   a. 60% of cases of MDR-TB worldwide were in India, China, and Russia.

   b. In some countries, the rate of MDR-TB among new cases is 9–32% and > 50% in those previously treated.

3. Suspect MDR-TB in patients previously treated for TB, in patients who are HIV positive, in close contacts of patients with MDR-TB, and in patients who have not responded to therapy.

4. 9% of MDR-TB cases are extensively drug resistant (XDR-TB).

5. DOT should be used for patients with MDR-TB.

6. Surgery is occasionally used for patients with localized disease and persistently positive sputums. Antituberculous therapy is continued.

7. Expert consultation is mandatory.

D. Treatment in patients at low risk for MDR-TB

1. Obtain baseline LFTs, CBC, basic metabolic panel, and uric acid. HIV testing is recommended. Tests for hepatitis B and C should be obtained in high-risk groups or patients with abnormal baseline LFTs. Ophthalmology evaluation is recommended for patients receiving ethambutol.

2. Obtain follow-up LFTs in symptomatic patients and those at high risk for isoniazid hepatotoxicity, including patients with risk factors for hepatitis (eg, alcohol consumption, pregnancy and postpartum, HIV-infection, chronic liver disease, or other hepatotoxic medication) and patients receiving pyrazinamide after the first 2 months.

3. Initiate therapy with isoniazid, rifampin, pyrazinamide, and ethambutol.

4. After 2 months, the regimen is simplified to isoniazid and rifampin, if the organism is fully susceptible, for an additional 4 months.

5. Patients with cavitary TB who have positive sputum culture at 2 months should receive isoniazid and rifampin for an additional 3 months (9 months of therapy altogether).

6. The median duration of fever after the institution of antituberculous drugs was 10 days but ranged from 1 to 109 days. For patients with tuberculous effusion, resorption can take 4 months.

E. Pleural fluid drainage does not improve outcome in patients with tuberculous effusions (nonempyema).

F. Latent TB

1. Definition of positive PPD test depends on the population.

2. The patients with the highest priority for treatment of latent TB include recent contacts of infectious TB, patients with HIV infection, and recent immigrants from areas with high prevalence of TB.

3. Prior to treatment for LTBI, active infection must be ruled out with a careful history, physical exam, and chest radiograph.

4. Expert consultation is recommended if exposure to drug-resistant TB is likely.

5. Isoniazid is most commonly used treatment option; other options exist for patients with isoniazid-resistant TB and in those intolerant of isoniazid.

6. Isoniazid

a. Dose is 300 mg/day for 9 months or 900 mg twice a week with DOT.

b. Side effects

(1) Hepatitis

(a) Reported incidence is 0.1–2.3%; may be higher in older patients.

(b) Alcohol consumption is the most important risk factor for isoniazid hepatitis. Patients who are taking isoniazid should avoid drinking alcohol.

(c) Monitor monthly for *clinical* symptoms of hepatitis.

(d) Obtain baseline and monthly LFTs in patients with risk factors for hepatitis (alcohol consumption, pregnant and postpartum patients, HIV-infected patients, patients with chronic liver disease or other hepatotoxic medications). Baseline LFTs are optional for patients without these risk factors.

(e) Obtain LFTs in symptomatic patients (right upper quadrant pain, anorexia, or nausea).

(f) Discontinue isoniazid in symptomatic patients with transaminase elevations > 3 times the upper limit of normal or in asymptomatic patients with elevations > 5 times the upper limit of normal.

(2) Peripheral neuropathy

(a) Develops in 2% of patients taking isoniazid

(b) Can be prevented with pyridoxine (25–50 mg/day); this is also advised for pregnant women and breastfeeding women taking isoniazid.

CASE RESOLUTION

Fortunately, Mr. P's HIV result was negative. His PPD and AFB smears were negative. On day 3 of his hospitalization, he became agitated, tachycardic, and complained of visual hallucinations. He was treated for delirium tremens with high doses of IV benzodiazepines. By day 5, he was improving. He was afebrile and his appetite improved. He was given a prescription for oral antibiotics and discharged to an outpatient alcohol treatment center.

 Patients with a history of alcohol abuse must be monitored for withdrawal during any hospitalization.

REVIEW OF OTHER IMPORTANT DISEASES

Influenza

Textbook Presentation

Although there is a wide range of severity of influenza symptoms, patients typically complain of a severe, febrile, respiratory illness that began abruptly. Complaints include an abrupt onset ("like being hit by a train"), severe myalgias (even their eyes hurt when they look around), diffuse pain (they may complain that their hair or skin hurts), respiratory symptoms (cough, rhinitis, pharyngitis), and fever that is often pronounced and peaks within 12 hours (occasionally as high as 40–41°C). Patients may have rigors (frankly shaking chills) and headache (Figure 10-4).

Disease Highlights

A. Pathogenesis

1. Influenza virus A or B infects respiratory epithelium.

2. Antigenic change in the virus surface glycoprotein (hemagglutinin or neuraminidase) renders populations susceptible to the virus. Antigenic shifts are most common with influenza virus A and are associated with epidemics.

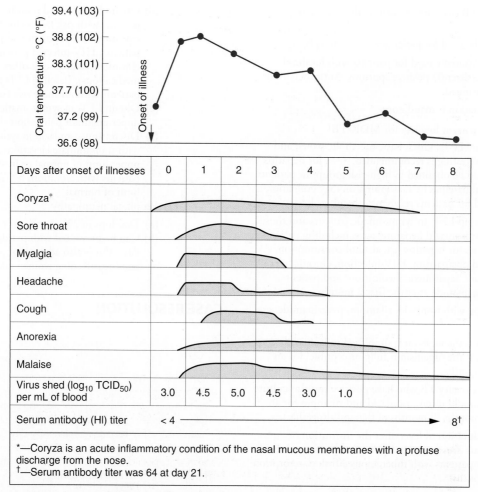

Days after onset of illnesses	0	1	2	3	4	5	6	7	8
Coryza*									
Sore throat									
Myalgia									
Headache									
Cough									
Anorexia									
Malaise									
Virus shed ($\log_{10}$ TCID$_{50}$) per mL of blood	3.0	4.5	5.0	4.5	3.0	1.0			
Serum antibody (HI) titer	< 4								8†

*—Coryza is an acute inflammatory condition of the nasal mucous membranes with a profuse discharge from the nose.
†—Serum antibody titer was 64 at day 21.

Figure 10-4. The typical clinical course of influenza. (Reproduced with permission from Montalto NJ. An office-based approach to influenza: Clinical diagnoses and laboratory testing. Am Fam Physician. 2003;67:111-8. Copyright © 2003. American Academy of Family Physicians.)

3. Adults are infectious from the day prior to the onset of symptoms until about 5 days later (10 days in children).

4. The incubation period is 1–4 days.

B. Epidemiology

1. Results in 200,000 hospitalizations per year in United States and 3000–49,000 deaths

2. Influenza typically occurs during the winter months in the Northern and Southern hemispheres (between December and May in the Northern Hemisphere).

3. Influenza occurs throughout the year in the tropics.

 Influenza is an unlikely diagnosis in the late spring, summer, or early fall.

4. Current prevalence of influenza helps determine likelihood and is updated (along with susceptibility patterns); see http://www.cdc.gov/flu/weekly/fluactivity.htm.

5. Spread is primarily airborne (inhalation of virus-containing large droplets aerosolized during coughing and sneezing).

C. Manifestations

1. History

   a. Onset is sudden in 75% of cases.

b. Fever

   (1) Present in 51% of cases

   (2) Peaks within 12–24 hours of onset of illness

   (3) Typically 38.0–40.0°C, occasionally 41.0°C

   (4) Typical duration is 3 days but may last 1–5 days

 High fever within 12–24 hours of symptom onset is typical of influenza but not other viral respiratory pathogens. Fever that increases over several days is not typical of influenza. When accompanied by cough, such a fever suggests bacterial pneumonia.

c. Prevalence of other symptoms in influenza

   (1) Headache, 58–81%

   (2) Cough, 48–94%

   (3) Sore throat, 46–70%

   (4) GI symptoms are not characteristic of influenza.

 Patients with significant diarrhea or vomiting should be evaluated for an alternative diagnosis.

d. Symptoms help distinguish influenza from acute bronchitis or pneumonia (Table 10-8).

e. Influenza may also present as a COPD or HF exacerbation (with or without fever) and severe febrile illnesses.

2. Crackles are seen in < 25% of patients.

D. Complications

1. Pneumonia

a. High-risk groups for pneumonia and death include

  (1) Elderly. Influenza mortality rates are 200 times greater in patients over age 65 than in patients aged 0–49 years.

  (2) HIV-infected patients also suffer a 100 times increase in mortality.

  (3) Other high-risk groups include patients with heart disease, lung disease, renal disease, diabetes mellitus, hemoglobinopathies, cancer, immunocompromised states, impaired handling of respiratory secretions, morbid obesity, and pregnancy (pre and postpartum) as well as Native Americans and residents of nursing homes facilities.

b. 2 types of pneumonia are seen in influenza patients: influenza pneumonia as a direct result of influenza infection and postinfluenza bacterial pneumonia.

c. Influenza pneumonia

  (1) Often develops within 1 day of onset of influenza

  (2) Most frequent in patients with underlying cardiopulmonary disease, diabetes mellitus, immunodeficiency states, and pregnancy.

  (3) Patients with influenza pneumonia complain of shortness of breath more often than patients with uncomplicated influenza (82% vs 17%).

Obtain a chest film in patients with influenza and shortness of breath to rule out pneumonia.

  (4) Associated with tachycardia, tachypnea, cyanosis, and crackles on pulmonary exam

  (5) Hypoxemia and leukocytosis may be seen

  (6) Chest film shows bilateral or lobar pulmonary infiltrates.

  (7) 29% mortality

d. Postinfluenza (secondary) bacterial pneumonia

  (1) Suspect when initial improvement is followed by relapse with worsening cough, purulent sputum, and increasing fever.

  (2) Among patients hospitalized for influenza pneumonia, 30% have concomitant bacterial pneumonia caused by *S pneumoniae, S aureus* (commonly MRSA), or group A streptococci.

  (3) Chest film may show either bilateral or lobar infiltrates.

  (4) *S pneumoniae* is most common (29–48%).

  (5) *S aureus* is next most common (7–40%), is highly destructive, and associated with significant incidence of empyema and death.

  (6) *Haemophilus* and *Moraxella* may also cause secondary pneumonia.

2. Exacerbation of asthma or COPD

3. Less common complications include HF, myositis, myocarditis, myocardial infarction, pericarditis, meningoencephalitis, Guillain-Barré syndrome

Evidence-Based Diagnosis

A. History, physical exam, and vaccination status. The summary of findings and likelihood ratios is presented in Table 10-9.

1. The negative LRs are modest, suggesting it is difficult to rule out influenza clinically. The absence of fever and cough helps decrease the likelihood of flu in patients of all ages, but less so in patients aged 60 years or older.

2. Fever and cough, particularly in older patients, increases the likelihood of influenza.

Table 10-9. Likelihood ratios for signs and symptoms in influenza.

Finding	Patients: All Ages		Patients ≥ 60 y	
	LR+	LR−	LR+	LR−
Fever	1.8	0.40	3.8	0.72
Cough	1.1	0.42	2.0	0.57
Chills	1.1	0.68	2.6	0.66
Fever and cough	1.9	0.54	5.0	0.75
Fever and cough and acute onset	2	0.54	5.4	0.77
Decision rule[1]	6.5	0.3		
Vaccine history	0.63	1.1		

[1] The negative LRs refer to the likelihood of pneumonia if both the vital signs and lung exam are normal

Table 10-8. Comparison of features in influenza, community-acquired pneumonia, and acute bronchitis.

Infection	High Fever[1]	Localized Lung Findings[2]	Shortness of Breath[3]	Season
Community acquired pneumonia	Common	Common	Variable	Anytime
Influenza	Common	Uncommon	Uncommon[4]	December–May
Acute bronchitis	Uncommon	Uncommon	Uncommon	Anytime

[1]Indication for chest film (unless flu season and patient has normal lung exam).
[2]Findings include crackles, dullness, bronchophony or egophony. All such findings indication for chest film.
[3]Indication for chest film.
[4]Unless influenza pneumonia.

3. A clinical prediction rule helps rule in influenza (fever ≥ 37.8°C with at least 2 of the following: headache, myalgia, cough, or sore throat and symptom onset within 48 hours. In addition, the rule requires at least 2 cases of confirmed influenza in the community).

B. Laboratory results

1. Confirmation is usually not required for affected outpatients but is recommended for all hospitalized patients with suspected influenza.

2. During influenza outbreaks, empiric therapy (see below) without laboratory confirmation is appropriate in patients with typical symptoms, clear lung fields, and no history of vaccination who present within 48 hours of symptom onset.

3. Testing is most appropriate in *non*influenza periods and may be particularly useful in identifying outbreaks to implement control measures.

   a. Various methods are available including reverse transcriptase PCR (RT-PCR), culture, immunofluorescence staining, and rapid influenza diagnostic tests (RIDT)

   b. RT-PCR is considered the gold standard and preferred when available. However, it is not widely available and results may be delayed.

   c. RIDT can provide results at the point of care often within 15 minutes.

   (1) Specificity

   (a) In general, the RIDTs are highly specific 98.2% (LR+ 34.5).

   (b) Positive tests help rule in influenza

   (c) Live attenuated influenza vaccine within the last 7 days can cause false-positive RIDTs.

   (2) Sensitivity

   (a) The tests are not terribly sensitive (62.3%) and cannot rule out influenza (LR– 0.38).

   (b) Test sensitivity is lower in adults than children (53.9% vs 66.6%), and lower in influenza B than influenza A (52.2% vs 64.6%)

   (c) The tests are most sensitive on days 2 and 3 compared with days 1 or 4 (≈ 75% vs 55%)

   (3) The source of the sample (throat vs nasopharyngeal swabs) does not affect sensitivity and specificity.

   (4) Antiviral therapy should not be withheld from patients with a negative RIDT result when the clinical suspicion is high (typical symptoms during influenza season).

   d. The CDC recommends testing hospitalized patients with immunofluorescence, RT-PCR or viral culture.

4. Institutionalized patients are at higher risk for respiratory syncytial virus, which can mimic influenza. Testing may be useful in such patients.

5. The IDSA recommends testing in patients in whom it will influence management, especially immunocompromised patients, immunocompetent patients at risk for severe illness, hospitalized patients with pneumonia during influenza season, elderly patients with fever of unknown origin, health care personnel, residents of or visitors to an institution.

Treatment

A. Prevention

1. The 2013 ACIP recommends annual influenza vaccination for all persons ≥ 6 months ideally by October of each year (in the Northern Hemisphere)

   a. A variety of vaccines are available, including

   (1) Inactivated influenza vaccine, which may be trivalent or quadrivalent,

   (2) Recombinant influenza vaccine, trivalent

   (3) Live attenuated intranasal influenza vaccine, quadrivalent

   b. Inactivated influenza vaccine

   (1) Uses inactivated (killed) viruses that are currently prevalent.

   (2) Updated and administered annually.

   (3) Vaccination results in 50% fewer cases of influenza, associated pneumonia, and hospitalizations.

   (4) 68% decrease in all cause mortality

   (5) Contraindications

   (a) Egg allergy: A subset of inactivated influenza vaccines can be used in patients with egg allergy (eg, Flucelvax)

   (b) Significant febrile illness at time of vaccination (Patients may be vaccinated during mild nonfebrile upper respiratory tract infections.)

   (c) History of Guillain-Barré syndrome following prior vaccination

   (6) Adverse effects

   (a) Soreness at injection site occurs in 10–64% of patients.

   (b) No increase in systemic symptoms (compared with placebo)

   (c) Guillain-Barré may increase by 1 case per million recipients.

   (d) Upper respiratory tract infection symptoms are *not* more common than placebo.

   (e) Inactivated influenza vaccine cannot *cause* influenza.

   c. Live attenuated intranasal vaccine

   (1) Uses live-attenuated strains administered intranasally that replicate poorly in the warmer lower respiratory tract.

   (2) Increases upper respiratory symptoms due to intranasal viral replication. Compared with placebo, live attenuated intranasal vaccine increases nasal congestion (45% vs 27%) and sore throat (28% vs 17%).

   (3) Persons vaccinated with live attenuated intranasal influenza vaccine can transmit the attenuated infection to other persons.

   (4) Should not be given to contacts of severely immunosuppressed individuals (ie, hematopoietic stem cell recipients).

   (5) Approved for *healthy* nonpregnant persons 2–49 years

   (6) Updated and administered annually

   (7) Should not be given to patients with significant nasal congestion that may impair delivery

   (8) Still under study in older adults

   (9) Contraindications include egg allergy, pregnancy, a prior history of Guillain-Barré syndrome, or underlying medical conditions that serve as an indication for inactivated influenza vaccination (heart or lung disease [including asthma but excluding hypertension]; immunocompromise;

renal, hepatic, or hematologic disease [including sickle cell disease]; neurologic or neuromuscular disease; pregnancy; immunosuppression; morbid obesity; and nursing home residents).

2. Chemoprophylaxis

   a. Significantly more costly than vaccination

   b. Oseltamivir and zanamivir are neuraminidase inhibitors active against influenza viruses A and B and are usually highly effective as chemoprophylaxis.

   c. Amantadine and rimantadine are not effective against influenza B (and often not against influenza A) and should not be used for chemoprophylaxis or treatment.

   d. Indications for chemoprophylaxis

      (1) Persons at high risk (or those who come in contact with such persons) who were vaccinated after exposure to influenza (continue treatment until 7 days after last exposure or 2 weeks after vaccination). Additionally, such patients should receive chemoprophylaxis if there was a poor match between the vaccine and circulating virus strain.

      (2) Persons with immune deficiencies who are unlikely to mount a response to vaccination (ie, those with advanced HIV disease) could also receive prophylaxis.

      (3) Persons with contraindications to vaccination.

      (4) Persons living in institutions during outbreaks (ie, nursing homes) regardless of vaccination status.

B. Treatment of influenza

   1. Zanamivir and oseltamivir

      a. When given within 48 hours of symptom onset, they reduce the symptom severity and the duration of symptoms approximately 1–2 days. Oseltamivir has also been demonstrated to reduce the incidence of pneumonia.

      b. A benefit may be present when started within 96 hours of symptoms in hospitalized patients.

      c. Safety during pregnancy is unknown.

      d. Studies suggest that empiric therapy is cost effective for several groups.

      e. RIDT is recommended if prevalence of influenza is low.

   2. Oseltamivir

      a. Route of administration is oral. Taking the drug with food decreases nausea and vomiting, which occurs in 10% of patients.

      b. Transient neuropsychiatric events have been recorded.

      c. Reduce the dose by 50% if creatinine clearance < 30 mL/min.

      d. Drug resistance

         (1) A strain of influenza A (H1N1) was discovered to be resistant to oseltamivir in the 2008–2009 season (99% of isolates).

         (2) The CDC has recommended combining oseltamivir with rimantadine or using zanamivir alone for this strain or if the influenza strain is unknown.

         (3) Oseltamivir alone is recommended for other strains of influenza (influenza B or influenza A, H3N2).

   3. Zanamivir

      a. Route of administration is inhalation; can cause bronchospasm. Other adverse side effects include diarrhea and nausea.

      b. Not recommended in patients with asthma or COPD.

   4. Indications for treatment in patients with suspected influenza

      a. All hospitalized patients, patients with severe influenza (pneumonia), and patients at high risk for complications including pregnant patients (see above Complications)

      b. Therapy should be started within 48 hours when possible but may still provide a benefit in severely sick patients when started within 5 days of symptom onset.

      c. In addition to antiviral therapy, patients with influenza pneumonia and postinfluenza pneumonia should receive anti-bacterial coverage that includes coverage for methicillin-resistant *S aureus* (MRSA).

      d. Consider for patients without risk factors for complications who present within 48 hours of symptom onset and wish to shorten the duration of illness.

Healthcare-Associated Pneumonia (HCAP)/ Hospital-Acquired Pneumonia (HAP) and Ventilator-Associated Pneumonia (VAP)

Textbook Presentation

Patients with HCAP present similarly to patients with CAP although they are often sicker due to a combination of greater comorbidities and an increased likelihood of colonization and infection with virulent pathogens. Those with HAP may be recovering from surgery when fever or delirium heralds the development of HAP.

Disease Highlights

A. A variety of clinical situations increase the likelihood that patients are colonized with multidrug resistant bacteria.

B. Pneumonia in such patients is often secondary to these multidrug resistant organisms and requires different antimicrobial coverage than patients with CAP.

C. Mortality in patients with HCAP is greater than for patients with CAP (19.8–24.6% vs 9.1–10%).

D. Risk factors include recent or current hospitalization, mechanical ventilation, nursing home and assisted-living residence, hemodialysis, infusion therapy or immunosuppression.

E. Classification

   1. HCAP: Pneumonia that develops in any of the following:

      a. A nonhospitalized patient within 90 days of a prior hospitalization

      b. Nursing home or long-term–care facility resident

      c. Patients receiving antibiotics or chemotherapy

      d. Patients who have received wound care within last 30 days

      e. Patients undergoing hemodialysis or home infusion

   2. HAP: Pneumonia that develops more than 48 hours after hospitalization.

   3. VAP: Pneumonia that was not present on admission and develops more than 48–72 hours after endotracheal intubation.

F. Patients with HCAP, HAP, or VAP are at markedly increased risk for infection with multidrug resistant organisms, including MRSA, gram-negative bacilli including *Pseudomonas aeruginosa* and *Acinetobacter baumanii*. They may also be infected with organisms that commonly cause CAP (*S pneumoniae* and *H influenzae*).

Evidence-Based Diagnosis

A. The diagnosis of pneumonia is typically made clinically by the presence of a new lung infiltrate and ≥ 2 of the following: fever > 38°C, leukocytosis or leukopenia, and purulent secretions.

B. The American Thoracic Society Guidelines recommend obtaining a lower respiratory tract culture in these patients. Samples may include endotracheal aspirate, or samples from bronchoscopy (BAL or protected brush specimen.)

C. Blood cultures are recommended for patients with VAP.

Treatment

A. Antimicrobial spectrum should be broadened to cover afore mentioned bacteria taking into account local resistance patterns and available culture data

B. Recent recipients of antibiotics should include antibiotics from a different class

C. Typically coverage includes antibiotics active against both MRSA and *Pseudomonas*. Infectious disease consultation is recommended.

Pertussis

Textbook Presentation

The typical adult with pertussis presents with "viral type" upper respiratory infection symptoms of nonproductive cough, rhinorrhea, sore throat, and sneezing. However, instead of resolving over 3–7 days the cough persists and is paroxysmal, often severe and occasionally even terminates in posttussive emesis. Whooping, a deep inspiration at the end of a cough, is unusual in adults.

Disease Highlights

A. The average incubation period is 7–10 days but may be 28 days or longer.

B. Half of pertussis cases occur in adolescents and adults.

C. Develops in about one-third of household contacts.

D. Typically occurs in 3 stages: catarrhal, paroxysmal, and chronic.

   1. Catarrhal stage lasts 1–2 weeks.

      a. Typical symptoms include rhinitis, lacrimation, sore throat, coughing, and sneezing.

      b. The cough is usually mild.

      c. Fever is absent or low grade.

   2. Paroxysmal phase begins in the second week with fits of 5–10 or more forceful coughs (paroxysms) in an otherwise well appearing patient.

      a. A deep inspiration may occur at the end of coughing (the "whoop").

      b. Emesis may occur at the end of coughing.

      c. Can last 2–3 months (the chronic phase).

      d. The cough may be severe and prevent sleeping.

      e. Unusual complications from coughing in adults include hernia, pneumothorax, rib fracture, and weight loss.

Evidence-Based Diagnosis

A. Among patients with cough of > 6–7 days the prevalence of pertussis is 3–20% but the likelihood increases in adult patients with acute cough > 3weeks 12–32%.

B. The median duration of cough is 42 days (27–66).

C. Clinical symptoms

   1. Absence of paroxysms or posttussive gagging makes pertussis unlikely.

      a. Paroxysmal cough: 100% sensitivity, 12% specificity, LR+ 1.1, LR– 0

      b. Posttussive gagging: 100% sensitive, 28.7% specific, LR+ 1.4, LR– 0

   2. No symptom is terribly specific or diagnostic.

      a. Whooping sensitivity 26%, specificity 85.4%, LR+ 1.8, LR– 0.9

      b. Posttussive emesis sensitivity 56%, specificity 68%, LR+ 1.7, LR– 0.65

   3. Productive cough makes pertussis unlikely (occurs in 3% of patients with pertussis)

 Pertussis is *unlikely* in patients with productive coughs.

   4. Other common causes of persistent cough include other infections, therapy with an ACE inhibitor, gastroesophageal reflux disease, asthma, and allergic cough.

   5. Testing options include culture, PCR, and serology.

      a. Culture is 30–60% sensitive, 100% specific, and takes 7–10 days.

      b. For patient with symptoms of 2–4 weeks, culture and PCR are recommended.

      c. For patients with symptoms > 4 weeks, serology is recommended (diagnosis is confirmed with a 4-fold change in titer or an IgG anti-PT level ≥ 100–125 EU/mL).

Treatment

A. Vaccination

   1. Childhood vaccination diminishes over 5–10 years and is rarely effective for more than 12 years.

   2. ACIP recommends a single Tdap vaccination for all adults.

B. Treatment

   1. Treatment usually started during the paroxysmal phase.

      a. Probably does not affect the course of illness

      b. Decreases spread to others. Without postexposure prophylaxis (see below) the secondary attack rate is > 80% among susceptible persons.

      c. Infected patients should avoid contact with young children and infants and working in healthcare facilities for at least 5 days after starting antibiotics.

   2. Azithromycin and clarithromycin are drugs of choice.

   3. Postexposure prophylaxis recommended for people in close contacts with pertussis regardless of the immunization status.

REFERENCES

Call SA, Vollenweider MA, Hornung CA, Simel DL, McKinney WP. Does this patient have influenza? JAMA. 2005;293(8):987–97.

Centers for Disease Control and Prevention. Guidance for Clinicians on the Use of Rapid Influenza Diagnostic Tests. www.cdc.gov/flu/professionals/diagnosis/clinician_guidance_ridt.htm.

Centers for Disease Control and Prevention. Updated Guidelines for Using Interferon Gamma Release Assays to Detect *Mycobacterium tuberculosis* Infection – United States, 2010. MMWR. 2010 June 25;59(5):1–25.

Chartrand C, Leeflang MMMG, Minion J et al. Accuracy of rapid influenza diagnostic tests. A meta-analysis. Ann Intern Med. 2012;156:500–11.

Cornia PB, Hersh AL, Lipsky BA, Newman TB, Gonzales R. Original article: does this coughing adolescent or adult patient have pertussis? In: Simel DL, Rennie D, eds. *The Rational Clinical Examination: Evidence-Based Clinical Diagnosis*. New York, NY: McGraw-Hill; 2012. http://www.jamaevidence.com/content/3498462.

Division of Tuberculosis Elimination, National Center for HIV/AIDS, Viral Hepatitis, STD, and TB Prevention, CDC. Updated Guidelines for the use of Nucleic Acid Amplification Tests in the Diagnosis of TB. MMWR. 2009 Jan 16;58(1):7–10.

Dosanjh DP, Hinks TS, Innes JA et al. Improved diagnostic evaluation of suspected tuberculosis. Ann Intern Med. 2008;148(5):325–36.

Kikawada M, Iwamoto T, Takasaki M. Aspiration and infection in the elderly: epidemiology, diagnosis and management. Drugs Aging. 2005;22(2):115–30.

Kunimoto D, Long R. Tuberculosis: still overlooked as a cause of community-acquired pneumonia—how not to miss it. Respir Care Clin N Am. 2005;11(1):25–34.

Mattoo S, Cherry JD. Molecular pathogenesis, epidemiology, and clinical manifestations of respiratory infections due to *Bordetella pertussis* and other *Bordetella* subspecies. Clin Micro Rev. 2005;18:326–82.

Metlay JP, Fine MJ. Testing strategies in the initial management of patients with community-acquired pneumonia. Ann Intern Med. 2003;138(2):109–18.

Metlay JP, Kapoor WN, Fine MJ. Does this patient have community-acquired pneumonia? Diagnosing pneumonia by history and physical examination. JAMA. 1997;278(17):1440–5.

Metlay JP, Schulz R, Li YH et al. Influence of age on symptoms at presentation in patients with community-acquired pneumonia. Arch Intern Med. 1997;157(13):1453–9.

Montalto NJ. An office-based approach to influenza: clinical diagnosis and laboratory testing. Am Fam Physician. 2003;67(1):111–8.

Moran GJ, Barrett TW, Mower WR et al. Decision instrument for the isolation of pneumonia patients with suspected pulmonary tuberculosis admitted through US emergency departments. Ann Emerg Med. 2009;53:625–32.

O'Brien WT Sr, Rohweder DA, Lattin GE Jr et al. Clinical indicators of radiographic findings in patients with suspected community-acquired pneumonia: who needs a chest x-ray? J Am Coll Radiol. 2006;3(9):703–6.

Onishi A, Sugiyama D, Kogata Y et al. Diagnostic accuracy of serum 1,3-β-D-glucan for *Pneumocystis jiroveci* pneumonia, invasive candidiasis, and invasive aspergillosis: systematic review and meta-analysis. J Clin Microbiol. 2012 January;50(1):7–15.

Pai M, Zwerling A, Menzies D. Systematic review: T-cell-based assays for the diagnosis of latent tuberculosis infection: an update. Ann Intern Med. 2008;149(3):177–84.

Rapid Diagnostic Testing for Influenza: Information for Health Care Professionals. (Accessed at http://www.cdc.gov/flu/professionals/diagnosis/rapidclin.htm.)

Role of Laboratory Diagnosis of Influenza. (Accessed at http://www.cdc.gov/flu/professionals/diagnosis/labrole.htm.)

Selwyn PA, Pumerantz AS, Durante A et al. Clinical predictors of *Pneumocystis carinii* pneumonia, bacterial pneumonia and tuberculosis in HIV-infected patients. AIDS. 1998;12(8):885–93.

Stein J, Louie J, Flanders S et al. Performance characteristics of clinical diagnosis, a clinical decision rule, and a rapid influenza test in the detection of influenza infection in a community sample of adults. Ann Emerg Med. 2005;46(5):412–9.

Strebel P, Nordin J. Population-based incidence of pertussis among adolescents and adults, Minnesota, 1995–1996. J Infect Dis. 2001;183:1353–9.

Tietjen PA. Clinical presentation and diagnosis of *Pneumocystis carinii (P. jiroveci)* infection in HIV-infected patients. In: UpToDate; 2008.

Woodring JH, Vandiviere HM, Fried AM et al. Update: The Radiographic Features of Pulmonary Tuberculosis. AJR. 1986;146:497–506.

I have a patient with delirium or dementia. How do I determine the cause?

CHIEF COMPLAINT

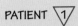

PATIENT

Mr. B is a previously healthy 70-year-old man who underwent right upper lobectomy for localized squamous cell lung cancer 5 days ago. On morning rounds, he comments that he is in a military barracks and that he is ready to go home.

What is the differential diagnosis of delirium and dementia? How would you frame the differential?

CONSTRUCTING A DIFFERENTIAL DIAGNOSIS

Delirium and dementia are both syndromes of neurologic dysfunction that present as a "change in mental status." Since the term "altered mental status" can be broad, categorizing the change as chronic or acute and then further classifying acute changes as fluctuating or nonfluctuating may be helpful (Figure 11-1). A patient whose mental status change is acute may have either fluctuating or nonfluctuating symptoms. A patient with acute, fluctuating mental status change is probably delirious. A patient with an acute but stable mental status change may have delirium but may also have a long list of other CNS insults (head trauma, CNS infection, hypoglycemia, CVA among others). Chronic mental change is caused by an irreversible change to the CNS, such as dementia, chronic psychiatric disease, or long-standing CNS injury.

Delirium and dementia are thus very different syndromes. Whereas delirium is acute, usually reversible and nearly always has an underlying, non-neurologic etiology, dementia is chronic and seldom reversible. The definition of delirium from the DSM-V is:

A. A disturbance in attention (ie, reduced ability to direct, focus, sustain, and shift attention) and awareness (reduced orientation to the environment).

B. The disturbance develops over a short period of time, represents a change from baseline attention and awareness, and tends to fluctuate in severity during the course of a day.

C. An additional disturbance in cognition (eg, memory deficit, disorientation, language, visuospatial ability, or perception).

D. The disturbances in Criteria A and C are not better explained by another preexisting, established, or evolving neurocognitive disorder and do not occur in the context of a severely reduced level of arousal, such as coma.

E. There is evidence from the history, physical exam, or laboratory findings that the disturbance is a direct physiologic consequence of another medical condition, substance intoxication or withdrawal, or exposure to a toxin, or is due to multiple etiologies.

The DSM V now defines dementia as a major neurocognitive disorder and then defines the many underlying diseases. The definition of a major cognitive disorder is:

A. Evidence of significant cognitive decline from a previous level of performance in 1 or more cognitive domains (complex attention, executive function, learning and memory, language, perceptual-motor, or social cognition) based on:

1. Concern of the individual, a knowledgeable informant, or the clinician that there has been a significant decline in cognitive function; and

2. A substantial impairment in cognitive performance, preferably documented by standardized neuropsychological testing or, in its absence, another quantified clinical assessment.

B. The cognitive deficits interfere with independence in everyday activities (ie, at a minimum, requiring assistance with complex instrumental activities of daily living [ADLs] such as paying bills or managing medications).

C. The cognitive deficits do not occur exclusively in the context of a delirium.

D. The cognitive deficits are not better explained by another mental disorder (eg, major depressive disorder, schizophrenia).

Because any illness can cause delirium in a susceptible patient, the differential diagnosis of delirium is long and needs to consider a broad range of illnesses, comorbidities, and medication effects. The differential diagnosis of dementia is more finite; disorders have been listed in order of their approximate prevalence as etiologic factors.

A. Delirium

  1. Metabolic

    a. Dehydration

    b. Electrolyte abnormalities

    c. Hyperglycemia or hypoglycemia

    d. Acidosis or alkalosis

    e. Liver disease

    f. Hypoxia or hypercarbia

    g. Uncontrolled thyroid disease

    h. Uremia

    i. Thiamine deficiency (Wernicke encephalopathy)

  2. Infectious disease

    a. CNS infection

    b. Systemic infection of any kind

  3. Cerebrovascular event

    a. Ischemic stroke

    b. Hemorrhagic stroke

    c. Vasculitis

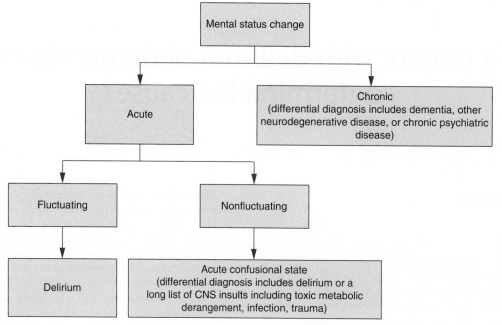

Figure 11-1. Schematic of mental status change.

4. CNS mass
   a. Tumor
   b. Subdural hematoma
5. Cardiovascular
   a. Myocardial infarction
   b. Heart failure
   c. Arrhythmia
6. Drugs
   a. Alcohol withdrawal
   b. Diuretics
   c. Anticholinergics
   d. Corticosteroids
   e. Digoxin
   f. Opioids
   g. Antidepressants
   h. Anxiolytics
7. Miscellaneous
   a. Fecal impaction
   b. Urinary retention
   c. Sensory deprivation
   d. Severe illness

B. Dementia
1. Alzheimer dementia
2. Dementia with Lewy bodies
3. Vascular dementia
4. Frontotemporal dementia
5. Alcohol-related
6. Uncommon dementias
   a. Subdural hematoma
   b. Hypothyroidism
   c. Vitamin B_{12} deficiency

d. Infectious
   (1) Syphilis
   (2) Prion disease
e. Normal-pressure hydrocephalus

 Almost any illness can cause delirium in a susceptible patient.

 Mr. B's only medical problem is mild chronic obstructive pulmonary disease. His surgery was complicated by transient hypotension and excessive blood loss. He was extubated on postoperative day 3. On postoperative day 4, his wife noted some confusion. The medical team did not detect any abnormalities when they evaluated him.

Today, postoperative day 5, he is more confused. He is oriented only to person. He is unable to answer any minimally complicated questions.

 At this point, what is the leading hypothesis, what are the active alternatives, and is there a must not miss diagnosis? Given this differential diagnosis, what tests should be ordered?

RANKING THE DIFFERENTIAL DIAGNOSIS

Based on his history, Mr. B's subacute mental status change appears to fulfill the definition of delirium. The pivotal points in this case are the waxing and waning symptoms and his disorientation and inattentiveness. His postoperative state, recent exposure to sedatives and pain medications (anesthesia), and fluid shifts are all potential causes of delirium. Although Mr. B does not have a history of

Table 11-1. Diagnostic hypotheses for Mr. B.

Diagnostic Hypotheses	Demographics, Risk Factors, Symptoms and Signs	Important Tests
Leading Hypothesis		
Delirium caused by postsurgical state, fluid and electrolyte abnormalities, hypoxia or hypercarbia, medications, or cardiac ischemia	Subacute onset and fluctuating course	Confusion Assessment Method Basic metabolic panel Pulse oximetry/ABG Urinalysis ECG/chest radiograph Review of medications
Active Alternative—Must Not Miss		
Delirium caused by alcohol withdrawal	History of alcohol use Predictable syndrome with systemic and neurologic symptoms	Clinical diagnosis
Other Alternatives		
Delirium caused by stroke, seizure, or meningitis	Focal neurologic exam Seizure activity Fever or meningismus	Rarely needed (see text) CNS imaging EEG Lumbar puncture

ABG, arterial blood gas; CNS, central nervous system; ECG, electrocardiogram; EEG, electroencephalogram.

alcohol abuse, alcohol withdrawal is always a possible diagnosis for acute mental status change in the hospital and is a "must not miss" hypothesis. Stroke and seizure, although commonly considered in the differential diagnosis of mental status change, actually are exceedingly rare causes of delirium. Table 11-1 lists the differential diagnosis.

On physical exam, Mr. B is lying in bed. He is irritable and hypervigilant. He becomes frustrated during questioning. His vital signs are temperature, 37.0°C; BP, 146/90 mm Hg; pulse, 80 bpm; RR, 18 breaths per minute. General physical exam reveals a healing surgical scar; lung, heart, and abdominal exams are normal. On neurologic exam, he scores a 3 out of 4 on the confusion assessment method (see below). The remainder of the neurologic exam is normal.

Initial laboratory data, including basic metabolic panel, liver function tests (LFTs), and urinalysis, are normal.

Is the clinical information sufficient to make a diagnosis? If not, what other information do you need?

Leading Hypothesis: Delirium

Textbook Presentation

Delirium commonly manifests as inattention and confusion. It is usually seen in older patients with severe illness. Clouding of consciousness has classically been used to describe a patient's symptoms.

Disease Highlights

A. Almost any illness can present as delirium in a susceptible patient.

B. Delirium often complicates medical or surgical hospitalizations.

C. The most important clue to delirium is the acuity of onset and fluctuation in course.

D. Delirium most commonly occurs in older persons and in patients with underlying neurologic disease.

There is always a cause of delirium. Clinicians must recognize delirium and identify the cause.

E. Several diseases are more likely to cause delirium than others.
   1. Severe illness
   2. Drug toxicity
   3. Fluid and electrolyte disturbances (hyponatremia and azotemia)
   4. Infections
   5. Hypothermia or hyperthermia

F. Delirium is very common in sick, hospitalized patients over the age of 65.
   1. 10% of emergency department patients
   2. 12–25% of medical patients
   3. 20–50% of surgical patients (highest in patients after hip replacement)

Most acutely ill, older patients, who have an acute deterioration in mental status are suffering from delirium.

G. The prognosis of delirium is poor.
   1. Although reliable data is difficult to obtain, delirium is a predictor of poor outcomes.
   2. A recent meta-analysis showed that, after controlling for age, sex, comorbid illness or illness severity, and baseline dementia, patients who experienced delirium had a higher risk of death, institutionalization, and dementia during follow-up.
      a. The mortality rate, over about 2 years, for patients in whom delirium developed was 38%.
      b. The rate of institutionalization, over about a year, was 33.4%.
      c. The rate of developing dementia over the next 4 years was 62.5%.
   3. In this same study, patients with dementia and delirium had the highest risk of death.

H. Delirium in often persistent. Many studies show that most patients in whom delirium develops have at least some persistent symptoms at discharge. These symptoms may be present for months.

Only a small percentage of patients with delirium have complete resolution of symptoms with treatment of the underlying disease and return home.

I. Delirium can occasionally "unmask" an underlying dementia. This occurs when a patient with a mild, undiagnosed dementia becomes delirious in the hospital and is then evaluated more fully for cognitive impairment.

Evidence-Based Diagnosis

A. Pretest probability

  1. Predictors of delirium have been identified. These help provide pretest probabilities.

  2. One study developed a model to determine a patient's risk of delirium developing while in the hospital. Predictors included:

    a. Vision impairment

    b. Severe illness

    c. Cognitive impairment

    d. High BUN/creatinine ratio

  3. In a patient population with a mean age of 78, the number of risk factors present correlated with the risk of developing delirium.

    a. No risk factors: 3% chance of delirium developing.

    b. 1 or 2 risk factors: 14% chance of delirium developing.

    c. 3 or 4 risk factors: 26% chance of delirium developing.

  4. Several predictors from another study, with ORs for association with delirium, are listed below:

    a. Abnormal sodium level (OR 6.2)

    b. Severe illness (OR 5.9)

    c. Chronic cognitive impairment (OR 5.3)

    d. Hypothermia or hyperthermia (OR 5.0)

    e. Moderate illness (OR 4.0)

    f. Psychoactive drug use (OR 3.9)

    g. Azotemia (OR 2.9)

Consider a patient's risk of delirium upon hospital admission; an accurate identification of risk can prompt intervention to lessen the likelihood of delirium and allow more rapid intervention if delirium does occur.

B. Diagnosis

  1. Doctors are generally not very good at recognizing delirium.

  2. A routine exam is specific but insensitive for the diagnosis of delirium.

  3. Multiple tools (such as the Confusion Assessment Method [CAM]) have been developed to diagnose delirium.

  4. The CAM is the best-validated and most widely used tools for diagnosing delirium.

  5. The CAM is considered positive when a patient fulfills both criteria a *and* b as well as either c *or* d:

    a. The mental status change is of acute onset and fluctuating course.

    b. There is inattention. The patient has difficulty focusing his attention (being easily distracted or having trouble following a conversation).

    c. There is disorganized thinking. The patient's thinking is disorganized or incoherent (such as rambling or irrelevant conversation, unclear or illogical flow of ideas, or unpredictable switching from subject to subject).

    d. There is an altered level of consciousness. This can be anything other than alert (vigilant, lethargic, stuporous).

  6. The test characteristics for the CAM are good and surpass those of an unaided physician assessment.

    a. CAM: sensitivity, 86%; specificity, 93%; LR+, 12.3; LR–, 0.15.

    b. Physician evaluation (in the emergency department): sensitivity, 17–35%; specificity, 98–100%; LR+, 8.5– ∞; LR–, 0.65–0.85.

C. Etiology

  1. Because delirium is a symptom and not a disease, once a diagnosis of delirium is made, it is necessary to identify the cause.

  2. The initial evaluation of the patient involves a review of the most common causes of delirium.

    a. Repeat a full physical exam, focusing on sources of infection.

    b. Review medications in detail, including reconciling home and hospital medications.

Medication toxicity, even at therapeutic doses, is a common cause of delirium and is particularly common in older patients. Review all medications, especially psychoactive ones.

    c. Always order basic laboratory tests, such as a CBC, basic metabolic panel, LFTs, and urinalysis.

    d. Consider other tests (based on the clinical situation) such as ECG, chest radiograph, pulse oximetry (with ABG if the patient is at risk for CO_2 retention), and blood and urine cultures.

  3. Uncommon causes

    a. A common question when evaluating a patient with delirium is: If the initial work-up is negative, is it reasonable to assume the delirium is related to the acute illness or should the patient be assessed for diseases that directly affect the CNS (eg, stroke, seizure, and meningitis or encephalitis)?

      (1) Stroke

        (a) Very rare cause of delirium

        (b) A very good study reported that only about 7% of cases of delirium are caused by stroke.

        (c) 97% of these patients had focal abnormalities on a careful neurologic exam.

      (2) Seizure

        (a) Nonconvulsive seizures, such as temporal lobe epilepsy, are usually recognized by their intermittent nature.

        (b) Nonconvulsive status epilepticus is very rare but is a potential cause of mental status change that could be confused with delirium. Patients with nonconvulsive status epilepticus almost always have risk factors for seizures or abnormal eye movements (eye jerking, hippus, repeated blinking, persistent eye deviation).

      (3) Meningitis: Fever and mental status change may be the only presenting symptoms.

b. When evaluating a delirious patient, consider neuroimaging, EEG, and lumbar puncture only in certain conditions.

   (1) **Neuroimaging** is only necessary if delirium is associated with a focal neurologic exam or if there is a very high suspicion of a cerebrovascular event.

   (2) **EEG** is only necessary if there is no other explanation for delirium **and** the patient has risk factors for, or signs of, seizures.

   (3) **Lumbar puncture** is only necessary if there is fever with no other source or a suspicion for a CNS infection.

Treatment

A. Prevention

  1. Because of its poor prognosis, delirium should be prevented when possible.

  2. Multidisciplinary interventions have been shown to prevent delirium. One study demonstrated a decrease in the rate of delirium from 15% to 9.9% (number needed to treat ≅ 20).

  3. Recently, the National Institute for Health and Clinical Excellence published a guideline for the prevention of delirium. Among the 13 recommendations were:

   a. Addressing cognitive impairment (such as stimuli to reorient patients)

   b. Paying attention to hydration status, constipation, and hypoxia

   c. Focusing on preventing, identifying, and treating infection

   d. Encouraging early mobility

   e. Addressing sensory impairments (use of glasses and hearing aids, cerumen disimpaction)

   f. Promoting good sleep patterns/sleep hygiene

B. Treatment

  1. Once delirium occurs, the causes must be addressed and then supportive measures must be instituted.

   a. Administer fluids to treat and prevent dehydration.

   b. Avoid sleep deprivation.

   c. Provide a quiet environment.

   d. Keep nighttime awakenings to a minimum.

   e. Protect from falls or self-inflicted injury.

    (1) "Sitters" are preferable to restraints as the latter can increase the risk of physical injury.

    (2) Sitters can also provide constant reorientation and reassurance.

    (3) Occasionally, medications such as low doses of neuroleptics can be used for sedation. Long-term use should be avoided whenever possible.

MAKING A DIAGNOSIS

 Review of Mr. B's medication list revealed that 0.5 mg doses of lorazepam ordered to be given as needed, were being given every 8 hours. Laboratory data was normal with the exception of an ABG: 7.36/46/80.

Have you crossed a diagnostic threshold for the leading hypothesis, delirium? Have you ruled out the active alternatives? Do other tests need to be done to exclude the alternative diagnoses?

By CAM criteria, Mr. B is delirious. He has recently undergone a major surgery, and he is taking medications known to cause delirium. Despite his intraoperative blood loss and hypotension, there are no signs of a stroke, cardiac ischemia, heart failure, or anemia.

Alternative Diagnosis: Alcohol Withdrawal

Textbook Presentation

A typical presentation of alcohol withdrawal in the inpatient setting is agitation, hypertension, and tachycardia occurring during the first 2 days after hospital admission. Seizures may soon follow with delusions and delirium occurring during the first 3–5 days.

Disease Highlights

A. Symptoms of alcohol withdrawal are stereotypical, occurring on a predictable time line as outlined in Figure 11-2.

B. The predominant symptoms of minor withdrawal are irritability, hypertension, and tachycardia.

C. Alcoholic hallucinosis

  1. Syndrome of hallucinations (usually visual)

  2. Patients with alcoholic hallucinosis usually have a clear sensorium (ie, they would perform well on CAM). This fact usually makes alcoholic hallucinosis easily distinguishable from delirium.

D. Major withdrawal is synonymous with delirium tremens.

  1. Occurs in patients with history of severe alcohol abuse.

  2. Confusion, disorientation, and autonomic hyperactivity are hallmarks.

  3. Delirium tremens can be fatal if not appropriately treated.

E. Wernicke encephalopathy

  1. Wernicke encephalopathy is not an alcohol withdrawal syndrome but is caused by thiamine deficiency.

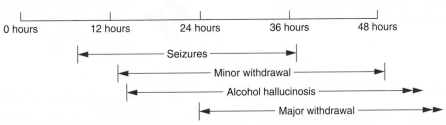

Figure 11-2. Symptoms of alcohol withdrawal (Virtual Naval Hospital. A Digital Library of Naval Medicine and Military Medicine. http://www.vnh.org/).

2. Alcohol abuse is the most common cause of thiamine deficiency.

3. Wernicke encephalopathy may occur when a patient, who is thiamine deficient, receives intravenous glucose.

4. Symptoms include the triad of confusion, disorders of ocular movement, and ataxia. The confusion commonly manifests as disorientation and indifference.

5. Korsakoff syndrome is the chronic form of Wernicke encephalopathy. Korsakoff syndrome presents with memory problems and resulting confabulation.

Evidence-Based Diagnosis

A. Delirium tremens and Wernicke encephalopathy are the alcohol-related syndromes most likely to be confused with nonalcohol-related delirium. Various features clearly differentiate these syndromes.

B. Wernicke encephalopathy
1. Generally requires long-term alcohol abuse. (Rare cases of Wernicke encephalopathy with hyperemesis gravidarum or after bariatric surgery do occur).

2. It is important to recognize that Wernicke encephalopathy usually presents with only 1 or 2 of the features of the classic triad.

3. Fluctuation that characterizes nonalcohol-related delirium is absent.

4. The diagnosis of Wernicke encephalopathy can be made if 2 of the following 4 signs are present:
   a. Dietary deficiencies (as evidenced by underweight, thiamine deficiency, or abnormal dietary history)
   b. Disorders of ocular movement (such as ophthalmoplegia, nystagmus or gaze palsy)
   c. Cerebellar signs
   d. Altered mental state or memory impairment

5. Wernicke encephalopathy is a difficult diagnosis to make in the setting of hepatic encephalopathy.

6. There are specific MRI findings that are seen in Wernicke encephalopathy.

C. Delirium tremens
1. Always preceded by minor withdrawal.
2. Minor withdrawal can be overlooked in the hospital if a patient is critically ill, sedated, or anesthetized.
3. History of heavy alcohol use required.
4. Adrenergic overactivity (hypertension, tachycardia, fever) is always present unless masked by medications.

 Every patient should have an alcohol history taken on admission. If a clinical syndrome suggestive of alcohol withdrawal occurs in a patient who denied alcohol use, information about alcohol use should be sought from other sources.

Treatment

A. Both Wernicke encephalopathy and delirium tremens are preventable.

B. Wernicke encephalopathy
1. Any patient in whom thiamine deficiency is suspected should receive 100 mg of IV thiamine prior to receiving glucose-containing fluids.

2. Patients in whom Wernicke encephalopathy is suspected should receive thiamine until symptoms resolve.

C. Alcohol withdrawal and delirium tremens
1. Supportive care
2. Benzodiazepines
   a. Benzodiazepines decrease the symptoms of withdrawal and can prevent delirium tremens, seizures, and death.
   b. Some patients can be treated for alcohol withdrawal with benzodiazepines as outpatients.
   c. Indications for inpatient therapy
      (1) Moderate to severe withdrawal
      (2) Prior history of seizures or delirium tremens
      (3) Patient unable to cooperate with outpatient therapy
      (4) Comorbid psychiatric or medical conditions
      (5) Unsuccessful outpatient detoxification
   d. Inpatient management
      (1) The optimal dose of benzodiazepines cannot be determined in advance and must be titrated to the particular needs of the patient.
      (2) Benzodiazepines may either be given on a fixed-scheduled or be given to treat symptoms. Both strategies require careful patient monitoring and medication adjustment.
      (3) The Addiction Research Foundation Clinical Institute Withdrawal Assessment for Alcohol (CIWA-Ar) developed a tool to predict the level of alcohol withdrawal.
         (a) The tool scores the severity of symptoms in various categories such as tremor, anxiety, and sensory disturbances.
         (b) A higher score (> 8–12) generally calls for active pharmacologic management, whether using a fixed-dose or symptom-triggered protocol.
         (c) Printable versions of the tool are available online.
      (4) Fixed-schedule therapy
         (a) Delivers regular fixed doses of benzodiazepines.
         (b) Careful monitoring is still required to avoid undertreatment or oversedation.
         (c) Fixed-schedule therapy may provide a slight margin of safety if careful monitoring cannot be performed adequately.
      (5) Symptom-triggered therapy
         (a) Avoids unnecessary medications in the group of patients who will not need them.
         (b) Careful monitoring is required to avoid withdrawal and delirium tremens.

 Careful monitoring and prompt patient-specific adjustment of benzodiazepine dose is the key to successful management of the alcoholic patient.

3. Beta-blockers
   a. Can decrease sympathetic overactivity in patients during withdrawal
   b. Are useful adjuncts but, because they can mask sympathetic signs that alert the clinician to increasingly severe withdrawal, they increase the risk of inadequate use of benzodiazepines.

CASE RESOLUTION

On the afternoon of the fifth postoperative day, Mr. B pulled out his IV and attempted to climb out of bed while his chest tube was still attached. Around the clock observation was ordered.

Further history revealed no history of alcohol use. Mr. B was placed on oxygen with near normalization of his blood gas. The benzodiazepines were discontinued.

(continued)

By postoperative day 8 (3 days after the onset of his delirium) Mr. B's mental status had returned nearly to baseline. He was still occasionally disoriented to time.

He was discharged on postoperative day 14. His wife noted him to still be occasionally "spacey" at the time of discharge. The patient was completely back to normal at a postoperative visit 14 days later.

The patient's delirium was severe for 3–4 days and persisted for at least 1 week. The delirium was assumed to be a symptom of the postsurgical state, and medication complication. No specific therapy was given. The patient's safety was ensured with a "sitter" and the reversible factors were addressed.

CHIEF COMPLAINT

PATIENT 2

Mr. R is a 70-year-old man who comes to see you in clinic accompanied by his wife because she is concerned that his memory is getting worse. She states that for the last few months he has been getting lost driving 20 miles from his home to his local VA hospital, where he volunteers. He has done this job twice a week for 25 years.

At this point, what is the leading hypothesis, what are the active alternatives, and is there a must not miss diagnosis? Given this differential diagnosis, what tests should be ordered?

RANKING THE DIFFERENTIAL DIAGNOSIS

Mr. R has had a decline in cognitive status. He has lost to the ability to do a higher-level task. Given the patient's advanced age, dementia—most commonly Alzheimer disease (AD)—has to be included in the differential diagnosis of his cognitive decline. The subacute onset of this patient's symptoms makes AD the leading hypothesis. Another common cause of dementia in older persons is vascular dementia (VaD). It will be important to determine whether this patient has risk factors for cerebrovascular disease. In an older person, clinicians also have to consider the normal cognitive decline that comes with aging. This, however, never causes functional compromise. An alternative diagnosis is mild cognitive impairment (MCI), a syndrome of memory loss more severe than normal, age-related cognitive decline. MCI also does not cause functional impairment. Delirium and depression should always be considered in an older patient with cognitive decline because they are highly treatable. Table 11-2 lists the differential diagnosis.

A patient who is unable to successfully live independently because of cognitive issues always has an abnormality.

PATIENT 2

Mr. R's past medical history is notable for chronic leg pain resulting from an injury during the war in Vietnam. He also has gout. Mr. R is a retired accountant. He completed 4 years of college. His physical exam reveals an alert, pleasant man.

(continued)

Table 11-2. Diagnostic hypotheses for Mr. R.

Diagnostic Hypotheses	Demographics, Risk Factors, Symptoms and Signs	Important Tests
Leading Hypothesis		
Dementia, most commonly Alzheimer type	Memory loss with impairments in instrumental activities of daily living	MMSE Neuropsychiatric testing
Active Alternative		
Vascular dementia	Risk factors for vascular disease	Evidence of vascular disease Positive ischemia score
Active Alternative—Must Not Miss		
Delirium	Altered level of consciousness with variation during the day	Confusion Assessment Method
Depression	May present as patient-reported memory loss	Fulfillment of DSM-V criteria

MMSE, Mini-Mental Status Exam.

His medications are

1. Paroxetine, 20 mg daily
2. Methadone, 20 mg 3 times daily
3. Meloxicam, 7.5 mg daily
4. Acetaminophen with codeine (300/60), 2 tablets 3 times daily
5. Allopurinol, 300 mg daily

On examination, his vital signs are normal. He answers about half the history questions himself but turns to his wife for assistance with details about doctors he has seen and the medications he takes. He and his wife deny any symptoms of depression, although they note this has been a problem in the past. He has taken paroxetine for years.

His physical exam is normal except for evidence of bilateral knee osteoarthritis. Except for his mental status, his initial neurologic exam, including motor, sensory, and reflex examination, is normal.

Is the clinical information sufficient to make a diagnosis? If not, what other information do you need?

Leading Hypothesis: AD

Textbook Presentation

Typically, a family member brings in an older patient because of confusion, memory loss, or personality change. The patient may deny that a problem exists. Detection of dementia during casual conversation may be difficult early in its course; more formal assessment is frequently necessary.

Disease Highlights

A. AD most commonly occurs after the age of 65, although earlier presentations are possible.

B. Language disturbances
   1. In addition to memory loss, behavioral or personality change, functional impairments, or social withdrawal, language disturbances are often present early in the course of disease and often become severe with time.
   2. These may include fluent aphasia, paraphasias, and word substitutions.

C. Later in the course of the disease, global cognitive impairment develops and patients become unable to independently accomplish the most basic ADLs.

Although present, memory loss may not be the presenting symptom in patients with AD; rather, behavioral or personality changes, functional impairments, social withdrawal, or language disturbances may be the initial symptoms.

D. AD accounts for about 67% of cases of dementia.

E. Strictly speaking, the diagnosis of AD can only be made pathologically. That said, the diagnosis of AD is always made clinically.

F. All definitions of AD include the deterioration in a person's ability to function independently. A patient's level of functioning can be evaluated by assessing his ability to do the instrumental ADLs.
   1. Instrumental ADLs include
      a. Cooking
      b. House cleaning
      c. Laundry
      d. Management of medications
      e. Management of the telephone
      f. Management of personal accounts
      g. Shopping
      h. Use of transportation
   2. Late in the disease, a patient's ability to perform the ADLs often becomes compromised. These ADLs are
      a. Bathing
      b. Eating
      c. Walking

d. Toileting and continence
e. Dressing
f. Grooming

G. The prognosis of AD is poor.
   1. Estimates of median survival have traditionally ranged from 5 to 9 years with more recent data suggesting median survival close to 3 years with a range of 2.7 to 4 years.
   2. Patients with advanced dementia do especially poorly. In 1 cohort of patients with advanced dementia who were monitored for 18 months, 54.8% died, 41.1% developed pneumonia and 85.8% developed an eating problem.
   3. Patients with AD also have a much worse prognosis after an acute illness. In the same cohort, the 6-month mortality rate for patients who had pneumonia was 46.7%.

Evidence-Based Diagnosis

A. Diagnosing AD can be challenging because patients often have subtle symptoms early in the disease course.
   1. AD presents with self-reported memory loss in only a minority of patients.
      a. Memory loss reported by a spouse, relative, or close friend is more predictive of dementia.
      b. Memory loss reported by a patient is more predictive of depression.
   2. Behavioral changes and mood changes are commonly recognized by family members.
   3. Clinicians may recognize behavioral changes, such as increased anxiety, increased somatic complaints, or delusional thinking regarding illness, as early symptoms of the disease.

Be aware that AD should be on the differential diagnosis of subtle behavioral changes in older patients.

B. The most efficient way to diagnose AD is to follow these 3 steps:
   1. Consider the probability that a patient has dementia.
   2. Diagnose dementia.
   3. Diagnose AD by ruling out other causes of dementia and ensuring that the patient's symptoms are consistent with AD.

C. Diagnosing dementia
   1. The prevalence of dementia in the older population is very high. The prevalence at different ages is given in Table 11-3.
   2. Screening tests
      a. Multiple tests are used to screen patients for dementia. Those most commonly used are the Mini-Mental Status Exam (MMSE), the Modified Mini-Mental

Table 11-3. Prevalence of dementia by age.

Age	Prevalence	
	Outpatient	Inpatient
65–75	2.1%	6.4%
>75	11.7%	13%
>85	—	31.2%

Status Exam (3MSE), the Mini-Cog, and the Memory Impairment Screen (MIS).

(1) 3MSE

(a) An expanded version of the MMSE

(b) It is scored out of 100 and takes 15–20 minutes to administer.

(2) Mini-Cog

(a) 3-item recall and clock drawing (which serves as the interference task)

(b) It is scored out of 5 (1 point for each item and 2 points for a normal clock) and takes about 3 minutes to administer.

(3) MIS

(a) 4-word recall after an interference task (counting by 3s).

(b) It is scored out of 8 (2 points for words spontaneously recalled and 1 point for words recalled with a clue) and takes about 4 minutes to administer.

b. A study showed these 3 tests have similar performance, with the Mini-Cog being almost as accurate as the more time-consuming 3MSE. The MIS was the most specific. Test characteristics are shown in Table 11-4.

3. Neuropsychiatric testing

a. Considered the clinical gold standard for diagnosing dementia

b. Neuropsychiatric testing can be very helpful when the diagnosis of dementia is especially difficult. Situations in which neuropsychiatric testing is commonly used are

(1) When there is disagreement between the clinical suspicion and in-office tests.

(2) To specifically gauge deficits in order to recommend ways of compensating.

(3) When present or suspected psychiatric disease (usually depression) complicates the diagnosis.

(4) When a more definitive diagnosis would be helpful for the patient or family members.

 Neuropsychiatric testing is especially useful when in office testing is negative despite a high clinical suspicion of dementia.

D. The diagnosis of AD is clinical, based on the diagnosis of dementia and the presence of features consistent with AD.

1. Various office-based tests are useful in making this diagnosis. The National Institute of Neurological and Communicative Disorders and Stroke and the Alzheimer's Disease and Related Disorders Association (NINCDS-ADRDA) criteria for probable AD are currently the most commonly used by specialists.

Table 11-4. Test characteristics for the MMSE, some of its components, and other tests in the diagnosis of dementia.

Test	Sensitivity	Specificity	LR+	LR−
3MSE (< 83)	86%	79%	4.06	0.18
Mini-Cog (< 3)	76%	73%	2.8	0.33
MIS (<5)	43%	93%	5.9	0.62

3MSE, Modified Mini-Mental Status Exam; MIS, Memory Impairment Screen; MMSE, Mini-Mental Status Exam.

2. Criteria for the clinical diagnosis of probable AD include all of the following:

a. Dementia

b. Deficits in 2 or more areas of cognition

(1) Orientation

(2) Registration

(3) Visuospatial and executive functioning

(4) Language

(5) Attention and working memory

(6) Memory

c. Progressive worsening of memory and other cognitive functions

d. No disturbance of consciousness

e. Onset between ages 40 and 90, most often after age 65

f. Absence of other disorders that could account for the symptoms

3. The test characteristics for these criteria are:

a. Sensitivity, 83%; specificity, 84%

b. LR+, 5.19; LR−, 0.2

4. The NINCDS-ADRDA also gives factors that support the diagnosis. These are very helpful clinically, although none are necessary to make the diagnosis. Some of these are included below:

a. Progressive deterioration of specific cognitive functions

(1) Aphasia

(2) Apraxia

(3) Agnosia

b. Impaired ADLs and altered patterns of behavior

c. Family history of dementia

d. Normal lumbar puncture, normal or nonspecific EEG findings, and cerebral atrophy on neuroimaging

5. Because these criteria are not perfect in the diagnosis of AD, patients in whom dementia or AD is suspected but who do not meet the criteria should be monitored closely or referred for more detailed neuropsychiatric testing.

E. Reversible dementias

1. An important issue when diagnosing AD is how much more of a work-up should be done? The concern is that when making a clinical diagnosis, potentially reversible dementias might be missed. These reversible dementias include:

a. CNS infections

b. Hypothyroidism

c. B_{12} deficiency

d. CNS masses

(1) Neoplasms

(2) Subdural hematomas

e. Normal-pressure hydrocephalus

f. Medications

2. Current practice is to order the following tests:

a. CBC

b. TSH

c. Basic metabolic panel and LFTs

d. Vitamin B_{12} level

e. Rapid plasma reagin

f. Consider neuroimaging (MRI or CT)

　(1) Imaging is not required in most patients with dementia.

　(2) In practice, most patients will undergo imaging both to assess for diagnoses other than AD and to detect brain atrophy that may support the diagnosis of AD.

Treatment

A. Counseling

1. When the diagnosis of AD is made, patients and families should be educated on course, complications, and prognosis of the disease.

2. Decisions need to be made regarding health care proxies, financial and estate planning, and end-of-life care.

3. It is crucial to make these decisions while the patient is still a competent decision maker. Referral to support services, such as the Alzheimer's Association, may be helpful.

B. Safety

1. As the disease progresses, patient safety often becomes an issue.

2. Driving, wandering, and cooking are often early concerns.

a. Driving is usually the most difficult to address because patients lack insight into the dangers they pose and resist the loss of independence that not driving brings.

b. Physicians should raise this issue since it is often difficult for caregivers to bring up.

c. Patients with even mild dementia should either be told to not drive or be required to undergo frequent performance evaluations.

d. Home safety checklists are available online that can help family members protect patients with dementia.

C. Behavioral

1. Caregivers should be told to expect behavioral and personality changes, and be instructed on how to respond.

2. Maintenance of routines is important.

3. Situations likely to be stressful to patients, such as those in which a patient's deficits interfere with his functioning, should be avoided.

D. Pharmacotherapy

1. Cholinesterase inhibitors

a. 4 cholinesterase inhibitors are approved for treatment

　(1) Donepezil

　(2) Tacrine

　(3) Rivastigmine

　(4) Galantamine

b. These medications have been shown to have modest effects on objective measures of dementia and functional status.

2. Memantine is an NMDA receptor antagonist also approved for the treatment of AD. It has similar efficacy to the drugs above and may be used in combination with cholinesterase inhibitors.

3. Associated neuropsychiatric symptoms

a. May include agitation (60–70%) or either delusions or hallucinations (30–60%)

b. Atypical neuroleptics, such as olanzapine and risperidone, are frequently used but the evidence base for their efficacy is poor and they have been associated with higher mortality. Neither of these drugs is approved for this indication.

4. Depression

a. Very common in patients with AD

b. Present in up to 50% of patients

c. All patients with AD should be screened for depression and treated if it is found.

5. Caregiver care

a. Taking care of a friend or relative with AD can be extremely challenging.

b. Caregivers should be counseled on the importance of taking time off and the availability of respite care.

c. They should be counseled that behavioral difficulties are a result of the disease and not the patient's anger or heartlessness.

d. Caregiver support groups can be extremely helpful.

MAKING A DIAGNOSIS

Mr. R's exam thus far reveals some difficulty with recalling recent events. Given his age, his baseline risk of dementia is at least 10%. The first step in his work-up would be to perform 1 of the screening tests for dementia. If this is positive, consider whether he fulfills the NINCDS-ADRDA criteria for probable AD.

Further history revealed that the patient's wife had taken over bookkeeping because a few bills had gone unpaid during the last 3 months.

The patient was given the Mini-Cog and scored a 2 out of 5. Consideration of the NINCDS-ADRDA criteria showed him to have dementia with deficits in 2 or more areas of cognition (orientation, visuospatial and executive functioning, attention and working memory, and memory). At the time of the visit, it was not clear whether his cognitive functioning was worsening, and there were no disturbances in consciousness.

The plan was made for initial laboratory work to be done and for a 3-month follow-up visit. Given that he was taking multiple psychoactive medications, his regimen was scaled back to the minimum doses necessary to control his pain.

Have you crossed a diagnostic threshold for the leading hypothesis, AD? Have you ruled out the active alternatives? Do other tests need to be done to exclude the alternative diagnoses?

Alternative Diagnosis: Multi-infarct Dementia (Vascular Dementia, VaD)

Textbook Presentation

A patient with VaD may have dementia that has an abrupt onset or is slowly worsening. The patient usually has risk factors for vascular disease or has previously diagnosed vascular disease. The patient often has difficulty walking during the neurologic exam.

Disease Highlights

A. Generally considered to be the most common cause of dementia after AD.

B. Most common in patients with risk factors for vascular disease or embolic stroke.

C. Patients have dementia and evidence that cerebrovascular disease has caused the dementia.

  1. A classic, but insensitive, clue is a "step-like deterioration" related to intermittent cerebrovascular accidents.

  2. Other clues are a focal neurologic exam or evidence of strokes, white matter changes, or atrophy on neuroimaging.

D. Symptoms of VaD include gait disturbance, urinary symptoms, and personality changes.

Evidence-Based Diagnosis

A. The DSM-V criteria for the clinical diagnosis of VaD are:

  1. The criteria are met for major or mild neurocognitive disorder.

  2. The clinical features are consistent with a vascular etiology, as suggested by either of the following:

    a. Onset of the cognitive deficits is temporally related to 1 or more cerebrovascular events.

    b. Evidence for decline is prominent in complex attention (including processing speed) and frontal-executive function.

  3. There is evidence of the presence of cerebrovascular disease from history, physical exam, and/or neuroimaging considered sufficient to account for the neurocognitive deficits.

  4. The symptoms are not better explained by another brain disease or systemic disorder.

B. Features consistent with the diagnosis of VaD are

  1. Exaggeration of deep tendon reflexes

  2. Extensor plantar response

  3. Gait abnormalities (consider history of unsteadiness and frequent, unprovoked falls)

  4. Pseudobulbar palsy (pathologic laughing, crying, grimacing; and weakness of the muscles associated with cranial nerves V, VII, IX, X, XI, and XII)

  5. Focal neurologic signs

C. The actual diagnosis of VaD is complicated by the presence of multiple different criteria.

D. The Hachinski Ischemic Score seems to be a clinically useful test for determining whether ischemic disease is playing a role in a patient's dementia.

  1. In the score, 2 points are given for each of the following features:

    a. Abrupt onset

    b. Fluctuating course

    c. History of stroke

    d. Focal neurologic signs and symptoms

  2. 1 point is given for each of the following features:

    a. Stepwise deterioration

    b. Nocturnal confusion

    c. Preservation of personality

    d. Depression

    e. Somatic complaints

    f. Emotional lability

    g. Hypertension

    h. Atherosclerosis

  3. A score of greater than 7 carries a LR+ of 8.3 for differentiating VaD from AD. The score performs less well for differentiating AD or VaD from a mixed dementia.

Treatment

A. Behavioral, pharmacologic, and surgical means of modifying risk factors for cerebrovascular disease and preventing recurrent vascular events should be used.

B. Behavioral interventions include smoking cessation and dietary intervention to decrease vascular risk.

C. Pharmacologic interventions include treatment of hypertension and diabetes mellitus, treatment of hypercholesterolemia (to an LDL < 100 mg/dL), aspirin therapy, and anticoagulation when indicated.

D. Surgical therapy includes carotid endarterectomy when indicated.

CASE RESOLUTION

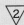

Initial laboratory evaluation, including CBC, TSH, basic metabolic panel and LFTs, vitamin B_{12} level, and rapid plasma reagin, was normal. He was able to wean his medications and felt like he had a little more energy. On a follow-up visit 3 months later, the patient's wife reported that he was no longer driving to his job as it had become too difficult. On physical exam, his language skills had worsened, and he frequently answered questions with short affirmative phrases and nods that were often contradicted by his wife. (He would subsequently agree with her.) A CT scan with contrast was ordered and showed only cerebral atrophy.

AD can be confidently diagnosed in this patient. He has no risk factors for VaD. His ischemia score is 1. Dementia was diagnosed at his previous visit; since his symptoms have progressed, he now fulfills the criteria for AD. Reversible causes of dementia are unlikely given the normal evaluation. The patient's functional limitations exclude MCI as a cause. The patient has no symptoms of delirium or depression.

REVIEW OF OTHER IMPORTANT DISEASES

Mild Cognitive Impairment (MCI)

Textbook Presentation

Usually presents in an older patient complaining of memory loss. Common complaints are difficulty remembering names and appointments or solving complex problems. Detailed testing shows abnormal memory, but patients have no functional impairment.

Disease Highlights

A. MCI is a diagnosis that stands between the normal, age-related decline in cognition and dementia.

B. The diagnosis can be difficult to make as memory complaints, and concern about dementia, are very common in older people.

C. 4 types of MCI are:

  1. Single domain amnestic MCI in which people have memory loss and no other deficits.

  2. Multiple domain amnestic MCI in which people have memory loss as well as other deficits.

  3. Single domain non-amnestic MCI in which people have impairment in a single, non–memory-related, cognitive domain.

4. Multiple domain non-amnestic MCI in which people have impairment in multiple, non–memory-related, cognitive domain.

D. Patients with this disorder are not neurologically normal.

1. For patients with amnestic types of MCI, their memory is worse than age-matched controls.

2. Patients with MCI have a higher rate of progression to dementia than age- matched controls.

Evidence-Based Diagnosis

The diagnosis of this disease is generally made by neuropsychiatric testing. Evaluation for reversible causes, as in patients with dementia, is appropriate.

Treatment

Presently, there is no proven treatment for MCI. Patients should be monitored closely for development of more severe cognitive or functional decline.

Dementia with Lewy Bodies (DLB)

Textbook Presentation

DLB is typically seen in a patient with Parkinson disease who has dementia. The predominant symptoms of the dementia are a fluctuating course and the presence of hallucinations. In patients without a previous diagnosis of Parkinson disease, motor symptoms similar to those seen in Parkinson disease are often present.

Disease Highlights

A. DLB is among the most common types of dementia after AD.

1. Lewy bodies are seen in the cortex of about 20% of patients with dementia.

2. Lewy bodies may be present in some patients with a clinical diagnosis of AD thus DLB may coexist with AD.

B. The most important features of DLB are included in the Evidence-Based Diagnosis section below.

C. Patients with DLB may have a fluctuating course.

1. Early in the disease patients may seem nearly normal at times and demented at other times.

2. Because of the fluctuation in symptoms, delirium needs to be included in the differential diagnosis.

D. Visual hallucinations are common in DLB, unlike in most other types of dementia.

E. Mild extrapyramidal motor symptoms (rigidity and bradykinesis) are often seen. These may occur late in the course of other dementias but occur early with DLB and worsen over time.

Evidence-Based Diagnosis

The diagnostic criteria for DLB are presented below.

A. There is dementia that might be mild at the onset of disease.

B. 2 of the following are essential for a diagnosis of probable DLB:

1. Fluctuating cognition with pronounced variations in attention and alertness

2. Recurrent visual hallucinations that are typically well formed and detailed

3. Spontaneous motor features of parkinsonism

C. The following features are supportive of the diagnosis of DLB:

1. Repeated falls

2. Syncope

3. Transient loss of consciousness

4. Neuroleptic sensitivity

5. Systematized delusions and hallucinations

Treatment

A. Supportive treatment of patients with DLB is the same as for patients with AD.

B. Cholinesterase inhibitors have also been shown to be effective.

C. Neuroleptics can be dangerous, potentially worsening symptoms.

 Patients with dementia with parkinsonian features, a fluctuating course, and visual hallucinations should be evaluated for DLB before they are treated with neuroleptics.

REFERENCES

Benbadis SR, Sila CA, Cristea RL. Mental status changes and stroke. J Gen Intern Med. 1994;9:485–7.

Black ER. Diagnostic strategies for common medical problems. Philadelphia: American College of Physicians; 1999:674.

Caine D, Halliday GM. Operational criteria for the classification of chronic alcoholics: identification of Wernicke's encephalopathy. J Neurol Neurosurg Psychiatry. 1997;62:51–60.

ElieM, Rousseau F, Cole M, Primeau F, McCusker J, Bellavance F. Prevalence and detection of delirium in elderly emergency department patients. CMAJ. 2000;163:977–81.

Francis J, Martin D, Kapoor WN. A prospective study of delirium in hospitalized elderly. JAMA. 1990;263:1097–101.

Holsinger T, Plassman BL et al. Screening for cognitive impairment: comparing the performance of four instruments in primary care. J Am Geriatr Soc. 2012;60:1027–36.

Husain AM, Horn GJ, Jacobson MP. Non-convulsive status epilepticus: usefulness of clinical features in selecting patients for urgent EEG. J Neurol Neurosurg Psychiatry. 2003;74:189–91.

Inouye SK. The dilemma of delirium: clinical and research controversies regarding diagnosis and evaluation of delirium in hospitalized elderly medical patients. Am J Med. 1994;97:278–88.

Inouye SK, Bogardus ST Jr, Charpentier PA et al. A multicomponent intervention to prevent delirium in hospitalized older patients. N Engl J Med. 1999; 340:669–76.

Inouye SK, Viscoli CM, Horwitz RI, Hurst LD, Tinetti ME. A predictive model for delirium in hospitalized elderly medical patients based on admission characteristics. Ann Intern Med. 1993;119:474–81.

Lewis LM, Miller DK, Morley JE, Nork MJ, Lasater LC. Unrecognized delirium in ED geriatric patients. Am J Emerg Med. 1995;13:142–5.

Mitchell SL, Teno JM. The clinical course of advanced dementia. N Engl J Med. 2009;361:1529–38.

Moroney JT, Bagiella E, Desmond DW et al. Meta-analysis of the Hachinski Ischemic Score in pathologically verified dementias. Neurology. 1997;49(4): 1096–105.

O'Mahony R, Murthy L. Synopsis of the National Institute for Health and Clinical Excellence Guideline for Prevention of Delirium. Ann Intern Med. 2011;154:746–51.

Rockwood K. The occurrence and duration of symptoms in elderly patients with delirium. J Gerontol. 1993;48:M162–6.

Siu AL. Screening for dementia and investigating its causes. Ann Intern Med. 1991;115:122–32.

Wiederkehr S, Simard M, Fortin C, van Reekum R. Comparability of the clinical diagnostic criteria for vascular dementia: a critical review. Part I. J Neuropsychiatry Clin Neurosci. 2008;20(2):150–61.

Witlox J, Eurelings LSM et al. Delirium in elderly patients and the risk of postdischarge mortality, institutionalization, and dementia: a meta-analysis. JAMA. 2010;304(4):443–51.

Wong CL, Holroyd-Leduc J. Does this patient have delirium?: value of bedside instruments. JAMA. 2010;304(7):779–86.

I have a patient who is concerned that she has diabetes. How do I confirm the diagnosis and treat patients with diabetes?

CHIEF COMPLAINT

PATICNT ∇ 1

Mrs. D is a 50-year-old African American woman who is worried she has diabetes.

 What is the differential diagnosis of diabetes? How would you frame the differential?

CONSTRUCTING A DIFFERENTIAL DIAGNOSIS

The differential diagnosis of diabetes mellitus (DM) is actually a classification of the different causes of diabetes:

A. Type 1 DM
   1. Of the persons with DM in Canada, the United States, and Europe, 5–10% have type 1.
   2. Caused by cellular-mediated autoimmune destruction of the pancreatic beta cells in genetically susceptible individuals, triggered by an undefined environmental agent
      a. Some combination of antibodies against islet cells, insulin, glutamic acid decarboxylase (GAD_{65}), or tyrosine phosphatases IA-2 and IA-2beta are found in 85–90% of patients.
      b. Strong HLA association
      c. Risk is 0.4% in patients without family history, 5–6% in siblings and children, and 30% in monozygotic twins.
      d. Patients are also prone to autoimmune thyroid disease, Addison disease, vitiligo, celiac sprue, autoimmune hepatitis, myasthenia gravis, and pernicious anemia.
   3. Occasionally occurs without a defined HLA association or autoimmunity in patients of African or Asian ancestry
   4. Insulin therapy is always necessary.
   5. Patients are at high risk for diabetic ketoacidosis (DKA).

B. Type 2 DM

C. Other, less common causes of diabetes
   1. Genetic defects of beta cell function or insulin action
   2. Exocrine pancreatic diseases (pancreatitis, trauma, infection, pancreatectomy, pancreatic carcinoma)
   3. Endocrinopathies (acromegaly, Cushing syndrome, glucagonoma, pheochromocytoma)
   4. Medications (especially corticosteroids)
   5. Infections

D. Gestational diabetes

Type 1 DM generally occurs in children, although approximately 7.5–10% of adults assumed to have type 2 DM actually have type 1, as defined by the presence of circulating antibodies. Type 2 DM is becoming more prevalent in teenagers and young adults, presumably related to the increased prevalence of obesity.

In most patients, the distinction between type 1 and type 2 DM is clear. Thus, the primary tasks of the clinician are to determine who should be tested for diabetes, who has diabetes, which complications to monitor, and how to treat the patient.

Mrs. D has worried about having diabetes since her father died of complications from the disease. Over the last couple of weeks, she has been urinating more often and notes larger volumes than usual. She is aware that excess urination can be a symptom of diabetes, so she scheduled an appointment.

 At this point, what is the leading hypothesis, what are the active alternatives, and is there a must not miss diagnosis? Given this differential diagnosis, what tests should be ordered?

RANKING THE DIFFERENTIAL DIAGNOSIS

Mrs. D's pretest probability of diabetes is high because of 2 pivotal points in her history, the polyuria and the positive family history. Excess fluid intake and diseases that cause true polyuria, defined as urinary output of > 3 L/day, should also be considered. Bladder dysfunction and urinary tract infection generally cause frequent, small volume urination. Since patients sometimes have trouble quantifying the amount of urine produced, causes of small volume urinary frequency should be kept in the differential. Table 12-1 lists the differential diagnosis.

Mrs. D has no dysuria or hematuria. She takes no medications, drinks 1 cup of coffee per day, and uses alcohol rarely. She has been trying to lose weight and has been drinking more water in an attempt to reduce her appetite.

On physical exam, she looks a bit tired. Vital signs are as follows: BP, 138/82 mm Hg; pulse, 96 bpm; RR, 16 breaths per minute. The remainder of the physical exam is normal. A random plasma glucose is 152 mg/dL.

 Is the clinical information sufficient to make a diagnosis? If not, what other information do you need?

Table 12-1. Diagnostic hypotheses for Mrs. D.

Diagnostic Hypotheses	Demographics, Risk Factors, Symptoms and Signs	Important Tests
Leading Hypothesis		
Type 2 diabetes mellitus	Family history Obesity Hypertension Ethnic group Polyuria Polydipsia	Fasting plasma glucose or HgbA$_{1c}$
Active Alternatives—Most Common		
Excess fluid intake	Polyuria Frequency	History
Other Hypotheses		
Primary polydipsia	Polyuria > 3 L/day Excess water intake	Water restriction test
Diabetes insipidus	Polyuria > 3 L/day	Water restriction test
Urinary tract infection	Urgency Frequency Hematuria	Urinalysis Culture
Bladder dysfunction	Urgency Frequency Incontinence	Postvoid residual Urodynamic testing

Leading Hypothesis: Type 2 DM

Textbook Presentation

Patients with type 2 DM can have the classic symptoms of polyuria, polydipsia, and weight loss. The presentation can also be more subtle, with patients complaining that they feel tired or "just not right." Many patients are asymptomatic; the diagnosis is made after plasma glucose testing. The complications of diabetes may already be present by the time patients seek medical attention.

Disease Highlights

A. Caused by a combination of impaired insulin secretion and insulin resistance with no evidence of autoimmunity

B. Accounts for 90–95% of cases of DM, with prevalence in the United States of about 13–14%; up to 50% of patients are unaware that they have DM.

C. The lifetime risk of diabetes developing in individuals born in 2000 is estimated to be 32.8% for males and 38.5% for females; rates are as high as 50% for African American and Hispanic women.

D. Strong genetic component

  1. In the United States, type 2 DM is 2–6 times more prevalent among African Americans, Native Americans, Pima Indians, and Latinos than among whites.

  2. 39% of patients have at least 1 parent with diabetes

  3. 60–90% concordance in monozygotic twins

  4. The lifetime risk of a first-degree relative of a patient with type 2 DM is 5–10 times higher than that of age- and weight-matched individuals without a family history.

E. The most important risk factor is obesity, which induces insulin resistance.

  1. The relative risk of diabetes developing in a woman who has a body mass index (BMI) > 35 kg/m^2 is 93, compared with a woman who has a BMI < 22 kg/m^2.

  2. The relative risk of diabetes developing in a man who has a BMI > 35 kg/m^2 is 42, compared with a man who has a BMI < 23 kg/m^2.

F. DKA develops less often in patients with type 2 DM than those with type 1; however, DKA can occur in persons with type 2 DM. Recent data show that two-thirds of patients with DKA have type 1 DM, and one-third have type 2 DM.

 Do not assume all patients with DKA have type 1 DM; DKA can develop in persons with type 2 DM.

G. Risk factors for type 2 DM include

  1. Age ≥ 45

  2. BMI ≥ 25 kg/m^2

  3. A first-degree relative with diabetes

  4. Physical inactivity

  5. Being a member of a high-risk ethnic group (African American, Latino, Native American, Asian American, Pacific Islander)

  6. Having delivered a baby weighing > 9 pounds or having had gestational DM

  7. Hypertension

  8. High-density lipoprotein [HDL] cholesterol < 35 mg/dL or triglycerides > 250 mg/dL

  9. Polycystic ovary syndrome

  10. Vascular disease

  11. Prediabetes (impaired glucose tolerance [IGT], impaired fasting glucose [IFG], or mildly elevated HgbA$_{1c}$; see Evidence-Based Diagnosis section for definitions)

    a. Patients with either IGT or IFG have a 5–10% annual risk of developing diabetes; those with both have a 10–15% annual risk.

    b. Patients with an HgbA$_{1c}$ in the prediabetes range have an annual risk of 5–10%.

    c. These annual risks are 10–20 times higher than in people without prediabetes.

H. Screening for diabetes

  1. American Diabetes Association (ADA) recommends screening patients beginning at age 45.

    a. Screening should be done at any age in patients with a BMI ≥ 25 and 1 of the additional risk factors listed above.

    b. Screening should be done every 3 years in patients with normal results, and every 1–2 years in patients with prediabetes.

  2. In 2008, the US Preventive Services Task Force recommended screening asymptomatic adults with sustained BP > 135/80 mm Hg. The Task Force concluded that evidence is insufficient to assess the benefits and harms of routine screening in asymptomatic patients with BP of 135/80 mm Hg or lower.

Evidence-Based Diagnosis

A. Table 12-2 lists the ADA diagnostic criteria for diabetes and prediabetes.

Table 12-2. American Diabetes Association diagnostic criteria for prediabetes and diabetes.

	Fasting Plasma Glucose	2-Hour Plasma Glucose (After 75-g Oral Glucose Load)	HgbA$_{1c}$
Normal	< 100 mg/dL	≤ 140 mg/dL	<5.7%
Prediabetes	100–125 mg/dL	140–199 mg/dL	5.7–6.4%
Diabetes[1]	≥ 126 mg/dL	≥ 200 mg/dL	≥ 6.5%

[1]A random plasma glucose ≥ 200 mg/dL also diagnoses diabetes.

B. The ADA recommends that all abnormal results be confirmed with repeat testing.

C. Most physicians screen with either the fasting plasma glucose (FPG), HgbA$_{1c}$, or both; the oral glucose tolerance test is used primarily to screen for gestational diabetes.

1. FPG is widely available and inexpensive; the primary disadvantage is the need for fasting at least 8 hours.

2. The HgbA$_{1c}$ is now globally standardized and does not require fasting.

   a. Falsely low values can occur in patients with hemoglobinopathies, active hemolysis, and stage 4 or 5 chronic kidney disease.

   b. Falsely high values can be seen in iron deficiency.

   c. African American patients tend to have slightly higher HgbA$_{1c}$ levels than white patients (0.2–0.3%).

D. Patients may have abnormal results on 1 or both tests; in 1 study, one-third of new diabetes cases were detected by FPG testing only, one-third by HgbA$_{1c}$ testing only, and one-third by both tests.

 Patients with normal HgbA$_{1c}$ levels may still have diabetes by fasting glucose criteria.

Treatment of Prediabetes

A. The goals are to prevent or delay the onset of diabetes and to optimize other cardiac risk factors.

B. Large randomized trials have shown that lifestyle modification or medication can prevent or delay diabetes.

1. Finnish patients with IGT were randomized to brief diet/exercise counseling or intensive individualized instruction.

   a. There was a 58% relative reduction in the development of diabetes in the intensive group, (NNT = 22 to prevent 1 case of DM over 1 year; NNT = 5 to prevent 1 case of DM over 5 years).

   b. The study cohort has been monitored for 10 years post intervention; the group of patients initially assigned to the intensive lifestyle intervention maintained a 43% relative risk reduction in the development of diabetes.

2. Patients in the United States (45% African American or Hispanic) were randomized to intensive diet/exercise program, metformin, or placebo.

   a. There was a 58% relative reduction in the development of DM in the intensive diet/exercise group and a 31% relative reduction in metformin group.

   b. NNT = 7 over 3 years to prevent 1 case of diabetes for the intensive diet/exercise group, and NNT = 14 for the metformin group.

   c. The patients initially assigned to the intensive diet/exercise program maintained a 43% relative risk reduction in the development of diabetes over 10 years.

3. Acarbose, orlistat, and pioglitazone have also been studied, but the ADA does not recommend their use in diabetes prevention.

 Lifestyle modification is the best way to prevent or delay the onset of diabetes.

C. Optimal lifestyle modification goals are 150 minutes of aerobic exercise weekly and losing 7% of the baseline body weight.

D. None of the drugs studied is FDA approved for diabetes prevention; the ADA recommends considering metformin in patients under 60 with a BMI > 35 and/or with progressive hyperglycemia.

E. The goal of hypertension therapy in patients with prediabetes is to achieve a BP < 140/90 mm Hg.

F. Lipids should be treated according to current guidelines for nondiabetic patients (see Chapter 23, Hypertension).

MAKING A DIAGNOSIS

 Mrs. D's random glucose is elevated but is not diagnostic of diabetes. She reports that when she reduces her fluid intake, she urinates less. You ask her to return for more testing:

FPG, 120 mg/dL
HgbA$_{1c}$, 6.0%

Urinalysis: negative for protein, glucose, and blood; no WBCs or bacteria; specific gravity, 1.015.

 Have you crossed a diagnostic threshold for the leading hypothesis, type 2 DM? Have you ruled out the active alternatives? Do other tests need to be done to exclude the alternative diagnoses?

Mrs. D does not meet diagnostic criteria for diabetes, but she does have prediabetes. This does not cause glycosuria of a degree sufficient to cause urinary frequency. A urinary tract infection is ruled out by the normal urinalysis. She has increased her water consumption, so excess fluid intake is a likely cause of her symptoms. Bladder dysfunction should be considered if her symptoms do not resolve with reduction in fluid intake. Diabetes insipidus and primary polydipsia are rare diseases that do not need to be considered unless she has a documented urinary output of more than 3 L/day. The next diagnostic test should be reducing her fluid intake.

CASE RESOLUTION

Mrs. D stops forcing herself to drink extra water, and her urination pattern returns to normal. She is very concerned about her elevated FPG and wants to know how to prevent progression to diabetes. Her BMI is 30 kg/m², and her fasting lipid panel shows total cholesterol of 220 mg/dL; HDL, 38 mg/dL; triglycerides, 250 mg/dL; and low-density lipoprotein (LDL), 132 mg/dL. You refer her to a dietician for dietary counseling and recommend that she walk 30 minutes per day 5 days a week. When she returns to see you 4 months later, she has lost 8 pounds. Her FPG is 112 mg/dL; total cholesterol 197 mg/dL, HDL, 42 mg/dL; triglycerides, 150 mg/dL; and LDL, 125 mg/dL.

FOLLOW-UP OF MRS. D

Mrs. D returns 5 years later, having lived in another city in the meantime. She reports that she did quite well with her diet and exercise program for several years, maintaining a 10% weight loss. However, over the last couple of years, she has not been able to continue her exercise program or be as careful about her diet because of the stresses of caring for her chronically ill mother as well as working and caring for her own family. Her mother died recently, so Mrs. D has moved back. She knows that she has gained weight and is especially worried about her blood sugar level because she did not have time to see a doctor herself during her mother's illness.

On physical exam, her BMI is now 34 kg/m² (up 4 kg/m² from her initial visit), and her BP is 155/88 mm Hg. Her lungs are clear, and on cardiac exam you hear an S₄ but no S₃ or murmurs. Abdominal exam is normal, and there is no peripheral edema. Her peripheral pulses are normal, and there are no ulcerations on her feet. She does have tinea pedis. Her point-of-care glucose measurement is 335 mg/dL.

 At this point, what is the leading hypothesis, what are the active alternatives, and is there a must not miss diagnosis? Given this differential diagnosis, what tests should be ordered?

RANKING THE DIFFERENTIAL DIAGNOSIS

Clearly, Mrs. D now has type 2 DM. At this point, in addition to starting treatment, the clinician should focus on identifying and managing diabetic complications and associated cardiovascular risk factors rather than ruling out other diagnoses (Table 12-3).

Mrs. D does not report any vision loss, numbness, edema, dyspnea, or chest pain.

 Is the clinical information sufficient to make a diagnosis? If not, what other information do you need?

Table 12-3. Diagnostic hypotheses for Mrs. D's follow-up.

Diagnostic Hypotheses	Demographics, Risk Factors, Symptoms and Signs	Important Tests
Leading Hypothesis: Diabetic Complications		
Retinopathy	Asymptomatic Decreased vision	Ophthalmologic exam
Nephropathy	Poor glycemic control Hypertension	Albumin/creatinine ratio
Peripheral neuropathy	Paresthesias	Monofilament test EMG
Diabetic foot ulcers	Neuropathy Peripheral arterial disease	Physical exam Ankle-brachial index
Vascular disease	Coronary artery disease Peripheral arterial disease Cerebrovascular disease	Stress test Ankle-brachial index Carotid duplex ultrasound
Active Alternatives that Increase Cardiovascular Risk—Must Not Miss		
Hypertension		Physical exam
Hyperlipidemia		Fasting lipid panel
Smoking		History
Obesity		Body mass index

EMG, electromyogram.

Leading Hypothesis: Diabetic Complications

1. Retinopathy

Textbook Presentation

Most patients with retinopathy are asymptomatic. Other patients experience either gradual or sudden vision loss.

Disease Highlights

A. Most common cause of new cases of blindness in adults aged 20–74 years

B. Incidence and risk of progression have declined over the past 30 years, with a 77% decrease in the annual incidence of retinopathy in patients with type 1 DM.

C. Stages of diabetic retinopathy (DR)

   1. Nonproliferative (NPDR)

     a. Earlier stage of DR

     b. Earliest signs are microaneurysms and retinal hemorrhages

     c. Progressive capillary nonperfusion leads to ischemia, manifested by increasing cotton wool spots, venous beading, and intraretinal vascular abnormalities.

   2. Proliferative diabetic retinopathy (PDR)

     a. Most advanced form of DR

     b. Progressive retinal ischemia causes formation of new blood vessels on the retina or optic disk.

     c. The new vessels bleed, leading to vision loss because of vitreous hemorrhage, fibrosis, or retinal detachment.

3. Diabetic macular edema (DME)

   a. Can develop at any stage of retinopathy

   b. Now the leading cause of vision loss in persons with diabetes

   c. Increased vascular permeability causes plasma leaks from the macular vessels, leading to swelling and formation of hard exudates at the central retina.

D. Risk factors

   1. Most consistently identified risk factors are duration of DM, elevated HgbA$_{1C}$ level, hypertension, hyperlipidemia, pregnancy, nephropathy.

   2. Less consistently identified risk factors include obesity, smoking, moderate alcohol consumption, physical inactivity.

Evidence-Based Diagnosis

A. Evaluation should include dilated indirect ophthalmoscopy or fundus photography, or both, by an ophthalmologist.

B. Patients with type 1 DM should have an exam within 5 years of disease onset, followed by at least annual exams.

C. Patients with type 2 DM should have an exam at the time of diagnosis, followed by at least annual exams.

 All patients with type 2 DM need eye exams by an ophthalmologist at least annually.

Treatment

A. Glycemic control

   1. In persons with type 1 DM *without* retinopathy, the risk of developing DR is reduced 76% by tight control (HgbA$_{1C}$ 7.2% vs 9.1% in the Diabetes Control and Complications Trial).

   2. In persons with type 1 DM *with* retinopathy, the risk of progression is reduced by 54% by tight control.

   3. In persons with type 2 DM, better control reduces the risk of microvascular complications (retinopathy and nephropathy) by 16–25%. (HgbA$_{1C}$ 7% vs 7.9% in the United Kingdom Prospective Diabetes Study [UKPDS] [1998]; HgbA$_{1C}$ 6.5% vs 7.2% in the ADVANCE trial [2008].)

   4. In persons with type 2 DM, there is a 35% reduction in the risk of microvascular complications for every percentage point decrease in HgbA$_{1C}$.

B. Better BP control reduces the risk of progression of retinopathy.

C. Aspirin neither improves nor worsens retinopathy; the presence of DR is not a contraindication to aspirin therapy.

D. Laser photocoagulation is indicated for PDR, DME, and selected cases of severe NPDR.

E. Anti-vascular endothelial growth factor, given by intraocular injection, improves vision in patients with DME.

F. Emerging therapies include intravitreal fluocinolone and possibly fenofibrate.

2. Neuropathy

Textbook Presentation

Diabetic peripheral neuropathy (DPN) can be focal but classically presents as paresthesias or burning pain in a "glove-stocking," symmetric distribution. Diabetic autonomic neuropathy can manifest in a variety of ways, including orthostatic dizziness, diarrhea, urinary incontinence, and gastroparesis.

Disease Highlights

A. Focal mononeuropathies

   1. Cranial (0.05% of mononeuropathies)

     a. Usually cranial nerve III or VI

     b. Usually acute and transient

     c. Caused by ischemia

   2. Thoracolumbar

   3. Limb

     a. Median nerve most common site (5.8% of mononeuropathies)

     b. Ulnar (2.1%), femoral, and peroneal also affected

B. Diabetic lumbosacral radiculoplexus neuropathy (also called diabetic amyotrophy): pain, severe asymmetric muscle weakness, and wasting of the iliopsoas and quadriceps muscles

C. Symmetric distal polyneuropathy (most common manifestation of DPN)

D. Epidemiology of symmetric distal polyneuropathy

   1. Prevalence ranges from 28% to 55%

     a. In 1 study, 55% of patients had DPN, but only about 14% were symptomatic

     b. Develops at a rate of 6.1 per 100 person years

   2. Severity is related to duration of disease, degree of glycemic control, and presence of hypertension and hyperlipidemia.

   3. DPN is an independent risk factor for foot ulceration and amputation; patients with neuropathy have a 15% lifetime risk of amputation.

E. Clinical manifestations of symmetric distal polyneuropathy

   1. History

     a. Frequently asymptomatic

     b. Burning, shooting, or lancinating pain

     c. Paresthesias, hyperesthesias

     d. Often worse at night

     e. When symptoms ascend to the knees, upper extremity symptoms start

   2. Physical exam

     a. Loss of vibration, pain, pressure, and temperature sensation

     b. Loss of ankle reflexes

     c. Distal muscle atrophy late in the course

   3. Charcot joints develop, usually in the tarsometatarsal region, in 10% of patients.

F. Differential diagnosis of symmetric distal polyneuropathy

   1. Cervical myelopathy, lumbar stenosis, tarsal tunnel syndrome, and digital neuropathies can all mimic DPN, and must be looked for on physical exam.

   2. Consider other causes of neuropathy if

     a. It develops before the onset of or early in the course of the diabetes

     b. Patient has a history of excellent glycemic control

     c. It is asymmetric

     d. Proximal or upper extremity involvement is disproportionate to distal lower extremity involvement

3. Be sure to check for other causes of peripheral neuropathy (eg, hypothyroidism, vitamin B$_{12}$ deficiency, monoclonal gammopathy), even in patients with long-standing diabetes.

 Think about other causes of neuropathy in diabetic patients.

G. Diabetic autonomic neuropathy can affect any organ innervated by the autonomic nervous system.

1. Cardiovascular autonomic neuropathy has many possible manifestations.

   a. Reduced heart rate variability; associated with increased risk of silent ischemia and cardiac death

   b. Fixed heart rate

   c. Resting sinus tachycardia

   d. Inadequate increase in heart rate/BP with exercise

   e. Postural hypotension with systolic BP drop of > 30 mm Hg, without an appropriate heart rate response

   f. Intraoperative cardiac instability

2. Gustatory sweating

   a. Facial sweating, often accompanied by flushing, that occurs after eating

   b. Generally occurs in patients with nephropathy or peripheral neuropathy

   c. Cause unknown

3. GI dysfunction

   a. Reduced esophageal motility

   b. Gastroparesis

      (1) Abnormality of gastric motility leading to delayed gastric emptying

      (2) Symptoms include nausea, vomiting, anorexia, postprandial fullness, early satiety.

      (3) Poor correlation between demonstrated motility abnormalities and symptoms

   c. Diabetic diarrhea

      (1) Characterized by intermittent, brown watery, voluminous stools, occasionally accompanied by tenesmus

      (2) Can be episodic, separated by periods of normal bowel movements or constipation

      (3) Rare in the absence of other manifestations of neuropathy, either peripheral or autonomic

   d. Constipation

      (1) Constipation specifically resulting from autonomic neuropathy occurs in 20% of patients with type 2 DM.

      (2) Caused by abnormality in autonomic neural control of colonic motility

   e. Anorectal dysfunction

      (1) Results in fecal incontinence, even in the absence of diarrhea

      (2) Patients can generally sense the presence of stool, but cannot prevent passage

4. Genitourinary dysfunction

   a. Bladder dysfunction

      (1) Initially motor function normal, but sensation of bladder distention impaired

      (2) Then, detrusor muscle hypocontractility occurs, leading to urinary retention and overflow incontinence.

   b. Erectile dysfunction

      (1) Present in 28–45% of diabetic men

      (2) Most common organic cause of erectile dysfunction

      (3) Risk factors include duration of DM, glycemic control, smoking, other diabetic complications.

Evidence-Based Diagnosis

A. Symmetric distal polyneuropathy

1. Nerve conduction studies and electromyographic studies are the gold standard.

2. A randomized trial showed that patients screened for DPN with a physical exam had lower amputation rates than those not screened

3. The ADA recommends *annual comprehensive foot exams* including inspection, assessment of pedal pulses, and testing for loss of protective sensation with a 10-g monofilament plus any 1 of the following: vibration using a tuning fork, pinprick sensation, ankle reflexes.

4. Although studies use variable physical exam techniques, the standards follow:

   a. Semmes-Weinstein monofilament examination

      (1) Apply a 5.07/10-g monofilament to a non-callused site on the dorsum of the first toe just proximal to the nail bed.

      (2) Repeat 4 times on both feet in an arrhythmic manner.

      (3) Add up the total number of times the monofilament is perceived by the patient (score range = 0–8).

      (4) Some studies test different sites with the monofilament: plantar surfaces of the first, third, and fifth toes; the first, third, and fifth plantar metatarsal heads, medial foot, lateral foot. One study showed that testing the third and fifth toes plus the first and third metatarsal heads identified 95% of the patients with abnormal results on 8-point testing.

   b. On–off vibration testing

      (1) Apply a vibrating 128-Hz tuning fork to the bony prominence at the dorsum of the first toe just proximal to the nail bed.

      (2) Repeat twice on each foot.

      (3) Add up the total number of times the patient perceives the application of the vibrating tuning fork and the cessation of the vibration (score range = 0–8).

   c. Timed vibration testing

      (1) Apply a vibrating 128-Hz tuning fork to the same location used for the on–off vibration test.

      (2) Ask the patient to report the time at which vibration diminished beyond perception, and compare with the number of seconds perceived by the examiner when the tuning fork is applied to the examiner's thumb.

      (3) Record number of times patient's perception time less than examiner's (score range = 0–8).

d. Superficial pain sensation

   (1) Apply a sterile sharp to the same sites used for the monofilament.

   (2) Repeat 4 times on each foot.

   (3) Add up the total number of times the patient did not perceive the painful stimulus (score range = 0–8).

5. Monofilament testing is more reproducible than timed vibration testing.

6. Table 12-4 lists the test characteristics.

 Patients with any abnormal neurologic exam findings in the foot are likely to have DPN and are at high risk for developing ulcerations; those with normal exams may have early DPN but have a lower risk of developing ulcerations.

B. Diabetic autonomic neuropathy

1. Cardiovascular autonomic neuropathy

   a. Cardiology consultation is necessary to evaluate heart rate variability.

   b. Postural change in systolic BP is used to diagnose orthostatic hypotension caused by diabetic autonomic neuropathy; the systolic BP is measured with the patient supine and again after 2 minutes of standing.

      (1) A drop of < 10 mm Hg is normal.

      (2) A drop of 10–29 mm Hg is borderline.

      (3) A drop of > 30 mm Hg is definitely abnormal.

2. Gustatory sweating is diagnosed by history.

3. GI dysfunction

   a. Esophageal dysmotility: Esophagogastroduodenoscopy and manometry

   b. Gastroparesis: Diagnosed clinically or by a "gastric emptying" study, consisting of double-isotope scintigraphy of either solids or liquids.

   c. Diabetic diarrhea: Rule out other causes of chronic diarrhea.

   d. Anorectal dysfunction: Anorectal manometry and defecography can be done to document abnormalities.

4. Genitourinary dysfunction

   a. Urinary bladder dysfunction: Ultrasound and urodynamic testing

   b. Erectile dysfunction: History

Table 12-4. Physical exam findings in diabetic peripheral neuropathy.

Test	Able to perceive stimulus ≥ 4 times (normal test)		Able to perceive stimulus ≤ 3 times (abnormal test)	
	Sensitivity (%)	LR–	Specificity (%)	LR+
Monofilament	77[1]	0.34	96	10.2
Timed vibration	80	0.33	98	18.5
Superficial pain	59	0.5	97	9.2
On-off vibration	53	0.51	99	26.6

[1]This is the sensitivity when 7/8 monofilament applications are correctly identified.

Treatment

A. Tight glycemic control

1. Definitely prevents and improves neuropathy in persons with type 1 DM (relative risk reduction of 60%, NNT of 15 to prevent 1 case of neuropathy in tightly controlled patients)

2. Possibly prevents and improves neuropathy in persons with type 2 DM

B. Otherwise, treatment is symptomatic.

1. Peripheral neuropathy

   a. Tricyclic antidepressants, gabapentin, and pregabalin have all been shown to effectively reduce neuropathic pain.

   b. Tramadol and opioids are also effective.

   c. Capsaicin is possibly effective.

   d. Nonsteroidal antiinflammatory drugs generally are not effective.

 All patients with DM should receive foot care education. Those with DPN or structural foot abnormalities should be referred to a podiatrist, and screening for peripheral arterial disease with an ankle-brachial index should be considered.

2. Autonomic neuropathy

   a. Cardiovascular

      (1) Orthostatic hypotension is usually the most disabling symptom.

         (a) Patients should raise head of bed, and rise slowly.

         (b) Patients can try an elasticized garment that extends from the feet to the costal margins.

         (c) Fludrocortisone is sometimes used but must beware of supine hypertension, and excessive salt and water retention.

      (2) Cardioselective beta-blockers are sometimes helpful.

   b. Sweating: no specific treatment available; clonidine may be effective.

   c. Esophageal dysmotility: can try prokinetic agents such as metoclopramide.

   d. Gastroparesis

      (1) Severe gastroparesis is very difficult to manage.

      (2) Small meals sometimes help.

      (3) Prokinetic agents, such as metoclopramide or erythromycin, sometimes are effective.

      (4) Gastric electrical stimulation is being studied for refractory cases.

   e. Constipation

      (1) Increase fiber.

      (2) Drug choices include lactulose, polyethylene glycol, stool softeners.

      (3) Avoid senna, cascara due to stimulant activity.

   f. Urinary bladder dysfunction

      (1) Bethanecol

      (2) Intermittent self-catheterization

   g. Erectile dysfunction: sildenafil and other similar agents

3. Nephropathy

Textbook Presentation

Diabetic nephropathy is asymptomatic until it is so advanced that the patient has symptoms of chronic kidney disease.

Disease Highlights

A. Occurs in 20–40% of patients with diabetes

B. The most common cause of end-stage renal disease (ESRD) in the United States

C. Definitions (based on spot collection and calculation of the albumin/creatinine ratio in mcg/mg)

  1. Normal < 30 mcg/mg

  2. Microalbuminuria = 30–299 mcg/mg

  3. Macroalbuminuria (overt nephropathy) ≥ 300 mcg/mg

D. Natural history: much better defined for type 1 than for type 2 DM

  1. Type 1 DM

    a. Renal enlargement and hyperfunction at onset of diabetes; continues for 5–15 years

    b. Microalbuminuria appears 10–15 years after onset of DM; glomerular filtration rate (GFR) and BP initially normal.

    c. Over the ensuing 10–15 years, 80% of patients progress to macroalbuminuria; GFR declines and hypertension develops.

    d. ESRD develops in 50% of patients with macroalbuminuria within 10 years and in 75% by 20 years.

  2. Type 2 DM

    a. Natural history is less well defined because onset of type 2 DM is usually not well defined, and other causes of kidney disease (such as hypertension and vascular disease) are common comorbidities.

    b. 20–40% of patients with microalbuminuria progress to macroalbuminuria.

    c. 20% have ESRD within 20 years of the onset of macroalbuminuria.

E. Risk factors for development of nephropathy

  1. Poor glycemic control

  2. Hypertension

  3. Long duration of DM

  4. Male sex

  5. Ethnic predisposition (Native American, African American, Hispanic [especially Mexican American])

F. Patients with any amount of albuminuria have an increased risk of cardiovascular events.

Evidence-Based Diagnosis

A. ADA recommends annual screening for microalbuminuria beginning at the time of diagnosis for patients with type 2 DM and starting at year 5 for patients with type 1 DM.

B. The recommended screening is a spot urinary albumin/creatinine ratio.

  1. There is diurnal variation, so first-void or early-morning specimens are best; otherwise, try to obtain confirmatory specimen at same time of day as initial specimen.

  2. Short-term hyperglycemia, exercise, urinary tract infection, marked hypertension, heart failure, and acute febrile illness can cause transient elevations in albumin excretion.

  3. Because of variability, 2–3 specimens in a 3- to 6-month period should be abnormal before diagnosing new or progressive diabetic nephropathy.

  4. For morning specimens, sensitivity ranges from 70% to 100% and specificity ranges from 91% to 98%.

  5. For random specimens, sensitivity ranges from 56% to 97% and specificity ranges from 81% to 92%.

C. It is not clear whether it is necessary to measure the albumin/creatinine ratio annually in patients being treated with an angiotensin-converting enzyme (ACE) inhibitor or angiotensin receptor blocker (ARB).

D. All patients should have a serum creatinine checked at least annually.

Treatment

A. Tight glycemic control reduces nephropathy.

  1. Type 1 DM: incidence of microalbuminuria is reduced by up to 43% and that of macroalbuminuria by 56%

  2. Type 2 DM

    a. Better control reduces the risk of microvascular complications (retinopathy and nephropathy) by 16–25%.

    b. NNT = 36 over 10 years in the UKPDS; NNT = 66 over 5 years in the ADVANCE trial

    c. The microvascular complication rate was 58% for patients with an $HgbA_{1C} \geq 10\%$ and 6.1% for patients with an $HgbA_{1C} < 6.0\%$ (UKPDS).

    d. Microvascular complication rate decreases by 37% for every 1% reduction in $HgbA_{1C}$.

B. BP control and choice of agents

  1. BP should be < 140/80 mm Hg; aiming for a systolic BP < 130 mm Hg is appropriate if it can be achieved without adverse medication effects.

  2. Either ACE inhibitors or ARBs should be used.

    a. ACE inhibitors have been shown to reduce

      (1) Progression to overt nephropathy in persons with type 1 and type 2 DM who have hypertension and microalbuminuria

      (2) Progression to microalbuminuria in persons with type 2 DM who have hypertension and normoalbuminuria

      (3) Cardiovascular events in patients with type 2 DM

    b. ARBs have been shown to reduce progression to overt nephropathy in persons with type 2 DM who have hypertension and albuminuria.

C. There are conflicting data regarding the efficacy of dietary protein restriction.

4. Diabetic Foot Ulcers

Textbook Presentation

A patient with peripheral neuropathy is unaware of minor trauma and the beginning of plantar ulceration. By the time the ulcer is discovered incidentally, it is often advanced, often with associated osteomyelitis.

Disease Highlights

A. Lifetime risk of developing an ulcer is about 15%.

B. Nearly all patients with ulcers have neuropathy, and over 50% have peripheral arterial disease, a strong predictor of nonhealing ulcers.

C. Tend to occur at pressure points, so plantar surface and sites of calluses are common locations

1. Venous ulcers generally occur above the medial or lateral malleolus.

2. Arterial ulcers generally occur on the toes, metatarsal heads, or shins.

D. Risk factors

1. Previous amputation or foot ulcer
2. Peripheral neuropathy
3. Foot deformity
4. Peripheral arterial disease
5. Visual impairment
6. Diabetic nephropathy (especially patients on dialysis)
7. Poor glycemic control
8. Smoking

E. Pathophysiology

1. Repetitive mechanical stress occurs as a result of altered biomechanics, foot deformities, ill-fitting shoes.

2. Peripheral neuropathy causes loss of protective sensation, so the patient is unaware of the incipient ulceration.

3. Ischemia, resulting from macrovascular peripheral arterial disease (commonly in the tibioperoneal vessels) or microvascular dysfunction from autonomic neuropathy, inhibits healing and promotes progression.

F. Classification of diabetic foot infections

1. Mild

   a. Local swelling or induration, erythema, local tenderness or pain, local warmth, purulent discharge
   b. Involves skin and subcutaneous tissue, with no involvement of deeper tissues and no systemic signs
   c. Erythema extends ≤ 2 cm from the ulcer

2. Moderate: signs of local infection, plus

   a. Erythema extends more than 2 cm from the ulcer, or deep structure involved (abscess, osteomyelitis, septic arthritis, fasciitis)
   b. No systemic inflammatory response signs (SIRS)

3. Severe: local infection plus at least 2 SIRS criteria (temperature > 38°C or < 36°C; pulse > 90 bpm; RR > 20 breaths/min or $PaCO_2$ < 32 mm Hg; WBC > 12,000 or < 4000 cells/mcL or ≥ 10% band forms)

G. Microbiology (see Table 12-5)

H. Osteomyelitis develops in up to 20% of patients with mild foot infections and 50–60% of those with moderate to severe infections.

 Osteomyelitis can still develop in patients with mild foot infections.

Evidence-Based Diagnosis

A. Patients with neuropathy should have a foot exam at every visit.

 You cannot examine the feet of your diabetic patients too often, and you cannot examine them with their shoes on!

B. All patients with ulcers should have an ankle-brachial index to look for peripheral arterial disease.

Table 12-5. Microbiology and treatment of diabetic foot infections.

Infection Severity	Usual pathogens	Initial Treatment
Mild	Staphylococcus aureus, Streptococcus spp	**Oral antibiotics** Cephalexin or amoxicillin-clavulanate if MSSA suspected Clindamycin if MRSA suspected[1] Add coverage for gram-negative organisms if the patient has received antibiotics within the past month
Moderate	S aureus, Streptococcus spp, Enterobacteriaceae, Anaerobes	**Usually parenteral antibiotics are used** Ampicillin-sulbactam[2] Cefoxitin[2] Piperacillin-tazobactam[2] if Pseudomonas aeruginosa suspected[3] **Sometimes oral antibiotics are used in the least serious moderate infections:** Clindamycin + levofloxacin, ciprofloxacin or moxifloxacin
Severe	S aureus, Streptococcus spp, Enterobacteriaceae, Anaerobes	**Parenteral antibiotics are always used:** Vancomycin + ceftazidime, cefepime, piperacillin-tazobactam, aztreonam, or a carbapenem

[1]Doxycycline and trimethoprim/sulfamethoxazole are active against MRSA and selected gram negative organisms but not usually streptococci
[2]All of these antibiotics cover MSSA; add vancomycin if MRSA is suspected
[3]In areas of high local prevalence of Pseudomonas aeruginosa, warm climates, frequent exposure of the foot to water
MRSA, methicillin-resistant S aureus; MSSA, methicillin-susceptible S aureus.

C. Culturing ulcers

1. Do not culture clinically uninfected ulcers.
2. Do not obtain a specimen by swabbing the wound or wound drainage.
3. Cleanse and debride the wound before obtaining a specimen.

   a. If purulent secretions are present, aspirate using a sterile needle or syringe.
   b. Obtain a tissue specimen by scraping the base of a debrided ulcer with a sterile scalpel or dermal curette.

D. Diagnosing complications

1. Cellulitis: clinical diagnosis (see Chapter 17, Edema)
2. Osteomyelitis (Table 12-6)

   a. Open bone biopsy with culture is the gold standard.
   b. Needle bone biopsy subject to sampling error (sensitivity, 87%; specificity, 93%; LR+, 12.4; LR–, 0.14)
   c. Being able to see bone or to probe the ulcer down to bone substantially increases the probability the patient has osteomyelitis.
   d. C-reactive protein, erythrocyte sedimentation rate, CBC, blood cultures not sufficiently sensitive or specific to diagnose osteomyelitis.

Table 12-6. Test characteristics for the diagnosis of osteomyelitis in patients with diabetic foot ulcers.

Diagnostic Findings	LR+	LR–
Bone exposure	9.2	0.7
Ulcer area > 2 cm²	7.2	0.48
Positive probe to bone	6.4	0.39
Ulcer inflammation (erythema, swelling, purulence)	1.5	0.84
ESR > 70 mm/h	11	0.34
MRI	5.1	0.12
Radiographs	2.3	0.63

ESR, erythrocyte sedimentation rate; MRI, magnetic resonance imaging.

e. MRI is the imaging procedure with the best test characteristics; bone scan and WBC scans are less specific but are sometimes done in patients who cannot undergo MRI.

MRI scan is the best imaging procedure to diagnose osteomyelitis in a patient with a diabetic foot ulcer.

A normal CBC, C-reactive protein, or erythrocyte sedimentation rate does not rule out osteomyelitis.

Treatment

A. Preventive foot care
   1. Improve glycemic control to reduce risk of neuropathy.
   2. Reduce vascular risk factors (smoking cessation, BP control, lipid management, glycemic control).
   3. Examine the feet of high-risk patients at every visit.
   4. Examine the feet of low-risk patients at least annually.
   5. Ensure patients wear well-fitted shoes.
   6. Educate patients regarding need for daily visual inspection of feet.
   7. Refer to podiatrist for débridement of calluses, assessment of bony deformities.

B. Treatment of ulcers
   1. Treat any infection (see Table 12-5).
   2. Determine need for revascularization, and revascularize as early as possible in patients with treatable peripheral vascular disease.
   3. Heal the ulcer.
      a. Off loading: use orthotics or fiberglass casts to remove pressure from the wound while allowing the patient to remain active.
      b. Débride ulcers (surgically or with débriding agents such as hydrogels).
      c. Control edema.
      d. Growth factors are being studied.

4. Institute preventive measures once the ulcer has healed.

A multidisciplinary approach, including internal medicine, vascular surgery, and podiatry is necessary for the optimal treatment of diabetic foot ulcers.

MAKING A DIAGNOSIS

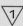

The ophthalmologist reports that Mrs. D has no retinopathy. Her neurologic exam, including monofilament testing, is normal. She does not complain of orthostatic dizziness or any GI or genitourinary symptoms. She has bilateral bunions but no calluses or ulcers. Her albumin–creatinine ratio is 50 mcg/mg, confirmed on repeat testing. Her HgbA$_{1C}$ is 9.1%.

Have you crossed a diagnostic threshold for the leading hypothesis, diabetic complications? Have you ruled out the active alternatives? Do other tests need to be done to exclude the alternative diagnoses?

The evaluation for diabetic complications is complete. Mrs. D has no evidence of retinopathy, neuropathy, or diabetic foot disease. She does have microalbuminuria. However, before formulating a treatment plan for Mrs. D, it is necessary to assess for the presence or absence of other cardiovascular risk factors and cardiovascular disease:

1. Dyslipidemia
2. Hypertension
3. Obesity
4. Smoking
5. Coronary artery disease (CAD)
6. Cerebrovascular disease
7. Peripheral vascular disease

Table 12-7 outlines a summary of testing that must be performed on all patients with diabetes.

CASE RESOLUTION

Mrs. D has no symptoms of vascular disease on careful questioning, and her exercise tolerance is more than 1 mile. Her fasting lipid panel shows total cholesterol of 230 mg/dL, HDL of 45 mg/dL, triglycerides of 200 mg/dL, and LDL of 145 mg/dL. You refer Mrs. D to a diabetes educator and a dietician for instruction about diet and exercise. You also prescribe metformin for the diabetes and atorvastatin for the hyperlipidemia. Because she has hypertension and microalbuminuria, you elect to start an ACE inhibitor, lisinopril, to treat her hypertension. You also recommend that she start taking aspirin, 81 mg daily. Over the next 12–18 months, Mrs. D loses 5 pounds. You increase the dose of metformin and add glipizide, and her HgbA$_{1C}$ decreases to 6.7%. After increasing the dose of lisinopril and adding hydrochlorothiazide, her BP is 128/80 mm Hg. Her LDL is now 85 mg/dL.

Table 12-7. Summary of testing and monitoring recommended by the ADA for patients with diabetes.

Condition	Required Test/Action
Retinopathy	Ophthalmologic exam[1]
Peripheral neuropathy and foot ulcers	Comprehensive foot exams (including inspection, assessment of pedal pulses, and testing for loss of protective sensation with a 10-g monofilament plus any 1 of the following: vibration using a tuning fork, pinprick sensation, ankle reflexes)[1]
Nephropathy	Albumin/creatinine ratio, serum creatinine[1]
Dyslipidemia	Fasting total cholesterol, HDL, triglycerides, LDL[1]
Hypertension	BP measurement[1]
Smoking	Obtain history and counsel cessation[1]
Obesity	Measure weight and calculate BMI[1]
Coronary artery disease	Assess for symptoms[1]
Cerebrovascular disease	Carotid duplex ultrasound in patients with TIA symptoms
Peripheral arterial disease	ABIs in patients over 50 and those under 50 with other vascular risk factors in addition to diabetes

[1]Should be performed at least annually and may need to be done more often in patients with abnormalities.
ABI, ankle-brachial index; ADA, American Diabetes Association; BP, blood pressure; BMI, body mass index; HDL, high-density lipoprotein; LDL, low-density lipoprotein; TIA, transient ischemic attack.

Treatment of Type 2 DM

The treatment of type 2 DM involves not only the treatment of the hyperglycemia but the management of associated complications and cardiovascular risk factors as well. According to survey data, only 51% of participants reach HgbA$_{1C}$ goals, 51% reach BP goals, and 57% reach cholesterol goals; only 14.3% reach all 3 goals.

 It is common for patients to require 6–7 medications to meet accepted treatment goals.

Treatment of Hyperglycemia

A. Treatment goals for patients with type 2 DM

1. The ADA recommends treating to a HgbA$_{1C}$ < 7.0% in most patients.

   a. HgbA$_{1C}$ levels < 7% have been clearly shown to reduce microvascular events in patients with type 2 DM (see data above).

   b. Intensive control has not been consistently shown to reduce macrovascular events; intensive control may be harmful in *older* diabetics *with* cardiovascular disease, and may be beneficial in younger persons in whom diabetes was recently diagnosed.

   (1) UKPDS (1998)

      (a) About 4200 persons with *newly* diagnosed type 2 DM without cardiovascular disease, mean age 53, randomized to conventional therapy (HgbA$_{1C}$ 7.9%) vs intensive therapy with sulfonylureas with or without insulin (HgbA$_{1C}$ 7.0%) and monitored for 10 years

   (b) Relative risk of myocardial infarction (MI) in the intensive group = 0.84 (95% CI, 0.71–1.00)

   (c) A separate study arm randomized obese patients to receive metformin or conventional therapy; there was a significant reduction in MI with metformin (relative risk = 0.61, 0.41–0.89)

(2) UKPDS 10-year follow up (2008)

   (a) About 3200 of the original 4200 patients were monitored for an additional 10 years after the intervention trial ended, with patients returning to their personal physicians for diabetes care.

   (b) End points included death from any cause, diabetes-related death, MI, stroke, peripheral arterial disease, microvascular disease, any diabetes-related end point.

   (c) The mean HgbA$_{1C}$ was about 8% in all groups (conventional, sulfonylurea/insulin, metformin) 1 year after the intervention trial ended.

   (d) Patients originally assigned to sulfonylurea/insulin had significant reductions in all end points measured (relative risk for MI 0.85, 95% CI 0.74–0.97; relative risk for death from any cause = 0.87, 0.79–0.96).

   (e) Patients originally assigned to metformin had significant reductions in any diabetes-related end point, death from any cause (relative risk = 0.73, 0.59–0.89), diabetes-related death, and MI (relative risk = 0.67, 0.51–0.89).

   (f) These results suggest a "legacy" effect from initial intensive therapy in type 2 DM, similar to that seen in long-term follow-up of type 1 diabetics.

(3) ADVANCE trial (2008)

   (a) About 11,000 type 2 diabetics with cardiovascular disease or multiple risk factors, mean age 66, randomized to intensive control with a sulfonylurea-based regimen (HgbA$_{1C}$ 6.5%) vs conventional control (HgbA$_{1C}$ 7.2%) and monitored for 5 years

   (b) No difference in macrovascular events (relative risk = 0.94, 0.84–1.06)

(4) ACCORD trial (2008)

   (a) About 10,000 type 2 diabetics with cardiovascular disease or multiple risk factors, mean age 62, randomized to intensive control (HgbA$_{1C}$ 6.4%) vs conventional control (7.5%) and monitored for 3.5 years

   (b) No difference in primary end point (nonfatal MI, nonfatal stroke, or cardiovascular death)

   (c) Increase in any cause death with intensive treatment (relative risk = 1.22 (1.01–1.46), NNH = 100)

   (d) Increase in cardiovascular death with intensive treatment (relative risk = 1.35 (1.04–1.76), NNH = 125)

   (e) Most patients in the intensive group received rosiglitazone, which is associated with increased risk of MI.

2. Goals should be modified for frail elderly, in whom avoidance of hypoglycemia and optimization of functional status may be more important than tight glycemic control.

3. Goals should be individualized based on the overall health and age of the patient (Figure 12-1).

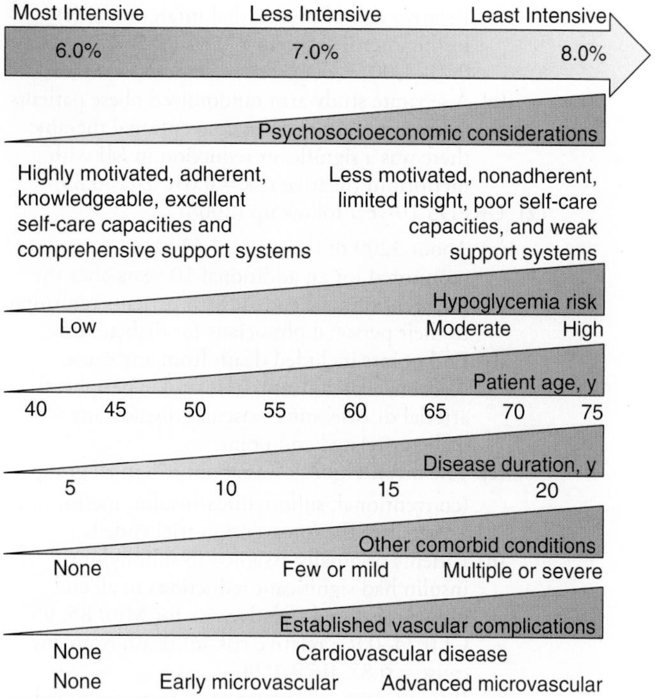

Most Intensive	Less Intensive	Least Intensive
6.0%	7.0%	8.0%

Psychosocioeconomic considerations

Highly motivated, adherent, knowledgeable, excellent self-care capacities and comprehensive support systems	Less motivated, nonadherent, limited insight, poor self-care capacities, and weak support systems

Hypoglycemia risk

Low		Moderate	High

Patient age, y

40	45	50	55	60	65	70	75

Disease duration, y

5	10	15	20

Other comorbid conditions

None	Few or mild	Multiple or severe

Established vascular complications

None	Cardiovascular disease	
None	Early microvascular	Advanced microvascular

Figure 12-1. Framework for determining HgbA$_{1c}$ targets. Reproduced, with permission, from Ismail-Beigi F, Moghissi E, Tiktin M et al. Individualizing glycemic targets in type 2 diabetes mellitus: implications of recent clinical trials. Ann Intern Med. 2011;154:554–9.

B. Monitoring
1. HgbA$_{1c}$ levels every 6 months in stable patients meeting goals; every 3 months in patients not meeting goals or undergoing changes in therapy
   a. Table 12-8 shows correlation between plasma glucose and HgbA$_{1C}$.
   b. 50% of HgbA$_{1c}$ is determined by glycemia during the month before the measurement, 25% from the 30–60 days before, and 25% from 60–90 days before.
2. Home glucose monitoring
   a. Patients taking multiple doses of daily insulin should test blood levels several times a day (fasting, before lunch, before dinner, and before bed); those taking bedtime long-acting insulin should test in the morning.
   b. Optimal frequency for patients taking oral agents is unclear; data regarding effects on control are mixed but show only slight improvement at best.

Table 12-8. Correlation between plasma glucose and HgbA$_{1c}$.

HgbA$_{1c}$ (%)	Mean Plasma Glucose (mg/dL)
6	126
7	154
8	183
9	212
10	240
11	269
12	298

C. Lifestyle modification
1. Weight loss (goal of at least 10% of body weight), diet modification, and exercise (goal of at least 150 minutes/week) are the foundations of all treatment for patients with type 2 DM.
2. Best instituted in conjunction with a certified diabetes educator or dietician

D. Oral hypoglycemics
1. Sulfonylureas
   a. Examples: glyburide, glipizide, glimepiride
   b. Increase insulin secretion.
   c. Average decrease in HgbA$_{1c}$ about 1–1.5%
   d. Side effects include weight gain (2–5 kg) and hypoglycemia, especially in the elderly, patients with reduced renal function, and those with erratic eating habits.
   e. Shown to reduce microvascular outcomes; no change in cardiovascular events.
   f. Can be used as monotherapy or in combination with insulin or other oral agents (except non-sulfonylurea secretagogues)
   g. May become less effective with time, as beta cell function decreases
2. Biguanides
   a. Example: metformin
   b. Reduce hepatic glucose production.
   c. Average decrease in HgbA$_{1c}$ about 1–2%
   d. Associated with weight loss (or at least no weight gain); hypoglycemia rare
   e. Most common side effects are GI (abdominal pain, nausea, diarrhea).
   f. Associated with an increased risk of vitamin B$_{12}$ deficiency
   g. Because of risk of lactic acidosis, relatively contraindicated in patients with creatinine ≥ 1.5 mg/dL, decompensated heart failure, significant hepatic dysfunction, metabolic acidosis, and alcoholism.

 Metformin should be withheld in patients with acute illness and those undergoing surgery or procedures using radiocontrast.

   h. Has been shown to decrease microvascular and macrovascular outcomes, and total mortality in obese patients with type 2 DM (UKPDS, 1998)
   i. Can be used as monotherapy or in combination with all other oral agents and insulin
3. Alpha-glucosidase inhibitors
   a. Example: acarbose
   b. Delay and decrease intestinal carbohydrate absorption, decreasing postprandial glucose swings
   c. About 50% less effective than sulfonylureas and metformin in reducing HgbA$_{1C}$ (average reduction 0.5–0.9%)
   d. Side effects include flatulence, abdominal discomfort, and diarrhea.
   e. No studies of effects on macrovascular or microvascular outcomes
   f. Can be used as monotherapy, but this is rarely done because of relatively poor efficacy; can also be used in combination with sulfonylureas

4. Thiazolidinediones

   a. Example: pioglitazone

   b. Increase insulin-stimulated glucose uptake by skeletal muscle cells and decrease hepatic glucose production

   c. Average decrease in HgbA$_{1c}$ about 0.5–1.4%

   d. Tend to increase HDL and decrease triglycerides

   e. Can take weeks or months to obtain maximum effect

   f. Side effects include weight gain (as great as or more so than that seen with sulfonylureas) and edema.

   g. Increased risk of heart failure (relative risk ~ 3)

   h. Current data do not show that pioglitazone increases the risk of cardiovascular events (as was shown with rosiglitazone).

 Do not use thiazolidinediones in patients with heart failure or edema.

   i. Can be used as monotherapy or in combination with sulfonylureas, metformin, and insulin.

5. Non-sulfonylurea secretagogues (meglitinides)

   a. Examples: repaglinide, nateglinide

   b. Because of short half-life, cause brief, episodic increases in insulin secretion

   c. Primarily reduce postprandial glucose, with less risk of hypoglycemia than with sulfonylureas

   d. Average decrease in HgbA$_{1c}$ 0.5–1%

   e. No long-term studies of effects on macrovascular or microvascular outcomes

   f. Must be dosed with every meal

   g. Should be used cautiously in patients with liver or kidney dysfunction

   h. Can be used as monotherapy or in combination with metformin

6. Dipeptidyl peptidase 4 (DPP4) inhibitors

   a. Incretins (glucose-dependent insulinotropic polypeptide [GIP] and glucagonlike peptide 1 [GLP-1]) are intestinal peptides that augment insulin secretion in the presence of glucose or nutrients in the gut; they are inactivated by the enzyme DPP4.

   b. Sitagliptin and vildagliptin are selective DPP4 inhibitors.

   c. Decrease HgbA$_{1c}$ by ~0.75%

   d. No GI side effects; average weight gain < 1 kg

   e. Less effective than metformin in a direct comparison

   f. No data on macrovascular or microvascular outcomes

E. GLP-1 receptor analogues

  1. Example: exenatide

  2. Given subcutaneously twice daily

  3. Decrease HgbA$_{1c}$ by 0.5–1.5%

  4. Most common side effects are nausea and vomiting.

  5. Average weight loss of ~1.5 kg when compared with placebo and of ~4.75 kg when compared with insulin

  6. No data on macrovascular or microvascular outcomes

F. Insulin

  1. Types of insulin (Table 12-9)

  2. Reduces HgbA$_{1c}$ by 1–2.5%

Table 12-9. Types of insulin.

	Onset of Action	Peak	Duration of Action
Rapid Acting			
Lispro (Humalog)	5–15 min	45–75 min	2–4 h
Aspart (Novolog)			
Short Acting			
Regular U100	~30 min	2–4 h	5–8 h
Intermediate Acting			
Isophane (NPH, Humulin N, Novolin N)	~2 h	4–10 h	10–16 h
Insulin zinc (Lente, Humulin L, Novolin L)	~2 h	4–12 h	12–18 h
Long Acting			
Glargine (Lantus)	~2 h	No peak	20 to > 24 h
Detemir (Levemir)	~2 h	No peak	6–24 h
Premixed			
Humulin 70/30 (70% NPH/30% regular)			
Humalog Mix 75/25 (75% NPL [neutral protamine lispro, similar to NPH]/25% lispro)			
Novolog Mix 70/30 (70% NPH/30% aspart)			

3. Adverse effects of insulin

   a. Hypoglycemia, especially with short-acting forms

   b. Weight gain of 2–4 kg

G. Choosing a medication to treat type 2 DM (Figure 12-2)

  1. Most studies compare an agent to placebo, so direct comparison data are limited.

  2. Sulfonylureas, metformin, and insulin have the best long-term outcome data.

  3. 75% of patients require more than 1 drug by 9 years; there is no evidence that any specific combination is better than another.

  4. Metformin is the preferred initial therapy in most patients with type 2 DM.

  5. Consider starting metformin plus a second agent in patients who present with an HgbA$_{1c}$ > 9%.

  6. Patients who present with DKA, hyperosmolar hyperglycemic state (HHS), or an HgbA$_{1c}$ > 10% should be given insulin as the initial therapy, although some patients may eventually be able to stop insulin and reach goal with oral agents.

  7. Using insulin to manage type 2 DM

   a. Beta cell function declines over time in type 2 DM, so many patients will eventually need insulin.

   b. The first step is to add long-acting basal insulin to oral agents, titrating the insulin dose to the fasting blood sugar.

     (1) There are fewer nocturnal hypoglycemic episodes with bedtime glargine than with bedtime NPH.

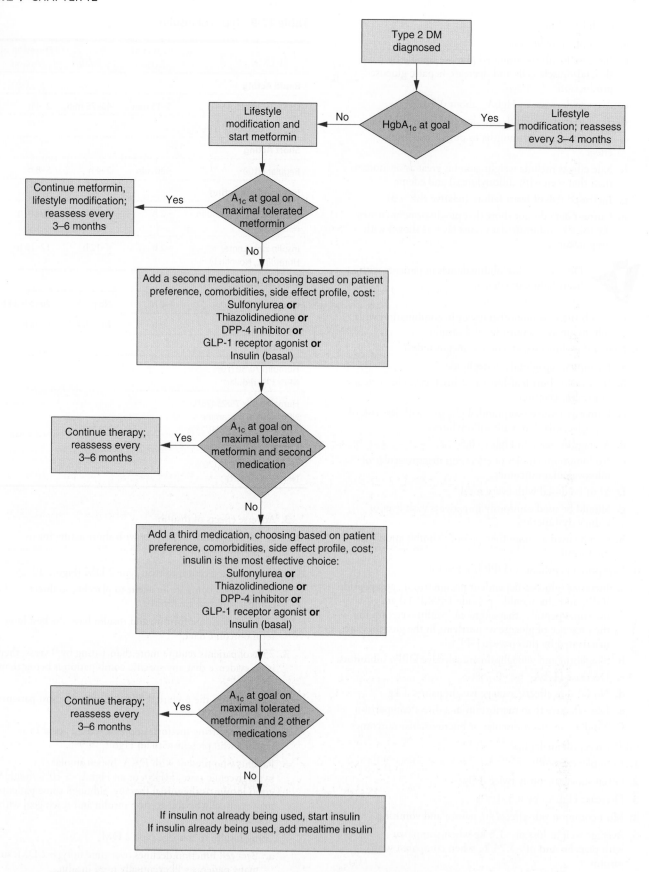

DM, diabetes mellitus; DPP4, dipeptidyl peptidase 4; GLP-1, glucagonlike peptide 1.

Figure 12-2. Approach to the treatment of type 2 DM.

(2) There is less weight gain with metformin and insulin than with sulfonylureas or thiazolidinediones and insulin.

c. If the HgbA$_{1c}$ target is not achieved, options include adding a short-acting insulin, such as lispro, with meals, or switching to twice daily biphasic insulin.

d. Sulfonylureas should be stopped when short-acting insulins are used because of increased hypoglycemia.

Treatment of Hypertension

The treatment goal is to achieve a BP < 140/80 mm Hg. See Nephropathy section and Chapter 23, Hypertension for details.

Treatment of Hypercholesterolemia

A. American Diabetes Association guidelines

1. Statin therapy should be used, *regardless of baseline lipid levels*, in diabetic patients with cardiovascular disease, and those without cardiovascular disease who are over age 40 and have at least 1 other cardiovascular risk factor (family history, hypertension, smoking, dyslipidemia, or albuminuria).

2. Low-risk patients (those under age 40 without overt cardiovascular disease) do not require statin therapy if their LDL is < 100 mg/dL, although it should be considered in patients with multiple risk factors.

3. The LDL goal is < 100 mg/dL for patients without overt cardiovascular disease.

4. The LDL goal is < 70 mg/dL for patients with overt cardiovascular disease.

5. Reduction of LDL by 40% is an alternative therapeutic goal in patients who cannot achieve targets on maximal tolerated doses of statins.

6. Combination lipid-lowering therapy has not been shown to further lower cardiovascular event rates when compared to statin therapy alone and is not recommended by the American Diabetes Association guidelines.

a. The ACCORD Lipid trial randomized 5518 patients with type 2 DM to simvastatin + fenofibrate vs. simvastatin + placebo; there were no differences in cardiovascular outcomes between the 2 groups.

b. The subgroup with the lowest HDL (≤ 34 mg/dL) and highest triglycerides (≥ 204 mg/dL) benefited from combination therapy (relative risk = 0.72, NNT = 20); addition of fenofibrate could be considered in such patients.

B. See Chapter 23, Hypertension (Table 23-7) for new ACC/AHA guidelines for treating cholesterol in patients with diabetes.

Antiplatelet Therapy

A. Low-dose aspirin (75–162 mg/day) is indicated for secondary prevention in all patients with cardiovascular disease.

B. Low-dose aspirin is indicated for primary prevention in patients with diabetes and increased cardiovascular risk (Framingham 10-year risk > 10%; see Chapter 2, Screening and Health Maintenance for information on calculating risk).

1. Patients with low cardiovascular risk (10-year risk < 5%) should not take aspirin for primary prevention; the risk of bleeding is higher than the potential benefit.

2. Aspirin should be considered in patients with intermediate risk (10-year risk of 5–10%).

C. Clopidogrel, 75 mg/day, should be used in patients with aspirin allergies.

CHIEF COMPLAINT

PATIENT 2

Mr. G is a 56-year-old African American man with diabetes, chronic hepatitis B, CAD status post MI 2 months ago, hypertension, and a history of stroke 1 year ago. He is taking many medications, including Humulin 70/30 20 units twice daily, metoprolol, aspirin, atorvastatin, lisinopril, furosemide, and ribavirin. Despite all of these problems, he has been slowly improving and reported at his last visit 3 weeks ago that he had recently given up his walker for a cane. Today you are paged by his sister, who reports that Mr. G is very weak and cannot get up; his home glucose monitor reading is "critical high." Mr. G's voice is barely recognizable over the phone, and he is unable to respond to your questions. You advise his sister to call 911.

 At this point, what is the leading hypothesis, what are the active alternatives, and is there a must not miss diagnosis? Given this differential diagnosis, what tests should be ordered?

RANKING THE DIFFERENTIAL DIAGNOSIS

The differential diagnosis at this point is very broad and difficult to organize. It is helpful to recognize that Mr. G appears to be suffering from the syndrome of delirium and to use the framework for delirium to organize your thinking (see Chapter 11, Delirium and Dementia). It is also reasonable to consider Mr. G's underlying chronic medical problems as important clinical clues and initially focus on the serious complications of these conditions; in other words, initially focus on diseases for which he has a high pretest probability:

1. Diabetes: DKA, HHS, infection with or without sepsis.

2. CAD: recurrent MI, possibly with HF or cardiogenic shock

3. Cerebrovascular disease: recurrent stroke

4. Chronic hepatitis B: hepatic encephalopathy

Table 12-10 lists the differential diagnosis.

 Mr. G could have any, or a combination, of these conditions. His critical high blood sugar makes a complication of diabetes the leading hypothesis; all of the other diagnoses are "must not miss" hypotheses.

When Mr. G arrives in the emergency department, he is barely responsive but able to move all 4 extremities. His BP is 85/50 mm Hg; pulse, 120 bpm; RR, 24 breaths per minute; temperature, 37.2°C. His lungs are clear, and cardiac exam shows an S$_4$ with no S$_3$ or murmurs. His abdomen

(continued)

Table 12-10. Diagnostic hypotheses for Mr. G.

Diagnostic Hypotheses	Demographics, Risk Factors, Symptoms and Signs	Important Tests
Leading Hypothesis		
Hyperosmolar hyperglycemic state (HHS)	Delirium/coma Polyuria Polydipsia Dehydration	Plasma glucose Serum/urine ketones
Active Alternatives—Must Not Miss		
Diabetic ketoacidosis	Delirium/coma Polyuria Polydipsia Dehydration	Plasma glucose Bicarbonate Serum/urine ketones pH
Sepsis	Hypotension Fever	Blood cultures Urinalysis Chest radiograph
Myocardial infarction	Chest pain Dyspnea	ECG Cardiac enzymes
Cerebrovascular accident	Hemiparesis Aphasia	Physical exam Head CT or MRI
Hepatic encephalopathy	Delirium Cirrhosis	Clinical diagnosis

is nontender, and there is no peripheral edema. He has no foot ulcers. Initial laboratory tests include the following:

Sodium, 140 mEq/L; K, 4.9 mEq/L; Cl, 110 mEq/L; HCO_3, 20 mEq/L; BUN, 99 mg/dL; creatinine, 4.3 mg/dL; glucose, 1246 mg/dL.
Arterial blood gases: pH 7.40; PO_2, 88 mm Hg; PCO_2, 35 mm Hg.
WBC is 8400/mcL, with 75% polymorphonuclear neutrophils, 3% bands, 18% lymphocytes, and 4% monocytes.
Albumin, 4.4 g/dL; total bilirubin, 0.3 mg/dL; alkaline phosphatase, 175 units/L; AST (SGOT), 40 units/L; ALT (SGPT), 56 units/L; INR, 1.1.
Serum ketones, negative

$$\text{Corrected serum Na} = \text{measured Na} + \frac{(1.6 \times [\text{glucose} - 100])}{100}$$

$$= 140 + 1.6(11) = 158$$

Urinalysis: 2+ protein, 4+ glucose, no ketones, 3–5 WBC/hpf, occasional bacteria

 Is the clinical information sufficient to make a diagnosis? If not, what other information do you need?

Leading Hypothesis: Hyperosmolar Hyperglycemic State

Textbook Presentation

Patients who have HHS are usually older type 2 diabetics with the gradual onset of polydipsia, polyuria, and lethargy. They become extremely dehydrated, with reduction in urinary output, and have very high serum glucose levels, accompanied by alterations in mental status.

Disease Highlights

A. Epidemiology
   1. Risk factors include older age, nursing home residence, inability to recognize thirst, and lack of access to fluids.

   2. Mortality rate is 5–20%, compared to 1–5% in patients with DKA.

B. Pathogenesis
   1. Reduced effective insulin concentrations and a concomitant increase in counterregulatory hormones lead to increased hepatic and renal glucose production and impaired glucose utilization in peripheral tissues.
   2. Glycosuria leads to an osmotic diuresis with loss of free water in excess of electrolytes, leading to hyperosmolality.
   3. As volume depletion occurs, urinary output drops, and hyperglycemia worsens.
   4. Insulin levels are higher than in DKA and are adequate to prevent lipolysis and ketogenesis.

C. Precipitating factors
   1. The 3 most common precipitants are infection, lack of compliance with insulin, and first presentation of diabetes.
   2. Other precipitants include postoperative state, cerebrovascular accident, MI, pancreatitis, alcohol abuse, trauma, thyrotoxicosis, and medications (eg, corticosteroids, antipsychotic drugs, total parenteral nutrition).

D. Clinical manifestations
   1. History
      a. Symptoms and signs usually evolve over several days or even weeks.
      b. Common findings include polyuria followed by decreased urinary output, polydipsia, fatigue, and weight loss.
      c. Abdominal pain generally does not occur in HHS, as it does in DKA.
      d. Neurologic manifestations
         (1) Lethargy and disorientation common
         (2) Focal neurologic findings, including seizures, can occur with hyperglycemia and resolve with normalization of serum glucose.
         (3) Changes in mental status correlate with the degree of hyperosmolarity.
            (a) 20–25% present with coma.
            (b) Coma is present in half of patients with effective serum osmolality of ≥ 320 mOsm/L.
            (c) Must search for another cause of altered mental status if osmolality < 320mOsm/L
   2. Physical exam
      a. Hypothermia often seen resulting from peripheral vasodilation
      b. Signs of dehydration often seen (see Chapter 28, Acute Kidney Injury)
      c. Tachycardia and hypotension suggest severe dehydration or underlying sepsis.

Evidence-Based Diagnosis

A. Typical total body water deficit is 20–25% (about 9 L).

B. See Table 12-11 for laboratory findings in HHS compared with DKA.

Treatment

A. Patients with HHS generally need more fluid and less insulin than those with DKA.

B. Figure 12-3 outlines the treatment approach.

Table 12-11. Laboratory findings in HHS and DKA.

Laboratory Parameter	HHS	DKA
Plasma glucose (mg/dL)	> 600	> 250
Arterial pH	> 7.30	< 7.3 (< 7.0 in severe DKA)
Serum bicarbonate (mEq/L)	> 18	< 18 (< 10 in severe DKA)
Urine ketones	Negative or small	> 3+
Serum ketones	Negative or small	Positive
Anion gap	Variable	> 12
Effective serum osmolality (mOsm/L)[1]	> 320	Variable

[1]Effective serum osmolality = 2 × Na (mEq/L) + glucose (mg/dL)/18.
HHS, hyperosmolar hyperglycemic state; DKA, diabetic ketoacidosis.

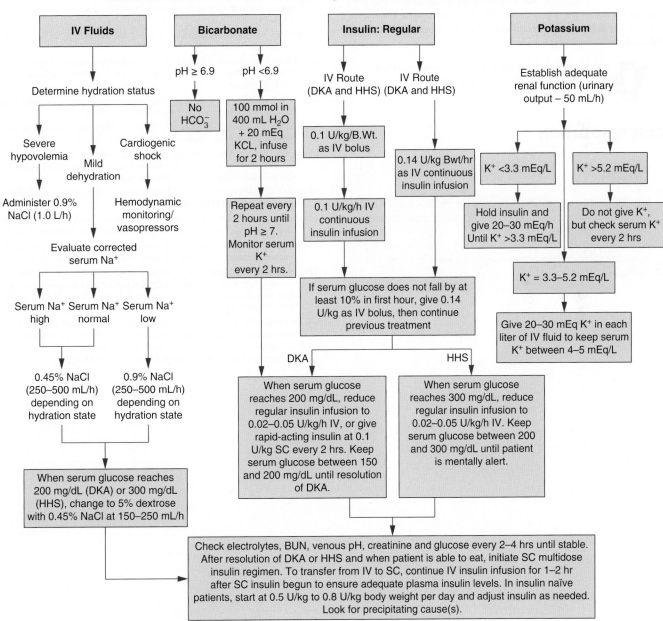

Bwt, body weight; IV, intravenous; SC, subcutaneous.

Figure 12-3. Management of adult patients with hyperosmolar hyperglycemic state (HHS). (Reproduced, with permission, from Kitabchi AE, Umpierrez GE, Miles JM, Fisher JN. Hyperglycemic crises in adult patients with diabetes. Diabetes Care. 2009;32:1339.)

MAKING A DIAGNOSIS

Mr. G's glucose is > 600 mg/dL, ketones are negative, and calculated serum osmolality is 345 mOsm/L (effective serum osmolality = 2 × measured Na + glucose/18 = (2 × 138) + 1246/18 = 345).

Have you crossed a diagnostic threshold for the leading hypothesis, HHS? Have you ruled out the active alternatives? Do other tests need to be done to exclude the alternative diagnoses?

Mr. G fulfills the diagnostic criteria for HHS. It is not necessary to consider other diagnoses, but it is essential to determine the precipitant for this event. Considering Mr. G's complicated history, he is at risk for many of the precipitants of HHS, especially infection, MI, and cerebrovascular accident.

Always look for the precipitant when patients present with either HHS or DKA.

CASE RESOLUTION

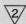

Mr. G's chest radiograph is clear, his urine and blood cultures are negative, his ECG shows no acute changes, and his cardiac enzymes are normal. He responds well to IV hydration and insulin therapy. When he becomes more alert, he reports that he had become depressed and had stopped taking his insulin.

REFERENCES

American Diabetes Association. Standard of medical care in diabetes—2013. Diabetes Care. 2013;36 (Supplement 1):S11–S66.

Bax JJ, Young LH, FryeRL et al. Screening for coronary artery disease in patients with diabetes. Diabetes Care. 2007;30:2729–36.

Bolen S, Feldman L, Vassy J et al. Systematic review: comparative effectiveness and safety of oral medications for type 2 diabetes mellitus. Ann Intern Med. 2007;147:386–99.

Boulton AJM, Vinik AI, Arezzo JC et al. Diabetic neuropathies. Diabetes Care. 2005;28:956–62.

Butalia S, Palda VA, Sargeant RJ et al. Does this patient with diabetes have osteomyelitis of the lower extremity? JAMA. 2008;299:806–13.

England JD, Gronseth GS, Franklin G et al. Distal symmetric polyneuropathy: a definition for clinical research. Neurology. 2005;64:199–207.

Holman RR, Paul SK, Bethel A et al. 10-year follow up of intensive glucose control in type 2 diabetes. N Engl J Med. 2008;359:1577–89.

Inzucchi SE. Diagnosis of diabetes. N Engl J Med. 2012;367:542–50.

Inzucchi SE, Bergenstal RM, Buse JB et al. Management of hyperglycemia in type 2 diabetes: a patient centered approach. Diabetes Care. 2012;35:1364–79.

Ismail-Beigi F. Glycemic management of type 2 diabetes mellitus. N Engl J Med. 2012;366:1319–27.

Ismail-Beigi F, Moghissi E, Tiktin M et al. Individualizing glycemic targets in type 2 diabetes mellitus: implications of recent clinical trials. Ann Intern Med. 2011;154:554–9.

Kapoor A, Page S, LaValley M et al. Magnetic resonance imaging for diagnosing foot osteomyelitis. Arch Intern Med. 2007;167:125–32.

Kitabchi AE, Umpierrez GE, Miles JM, Fisher JN. Hyperglycemic crises in adult patients with diabetes. Diabetes Care. 2009;32:1335–43.

Lipsky BA, Berendt AR, Cornia PB et al. 2012 Infectious Diseases Society of America clinical practice guideline for the diagnosis and treatment of diabetic foot infections. Clin Infect Dis. 2012;54:132–73.

Mohamed Q, Gillies MC, Wong TY. Management of diabetic retinopathy: a systematic review. JAMA. 2007;298:902–16.

The Action to Control Cardiovascular Risk in Diabetes Study Group. Effects of intensive glucose lowering in type 2 DM. N Engl J Med. 2008;358:2545–59.

The ADVANCE Collaborative Group. Intensive blood glucose control and vascular outcomes in patients with type 2 diabetes. N Engl J Med. 2008;358:2560–72.

The Diabetes Control and Complications Trial Research Group. The effect of intensive treatment of diabetes on the development and progression of long-term complication in insulin-dependent diabetes mellitus. N Engl J Med. 1993;329:977–86.

UK Prospective Diabetes Study (UKPDS) Group. Intensive blood-glucose control with sulphonylureas or insulin compared with conventional treatment and risk of complications in patients with type 2 diabetes. (UKPDS 34) UK Prospective Diabetes Study Group. Lancet. 1998;352:837–53.

13

I have a patient with acute diarrhea. How do I determine the cause?

CHIEF COMPLAINT

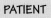

PATIENT 1

Mr. C is a 35-year-old man who comes to your outpatient office complaining of 1 day of diarrhea.

 What is the differential diagnosis of diarrhea? How would you frame the differential?

CONSTRUCTING A DIFFERENTIAL DIAGNOSIS

Clinically, it is probably most useful to define acute diarrhea as diarrhea (bowel movements of a looser consistency than usual that occur more than 3 times a day) that develops over a period of 1–2 days and lasts for less than 4 weeks. The differential diagnosis below uses pivotal points in a patient's presenting symptoms to organize potential diagnoses into 3 categories: noninfectious, gastroenteritis, and infectious colitis. Noninfectious diarrhea is recognized by the lack of constitutional symptoms. Infectious diarrhea that presents with large volume (often watery) stool, constitutional symptoms, nausea and vomiting, and often abdominal cramps can be categorized as gastroenteritis. Infectious colitis presents with fever, tenesmus, and dysentery (stools with blood and mucus). This structure is easy to remember, focuses history taking, allows prognosticating, and is also a good framework on which to consider therapy. Figure 13-1 uses this framework to suggest therapy.

A. Noninfectious diarrhea
1. Medications and other ingestible substances (some with osmotic effect)
   a. Sorbitol (gum, mints, pill fillers)
   b. Mannitol
   c. Fructose (fruits, soft drinks)
   d. Fiber (bran, fruits, vegetables)
   e. Lactulose
2. Magnesium-containing medications
   a. Nutritional supplements
   b. Antacids
   c. Laxatives
3. Malabsorption
   a. Lactose intolerance
   b. Pancreatitis
4. Medications causing diarrhea through nonosmotic means
   a. Metformin
   b. Antibiotics

c. Colchicine
d. Digoxin
e. Selective serotonin reuptake inhibitor antidepressants

B. Infectious diarrhea: gastroenteritis
1. Viral (most common)
   a. Caliciviruses (including Norovirus)
   b. Rotovirus
2. Bacterial
   a. *Vibrio cholera*
   b. *Escherichia coli*
   c. *Shigella* species
   d. *Salmonella* species
   e. *Campylobacter* species
   f. *Yersinia enterocolitica*
3. Toxin-mediated
   a. *Staphylococcus aureus*
   b. *Clostridium perfringens*
   c. *Bacillus cereus*

C. Infectious diarrhea: inflammatory colitis
1. *Shigella* species
2. *E coli*
3. *Campylobacter* species
4. *Salmonella* species
5. *Y enterocolitica*
6. *Clostridium difficile*
7. *Klebsiella oxytoca*

 1

The first symptom the patient noted was loss of appetite while eating breakfast. He was unable to finish his usual cup of coffee and a bowl of cereal. During his 20-minute drive to work he developed nausea and diaphoresis. Upon arriving at work he developed low-grade fever, abdominal cramping, and vomiting. Over the next 12 hours, diarrhea developed. He describes the stool being watery and brown without any blood.

 At this point, what is the leading hypothesis, what are the active alternatives, and is there a must not miss diagnosis? Given this differential diagnosis, what tests should be ordered?

217

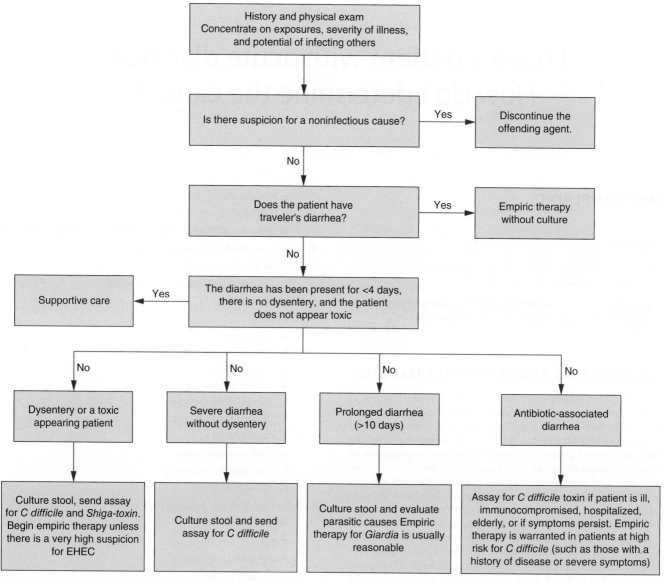

EHEC, enterohemorrhagic *escherichia coli*.

Figure 13-1. Diagnostic approach: diarrhea.

RANKING THE DIFFERENTIAL DIAGNOSIS

The pivotal point in this case presentation is the acute onset of watery diarrhea. The early predominance of nausea will also help in making a diagnosis. This presentation certainly speaks for an infectious cause. The low-grade fever and absence of dysentery make it likely that the diagnosis is in the category of gastroenteritis. Table 13-1 lists the differential diagnosis.

Mr. C is otherwise in good health. He reports no recent illnesses or antibiotic exposures. There have been no recent

(continued)

changes in his diet and he has eaten only food prepared at home for the last week. He lives with his wife and reports no known sick contacts. He works as a bus driver. He has not traveled out of New York City, where he lives and works.

The physical exam is notable for temperature, 38.2°C; BP is 110/80 mm Hg and pulse is 100 bpm while lying down; BP is 90/72 mm Hg and pulse is 126 bpm while standing; RR, 12 breaths per minute. Sclera and conjunctiva are normal. The abdomen is soft and diffusely tender with hyperactive bowel sounds. The rectal exam shows brown, heme-negative stool.

 Is the clinical information sufficient to make a diagnosis? If not, what other information do you need?

Table 13-1. Diagnostic hypotheses for Mr. C.

Diagnostic Hypotheses	Demographics, Risk Factors, Symptoms and Signs	Important Tests
Leading Hypothesis		
Norovirus virus	Hyperacute onset Vomiting usually present	Resolution in 24–48 hours
Active Alternatives		
Toxin-mediated gastroenteritis, such as *Staphylococcus aureus*	Common food poisoning Onset 1–8 hours after exposure Vomiting is predominant	Rapid resolution, within 12 hours
Bacterial gastroenteritis, such as *Salmonella* infection	Usually food-borne Fairly specific clinical syndromes High fevers possible	Stool cultures can be diagnostic
Other Alternative		
Rotavirus	Contact with children Vomiting common and constitutional signs present	Resolution in 24–72 hours

Leading Hypothesis: Norovirus

Textbook Presentation

Acute vomiting is usually the presenting symptom. The onset of diarrhea follows the vomiting. Mild abdominal cramping is common. Low-grade fever is common. All symptoms resolve completely by 3 days.

Disease Highlights

A. Caliciviruses, of which Norovirus and closely related viruses such as Sapovirus are the most common, account for about 80% of adult viral gastroenteritis.

B. Most commonly occurs in winter.

C. Transmission

1. Norovirus is easily transmissible via the fecal-oral route, in air-borne droplets, via food, and through fomites.

2. Norovirus is probably the most common cause of food-borne diarrhea.

3. Attack rates as high as 50% have been documented.

D. Incubation period is 1–2 days.

Evidence-Based Diagnosis

There are no diagnostic tests for norovirus available for routine clinical use; diagnosis is made by clinical presentation.

Treatment

A. Supportive care

1. Most patients with acute diarrhea require only supportive care. Supportive care is meant to provide rehydration and symptom relief.

2. Rehydration

   a. Oral rehydration is generally sufficient.

   b. For patients with mild diarrhea and little volume depletion, any oral fluids are appropriate rehydration. (Sports drinks, Pedialyte, and chicken soup are commonly prescribed.)

   c. For patients with more significant volume depletion, oral rehydration solutions should contain NaCl, KCl, HCO_3 or citrate, and glucose. The World Health Organization oral rehydration solution has the following composition:

   (1) Sodium: 75 mmol/L

   (2) Chloride: 65 mmol/L

   (3) Glucose: 75 mmol/L

   (4) Potassium: 20 mmol/L

   (5) Citrate: 10 mmol/L

   d. If this solution is not available, patients can be instructed to mix the following in 1 L of water

   (1) One-half teaspoon of salt

   (2) One-quarter teaspoon of baking soda

   (3) 8 teaspoons of sugar

   e. In patients who cannot tolerate oral rehydration or who are very volume depleted, IV fluids (lactated Ringer solution or normal saline) are indicated.

3. Antidiarrheals (such as loperamide) are safe and effective for patients without dysentery. Using antidiarrheals in a patient with dysentery is not considered safe because evidence suggests they can:

   a. Cause prolonged fever

   b. Cause toxic megacolon and perforation

   c. Possibly increase the risk of hemolytic uremic syndrome (HUS) in patients with *Shiga* toxin–producing *E coli* (STEC).

4. Antiemetics

5. Diet

   a. BRAT diet (banana, rice, applesauce, toast) is often recommended.

   b. Dairy products should be avoided. (See discussion below).

B. Antimicrobial therapy

1. Treatment other than supportive care is not necessary for norovirus-like illnesses.

2. Empiric antimicrobial therapy is recommended for diarrheal infections only in limited circumstances. These circumstances never occur in patients with noninfectious diarrhea and almost never in patients with gastroenteritis. Specific circumstances are discussed throughout the chapter; general circumstances include the following:

   a. Dysentery

   b. Severe disease (profuse diarrhea with hypovolemia, high fever, severe abdominal pain, high band count)

   c. High suspicion for *C difficile*

   d. Travelers' diarrhea

 Empiric antimicrobial therapy for diarrhea is reasonable for patients with severe symptoms.

MAKING A DIAGNOSIS

At the time of the patient's visit he was beginning to feel better. He still noted an "upset stomach" and was having soft watery diarrhea every 2–3 hours. He had not had any vomiting in about 6 hours and was able to tolerate fluids.

Have you crossed a diagnostic threshold for the leading hypothesis, Norovirus? Have you ruled out the active alternatives? Do other tests need to be done to exclude the alternative diagnoses?

Most patients with acute diarrhea do not need diagnostic testing as the illness usually resolves without treatment and work up is usually unrewarding. (A detailed discussion of when evaluation is necessary appears in case 2). Data that support this are that only 2–12% of stool cultures are positive and 0.4–0.7% of tests for ova and parasites are positive in preselected populations. Patients and settings that indicate need for evaluation include:

A. Patients with bloody diarrhea (tests should include assay for *Shiga* toxin and *C difficile* toxin).

B. If an outbreak is suspected.

C. Patients at high risk for infecting others.
   1. Residents of long-term–care facilities
   2. Daycare workers
   3. Food service workers
   4. Healthcare workers

D. Patients with severe disease (dehydration, toxic appearance) or risk factors for poor outcome (immunosuppression, severe comorbid illnesses).

E. Patients with prolonged diarrhea (> 7 days) should be tested for parasitic causes (stool for ova and parasites).

Mr. C present is presenting with a clinical syndrome that is consistent with viral gastroenteritis. By recognizing this syndrome, you are able to reassure him that he should be better in the next 24–48 hours. Even if a diagnostic test for norovirus were available for routine use, the usefulness would be low because treatment is only supportive.

In most patients with an acute diarrheal illness, diagnostic testing is not helpful to the patient but may be important from a public health standpoint.

Alternative Diagnosis: Toxin-Mediated Gastroenteritis

Textbook Presentation

The presentation of this syndrome, most commonly caused by *S aureus* or *C perfringens,* usually includes acute-onset vomiting and crampy abdominal pain. Vomiting is the predominant symptom with diarrhea being mild and watery and fever being low grade. Because of the very short lag between ingestion and illness (2–8 hours), the culpable meal is usually the last one eaten. Recovery is very rapid (12–48 hours).

Disease Highlights

A. Toxin-mediated gastroenteritis (often referred to as food poisoning) is not an infection – it occurs when a preformed toxin, produced by bacteria, is ingested.

B. *S aureus, C perfringens,* or *B cereus* are the most common causes.

C. Although these organisms are the most common causes of food poisoning, they account for only about 1% of food-borne diarrheal illnesses.
   1. Viral causes probably account for most food-borne infections.
   2. *Salmonella, Campylobacter, and E coli* are the most common bacterial causes of food-borne infections.
   3. Table 13-2 presents recent data on the incidence of food-borne illnesses.

D. *S aureus, C perfringens,* and *B cereus* can often be recognized by the clinical and exposure history. Table 13-3 describes the clinical syndromes of these infections.

Illnesses presenting with the acute onset of vomiting and constitutional symptoms, often with abdominal cramping, are usually caused by viruses or bacteria that elaborate toxins.

Evidence-Based Diagnosis

A. There are no diagnostic tests for toxin-mediated gastroenteritis available for routine clinical use.

B. Toxin-mediated gastroenteritis should be considered in any patient with acute gastrointestinal symptoms and recent, suspect food intake.

Treatment

Treatment is supportive care.

Table 13-2. Causes of food-borne illness in the United States.

Organism	Estimated Annual Number of Cases[1]	% Infections that are Food-Borne
Norovirus	5.46 million	26
Salmonella	1.02 million	94
Campylobacter	850,000	80
EHEC	180,000	76
Shigella	130,000	31
Giardia	80,000	7
Cryptosporidium	60,000	8
Vibrio	50,000	65
Staphylococcus	240,000	100
Clostridium	970,000	100

[1] Rounded to nearest 10,000.
EHEC, enterohemorrhagic *Escherichia coli.*

Table 13-3. Clinical syndromes of toxin-mediated gastroenteritis.

Organism	Pathogenesis	Incubation	Source	Clinical Syndrome
Staphylococcus aureus	Preformed toxin	1–6 hours	Protein rich food	Acute onset Vomiting predominant Resolves within 2 hours
Clostridium perfringens	Elaborated toxin	8–16 hours	Meats	Diarrhea with abdominal cramping Lasts 1–2 days
Bacillus cereus	Preformed toxin	1–6 hours	Grains	Very similar to *S aureus*

Alternative Diagnosis: Gastroenteritis Caused by *Salmonella* Species

Textbook Presentation

The onset of disease is usually subacute with nausea, fever, and diarrhea. Fever and nausea often resolve over 1–2 days while diarrhea persists for 5–7 days. Patients usually have watery diarrhea with 6–8 bowel movements each day. Salmonella gastroenteritis may cause higher fevers than viral or preformed toxin disease. Dysentery may occur.

Disease Highlights

A. *Salmonella* species cause 3 major types of disease.

   1. Diarrheal illnesses

      a. Gastroenteritis

      b. Dysentery (discussed later in the chapter)

   2. Bacteremia

      a. Bacteremia develops in ~5% of patients.

      b. Usually a complication of gastroenteritis.

      c. Endovascular infections and osteomyelitis may complicate bacteremia.

   3. Typhoid fever

      a. A systemic illness characterized by fever and abdominal pain caused by *Salmonella typhi.*

      b. Typhoid fever is distinct from gastroenteritis, which is caused by non-typhi *Salmonella* species.

      c. Although not generally considered a diarrheal illness, some patients have diarrhea as a predominant symptom.

      d. Although typhoid fever is a major problem worldwide, it is seen predominantly in the United States in unvaccinated travelers.

         (1) Recent data show that 79% of American patients with typhoid had returned from foreign travel within the previous 30 days.

         (2) Only 5% of the patients had received the typhoid vaccine.

      e. Typhoid fever should be considered in the differential diagnosis of a traveler with a febrile illness.

B. Gastroenteritis is the most common *Salmonella*-related disease in the United States. The estimated annual incidence of *Salmonella* is 1.23 million cases.

C. *Salmonella* is transmitted by:

   1. Food

      a. Eggs and poultry are most common sources.

      b. There are reports of infection from almost any type of food.

   2. Fecal-oral contact with infected patients

      a. Person-to-person transmission is less common than infection from contaminated food.

      b. Bacteria commonly remain in the stool for 4–5 weeks after infection.

   3. Animals also carry salmonella (reptiles most classically).

Evidence-Based Diagnosis

A. The gold standard for diagnosis of salmonella gastroenteritis remains stool culture.

B. There are tests with greater sensitivity, but none are used in routine clinical practice.

Treatment

A. Prevention: Because salmonella is heat sensitive, cooking food well and good hand washing practices prevent most infections.

B. Treatment

   1. Most salmonella infections require no treatment.

   2. The patients who should receive therapy beyond supportive care are those who have

      a. Severe disease (dehydration, dysentery, high fever)

      b. Immunocompromised status, including patients older than 65 years

      c. Elevated risk of focal infection

         (1) Bacteremia

         (2) Prosthetic joints or hardware

         (3) Sickle cell anemia

      d. Typhoid fever

   3. Although most patients shed bacteria for weeks after infection, antibiotics should not be used in attempts to prevent transmission. Antibiotics do not shorten the duration of carriage and may prolong it.

CASE RESOLUTION

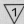

Mr. C was sent home with directions for oral rehydration. He reported sleeping for most of the afternoon and was well enough to return to work the next day. By the following day (day 4 of the presentation), the patient was completely better. He reported that none of his close contacts became ill.

The patient's symptoms lasted 48–72 hours. He required no specific therapy. There were no suspicious food exposures and nobody else became ill. The case is consistent with a viral gastroenteritis such as that caused by norovirus. The lack of a suspicious diet history makes a toxin-induced food-borne illness (food poisoning) less likely.

FOLLOW-UP OF MR. C

Two weeks later Mr. C comes to see you again. He attributes his recovery to antibiotics that he took on the day he saw you. (The antibiotics were left over from a prescription he was given for a dental infection). About 5 days after his recovery, he began to feel poorly again. For the last 10 days he has had diarrhea, abdominal bloating, and belching. He denies fever, chills, nausea, vomiting, or tenesmus. There has been no blood in his stool.

At this point, what is the leading hypothesis, what are the active alternatives, and is there a must not miss diagnosis? Given this differential diagnosis, what tests should be ordered?

RANKING THE DIFFERENTIAL DIAGNOSIS

The pivotal point in this presentation is the duration of the symptoms: 10 days. Other important features are the recent infectious gastrointestinal illness and recent exposure to antibiotics.

Because 10 days is prolonged when considering acute infectious diarrhea, noninfectious causes should be considered. Both the duration of symptoms and the recent gastroenteritis should raise the possibility of lactose intolerance. Lactose intolerance is common after gastroenteritis due to injury to the small bowel mucosa. Other potential diagnoses include recurrent gastroenteritis or antibiotic-associated diarrhea. Recurrent infectious gastroenteritis can occur since many of the bacteria that cause diarrhea can persist in the stool after clinical symptoms have resolved. This prolonged bacterial shedding also accounts for spread of the illness. This is especially common with *Salmonella* and *Campylobacter*. Antibiotic-associated diarrhea is another common entity, complicating between 2% and 25% of courses of antibiotics. The level of risk varies with the specific antibiotic. The prolonged nature of the illness should prompt consideration of the less typical pathogens, such as parasites; could our initial diagnosis have been incorrect? Table 13-4 lists the differential diagnosis.

The patient describes 3–4 soft bowel movements a day. He also has abdominal discomfort. There is no real pain, but there is bloating and belching. He says he goes to the bathroom 3 or 4 additional times each day just to pass gas.

The patient took 3 doses of amoxicillin on the day he first came to see you. He ran out after these 3 doses. He has not traveled since his infection and does not note any unusual exposures. He reports that his diet has been a little more simple than usual with a lot of cereal, rice, potatoes, and milk to "soothe his stomach."

Is the clinical information sufficient to make a diagnosis? If not, what other information do you need?

Table 13-4. Diagnostic hypotheses for Mr. C's repeat visit.

Diagnostic Hypotheses	Demographics, Risk Factors, Symptoms and Signs	Important Tests
Leading Hypothesis		
Lactose intolerance	Ethnic predisposition Recent illness Relation to diet	Resolution with dietary changes
Active Alternatives		
Antibiotic-associated diarrhea	Only caused by *Clostridium difficile* about 15–20% of time	Usually resolves with discontinuation of antibiotic Specific tests for *C difficile* toxin
Recurrent infection	Similar symptoms as initial illness Most common with bacterial pathogen	Stool cultures
Other Alternative		
Parasitic infection	Exposure history common (often with travel) Consider especially in immunosuppressed patients	Stool ova and parasites may be diagnostic

Leading Hypothesis: Lactose Intolerance

Textbook Presentation

Lactose intolerance commonly presents as chronic symptoms of belching, bloating, flatulence, diarrhea, or abdominal pain in a person of susceptible ethnic background. The symptoms may be subacute or acute in the setting of infection or dietary changes. A suspicious dietary history should be present.

Disease Highlights

A. Most mammals become lactose intolerant after weaning. It is thought that some ethnicities evolved persistent lactase activity because of the importance of milk products as a calorie source in their environments.

B. Lactose intolerance is thus very common and predictable by ethnic background. It also worsens with age.

C. Episodes of small bowel infection can cause transient lactose intolerance. This is more common in people with low levels of lactase activity at baseline.

It is common to see transient lactose intolerance after episodes of gastroenteritis.

D. Ethnic groups and native populations most likely to have low levels of lactase activity come from the following regions:

1. Middle East and Mediterranean

2. East Asia

3. Africa

4. Native American

E. Milk, ice cream, and yogurt have the highest levels of lactose.

F. Foods with high lactose and low fat (skim milk) tend to cause the most symptoms as these foods deliver lactose to the small intestine the fastest.

Evidence-Based Diagnosis

A. The diagnosis of lactose intolerance is generally a clinical one based on a suspicious history, in a patient with a susceptible background, whose symptoms resolve on a lactose-free diet.

B. More definitive tests, the lactose tolerance test or lactose breath hydrogen test, can be performed in patients in whom the diagnosis is likely but not clear historically.

Treatment

A. In general, lactose intolerance is treated by decreasing lactose intake.

B. Because people have variable levels of lactase activity, levels of tolerance differ from person to person.

C. Enzyme supplements are often helpful.

D. In acquired illness (eg, post gastroenteritis), lactase levels will eventually recover when the intestinal brush border regenerates.

E. Because of the high prevalence of mild lactose intolerance and the frequent exacerbation following gastroenteritis, patients with acute gastroenteritis should be advised to avoid dairy products for 2 weeks after recovery.

MAKING A DIAGNOSIS

On exam he appears well. Vital signs are all normal. His abdominal exam reveals hyperactive bowel sounds with minimal distention. It is soft and nontender. Rectal exam reveals soft, brown, heme-negative stool.

Have you crossed a diagnostic threshold for the leading hypothesis, lactose intolerance? Have you ruled out the active alternatives? Do other tests need to be done to exclude the alternative diagnoses?

The patient does not appear to have an infectious cause of his diarrhea—at least not a bacterial or viral cause. This fact makes recurrence of his previous infection very unlikely. Antibiotic-associated diarrhea or diarrhea caused by a parasitic infection are still possible.

Alternative Diagnosis: Antibiotic-Associated Diarrhea

Textbook Presentation

Patients with antibiotic-associated diarrhea usually have symptoms of gastroenteritis or dysentery during antibiotic therapy. Upper abdominal symptoms of nausea and vomiting are rare.

Disease Highlights

A. There are really 2 distinct types of antibiotic-associated diarrhea: diarrhea related to an enteric pathogen (primarily *C difficile*) and diarrhea related to other effects of antibiotics.

B. Although any antibiotic can be associated with antibiotic-associated diarrhea, those most commonly responsible for both types of diarrhea are:

1. Clindamycin
2. Cephalosporins
3. Ampicillin, amoxicillin, and amoxicillin-clavulanate

C. *C difficile*

1. Accounts for 10–20% of antibiotic-associated diarrhea
2. *C difficile* causes diarrhea via toxin-mediated effects on the large bowel. This can present as severe diarrhea, often with symptoms of colonic inflammation and a high WBC count.
3. Risk factors for *C difficile* include advanced age, hospitalization, and exposure to antibiotics.
4. *C difficile* has been reported up to 6 months after a course of antibiotics.
5. The incidence of community-acquired *C difficile* is rising. This may be related to increasing use of antibiotics as well as, possibly, to proton pump inhibitors and nonsteroidal antiinflammatory drugs.
6. Recent reports also speak to the increasing severity of *C difficile* related to changes in the genetics dictating toxin production.

D. *K oxytoca*

1. Newly recognized cytotoxin-producing bacteria capable of causing antibiotic-associated hemorrhagic colitis.
2. Much less common than *C difficile*.

E. Patients with antibiotic-associated diarrhea not related to *C difficile* usually have mild disease that occurs either during or immediately after a course of antibiotics. Possible causes of this type of diarrhea are numerous:

1. Change in intestinal flora
2. Nonantimicrobial effect of antibiotics such as the promotility effects of erythromycin
3. Enteric infections other than *C difficile*

Evidence-Based Diagnosis

A. Certain features make the diagnosis of antibiotic-associated diarrhea not associated with *C difficile* likely.

1. History of previous antibiotic-associated diarrhea not associated with *C difficile*.
2. Mild to moderate symptoms

B. *C difficile* colitis

1. Diagnosed by identification of either the toxin in the stool or by demonstration of the classic pseudomembranous colitis on endoscopy.
2. Culture, although highly sensitive and specific, is not frequently used because it is slow and because there are nontoxin-producing strains of *C difficile* that are not clinically important.
3. Polymerase chain reaction (PCR) has become the diagnostic standard: sensitivity, ≥ 90%; specificity, ≥ 97%.

C. If a clinical syndrome consistent with *C difficile* colitis persists despite negative PCR, sigmoidoscopic exam of the colon is recommended. If symptoms do not resolve and evaluation for *C difficile* is negative, stool cultures to rule out another antibiotic-associated enteric infection are reasonable.

Treatment

A. Antibiotic-associated diarrhea not related to *C difficile* infection usually resolves with discontinuation of antibiotics. Other useful treatments include:

   1. Probiotic agents reduce the risk of antibiotic-associated diarrhea and probably shorten an episode once it has occurred.

   2. Antidiarrheals

B. The treatment of *C difficile* is as follows:

   1. Avoid antidiarrheals

   2. When possible, patients with *C difficile* infection should discontinue the causative antibiotic.

   3. Infection control practices should be instituted to limit spread of the infection.

   4. Antibiotics

   a. First-line therapy for patients without severe disease is oral metronidazole. This is the case for an initial infection or a recurrence.

   b. First-line therapy for severe disease is oral vancomycin. For patients with the most severe disease, IV vancomycin can be added to oral vancomycin. Intracolonic vancomycin has been used in patients with severe ileus.

   c. Vancomycin is also suggested for patients with a second recurrence.

   d. Surgical therapy (colectomy) is sometimes necessary for patients with perforation, toxic megacolon, or severe ileus.

   5. Relapse complicates 20–25% of cases of treated *C difficile*.

   6. Treatment with donor feces, given by enema or nasojejunal infusion has been shown to be effective in patients with multiple relapses.

Alternative Diagnosis: *Giardia lamblia*

Textbook Presentation

Giardiasis can present as either acute or chronic diarrhea. It usually occurs in patients with exposure to infected water supplies, although person-to-person transmission can occur. Symptoms usually include diarrhea, nausea, abdominal cramps, bloating, flatulence, and foul-smelling stools.

Disease Highlights

A. *Giardia* is the most common parasitic cause of diarrhea in the United States.

B. Most infections in the United States result from ingestion of contaminated water (from streams and lakes).

C. Cases most commonly occur in children age 1–9 or adults age 30–39.

D. Incidence peaks annually during the summer and early fall when people most commonly participate in water sports and camping.

E. Although usually sporadic, there are occasional outbreaks related to contamination of bodies of water used for recreation and drinking supplies.

F. Common symptoms

   1. Diarrhea occurs in 96% of cases.

   2. Weight loss is present in 62% of cases.

   3. Abdominal cramps occur in 61% of cases.

   4. Greasy stools are present in 57% of cases.

   5. Belching, flatulence, and foul-smelling stools are commonly reported.

G. Fever is uncommon.

H. Chronic infection occurs in about 10% of untreated patients.

I. If evaluation for *Giardia* is negative and there is no response to empiric therapy, other organisms should also be considered.

   1. This is especially true in patients who are immunocompromised.

   2. Other organisms that may cause disease are:

   a. *Cryptosporidium*

   b. *Cyclospora cayetanensis*

   c. *Isospora belli*

Evidence-Based Diagnosis

A. *G lamblia*

   1. Sensitivity of stool ova and parasites for *Giardia* is 50–70% for 1 stool sample.

   2. Sensitivity is over 90% for 3 samples.

   3. Antigen assays sensitive to over 90%.

B. Other organisms

   1. *Cryptosporidium* can be identified on stool antigen assay.

   2. *C cayetanensis* and *I belli* can be identified on acid-fast stain.

Treatment

A. The treatment of choice for *G lamblia* infection is oral metronidazole.

B. Empiric therapy is often recommended.

CASE RESOLUTION

A lactose-free diet was recommended for the patient. PCR for *C difficile* was negative. The suspicion for a recurrent bacterial infection or a parasitic infection was very low.

The patient began a lactose-free diet and was better within 3 days. After 2 weeks, he slowly reintroduced his usual diet without symptoms.

CHIEF COMPLAINT

PATIENT 2

Ms. V is a 45-year-old woman who comes to see you in the office; she complains of 4 days of diarrhea. She reports feeling tired and weak. She is moving her bowels about 6–8 times a day. She says that she has significant abdominal pain. She came in today because she has begun to pass bloody stools.

On physical exam, her vital signs are temperature, 38.3°C; BP, 130/84 mm Hg; pulse, 90 bpm; RR, 12 breaths per minute. She is orthostatic.

Her abdomen has hyperactive bowel sounds. It is diffusely tender, without peritoneal signs. Her stool is a mixture of soft brown stool and blood.

At this point, what is the leading hypothesis, what are the active alternatives, and is there a must not miss diagnosis? Given this differential diagnosis, what tests should be ordered?

Ranking the Differential Diagnosis

The pivotal points in this case are the presence of bloody stools, abdominal pain, and fever. This symptom complex makes diarrhea caused by a bacterial infection likely. The organisms that commonly cause bloody diarrhea are *Shigella* species, *Campylobacter* species, and *E coli*. *Salmonella* species, *Y enterocolitica,* and *C difficile* also may cause bloody diarrhea. Noninfectious causes, such as ischemia or ulcerative colitis, should also be considered.

Clinically, it is impossible to differentiate between the different causes of bacterial diarrhea. That said, it is important to know organisms' recognizable symptom complexes because these can give clues to the causative organism and guide empiric therapy. Table 13-5 lists the differential diagnosis.

Table 13-5. Diagnostic hypotheses for Ms. V.

Diagnostic Hypotheses	Demographics, Risk Factors, Symptoms and Signs	Important Tests
Leading Hypothesis		
Bacterial diarrhea caused by *Campylobacter* infection	Constitutional prodrome Diarrhea with significant abdominal pain Occasional dysentery	Stool culture
Active Alternative		
Bacterial diarrhea, caused by infection with *Shigella* species	Varies by species but classically colonic predominant symptoms—dysentery	Stool culture High bandemia common
Active Alternatives—Must Not Miss		
Bacterial diarrhea, caused by infection with *Shiga* toxin–producing *Escherichia coli* O157	Diarrhea, usually bloody Fever uncommon Right-sided abdominal pain	Culture and toxin assay
Other Alternative		
Ulcerative colitis	Usually subacute to chronic	Endoscopic diagnosis

The patient's first symptoms, 4 days ago, were fever and lethargy. She felt terrible for the entire day and thought she was getting the flu. The following day, she began to have diarrhea and diffuse abdominal pain. Two days later, the day she comes to your office, she began to have blood in her stool.

She reports that her husband is also sick with similar symptoms. His diarrhea developed the day before hers did but he has not noticed blood in his stool. He refused to come in because he figured it was "just a virus."

Is the clinical information sufficient to make a diagnosis? If not, what other information do you need?

Leading Hypothesis: *Campylobacter* Infection

Textbook Presentation

Presenting symptoms of *Campylobacter* infection are usually diarrhea and abdominal pain. The diarrhea is often profuse and watery and associated abdominal pain can be severe, sometimes mimicking appendicitis. The fever usually resolves over the first 2 days of the illness, while the diarrhea and abdominal pain may last 4–6 days.

Disease Highlights

A. *Campylobacter* species are among the most commonly isolated pathogens in patients with diarrhea and are a common cause of bloody stool.

B. The incidence of *Campylobacter* diarrhea is generally about 13/100,000 persons with about 2.4 million persons affected each year.

C. In 1 recent study of patients arriving at emergency departments with bloody diarrhea, the breakdown of diagnoses were:
  1. *Shigella* in 15.3% of patients
  2. *Campylobacter* in 6.2% of patients
  3. *Salmonella* in 5.2% of patients
  4. *Shiga* toxin–producing *E coli* in 2.6% of patients
  5. Other cause in 1.6% of patients

D. Common aspects of the presentation are
  1. Constitutional symptoms before gastrointestinal disease
  2. Bloody diarrhea beginning after 2–3 days of watery diarrhea

E. *Campylobacter* infection can (rarely) be associated with extraintestinal complications.
  1. Reactive arthritis
  2. Guillain-Barré syndrome

F. Bacteria commonly remain in the stool for 4–5 weeks and reinfection can occur.

Evidence-Based Diagnosis

A. Although stool cultures are most likely to be negative (even in patients with bloody diarrhea), they can be useful in some circumstances.
  1. *Campylobacter* and *Shigella* infections clearly benefit from treatment.

2. Inappropriate treatment of salmonella (treating mild or moderate non-typhi infection) is not helpful and may lead to prolonged carriage.

3. Culture results can be very useful from a public health standpoint.

B. Stool cultures are the only way to distinguish organisms as many studies of the clinical characteristics of patients with diagnostic stool cultures demonstrate the overlap of the clinical syndromes.

 Even organisms that are generally considered to be common causes of dysentery (*Shigella, Campylobacter, Salmonella*) are at least as likely to cause non-bloody diarrhea and a gastroenteritis-type illness.

C. The decision making regarding whether to send stool cultures considers ways to increase the yield of the cultures (both in terms of positive results and clinical utility). Consider the following questions:

1. Is there a clinical suspicion for a specific disease that requires treatment?

   a. Severely ill patient (fever, dysentery, abdominal pain); about 30% of patients with dysentery have positive cultures (compared with 1–6% of all patients).

   b. Suspicious exposure (travel, high-risk sexual behavior, antibiotics)

      (1) Traveler's diarrhea (usually *E coli*) can usually be treated empirically.

      (2) Other infections associated with travel (*Entamoeba histolytica, G lamblia*) benefit from treatment.

2. Does the patient have an underlying disease that makes treatment more necessary?

   (1) Immunosuppression

   (2) Inflammatory bowel disease

3. Are there public health reasons that a diagnosis needs to be made?

   (1) Possible outbreak of food-borne illness

   (2) Patient might potentially spread disease (healthcare worker, daycare worker, food handler).

4. Is there a reason not to culture?

   (1) Stool cultures and ova and parasite exams of patients in whom diarrhea develops after being hospitalized for another cause are particularly unrevealing.

   (2) Consider limiting in-hospital cultures to the following circumstances:

      (a) Onset of diarrhea within 3 days of admission

      (b) Onset > 3 days but

         (i) Patient is older than 65 years and has comorbidities.

         (ii) Patient has HIV infection.

         (iii) Neutropenia is present.

         (iv) Extraintestinal manifestations are present.

         (v) There is an outbreak of diarrhea in the hospital.

   (3) Testing for *C difficile* as a cause of diarrhea in the hospital is always appropriate.

D. Patients with more severe clinical presentations, including high fever, abdominal pain, and dysentery, should always have stool cultures sent.

E. Diagnostic tests other than stool cultures are useful in certain situations.

1. *C difficile* toxin for patients exposed to antibiotics or proton pump inhibitors

2. *Shiga* toxin to identify enterohemorrhagic *E coli* (EHEC) in all patients with bloody diarrhea

3. Fecal leukocytes may be helpful in deciding which patients are more likely to have positive stool cultures.

   a. Sensitivity, 73%; specificity, 84%

   b. LR+, 4.56; LR–, 0.32

4. WBC

   a. WBC is neither sensitive nor specific for the presence of invasive bacterial infections.

   b. A marked left shift, at least if the band count is > neutrophil count, suggests bacterial etiology in general and *Shigella* in particular.

Treatment

A. Severe diarrhea with blood should be treated empirically while cultures are pending.

B. Empiric therapy is generally with a quinolone.

C. Some very important caveats should be kept in mind when empirically treating suspected bacterial diarrhea or dysentery.

1. Antibiotics shorten the course of diarrhea caused by *Shigella* and *Campylobacter*.

2. There is quinolone resistance in some strains of *Campylobacter*, so empiric therapy should be broadened to include a macrolide if the suspicion for *Campylobacter* is high or if the patient is very ill.

3. Antibiotics should probably be withheld if the patient is at high risk for EHEC (see below).

4. Antibiotics are only beneficial for salmonella infections in the case of typhoid or severe disease.

 Remember that antidiarrheals should never be used for patients with dysentery or signs of invasive infection (tenesmus, blood or mucus in stool, high fever, and severe abdominal pain).

MAKING A DIAGNOSIS

 The patient is given IV fluids in the office. After receiving acetaminophen and 2 L of fluid she is feeling somewhat better. Stool cultures are sent. A CBC and Chem-7 are normal.

 Have you crossed a diagnostic threshold for the leading hypothesis, *Campylobacter* infection? Have you ruled out the active alternatives? Do other tests need to be done to exclude the alternative diagnoses?

Alternative Diagnosis: *Shigella* Infection

Textbook Presentation

Shigella infection often begins with fever and constitutional symptoms. Diarrhea is initially watery and may become bloody. The diarrhea can be very frequent. Tenesmus is often prominent.

Disease Highlights

A. Although there is a spectrum of disease (some *Shigella* species can cause milder disease), a patient who is systemically ill with classic dysentery (frequent bloody stools with tenesmus) is most likely to have *Shigella* infection.

B. Incidence is estimated at about 6 cases/100,000 people.

C. *Shigella* is a highly infectious organism with as few as 10 organisms causing disease.

Evidence-Based Diagnosis

A. Because of the highly invasive nature of *Shigella*, some of the tests that reveal colonic inflammation are more useful in detecting *Shigella* than other organisms.

  1. Sensitivity of band count > 1% = 85%.

  2. Sensitivity of fecal leukocytes is at least 70%.

B. Stool culture is gold standard.

Treatment

A. *Shigella* dysentery clearly benefits from treatment.

B. The drug of choice is oral ciprofloxacin.

Alternative Diagnosis: Enterohemorrhagic *E coli* (EHEC)

Textbook Presentation

The presentation of *E coli* depends on the type. EHEC usually presents with diarrhea and abdominal pain. The pain is often worse in the right lower quadrant. Bloody diarrhea is very common, while nausea, vomiting, and fever are not.

Disease Highlights

A. Nomenclature

  1. EHEC is a group of *E coli* that elaborates *Shiga* toxin. The associated disease is caused by the effects of the toxin.

  2. EHEC is also called "*Shiga* toxin–producing" *E coli*, (STEC) or verocytotoxigenic *E coli* (VTEC).

  3. Common strains of EHEC are O104:H4 and O157:H7 (the most common strain in the United States).

  4. Other than EHEC, there are 4 types of *E coli* that cause diarrheal illness in adults. Information about the *E coli* diseases other than EHEC is listed in Table 13-6.

Table 13-6. Diarrhea-producing *E coli* other than enterohemorrhagic *E coli* (EHEC, *Shiga* toxin–producing *E coli*).

Type	Common Abbreviation	Characteristics
Enterotoxigenic *Escherichia coli*	ETEC	Symptoms caused by toxin Watery diarrhea Common cause of traveler's diarrhea
Enteropathogenic *E coli*	EPEC	Common cause of diarrhea in adults and children
Enteroinvasive *E coli*	EIEC	Causes bloody diarrhea with tenesmus similar to *Shigella*
Enteroaggregative *E coli*	EAEC	Common cause of diarrhea in children and traveler's diarrhea May be *Shiga* toxin–producing

B. Symptoms of EHEC include bloody diarrhea (seen in most infected patients), severe abdominal pain, and absence of fever.

C. Incidence varies year to year but is generally 1–2 cases/100,000 people.

D. EHEC is associated with the HUS.

  1. HUS is the simultaneous presence of a microangiopathic hemolytic anemia, thrombocytopenia, and acute kidney injury.

  2. HUS occurs mainly in children and affects 5–10% of children infected with EHEC.

  3. About 5% of cases HUS/thrombotic thrombocytopenic purpura in adults are related to EHEC.

Evidence-Based Diagnosis

A. Patients infected with EHEC are significantly more likely than patients infected with other pathogens to

  1. Report bloody diarrhea

  2. Provide visibly bloody specimens

  3. Not report fever

  4. Have abdominal tenderness

  5. Have a WBC > 10,000/mcL

  6. Have any fecal leukocytes in their specimen (70.5% vs. 39.5%)

B. If an organism is isolated from a patient with bloody diarrhea, it is most likely to be *Shigella* or *Campylobacter*. On the other hand, a patient infected with EHEC is more likely to have bloody diarrhea than a patient with *Shigella* or *Campylobacter* infection.

C. Positive culture or detected *Shiga* toxin are considered diagnostic.

D. Culture/toxin testing for EHEC often must be specifically requested.

Treatment

A. Treatment of EHEC is controversial.

B. Studies have reported no effect, an increase in risk of HUS, and beneficial effects with antibiotics.

C. Antibiotics are generally thought to not be indicated in the treatment of EHEC.

CASE RESOLUTION

The patient was treated with supportive therapy. Anti-diarrheals were withheld because of her bloody diarrhea. Ciprofloxacin was prescribed empirically. Her stool was sent for culture.

Her stool cultures were negative, and her symptoms resolved within 3 days.

The resolution of this case is not surprising. The decision to treat the patient was based on her ill appearance and the fact that her presentation was thought to be consistent with *Campylobacter* infection. Even though stool cultures have the highest yield in patients with bloody stool, about two-thirds of the cultures will still be negative. Also not surprising is her rapid improvement.

REVIEW OF OTHER IMPORTANT DISEASES
Travelers' Diarrhea

Textbook Presentation

Patients with traveler's diarrhea usually become ill in the first 5 days of their trips from a temperate climate to a tropical one. They usually have mild symptoms of a gastroenteritis-like illness. Patients are often better by the time they return home.

Disease Highlights

A. Up to 10 million cases yearly

B. The highest risk destinations for traveler's diarrhea are in Asia, Africa, and South and Central America.

C. Disease usually occurs in the first 5 days (with a peak onset at 4 days) and resolves in 1–5 days.

D. Symptoms are usually of mild to moderate diarrhea but more severe symptoms can occur.

E. Although the predominant cause of traveler's diarrhea is enterotoxigenic *E coli* (ETEC), any bacteria, virus, or parasite can be causative. It is important to consider infections particularly common in certain locations.

   1. St. Petersburg: *G lamblia*

   2. Wilderness streams in Western United States: *G lamblia*

   3. Nepal: *Cyclospora, G lamblia*

   4. India: *E histolytica*

F. Because these infections usually occur far from the patient's physician, the doctor's role is usually advisory.

   1. Prevention

     a. Ensure clean water

       (1) Boiled, filtered, or chemically purified local water.

       (2) Carbonated beverages and bottled water

     b. Gastric acidity is natural prevention; temporarily discontinue proton pump inhibitors or H$_2$-blockers if safe to do so.

     c. Antibiotics

       (1) Only recommended for traveler at particularly high risk for complications or for very high stakes trips.

       (2) Rifaximin is the most commonly recommended agent.

       (3) Bismuth is also effective, taken before meals and at bedtime.

     d. CDC Web site has very useful information for patients.

   2. Advise patients of common mistakes.

     a. Ice and mixed drinks are often made with contaminated water.

     b. Ensure bottled water is sealed and not just bottled tap water.

     c. As the parasitologist B. H. Kean once said, "The only way to clean lettuce is with a blowtorch."

     d. Any food heated for a prolonged time is potentially dangerous.

     e. Fruit is only safe if the traveler peels it.

     f. A recent study reported that among table top sauces collected from restaurants in Guadalajara and tested for diarrheogenic *E coli*, 4 of 43 contained ETEC and 14 of 32 contained enteroaggregative *E coli* (EAEC).

Treatment

A. Supportive care

B. Avoid antidiarrheals if dysentery is present.

C. Antibiotics are warranted.

   1. Ciprofloxacin, azithromycin, and rifamaxin are the preferred agents.

   2. Consider causes of traveler's diarrhea other than ETEC (such as giardiasis, amebiasis), which require different therapies.

REFERENCES

Adachi JA, Mathewson JJ, Jiang ZD, Ericsson CD, DuPont HL. Enteric pathogens in Mexican sauces of popular restaurants in Guadalajara, Mexico, and Houston, Texas. Ann Intern Med. 2002;136(12):884–7.

Bartlett JG. Clinical practice. Antibiotic-associated diarrhea. N Engl J Med. 2002;346(5):334–9.

Brodsky RE, Spencer HC Jr, Schultz MG. Giardiasis in American travelers to the Soviet Union. J Infect Dis. 1974;130(3):319–23.

Dupont HL. Bacterial diarrhea. N Engl J Med. 2009;261:1560–9.

Guerrant RL, Van Gilder T, Steiner TS et al. Practice guidelines for the management of infectious diarrhea. Clin Infect Dis. 2001;32(3):331–51.

Hatchette RG, Farina D. Infectious diarrhea: when to test and when to treat. CMAJ. 2011;183:339–44.

Hogenauer C, Langner C, Beubler E et al. *Klebsiella oxytoca* as a causative organism of antibiotic-associated hemorrhagic colitis. N Engl J Med. 2006;355(23):2418–26.

Lynch MF, Blanton EM, Bulens S et al. Typhoid fever in the United States, 1999–2006. JAMA. 2009;302(8):859–65.

Musher DM, Musher BL. Contagious acute gastrointestinal infections. N Engl J Med. 2004;351(23):2417–27.

Scallan E, Hoekstra RM, Angulo FJ et al. Foodborne illness acquired in the United States—major pathogens. Emerg Infect Dis. 2011 Jan;17(1):7–15.

Slutsker L, Ries AA, Greene KD, Wells JG, Hutwagner L, Griffin PM. *Escherichia coli* O157:H7 diarrhea in the United States: clinical and epidemiologic features. Ann Intern Med. 1997;126(7):505–13.

Talan D, Moran GJ, Newdow M et al. Etiology of bloody diarrhea among patients presenting to United States emergency departments: prevalence of *Escherichia coli* O157:H7 and other enteropathogens. Clin Infect Dis. 2001;32(4):573–80.

Thielman NM, Guerrant RL. Clinical practice. Acute infectious diarrhea. N Engl J Med. 2004;350(1):38–47.

Yoder JS, Beach MJ. Giardiasis surveillance—United States, 2003–2005. MMWR Surveill Summ. 2007;56(7):11–8.

I have a patient with dizziness. How do I determine the cause?

CHIEF COMPLAINT

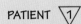

PATIENT 1

Mr. J is a 32-year-old man who comes to your office complaining of dizziness.

What is the differential diagnosis of dizziness? How would you frame the differential?

CONSTRUCTING A DIFFERENTIAL DIAGNOSIS

The differential diagnosis for dizziness is extensive, encompassing diseases of the inner ear, central and peripheral nervous system, cardiovascular system and psychiatric disease. Fortunately, an organized approach greatly simplifies evaluating the dizzy patient. The first step recognizes that most patients who complain of dizziness are actually complaining of 1 of 4 distinct symptoms: vertigo, near syncope, disequilibrium, and ill-defined lightheadedness. Each of these symptoms has its own particular differential diagnosis and evaluation.

The first pivotal step in evaluating the dizzy patient is to clarify which symptom the patient is experiencing, since this limits the differential diagnosis and focuses the evaluation on the appropriate set of diagnostic possibilities for that particular symptom. Therefore, the first and most important pivotal question is "What does it feel like when you are dizzy?" At this point, patients must be given enough time, *without interruptions or suggestions*, to describe their dizziness as clearly as possible (Figure 14-1). Commonly used descriptions, their precipitants, and differential diagnosis are listed in Table 14-1.

In practice, many patients often have difficulty describing their symptom and have ill-defined lightheadedness. Therefore, the second pivotal step in those patients is to search for neurologic and cardiovascular clues (signs and symptoms) that point to the involved system. For instance, dizzy patients with other CNS symptoms or signs (new headache, double vision, ataxia or diplopia) almost certainly have CNS disease whereas patients who note dizziness immediately on standing associated with a drop in their BP almost certainly have orthostatic hypotension causing their dizziness. These clues can be particularly useful in patients who are having trouble describing their dizziness. The approach to patients with ill-defined lightheadedness is illustrated in Figure 14-2.

Differential Diagnosis of Dizziness

A. Vertigo is the most common cause of dizziness. Vertigo arises from diseases of the inner ear (peripheral) or diseases of the

brainstem (central). Central vertigo is less common than peripheral (≈ 10% vs. 90%) but far more serious.

1. Peripheral
   a. Benign paroxysmal positional vertigo (BPPV)
   b. Labyrinthitis or vestibular neuritis
   c. Meniere disease
   d. Uncommon etiologies: head trauma, herpes zoster
2. Central
   a. Cerebrovascular disease
      (1) Vertebrobasilar insufficiency (VBI)
      (2) Cerebellar or brainstem stroke
      (3) Cerebellar hemorrhage
      (4) Vertebral artery dissection (VAD)
      (5) Brainstem aneurysm
   b. Cerebellar degeneration
   c. Migraine
   d. Multiple sclerosis (MS)
   e. Alcohol intoxication
   f. Phenytoin toxicity
   g. Inhalant abuse
   h. Tumors of the brainstem or cerebellum

B. Near syncope is a common cause of severe dizziness, particularly in the elderly. It can be caused by a variety of life-threatening diseases. (See Chapter 31, Syncope.)

C. Dysequilibrium
1. Multiple sensory deficits
2. Parkinson disease
3. Normal-pressure hydrocephalus
4. Cerebellar disease (degeneration, tumor, infarction)
5. Peripheral neuropathy (ie, diabetes)
6. Dorsal column lesions
   a. B$_{12}$ deficiency
   b. Syphilis
   c. Compressive lesions
7. Drugs (alcohol, benzodiazepines, anticonvulsants, aminoglycosides, antihypertensives, muscle relaxants, cisplatin)

D. Nonspecific dizziness
1. Psychological
   a. Major depression
   b. Anxiety, panic disorder
   c. Somatization disorder

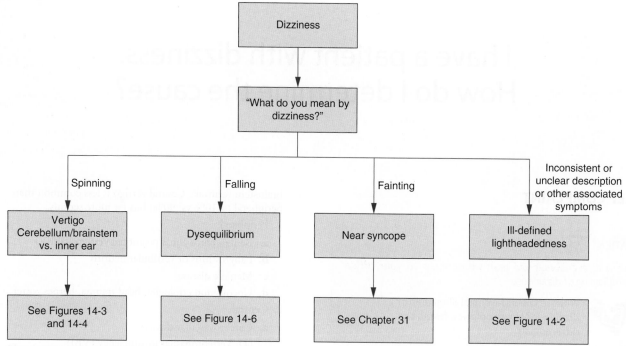

Figure 14-1. Step 1: Approach to the patient with dizziness.

Table 14-1. Classification and characteristics of dizziness.

	Vertigo	Near Syncope	Dysequilibrium	Nonspecific Dizziness
Chief complaint	Spinning or sensation of self motion (when none is occurring)	Sense of impending loss of consciousness	Unstable while seated, standing or walking	Floating, vague
Typical precipitants	Turning over in bed Looking up to shelf Moving the head	Standing	Walking	Stress
Important historical features	*CNS signs or symptoms* (eg, dysarthria, ataxia, diplopia, headache, neck pain) Attack duration Peripheral symptoms (eg, hearing loss, tinnitus)	Tunnel vision Cognitive impairment CAD, HF Syncope during exercise Palpitations Medications Melena or rectal bleeding	Diabetes Neuropathy Visual problems Imbalance Medications	Multiple somatic complaints Feeling down or hopeless Anhedonia
Key physical exam findings	Cranial nerve exam Gait Finger-to-nose exam Romberg Dix-Hallpike maneuver	Orthostatic blood pressure and pulse Cardiac exam for murmur or S3	Gait Romberg Position sense Sensation Cranial nerve exam Finger-to-nose exam	
Differential diagnosis	**Peripheral:** BPPV Vestibular neuritis Meniere disease **Central:** Cerebrovascular disease, MS, cerebellar hemorrhage, migraine, brainstem tumors	Dehydration Hemorrhage Orthostatic hypotension Vasovagal Arrhythmias Hypoglycemia Aortic stenosis PE	Multiple sensory deficits Parkinson disease Cerebellar degeneration or stroke B_{12} deficiency Tabes dorsalis Myelopathy Normal pressure hydrocephalus	Depression Generalized anxiety disorder Panic attacks Somatization disorder Medications

BPPV, benign paroxysmal positional vertigo; CAD, coronary artery disease; CVA, cerebrovascular accident; HF, heart failure; MS, multiple sclerosis; PE, pulmonary embolism.

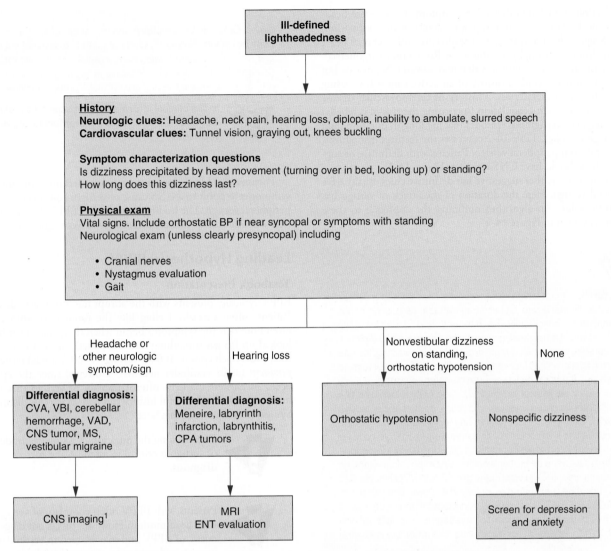

Figure 14-2. Step 2: Approach to the patient with ill-defined lightheadedness.

Within the flowchart:

Ill-defined lightheadedness

History
Neurologic clues: Headache, neck pain, hearing loss, diplopia, inability to ambulate, slurred speech
Cardiovascular clues: Tunnel vision, graying out, knees buckling

Symptom characterization questions
Is dizziness precipitated by head movement (turning over in bed, looking up) or standing?
How long does this dizziness last?

Physical exam
Vital signs. Include orthostatic BP if near syncopal or symptoms with standing
Neurological exam (unless clearly presyncopal) including

- Cranial nerves
- Nystagmus evaluation
- Gait

Branch 1 — Headache or other neurologic symptom/sign:
Differential diagnosis: CVA, VBI, cerebellar hemorrhage, VAD, CNS tumor, MS, vestibular migraine → CNS imaging[1]

Branch 2 — Hearing loss:
Differential diagnosis: Meniere, labryinth infarction, labrynthitis, CPA tumors → MRI, ENT evaluation

Branch 3 — Nonvestibular dizziness on standing, orthostatic hypotension:
Orthostatic hypotension

Branch 4 — None:
Nonspecific dizziness → Screen for depression and anxiety

[1]Consider emergent head CT if cerebellar hemorrhage is being considered. Follow-up MRI is recommended. CT angiography, magnetic resonance angiography, or angiography should be considered in stroke patients or patients with neck pain who may have VAD.

BP, blood pressure; CNS, central nervous system; CPA, cerebellopontine angle; CVA, cerebrovascular accident; ENT, ear nose and throat; MRI, magnetic resonance imaging; VAD, vertebral artery dissection; VBI, vertebrobasilar insufficiency.

---

2. Recently corrected vision (new glasses, cataract removal)
3. Medication side effect

Mr. J reports that when he is dizzy, it feels as though the room is spinning. His first episode occurred 3 days ago when he rolled over in bed. The spinning sensation was very intense, causing nausea and vomiting. It lasted less than 1 minute.

At this point, what is the leading hypothesis, what are the active alternatives, and is there a must not miss diagnosis? Given this differential diagnosis, what tests should be ordered?

RANKING THE DIFFERENTIAL DIAGNOSIS

Clearly, Mr. J is describing vertigo, the most common complaint in patients with dizziness. Patients with vertigo complain that either they or their surroundings are spinning. A recent consensus panel defined vertigo as a sense of self-motion (when there is no real movement). Recognizing that Mr. J is suffering from vertigo allows the examiner to limit the differential diagnosis to the subset of diseases that cause vertigo. Diseases of the peripheral nervous system (inner ear) and central nervous system (brainstem) can cause vertigo. Central vertigo is less common but is a must not miss possibility since central vertigo may be caused by stroke, hemorrhage, tumors, and MS. Therefore, the next **pivotal step** in the evaluation of patients with vertigo is to look for clues on history and neurologic exam that suggest CNS disease. The neurologic exam should focus on the cranial nerve and cerebellar exam, (including gait) and the Dix-Hallpike maneuver. Clues that *definitively* point to a CNS etiology include other CNS symptoms (new severe head-ache or neck pain, dysarthria, diplopia, ataxia or incoordination) or CNS signs (dysconjugate gaze, papilledema, other cranial nerve abnormalities, abnormal gait, abnormal Romberg, or dysmetria). Risk factors and other symptoms that may *suggest* CNS disease but are less definitive include a history of an active cancer (increasing the risk for brain metastases), a history of cerebrovascular disease or its risk factors, anticoagulation (increasing the risk of cerebellar hemorrhage) or vertiginous episodes that are long in duration (and may suggest stroke). Table 14-2 contrasts the features distinguish-ing central from peripheral vertigo. Patients with definitive or sug-gestive clues should have CNS imaging (Figure 14-3).

Patients with neither suggestive nor definitive clues usually have peripheral vertigo. Here the duration of the attack of vertigo has diagnostic value. An algorithm outlining the approach to these patients is shown in Figure 14-4.

On further questioning, Mr. J reports that he had a similar episode 5 years ago. Other than nausea, he has no other symptoms. Specifically, he has not had definitive CNS symptoms like new severe headache or neck pain, diplopia, numbness, weakness, dysarthria, or trouble walking. He has no risk factors that increase the likelihood of central vertigo such as diabetes mellitus, hypertension, coronary artery disease or peripheral vascular disease (which increase the likelihood of cerebrovascular disease), no history of active cancer, and he is not taking any anticoagulants (which increase the likelihood of CNS hemorrhage). He has no prior history of neurologic complaints (eg, unilateral vision loss of optic neuritis or motor weakness). On physical exam, he appears anxious. His vital signs are BP, 110/70 mm Hg; RR, 16 breaths per minute; pulse, 84 bpm; temperature, 37.0°C. HEENT exam reveals extraocular muscles intact with 15 beats of horizontal nystagmus on left lateral gaze. This stops after repeating the maneuver several

times. Optic disks are sharp and visual fields are intact to confrontation. Cardiac, pulmonary, and abdominal exams are normal. On neurologic exam, cranial nerves are intact (except for nystagmus). Hearing is grossly normal. Gait and finger-to-nose testing are normal. Romberg is negative.

 Is the clinical information sufficient to make a diagnosis? If not, what other information do you need?

Fortunately, Mr. J does not have any definitive or suggestive symptoms to point to a CNS cause of vertigo. You strongly suspect peripheral vertigo. The leading hypothesis is BPPV. Vestibular neu-ritis and Meniere disease are active alternatives (Table 14-3).

Leading Hypothesis: BPPV

Textbook Presentation

BPPV typically presents with the abrupt onset of severe dizziness. Patients often describe feeling like the room is spinning. They often note that the symptoms began when they rolled over in bed, looked up (to get something out of a closet), or bent down to tie their shoe. Each episode is *brief* (lasting 10–20 seconds) rather than *persistent* (as in vestibular neuritis). However, since the episodes occur in clusters, patients often complain of vertigo that occurs for days or weeks. A careful history can help make this distinction. Symptoms may recur years later.

 Determining the duration of a single episode of vertigo is critical to establish the correct diagnosis.

 Patients with BPPV often complain of vertigo with head motion. However, this is not diag-nostic of BPPV and may be seen in vestibular neuritis and vertigo from central etiologies.

Table 14-2. Features distinguishing central from peripheral vertigo.

Finding	Peripheral Vertigo	Central Vertigo
CNS symptoms and signs (eg, headache, dysarthria, diplopia, ataxia, cranial nerve palsies)	Rare	Common
Imbalance	Mild to moderate[1]	Severe
Nystagmus characteristics	Inhibited by fixation Unidirectional Latent period 2–20 seconds before nystagmus starts Horizontal with torsional component Lasts < 1 minute Fatigues with repetition	Not inhibited by fixation May change direction No latency May be purely vertical, down beating or torsional Lasts > 1 minute Does not fatigue
Duration of single episode	Depends on etiology	Depends on etiology
Risk factors for vascular disease	May be present or absent	Commonly present
Nausea and vomiting	Severe	Variable, may be minimal
Severity of vertigo	Severe	Less severe to none
Hearing loss	May occur in Meniere disease	May occur in labyrinth and pontine infarctions

[1]Patients with peripheral lesions can usually walk, whereas those with central lesions may have great difficulty.

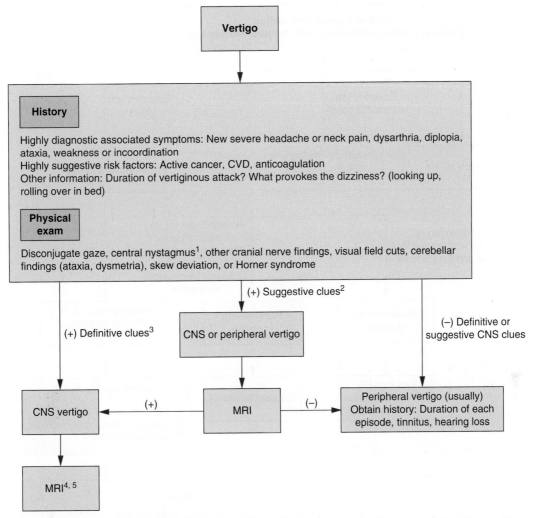

[1]Central nystagmus includes nystagmus that is either persistent (lasts >1 minute), fails to extinguish, is vertical, not suppressed by visual fixation or occurs looking to both directions.

[2]Suggestive clues include history of active cancer, cerebrovascular disease or its risk factors (hypertension, hyperlipidemia, tobacco use, diabetes, peripheral vascular disease, atrial fibrillation, hypercoagulable state, recent cervical trauma, or coronary artery disease), anticoagulation, vertigo of long duration (days), hearing loss. A prior history of unexplained neurologic symptoms (like optic neuritis) can suggest multiple sclerosis.

[3]Definitive clues include new or severe headache/neck pain numbness, weakness, dysarthria, diplopia, papilledema, ataxia, abnormal Romberg, incoordination, cranial nerve findings, Horner syndrome, skew deviation or central nystagmus.

[4]Consider emergent head CT if cerebellar hemorrhage is being considered; follow-up MRI is recommended. CTA, MRA, or angiography should be considered in patients with stroke or patients with neck pain who may have vertebral artery dissection.

[5]The sensitivity of the MRI is approximately 88% for acute posterior fossa strokes, and strokes should not be considered ruled out if there is a high clinical suspicion and normal MRI.

CNS, central nervous system; CVD, cerebrovascular disease; MRI, magnetic resonance imaging.

Figure 14-3. Approach to the patient with vertigo, part 1.

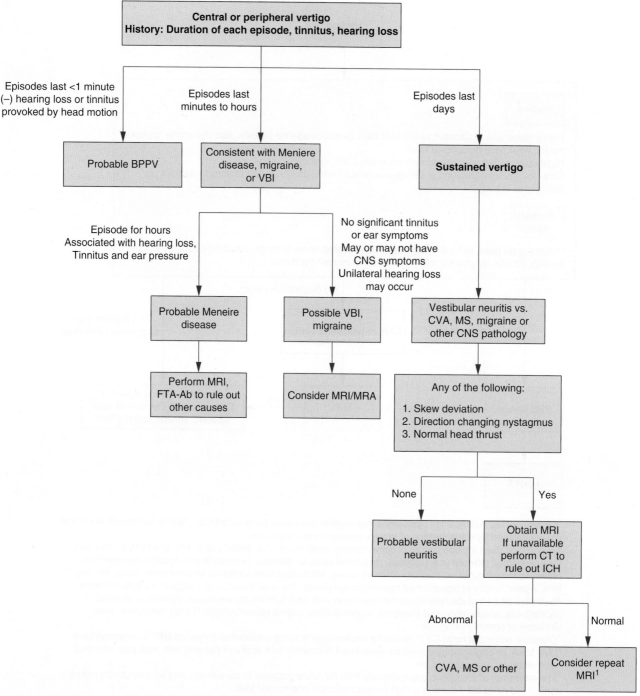

[1]The sensitivity of MRI is approximately 88% for acute posterior fossa strokes, and strokes remain in the differential if there is a high clinical suspicion and negative MRI.

BPPV, benign paroxysmal positional vertigo; CNS, central nervous system; CT, computed tomography; CVA, cerebrovascular accident; FTA-Ab, fluorescent treponemal antibody; ICH, intracranial hemorrhage; MRI/MRA magnetic resonance imaging, magnetic resonance angiography; MS, multiple sclerosis; VBI vertebrobasilar insufficiency.

Figure 14-4. Approach to the patient with vertigo, part 2.

Table 14-3. Diagnostic hypotheses for Mr. J.

Diagnostic Hypotheses	Demographics, Risk Factors, Symptoms and Signs	Important Tests
Leading Hypothesis		
Benign paroxysmal positional vertigo	Vertigo lasts seconds, precipitated by rolling over in bed or looking up to shelf Peripheral type nystagmus	Thorough neurologic history and physical exam (to exclude CNS lesions)
Active Alternatives—Most Common		
Vestibular neuritis	Vertigo lasts for days Peripheral type nystagmus	Thorough neurologic history and physical exam (to exclude CNS lesions) Consider MRI
Meniere disease	Vertigo lasts for minutes to hours Tinnitus, intermittent hearing loss Peripheral type nystagmus	Thorough neurologic history and physical exam Audiogram

Disease Highlights

A. Most common cause of vertigo

B. Vertigo precipitated by positional changes

C. Vertigo is brief, usually lasting < 15 seconds but may last as long as 90 seconds.

D. Patients typically have clusters of attacks over several weeks to 1 month and then remission. Recurrent clusters occur in about half of patients.

E. Secondary to a free-floating canalith usually within 1 of the semicircular canals. The canalith creates turbulent flow within the endolymph resulting in the sensation of motion (vertigo). The precipitant is usually unknown, although BPPV may also be caused labyrinthitis or head trauma.

Evidence-Based Diagnosis

 A. Patients with all 4 of the following criteria usually have BPPV (88% sensitive, 92% specific; LR+ 11, LR– 0.13):

1. Recurrent vertigo

2. Duration of attack < 1 minute

3. Symptoms invariably provoked by changing head position

   a. Lying down or turning over in bed *or*

   b. 2 of the following: Reclining the head, rising from supine, or bending forward

4. Not attributable to another disorder

B. One study reported the following symptoms in patients with BPPV:

1. All patients with BPPV complained that turning over in bed provoked the vertigo.

2. 50% of patients complained of imbalance but falling was rare (only 1/61). Given the rarity of falling, this should raise the concern for another disorder.

C. Positional nystagmus has a mixed rotary and horizontal component and can be precipitated by the Dix-Hallpike maneuver.

1. Nystagmus usually begins after a few seconds, is brief (< 30 seconds), and fatigues with repetition of maneuver.

2. Sensitivity, 42–78%; specificity 94%

3. Features that suggest a central (brainstem) disorder include nystagmus that begins immediately, lasts longer than 1 minute, fails to fatigue, is not suppressed by visual fixation or is purely vertical.

D. CNS imaging should be performed in patients with findings that suggest central disease and in patients with *atypical* findings for BPPV including patients with symptoms that persist or progress.

Treatment

A. Most patients recover regardless of therapy; however, spontaneous resolution can take weeks to months.

B. The Epley maneuver is a complex rotational maneuver that repositions the canalith and is 80–95% effective at stopping vertigo.

C. Vestibular suppressants (meclizine and benzodiazepines) may cause drowsiness, worsen imbalance and delay CNS adaptation and should be used only when necessary for patients with frequent intolerable spells.

D. Surgical options are available for patients with refractory symptoms but are rarely necessary.

MAKING A DIAGNOSIS

Mr. J's history is characteristic of BPPV. At this point, the Dix-Hallpike maneuver should be performed to evaluate positional nystagmus.

Mr. J reports intense vertigo with the maneuver. Horizontal nystagmus with a rotary component is noted, which lasts for 20 seconds. After repeating the maneuver, the nystagmus disappears.

 Have you crossed a diagnostic threshold for the leading hypothesis, BPPV? Have you ruled out the active alternatives? Do other tests need to be done to exclude the alternative diagnoses?

The clinical history, exam, and lack of risk factors for CNS disease or CNS signs all point to peripheral rather than central vertigo. The brief episodes strongly suggest BPPV. Other peripheral causes of vertigo should be considered.

Alternative Diagnoses: Acute Vestibular Neuritis

Textbook Presentation

Acute vestibular neuritis typically presents abruptly with severe *constant* vertigo and nausea made worse by head turning that lasts for days. The vertigo is often exacerbated by head motion (as in BPPV or stroke). Subsequently, patients may complain of *intermittent* vertigo that occurs for weeks to months and is precipitated by head movement.

Disease Highlights

A. Acute vestibular neuritis may follow viral infection involving the vestibular nerve and the labyrinth.

B. Patients often have spontaneous vestibular nystagmus that is unilateral, horizontal, or horizontal and torsional and suppressed by visual fixation.

C. Nausea and vomiting are common.

D. Gait instability may be present, but patients maintain the ability to ambulate.

E. Severe vertigo typically lasts 2–3 days and may last up to 1 week.

F. Ramsay Hunt syndrome is a variant of vestibular neuritis.

1. Varicella zoster reactivation involving cranial nerves VII and VIII produces vestibular neuritis *with* hearing loss and facial weakness.

2. Vesicles are seen in the external auditory canal.

Evidence-Based Diagnosis

A. Diagnosis is usually made clinically.

B. Exclusion of serious CNS diseases that mimic vestibular neuritis is critical before making this diagnosis. Acute persistent vertigo may also be due to posterior fossa strokes (usually ischemic but may be hemorrhagic), MS, and posterior fossa tumors.

> One must carefully exclude posterior fossa strokes before diagnosing vestibular neuritis. A careful neurologic exam must be performed in all patients with select use of MRI (see below).

C. The neurologic exam should include a cranial nerve exam with particular emphasis on extraocular movements, a cerebellar exam (including gait), and Romberg sign.

1. Significant CNS signs or symptoms suggest central vertigo and the need for neuroimaging (see below). Key CNS symptoms and signs include headache, neck pain, dysarthria, diplopia, weakness, inability to ambulate, dysmetria, cranial nerve findings, Horner syndrome, central type nystagmus, or persistence of severe vertigo beyond a few days.

2. However, 49% of patients with persistent vertigo due to stroke lack obvious neurologic abnormalities (or only had truncal ataxia defined as inability to sit with arms crossed unaided). Additional specific maneuvers are very accurate in identifying strokes in these patients (Table 14-4). Specifically *any* of the following suggest stroke: (1) direction changing nystagmus, (2) skew deviation, and (3) a *normal* head thrust. The absence of all 3 criteria make stroke very unlikely: sensitivity, 98%; specificity, 85%; LR+, 6.5; LR–, 0.02. These findings were in fact even more sensitive than initial diffusion-weighted MRI (DW-MRI).

   a. Skew deviation: A condition in which the eyes move in different directions with upward gaze. More easily identified during a cover-uncover test. See http://emcrit.org/misc/posterior-stroke-video/

   b. Head thrust test

   (1) In this maneuver the examiner holds the patients head in their hands and asks the patient to focus on the examiner's stationary nose. The examiner then rapidly turns the patient's head while the patient

Table 14-4. Findings in central vertigo versus vestibular neuritis

	Central Vertigo			Vestibular neuritis
	Frequency	LR+	LR–	Frequency
Head thrust: Normal	85%	17	0.16	5%
Skew deviation	30%	15	0.71	2%
Direction changing nystagmus[1]	38%	4.75	0.67	8%
Any 1/3: Negative head thrust, skew deviation or direction changing nystagmus	98%	6.5	0.02	15%
Abnormality on careful neurologic exam[2]	93%	15.5	0.07	6%
Severe truncal ataxia	33%	∞	0.67	0%
Headache or neck pain	≈ 40%	3.3	0.7	12%
Obvious neurologic abnormalities: gaze palsy, weakness, vertical nystagmus)	51%	∞	0.49	0%

[1]Direction changing nystagmus (ie, right beating on right gaze and left beating on left gaze.
[2]Including cranial nerves, extraocular movements, gait, Romberg, finger to nose, head thrust, and skew deviation.

tries to maintain eye contact with the examiner's nose. In health, a patient is able to maintain eye contact with the examiner's nose despite the head thrust. See http://www.youtube.com/watch?v=CZXDNLLGG8k

(2) In vestibular neuritis, the vestibular-ocular reflex is impaired and the eyes move with the head and are unable to maintain eye contact with the examiner's nose. The patient's eyes have saccade movements to return the nose to focus. This is referred to as a positive head thrust test. Thus, such a finding suggests a peripheral etiology.

(3) In posterior fossa strokes, the vestibular-ocular reflex is intact and patients *are* able to maintain focus on the examiner's finger or nose when their head is turned. Therefore, a *negative (normal)* head thrust in a patient with persistent vertigo suggests a central lesion rather than vestibular neuritis.

c. A careful neurologic exam that included head thrust and skew deviation was found to be 93% sensitive and 94% specific in another study.

> A normal head thrust test, skew deviation, or direction changing nystagmus are very sensitive for the diagnosis of stroke in patients with persistent vertigo.

3. Hearing loss may be seen with vestibular neuritis and with posterior circulation infarcts and is not helpful diagnostically.

D. CT scan is insensitive to the diagnosis of ischemic stroke (16%) (see Table 14-7).

E. DW-MRI is superior to CT but imperfect at detecting pontine infarcts (sensitivity 80% in first 24 hours). Repeat examination should be considered when the clinical exam suggests stroke.

F. In summary, a careful neurologic exam including testing of the head thrust, skew deviation, and direction changing nystagmus is very sensitive for the diagnosis of cerebrovascular accident. Patients with any abnormality suggestive of central vertigo should undergo DW-MRI. If clinical uncertainty exists, MRI should be performed, and if unavailable a CT should be done to rule out hemorrhage.

G. An approach to the diagnosis of patients with persistent vertigo is shown in the bottom right section of Figure 14-4.

Treatment

A. Meclizine (antihistamine), dimenhydrinate, and scopolamine (anticholinergic) are drugs of choice in most patients.

B. Promethazine (especially for severe nausea, vomiting)

C. Benzodiazepines have also been used.

D. Medications are sedating. Driving should be avoided.

E. Corticosteroids have been demonstrated to improve vestibular recovery, although symptomatic and functional improvements have not been demonstrated. Their use is controversial.

F. Antiviral medications have not been demonstrated to be useful.

G. Vestibular rehabilitation using exercises that stimulate the labyrinth can promote CNS adaptation.

Alternative Diagnosis: Meniere Disease

Textbook Presentation

Patients complain of intermittent spells of vertigo. They may note associated ear fullness, unilateral hearing loss, and tinnitus. Spells typically last for minutes to hours (rarely longer than 4–5 hours) and occasionally up to a day.

Disease Highlights

A. Associated with excess fluid (hydrops) in the endolymphatic spaces of the inner ear.

B. The disease may be unilateral or bilateral.

C. Patients have both episodic sensorineural hearing loss and vertigo. Patients may also experience tinnitus.
1. Vertigo lasts 20 minutes to 24 hours.
2. The hearing loss typically affects lower frequencies initially and then progresses.
3. Tinnitus is often described as low pitch.

Evidence-Based Diagnosis

A. There are no tests that definitely confirm Meniere disease. The disease is diagnosed clinically.

B. Diagnostic criteria of the American Academy of Otolaryngology and Head and Neck Surgery require the following for a definite clinical diagnosis:
1. Two spontaneous episodes of vertigo lasting > 20 minutes
2. Confirmed sensorineural hearing loss
3. Tinnitus or perception of aural fullness, or both
4. Other causes excluded. The utilization of other tests is controversial. A recent review recommended an MRI to rule out other causes (ie, acoustic neuroma, cerebrovascular accident or MS) before confirming the diagnosis.

 Hearing loss may accompany Meniere disease or posterior circulation ischemia (due to infarction of the labyrinth) but does not confirm the diagnosis of Meniere disease.

C. Audiometry should be performed.
1. Early Meniere disease is characterized by low frequency sensorineural hearing loss.
2. Hearing can be normal between attacks.

D. Test should be done to rule out syphilis (fluorescent treponemal antibody absorption [FTA-Ab]).

E. Specialized testing is available (eg, electronystagmogram).

Treatment

A. Specialty consultation is advised.

B. Anecdotal evidence suggests low-salt diet and restriction of caffeine, alcohol, and tobacco.

C. Diuretics and corticosteroids (both oral and intratympanic) have been used but their utility is unclear. Diuretics are frequently used when lifestyle changes are inadequate.

D. Surgical therapies are available for patients with refractory incapacitating symptoms.

CASE RESOLUTION

Mr. J's history, physical exam, and response to Dix-Hallpike maneuver are entirely consistent with peripheral vertigo. There are no alarm features to suggest central vertigo. The duration of each vertiginous episode suggests BPPV rather than vestibular neuritis or Meniere disease. There is no tinnitus or hearing loss to suggest Meniere disease. Further testing is not indicated.

An Epley maneuver is performed resulting in resolution of Mr. J's symptoms. One month later he returns and is feeling well.

CHIEF COMPLAINT

PATIENT 2

Mr. D is a 29-year-old white man who complains of dizziness. Detailed questioning reveals that he has had a constant spinning sensation for the last 3–4 days. He has no history of similar episodes or hearing loss. Although head movement exacerbates the symptom, it is persistent even when he is still.

At this point, what is the leading hypothesis, what are the active alternatives, and is there a must not miss diagnosis? Given this differential diagnosis, what tests should be ordered?

RANKING THE DIFFERENTIAL DIAGNOSIS

Again, the first task in evaluating the dizzy patient is to properly identify whether the patient has vertigo, near syncope, dysequilibrium, or nonspecific dizziness. Mr. D is clearly suffering from vertigo. Peripheral vertigo is more common and of these, only vestibular neuritis causes continuous vertigo that lasts for days. This is the leading hypothesis. The next pivotal step searches for any definitive or suggestive symptoms or signs that point to the less common but more serious causes of central vertigo. Central causes include migraine with vertigo, MS, cerebrovascular disease, and intracranial neoplasms.

2

Mr. D denies any history of significant headaches. He denies any history of prior or current neurologic complaints such as diplopia, visual loss, ataxia, or unexplained motor or sensory symptoms. He has no risk factors for cerebrovascular disease (history of hypertension, diabetes mellitus, tobacco use, atrial fibrillation, or cocaine use). He has no prior history of cancer.

Fortunately Mr. D denies any worrisome CNS symptoms. His lack of headache history makes migraine with vertigo (vestibular migraine) very unlikely. In addition, he lacks any risk factors for cerebrovascular disease. He has not had any prior symptoms suggestive of MS (eg, diplopia, dysarthria, weakness) but this could still represent his initial presentation. Finally, he has no history of cancer making metastatic disease unlikely but a primary CNS neoplasm remains possible. Table 14-5 summarizes the differential diagnosis.

Is the clinical information sufficient to make a diagnosis? If not, what other information do you need?

Leading Hypothesis: Vestibular Neuritis

See above.

Table 14-5. Diagnostic hypotheses for Mr. D.

Diagnostic Hypotheses	Demographics, Risk Factors, Symptoms and Signs	Important Tests
Leading Hypothesis		
Vestibular neuritis	Vertigo lasts for days Absent skew, abnormal head thrust, and peripheral type nystagmus	Thorough neurologic history and physical exam (to exclude CNS lesions) Consider MRI
Active Alternatives—Most Common		
Multiple sclerosis	CNS lesions developing at different times and places: prior episodes of visual loss (optic neuritis), weakness, diplopia	Brain MRI Oligoclonal bands in cerebrospinal fluid
Posterior fossa tumor	Prior malignancy Headache, papilledema, focal neurologic deficit	Head CT scan or MRI/ MRA

MAKING A DIAGNOSIS

As noted above, Mr. D's duration of vertigo is consistent with vestibular neuritis, a relatively benign cause of vertigo. Recognizing that a pivotal issue in vertigo is the identification of the less common but more serious CNS causes of vertigo, you perform a detailed neurologic exam, searching for clues that would suggest a serious CNS etiology.

2

On physical exam his vital signs are BP, 126/82 mm Hg; pulse, 74 bpm; RR, 16 breaths per minute; temperature, 37.0°C. HEENT exam reveals horizontal nystagmus on leftward and rightward gaze that lasts 1–2 minutes. The nystagmus does not fatigue with repetition of the maneuver. Pupils are equal, round, react to light and accommodation. Cardiac, pulmonary, and abdominal exams are normal. Neurologic exam reveals normal gait, motor strength, sensation, negative Romberg sign, and intact cranial nerves with the exception of the nystagmus noted above. His head thrust test is normal.

Have you crossed a diagnostic threshold for the leading hypothesis, vestibular neuritis? Have you ruled out the active alternatives? Do other tests need to be done to exclude the alternative diagnoses?

While the bulk of his neurologic exam is normal, a number of findings strongly suggest a central cause of his symptoms. The duration of his nystagmus and the fact that it fails to fatigue are findings seen with central causes. In addition, his head thrust test was normal, arguing strongly against vestibular neuritis. These findings refocus the diagnostic search on CNS causes. Reconsidering your hypotheses, you recognize that Mr. D is the right age for MS (but is at lower risk given his gender and unusual presentation). A primary intracranial neoplasm is also possible and given these alternative hypotheses neuroimaging is required and an MRI is ordered.

The MRI reveals multiple periventricular white matter plaques in addition to 1 in the brainstem, highly suggestive of MS.

Alternative Diagnosis: Multiple Sclerosis

Textbook Presentation

MS typically affects young women of Western European descent who experience *attacks* of CNS dysfunction that develop over days to weeks and then remit partially or completely. New attacks at different times and in different CNS locations are the hallmark of MS.

Disease Highlights

A. Etiology
   1. MS develops secondary to an inflammatory autoimmune disease triggered by environmental agents in genetically susceptible patients resulting in multifocal CNS demyelination.
   2. Demyelination may result in neurologic deficits, which can be transient if remyelination or axonal adaptation occurs.
   3. *Axonal* injury may result in irreversible injury.

B. Epidemiology
   1. The most common cause of nontraumatic neurologic disability in young adults
   2. Women are affected 2–3 times more than men.
   3. Patients are usually between the ages of 18 and 45 years at onset.
   4. Several studies suggest that late infection (ie, in adolescence) with Epstein-Barr virus may predispose patients to MS.

C. Presentation: Although MS evolves with time into a multifocal disease, 85% of patients present with 1 of several clinically isolated syndromes (CIS). Common initial syndromes include:
   1. Partial spinal cord syndromes
      a. Band like sensation
      b. Varying degrees of pain, light touch, and proprioceptive loss
      c. Bilateral sensory loss caudal to a level
      d. Weakness associated with spasticity, extensor plantar responses, hyperreflexia, and clonus
      e. Electrical sensation from spine into the limbs that occurs with neck flexion (Lhermitte sign)
   2. Optic neuritis
      a. Presenting complaint in 15–20% of patients
      b. Patients complain of monocular visual loss, monocular visual field loss (scotoma), and difficulty discerning color that evolves over hours to days.
      c. Pain with extraocular movement is common (92%).
      d. Afferent pupillary defect (Marcus Gunn pupil) is almost always seen.
      e. Fundoscopic exam is normal in two-thirds of patients. Swelling of the optic nerve may be seen but hemorrhages are rare.
      f. With long-term follow-up, MS develops in 15–75% of patients with optic neuritis (50–80% if the MRI

scan is abnormal versus 6–22% if the MRI scan lacks disseminated features of MS).
   3. Intranuclear ophthalmoplegia (INO)
      a. The medial longitudinal fasciculus coordinates conjugate eye movement such that on lateral gaze 1 eye adducts while the other abducts.
      b. An INO develops when a lesion interrupts the medial longitudinal fasciculus pathway.
      c. On lateral gaze, abduction occurs but adduction is impaired producing diplopia. Nystagmus develops in the abducting eye.
      d. Adduction during convergence is maintained, distinguishing an INO from a third nerve palsy.
      e. INO is seen in 33–50% of patients with MS.
      f. INO is not specific for MS; it may develop secondary to vascular disease.
   4. Vertigo is the presenting symptom in 5% of patients with MS and is reported in 30–50% of patients with MS; it is commonly associated with other cranial nerve dysfunction.
   5. Up to 33% of patients presenting with a "first" demyelinating event are discovered to have had prior symptoms suggestive of prior events on careful questioning.

D. Other common symptoms include a variety of sensory symptoms, gait disturbance, urinary incontinence, fatigue (in 90%), depression, and cognitive dysfunction.

E. Uhthoff phenomenon may also be observed: worsening of MS symptoms in warm environments (eg, in the shower and during exercise); believed to be due to decreased nerve conduction in heat.

F. Atypical findings that suggest alternative diagnoses include atypical age of presentation, rapid development of neurologic symptoms (within minutes), early dementia, delirium, cortical defects (eg, aphasia), seizures, a single brain lesion, or a spinal lesion without brain lesion.

G. The clinical course is variable and patients with different patterns may respond differently to therapeutic interventions.

H. Infections (viral or bacterial) and live attenuated virus vaccinations may trigger attacks. (Inactivated vaccines are safe.)

I. Prognosis at 10 years
   1. 50% of patients require a cane
   2. 15% of patients are wheelchair-dependent

Evidence-Based Diagnosis

A. Diagnosis requires the demonstration of ≥ 2 attacks of ≥ 24 hours (in the absence of fever or infection), separated in time and in space (different CNS locations).
   1. The McDonald criteria use either clinical findings alone or a combination of clinical and MRI findings to fulfill the necessary requirement of CNS lesions that are separated by time and space. These criteria are complex. The most recent revision took place in 2010.
      a. Alternative diagnoses must be considered and excluded.
      b. These criteria were developed for patients with a CIS. They should not be applied to asymptomatic individuals with MRI abnormalities.
   2. Cerebrospinal fluid (CSF) positive oligoclonal bands or an elevated IgG index can support the diagnosis.
   3. The exact sensitivity and specificity of the tests varies depending on whether the patient has a CIS or multiple

symptoms, the duration of follow-up, and the criteria of a positive result.

B. Brain MRI is the test of choice.

1. Useful to predict, diagnose, and determine disease activity in MS.

2. Demonstrates periventricular white matter lesions (lesions may also be seen in other white matter locations).

3. Sensitivity, ≈ 81–90%; specificity, 71–96%

4. Gadolinium enhancement suggests active plaques.

5. In patients with a CIS, MRI can be used to predict or diagnose MS.

    a. Asymptomatic MRI lesions compatible with MS can suggest additional CNS plaques and increases the likelihood of MS.

    b. The McDonald criteria utilize MRI findings to diagnose MS in patients with a CIS (who by definition do not meet *clinical* criteria for MS since they have had only 1 clinical event).

C. Spinal MRI has similar sensitivity (75–83%) to brain MRI but is more specific (97%).

D. Evoked potentials

1. Visual evoked potentials are 65–85% sensitive but not specific for MS.

2. Somatosensory evoked potentials

    a. 69–77% sensitive

    b. Abnormal in 50% of patients with MS without sensory signs or symptoms

E. CSF can be useful in patients in whom the diagnosis is uncertain.

1. Cell counts are usually normal.

2. Oligoclonal bands, a subclass of antibodies, may be elevated. These are considered significant only if they are different from such bands in the serum (and represent CSF IgG production).

    a. Elevated in 60–70% of patients with CIS and 90–98% of patients with MS; 92% specific

    b. LR+, 11.8; LR– 0.07

    c. 25% of patients with oligoclonal bands and 1 event progressed to MS, compared with 9% without bands (at 3 years)

    d. Other diagnoses should also be pursued in patients without oligoclonal bands, which may be especially important in patients with nonspecific white matter changes on MRI.

3. CSF IgG production is usually elevated in MS. The IgG index evaluates the CSF IgG compared with the CSF albumin. The index is elevated in 90% of MS patients.

Treatment

A. Acute exacerbations can be treated with high-dose IV corticosteroids, or plasma exchange

B. A variety of immunomodulatory agents have been used in MS as disease-modifying treatments, including interferon beta, glatiramer, fingolimod, teriflunomide, mitoxantrone, and anti-integrin antibodies (natalizumab).

C. Monthly IV corticosteroids, cyclophosphamide, and methotrexate have also been used.

D. Neuropathic pain can be treated with gabapentin, carbamazepine, and valproic acid.

E. Bone mineral density should be monitored in patients with diminished activity and in those requiring corticosteroids.

F. Other complications such as tremor, mood disorders, cognitive impairment, spasticity, bladder and bowel dysfunction can benefit from specific therapies.

G. Specialty consultation is advised.

Alternative Diagnosis: Intracranial Neoplasm

See Chapter 20, Headache.

CASE RESOLUTION

The MRI is highly suggestive of MS. A variety of tests can help confirm the diagnosis including examination of the CSF for oligoclonal bands.

Despite encouragement from you to continue the evaluation, Mr. D refuses and is lost to follow-up. One year later he presents with urinary incontinence, and a spinal MRI reveals new enhancing white matter plaques. He thus has evidence of lesions distributed in time and space and fulfills criteria for MS. He is referred to neurology for treatment.

Although CNS causes of vertigo are less common, they must be considered in patients with vertigo and both symptoms and signs can be critical clues that focus the diagnostic search. Mr. D had 2 highly diagnostic signs that were discovered on careful neurologic exam, which correctly led to an evaluation of the CNS and the eventual diagnosis of a disease that at first glance seemed improbable, MS.

CHIEF COMPLAINT

PATIENT

Mrs. S is a 70-year-old woman with a history of depression and anxiety who complains of dizziness. Over the last 1–2 months she notes increasing intermittent dizziness. When asked to describe her dizziness in more detail, she has trouble and describes neither vertigo nor near syncope. She does mention that it seems to be worse while standing. Mrs. S has also been under more stress than usual. Her daughter died several years ago and her husband has been chronically ill and is scheduled for surgery next month.

At this point, what is the leading hypothesis, what are the active alternatives, and is there a must not miss diagnosis? Given this differential diagnosis, what tests should be ordered?

RANKING THE DIFFERENTIAL DIAGNOSIS

Mrs. S has described ill-defined lightheadedness. Her psychiatric history and social stressors clearly suggests that she may be suffering from nonspecific dizziness due to depression, anxiety, or her social stressors. This is the leading hypothesis. Mrs. S also mentioned that her symptoms are worse while standing, which raises the possibility of orthostatic hypotension. Finally, nonspecific dizziness is frequently caused by medications. Table 14-6 lists the differential diagnosis.

Mrs. S readily admits to a loss of interest in her activities and anhedonia, increasing your suspicion that she has active depression. Her only medication is a bisphosphonate for her osteoporosis that she has been taking for years and is unlikely to be related to her dizziness.

Is the clinical information sufficient to make a diagnosis? If not, what other information do you need?

Table 14-6. Diagnostic hypotheses for Mrs. S.

Diagnostic Hypotheses	Demographics, Risk Factors, Symptoms and Signs	Important Tests
Leading Hypothesis		
Nonspecific dizziness	Psychiatric history, ill-defined dizziness, other symptoms of anxiety	Depression screen Anxiety screen (See Chapter 32, Unintentional Weight Loss)
Active Alternatives—Most Common		
Orthostatic hypotension	Near syncope upon standing; tunnel vision	Orthostatic hypotension or tachycardia on standing
Medication side effect	New medications	Review of medication lists and start dates

Leading Hypothesis: Nonspecific Dizziness

Textbook Presentation

Patients with a variety of psychiatric disorders including panic disorder, generalized anxiety disorder, depression, and somatization disorder may complain of ill-defined dizziness. The dizziness is often of long duration (years) and poorly defined. Patients may complain of fogginess, feeling woozy, mental fuzziness, loss of energy, or a wobbly or a floating sensation. Patients may complain of other associated symptoms particularly if they have panic attacks including chest pain, shortness of breath, impending sense of doom, palpitations, perioral paresthesias, tingling in the hands and feet, and lightheadedness.

Disease Highlights

A. 20–38% of patients attending a clinic specializing in dizziness demonstrated panic disorder.

B. Psychiatric symptoms may develop without any identifiable organic cause or develop after episodes of true vertigo or syncope.

C. Symptoms are in part secondary to hyperventilation, which leads to hypocapnia resulting in decreased cerebral blood flow.

D. Patients may complain of lightheadedness or near syncope.

E. Depression is reviewed in Chapter 32, Unintentional Weight Loss.

F. Milder variants of somatization disorder are more common than the full-blown entity. Such variants may be precipitated by stress or minor physiologic disturbances. Paradoxically, such patients are often disturbed by negative test results rather than reassured.

Evidence-Based Diagnosis

A. *Continuous sensation of vertigo > 1–2 weeks* without daily variation is likely psychogenic. This is to be distinguished from intermittent vertigo, recurring for weeks, precipitated by motion.

B. One study reported 62% of patients with hyperventilation had other significant psychiatric disorders.

C. Symptom reproduction by induced hyperventilation is nonspecific.

D. Care must be taken before ascribing dizziness to a psychiatric etiology.

1. Multiple studies have demonstrated a high prevalence of anxiety (22–67%) among patients with well-defined *organic* etiologies of their dizziness.

2. Anxiety scores are as high in patients with acute labyrinthine failure and vestibular dysfunction as among patients with no vestibular diagnosis.

3. This suggests that dizziness from an organic etiology leads to significant psychiatric distress in many patients and that the psychiatric symptoms may be sequelae of the dizziness rather than the cause of the dizziness.

E. Certain physical findings suggest a psychogenic etiology.

1. Moment-to-moment fluctuations in impairment

2. Excessive slowness or hesitation

3. Exaggerated sway on Romberg, improved by distraction

4. Sudden buckling of knee, typically without falling

5. A cautious "walking on ice" pattern

Treatment

A. Appropriate evaluation considers organic etiologies and evaluates appropriate possibilities.

B. Discuss patient's concerns and fears about the diagnosis.

C. Educate the patient not to overly restrict physical activities since this impairs CNS compensation and may worsen the physical symptoms.

D. Selective serotonin reuptake inhibitors (SSRIs) and benzodiazepines are used in patients with panic attacks and anxiety disorders. SSRIs are preferred due to potential problems with benzodiazepines (eg, dependence, tolerance, exacerbation of symptoms on discontinuation, sedation, interference with cognition in the elderly, and exacerbation of depression).

E. Cognitive and behavioral therapy have also been effective.

MAKING A DIAGNOSIS

Mrs. S confirms your suspicion that she is depressed and you feel that this is the likely cause of her nonspecific dizziness. You still wonder if she might have orthostatic hypotension.

Have you crossed a diagnostic threshold for the leading hypothesis, nonspecific dizziness? Have you ruled out the active alternatives? Do other tests need to be done to exclude the alternative diagnoses?

Alternative Diagnosis: Orthostatic Hypotension

Orthostatic hypotension is covered in detail in Chapter 31, Syncope. This section will briefly cover aspects of orthostatic hypotension as it pertains to patients with complaints of dizziness.

Textbook Presentation

Patients with orthostatic hypotension classically complain of near syncope or faintness upon standing. They may describe blurring or graying of the visual field or the need to hold on to an object.

Disease Highlights

A. Many patients complain of dizziness upon standing (orthostatic dizziness, OD), which may or may not be associated with orthostatic hypotension.

  1. Criteria for OD include nonvestibular dizziness, which is precipitated by standing and lasts from seconds to < 5 minutes.

  2. Lifetime prevalence of OD in the adult population is 8.5% and accounts for 55% of nonvestibular dizziness.

  3. Consequences of OD include

   a. Syncope, 18.5%

   b. Falls, 17.3%

   c. Trauma, 5%

   d. Fear of falling, 32.9%

   e. Moderate to severe impact on daily living, 27%

   f. Physician consultation, 45%

  4. Etiologies of OD include neuropathy, impaired vision, orthostatic hypotension, or *initial* orthostatic hypotension.

B. Orthostatic hypotension

  1. Prevalence exceeds 50% in some populations (elderly patients in rehabilitation unit)

  2. Symptoms include

   a. Light-headedness, 88%

   b. Leg weakness, 72%

   c. Blurred vision or tunnel vision, 47%

   d. Cognitive difficulties (including disorientation and mental slowing on standing), 47%

   e. Syncope, 42%

   f. Palpitations or tachycardia, 26%

  3. Patients may also be asymptomatic or have atypical symptoms (headache, backache, or focal neurologic symptoms).

  4. Aggravating factors include warm environments, hot baths, and climbing stairs.

C. Patients with OD may also have *transient initial* orthostatic hypotension that is difficult to document.

  1. BP falls and recovers rapidly upon standing

  2. In healthy adults over age 50, the systolic BP nadir (at < 40 seconds) was 30–40 mm Hg < baseline but recovered rapidly (within 20–60 seconds). Patients older than 70 years had larger drops than patients between the ages of 50 and 59.

  3. Some patients have an exaggerated transient initial orthostatic hypotension.

Consider orthostatic hypotension as a cause of dizziness when patients complain of symptoms upon standing. Symptoms may include impending faint, lightheadedness, falling, or changes in vision (blurring, seeing black spots, etc).

Evidence-Based Diagnosis

A. Orthostatic hypotension is defined as a drop in systolic BP ≥ 20 mm Hg or a drop in diastolic BP ≥ 10 mm Hg within 3 minutes of standing. A criterion of a drop in systolic BP of ≥ 30 mm Hg may be more appropriate in patients who have hypertension while supine.

  1. This definition fails to consider pulse changes, which may decrease its sensitivity.

  2. Experimental studies document that patients with acute blood loss of up to 500 mL rarely have BP changes of this magnitude, with an average drop of 14 mm Hg in systolic BP and of 7 mm Hg in diastolic BP with standing. However, the pulse increased 36–40%.

B. *Transient* orthostatic hypotension is defined as a drop in systolic BP > 40 mm Hg or diastolic BP > 20 mm Hg within 15 seconds of standing.

  1. Due to its rapid improvement this cannot be detected without beat-to-beat BP measurements, but patients may be symptomatic nonetheless.

  2. One study documented that 27% of patients with OD but without demonstrable orthostatic hypotension had a history of syncope, suggesting that many of these patients had transient or intermittent orthostatic hypotension that was undetected. Another study documented that this accounted for 8% of syncope cases among young adults.

Treatment

See Orthostatic Hypotension in Chapter 31, Syncope.

CASE RESOLUTION

Orthostatic hypotension is unlikely since Mrs. S has a normal BP, without change of either BP or pulse. You elect to initiate treatment for her depression with an SSRI, refer her to psychiatry for counseling and see her back in 1 month. You hope her symptoms will have improved at that time.

Mrs. S returns 1 month later even more distressed than at the time of her last visit. She reports her dizziness is worse, and that she is now having trouble walking and driving. When asked to elaborate, she reports that she feels unsteady on her feet and is scared that she will fall.

RANKING THE DIFFERENTIAL DIAGNOSIS

Mrs. S's complaints are clearly worrisome. Her symptoms have evolved and she is no longer describing ill-defined lightheadedness but rather dysequilibrium. Dysequilibrium can arise from abnormalities of the brain, cerebellum, spinal cord, or peripheral nerves. Causes include Parkinson disease, normal-pressure hydrocephalus, cerebellar degeneration (eg, alcoholic cerebellar degeneration), cerebellar stroke, VBI, B_{12} deficiency, tabes dorsalis, and multiple sensory deficits. The cranial nerve exam, gait, and sensory exams may provide critical clues to the diagnosis. Gait disturbances may suggest Parkinson disease (shuffling gait) or cerebellar disease (wide-based gait). Stocking glove sensory deficits are typical of diabetic neuropathy, whereas loss of proprioception suggests posterior column disease (ie, B_{12} deficiency, tabes dorsalis, and some compressive spinal lesions). A diagnostic approach is illustrated in Figure 14-5.

Mrs. S denies headache, numbness or weakness. However, she reports that she no longer trusts herself driving because of her double vision. Surprised by this comment you ask her to describe her double vision and she reports that she sees two lines on the road in areas where there is only one. On neurologic exam her cranial nerves are intact, there is no obvious diplopia, and her gait appears mostly normal, perhaps slightly unsteady.

Despite the lengthy differential diagnosis for dysequilibrium, Mrs. S's complaint of diplopia is a highly specific pivotal clinical clue that focuses the differential diagnosis on diseases affecting the brainstem. Neither diseases of the dorsal column, peripheral nerves, multiple sensory deficits nor her depression would cause diplopia. You revise your leading hypothesis to diseases affecting that region of the brain (eg, cerebrovascular disease or posterior fossa tumor).

Leading Hypothesis: Cerebrovascular Disease

Textbook Presentation

Cerebrovascular disease encompasses a multitude of diseases in which disordered blood supply results in CNS dysfunction. The neurologic symptoms may be transient (typically < 1 hour) if blood supply is reestablished quickly (transient ischemic attack [TIA]) or permanent if blood flow is not reestablished within this period (stroke). Patients with symptoms lasting > 1 hour but < 24 hours often have subclinical infarction. The location of ischemia within the brain and the mechanism of the event determine the type of

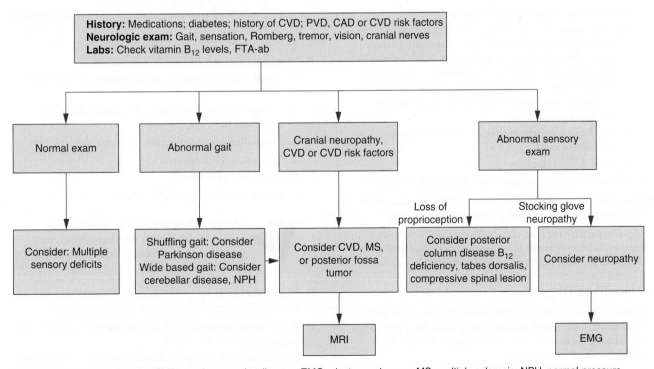

CAD, coronary artery disease; CVD, cerebrovascular disease; EMG, electromyelogram; MS, multiple sclerosis; NPH, normal-pressure hydrocephalus; PVD, peripheral vascular disease.

Figure 14-5. A diagnostic approach to dysequilibrium.

symptoms, their rapidity of onset, and severity. After a brief review of the mechanisms of cerebrovascular disease, this discussion will focus on those CVD syndromes associated with vertigo or dysequilibrium; VBI and lacunar infarction of the pons and cerebellum. Other causes, cerebellar hemorrhage and VAD are discussed later in the chapter.

Disease Highlights

A. Thrombosis

1. Large intracranial or extracranial vessels (ie, middle cerebral artery, carotid artery, vertebral artery)

   a. Risk factors include older age, hypertension, tobacco use, and diabetes.

   b. Occasionally, secondary to hypercoagulable states, heparin-induced thrombocytopenia, vasculitis (ie, Takayasu arteritis, giant cell arteritis), or sickle cell anemia

2. Small penetrating vessels: Small arteries that penetrate at right angles may be obstructed, resulting in small cavitary infarcts (lacunar infarcts—see below); usually involve basal ganglia, internal capsule, thalamus and pons.

3. May progress in stuttering manner

4. Unusual in patients younger than age 40

5. Headache *unusual* at onset of symptoms (< 20%)

B. Embolization

1. Sources include left atrium (particularly in patients with atrial fibrillation), left ventricle (in patients with myocardial infarction, heart failure), heart valves, aortic arch, and carotid or vertebral arteries.

2. Symptoms are maximal at onset and may involve multiple vascular territories.

C. Hemorrhage (≈20%)

1. Intraparenchymal hemorrhage

   a. Usually secondary to hypertension

   b. Other causes include trauma, amyloid angiopathy, bleeding diathesis (warfarin), vascular malformations or cocaine or methamphetamine use. (Cocaine may be associated with spasm and thrombosis or intracranial hemorrhage.)

   c. Neurologic symptoms and headache progress over minutes to hours.

   d. Headache is present at the onset of symptoms in 50–60% of cases.

   e. Focal deficits common

2. Subarachnoid hemorrhage: (See Chapter 20, Headache)

D. Dissection of the carotid or vertebral arteries can cause ischemia due to thrombosis, embolization, or hemorrhage.

E. *Hypotension* may result in symmetric damage to watershed areas including occipital cortex (resulting in blindness) and motor strips (resulting in shoulder and hip weakness).

Evidence-Based Diagnosis

A. Initial evaluation should include serum glucose, basic metabolic panel, CBC, prothrombin time, partial thromboplastin time, an ECG (to look for atrial fibrillation or myocardial infarction), and neuroimaging.

B. Neuroimaging: MRI is far superior to CT scan for the diagnosis of ischemic stroke and almost identical for the diagnosis of hemorrhagic stroke (Table 14-7).

Table 14-7. Sensitivity for diagnosis of acute stroke.

Imaging Method	All Strokes	Ischemic Strokes	Hemorrhagic Strokes	Ischemic Strokes < 3 h
CT (noncontrast)	26%	16%	93%	12%
MRI	83%	83%	85%	73%

1. Vertebrobasilar Insufficiency (VBI)

Textbook Presentation

The classic presentation of VBI is an elderly patient with diabetes, hypertension, or both who complains of intermittent spells of vertigo associated with other neurologic symptoms, such as diplopia, dysphagia, dysarthria, weakness, numbness, or ataxia.

Disease Highlights

A. Risk factors include hypertension (58–70%), tobacco use (42%), diabetes (25%), and hyperlipidemia (19%). Common comorbidities include coronary artery disease (42%) and peripheral vascular disease (11%).

B. Atherosclerosis is often present in the vertebral and the basilar arteries. Symptoms may be caused by low flow, embolism (artery to artery), or thrombosis. VAD is another important cause in young patients (see below). Cardiac sources of embolism may also cause posterior strokes or TIAs.

C. Dizziness in patients with VBI may be described as tilting rather than spinning.

D. Symptoms may last for minutes or hours with VBI (but may persist in patients with stroke or cerebellar hemorrhage).

Evidence-Based Diagnosis

A. 50% of patients have a normal neurologic exam between the episodes. Attacks can last seconds to hours but usually last minutes (if they were not associated with infarction).

B. Manifestations of VBI and their frequency

1. Visual changes (diplopia, hallucinations, or field defects), 69% of cases

2. Vertigo, 58% of cases (isolated without other CNS symptoms in 7.5–29%)

3. Unsteadiness-incoordination, 21% of cases

4. Confusion, 17% of cases

5. Headache, 14% of cases

6. Loss of consciousness, 10% of cases

 Basilar ischemia should be considered in patients with vertigo who have significant cerebrovascular disease risk factors (eg, diabetes mellitus).

C. Most common symptom is visual dysfunction (eg, diplopia, visual field defects, hallucinations, and blindness).

D. Transcranial Doppler, MRA, CT angiography (CTA), and angiography have been used.

1. MRI with MRA is procedure of choice; 83–89% sensitive, 87–98% specific

2. CTA can be used in patients with contraindications to MRI/MRA; 58–68% sensitive, 92–93% specific

3. Transcranial Doppler is less sensitive (44%), but 95% specific.

4. Angiography is invasive but the gold standard.

5. Echocardiography is useful in patients with suspected embolic disease, particularly those without evidence of basilar or vertebral artery disease on neuroimaging and in those with isolated cerebellar infarcts or infarcts in multiple vascular territories.

Treatment

A. Recurrent TIAs and strokes are very common in patients with VBI (28% recurrent TIA or stroke within 90 days). The highest risk of stroke is within the subsequent 48 hours with 49% of subsequent strokes occurring in the next 2 days.

B. Emergent neuroimaging, including MRA or CTA and neurology consultation is advised.

C. Patients with new strokes should be treated as outlined under Lacunar Infarction of the Pons and Cerebellum (see below).

D. Angioplasty, stenting, and surgical reconstruction have been used in addition to medical management in patients with vertebral and basilar artery stenosis.

2. Lacunar Infarction of the Pons or Cerebellum

Textbook Presentation

Typically, the presenting symptoms are rapid onset of hemiparesis, sensory symptoms, or ataxia.

Disease Highlights

A. Small, deep, non-cortical white matter infarcts secondary to obstruction of the small penetrating arteries

B. Common causes of lacunar infarcts

1. Hyalinosis of the small penetrating artery with subsequent thrombosis is the most common cause. The hyalinosis is a long-term complication of hypertension.

2. The small penetrating arteries may also be obstructed by thrombosis or embolization arising from the parent artery (middle cerebral artery or basilar artery), which feeds the small penetrating artery. The recurrence rate in patients with parent arterial lesions is much higher than in patients without such lesions (16% vs 1%) and similar to patients with large artery infarcts (17%).

3. Cardioembolism

C. Hypertension, diabetes mellitus, and smoking are risk factors.

D. Incidence in the black population is approximately twice that in the white population.

E. Typically involves basal ganglia, internal capsule, thalamus, and pons

F. Cortical signs (aphasia, agnosia, apraxia, and hemianopsia) are absent.

G. Symptoms depend on stroke location.

H. Pontine/cerebellar strokes may be associated with vertigo, ipsilateral weakness, ataxia, dysarthria, and nystagmus.

1. The dizziness may be described as vertigo, tilting, or swaying.

2. It is estimated that 25% of patients with acute persistent vertigo have suffered a stroke.

3. Deterioration occurs in 10–20% of patients in the first 3 days, which may result in brainstem compression and death without neurosurgical intervention. Therefore, a detailed neurologic evaluation, frequently accompanied by neuroimaging is required to exclude a stroke.

4. 25% of these strokes occur in patients < 50 years

   a. Although cerebrovascular risk factors increase the probability of stroke, these strokes may be secondary to VAD.

   b. Thus, they are commonly missed in young patients without traditional risk factors.

Evidence-Based Diagnosis

A. Similar to BPPV and vestibular neuritis, vertigo may be exacerbated by head motion.

Vertigo exacerbated by motion is not diagnostic of BPPV.

B. The vertigo in pontine and cerebellar infarction often lasts for days and may mimic vestibular neuritis, which is frequently misdiagnosed in patients with cerebellar/pontine infarction (see Table 14-4 and Figure 14-4). Neuroimaging with DW-MRI should be done in patients with any of the following:

1. Headache

   a. Although insensitive (40% overall), headaches are an important clue to the diagnosis of cerebellar infarction

   b. In 1 case series, headaches were present in 13 of 15 patients in whom the diagnosis was missed.

2. Multiple cerebrovascular risk factors

3. Other CNS signs or symptoms

   a. Neck pain, persistence of severe vertigo beyond a few days, dysarthria, diplopia, weakness, inability to ambulate, difficulty sitting upright without support, dysmetria, cranial nerve findings, visual field deficits, Horner syndrome or central type nystagmus

   b. Oscillopsia (in which objects appear to vibrate)

   c. Facial or limb pain

4. Normal head thrust test, skew deviation, or direction changing nystagmus

5. If clinical uncertainty exists, MRI should be performed, and if unavailable a CT should be done to rule out hemorrhage.

C. Neuroimaging

1. Overall, CT scanning has low sensitivity (16%). However, it can be useful in acute cases to rule out hemorrhagic but not ischemic strokes.

2. DW-MRI is superior to CT but still imperfect at detecting pontine infarcts (80% sensitivity in first 24 hours). Repeat MRI should be considered when the clinical exam suggests stroke.

3. MRA or CTA should be performed to evaluate patients for vertebral artery or basilar artery stenosis, VAD, or emboli. Studies suggest that risk factors do not reliably separate patients with lacunar infarctions due to disease of the small penetrating arteries from patients with large vessel disease.

D. Echocardiogram (to look for embolic etiology) and erythrocyte sedimentation rate (elevated in certain vasculitides) may be useful

Treatment

A. Neurology consultation is recommended.

B. IV recombinant tissue-type plasminogen activator (rt-PA) improves outcomes in carefully selected stroke patients only if given within 4.5 hours of symptom onset. For patients ineligible for IV rt-PA due to recent surgery who have proximal cerebral arterial occlusions, intra-arterial rt-PA can be given up to 6 hours after symptom onset. Guidelines for the use of rt-PA have been published and must be followed carefully to minimize the risk of intracranial hemorrhage.

C. Appropriate use of antihypertensive therapy during an acute stroke is controversial. Due to the loss of cerebral autoregulation, lowering BP may decrease cerebral perfusion and increase ischemia, whereas higher blood pressures may increase the risk of intracranial hemorrhage in patients who receive thrombolytics or worsen hemorrhage in those with a hemorrhagic stroke.

D. Early aspirin (160–325 mg) is recommended for patients with acute ischemic stroke or TIA. It is not recommended in the first 24 hours for patients receiving thrombolytic therapy.

E. Secondary prevention with antiplatelet therapy is recommended.

   1. Options include aspirin (75–100 mg/day), clopidogrel (75 mg/day), or the combination of extended-release dipyridamole/aspirin 200/25 mg twice daily

   2. Extended-release dipyridamole/aspirin 200/25 mg twice daily or clopidogrel is recommended over other alternatives.

F. In patients with atrial fibrillation and stroke, oral anticoagulation therapy is recommended over antiplatelet therapy. Recent ACCP guidelines recommend oral dabigatran over vitamin K antagonists (eg, warfarin).

G. Long-term antihypertensive therapy reduces stroke 35–40%. BP reduction is recommended for all such patients for whom it is appropriate.

H. Risk factor management includes control of diabetes mellitus, statin therapy for ischemic but not hemorrhagic stroke (target LDL ≤ 70 mg/dL), avoidance of heavy drinking, regular moderate physical exercise (for those who are able), and smoking cessation.

MAKING A DIAGNOSIS

An MRI is performed on Mrs. S and reveals a large 2-cm aneurysm at the distal right vertebral artery, compressing the medulla, with surrounding edema (Figure 14-6)

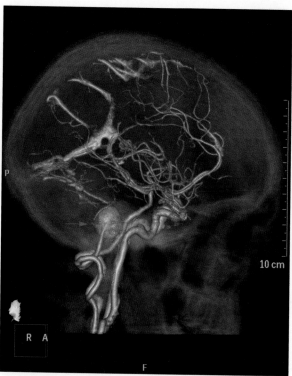

Figure 14-6. Mrs. S's MRA. The red arrow shows a large vertebral artery aneurysm.

CASE RESOLUTION

Mrs. S was referred to neurosurgery and underwent surgical clipping of her aneurysm. Over time her symptoms resolved and she returned to full function.

Mrs. S's case demonstrates several key features. First, that depressed patients often have other serious medical issues and care must be taken not to assume their symptoms are always due to their depression. Second, highly specific neurologic symptoms (in this case diplopia) can be critical clues to CNS disease. They must be actively sought and carefully evaluated.

 Depression is common and can cause a multitude of somatic complaints, including dizziness. However, depression is not always causal. Some patients have other medical illness *and* depression while others have depression *caused* by their illness. Clinicians should be careful when ascribing a patient's symptoms to depression and use careful clinical judgment and follow-up to avoid overlooking other serious medical illnesses in such patients.

CHIEF COMPLAINT

PATIENT 4

Mr. W is a 29-year-old man who arrives at the emergency department with a chief complaint of dizziness. He reports that he was in his usual state of excellent health until about 1 hour ago. At that time he experienced a fairly intense sensation of dizziness. He describes the sensation as spinning. He also complains of a severe headache with neck pain.

At this point, what is the leading hypothesis, what are the active alternatives, and is there a must not miss diagnosis? Given this differential diagnosis, what tests should be ordered?

RANKING THE DIFFERENTIAL DIAGNOSIS

As noted in Figure 14-1, the first pivotal decision in patients with dizziness is to determine whether the patient is experiencing vertigo, dysequilibrium, near syncope, or ill-defined lightheadedness. Mr. W has a sensation of motion and therefore has vertigo. The second pivotal point in patients with vertigo is to search for suggestive or definitive clues that suggest that the pathologic process is coming from the brainstem or cerebellum (Figure 14-3). His headache makes this an obvious consideration. The subset of diseases that cause vertigo *and* headache include migraine with vertigo (vestibular migraine), cerebellar hemorrhage, intracranial neoplasm, and VAD. Clearly, several of these are potentially life-threatening.

4

Mr. W reports that he has never experienced vertigo before. He has an occasional headache that resolves with ibuprofen and has never been associated with an aura. He has no known vascular disease and does not have a history of hypertension, diabetes, tobacco use, coagulopathy, atrial fibrillation, or cocaine use. He has no known malignancy. Finally, although he feels that it is unrelated, he mentions that he saw a chiropractor for cervical adjustment about 1 hour before his symptoms started. He reports that he sees his chiropractor regularly and has never had any symptoms subsequently.

On exam he looks fairly uncomfortable. His vital signs are normal except for mild hypertension 140/90 mm Hg. His cranial nerve exam and gait are normal. He has no nystagmus or dysmetria. The remainder of his exam is unremarkable.

Given Mr. W's young age and overall health, you wonder if he is presenting with a migraine and vertigo. However, all of the alternative hypotheses are potentially life-threatening and must not miss hypotheses. Table 14-8 lists the differential diagnosis.

Leading Hypothesis: Vestibular Migraine

Textbook Presentation

Classically, migraine sufferers complain of intermittent attacks of severe unilateral throbbing headache associated with photophobia, phonophobia, nausea and vomiting (see Chapter 20, Headache).

Table 14-8. Diagnostic hypotheses for Mr. W.

Diagnostic Hypotheses	Demographics, Risk Factors, Symptoms and Signs	Important Tests
Leading Hypothesis		
Vestibular migraine	History of recurring throbbing headaches with or without aura. Temporal association of headache and vertigo	Thorough neurologic history and exam to exclude CNS lesions. MRI
Active Alternatives—Must Not Miss		
Cerebellar hemorrhage	Hypertension, cocaine use, anticoagulant therapy. Severe headache at onset, vomiting, ataxia	Head CT scan or MRI/MRA
Vertebral artery dissection	Trauma or spinal manipulation. Severe headache or neck pain at onset, progressive neurologic deficit with cranial neuropathies, ataxia, weakness	MRA or angiogram
Intracranial neoplasm	Known malignancy. Focal neurologic deficit. Seizures	Neuroimaging

Headaches may be preceded by a visual aura (scotoma or scintillating lights). Occasionally, an associated symptom is vertigo. This discussion will be limited to migraine and vertigo.

Disease Highlights

A. Dizziness or vertigo is common during a migraine attack, affecting as many as 24.5% of patients with migraine accompanied by aura and up to 47.5% of patients with severe migraine pain (≥ 7/10).

B. Characteristics of the vertigo in vestibular migraine include
   1. Vertigo lasts seconds to a week
   2. The vertigo is constant in 30% of patients and positional (brought on by head movement) in 60% of patients.
   3. May precede, be concurrent with, follow, or be temporally unrelated to headache.

C. A history of migraines preceded the development of vertigo in 95% of patients (by an average of 8–20 years.)

Migraines almost always precede the development of vestibular migraine. New-onset migraines with vertigo are very unusual. Other diagnoses should be explored in patients with vertigo and new headache.

Evidence-Based Diagnosis

A. Criteria for *definite* vestibular migraine include:
   1. Recurrent episodic vertigo
   2. Current or prior history of migraine
   3. Migrainous symptoms during at least 2 vertiginous attacks (ie, migrainous headache, photophobia, phonophobia, visual or other aura)
   4. Other causes ruled out by appropriate diagnostic studies

B. Patients that satisfy the first and last criteria above but only 1 of the other 2 are classified as having *probable* vestibular migraine.

C. These criteria are helpful but imperfect.

1. The diagnosis of vestibular migraine was confirmed at 12.7 year follow-up in 85% of patients with *definitive* vestibular migraine but only 50% of patients with *probable* vestibular migraine.

2. 49% of patients with *definitive* vestibular migraine had other cochlear symptoms (tinnitus, aural fullness or hearing loss) at follow-up raising the possibility of other diagnoses (eg, Meniere disease).

D. Vertigo was regularly associated with headache in 45% of patients and occurred with *and* without headache in 48% of patients. In 6% of patients, vertigo and migraine did not occur together.

E. Other common symptoms during the attack include nausea (95%), photophobia (70%), headache (65%), phonophobia (10%), and aura (10%).

F. Nystagmus may be pathologic during the attack.

G. One study evaluated patients during an attack. Physical findings included

1. All patients had a normal finger to nose, heel to shin, and no diadochokinesis.

2. 65% of patients had disturbances of gait, but only 5% were unable to stand and walk.

3. 70% of patient had an abnormal Romberg sign.

 Patients with vestibular migraine typically maintain the ability to ambulate. Patients unable to do so should be evaluated with MRI for other diagnoses.

H. Brainstem signs are rare.

Treatment

See Chapter 20, Headache.

MAKING A DIAGNOSIS

Mr. W's prior headache disorder does not sound migrainous nor does he have a prior history of headaches associated with vertigo, making vestibular migraine unlikely. Coupled with the life-threatening nature of the alternatives, his evaluation needs to continue. In particular, cerebellar hemorrhage is imminently life-threatening and must be excluded.

 Cerebellar hemorrhage is a must not miss possibility that *must* be considered in all patients with headache and vertigo.

 Have you crossed a diagnostic threshold for the leading hypothesis, vestibular neuritis? Have you ruled out the active alternatives? Do other tests need to be done to exclude the alternative diagnoses?

Alternative Diagnosis: Cerebellar Hemorrhage

Textbook Presentation

The textbook presentation of cerebellar hemorrhage is the abrupt onset of headache associated with vomiting, ataxia, and vertigo.

Brainstem compression may produce weakness, cranial nerve abnormalities, coma, and death. Patients with cerebellar infarctions have similar symptoms.

Disease Highlights

A. Cerebellar hemorrhage accounts for 5–16% cases of intracerebral hemorrhages.

B. Etiologies are heterogeneous:

1. Most common: Hypertensive hemorrhage is the most common cause. Other common causes include subarachnoid hemorrhage, amyloid angiopathy, and arteriovenous malformations.

2. Less common: Blood dyscrasias, hemorrhagic infarction, septic emboli, anticoagulant and thrombolytic therapy, neoplasms, herpes simplex virus encephalitis, vasculitis, and cocaine and amphetamine use.

C. Demographics

1. Mean age is 61–73 years, 36% have diabetes mellitus, 32–73% have hypertension, 14% have coagulopathies

2. Frequency: Asians > Blacks > Hispanics > Whites

D. Clinical course

1. Rapid progression within minutes to hours is common.

   a. 26% of patients demonstrate an increase in the hematoma on repeat CT scan 1 hour after the initial scan.

   b. Hematoma expansion is associated with a 5-fold increase in poor outcomes and death.

   c. Both hematoma expansion and edema contribute to an increase in intracranial pressure and brainstem herniation.

E. Complications

1. Hydrocephalus (48%)

2. Chronic disability

3. Herniation and death (42%)

4. Other: Pneumonia, myocardial infarction, and ventricular arrhythmias

F. Poor prognostic factors include

1. Marked hydrocephalus

2. Deteriorating consciousness

3. Stupor and coma (100% mortality without surgery)

4. Fever (correlates with ventricular extension of bleeding)

Evidence-Based Diagnosis

A. Clinical findings

1. The most common clinical symptoms were headache, vomiting, and altered consciousness.

2. Brainstem findings were universal in 1 study (Table 14-9).

 Cerebellar hemorrhage must be considered in patients who complain of acute headache and vertigo.

B. Laboratory evaluation should include CBC, platelet count, international normalized ratio, partial thromboplastin time, basic metabolic panel, ECG, chest radiograph, glucose and toxicology screen in young and middle-aged patients.

Table 14-9. Clinical findings in cerebellar hemorrhage.

Findings	Frequency
Brainstem findings	100%
Headache	72–80%
Vomiting	77%
Vertigo	59%
Altered consciousness	60–73%
Extensor plantar responses	55%
Nuchal rigidity	50%
Inability to stand	40%
Dysarthria	22%

C. Prompt cross sectional imaging is critical.

1. Rapid neuroimaging with CT or MRI is recommended to identify hemorrhage.

2. In patients with cerebellar hemorrhage, arteriovenous malformations and aneurysms should be considered when there is a low likelihood that the hemorrhage was secondary to hypertension (ie, patients < 60 years old who do not have a convincing history of hypertension).

3. Patients with a history of cocaine use also have a higher risk of aneurysms.

4. Aneurysms can be identified with CTA, contrast-enhanced CT, contrast-enhanced MRI or MRA.

5. Abnormal results on MRA can be evaluated with cerebral angiography.

Treatment

A. Cerebellar hemorrhages can compress vital brainstem structures and surgical evacuation can be lifesaving, particularly in large hemorrhages (> 3 cm) or those with brainstem compression or hydrocephalus.

1. Surgical evacuation of these hematomas is recommended.

2. Emergent neurosurgical consultation is advised.

B. ICU monitoring is critical.

C. Anticoagulation should be reversed, if present.

D. Antiplatelet therapy should be held.

E. Platelets should be administered to patient with severe thrombocytopenia.

F. Guidelines of potential therapies to treat intracerebral hemorrhage, the associated hypertension, venous thromboembolism prophylaxis, and increased intracranial pressure were published in 2010.

An emergent head CT without contrast is performed and normal.

The normal head CT is reassuring because it markedly decreases the likelihood of 1 of the life-threatening hypotheses, cerebellar hemorrhage (sensitivity 93%). However, a diagnosis has not been established and the evaluation must continue.

On reevaluation, Mr. W complains of weakness on his left side. Neurologic exam reveals a new flaccid paralysis on the left side.

The new neurologic findings coupled with the vertigo, headache, neck pain and recent neck trauma (chiropractic manipulation) make you revise your leading hypotheses to VAD.

Revised Leading Hypothesis: Vertebral Artery Dissection (VAD)

Textbook Presentation

Unlike patients with atherosclerotic disease, patients with VAD are usually younger (mean age 46) and often complain of severe neck pain, occipital headache, and evolving neurologic symptoms due to progressive involvement of the brainstem. Numbness, hemiparesis, quadriparesis, coma, a locked-in syndrome, or death can result from this uncommon but occasionally devastating illness.

Disease Highlights

A. The vertebral artery passes through the transverse process of C1–C6. As C1 rotates on C2, the vertebral artery can be stretched and can be injured initiating dissection and subsequent thrombosis or aneurysm formation (which may be complicated by subarachnoid hemorrhage). The dissection can be intracranial or extracranial. Thrombosis is more common and may extend to involve the basilar artery compromising the entire brainstem.

B. VAD is the leading cause of posterior circulation strokes among young adults. One study found that 42% of strokes associated with vertigo in patients younger than 50 were due to VAD.

C. Stroke develops in 63% of patients. A good outcome was reported in 69%, fair outcome in 18%, and poor outcome in 10%

D. Risk factors *differ* from patients with typical ischemic stroke. VAD may occur following sporting activities (15% of cases), minor trauma, chiropractic manipulation (16% of cases) or spontaneously (> 50%).

1. Examples of sporting activities include jogging, horseback riding, tennis, skiing, and others. Given the frequency with which individuals engage in these activities, it is unclear if this relationship is causal.

2. It is also unclear if chiropractic manipulation causes VAD or if these dissections were already present and patients were seeking relief of pain when visiting their chiropractors. When associated with chiropractic manipulation, symptoms develop within 1 hour of procedure in 85% of patients.

E. Pain (from the dissection) is a common feature (see below).

Evidence-Based Diagnosis

A. Clinical findings

1. The most common symptoms are headache (51%), neck pain (46%) and dizziness/vertigo (58%).

   a. These symptoms are usually sudden, severe, and persistent until other neurologic signs develop.

   b. Headache preceded other neurologic signs and symptoms by 1–14 days.

In patients who complain of vertigo *and headache*, diagnostic possibilities include migraine, subarachnoid hemorrhage, cerebellar hemorrhage, and VAD.

2. Other symptoms include ataxia (38%), change in vision (36%), nausea/vomiting (35%).

3. Signs include nystagmus (29%), Horner syndrome (22%), and cranial nerve palsies (21%).

4. Isolated vertigo and headache are present in 12% of cases.

B. Neuroimaging: VAD can be visualized with MRA, CTA, and conventional angiography.

1. MRA and CTA are highly accurate.

2. Ultrasound with color Doppler is less sensitive for VAD (66%).

3. Neuroimaging: Infarction is seen in 65% of scans.

Treatment

A. For patients with VAD and thrombosis, anticoagulation is the currently recommended therapy. Anticoagulation has been associated with lower mortality than placebo in uncontrolled trials. In 10% of patients, however, VAD is complicated by subarachnoid hemorrhage for which anticoagulation would be contraindicated. Consultation is recommended.

B. For patients with aneurysm formation, endovascular repair and surgery have been used.

CASE RESOLUTION

An emergent MRA is performed and reveals a VAD with new evidence of thrombosis in the left vertebral artery.

The MRA confirms VAD. This unusual but very dangerous condition must be treated immediately.

Despite anticoagulation, the neurologic deficit progresses. Within 24 hours, a major brainstem infarction occurred resulting in quadriparesis and loss of multiple cranial nerve functions. The patient is unable to speak, look around, or move. He has locked-in syndrome. At follow-up 5 years later, he has not improved and will spend the remainder of his life in a nursing home.

Although CNS causes of vertigo are less common, they must be carefully considered in patients with vertigo and neurologic symptoms. A careful neurologic history and exam are of paramount importance. Mr. W had a less common but life-threatening cause of vertigo, which illustrates the need for careful diagnostic reasoning.

REVIEW OF OTHER IMPORTANT DISEASES
Multiple Sensory Deficits

Textbook Presentation

The typical patient is an elderly diabetic who complains of symptoms when arising from their bed during the night. Patients may fall or simply feel as though they are going to fall. Multiple sensory losses and physical deconditioning create imbalance and an unsteady gait.

Orthostatic hypotension (aggravated by many medications) and benzodiazepines for sleep may contribute to the symptoms.

Disease Highlights

A. Multiple systems are involved.

B. Typically, at least 2 or more of the following are present:

1. Visual loss

   a. May develop secondary to myopia, presbyopia, cataracts, macular degeneration

   b. The average 80-year-old requires 3 times the lighting to see like a 20-year-old.

   c. Age-related changes in the lens decrease color perception, decreasing the ability to discriminate objects of similar color and increase the risk of falls.

   d. Glare and accommodation to variations in light intensity also worsen with age.

2. Proprioceptive loss (eg, neuropathy from diabetes, myelopathy from cervical spondylosis)

3. Chronic bilateral vestibular damage (eg, from ototoxic drugs)

4. Orthopedic disorders impairing ambulation

Evidence-Based Diagnosis

A. Ataxia is uncommon (0/14 in 1 series).

B. Patients with significant ataxia or cerebellar findings should undergo MRI to exclude alternative diagnoses.

Treatment

A multifaceted approach is often necessary; elements include:

A. Visual correction

B. Night lighting

C. Amplify visual contrast by juxtaposing objects of distinctly different colors to highlight boundary zones (eg, floor coverings).

D. Instructing patients to sit at the edge of the bed prior to standing.

E. Modifying medications to minimize orthostatic hypotension (ie, alpha-blockers, diuretics)

F. When possible, eliminate benzodiazepines, neuroleptics, and any unnecessary medications.

G. Home visits can identify fall risks (electric and telephone cords, loose rugs, etc).

H. Lower limb strength training and balance training have been demonstrated to reduce falls.

I. Bisphosphonates reduce the risk of fractures in patients with osteoporosis.

REFERENCES

Balcer LJ. Clinical practice. Optic neuritis. N Engl J Med. 2006;354(12):1273–80.

Broderick J, Connolly S, Feldmann E et al. Guidelines for the management of spontaneous intracerebral hemorrhage in adults: 2007 update: a guideline from the American Heart Association/American Stroke Association Stroke Council, High Blood Pressure Research Council, and the Quality of Care and Outcomes in Research Interdisciplinary Working Group. Stroke. 2007;38(6):2001–23.

Chalela JA, Kidwell CS, Nentwich LM et al. Magnetic resonance imaging and computed tomography in emergency assessment of patients with suspected acute stroke: a prospective comparison. Lancet. 2007;369(9558):293–8.

Cnyrim CD, Newman-Toker D, Karch C, Brandt T, Strupp M. Bedside differentiation of vestibular neuritis from central "vestibular pseudoneuritis." J Neurol Neurosurg Psychiatry. 2008;79(4):458–60.

Fan CW, Savva GM, Finucane C, Cronin H, O'Regan C, Kenny RA; Irish Longitudinal Study on Ageing. Factors affecting continuous beat-to-beat orthostatic blood pressure response in community-dwelling older adults. Blood Press Monit. 2012;17:160–8.

Furman JM, Cass SP. Benign paroxysmal positional vertigo. N Engl J Med. 1999;341(21):1590–6.

Gomez CR, Cruz-Flores S, Malkoff MD, Sauer CM, Burch CM. Isolated vertigo as a manifestation of vertebrobasilar ischemia. Neurology. 1996;47(1):94–7.

Gomez-Moreno M, Diaz-Sanchez M, Ramos-Gonzalez A. Application of the 2010 McDonald criteria for the diagnosis of multiple sclerosis in a Spanish cohort of patients with clinically isolated syndromes. Mult Scler. 2012;18(1):39–44.

Gottesman RF, Sharma P, Robinson KA et al. Clinical characteristics of symptomatic vertebral artery dissection. Neurologist. 2012;18:245–54.

Lee H, Sohn SI, Cho YW et al. Cerebellar infarction presenting isolated vertigo: frequency and vascular topographical patterns. Neurology. 2006;67(7):1178–83.

Morgenstern LB, Hemphill JC 3rd, Anderson C et al; American Heart Association Stroke Council and Council on Cardiovascular Nursing. Guidelines for the management of spontaneous intracerebral hemorrhage: a guideline for healthcare professionals from the American Heart Association/American Stroke Association. Stroke. 2010;41:2108–29.

Neuhauser H, Leopold M, von Brevern M, Arnold G, Lempert T. The interrelations of migraine, vertigo, and migrainous vertigo. Neurology. 2001;56(4):436–41.

Polman CH, Reingold SC, Banwell B et al. Diagnostic Criteria for Multiple Sclerosis: 2010 Revisions to the McDonald Criteria. Ann Neurol. 2011;69:292–302.

Radtke A, Lempert T, von Brevern M, Feldmann M, Lezius F, Neuhauser H. Prevalence and complications of orthostatic dizziness in the general population. Clin Auton Res. 2011;21:161–8.

Rajajee V, Kidwell C, Starkman S et al. Diagnosis of lacunar infarcts within 6 hours of onset by clinical and CT criteria versus MRI. J Neuroimaging. 2008;18(1):66–72.

Semaan MT, Megerian CA. Meniere's Disease: A Challenging and Relentless Disorder. Otolaryngol Clin N Am. 2011;44:383–403.

Shenkin HA, Cheney RH et al. On the Diagnosis of Hemorrhage in Man *The American Journal of the Medical Sciences* October 1944 V. 208 No 4. 421–436.

Thacker EL, Mirzaei F, Ascherio A. Infectious mononucleosis and risk for multiple sclerosis: a meta-analysis. Ann Neurol. 2006;59(3):499–503.

van der Worp HB, van Gijn J. Clinical practice. Acute ischemic stroke. N Engl J Med. 2007;357(6):572–9.

15

I have a patient with dyspnea. How do I determine the cause?

CHIEF COMPLAINT

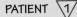

PATIENT

Mr. C is a 64-year-old man who comes to see you complaining of shortness of breath.

✓ What is the differential diagnosis of dyspnea? How would you frame the differential?

CONSTRUCTING A DIFFERENTIAL DIAGNOSIS

Heart disease, lung disease, and anemia are the most common causes of dyspnea. Neuromuscular disease and anxiety are less common causes. The simplest approach to the differential diagnosis is to consider the *anatomical* components of each of these systems. This allows us to develop a fairly comprehensive differential diagnosis of dyspnea.

Differential Diagnosis of Dyspnea

A. Heart
 1. Endocardium: Valvular heart disease (ie, aortic stenosis, aortic regurgitation, mitral regurgitation, and mitral stenosis)
 2. Conduction system
  a. Bradycardia (sick sinus syndrome, atrioventricular block)
  b. Tachycardia
   (1) Atrial fibrillation and other supraventricular tachycardias
   (2) Ventricular tachycardia
 3. Myocardium: Heart failure (HF)
  a. Systolic failure (coronary artery disease [CAD], hypertension, alcohol abuse)
  b. Diastolic failure (hypertension, aortic stenosis, hypertrophic cardiomyopathy)
 4. Coronary arteries (ischemia)
 5. Pericardium (tamponade, constrictive pericarditis)

B. Lung
 1. Alveoli
  a. Pulmonary edema (HF or acute respiratory distress syndrome)
  b. Pneumonia
 2. Airways
  a. Suprathoracic airways (ie, laryngeal edema)
  b. Intrathoracic airways

   (1) Asthma
   (2) Chronic obstructive pulmonary disease (COPD) (see Chapter 33, Wheezing & Stridor)
 3. Blood vessels
  a. Pulmonary emboli
  b. Primary pulmonary hypertension
 4. Pleural
  a. Pneumothorax
  b. Pleural effusions
   (1) Transudative
    (a) HF
    (b) Cirrhosis
    (c) Nephrotic syndrome
    (d) Pulmonary embolism (PE)
   (2) Exudative
    (a) Tuberculosis
    (b) Cancer
    (c) Parapneumonic effusions
    (d) Connective tissue diseases
    (e) PE
 5. Interstitium
  a. Edema
  b. Inflammatory
   (1) Organic exposures (eg, hay, cotton, grain)
   (2) Mineral exposures (eg, asbestos, silicon, coal)
   (3) Idiopathic diseases (eg, sarcoidosis, scleroderma, systemic lupus erythematosus, granulomatosis with polyangiitis [formerly Wegener granulomatosis])
  c. Infectious

C. Anemia

The extensive differential diagnosis for dyspnea necessitates a careful and detailed history, physical exam and review of basic laboratory examinations including chest film, ECG, and hematocrit. The history should detail the time course of the complaint, its severity, associated symptoms, and the patient's past medical history. The physical exam should include vital signs, a detailed cardiac and pulmonary exam, and a search for signs suggestive of anemia (conjunctival pallor or palmar crease pallor). This process often suggests the diagnosis. However, when the diagnosis is not straightforward, certain pivotal findings can narrow the differential diagnosis and focus the diagnostic search (Figure 15-1). One such pivotal clue is fever. Fever is typically seen in pneumonia but could also be seen in asthma or COPD with concomitant infection. Less common causes of fever and dyspnea include valvular heart disease due to endocarditis, pulmonary emboli, acute respiratory distress syndrome, or interstitial lung disease. Chest pain (covered extensively

253

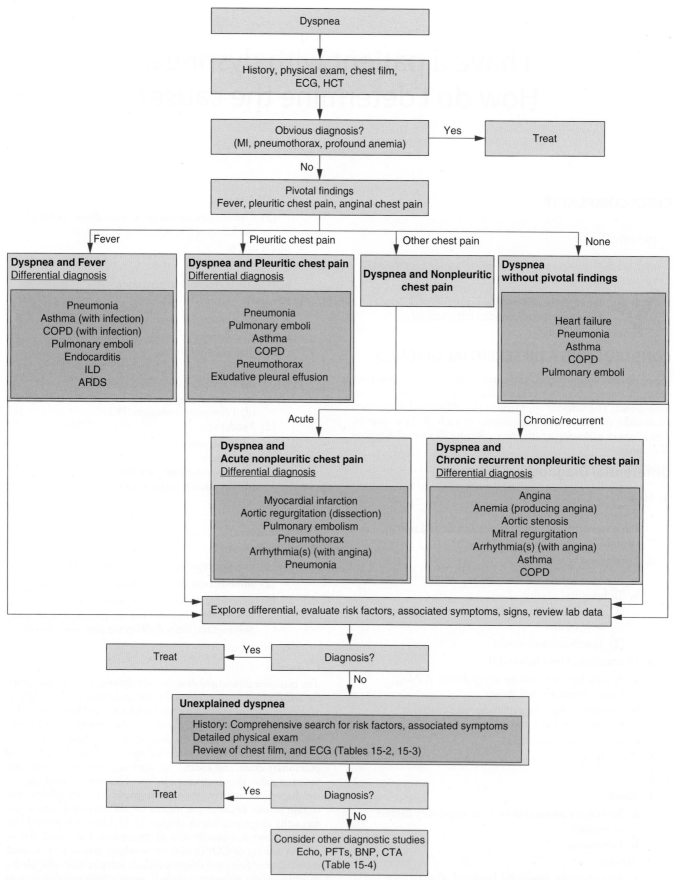

Figure 15-1. A diagnostic approach to dyspnea.

Table 15-1. Differential diagnosis of dyspnea and chest pain.

Pleuritic Chest Pain	Nonpleuritic Chest Pain	
	Acute	**Chronic/Recurrent**
Pneumonia	Myocardial infarction	Angina (CAD)
Pulmonary emboli	Aortic dissection	Angina (aortic stenosis)
Asthma	Pulmonary embolism	Angina (anemia)
COPD	Pneumonia	Arrhythmia(s) (if associated with ischemia)
Pneumothorax	Arrhythmia(s) (if associated with ischemia)	Asthma
Pleural effusion, exudative	Pneumothorax	COPD

CAD, coronary artery disease; COPD, chronic obstructive pulmonary disease.

in Chapter 9) is another pivotal clue in patients with dyspnea. Chest pain may be pleuritic or nonpleuritic and acute or chronic/recurrent. Each of these features can help focus the differential diagnosis (see Figure 15-1, Table 15-1). In brief, common causes of dyspnea and pleuritic chest pain are pneumonia, PE, pneumothorax, asthma, and COPD. On the other hand, many diseases may cause nonpleuritic chest pain (including those diseases already mentioned that may cause pleuritic chest pain). In these patients, the acuity of the chest pain can help narrow the differential diagnosis. Common causes of dyspnea associated with acute chest pain include myocardial infarction (MI), aortic dissection, PE, pneumothorax, arrhythmias (causing angina), and pneumonia. Common causes of dyspnea associated with chronic/recurrent chest pain include angina (caused by CAD, severe anemia, or aortic stenosis), asthma or COPD (which are often associated with chest tightness), and recurrent intermittent arrhythmias.

In patients with any of of any of the aforementioned pivotal clues (fever, chest pain), a search for risk factors, associated symptoms and signs of those diseases can help rank the differential diagnosis. Table 15-2 lists the highly suggestive risk factors as well as associated symptoms and signs of common diseases causing dyspnea.

When these pivotal clues are absent, it is appropriate to evaluate the most common causes of dyspnea, namely HF, pneumonia, asthma, COPD, and pulmonary emboli. Once again, looking for their respective risk factors, associated symptoms and specific signs can help determine their likelihood. Features that suggest HF include a history of MI, CAD risk factors, long-standing uncontrolled hypertension, or alcohol abuse. Furthermore, an S_3 gallop or jugular venous distention (JVD) are fingerprints for HF. Fever and cough raise the possibility of pneumonia and a significant smoking history ($\geq$ 20 pack years) raises the possibility of COPD. Wheezing—defined as a multi-pitched sound on *exhalation*—suggests COPD or asthma. Finally, PE can be obvious or subtle and should be considered in patients with risk factors such as recent immobilization, surgery, a history of cancer, or use of estrogen, or suggestive signs (eg, unilateral leg swelling).

Some patients remain difficult to diagnose. For such patients a more comprehensive review of risk factors, associated symptoms and signs (Table 15-2) as well as a careful review of their chest film findings may be helpful (Table 15-3). A normal chest radiograph makes pneumonia, interstitial lung disease, and acute respiratory

distress syndrome unlikely and rules out pneumothorax. Focal infiltrate(s) suggest pneumonia and can also be seen with COPD or asthma due to atelectasis or superimposed infection. Diffuse infiltrates or edema may be seen in a variety of settings including any cause of HF, acute respiratory distress syndrome, and certain pneumonias. The presence of a pleural effusion is a critical clue that should be evaluated.

Other diagnostic testing that is often necessary includes echocardiography, pulmonary function tests, B-type natriuretic peptide (BNP), and CT angiography (CTA). Echocardiography can reveal unsuspected HF or valvular heart disease. Pulmonary function tests can help determine whether the patient has obstructive, restrictive, or vascular lung disease (Table 15-4). Figure 15-1 summarizes a diagnostic approach to patients with dyspnea.

Over the last 2 years, Mr. C has noticed worsening dyspnea on exertion. He complains of shortness of breath with minimal exertion. He is unable to walk around his house without resting. Several years ago, Mr. C could walk several blocks without any difficulty. He notes that he is unable to sleep lying flat due to shortness of breath (orthopnea), and he has slept on a recliner for the last 6 months. Occasionally, he awakes from sleep acutely short of breath (paroxysmal nocturnal dyspnea). He complains that his feet are swollen.

 Always quantify the increase in dyspnea *from baseline*. Significant changes suggest serious disease and warrant thorough evaluations.

Past medical history is notable for an MI 2 years ago. Vital signs are temperature, 37.0°C; RR, 24 breaths per minute; pulse, 110 bpm; BP, 120/78 mm Hg. His pulse is regular with an occasional irregularity. Cardiac exam reveals JVD to the angle of the jaw in the upright position, a grade II/VI systolic murmur at the apex, and a positive S_3 gallop. Lung exam reveals crackles half of the way up from the bases bilaterally. He has 2+ pretibial edema to the knees.

 At this point, what is the leading hypothesis, what are the active alternatives, and is there a must not miss diagnosis? Given this differential diagnosis, what tests should be ordered?

RANKING THE DIFFERENTIAL DIAGNOSIS

Although the differential diagnosis of dyspnea is broad, the patient's risk factors, symptoms and signs point to a cardiac etiology and immediately focus the differential diagnosis. His past history of MI is a clear risk factor for HF. Furthermore, the JVD, S_3 gallop, and peripheral edema are all very suggestive of HF making this the leading hypothesis. His physical exam also reveals a heart murmur raising several alternative diagnoses (ie, mitral regurgitation, aortic stenosis, or aortic regurgitation). This particular murmur is most consistent with mitral regurgitation. Mr. C's irregular pulse also raises the possibility of atrial fibrillation. Finally, cardiac ischemia presenting as dyspnea rather than pain is a must not miss possibility. Table 15-5 lists the differential diagnosis.

Table 15-2. Common causes of dyspnea: highly suggestive risk factors, associated symptoms, signs, and tests.

Etiologies	Diagnostic Hypothesis	Highly Suggestive Risk Factors or Associated Symptoms	Suggestive Signs	Tests
Cardiac	Valvular heart disease	Rheumatic heart disease Fever Injection drug use (endocarditis)	Significant murmur	Echocardiography Blood cultures if endocarditis suspected
	Aortic regurgitation	Chest pain (dissection) Bicuspid aortic valve Marfan syndrome	Any diastolic murmur	
	Aortic stenosis	Bicuspid aortic valve	Significant systolic murmur	
	Mitral regurgitation	Mitral valve prolapse	Holosystolic murmur	
	Mitral stenosis		Any diastolic murmur	
	Arrhythmia	Palpitations History of heart failure, CAD	Irregular pulse	ECG Holter, event monitor
	Heart failure	CAD or risk factors Uncontrolled hypertension Alcohol abuse PND	S_3, JVD, crackles on lung exam	Chest film BNP Echocardiography
	Acute coronary syndrome	Chest pain CAD or risk factors PVD	S_3, JVD, crackles on lung exam	ECG Troponin, stress test Angiography
Pulmonary	COPD	≥ 20 pack years tobacco	↓ breath sounds, wheezing	Chest radiography PFTs
	ARDS	Sepsis Pancreatitis Severe injury Smoke inhalation Aspiration	Diffuse crackles	Chest radiography
	Asthma	Cold ± exercise → symptoms; Family history of asthma	Wheezing	PFTs Bronchodilator response Methacholine induced
	Pulmonary embolism	Sudden onset of dyspnea Pleuritic chest pain Cancer Surgery, immobilization Estrogen therapy	Unilateral leg swelling Pleural rub	D Dimer CT angiography V/Q scan Leg duplex
	Pneumonia (CAP, TB, PCP, aspiration)	Fever, productive cough High risk sexual exposures Injection drug use TB exposure	Crackles Thrush, Kaposi sarcoma Skin pop marks	Chest radiography HIV CD4
	Pneumothorax	Pleuritic chest pain	Pleural rub or decreased breath sounds	Chest radiography
	ILD	Known connective tissue disease Raynaud phenomenon Vocational, occupational exposure	Diffuse lung crackles	PFTs High resolution chest CT
Hematologic	Anemia	Menorrhagia Melena Rectal bleeding	Pale conjunctiva	Hematocrit

ARDS, acute respiratory distress syndrome; BNP, brain natriuretic peptide; CAD, coronary artery disease; CAP, community-acquired pneumonia; COPD, chronic obstructive pulmonary disease; ILD, interstitial lung disease; JVD, jugular venous distention; PCP, *Pneumocystis jirovecii* pneumonia; PFTs, pulmonary function tests; PND, paroxysmal nocturnal dyspnea; PVD, peripheral vascular disease; TB, tuberculosis.

Table 15-3. Typical radiographic patterns found in dyspneic patients.

	Normal	Focal infiltrate(s)	Diffuse infiltrates or edema	Pleural effusion(s)
Aortic stenosis	√	x	√**	√**
Aortic regurgitation	√	x	√**	√**
Mitral regurgitation	√	x	√**	√**
Mitral stenosis	√	x	√**	√**
Bradyarrhythmia*	√	x	√**	√**
AV heart block	√	x	√**	√**
Atrial fibrillation	√	x	√**	√**
Atrial flutter	√	x	√**	√**
Paroxysmal reenterant nodal tachycardia	√	x	x	x
Ventricular tachycardia	√	x	√**	√**
Heart failure, systolic	√	x	√	√
Heart failure, diastolic	√	x	√	√
Angina	√	x	√**	√**
Myocardial infarction	√	x	√**	√**
Acute respiratory distress syndrome	x	x	√	√
Pneumonia	x	√	√	√
Laryngeal edema	√	x	x	x
Asthma	√	x	x	x
COPD	√	√	x	x
Pulmonary emboli	√	√	x	√
Primary pulmonary hypertension	√	x	x	x
Pneumothorax	x	x	x	x
Pleural effusion, transudative	x	x	√	√*
Pleural effusion, exudative	x	√	√	√*
ILD	√	x	√	√
Anemia	√	x	√**	√**

*For example, sick sinus syndrome, second- or third-degree AV block.
√Possible chest film pattern; x chest film pattern not consistent with this diagnosis.
**May be associated with concomitant heart failure.
AV, atrioventricular; COPD, chronic obstructive pulmonary disease; ILD, interstitial lung disease.

Pursue highly specific positive physical findings (in this case the S₃ gallop and JVD); they should help drive the diagnostic search.

A chest radiograph, HCT, and ECG are performed.

Is the clinical information sufficient to make a diagnosis of HF? If not, what other information do you need?

Leading Hypothesis: HF

Textbook Presentation

Patients typically have fatigue, dyspnea on exertion, orthopnea, paroxysmal nocturnal dyspnea, and edema. Often, there is an antecedent history of either MI or poorly controlled hypertension.

Disease Highlights

A. HF refers to any cardiac pathology that impairs left ventricular filling or ejection, which may arise from diseases of the pericardium, myocardium, or valves. The remainder of this discussion will focus on myocardial causes of HF. Valvular heart disease is discussed separately.

B. Affects 5.8 million patients in the United States and accounts for 1 million hospitalizations and 53,000 deaths annually. Each year, HF is diagnosed in 670,000 patients.

C. Pathophysiologic classification: HF may occur in patients with impaired emptying (and an ejection fraction ≤ 40%) or impaired filling (with a preserved ejection fraction ≥ 50%). The distinction is important because both the etiologies and treatments of these 2 groups are different. HF may also be classified based on whether the primary process affects the left ventricle (LV) or the right ventricle (RV).

Table 15-4. Pulmonary function test (PFT) abnormalities in lung disease.

Mechanism	Key PFT Abnormality	Other PFT Findings
Obstruction (all types)	↓ Flows ↓ FEV$_1$/FVC	TLC N/↑ RV ↑
COPD (chronic bronchitis)	As above	
COPD (emphysema)	As above	DLCO ↓
Asthma	Above and Bronchodilator produces an increase of ≥ 12% ↑ Methacholine produces a decrease of ≥ 20% ↓	
Restriction (all types)	Volumes ↓, TLC ↓	
Interstitium (eg, pulmonary fibrosis)	As above	RV ↓ DLCO ↓ FEV$_1$% N/↑
Chest wall (eg, pleural effusion, obesity)	As above	DLCO WNL RV N FEV$_1$% N
Neuromuscular (eg, myasthenia)	As above	RV ↑, MVV ↓, NIF ↓, PIF ↓
Vascular (ie, pulmonary embolism)	DLCO ↓	Other PFTs often normal

DLCO, diffusing capacity of carbon monoxide; FEV$_1$, forced expiratory volume in 1 second; FEV$_1$%, FEV$_1$/FVC; FVC, forced vital capacity; MVV, maximal minute ventilation; NIF, negative inspiratory force; PIF, positive inspiratory force; RV, residual volume; TLC, total lung capacity.

Table 15-5. Diagnostic hypotheses for Mr. C.

Diagnostic Hypothesis	Demographics, Risk Factors, Symptoms and Signs	Important Tests
Leading Hypothesis		
Heart failure	History of myocardial infarction, poorly controlled hypertension, PND, S$_3$ gallop, JVD Crackles on lung exam Peripheral edema	Echocardiogram ECG BNP
Active Alternatives—Most Common		
Mitral regurgitation	Blowing systolic murmur at apex radiating to axilla	Echocardiogram
Aortic stenosis	Systolic murmur at right upper sternal border radiating to neck Loss of A2	Echocardiogram
Aortic regurgitation	Early diastolic murmur left sternal border	Echocardiogram
Atrial fibrillation	Irregularly irregular pulse	ECG Echocardiogram
Active Alternatives—Must Not Miss		
Angina	Exertional symptoms History of CAD or risk factors (diabetes mellitus, male sex, tobacco use, hypertension, hypercholesterolemia)	ECG Stress test Coronary angiogram

CAD, coronary artery disease; BNP, brain natriuretic peptide; JVD, jugular venous distention; PND, paroxysmal nocturnal dyspnea.

1. Heart failure with reduced ejection fraction (HF*r*EF)
   a. Previously called systolic HF or systolic dysfunction, HF*r*EF accounts for approximately 50% of cases of HF.
   b. HF*r*EF develops when systolic dysfunction impairs LV emptying.
   c. CAD accounts for 66% of all cases of HF*r*EF.
   d. Other common causes include long-standing hypertension and alcohol abuse.
   e. Less common causes include viral cardiomyopathy, postpartum cardiomyopathy, drug toxicity (ie, adriamycin), and idiopathic cardiomyopathy.
   f. Most patients with HF*r*EF (impaired emptying) also have diastolic dysfunction (impaired filling).
2. Heart failure with preserved ejection fraction (HF*p*EF)
   a. Previously referred to as diastolic HF, HF*p*EF accounts for approximately 50% of all HF cases.
   b. HF*p*EF develops when an increase in myocardial muscle mass (thickness), infiltration, or fibrosis decreases LV compliance.

   (1) Decreased LV compliance impairs LV filling.
   (2) Note that although LV filling is compromised, contractility is preserved and the ejection *fraction* is normal.
   c. The most common cause of HF*p*EF is hypertension. Less common causes include aortic stenosis, hypertrophic cardiomyopathy, and infiltrative cardiomyopathies (eg, hemochromatosis, amyloidosis).
3. The mortality in patients with HF*r*EF and HF*p*EF are similar.
4. Patients with ejection fraction of 41–49% are classified as HF*p*EF, borderline. Their treatment and outcomes appear similar to patients with HF*p*EF.
5. Right- versus left-sided HF
   a. HF may involve the LV, the RV, or both.
   b. Common causes of LV failure include CAD, hypertension, and alcoholic cardiomyopathy.
   c. Common causes of RV failure include severe pulmonary disease (especially COPD) and advanced LV failure.
   d. Peripheral edema, JVD, and fatigue may be seen in LV or RV failure. Pulmonary edema may also be seen in LV failure but not isolated RV failure.

6. Progression

   a. HF triggers maladaptive neurohormonal changes including increased activation of the renin-angiotensin-aldosterone system and the sympathetic nervous system.

   b. These neurohormonal responses promote sodium retention, increase afterload, and contribute to edema and progressive HF.

   c. Therapies that interrupt these responses reduce mortality (see below).

D. Classifications of HF

  1. New York Heart Association functional classification is descriptively useful but is limited by the ability of patients to move from 1 class to another with therapy.

   a. Class I: Asymptomatic (ie, symptoms only at levels of exertion that would make healthy patients dyspneic)

   b. Class II: Slight limitation of physical activity (eg, climbing stairs)

   c. Class III: Marked limitation of physical activity (eg, walking on flat surface)

   d. Class IV: Symptoms at rest or with any physical activity

  2. American College of Cardiology Foundation/American Heart Association (ACCF/AHA) stages of HF were developed to facilitate identifying stage-specific therapies.

   a. Stage A: Patients at high risk for HF without structural heart disease or symptoms (eg, patients with hypertension or CAD but normal LV function).

   b. Stage B: Patients with structural heart disease (eg, LV hypertrophy or decreased ejection fraction) without signs or symptoms of HF.

   c. Stage C: Structural heart disease and prior or current symptoms.

   d. Stage D: Refractory HF symptoms despite therapy.

E. Complications of HF

  1. Electrical: Heart block, ventricular tachycardia, atrial fibrillation, sudden death

  2. Pulmonary edema

  3. Stroke and thromboembolism

   a. 2–4% annual incidence

   b. Risk increases if atrial fibrillation coexists

  4. Mitral regurgitation (LV dilatation may lead to sufficient dilatation of the mitral annulus that it causes secondary mitral regurgitation [see below])

  5. Death

   a. Symptomatic mild to moderate HF: 20–30% per year

   b. Symptomatic severe HF: up to 50% per year

   c. Mechanism of death

    (1) Sudden in 50% (secondary to ventricular tachycardia or asystole)

    (2) Progressive HF in 50%

Evidence-Based Diagnosis

A. The history should assess risk factors for HF, including hypertension, CAD, alcohol abuse, illicit drug use, and adriamycin exposure.

B. Common symptoms include dyspnea on exertion, orthopnea and paroxysmal nocturnal dyspnea (Table 15-6).

Table 15-6. Accuracy of clinical findings in heart failure.

Finding	Sensitivity (%)	Specificity (%)	LR+	LR−
S$_3$	13	99	**11**	0.88
Jugular venous distention	39	92	**5.1**	0.66
Crackles	60	78	2.8	0.51
Paroxysmal nocturnal dyspnea	41	84	2.6	0.7
Edema	50	78	2.3	0.64
Orthopnea	50	77	2.2	0.65
Dyspnea on exertion	84	34	1.3	0.48

C. Physical exam

  1. Clinical signs and symptoms are affected by

   a. Patient's *current* volume status

   b. Chronicity. In *chronic* HF, signs and symptoms are frequently absent despite marked impairment of LV function *and* marked volume overload.

  2. S$_3$ gallop

   a. An S$_3$ gallop occurs when a large volume of blood rushes from the left atrium (LA) into the LV at the start of diastole (just after S$_2$).

   b. Virtually pathognomonic of volume overload and occurs most commonly in patients with decompensated HF.

  3. S$_4$ gallop

   a. Occurs when the LA contracts and sends blood into the LV (just before S$_1$).

   b. An S$_4$ gallop may be heard in some normal patients and in many patients with LV hypertrophy due to hypertension or other causes.

   c. S$_4$ is *not* specific for HF.

  4. JVD

   a. Defined as > 3 cm of elevation above the sternal angle (Figure 15-2).

   b. Highly specific for HF (> 95%); may occur in RV or LV failure.

  5. Table 15-6 summarizes the sensitivities, specificities, and LRs of clinical findings for HF in patients with dyspnea.

   a. Classic signs and symptoms (orthopnea, paroxysmal nocturnal dyspnea, crackles, gallops and edema) are not sensitive for HF and their absence does not rule out HF. Indeed, even in severe chronic HF (mean ejection fraction 18%, pulmonary capillary wedge pressure [PCWP] > 22 mm Hg), 42% of patients did not have crackles, increased JVP, or edema.

Signs of HF are commonly absent even in advanced HF.

   b. However, certain findings are highly specific and significantly increase the likelihood of HF when present. An S$_3$ (but not an S$_4$) and JVD strongly suggest HF.

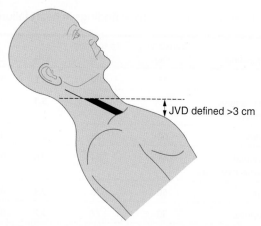

Figure 15-2. Measurement of jugular venous distention (JVD). Modified from McGee S. Evidence Based Physical Diagnosis, p. 402. Copyright ©2001. With permission from Elsevier.

c. Other classic symptoms, like orthopnea, paroxysmal nocturnal dyspnea, and crackles, are not specific for HF.

D. Chest radiography

1. Cardiomegaly is the most sensitive finding on chest film (74% sensitive, 78% specific), and its absence modestly decreases the likelihood of HF (LR– 0.33).

2. Pulmonary venous congestion and interstitial edema are highly specific (96–97%) and when present strongly suggest HF (LR+ 12).

3. Pleural effusions are seen in 26% of patients with HF.

   a. The effusions are usually small to moderate in size and unilateral or bilateral.

   b. These effusions are transudative.

   c. When due to HF, pleural effusions are usually accompanied by cardiomegaly, pulmonary vascular redistribution, or edema.

   d. The absence of these findings or the presence of massive pleural effusions suggests some other etiology and warrants further evaluation.

4. Table 15-7 summarizes the accuracy of the chest radiograph in the diagnosis of HF.

E. ECG, though not diagnostic for HF, can be suggestive if signs of prior MI or LV hypertrophy are present.

F. BNP

1. Secreted by LV or RV in response to increased volume, pressure, or both.

Table 15-7. Accuracy of chest radiography in heart failure.

Finding	Sensitivity	Specificity	LR+	LR–
Pulmonary venous congestion	54%	96%	12.0	0.48
Interstitial edema	34%	97%	12.0	0.68
Alveolar edema	6%	99%	6	0.95
Cardiomegaly	74%	78%	3.3	0.33
Pleural effusions	26%	92%	3.2	0.81

Table 15-8. Accuracy of BNP in heart failure.

BNP Cutoff	Sensitivity	Specificity	LR+	LR–
< 50 pg/mL	97%	62%	2.6	0.05
< 100 pg/mL	87–93%	66–72%	2.7–3.1	0.11–0.12
< 250 pg/mL	89%	81%	4.6	0.14

BNP, brain natriuretic peptide.

2. May be elevated in systolic or diastolic HF

3. Levels increase proportionately to the degree of HF

4. Low BNP levels decrease the likelihood of HF in patients with dyspnea.

5. High levels of BNP increase the likelihood of HF but are still not entirely specific.

6. The accuracy of the BNP is summarized in Table 15-8.

7. BNP is also elevated in many patients with pulmonary embolus (average 702 ng/L, and 1876 ng/L in patients with central PE).

8. The ACCF/AHA concluded that elevated BNP levels lend weight to a diagnosis of HF but should not be used in isolation to confirm or exclude HF.

G. Two-dimensional echocardiogram is the test of choice to diagnose HF and is recommended for all patients with known or suspected HF.

1. Systolic and diastolic function can be evaluated.

2. Regional systolic dysfunction suggests an ischemic etiology.

3. Valve function can be assessed.

4. Bedside hand-carried ultrasound accurately identifies patients with ejection fraction < 40% when performed by internal medicine residents with limited training (sensitivity, 94%; specificity, 94%; LR+, 15.7; LR– 0.06).

H. Radionuclide tests can quantify ejection fraction but cannot assess LV wall thickness or valvular abnormalities.

I. Cardiac MR, although more costly and difficult to perform than echocardiography, is another option for the evaluation of HF.

1. Cardiac MR can accurately measure ejection fraction and LV volume as well as assess myocardial perfusion, viability, and fibrosis.

2. Appropriate in the initial evaluation of patients with new or suspected HF.

3. Cardiac MR combined with magnetic resonance angiography and gadolinium enhancement can detect underlying CAD and ischemia (sensitivity 100%, specificity 96% in patients in sinus rhythm).

J. HF and COPD

1. HF is frequently present but unsuspected in patients in whom COPD is diagnosed.

2. Diagnosis is more difficult in these patients.

   a. Studies report unsuspected HF in ≈25% of patients with COPD. These patients had fewer pack years of tobacco use than patients without HF (9.6 vs 22.7).

   b. Pleural fluid, pulmonary revascularization, and edema were uncommon even in the subgroup with HF (9.1%) but when present strongly suggested HF (LR+ 9.1).

   c. BNP is less sensitive in patients with COPD (sensitivity, 35%; specificity, 90%; LR+, 3.5; LR–, 0.72).

Clinicians should have a low threshold for checking an echocardiogram in patients with COPD and dyspnea.

Treatment

A. Prevention: Hypertension therapy decreases the incidence of HF by 30–50%.

B. Evaluation

   1. Initial history and physical exam should assess functional capacity and volume status (weight, vital signs, lung exam, JVD, S_3 gallop and edema).

   2. Routine laboratory tests recommended by the ACCF/AHA

     a. CBC

     b. Urinalysis, blood urea nitrogen (BUN), creatinine

     c. Electrolytes

     d. Lipid panel, glycohemoglobin, liver function tests

     e. Thyroid-stimulating hormone

     f. Chest radiograph

     g. ECG

     h. Echocardiogram

   3. Evaluation of CAD

     a. HF develops secondary to ischemia in approximately two-thirds of patients with HFrEF.

     b. Identifying underlying CAD allows clinicians to optimize medical therapy and identify which patients can benefit from revascularization.

     c. CAD should be suspected in patients with chest pain, CAD risk factors, ischemic ECG findings, or regional wall motion abnormalities on noninvasive imaging.

     d. Stress test or angiography can be used depending on the pretest probability of CAD.

C. Treatment

   1. Certain treatments benefit all patients with HF whereas others have greater proven efficacy in patients with HFrEF.

   2. All HF patients

     a. Sodium restriction is recommended for all HF patients. A high sodium diet is associated with a marked increase in acute decompensated HF (an absolute increased risk 31–34%, NNH ≈ 3), hospitalizations, and all-cause mortality.

     b. Diuretics (loop or thiazides)

       (1) Mainstay of therapy to treat edema and pulmonary congestion (should be used in combination with salt restriction)

       (2) The clinical assessment of volume status is critical. Increasing weight, edema, JVD, pulmonary edema, or an S_3 gallop suggests patients are volume overloaded.

       (3) However, multiple studies demonstrate that despite severe chronic HF and marked volume overload (measured by PCWP) patients may not have signs of HF.

       (4) Therefore, dyspneic HF patients should undergo aggressive diuresis while monitoring renal function.

       (5) LV filling pressures can also be indirectly estimated using hand carried ultrasound evaluation of the inferior vena cava (IVC).

         (a) Hand carried devices can measure IVC diameter and collapsibility with inspiration.

         (b) HF (right or left) is associated with an increase in IVC diameter and a decrease in the normal collapsibility with inspiration.

         (c) IVC diameter > 2.0 cm suggests elevated PCWP ≥ 17 mm Hg (75% sensitive, 83% specific, LR+ 4.4, LR– 0.3).

         (d) IVC collapsibility < 45% suggests elevated PCWP ≥ 17 mm Hg (83% sensitive, 71% specific, LR+ 2.9, LR– 0.24).

         (e) IVC measurements may prove useful as an adjunct to determine the need for further diuresis. Larger IVC diameters and less collapsibility on discharge predicted the subsequent need for readmission.

       (6) Input and output, daily weights, lung and cardiac exam, electrolytes, BUN and creatinine should be monitored daily in hospitalized patients.

     c. Control of hypertension

     d. CAD revascularization: Coronary artery bypass surgery can improve cardiovascular outcomes in select patients with CAD and HF. Recommendations include the following:

       (1) Coronary artery bypass surgery should be considered in patients who have HF (HFrEF or HFpEF) with angina and left main stenosis or left main equivalent disease.

       (2) Coronary artery bypass surgery is also recommended for select patients with HFrEF and multivessel or proximal LAD disease

     e. Influenza and pneumococcal vaccination

     f. Nonsteroidal antiinflammatory drugs and thiazolidinediones increase fluid retention and have been associated with worsening and precipitating HF and should be avoided.

   3. Patients with HFrEF

     a. Therapy with angiotensin-converting enzyme (ACE) inhibitors, beta-blockers, aldosterone antagonists, and hydralazine combined with nitrates have been shown to reduce morbidity and mortality in patients with HFrEF.

     b. ACE inhibitors

       (1) Indicated in patients with HFrEF or patients with a prior MI

       (2) Angiotensin receptor blockers (ARBs) may be used in place of ACE inhibitors when a troublesome cough develops in patients taking ACE inhibitors.

       (3) ARBs may cause angioedema in patients who had angioedema while taking ACE inhibitors.

     c. Beta-blockers

       (1) Beta-blockers reduce morbidity and mortality in all stages of HF, including severe HF (ejection fraction < 25%)

       (2) Indicated in patients with HFrEF or patients with a prior MI. Beta-blockers with proven efficacy include carvedilol, sustained-release metoprolol and bisoprolol.

       (3) Initiate therapy at low doses, when patients are euvolemic and not requiring inotropes.

       (4) Beta-blockers can precipitate fatal asthma and should be avoided in patients with severe or decompensated reactive airway disease. Selective beta-1-agonists can be used with caution in patients with controlled reactive airway disease.

d. Aldosterone antagonist (eg, spironolactone)

    (1) Reduces mortality in patients with class II–IV HF and ejection fraction ≤ 35% (< 40% with prior MI)

    (2) Should be avoided in patients with a glomerular filtration rate ≤ 30 mL/min, K+ ≥ 5.0 mEq/dL, or patients who cannot have their serum potassium adequately monitored

e. Statins should be used in patients with HF*r*EF and prior MI.

f. Hydralazine and nitrates, in addition to ACE inhibitors and beta-blockers, have been demonstrated to reduce mortality in black patients with class III or IV HF. They may also be useful in patients who are unable to tolerate ACE inhibitors/ARBs.

g. Digoxin

    (1) Reduces hospitalizations but not mortality

    (2) Low serum concentrations (0.5–0.8 mg/dL) are as effective as higher concentrations.

    (3) ACCF/AHA guidelines recommend digoxin only in *symptomatic* patients with HF*r*EF.

    (4) Digoxin may *increase* mortality in women and is not advised for women by some authorities.

h. Cardiac resynchronization therapy: Some patients with HF have prolonged QRS intervals, associated with prolonged and dyssynchronous depolarization. This nonuniform depolarization results in poorly organized contraction and contributes to LV dysfunction. In addition, it contributes to mitral regurgitation and LV remodeling.

    (1) In cardiac resynchronization, wires are implanted in the atria and both ventricles to allow precise and coordinated depolarization of the atria and left and right ventricles.

    (2) Cardiac resynchronization therapy improves ejection fraction, quality of life, and functional status, and it reduces hospitalizations and mortality in select patients.

    (3) Indications are complex and detailed but include patients with symptomatic HF despite optimal medical therapy, an ejection fraction ≤ 35% and a QRS ≥ 0.15 s (and in certain patients ≥ 0.12s).

i. Implantable cardiac defibrillator

    (1) A substantial proportion of patients with HF experience sudden death (30% in dilated cardiomyopathy), presumably secondary to ventricular tachycardia and ventricular fibrillation.

    (2) Implantable cardiac defibrillators are recommended in the following select HF patients:

        (a) Patients who have survived cardiac arrest, ventricular fibrillation, or hemodynamically destabilizing ventricular tachycardia

        (b) Symptomatic HF patients (NYHA class II–III) with ischemic or nonischemic HF*r*EF with ejection fraction ≤ 35%, at least 40 days post MI while taking appropriate therapy

        (c) Asymptomatic patients with ischemic HF and an ejection fraction ≤ 30%, at least 40 days post MI while taking appropriate medical therapy

        (d) Placement could be considered in HF patients with unexplained syncope.

j. Heart transplantation is an option for a few patients with severe HF refractory to intensive medical therapy.

4. Patients with HF*p*EF

    a. Systolic and diastolic hypertension should be controlled.

    b. Diuretics can be used to treat pulmonary congestion or edema.

    c. Digoxin has no proven benefit.

    d. Control ventricular rate for patients with atrial fibrillation.

    e. The effectiveness of ACE inhibitors, beta-blockers, or ARBs is less well established. Recent studies suggest ARBs decrease hospitalizations in patients with HF*p*EF.

5. See ACCF/AHA guidelines for the treatment of patients with refractory HF and cardiogenic shock.

MAKING A DIAGNOSIS

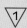

Mr. C has several features that are highly specific for HF. His history of prior MI, orthopnea, and most importantly the clinical findings of JVD and an S₃ gallop are highly specific for HF.

Have you crossed a diagnostic threshold for the leading hypothesis, HF? Have you ruled out the active alternatives? Do other tests need to be done to exclude the alternative diagnoses?

Alternative Diagnosis: Chronic Mitral Regurgitation

Textbook Presentation

Patients with mitral regurgitation may be identified by hearing a holosystolic murmur at the apex in an asymptomatic patient or during an evaluation of shortness of breath, dyspnea on exertion, edema, orthopnea, and fatigue. Alternatively, it may be discovered during the evaluation of patients with atrial fibrillation.

Disease Highlights

A. Trivial asymptomatic mitral regurgitation is commonly discovered on echocardiogram. The remainder of the discussion will focus on patients with more significant regurgitation.

B. Etiologies: Mitral regurgitation develops secondary to damaged mitral leaflets (primary) or a dilated mitral annulus (secondary).

    1. Primary mitral regurgitation

        a. Etiologies: mitral valve prolapse, rheumatic heart disease, and endocarditis.

        b. Although most patients with mitral valve prolapse never require valve replacement, it is the most common cause of mitral regurgitation and the need for valve replacement/repair.

    2. Secondary mitral regurgitation

        a. HF: LV dilatation leads to mitral annular dilatation and mitral regurgitation.

        b. Ischemic mitral regurgitation: Leaflet tethering shortens the mitral apparatus, resulting in mitral regurgitation.

C. Pathophysiology

    1. Compensated mitral regurgitation: Mitral regurgitation leads to LA dilatation, and compensatory LV dilatation.

If systolic function is maintained, ejection fraction remains normal to high and LV end-systolic volume remains low because mitral regurgitation reduces LV afterload.

2. Decompensated mitral regurgitation: Systolic function may fail leading to increased LV end systolic volume, decreased stroke volume, and decreased ejection fraction. This may be irreversible.

3. LA dilatation may lead to atrial fibrillation.

D. Disease progression is slow. Average delay from diagnosis to symptoms is 16 years. However, in patients with severe mitral regurgitation, the annual mortality is 5%.

E. Complications include dyspnea, pulmonary edema, atrial fibrillation, and sudden death.

Evidence-Based Diagnosis

A. Physical exam: The typical murmur is a blowing, holosystolic murmur heard at the apex that radiates to the axilla. S_2 may be inaudible.

1. Grade 3 or louder systolic murmur
   a. 85% sensitive, 81% specific for moderate to severe mitral regurgitation
   b. LR+, 4.5; LR−, 0.19

2. S_3 gallop may be heard due to increased flow across the mitral valve.

B. ECG may demonstrate LA enlargement or LV hypertrophy, neither sensitive nor specific for the diagnosis.

C. Chest radiograph may demonstrate LA or LV enlargement, neither sensitive nor specific for the diagnosis.

D. Echocardiography is the test of choice to diagnose and quantify mitral regurgitation and is recommended in all patients with suspected mitral regurgitation. Transesophageal echocardiography provides more precise details on valve anatomy and may help determine whether valve repair (versus replacement) is an option.

Treatment

A. Serial echocardiography

1. Serial echocardiography is important to detect signs of *LV dysfunction, which may occur despite the absence of symptoms.*

2. Echocardiography is recommended annually or semiannually in patients with moderate to severe mitral regurgitation and after a change in signs or symptoms in patients with any degree of mitral regurgitation.

3. Serial echocardiography is not recommended for asymptomatic patients with mild mitral regurgitation with normal LV size and function.

B. Valve repair versus replacement

1. Valve repair is superior to valve replacement (when technically feasible).

2. Valve repair is associated with substantially decreased operative mortality (2% vs 6%), a lower rate of endocarditis, and is associated with a significantly better ejection fraction. Importantly, valve repair does not require subsequent anticoagulation.

C. ACCF/AHA guidelines for valve repair are summarized below.

1. Mitral valve repair is reserved for patients with severe mitral regurgitation and any of the following:
   a. Symptoms
   b. Atrial fibrillation

c. Pulmonary hypertension
d. Likelihood of success > 90%
e. Mild to moderate LV dysfunction: (ejection fraction 30 − 60%, LV end-systolic diameter 40–55 mm)

2. Decisions in patients with severe LV dysfunction (ejection fraction < 30%, LV end-systolic diameter > 55 mm) and severe mitral regurgitation are complex.
   a. Mitral valve repair or replacement increases afterload (by preventing ejection of blood from the LV to the LA) and may worsen HF.
   b. Consultation is recommended. HF therapy should be optimized.

3. Isolated mitral valve surgery is not indicated in patients with mild to moderate mitral regurgitation.

D. Medical therapy of mitral regurgitation

1. Chronic primary asymptomatic mitral regurgitation with preserved LV function: No medical therapy has been demonstrated to be useful.

2. Secondary mitral regurgitation: Optimize HF regimen. ACE inhibitors, beta-blockers (particularly carvedilol), diuretics, and digoxin can be useful. Biventricular pacing reduces the severity of mitral regurgitation.

3. Mitral regurgitation with hypertension: Treat hypertension with ACE inhibitors, diuretics, or beta-blockers.

4. Treat underlying ischemia.

5. Endocarditis prophylaxis is recommended for patients following mitral valve replacement with a mechanical or bioprosthetic device and for repairs utilizing a bioprosthetic annuloplasty ring. It is also recommended for patients with a history of endocarditis.

Alternative Diagnosis: Chronic Aortic Regurgitation

Textbook Presentation

Patients with chronic aortic regurgitation typically complain of progressive dyspnea on exertion or the sensation of a pounding heart. Alternatively, the patient may be asymptomatic, and the diagnosis may be suspected when a careful examiner detects an early diastolic murmur.

Disease Highlights

A. Secondary to damaged aortic leaflets or dilated aortic root

B. Etiologies

1. Valvular abnormalities: Rheumatic carditis, bacterial endocarditis, collagen vascular disease, calcific degeneration, fenfluramine and phentermine

2. Aortic root dilatation: Hypertension, ascending aortic aneurysm, Marfan syndrome, aortic dissection, syphilitic aortitis

3. Bicuspid aortic valve disease
   a. Most common form of congenital heart disease affecting 1% of population, and transmitted in an autosomal dominant pattern.
   b. Affects the aortic valve (AV) and the aorta.
   c. Aortic regurgitation may occur due to valve changes or dilation of the proximal aorta.
   d. Dilation of the proximal ascending aorta is due to associated changes in the aortic media independent of the AV function.

e. Complications include aneurysms, aortic regurgitation, and dissection.

C. Pathophysiology

  1. Regurgitation results in LV remodeling and eccentric and concentric LV hypertrophy to maintain wall stress. LV end-diastolic volume increases to augment the stroke volume so that forward flow remains in the normal range despite the regurgitant volume. During the compensated stage the ejection fraction is normal.

  2. The increasing preload and afterload may eventually result in LV systolic dysfunction, and the LV end-systolic volume increases and ejection fraction decreases. LV end-diastolic pressure increases and pulmonary congestion and dyspnea result. Exertional angina may also occur.

  3. Significant LV dysfunction can become irreversible. Valve replacement should be performed before irreversible LV dysfunction and HF develop (see below).

  4. Progression to symptoms or LV dysfunction in patients with normal LV function develops in 4% of patients per year. Sudden death occurred in 0.2% per year.

Evidence-Based Diagnosis

A. The pulse pressure (systolic–diastolic BP) is often wide in aortic regurgitation due to 2 processes. First, the large stroke volume increases the systolic BP, and second, the regurgitation of blood back into the LV rapidly lowers the diastolic BP.

  1. The wide pulse pressure causes many of the classic physical findings, such as bounding pulses and head bobbing.

  2. Wide pulse pressures (typically defined as systolic BP – diastolic BP ≥ 50% of systolic BP) are not specific for aortic regurgitation. Other causes include anemia, fever, pregnancy, large arteriovenous fistula, cirrhosis, thyrotoxicosis, and patent ductus arteriosa. Elderly patients with systolic hypertension commonly have a widened pulse pressure.

B. Auscultation

  1. May demonstrate an early decrescendo *diastolic* murmur following S₂. Best heard at the left sternal border.

    a. Auscultation is more sensitive for moderate to severe aortic regurgitation.

    b. Sensitivity is 0–64% among students and residents.

    c. Sensitivity is 80–95% among experienced cardiologists.

    d. Another study reported that the diastolic murmur of mild to moderate aortic regurgitation was rarely detected by attending noncardiologists (sensitivity 4% mild aortic regurgitation, 14% moderate aortic regurgitation).

    e. However, the finding of a diastolic murmur is highly specific (98%).

    A diastolic murmur is always abnormal and warrants evaluation (echocardiography).

  2. A systolic murmur suggesting aortic stenosis may be heard.

    a. Regurgitation results in increasing end-diastolic volumes.

    b. Stroke volumes increase to maintain forward flow.

    c. The increased cardiac output may exceed the capacity of even a normal aortic valve to accommodate flow, resulting in a high flow systolic murmur across the aortic valve. One study reported that 51% of patients with mild to moderate aortic regurgitation had a *systolic* murmur (86% in moderate aortic regurgitation and 50% in mild aortic regurgitation).

    Although a diastolic murmur strongly suggests aortic regurgitation, *systolic* murmurs are often the *only* murmur heard in patients with aortic regurgitation.

  3. Austin Flint murmur

    a. Aortic regurgitant streams may impact the mitral valve leaflets during diastole resulting in functional mitral stenosis and a late diastolic murmur over the apex.

    b. Sensitivity varies from 0% to 100%.

C. Doppler echocardiography is the test of choice and should be performed in all patients with a diastolic murmur and in those patients with a dilated aortic root.

D. Patients with biscuspid valves in whom the aortic root is not adequately visualized with transthoracic echocardiography should undergo additional imaging to evaluate the aortic root (eg, transesophageal echocardiography or cardiac MR).

E. Exercise testing can help assess LV function during stress.

Treatment

A. Serial echocardiography is important to detect signs of *LV dysfunction, which may occur in patients without symptoms*. It should be performed 3 months after the initial study to ensure stability and then periodically and whenever there is a change of symptoms.

B. AV replacement

  1. LV dysfunction and death are more common in symptomatic patients and those with depressed ejection fraction or an increased LV systolic volume.

    a. Mortality in symptomatic patients without surgery is 10–20% per year.

    b. Outcomes are worse in medically treated asymptomatic patients with a LV end-systolic diameter > 50 mm. Symptoms, LV dysfunction, and death develop at 19% per year, compared with 6% per year with a LV end-systolic diameter 40–50 mm and none with a LV end-systolic diameter < 40 mm.

  2. AV replacement is recommended for select groups with severe aortic regurgitation.

    a. All symptomatic patients

    b. Asymptomatic patients with an ejection fraction ≤ 50%

    c. Asymptomatic patients with a LV end-diastolic diameter > 75 mm or a LV end-systolic diameter > 55 mm

    d. When aortic regurgitation is secondary to dilatation of the aortic root, valve repair is recommended in patients with aortic regurgitation of any severity associated with an aortic root > 4.5–5 cm.

C. Replacement valves may be either mechanical or bioprosthetic (eg, porcine valves).

  1. Mechanical valves are more durable and are often chosen for young patients to minimize the need for subsequent AV replacement. However, patients with mechanical valves require lifelong anticoagulation.

  2. Bioprosthetic valves are used more often in older patients (> 70 years) with shorter life expectancies and patients at greater risk for bleeding while receiving anticoagulation therapy.

3. Endocarditis prophylaxis is recommended for patients following AV replacement with a mechanical or bioprosthetic device and for repairs utilizing a bioprosthetic material. It is also recommended for patients with a history of endocarditis.

D. Afterload reduction

1. Should not be substituted for AV replacement in patients with an indication for valve replacement

2. Indications

  a. Severe aortic regurgitation

    (1) Symptomatic patients or those with LV dysfunction as short-term preoperative therapy to improve their hemodynamic function.

    (2) Symptomatic patients or those with LV dysfunction who are not surgical candidates

    (3) For asymptomatic patients with LV dilatation but normal systolic function, the ACCF/AHA concluded that vasodilators "may be considered." The evidence is inconclusive.

  b. Recommended for patients with any degree of aortic regurgitation and hypertension

3. Not indicated in asymptomatic, normotensive patients with normal systolic function and mild to moderate aortic regurgitation

E. Beta-blockers are relatively contraindicated. Prolonged diastole increases regurgitation and accelerates progression.

Alternative Diagnosis: Aortic Stenosis

See Chapter 31, Syncope.

Alternative Diagnosis: Atrial Fibrillation

Textbook Presentation

Classically, patients with atrial fibrillation seek medical care for palpitations. The abrupt onset often prompts patients to be seen emergently. Patients may also complain of shortness of breath and dyspnea on exertion. Occasionally, atrial fibrillation is detected during a routine office visit when an irregularly irregular pulse is discovered and evaluated.

Disease Highlights

A. Atrial fibrillation is the most common clinical arrhythmia; its incidence increases with age (3.8% of patients ≥ 60 years old to 9% in those ≥ 80 years old).

B. May be episodic or persistent

C. Secondary to multiple wavelets of excitation that meander around the atria

D. Etiologies

1. Most common etiologies are hypertension, CAD, and HF.

2. Acute coronary syndrome: In 2–5% of patients presenting to the emergency department with new-onset atrial fibrillation, it is secondary to an acute MI.

3. Other etiologies include alcoholic heart disease, valvular heart disease, cor pulmonale, thyrotoxicosis, and PE.

E. Complications

1. Stroke: Stasis promotes thrombus formation within the atria. Subsequent embolization results in stroke and other systemic emboli.

  a. Atrial fibrillation accounts for one-sixth of all strokes.

  b. Stroke is more common in patients with atrial fibrillation who have other clinical risk factors:

    (1) Valvular heart disease

    (2) Prior transient ischemic attack or stroke

    (3) Increasing age

    (4) Hypertension

    (5) Diabetes

    (6) HF

    (7) Sex (women affected 1.5–3.0 times more than men)

  c. The annual stroke rate in atrial fibrillation patients not receiving anticoagulation is 4.1% per year. However, there is substantial variation depending on the presence or absence of these other risk factors. For the subgroup of patients with a prior transient ischemic attack or stroke, the annual stroke rate increases to 13% per year.

2. Worsening HF due to loss of atrial kick; especially important in patients with stiff LV (ie, diastolic dysfunction)

Evidence-Based Diagnosis

A. Easily recognized on ECG (Figure 15-3)

B. Episodic atrial fibrillation can be detected with Holter monitoring or event recorders.

Treatment

A. Evaluation

1. ECG can document atrial fibrillation, as well as suggest underlying etiologies (ischemia or right heart strain in PE.)

2. Baseline echocardiogram to assess LV function and stroke risk

3. Thyroid function tests, electrolytes, BUN and creatinine are recommended.

4. Consider evaluation for other etiologies (eg, MI, PE).

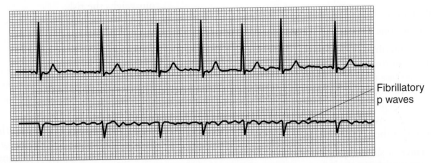

Figure 15-3. ECG of atrial fibrillation demonstrating irregularly spaced QRS complexes and fibrillatory p waves.

B. Rhythm control versus rate control

1. Cardioversion should be performed immediately in unstable patients (with ischemia, hypotension, or HF).

2. In stable patients, 2 options exist: rhythm control or rate control.

   a. Rhythm control attempts to restore normal sinus rhythm using cardioversion and antiarrhythmic agents.

   b. Rate control allows persistent atrial fibrillation. The *ventricular* response is controlled with atrioventricular nodal blocking agents (eg, beta-blockers, diltiazem, verapamil, or digoxin). Anticoagulation is used to prevent stroke.

   c. Studies show that rhythm control and rate control results in similar mortality and stroke rates, even in patients with underlying HF.

   d. Long-term anticoagulation: The American College of Chest Physicians (ACCP) recommends continuing long-term antithrombotic therapy in patients managed with a rate or rhythm control strategy based on their risk factors regardless of the appearance of persistent normal sinus rhythm (see below).

   e. Rate control is the recommended strategy in most patients. (Patients with their first episode of atrial fibrillation or with symptoms or exercise intolerance may choose rhythm control.)

      (1) A resting HR of < 110 bpm is recommended.

      (2) Uses beta-blockers, diltiazem, verapamil, or digoxin

      (3) Beta-blockers, diltiazem, and verapamil should be avoided in patients with decompensated HF.

      (4) Digoxin

         (a) Less effective at controlling ventricular response during activity and in paroxysmal atrial fibrillation

         (b) Should not be used as the sole agent for patients with paroxysmal atrial fibrillation

         (c) Useful in patients with HF*r*EF

         (d) Second-line drug

      (5) Combination therapy

         (a) Verapamil and beta-blockers should not be used concurrently in the same patient due to a high frequency of complications (bradycardia or HF).

         (b) Digoxin and beta-blockers or digoxin and diltiazem or verapamil may be used concurrently to achieve HR control.

      (6) AV ablation can be used to achieve rate control when pharmacologic therapy is unsuccessful or not tolerated.

      (7) Amiodarone can be used for HR control if other measures fail.

   f. Rhythm control therapy

      (1) Cardioversion options

         (a) Flecainide, dofetilide, propafenone, ibutilide, amiodarone, or direct current cardioversion can be used to restore normal sinus rhythm.

         (b) Electrical cardioversion is contraindicated in patients with hypokalemia or digoxin toxicity.

      (2) The probability of conversion to normal sinus rhythm decreases the longer the atrial fibrillation lasts.

      (3) The maintenance of sinus rhythm is complex and beyond the scope of this text.

      (4) Cardiology consultation is recommended.

      (5) Anticoagulation therapy for cardioversion.

         (a) Anticoagulation is often used preceding and following cardioversion (whether electrical or chemical) to decrease the risk that preexistent or new thrombi form or embolize.

         (b) Cardioversion should not be delayed in unstable patients. If the atrial fibrillation was < 48 hours in duration they should undergo cardioversion without delay. If the duration of atrial fibrillation was ≥ 48 hours or unknown, patients should undergo cardioversion while concurrently receiving an unfractionated heparin bolus and maintenance therapy to achieve an activated partial thromboplastin time of 1.5–2 times control until warfarin increases the INR to 2.0-3.0.

         (c) Anticoagulation for 3 weeks prior to cardioversion is recommended in stable patients with atrial fibrillation ≥ 48 hours or of unknown duration. For patients with atrial fibrillation < 48 hours, anticoagulation decisions may be based on other patient risk factors, (eg, mitral valve disease, HF, or prior embolism).

         (d) Low-risk patients (without the aforementioned risk factors) and atrial fibrillation of recent onset (< 48 hours) can undergo cardioversion without delay.

         (e) Alternatively, a transesophageal echocardiography can be performed to look for thrombi. Patients without thrombi can receive unfractionated heparin and then undergo cardioversion. Patients with thrombi should receive 3 weeks of anticoagulation therapy prior to cardioversion.

         (f) Patients typically receive a vitamin K antagonist (target INR 2.0–3.0) for 4 weeks following cardioversion. Patients with left atrial thrombi seen on a transesophageal echocardiogram should probably receive anticoagulation therapy longer.

C. Stroke prevention

1. Antithrombotic therapy with anticoagulants, typically using vitamin K antagonists, or antiplatelet agents (typically aspirin) has been used to prevent strokes in atrial fibrillation patients.

2. The 2 most widely studied therapies are warfarin and aspirin.

   a. Multiple studies suggest that warfarin is superior to aspirin at preventing stroke with a relative risk reduction of 64% compared to 19% for aspirin. In the absence of contraindications, the benefit of warfarin usually outweighs the risk.

   b. The standard INR target is 2.0–3.0.

   c. The absolute benefit of warfarin increases as the risk of stroke increases.

   d. Warfarin reduces the absolute rate of stroke on average by 2.7% per year, but in patients with prior transient ischemic attack/cerebrovascular accident, the absolute risk reduction is 8.4% per year.

   e. Contraindications to warfarin therapy include recent gastrointestinal or central nervous system hemorrhage, recent trauma or surgery, uncontrolled hypertension, noncompliance, syncope, or alcoholism.

Table 15-9. Recommendations to prevent stroke in patients with persistent or paroxysmal atrial fibrillation.

Risk Category	Definition	Therapeutic Recommendations
Highest risk	Mechanical heart valves or rheumatic mitral stenosis	VKA
High risk	Prior TIA/CVA or systemic embolization	Anticoagulant therapy[1]
Moderate risk	≥ 2 risk factors[2]	Anticoagulant therapy[1]
Low risk	1 risk factor[2]	Anticoagulant therapy[1, 3] or antiplatelet therapy[4]
Lower risk	≥ 1 less-validated risk factors: age 65–74, women, CAD	Anticoagulant therapy[1] or antiplatelet therapy[4]
Lowest risk Lone atrial fibrillation	Age ≤ 60, no heart disease, no hypertension or risk factors	Uncertain[5]

[1]Anticoagulant therapies include VKA or dabigatran. For VKA the target INR is 2.5–3.5 for patients with mechanical heart valves and 2.0–3.0 for other patients. Dabigatran is not recommended in patients with mechanical heart valves, hemodynamically significant valve disease, CAD, acute or chronic kidney disease (Cr Cl < 15 mL/min), or advanced liver disease.
[2]Risk factors include history of hypertension, heart failure, age ≥ 75 years, diabetes mellitus.
[3]The ACCF/AHA recommends either anticoagulant or antiplatelet therapy. The ACCP recommends anticoagulant therapy in these patients over antiplatelet therapy. If antiplatelet therapy is chosen, they recommend combined aspirin/clopidogrel.
[4]Aspirin (81–325mg/d) is recommended. Clopidogrel can be added (see text).
[5] Patients with lone atrial fibrillation are at low risk for events. VKAs are not recommended and the utility of aspirin is uncertain.
CAD, coronary artery disease; TIA/CVA, transient ischemic attack/cerebrovascular accident; VKAs, vitamin K antagonists.

    f. The ACCF/AHA have published guidelines for stroke prevention in persistent or paroxysmal atrial fibrillation (Table 15-9).

  3. Two special groups are worth mentioning.

    a. Although physicians worry about bleeding complications in the elderly, studies show that elderly patients with atrial fibrillation are at high risk for stroke and benefit from anticoagulation if they are carefully selected.

    b. Patients with lone atrial fibrillation (age < 60 years, no heart disease, hypertension or risk factors) are at the lowest risk for stroke (< 1% per year when treated with aspirin).

      (1) The absolute risk reduction from warfarin is very small and similar in magnitude to the risk of hemorrhage from warfarin.

      (2) The AHA/ACC/ACCP does not recommend warfarin in these patients.

      (3) The utility of aspirin is uncertain and the AHA/ACC concluded that the effectiveness of aspirin for this population has not been established.

  4. New oral anticoagulants provide alternatives to vitamin K antagonist.

    a. The new anticoagulants directly inhibit thrombin (dabigatran) or factor Xa (rivaroxaban and apixaban).

    b. Rivaroxaban and dabigatran accumulate in renal impairment.

    c. Compared with warfarin, dosing is easier, anticoagulation does not require monitoring, and there are fewer drug and food interactions.

    d. However, unlike warfarin, antidotes are not available to reverse anticoagulation in hemorrhaging patients.

      (1) Vitamin K and fresh frozen plasma are ineffective.

      (2) Preliminary data suggest that prothrombin complex concentrate may reverse anticoagulation due to Xa inhibitors (eg, rivaroxaban).

    e. The precise role of these agents compared with vitamin K antagonist remains an area of active clinical research.

  5. Aspirin combined with clopidogrel has been compared with either aspirin or warfarin monotherapy in the prevention of stroke in patients with atrial fibrillation.

    a. Combination therapy is less effective than warfarin at stroke prevention but associated with the same rate of major bleeding. Annual event rate on combination therapy of 5.6% vs 3.9% on warfarin.

    b. Combination therapy was slightly more effective than aspirin alone at preventing stroke, (0.9% per year absolute risk reduction), but associated with a 0.7% per year absolute increase in the rate of major bleeding.

Alternative Diagnosis: CAD

See Chapter 9, Chest Pain.

CASE RESOLUTION

Mr. C undergoes an ECG, chest film, CBC, and transthoracic echocardiogram. His CBC is normal and his chest film reveals cardiomegaly. His ECG demonstrates normal sinus rhythm with pathologic Q waves in leads V1–V4, and his echocardiogram reveals marked systolic dysfunction and an ejection fraction of 18%. There are regional wall motion abnormalities and the anterior wall is akinetic. There is no significant aortic stenosis or aortic regurgitation. Mitral regurgitation is mild.

Mr. C's echocardiogram confirms HF and rules out significant valvular heart disease as the primary etiology of his dyspnea. Similarly his ECG does not demonstrate atrial fibrillation. The likely etiology of his HF*r*EF is ischemia given his history of MI, ECG, and regional wall motion abnormalities on echocardiogram. An angiogram would be recommended by the AHA/ACC guidelines if not already performed.

An angiogram is performed. This reveals an unobstructed right coronary artery and circumflex but an occluded left anterior descending artery supplying the area of his large prior MI. The ejection fraction is 20%.

The angiogram confirms CAD as the cause of Mr. C's HF.

1

Mr. C is admitted for treatment of his HF. He starts a salt-restricted diet and is given diuretics, ACE inhibitors, beta-blockers (when his HF is controlled) and an aldosterone

antagonist. The diuresis results in a 20-pound weight loss, and his dyspnea on exertion improves markedly. His orthopnea resolves. He declines discussing the possibility of coronary artery bypass surgery but agrees to an implantable cardiac defibrillator. He remains stable at follow-up 5 years later.

CHIEF COMPLAINT

PATIENT 2

Mrs. L is a 58-year-old woman who arrives at the emergency department with a chief complaint of shortness of breath. She reports that this has developed gradually over the last 3–6 months. Six months ago, she was able to walk as far as she wanted without any shortness of breath. Now she is experiencing dyspnea even walking around her house. She denies any episodes of acute shortness of breath, fever, chest pain, or hemoptysis. She denies wheezing. She has no history of MI, hypertension, or known heart disease. She smoked 1 pack of cigarettes per day for 10 years and quit when she was 28 years old. She has no history of prior venous thromboembolism (VTE), cancer or immobilization. She drinks 1 glass of wine per week. She works as an accountant and spends her free time with her grandchildren. She has no unusual hobbies.

At this point, what is the leading hypothesis, what are the active alternatives, and is there a must not miss diagnosis? Given this differential diagnosis, what tests should be ordered?

RANKING THE DIFFERENTIAL DIAGNOSIS

Mrs. L's shortness of breath is not only severe but markedly worse than baseline. Both of these features should prompt a thorough investigation. Unfortunately, the clinical information does not suggest a specific diagnosis (Figure 15-1). She has no pivotal clues that can help limit the differential diagnosis (fever, pleuritic chest pain, or other chest pain.) Furthermore, there are no clues that might suggest one of the common causes of dyspnea: No risk factors for HF (CAD, hypertension, or alcohol abuse that commonly cause HF), no history of wheezing or smoking to suggest asthma or COPD, no fever or cough to suggest pneumonia, and no associated symptoms or risk factors to suggest PE (chest pain, cancer, immobilization, prior VTE). A careful exam is vital to look for helpful clues.

2

On physical exam, the patient appears comfortable at rest but becomes markedly dyspneic with ambulation. Vital signs are BP, 140/70 mm Hg; pulse, 72 bpm; temperature, 37.1°C; RR, 20 breaths per minute. Conjunctiva are pink. Lung exam is clear to percussion and auscultation. There are no crackles or wheezes. Cardiac exam reveals a regular rate and rhythm. S_1 and S_2 are normal. There is no JVD, S_3, S_4, or murmur. There is only trace peripheral edema. Abdominal exam is normal. A chest radiograph, ECG, and CBC are normal.

Despite a thorough exam, the leading diagnosis is unclear. In such cases, it is particularly important to systematically review the differential diagnosis in order to arrive at the correct diagnosis (Table 15-2). Each item on the list should be reviewed in light of the history and physical to determine whether it remains in the differential and should be explored further, or whether the existing information makes it highly unlikely.

Reviewing Table 15-2, the absence of a murmur makes mitral regurgitation and aortic stenosis unlikely, since the clinical exam is 85–90% sensitive for these conditions. The clinical exam is less sensitive for aortic regurgitation (see above). Therefore, aortic regurgitation remains on the differential diagnosis. An arrhythmia is essentially ruled out by the patient's normal heart rate *during* symptoms. HF is not particularly suggested by the history and physical exam, but it cannot be excluded given the low sensitivity of the S_3 gallop and JVD. The patient denies any history of chest pain, but dyspnea is occasionally an anginal equivalent, thus CAD remains a possibility. Pneumonia is highly unlikely given the normal chest film and the lack of fever and cough. Asthma remains a possibility although this is not particularly suggested by the history or physical exam. COPD is effectively ruled out by the trivial smoking history. PE cannot be excluded by the current information and remains on the list, although the presentation is not particularly classic for PE. Since PE is associated with a high mortality, it should be considered a must not miss possibility. A significant pleural effusion and pneumothorax are ruled out by the normal chest radiograph, which also makes interstitial disease unlikely (although not impossible). Anemia is ruled out by the normal CBC. We can now focus on the clinical clues and diagnostic tests for these remaining possible diagnoses (aortic regurgitation, HF, CAD, asthma, and PE). Table 15-10 lists the differential diagnosis.

A methodical approach to the differential diagnosis is vital whenever the leading diagnosis is unclear or when the leading hypothesis cannot be confirmed.

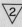

2

In terms of CAD, she denies any history of exertional chest pain or pressure and has minimal coronary risk factors. (Her last cholesterol level was normal [180 mg/dL] with an HDL of 70 mg/dL. She has no history of diabetes mellitus, no family history of CAD, and no recent tobacco use.) With respect to asthma, she denies any history of wheezing or worsening cough associated with cold, exercise, pets, or dust. With respect to PE, she denies sudden onset of chest pain, chest pain with inspiration, hemoptysis, immobilization, cancer, surgery, family history of VTE or leg swelling. She does take hormone replacement therapy.

An echocardiogram reveals normal LV function and a normal aortic valve. Pulmonary function tests reveal normal total lung capacity, forced expiratory volume in 1 second (FEV$_1$), and single-breath diffusing capacity (DLCO). A methacholine challenge test is also normal.

Table 15-10. Diagnostic hypotheses for Mrs. L.

Diagnostic Hypothesis	Demographics, Risk Factors, Symptoms and Signs	Important Tests
Active Alternatives—Most Common		
Heart failure	Poorly controlled hypertension or history of myocardial infarction S₃ gallop, JVD, PND Crackles on lung exam Peripheral edema	Echocardiogram BNP
Coronary artery disease	History of symptoms with exertion (eg, chest pain, pressure) Risk factors for coronary artery disease	ECG Exercise stress tests
Aortic regurgitation	Early diastolic murmur left sternal border	Echocardiogram
Asthma	History of wheezing Chest tightness Worsening cough with cold, exercise, pets, mold	Peak flow Pulmonary function tests Methacholine challenge Response to treatment
Active Alternatives—Must Not Miss		
Pulmonary embolism	Pleuritic chest pain Risk factors (immobilization, postoperative or postpartum states, estrogen therapy, cancer, thrombophilia)	CTA D-dimer Duplex leg exam Ventilation perfusion (V/Q) scan Pulmonary angiography

BNP, brain natriuretic peptide; CTA, CT angiography; JVD, jugular venous distention; PND, paroxysmal nocturnal dyspnea.

Considering each diagnosis in turn, the patient's physical exam and echocardiogram exclude HF and aortic regurgitation. The patient's pretest probability of CAD is quite low given her age, sex, and risk factors (3.2%; see Chapter 9, Chest Pain). In addition, the Framingham data suggest the likelihood of a coronary event in a female patient with these CAD risk factors to be < 1% over the ensuing 8 years. The history and normal pulmonary function tests with methacholine challenge make asthma very unlikely. Although her history sounds atypical for PE, she is taking hormone replacement therapy, a known risk factor for VTE. Given the exclusion of the other diagnoses, PE becomes more probable. You revise your differential diagnosis and make PE both your leading and must not miss diagnosis.

 Is the clinical information sufficient to make a diagnosis of PE? If not, what other information do you need?

Leading Hypothesis: PE

Textbook Presentation

Classically, patients with PE experience the sudden onset of shortness of breath and severe chest pain that increases with inspiration. Patients may complain of hemoptysis and associated unilateral leg swelling.

Disease Highlights

A. Pathophysiology: Most commonly occurs when a lower extremity venous thrombosis embolizes to the lung. Upper extremity thrombi may also cause PE.

  1. 80% of patients with PE have deep venous thrombosis (DVT).

  2. 48% of patients with DVT have PE (often asymptomatic).

B. Symptoms vary markedly. Massive obstruction may result in RV failure and death, whereas lesser obstruction may be asymptomatic.

C. 3-month mortality is 17.5%

D. Risk factors

  1. A variety of risk factors increase the odd ratio for VTE including a personal history of VTE (2.9), estrogen use (2.3), surgery within the last 4 weeks (2.3), personal history of thrombophilia (2.0), active or metastatic cancer (1.9), immobilization (1.7), age over 50 (1.5).

  2. Thrombophilia

    a. Antiphospholipid antibodies: Present in 2–8.5% of patients with VTE

    b. Factor V Leiden

      (1) Most common thrombophilia

      (2) Mutation in factor V causes resistance to cleavage by activated protein C

      (3) 11% of patients with DVT

      (4) Confers a 2.7 × increased risk of VTE

      (5) Combined with oral birth control pill, mutation increases risk 35 times

    c. Prothrombin gene mutation

    d. Protein C or S deficiency (rare)

      (1) Protein C and S are naturally occurring anticoagulants

      (2) Deficiency is associated with hypercoagulability.

      (3) Synthesis of protein C and S requires vitamin K.

      (4) Warfarin decreases synthesis of both factors.

      (5) Assays for protein C and S must be performed while patients are not taking warfarin.

    e. Antithrombin III deficiency (also rare): Assay must be done while patient is not taking heparin.

    f. Hyperhomocysteinemia: 3 × increased risk of VTE

    g. Increased factor VIII: 6 × increased risk

E. PE commonly presents as a "COPD exacerbation."

  1. Studies have reported that 16% of patients with a COPD exacerbation have pulmonary emboli.

  2. The rate was 25% among patients with an unexplained exacerbation of COPD, compared with 8% in those with an exacerbation of known etiology.

  3. Unexplained exacerbation was defined as patients without parenchymal consolidation on chest radiograph without fever or chills (ie, not obviously due to pneumonia) and

patients who lacked the common factors precipitating COPD exacerbations:

a. Lower respiratory tract infection (increased sputum, purulence, fever, cold or sore throat)

b. Exposure to noxious irritants

c. Objective signs of HF

d. Noncompliance

 Consider pulmonary emboli in patients with a COPD exacerbation that is unexplained.

Evidence-Based Diagnosis of PE

A. Clinical presentation: The diagnosis of pulmonary emboli is complicated because patients may present in a variety of ways and signs and symptoms are neither sensitive nor specific.

1. Although dyspnea and chest pain are the most common symptoms, neither is sufficiently sensitive to rule out the diagnosis when absent nor sufficiently specific to rule in pulmonary emboli when present.

2. The accuracy of the signs and symptoms are shown in Table 15-11.

3. The HR and RR are similar in patients with and without PE and neither confirm nor rule out PE.

 The classic presentation of PE is actually the exception. Patients may have very few symptoms. A high index of suspicion must be maintained for the diagnosis of PE.

B. The chest film, arterial blood gas level, and ECG cannot reliably rule out PE.

1. Chest film: May reveal focal oligemia (45%), wedge-shaped infiltrate (15%), or pleural effusions (45%) but is normal in 12–50% of patients with PE.

2. Arterial blood gas measurement: May demonstrate hypoxemia and hypocarbia, but findings are neither sensitive nor specific for PE. $PaO_2 < 80$ mm Hg: sensitivity 58–74%; LR+ 1.2, LR– 0.8

Table 15-11. Accuracy of symptoms and signs in PE.

Symptoms and Signs	Sensitivity	Specificity	LR+	LR–
Dyspnea	59–84%	51%	1.7	0.3
Dyspnea, sudden onset	73–81%	71%	2.7	0.3
Pleuritic chest pain	32–74%	70%	1.5	0.8
Cough	11–51%	85%	0.7	1.0
Hemoptysis	7–30%	95%	1.8	1.0
Syncope	5–26%	87%	2.0	0.9
Tachycardia	24–70%	77%	1.0	1.0
Crackles	18–58%	74%	0.7	1.1
Wheezes	4–21%	87%	0.3	1.1
Fever (>38°C)	7%	79%	0.3	1.2
Pleural rub	3–18%	96%	1	1
Leg swelling	17–41%	91%	1.9	0.9

 Patients with PE may *not* be hypoxic. Therefore, normal arterial oxygen does not rule out PE. On the other hand, unexplained hypoxia, particularly in the company of a normal chest radiograph, should increase the suspicion of PE.

3. ECG

a. Useful to diagnose other conditions (ie, MI).

b. Certain findings suggest PE but are unusual: S1Q3T3 (19–50% sensitive), transient right bundle-branch block (6–67% sensitive).

c. T wave inversions in V1–V4 when seen in conjunction with T wave inversions in lead III strongly suggests PE (88% sensitive, 99% specific; LR+ 88, LR– 0.12).

C. Decision rules and D-dimer testing

1. Decision rules and D-dimer testing are useful in combination but should not be used separately to rule out PE.

a. Wells, Geneva, and others decision rules have been developed to estimate the pretest probability of PE. (See below) A recent meta-analysis demonstrated that they are not sufficiently accurate to rule in or rule out PE without additional testing (LR+ 1.4–3; LR– 0.24–0.5).

b. PERC rule

(1) The PERC rule is a recently developed clinical decision rule designed to use clinical criteria to rule out PE without other objective testing (D-dimer or CTA)

(2) Criteria include age < 50 years, HR < 100 bpm, $SaO_2 > 94\%$ on room air, no prior history of VTE, no trauma or surgery in the last 4 weeks, no hemoptysis, no exogenous estrogen, and no unilateral leg swelling.

(3) Patients with none of the criteria are classified as PERC–.

(4) One large study suggested that PERC– patients are at low risk for PE (1%) and could safely avoid further testing for PE (D-dimer or CTA). However, the diagnostic protocol for PE in this study was not rigorous and may have missed patients with PE.

(5) A more recent study found the incidence of PE in PERC– patients to be 5.4% (95% CI, 3.1 – 9.3%).

(6) Should not be used as a stand-alone tool to rule out PE.

c. D-dimers

(1) D-dimers are fibrin breakdown products that are often elevated in patients with VTE but are nonspecific and elevated in many other conditions: surgery, trauma, cancer, and end-stage renal disease.

(2) Enzyme-linked immunosorbent assay (ELISA) and quantitative rapid ELISA are more sensitive than other assays (95–98%; LR– 0.05–0.11).

(3) Need to be used in conjunction with decision rules since not sufficiently sensitive to rule out PE in patients at high risk.

2. Decision rules combined with D-dimer testing

a. The precise rule is dependent on the sensitivity of the D-dimer assay used.

(1) A negative quantitative D-dimer assay in a patient with a Wells score of ≤ 4 has a failure rate (missed diagnoses) of 0.5%.

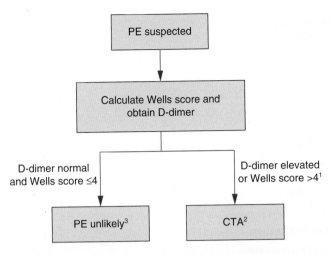

¹A cutoff of ≥2 should be used if a qualitative D-dimer assay is used.
²A ventilation-perfusion scan can be used in patients with contraindications to CTA (eg, renal insufficiency or contrast allergy).
³Failure rate <1%.

CTA, CT angiography; PE, pulmonary embolism.

Figure 15-4. Approach to diagnostic testing in patients with suspected pulmonary emboli.

  (2) A qualitative D-dimer assay in a patient with a Wells score of ≤ 2 has a failure rate of 0.9%.

  (3) Patients with an elevated D-dimer value or a Wells score > cutoff (2 or 4) should be evaluated with a CTA (or a ventilation-perfusion [V/Q] scan if CTA is contraindicated) (Figure 15-4).

D. CTA

 1. Test of choice in moderate- to high-risk patients

 2. May demonstrate filling defects in proximal pulmonary arteries

 3. Makes alternative diagnosis in 25% of patients (lymphadenopathy, tumor, aortic dissection)

 4. Accuracy

  a. A wide range of sensitivities and specificities have been published due to variations in CT methodology (single vs multidetector), standard for diagnosis, duration of follow-up and differing patient populations (sensitivity, 83–90%; specificity, 94–100%).

  b. Follow-up studies of patients with negative CTA have documented subsequent VTE in 1.3–5.3%. Rates are higher in patients with a high pretest probability of disease.

  c. The PIOPED II study reported on the accuracy of multidetector CT using stringent diagnostic criteria.

   (1) Multidetector CTA was 83% sensitive and 96% specific for PE (LR+ 19.6, LR– 0.18).

   (2) The negative predictive value was 96% in low-risk patients (Wells score < 2), 89% in intermediate-risk patients (Wells score 2–6) and only 60% in high-risk patients (Wells score > 6).

E. V/Q scan

 1. Radionuclear study used less frequently since advent of CTA

 2. Radio-isotope infused and inhaled. V/Q images are compared yielding the following potential results:

  a. *High probability scan*

   (1) Multiple areas of normal ventilation but no perfusion

   (2) Effectively rules in PE

    (a) 60% sensitive, 96% specific

    (b) LR+ 15, LR– 0.4

  b. *Normal or near normal perfusion scan* effectively rules out PE. (Normal scans are seen in 0–2% of patients with PE.)

  c. *Nondiagnostic scan (low or intermediate probability)*

   (1) Matched areas of ventilation and perfusion abnormalities

   (2) 67% of patients who undergo V/Q testing have this pattern

   (3) Neither rules in or out PE

F. Angiography

 1. Gold standard

 2. Invasive and rarely used; serious complications occur in 0–3% of patients.

G. Strategy

 1. First use the Wells score to estimate the patients' probability of disease.

  a. Clinical signs and symptoms of DVT: 3 points

  b. PE is as likely or more likely than alternative diagnoses: 3 points

  c. Heart rate > 100: 1.5 points

  d. Immobilization ≥ 3 days or recent surgery (< 4 weeks): 1.5 points

  e. Prior VTE (DVT or PE): 1.5 points

  f. Hemoptysis: 1 point

  g. Active cancer (treated in last 6 months or palliative): 1 point

 2. A negative D-dimer in conjunction with a low pretest probability of PE effectively rules out PE (Figure 15-4). All other patients should have CTA unless contraindicated.

  a. Positive CTA: effectively confirms the diagnosis of PE

  b. Negative CTA

   (1) Effectively rules out PE in low- to moderate-risk patients

   (2) Additional testing may be appropriate in intermediate-risk patients.

   (3) Additional testing is recommended in high-risk patients (Wells > 6).

   (4) Options for additional testing include duplex leg ultrasonography, indirect CT of the leg veins CT venography, V/Q scanning, and pulmonary angiography.

    (a) Since a diagnosis of DVT is taken as a surrogate marker for the diagnosis of PE, duplex leg ultrasonography is the most commonly used test in this situation.

    (b) Another alternative to rule out DVT is CT venography, which can be performed at the same time as CTA. However, some studies suggest that it is less sensitive than leg ultrasound (sensitivity 60–100%, specificity 93–100%).

    (c) A combined strategy of CTA and duplex leg ultrasonography has an excellent negative predictive value (≈100%) and is advisable for patients with a high likelihood of PE.

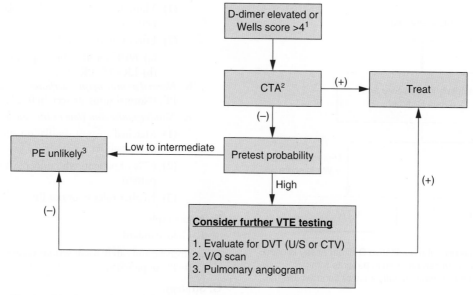

^{1}A cutoff of ≥2 should be used if a qualitative D-dimer assay is used.
^{2}A ventilation-perfusion scan can be used in patients with contraindications to CT angiography (eg, acute or chronic kidney disease or contrast allergy).
^{3}Failure rate <1%.

CTA, CT angiography; CTV, CT venography; PE, pulmonary embolism; U/S, ultrasound; V/Q ventilation-perfusion.

Figure 15-5. Diagnostic algorithm for suspected pulmonary emboli.

3. In patients with acute or chronic kidney disease or contrast allergy, V/Q scanning can be considered in place of CTA (see below).

4. Pulmonary angiography is rarely used.

5. The approach is illustrated in Figure 15-5.

Evidence-Based Diagnosis of DVT

A. Given the overlap of PE and DVT (and the same therapy), the diagnosis of DVT is often taken as evidence of concomitant PE.

B. Several clinical features modestly increase the likelihood of DVT including malignancy (LR+ 2.7), prior DVT (LR+ 2.3), immobilization (LR+ 2.0), and recent surgery (LR+ 1.8).

C. Signs and symptoms are not very helpful at ruling DVT in or out. Leg swelling is only 32% sensitive, LR+ 1.45, LR– 0.67; leg pain LR+ 1.08, LR– 0.9; Homan sign LR+ 1.4, LR– 0.87.

 The clinical exam for DVT is insensitive. Clinicians must have a low threshold for ordering D-dimer or duplex studies.

D. The diagnostic strategy for DVT integrates the pretest probability of DVT with diagnostic tests of appropriate sensitivity to achieve a satisfactory negative predictive value. In short, as the probability of DVT increases, strategies utilize more sensitive testing strategies to rule out DVT.

1. The Wells score can help predict risk of DVT.

   a. Patients are assigned 1 point for each of the following: active cancer, immobilization of the lower extremity, recently bedridden (≥ 3 days) or surgery within the last 12 weeks requiring general anesthesia, tenderness along the deep venous system, swelling of the entire leg, calf swelling ≥ 3 cm larger than the unaffected leg, pitting edema of the symptomatic leg, collateral superficial veins, and prior DVT.

   b. 2 points are subtracted if an alternative diagnosis is at least as likely as a DVT.

   c. The prevalence of DVT is 5% for patients with low probability score (≤ 0), 17% for patients with a moderate probability score (1–2), and 53% for patients with a high probability score (≥ 3).

2. Diagnostic tests

   a. D-dimer

      (1) D-dimers are very sensitive for VTE but not specific (88–92% sensitive, 45–72% specific).

      (2) Used in strategies to help rule out DVT when negative.

      (3) In patients with a low clinical risk, the negative predictive value of a negative D-dimer is 99%.

      (4) D-dimer never confirms DVT. When elevated, ultrasonography is indicated.

   b. Duplex ultrasonography

      (1) Ultrasonography may visualize the whole leg or be limited to the proximal leg.

         (a) Proximal ultrasonography can rule out proximal DVT but will not detect distal DVT (that rarely embolize but can extend and then embolize).

         (b) 89–96% sensitive for symptomatic proximal DVT, 94–99% specific; LR+, 24; LR–, 0.05

         (c) Even whole leg ultrasound less sensitive for distal (below the knee) DVT 73–93%

   c. Other options include venography (invasive) and magnetic resonance direct thrombus imaging (accurate but costly).

3. Diagnostic strategy

   a. In short, DVT is ruled in by a positive ultrasound.

b. DVT may be ruled out in the following situations:

    (1) Low probability Wells score: Negative D-dimer test

    (2) Moderate probability Wells score: Negative highly sensitive D-dimer test

    (3) High probability Wells score: Negative whole leg ultrasound or negative proximal leg ultrasound *and* negative D-dimer

    (4) In patients with a negative proximal leg ultrasound and a positive D-dimer, repeat ultrasound is often recommended to ensure a distal DVT has not extended.

c. Figure 15-6 illustrates the testing strategy recommended by the ACCP for evaluating patients for their first DVT.

Treatment

A. Oxygen should be administered to patients with hypoxemia.

B. Options include anticoagulation (with a variety of agents) or thrombolytic therapy.

C. Thrombolytic therapy is rarely used but recommended in hemodynamically unstable patients in whom the benefits outweigh the risks. If such patients have contraindications to thrombolysis, surgical embolectomy is recommended.

D. Anticoagulation: Overview

    1. A variety of options for anticoagulation exist, including intravenous unfractionated heparin, subcutaneous low-molecular-weight heparin (LMWH), oral vitamin K antagonists (eg, warfarin), oral thrombin inhibitors (dabigatran), and oral factor Xa inhibitors (rivaroxaban and apixaban). See overview of anticoagulants in section above (Atrial Fibrillation, Prevention of Stroke).

    2. Research is ongoing to determine optimal therapy and the choice of anticoagulants is likely to evolve rapidly. Two recent studies suggest apixaban and rivaroxaban are as effective and safer than vitamin K antagonists in patients with VTE. Further studies are needed.

E. 2012 ACCP Clinical Practice Guidelines for treatment of VTE

    1. Initiation of anticoagulation

        a. Initial treatment with either LMWH or fondaparinux followed by vitamin K antagonist (target INR 2.0–3.0).

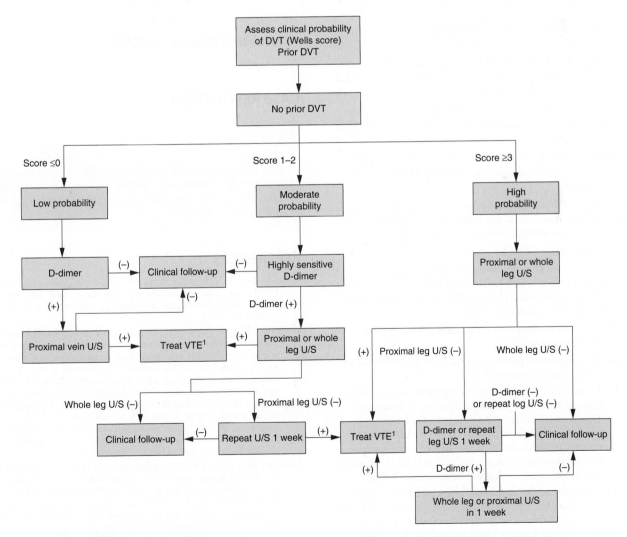

[1]For patients with isolated distal DVT, see text.

DVT, deep venous thrombosis; U/S, ultrasound; VTE, venous thromboembolism.

Figure 15-6. Diagnostic approach to DVT.[1]

b. Anticoagulation should be continued for a minimum of 5 days and until the INR is > 2.0 for ≥ 24 hours.

2. Isolated distal DVT (below the knee)

   a. Hold anticoagulation and repeat imaging over 2 weeks to rule out extension.

   b. Initiate anticoagulation (3 months) if patient has severe symptoms, extension of clot (even if still distal), or risk factors for extension (active cancer, recent surgery or transient risk factor), prior VTE, inpatient status, extensive thrombosis).

3. Acute proximal DVT or PE

   a. Duration of anticoagulation

     (1) Modified by the bleeding risk and inciting cause of the DVT or PE.

     (2) Anticoagulation is effective *during* therapy. After discontinuation, patients with persistent risk factors or idiopathic VTE are at increased risk for recurrence.

     (3) Surgery provoked: 3 months.

     (4) Nonsurgical transient risk factor: 3 months

     (5) Unprovoked:

       (a) Patient at substantial risk for bleeding: 3 months

       (b) Patient at low to moderate risk for bleeding: Extended therapy

     (6) Recurrent DVT/PE: Extended therapy unless the patient is at high risk for bleeding.

     (7) DVT/PE associated with active cancer: Extended therapy is recommended. LMWH is recommended over vitamin K antagonist.

F. DVT/PE in patients with a contraindication to anticoagulation or in whom anticoagulation therapy has failed: IVC filter is recommended.

G. Symptomatic DVT: Compression stockings are also recommended for 2 years to decrease the likelihood of postthrombotic syndrome.

H. Work-up for thrombophilia: Guidelines for routine testing have not been determined. Consider tests for thrombophilic states in patients without clear precipitant of VTE.

I. *Primary* prevention of VTE

1. 25% of venous thromboembolic events are associated with hospitalization. At particularly high risk are patients undergoing hip fracture surgery, hip or knee replacement, and those with spinal cord injury.

2. Hospitalized medical patients account for 50–75% of hospital-associated VTE.

   a. Anticoagulation prophylaxis has been demonstrated to reduce fatal and nonfatal VTE.

   b. At particularly high risk include patients who are older than 40 years, who are hospitalized for ≥ 3 days with limited mobility, and who have ≥ 1 of the following: Acute infectious disease, class III or IV HF, acute MI, cerebrovascular accident, active cancer, acute respiratory disease, rheumatic disease, body mass index > 30, recent surgery or trauma, thrombophilia, or prior VTE.

3. The intensity of the prophylaxis depends on the specific clinical situation. Options include compression stockings, pneumatic compression devices (particularly useful in patients who have active bleeding or are at high risk), and anticoagulation. The ACCP updates guidelines frequently.

MAKING A DIAGNOSIS

You review the patient's Wells score and assign her 3 points since PE is the most likely diagnosis. She also takes hormone replacement therapy, which is a risk factor for PE. Although there is some debate about the use of D-dimer to rule out PE in a patient with a score of 3, you elect to perform a CTA rather than a D-dimer because PE is the most likely diagnosis.

The CTA reveals multiple small pulmonary emboli.

Have you crossed a diagnostic threshold for the leading hypothesis, PE? Have you ruled out the active alternatives? Do other tests need to be done to exclude the alternative diagnoses?

The CTA is highly specific for PE. At this point, PE is ruled in and further confirmation is unnecessary. There is no need for further testing to exclude alternative diagnoses.

Alternative Diagnosis: Asthma

See Chapter 33, Wheezing and Stridor.

Alternative Diagnosis: CAD

See Chapter 9, Chest Pain.

CASE RESOLUTION

Mrs. L's hormone replacement therapy is stopped and she is started on LMWH and warfarin. At follow-up 6 months later, she reports feeling better. Her anticoagulation therapy has been uncomplicated.

REFERENCES

Alonso-Martinez JL, Urbieta-Echezarreta M, Aniccherico-Sánchez FJ, Abínzano-Guillén ML, Garcia-Sanchotena JL. N-terminal pro-B-type natriuretic peptide predicts the burden of pulmonary embolism. Am J Med Sci. 2009;337(2):88–92.

American College of Cardiology; American Heart Association Task Force on Practice Guidelines (Writing Committee to revise the 1998 guidelines for the management of patients with valvular heart disease); Society of Cardiovascular Anesthesiologists, Bonow RO, Carabello BA, Chatterjee K et al. ACC/AHA 2006 guidelines for the management of patients with valvular heart disease: a report of the American College of Cardiology/American Heart Association Task Force on Practice Guidelines (writing Committee to Revise the 1998 guidelines for the management of patients with valvular heart disease) developed in collaboration with the Society of Cardiovascular Anesthesiologists endorsed by the Society for Cardiovascular Angiography and Interventions and the Society of Thoracic Surgeons. J Am Coll Cardiol. 2006;48(3):e1–148.

American College of Cardiology Foundation; American Heart Association; European Society of Cardiology; Heart Rhythm Society; Wann LS, Curtis AB, Ellenbogen KA et al. Management of patients with atrial fibrillation (compilation of 2006 ACCF/AHA/ESC and 2011 ACCF/AHA/HRS recommendations): a report of the American College of Cardiology/American Heart Association Task Force on practice guidelines. Circulation. 2013;127:1916–25.

Assomull RG, Shakespeare C, Kaira PR et al. Role of cardiovascular magnetic resonance as a gatekeeper to invasive coronary angiography in patients presenting with heart failure of unknown etiology. Circulation. 2011;124:1351–60.

Bates SM, Jaeschke R, Stevens SM et al; American College of Chest Physicians. Diagnosis of DVT. Antithrombotic Therapy and Prevention of Thrombosis, 9th ed: American College of Chest Physicians Evidence-Based Clinical Practice Guidelines. Chest. 2012;141(2 Suppl):e351S–418S.

Battaglia M, Pewsner D, Juni P, Egger M, Bucher HC, Bachmann LM. Accuracy of B-type natriuretic peptide tests to exclude congestive heart failure: systematic review of test accuracy studies. Arch Intern Med. 2006;166(10):1073–80.

Bell WR, Simon TL, DeMets DL. The clinical features of submassive and massive pulmonary emboli. Am J Med. 1977;62(3):355–60.

Blair JE, Brennan JM, Goonewardena SN, Shah D, Vasaiwala S, Spencer KT. Usefulness of hand-carried ultrasound to predict elevated left ventricular filling pressure. Am J Cardiol. 2009;103:246–7.

American College of Cardiology/American Heart Association Task Force on Practice Guidelines; Society of Cardiovascular Anesthesiologists; Society for Cardiovascular Angiography and Interventions; Society of Thoracic Surgeons; Bonow RO, Carabello BA, Kanu C et al. ACC/AHA 2006 Guidelines for the Management of Patients with Valvular Heart Disease: A Report of the American College of Cardiology/American Heart Association Task Force on Practice Guidelines. Circulation. 2006;114:e84–e231.

Chunilal SD, Eikelboom JW, Attia J et al. Does this patient have pulmonary embolism? JAMA. 2003;290:2849–58.

European Heart Rhythm Association; Heart Rhythm Society, Fuster V, Rydén LE, Cannom DS et al; American College of Cardiology; American Heart Association Task Force on Practice Guidelines; European Society of Cardiology Committee for Practice Guidelines; Writing Committee to Revise the 2001 Guidelines for the Management of Patients With Atrial Fibrillation. ACC/AHA/ESC 2006 guidelines for the management of patients with atrial fibrillation–executive summary: a report of the American College of Cardiology/American Heart Association Task Force on Practice Guidelines and the European Society of Cardiology Committee for Practice Guidelines (Writing Committee to Revise the 2001 Guidelines for the Management of Patients With Atrial Fibrillation). J Am Coll Cardiol. 2006;48(4):854–906.

Falck-Ytter Y, Francis CW, Johanson NA et al; American College of Chest Physicians. Prevention of VTE in orthopedic surgery patients: Antithrombotic Therapy and Prevention of Thrombosis, 9th ed: American College of Chest Physicians Evidence-Based Clinical Practice Guidelines. Chest. 2012;141(2 Suppl):e278S–325S.

Fesmire FM, Brown MD, Espinosa JA, Shih RD, Silvers SM, Wolf SJ, Decker WW; American College of Emergency Physicians. Critical issues in the evaluation and management of adult patients presenting to the emergency department with suspected pulmonary embolism. Ann Emerg Med. 2011;57(6):628–52.

Goodacre S, Sutton AJ, Sampson FC. Meta-analysis: The value of clinical assessment in the diagnosis of deep venous thrombosis. Ann Intern Med. 2005;143(2):129–39.

Goonewardena SN, Gemignani A, Ronan A et al. Comparison of hand-carried ultrasound assessment of the inferior vena cava and N-terminal pro-brain natriuretic peptide for predicting readmission after hospitalization for acute decompensated heart failure. JACC Cardiovasc Imaging. 2008;1(5):595–601.

Gould MK, Garcia DA, Wren SM et al. Prevention of VTE in nonorthopedic surgical patients: Antithrombotic Therapy and Prevention of Thrombosis, 9th ed: American College of Chest Physicians Evidence-Based Clinical Practice Guidelines. Chest. 2012;141(2 Suppl):e227S–277S.

Hart RG, Pearce LA, Aguilar MI. Meta-analysis: antithrombotic therapy to prevent stroke in patients who have nonvalvular atrial fibrillation. Ann Intern Med. 2007;146(12):857–67.

Heidenreich PA, Schnittger I, Hancock SL, Atwood JE. A systolic murmur is a common presentation of aortic regurgitation detected by echocardiography. Clin Cardiol. 2004;27(9):502–6.

Hugli O, Righini M, Le Gal G et al. The pulmonary embolism rule-out criteria (PERC) rule does not safely exclude pulmonary embolism. J Thromb Haemost. 2011;9:300–4.

Kahn SR, Lim W, Dunn AS et al; American College of Chest Physicians. Prevention of VTE in nonsurgical patients: Antithrombotic Therapy and Prevention of Thrombosis, 9th ed: American College of Chest Physicians Evidence-Based Clinical Practice Guidelines. Chest. 2012;141(2 Suppl):e195S–226S.

Kline JA, Courtney DM, Kabrehel C et al. Prospective multicenter evaluation of the pulmonary embolism rule-out criteria. J Thromb Haemost. 2008;6:772–80.

Lucassen W, Geersing GJ, Erkens PM et al. Clinical decision rules for excluding pulmonary embolism: a meta-analysis. Ann Intern Med. 2012;155:448–60.

Marcus GM, Gerber IL, McKeown BH et al. Association between phonocardiographic third and fourth heart sounds and objective measures of left ventricular function. JAMA. 2005;293(18):2238–44.

Miniati M, Prediletto R, Formichi B et al. Accuracy of clinical assessment in the diagnosis of pulmonary embolism. Am J Respir Crit Care Med. 1999;159(3):864–71.

Miniati M, Cenci C, Monti S, Poli D. Clinical presentation of acute pulmonary embolism: survey of 800 cases. PLos ONE. 2012;7(2):1–7.

Oudega R, Moons KG, Hoes AW. Limited value of patient history and physical examination in diagnosing deep vein thrombosis in primary care. Fam Pract. 2005;22(1):86–91.

Page RL. Clinical practice. Newly diagnosed atrial fibrillation. N Engl J Med. 2004;351(23):2408–16.

Patel MR, White RD, Abbara S, American College of Radiology Appropriateness Criteria Committee; American College of Cardiology Foundation Appropriate Use Criteria Task Force. 2013 ACCF/ACR/ASNC/SCCT/SCMR appropriate utilization of cardiovascular imaging in heart failure. A joint report of the American College of Radiology Appropriateness Criteria Committee and the American College of Cardiology Foundation Appropriate Use Criteria Task Force. JACC. 2013;61(21):2207–31.

Qaseem A, Snow V, Barry P et al. Current diagnosis of venous thromboembolism in primary care: a clinical practice guideline from the American Academy of Family Physicians and the American College of Physicians. Ann Fam Med. 2007;5:(1):57–62.

Razi R, Estrada JR, Doll J, Spencer KT. Bedside hand-carried ultrasound by internal medicine residents versus traditional clinical assessment for the identification of systolic dysfunction in patients admitted with decompensated heart failure. J Am Soc Echocardiogr. 2011;24(2):1319–24.

Segal JB, Streiff MB, Hofmann LV, Thornton K, Bass EB. Management of venous thromboembolism: a systematic review for a practice guideline. Ann Intern Med. 2007;146(3):211–22.

Snow V, Qaseem A, Barry P et al. Management of venous thromboembolism: a clinical practice guideline from the American College of Physicians and the American Academy of Family Physicians. Ann Intern Med. 2007;146(3):204–10.

Tillie-Leblond I, Marquette CH, Perez T et al. Pulmonary embolism in patients with unexplained exacerbation of chronic obstructive pulmonary disease: prevalence and risk factors. Ann Intern Med. 2006;144(6):390–6.

Stein PD, Fowler SE, Goodman LR et al. Multidetector computed tomography for acute pulmonary embolism. N Engl J Med. 2006;354(22):2317–27.

Stein PD, Willis PW 3rd, DeMets DL. History and physical examination in acute pulmonary embolism in patients without preexisting cardiac or pulmonary disease. Am J Cardiol. 1981;47(2):218–23.

Studler U, Kretzschmar M, Christ M et al. Accuracy of chest radiographs in the emergency diagnosis of heart failure. Eur Radiol. 2008;18:1644–52.

Tapson VF. Acute pulmonary embolism. N Engl J Med. 2008;358(10):1037–52.

Wang CS, FitzGerald JM, Schulzer M, Mak E, Ayas NT. Does this dyspneic patient in the emergency department have congestive heart failure? JAMA. 2005;294(15):1944–56.

Wells PS, Owen C, Doucette S, Fergusson D, Tran H. Does this patient have deep vein thrombosis? JAMA. 2006;295(2):199–207.

Whitlock RP, Sun JC, Fremes SE, Rubens FD, Teoh KH; American College of Chest Physicians. Antithrombotic therapy for valvular disease: Antithrombotic Therapy and Prevention of Thrombosis, 9th ed: American College of Chest Physicians Evidence-Based Clinical Practice Guidelines. Chest. 2012;141(2 Suppl):e576S–e600S.

Yancy CW, Jessup M, Bozkurt B et al. 2013 ACCF/AHA guideline for the management of heart failure: executive summary: a report of the American College of Cardiology Foundation/American Heart Association Task Force on practice guidelines. Circulation. 2013 Oct 15;128(16):1810–52.

You JJ, Singer DE, Howard PA et al; American College of Chest Physicians. Antithrombotic therapy for atrial fibrillation: Antithrombotic Therapy and Prevention of Thrombosis, 9th ed: American College of Chest Physicians Evidence-Based Clinical Practice Guidelines. Chest. 2012;141(2 Suppl):e531S–75S.

I have a patient with dysuria. How do I determine the cause?

CHIEF COMPLAINT

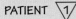

PATIENT 1

Ms. D is a 33-year-old woman who complains of dysuria for 4 days.

What is the differential diagnosis of dysuria? How would you frame the differential?

CONSTRUCTING A DIFFERENTIAL DIAGNOSIS

Dysuria is pain or burning with or after urination. Most patients with dysuria have a urinary tract infection (UTI). When considering this symptom, pivotal points are history and physical exam findings that suggest more serious or complicated etiologies. Important historical features include vaginal or penile discharge, flank pain, rectal/perineal pain, nausea or vomiting, fever, hematuria, urinary hesitancy, urinary urgency, nocturia, and urinary frequency. On the physical exam, vital signs including temperature and sometimes orthostatics are important as are abdominal and costovertebral-angle (CVA) tenderness. A pelvic exam should be performed in any woman with discharge. A prostate exam should be performed in any man in whom cystitis is suspected, especially those with symptoms of nocturia, hesitancy, or rectal pain. When approaching the differential diagnosis for dysuria, an anatomic approach to the genitourinary tract is helpful for organization.

A. Skin: rash causing irritation with urination
1. Herpes
2. Irritant contact dermatitis
3. Syphilitic chancre
4. Erosive lichen planus

B. Urethra (urethritis from sexually transmitted infections [STIs])
1. Gonorrhea
2. Chlamydia
3. Trichomoniasis

C. Male genital structures
1. Epididymis: epididymitis
2. Testes: orchitis
3. Prostate
a. Benign prostatic hypertrophy (BPH)
b. Acute prostatitis
c. Chronic prostatitis

D. Female genital structures
1. Vagina
a. Trichomoniasis
b. Bacterial vaginosis
c. Candidal infections
d. Atrophic vaginitis
2. Uterine/bladder prolapse
3. Cervix
a. *Neisseria gonorrhoeae* infection
b. *Chlamydia trachomatis* infection

E. Bladder
1. Acute cystitis
a. Uncomplicated (healthy women with no urinary tract abnormality)
b. Complicated (men or patients with any of the following: urinary obstruction; pregnancy; neurogenic bladder; concurrent kidney stone; immunosuppression; indwelling Foley catheter; systemic infection, such as bacteremia or sepsis)
2. Interstitial cystitis

F. Kidney: pyelonephritis

1

Ms. D noted the gradual onset of dysuria 4 days ago. She also has increased urinary frequency. She denies flank pain, fever or chills, nausea or vomiting, vaginal discharge, genital rash, or hematuria. Her last menstrual period ended 5 days ago, and she takes an oral contraceptive pill regularly for contraception.

At this point what is the leading hypothesis, what are the active alternatives, and is there a must not miss diagnosis? Given this differential diagnosis, what tests should be ordered?

PRIORITIZING THE DIFFERENTIAL DIAGNOSIS

Ms. D is a healthy young woman with symptoms consistent with cystitis. The pivotal points in this case are the absence of flank pain, vaginal discharge, nausea, vomiting, or fever. Vaginitis is a common disease that can cause similar symptoms, and pyelonephritis is a must not miss diagnosis. These diagnoses must be explored as part of the limited differential diagnosis (Table 16-1).

Table 16-1. Diagnostic hypotheses for Ms. D.

Diagnostic Hypotheses	Demographics, Risk Factors, Symptoms and Signs	Important Tests
Leading Hypothesis		
Uncomplicated cystitis	Dysuria or suprapubic pain or both with or without hematuria, frequency, urgency	Urine dipstick or urinalysis
Active Alternative—Most Common		
Vaginitis	Dysuria with vaginal irritation and discharge	Pelvic exam with discharge examination by saline wet mount, whiff test, and KOH wet mount
Active Alternative—Must Not Miss		
Pyelonephritis	Fever, chills, nausea or vomiting, flank pain, CVA tenderness	Urine dipstick or urinalysis Urine culture CT scan or ultrasound (if concern for obstruction or lack of clinical response)

Physical exam demonstrates normal vital signs, normal temperature, and absence of abdominal or CVA tenderness.

Is the clinical information sufficient to make a diagnosis? If not, what other information do you need?

Leading Hypothesis: Cystitis

Textbook Presentation

Cystitis typically presents with dysuria or suprapubic pain or both. Often, there is associated urinary frequency, urgency, or hematuria. There is usually no penile or vaginal discharge, CVA tenderness, nausea, vomiting, or fever.

Disease Highlights

A. Cystitis is an infection of the bladder.

B. Most common bacterial pathogens include enteric flora such as:

1. Gram negatives: *Escherichia coli* (75–95%), *Klebsiella pneumoniae*, and *Proteus mirabilis*.

2. Gram positives: *Staphylococcus saprophyticus*, *Enterococcus faecalis*, and group B streptococcus.

C. Risk factors for cystitis

1. Sexual intercourse

2. Use of spermicides

3. Previous UTI

4. A new sexual partner in the past year

D. Cystitis in the elderly

1. Elderly patients often have atypical presentations of cystitis; many have chronic symptoms of frequency and incontinence.

2. Delirium, functional decline, or acute confusion may be the presenting symptoms of cystitis in elderly patients.

Cystitis frequently presents in atypical ways in the elderly. UTIs should be on the differential for delirium or functional decline.

Evidence-Based Diagnosis

A. History

1. Dysuria or suprapubic pain with or without frequency, hematuria, or urgency.

2. The symptoms of vaginal discharge (LR– 0.3) or vaginal irritation (LR– 0.2) decrease the probability of cystitis in a woman.

3. The probability of cystitis is over 90% in women with dysuria and frequency without vaginal discharge or irritation.

B. Laboratory testing

1. Women with classic uncomplicated cystitis (dysuria with or without frequency and without vaginal discharge) may be treated without any testing.

2. Urinalysis or urine dipstick findings suggestive of cystitis

   a. Leukocyte esterase is an enzyme released by leukocytes and signifies pyuria. LR+ 12.3-48

   b. The presence of nitrites indicates the presence of bacteria that convert urinary nitrates to nitrites.

   c. White blood cells on urine microscopy

   d. Hematuria demonstrated by positive blood on dipstick or RBCs on microscopy

   e. Table 16-2 shows the sensitivity, specificity, and LRs of urinalysis and microscopy findings.

   f. The negative likelihood ratio of leukocyte esterase and urine nitrite is only 0.3. Absence of these findings does not rule out cystitis.

The diagnosis of cystitis should not be ruled out by a urinalysis that is negative for both leukocyte esterase and nitrites in the presence of a convincing clinical presentation.

Table 16-2. Test characteristics of urinalysis and microscopy.

Test Finding	Sensitivity	Specificity	LR+	LR–
Leukocyte esterase	74–96%	94–98%	12.3–48	0.04–0.3
Nitrite	45–60%	85–98%	3–30	0.4–0.6
Leukocyte esterase or nitrite	75%	82%	4.2	0.3
White blood cells (> 5 per high powered field)	72–95%	48–82%	1.4–5.6	0.06–0.6

3. Urine culture

    a. Used as a confirmatory test in the setting of diagnostic uncertainty or the need to identify a specific bacterial pathogen and the antimicrobial susceptibility (such as in the setting of recurrent cystitis).

    b. The definition of a positive urine culture is $> 10^5$ colony-forming units (CFU) of bacteria per milliliter.

    c. Women with clinical symptoms of cystitis and lower concentrations of bacteria may still have cystitis. One study demonstrated 30–50% of women with cystitis had CFU counts of 10^2 to 10^4.

Treatment

A. Prevention

    1. Factors that have *not* been found to be associated with cystitis

        a. Precoital or postcoital voiding patterns

        b. Daily beverage consumption

        c. Tampon use

        d. Douching

        e. Hot tub use

        f. Underwear type

        g. Body mass index

        h. Wiping patterns

    2. There are no data supporting that changing the above factors prevents recurrent cystitis.

B. Antibiotics

    1. Antibiotic choice is empiric, covering enteric organisms.

    2. First-line options include nitrofurantoin and trimethoprim-sulfamethoxazole (TMP-SMX).

    3. Other options include ciprofloxacin, levofloxacin, amoxicillin-clavulanate, and other beta-lactams.

    4. There is increasing resistance of *E coli* to TMP-SMX and fluoroquinolones. Once resistance in a treatment region exceeds 20% that antibiotic is no longer recommended.

    A urine culture is unnecessary in a patient with uncomplicated cystitis and no history of recurrent infections or recent treatment failure.

C. Treatment duration is based on whether the patient has uncomplicated or complicated cystitis.

    1. Uncomplicated cystitis is defined as cystitis in healthy women with no urinary tract abnormalities.

    2. Complicated cystitis is defined as cystitis occurring in:

        a. Pregnant women

        b. Men

        c. Patients with urinary tract abnormalities (such as obstruction, neurogenic bladder, kidney stones), or an indwelling Foley catheter

        d. Patients with immunosuppression or chronic kidney disease

    3. In uncomplicated cystitis, a shorter duration of antibiotics (1-5 days) is effective and recommended.

    4. In complicated cystitis, a longer duration of antibiotics (7-10 days) is recommended.

    5. In patients with complicated cystitis and previous or recurrent cystitis, it is helpful to review old cultures for previous resistance patterns when choosing empiric therapy.

D. Work-up for secondary causes

    1. Imaging (pre- and post-contrast CT) should be considered in women with multiple episodes of cystitis with the same pathogen.

    2. Patients with hematuria during cystitis should have repeat urinalysis after resolution to determine whether hematuria persists and further work-up is warranted.

    3. Men without a clear predisposition for cystitis (ie, Foley catheter, known BPH) should be considered for further urologic evaluation.

E. Recurrent cystitis

    1. If symptoms continue or return within 2 weeks after treatment for cystitis, relapse or antimicrobial resistance is likely. Antibiotics should be broadened and urine culture performed.

    2. If cystitis recurs beyond 1 month after successful treatment, then standard treatment may be used.

    3. Antimicrobial prophylaxis (continuous or postcoital) may reduce the risk of recurrence by 95% for women with 3 or more infections in 12 months.

MAKING A DIAGNOSIS

A clinical diagnosis of uncomplicated cystitis is made. Urine dipstick is positive for leukocyte esterase only.

    Have you crossed a diagnostic threshold for the leading hypothesis, uncomplicated cystitis? Have you ruled out the active alternatives? Do other tests need to be done to exclude the alternative diagnoses?

The results of the urine dipstick fit with the diagnosis of uncomplicated cystitis. The patient has neither discharge to suggest vaginitis nor flank pain, fever, nausea, or vomiting to suggest pyelonephritis.

Alternative Diagnosis: Vaginitis

Textbook Presentation

Vaginitis typically presents with abnormal vaginal discharge, odor, irritation, itching, dysuria, or dyspareunia.

Disease Highlights

A. Common infectious causes of vaginitis are bacterial vaginosis, trichomoniasis, and candidiasis.

B. Bacterial vaginosis occurs when the normal flora of the vagina are replaced with anaerobic bacteria most commonly, *Gardnerella vaginalis*.

C. Trichomoniasis is an STI caused by the flagellated protozoan, *Trichomonas vaginalis*. It can also infect men, causing urethritis or silent infection.

D. Vulvovaginal candidiasis is caused by various *Candida* species. It often occurs when changes in the vaginal environment precipitate pathologic activity, such as, high estrogen states (menses, pregnancy), antibiotic use, immunosuppression, uncontrolled diabetes.

E. Atrophic vaginitis occurs because of estrogen deficiency (most often postmenopausal) when the vaginal mucosa thins and becomes dry. In addition to being symptomatic itself, it may increase the risk of recurrent cystitis and treatment may be helpful.

F. Cervical infections often present with vaginal discharge. Although the discharge originates from the cervical os, the presentations may be similar. These infections are discussed later in the chapter.

Evidence-Based Diagnosis

A. The primary diagnostic test for vaginitis is examination of the discharge. The test characteristics for many of the tests are discussed in Table 16-3.

1. pH testing is done of discharge from the vaginal sidewall.

2. Saline wet mount viewed at high and low power through a microscope looking for clue cells, candida, or trichomonads.

3. The whiff test (performed by adding 10% potassium hydroxide (KOH) to the discharge and sniffing the sample for a fishy amine odor).

4. A KOH wet mount should be performed to look for findings of candidiasis.

B. Bacterial vaginosis

1. Presents with malodorous (typically fishy) white or gray discharge without pain or itching.

2. Bacterial vaginosis is diagnosed by the Amsel criteria (see Table 16-3).

C. Trichomoniasis

1. Presents with thin yellow or green frothy discharge, irritation, dysuria, and dyspareunia

2. May be asymptomatic

3. On physical exam punctate hemorrhages may be present on the cervix (strawberry cervix) or vaginal walls.

4. Diagnosis usually made by seeing motile trichomonads on saline wet mount.

5. Visualization of leukocytes being more prevalent than epithelial cells on wet mount also suggests trichomoniasis.

6. The whiff test may also be positive with trichomoniasis.

D. Vulvovaginal candidiasis

1. Presents with itching, irritation, dysuria, dyspareunia and thick white "curd-like" discharge without odor. Lack of itching argues against the disease.

2. Women are effective at self-diagnosis. Clinicians whose patients report "I have another yeast infection" can usually rely that it is an accurate diagnosis.

3. On exam, inflammation of the vulva and lack of odor increases the likelihood of candidiasis. A thick, curdy, white discharge argues for candidiasis while a watery discharge argues against it.

4. The presence of budding yeast or branching mycelia on KOH preparation of discharge is highly suggestive.

E. Atrophic vaginitis

1. Dryness is the most common symptom

2. Other symptoms that may occur include pruritus, irritation, discharge, dysuria and dyspareunia.

3. On exam, vaginal mucosa is thin and dry, and inflammation may be present.

4. Diagnosis is based on presentation and exam and lack of findings suggestive of infection.

F. Inconclusive evaluation

1. About 30% of women with vaginal complaints do not have a clear diagnosis after a complete evaluation.

2. Options include

   a. Empiric treatment for the most likely cause

   b. Further testing with culture or rapid diagnostic tests

   c. Testing for cervical infection

   d. Observation

Table 16-3. Test characteristics of diagnostic tests for vaginitis.

Diagnosis	Test Finding	Sensitivity	Specificity	LR+	LR−
Bacterial vaginosis	pH > 4.5	89%	74%	3.4	0.15
	Positive whiff test	67%	93%	22	0.35
	Clue cells > 20% on wet mount	74%	86%	5.3	0.30
	Thin homogeneous discharge	79%	54%	1.7	0.39
	At least 3 of 4 Amsel criteria (criteria are 4 findings above)	69%	93%	9.9	0.33
Trichomonas	Leukocytes > Epithelial cells	58–85%	70–98%	3.87–43.5	0.15–0.49
Candidiasis	Itching			1.4–3.3	0.18–0.79
	Self diagnosis			3.3	
	Vulvar inflammation	4–91%	77–99%	2.1–8.4	0.56–0.96
	Lack of odor on exam			2.9	
	Curdlike discharge described by patient			2.4	
	Curdlike discharge on exam	16–72%	97–100%	6.1–130	0.28–0.86
	Watery discharge described by patient			0.12	
	Budding yeast or branching mycelia	65–85%	77–99%	2.83–85	0.15–0.45

Treatment

A. Bacterial vaginosis in nonpregnant women is treated with oral metronidazole or intravaginal metronidazole or clindamycin.

B. The recommended treatment for trichomoniasis in nonpregnant women is tinidazole or metronidazole. Treatment of sexual partners is necessary and sexual intercourse should not be resumed until both partners are treated and symptoms resolve.

C. The recommended treatment for uncomplicated vulvovaginal candidiasis is a short course of topical over-the-counter anti-fungals or a single dose of oral fluconazole.

D. Complicated infection (immunosuppression, pregnancy, diabetes, severe infection, 4 or more annual episodes) should be treated with longer durations of topical or oral therapies.

E. Atrophic vaginitis is treated with intravaginal estrogen.

Alternative Diagnosis: Pyelonephritis

Textbook Presentation

Pyelonephritis typically presents with dysuria and flank or back pain, fever, chills, malaise, nausea and vomiting.

Disease Highlights

A. Pyelonephritis is an upper UTI affecting the parenchyma of the kidney.

B. Bacterial pathogens are the same as those for cystitis.

C. Uncomplicated pyelonephritis occurs in immunocompetent women with normal urinary tracts and without reduced kidney function.

D. Complicated pyelonephritis is present if the patient is male, pregnant, or immunosuppressed or has urinary obstruction, nephrolithiasis, foreign-body/catheters, or kidney dysfunction.

Evidence-Based Diagnosis

A. History often includes symptoms of cystitis with flank or back pain, fever, chills, malaise, and nausea or vomiting.

B. CVA tenderness on physical exam suggests pyelonephritis but is surprisingly nondiagnostic (LR+ 1.1-2.5 and LR− 0.78-0.96).

C. Urinalysis or urine dipstick testing also aids diagnosis with the same findings as cystitis.

D. Urine culture is indicated for all patients with suspected pyelonephritis. Urine culture is positive in 90% of patients with pyelonephritis.

E. Imaging (CT or ultrasound) is indicated if there is concern for concomitant nephrolithiasis or obstruction or if the diagnosis is uncertain.

Treatment

A. Many patients with pyelonephritis can be treated as outpatients.

B. Indications for admission include the following:

1. Unstable vital signs
2. Inability to tolerate oral medications
3. Concern for nonadherence
4. Pregnancy
5. Immunocompromised state
6. Concern for urinary tract obstruction or nephrolithiasis

C. Outpatient management

1. The first-line empiric therapy is a fluoroquinolone (if local *E coli* resistance does not exceed 20%).
2. A single IV dose of ceftriaxone or a long-acting aminoglycoside is recommended before outpatient therapy if fluoroquinolone resistance exceeds 10%.
3. Treatment should be adjusted once antimicrobial susceptibility results are available.
4. Duration of antibiotic therapy
    a. 7–10 days for uncomplicated pyelonephritis
    b. 14 days for complicated pyelonephritis
5. Follow-up
    a. Patients should be seen in 24–72 hours to ensure clinical improvement.
    b. If fever persists beyond 48–72 hours of appropriate antibiotics or illness worsens, the patient should be admitted for IV antibiotics and further evaluation.

D. Inpatient management

1. Patients who are admitted for treatment should be given IV antibiotics (a fluoroquinolone, ceftriaxone, or an aminoglycoside with or without ampicillin).
2. Treatment duration should be for 14 days.
3. If fever, pain, or vomiting has not improved in 48–72 hours of appropriate therapy, the following 2 options should be considered:
    a. Obtain imaging (CT scan or ultrasound) to evaluate for complications such as a perinephric abscess, kidney stone, or obstruction.
    b. Broaden antibiotic coverage to cover for resistant organisms if susceptibility data has not returned.

CASE RESOLUTION

No additional testing or urine culture was performed for Ms. D since she had no history of recurrent UTI or other complicating factors. She was given empiric antibiotics of nitrofurantoin 100 mg twice daily for 5 days based on the regional *E coli* resistance patterns. Her symptoms resolved with treatment.

It is important to know local *E coli* resistance patterns when prescribing empiric antibiotics for cystitis because resistance to fluoroquino-lones and TMP-SMX is not uncommon.

CHIEF COMPLAINT

PATIENT

Mr. C is a 57-year-old man who complains of dysuria that started suddenly 5 days ago. He reports the pain seems to radiate to his low back and perineum. He has felt "achy" and had chills but has not measured his temperature. He denies any penile discharge, rash, nausea, vomiting, or flank pain. He has had more difficulty urinating with a weaker urinary stream for the past few days. He also feels some dizziness upon standing.

At this point what is the leading hypothesis, what are the active alternatives, and is there a must not miss diagnosis? Given this differential diagnosis, what tests should be ordered?

PRIORITIZING THE DIFFERENTIAL DIAGNOSIS

Mr. C is a man experiencing dysuria with radiation to the perineum and associated urinary hesitancy. His gender and the radiation of the pain are pivotal points in this history suggesting possible acute prostatitis. Acute prostatitis is a life-threatening cause of dysuria in a male and must be considered. Urosepsis is another must not miss diagnosis given the systemic symptoms and orthostasis. The absence of penile discharge is important in limiting the list of diagnoses. Other common but less dangerous alternatives include urethritis from an STI and complicated cystitis. Pyelonephritis should also be considered. Table 16-4 lists the differential diagnosis.

Mr. C is sexually active with several female partners and does not use condoms or other barrier protection. He has no active medical problems but has noted nocturia over the past few months.

Temperature is 38.2°C, pulse 80 bpm, RR 12 breaths per minute, BP 142/78 mm Hg, and orthostatic vital signs are negative. Abdominal exam demonstrates suprapubic tenderness without rebound or guarding and the absence of CVA tenderness. Genital exam is normal, but there is tenderness on gentle prostate exam without any palpable masses.

Is the clinical information sufficient to make a diagnosis? If not, what other information do you need?

Leading Hypothesis: Acute Prostatitis

Textbook Presentation

Acute prostatitis typically presents with dysuria, low back pain, perineal pain or ejaculatory pain with fever, chills, and myalgias. Patients often have associated urinary symptoms including frequency, urgency, or obstruction.

Disease Highlights

A. Acute bacterial prostatitis is an infection of the prostate gland that occurs from an ascending urethral infection or through reflux of infected urine into the prostate through the ejaculatory or prostatic ducts.

Table 16-4. Diagnostic hypotheses for Mr. C.

Diagnostic Hypotheses	Demographics, Risk Factors, Symptoms and Signs	Important Tests
Leading Hypothesis		
Acute prostatitis	Pain radiating to the low back, rectum or perineum Malaise, fevers, chills, hesitancy	Digital rectal exam with gentle prostate exam Urinalysis Urine Culture Urine GC PCR BMP
Active Alternative—Most Common		
Complicated cystitis	Dysuria without radiation or flank pain	Urinalysis or dipstick Urine culture
Urethritis from STI	Dysuria, penile discharge, pain with intercourse, testicular pain	Examination for penile discharge Urine GC PCR
Active Alternative—Must Not Miss		
Urosepsis	Signs of cystitis accompanied with lethargy, confusion, orthostasis, and SIRS	CBC Urinalysis Urine culture SIRS criteria
Pyelonephritis	Fever, chills, nausea or vomiting, flank pain, CVA tenderness	Urine dipstick or urinalysis Urine culture CT scan or ultrasound (if concern for obstruction or lack of clinical response)

Urine GC PCR, polymerase chain reaction of urine sample for *Neisseria gonorrhoeae* and *Chlamydia trachomatis*.

B. Frequent pathogens include gram-negative coliform bacteria, *Klebsiella, Proteus,* enterococci, and *Pseudomonas.*

C. Sexually transmitted bacteria, such as *Chlamydia,* may also be the cause.

Evidence-Based Diagnosis

A. Although prostatitis may present with classic symptoms of low back pain, dysuria, and perineal pain, the disease may also present with nonspecific symptoms such as myalgias, malaise, or nausea and vomiting.

B. On physical exam, the prostate gland may be tender, warm, swollen, or firm.

C. Theoretically, infection may be induced or worsened by rigorous digital rectal exam so this is not recommended if acute bacterial prostatitis is suspected.

D. Prostate massage

    1. Traditionally, prostatic massage to examine prostatic secretions for white blood cells and bacteria has been advocated.

    2. This test has not been validated, and it is not recommended because it is difficult to perform, painful, and may worsen infection.

E. Urinalysis or urine dipstick

1. May show signs consistent with cystitis (eg, leukocyte esterase, nitrites or white blood cells)

2. May also be normal

F. Often the pathogen will be identified by urine culture; however, urine culture can be negative in acute prostatitis.

G. A urine sample should be sent for PCR testing for gonorrhea and chlamydia if a sexually transmitted pathogen is suspected.

H. Renal function should be assessed in patients who may have obstruction.

I. Diagnosis is made based on a combination of the history, physical exam, and urine studies. No single test is diagnostic for acute prostatitis.

Treatment

A. First-line antibiotics include a fluoroquinolone or TMP-SMX. If an STI is likely, treatment for *Chlamydia* should also be given.

B. While nitrofurantoin is used to treat cystitis, it is ineffective in prostatitis because it does not have good prostate penetration.

C. The duration of antibiotics is at least 3–4 weeks.

D. Supportive treatment for pain and stool softeners are also helpful.

E. Patients with severe infection or medically complex patients should be admitted for IV antibiotic therapy.

F. Patients who do not respond to treatment should be evaluated for a prostatic abscess. Although a prostatic abscess may be palpable on exam, it requires imaging by CT, MRI, or transrectal ultrasound to confirm diagnosis. Drainage or resection can be necessary.

G. Prostatitis will elevate prostate-specific antigen (PSA) levels.

MAKING A DIAGNOSIS

Mr. C's urinalysis is positive for leukocyte esterase, 10 WBCs per high power field, and occasional blood with 5 RBCs per high power field. His CBC shows a WBC count of 8.0 K/mcL and basic metabolic panel shows a creatinine of 1.0, similar to his previous baseline.

Have you crossed a diagnostic threshold for the leading hypothesis, acute prostatitis? Have you ruled out the active alternatives? Do other tests need to be done to exclude the alternative diagnoses?

The findings on urinalysis together with the tender prostate on physical exam support the presumed diagnosis of acute prostatitis as opposed to complicated cystitis or urethritis. Urosepsis is less likely given the reassuring vital signs and absence of systemic inflammatory response syndrome (SIRS) criteria (presence of 2 of the following: WBC > 12,000 K/mcL, WBC < 4000 K/mcL, fever > 38.0°C, hypothermia < 36.0°C, tachycardia > 90 bpm, or tachypnea > 20 breaths per minute). Diagnosis could be confirmed by culture of prostatic fluid but rigorous examination in the patient would be contraindicated because it could increase the severity of infection. Urine culture and GC PCR testing helps identify the bacterial pathogen.

Alternative Diagnosis: Urethritis from STIs (Cervicitis in Women)

Textbook Presentation

Urethritis in men typically presents with dysuria, urethral pruritus, and penile discharge. Patients may also have dyspareunia, abdominal pain, or testicular pain. Women with cervicitis typically have cervical discharge, dysuria, and dyspareunia. They may also have spontaneous or postcoital vaginal bleeding.

Disease Highlights

A. Urethritis and cervicitis are usually due to an STI.

B. The 2 main sexually transmitted pathogens causing cervicitis and urethritis are *N gonorrhoeae* and *C trachomatis*.

C. Other less common causes include *Mycoplasma genitalium*, *Trichomonas*, herpes simplex virus, and adenovirus. Herpes simplex virus may also cause cervicitis.

Evidence-Based Diagnosis

A. Urethritis can be diagnosed based on the following:

1. Discharge on physical exam

2. Microscopy of discharge showing > 5 WBCs per oil immersion field (sensitivity, 26%; specificity, 95%; LR+, 2.7)

3. Positive leukocyte esterase on first-void urine

4. Microscopy of first-void urine showing > 10 WBCs per high power field

5. Gram stain of discharge or urine culture that identifies organisms

B. Cervicitis can be diagnosed based on mucopurulent endocervical discharge on pelvic exam. Sustained cervical bleeding caused by gentle passage of a swab in the cervical os may also be seen.

C. PCR

1. To confirm the diagnosis of urethritis or cervicitis, an endocervical, vaginal, urine or urethral sample should be sent for PCR testing for gonorrhea and chlamydia.

2. Urine PCR is the preferred test for males (sensitivity and specificity 90–100% and 97–100% respectively).

3. Although urine testing may be equivalent, vaginal swabs are preferred for women (sensitivity and specificity of 96% and 99%, respectively).

Treatment

A. Patients should be treated empirically prior to confirmation of a pathogen.

B. The first-line treatment for chlamydia is a 1-time dose of 1 g of oral azithromycin or a 1-week course of 100 mg of doxycycline given twice daily.

C. Concurrent treatment for gonorrhea should be given if clinical suspicion or gonorrhea prevalence in the patient population is high.

D. The first-line treatment for gonorrhea is a 1-time injection of ceftriaxone 125 mg intramuscularly.

E. Given the high incidence of coinfection with chlamydia, patients treated for gonorrhea should always be treated for coexisting chlamydia infection unless testing for it is negative.

F. Patients should abstain from intercourse until 1 week after a single-dose treatment or until completion of a 1-week regimen (assuming symptoms have also resolved).

G. Partners

    1. Sexual partners of all patients infected with an STI should be evaluated and treated.

    2. If partners are unable to be seen at a health practice, the CDC recommends expedited partner treatment (the physician gives the patient a prescription for their partner). The laws regarding this practice vary by state.

H. Repeat testing to establish cure is not necessary unless symptoms persist or reinfection or nonadherence is suspected.

I. Due to the high risk of repeat infections, it is recommended all patients be re-tested 3–12 months after initial infection.

Alternative Diagnosis: Urosepsis

Textbook Presentation

Sepsis is covered extensively in Chapter 25, Hypotension. This section will focus on urosepsis specifically. Urosepsis typically presents with fever, chills, and lethargy or altered mental status. Symptoms of the underlying infection, such as dysuria or flank pain, are often present.

Disease Highlights

A. Sepsis is defined as a suspected or proven infection with the presence of the SIRS criteria.

B. Severe sepsis occurs when there is target organ dysfunction, such as hypotension, hypoxemia, oliguria, metabolic acidosis, thrombocytopenia, or obtundation.

C. Urosepsis occurs when the infectious source of sepsis is an infection of the urinary or male genital tract.

D. It is estimated one-quarter of sepsis cases are due to a urogenital infection.

Evidence-Based Diagnosis

Diagnosis is made based on SIRS criteria (see above) and the confirmation of a genitourinary infection.

Treatment

A. All patients with suspected urosepsis should be hospitalized. Admission to the ICU is often necessary.

B. Early empiric IV antibiotics and aggressive volume resuscitation with IV fluids should be initiated to prevent worsening sepsis.

CASE RESOLUTION

Mr. C was treated empirically with ciprofloxacin, 500 mg twice daily, and azithromycin, 1 g for 1 dose, for acute bacterial prostatitis. Results of the urine culture showed 150,000 colony forming units of *E coli* susceptible to fluoroquinolones. The urine PCR for gonorrhea and chlamydia was negative. Treatment with ciprofloxacin was continued for 21 days, and his symptoms resolved. He continued to have nocturia and treatment for benign prostatic hypertrophy was started.

REFERENCES

Anderson MR, Klink K, Cohrssen A. Evaluation of vaginal complaints. JAMA. 2004;291(11):1368–79.

Bent S, Nallamothu BK, Simel DL, Fihn SD, Saint S. Does this woman have an acute uncomplicated urinary tract infection? JAMA. 2002;287:2701–10.

Black ER. *Diagnostic Strategies for Common Medical Problems.* 2nd ed. Philadelphia: American College of Physicians; 1999.

Centers for Disease Control and Prevention. Sexually transmitted diseases treatment guidelines 2006: diseases characterized by urethritis and cervicitis. http://www.cdc.gov/STD/treatment/2006/urethritis-and-cervicitis.htm. Accessed September 14, 2013.

Chernesky MA, Martin DH, Hook EW et al. Ability of new APTIMA CT and APTIMA GC *assays to detect Chlamydia trachomatis* and *Neisseria gonorrhoeae* in male urine and urethral swabs. J Clin Microbiol. 2005;43(1):127–31.

Deville WL, Yzermans JC, van Duijn NP, Bezemer PD, van der Windt DA, Bouter LM. The urine dipstick test useful to rule out infections. A Meta-analysis of the accuracy. BMC Urol. 2004;4:4.

Gutman RE, Peipert JF, Weitzen S, Blume J. Evaluation of clinical methods for diagnosing bacterial vaginosis. Obstet Gynecol. 2005;105(3):551–6.

Hainer BL, Gibson MV. Vaginitis: Diagnosis and Treatment. Am Fam Physician. 2011;83(7):807–15.

Hooton TM. Clinical practice. Uncomplicated urinary tract infection. N Engl J Med. 2012;366:1028–37.

Hooton TM, Scholes D, Hughes JP et al. A prospective study of risk factors for symptomatic urinary tract infection in young women. N Engl J Med. 1996;335:468–74.

Kalra OP, Raizada A. Approach to a patient with urosepsis. J Glob Infect Dis. 2009;1(1):57–63.

Liang SY, Mackowiak PA. Infections in the elderly. Clin Geriatr Med. 2007;23(2):441–56.

Orellana MA, Gómez-Lus ML, Lora D. Sensitivity of Gram stain in the diagnosis of urethritis in men. Sex Transm Infect. 2012 Jun;88(4):284–7.

Ramakrishnan K, Scheid DC. Diagnosis and management of pyelonephritis in adults. Am Fam Physician. 2005;71(5):933–42.

Russell JA. Management of sepsis. N Engl J Med. 2006;355:1699–1713.

Sarma AV, Wei JT. Benign prostatic hypertrophy and lower urinary tract symptoms. N Engl J Med. 2012;367:248–57.

Schachter J, Chernesky MA, Willis DE et al. Vaginal swabs are the specimens of choice when screening for *Chlamydia trachomatis* and *Neisseria gonorrhoeae*: results from a multicenter evaluation of the APTIMA assays for both infections. Sex Transm Dis. 2005;32(12):725–8.

Scholes D, Hooton TM, Roberts PL, Stapleton AE, Gupta K, Stamm WE. Risk factors for recurrent urinary tract infection in young women. J Infect Dis. 2000;182:1177–82.

Stamm WE, Counts GW, Running KR, Fihn S, Turck M, Holmes KK. Diagnosis of coliform infection in acutely dysuric women. N Engl J Med. 1982;307:463–8.

Stevermer JJ, Easley SK. Treatment of prostatitis. Am Fam Physician. 2000;61(10):3015–22.

Van Vranken M. Prevention and treatment of sexually transmitted diseases: an update. Am Fam Physician. 2007;76(12):1827–32.

Workowski KA, Berman S. Sexually transmitted diseases treatment guidelines, 2010. MMWR Recomm Rep. 2010;59(RR-12):1–110.

I have a patient with edema. How do I determine the cause?

CHIEF COMPLAINT

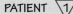

PATIENT 1

Mrs. V is 62-year-old woman with leg edema for the past 2 weeks.

What is the differential diagnosis of edema? How would you frame the differential?

CONSTRUCTING A DIFFERENTIAL DIAGNOSIS

Edema is defined as an increase in the interstitial fluid volume and is generally not clinically apparent until the interstitial volume has increased by at least 2.5–3 L. It is useful to review some background pathophysiology before discussing the differential diagnosis:

A. Distribution of total body water

1. 67% intracellular; 33% extracellular

2. Extracellular water: 25% intravascular; 75% interstitial

B. Regulation of fluid distribution between the intravascular and interstitial spaces

1. There is a constant exchange of water and solutes at the arteriolar end of the capillaries.

2. Fluid is returned from the interstitial space to the intravascular space at the venous end of the capillaries and via the lymphatics.

3. Movement of fluid from the intravascular space to the interstitium occurs through several mechanisms:

a. Capillary hydrostatic (hydraulic) pressure pushes fluid out of the vessels.

b. Interstitial oncotic pressure pulls fluid into the interstitium.

c. Capillary permeability allows fluid to escape into the interstitium.

4. Movement of fluid from the interstitium to the intravascular space occurs when opposite pressures predominate.

a. Intravascular (plasma) oncotic pressure from plasma proteins pulls fluid into the vascular space.

b. Interstitial hydrostatic pressure pushes fluid out of the interstitium.

5. In skeletal muscle, the capillary hydrostatic pressure and the intravascular oncotic pressure are the most important factors.

6. There is normally a small gradient favoring filtration out of the vascular space into the interstitium; the excess fluid is removed via the lymphatic system.

C. Edema formation occurs when there is

1. An increase in capillary hydrostatic pressure (for example, increased plasma volume due to renal sodium retention).

2. An increase in capillary permeability (for example, burns, angioedema).

3. An increase in interstitial oncotic pressure (for example, myxedema).

4. A decrease in plasma oncotic pressure (for example, hypoalbuminemia).

5. Lymphatic obstruction.

Although it is possible to construct a pathophysiologic framework (Figure 17-1) for the differential diagnosis of edema, it is more useful clinically to use the *distribution of the edema* as the pivotal point:

A. Bilateral leg edema

1. Due to a systemic cause (with or without presacral edema, ascites, pleural effusion, pulmonary edema, periorbital edema)

a. Cardiovascular

(1) Systolic or diastolic heart failure (HF)

(2) Constrictive pericarditis

(3) Pulmonary hypertension

b. Hepatic (cirrhosis)

c. Renal

(1) Advanced kidney disease of any cause

(2) Nephrotic syndrome

d. Hematologic: anemia

The most common systemic causes of edema are cardiac, hepatic, and renal diseases.

e. GI

(1) Nutritional deficiency or malabsorption leading to hypoalbuminemia

(2) Refeeding edema

f. Medications

(1) Antidepressants: Monoamine oxidase inhibitors

(2) Antihypertensives

(a) Calcium channel blockers, especially dihydropyridines

(b) Direct vasodilators (hydralazine, minoxidil)

(c) Beta-blockers

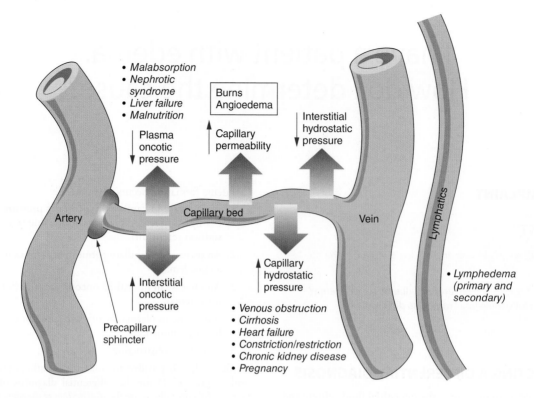

Figure 17-1. Pathophysiology of edema. (Adapted with permission from Cho S et al. Peripheral edema. Am J Med. 2002;V113:581. Copyright © 2002 *Excerpta Medica*, Inc.)

(3) Hormones

    (a) Estrogens/progesterones

    (b) Testosterone

    (c) Corticosteroids

(4) Nonsteroidal antiinflammatory drugs (NSAIDs)

(5) Thiazolidinediones

  g. Endocrine: myxedema

2. Due to a venous or lymphatic cause

  a. Venous obstruction

    (1) Bilateral deep venous thrombosis (DVT) (see Chapter 15, Dyspnea, for a full discussion of lower extremity DVT)

    (2) Bilateral pelvic or retroperitoneal lymphadenopathy or mass

  b. Venous insufficiency

  c. Lymphatic obstruction (lymphedema)

    (1) Primary (idiopathic, often bilateral)

      (a) Congenital

      (b) Lymphedema praecox (onset in puberty) or tarda (onset after age 20)

    (2) Secondary (more common; generally unilateral—see below)

B. Unilateral limb edema

  1. Venous obstruction

    a. Unilateral DVT

    b. Unilateral lymphadenopathy or mass

  2. Venous insufficiency (more often bilateral)

  3. Lymphedema (secondary)

    a. Neoplasm

    b. Surgery (especially following mastectomy)

    c. Radiation therapy

    d. Miscellaneous (tuberculosis, recurrent lymphangitis, filariasis)

  4. Cellulitis/erysipelas (can also be localized)

  5. Baker cyst (leg only)

C. Localized edema

  1. Burns

  2. Angioedema, hives

  3. Trauma

  4. Cellulitis, erysipelas

Figure 17-2 outlines the diagnostic approach to edema.

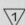

Mrs. V was well until a couple of months ago when she began feeling a bit more tired than usual, despite continuing to sleep well. She has had no shortness of breath or chest pain. She has noted intermittent vague abdominal pain, not related to eating, position, or bowel movements. She has been a bit constipated and feels bloated. Over the last 2 weeks, she has noted swelling in her feet and lower legs and has not been able to wear her regular shoes. As she tells you this, you note that she is wearing house slippers, and that her socks have produced a significant indentation above her ankles.

Her past medical history is notable for hypertension and diabetes, both well controlled. She had a blood transfusion

(continued)

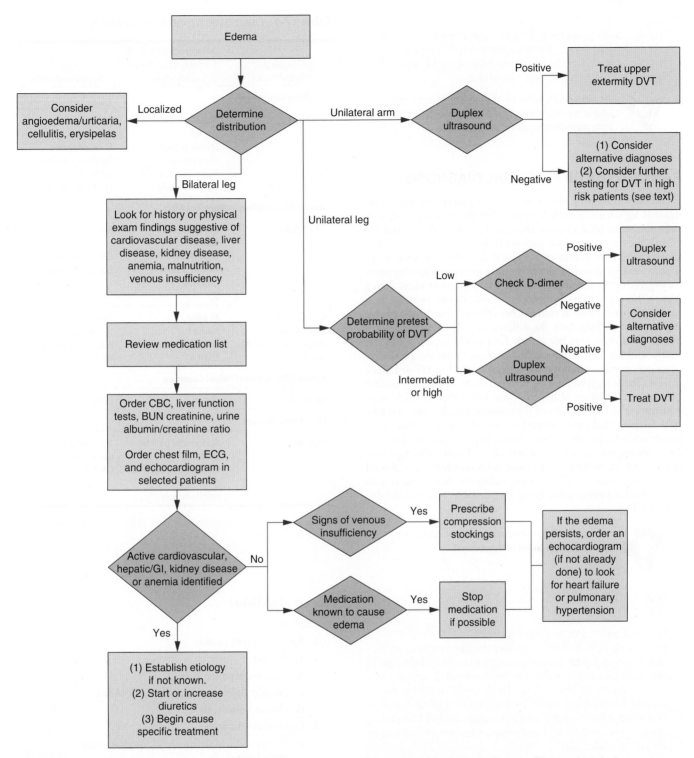

BUN, blood urea nitrogen; CBC, complete blood count; DVT, deep venous thrombosis; ECG, electrocardiogram; GI, gastrointestinal.

Figure 17-2. Diagnostic approach: edema.

during a cholecystectomy 25 years ago. Her current medications include hydrochlorothiazide, lisinopril, pioglitazone, simvastatin, and aspirin. She has no history of heart or kidney disease, or tobacco or alcohol use.

At this point, what is the leading hypothesis, and what are the active alternatives? What other tests should be ordered?

RANKING THE DIFFERENTIAL DIAGNOSIS

Even before examining Mrs. V, you can see that she has significant bilateral leg edema, a pivotal point in her presentation. Although there are some local diseases that can present with bilateral leg edema, the first step in such patients is always to look for systemic causes. While the history and physical are often not sensitive or specific enough to make a diagnosis, they are a good starting point for organizing the differential. So the first question to ask is, "Does Mrs. V have any signs, symptoms, or risk factors pointing to a cardiac, hepatic, or renal cause of her edema?" The results of this exploration will help rank the differential. Mrs. V's history of a blood transfusion puts her at risk for chronic hepatitis and cirrhosis, and her vague abdominal complaints raise the possibility of ascites, more commonly seen with cirrhosis than HF or kidney disease. She is certainly at risk for both heart and kidney disease because of her history of hypertension and diabetes. While most patients with HF complain of shortness of breath, some describe only fatigue. Medication should be considered as a cause, since pioglitazone frequently causes edema; hypothyroidism does not cause pitting edema, and so is not likely. Finally, although it is uncommon for obstruction to cause bilateral edema, you should think about ovarian cancer causing malignant ascites and venous obstruction if another cause is not found. Table 17-1 lists the differential diagnosis.

Always look for systemic causes of edema in patients with bilateral leg edema.

In general, Mrs. V appears fatigued. Her BP is 100/60 mm Hg, pulse is 92 bpm, and RR is 16 breaths per minute. Sclera are anicteric, jugular venous pressure is normal, and lungs are clear. On cardiac exam, she has a normal S_1 and S_2, a soft S_4, and no S_3 or murmurs. Her abdomen is slightly distended, but soft and nontender; there is a fluid wave. Her liver is not enlarged, but the spleen is palpable. Rectal exam shows hemorrhoids and guaiac-negative stool. She has 2+ edema bilaterally.

Is the clinical information sufficient to make a diagnosis? If not, what other information do you need?

Leading Hypothesis: Cirrhosis

Textbook Presentation

Patients with cirrhosis can be asymptomatic or have mild symptoms, such as fatigue. Some patients have the classic manifestations of portal hypertension: ascites, edema, variceal bleeding, encephalopathy, or hypersplenism.

Table 17-1. Diagnostic hypotheses for Mrs. V.

Diagnostic Hypotheses	Demographics, Risk Factors, Symptoms and Signs	Important Tests
Leading Hypothesis		
Cirrhosis	Hepatitis risk factors Ascites Spider angiomata Gynecomastia Normal or low JVP Splenomegaly	Ultrasound Bilirubin Liver enzymes Prothrombin time Albumin Liver biopsy
Active Alternatives—Must Not Miss		
Heart failure	Cardiovascular risk factors Dyspnea Elevated JVP Crackles S_3	ECG Chest radiograph Echocardiogram
Renal disease (chronic kidney disease or nephrotic syndrome)	Malaise Nausea Dyspnea Edema	BUN/creatinine Urinalysis Albumin/creatinine ratio
Active Alternatives—Most Common		
Medication	History	History
Other Hypotheses		
Ovarian cancer	Abdominal pain or bloating Increased abdominal girth Family history	Transvaginal ultrasound CA-125

BUN, blood urea nitrogen; CA-125, cancer antigen-125; ECG, electrocardiogram; JVP, jugular venous pressure.

Disease Highlights

A. Etiology

1. More common causes

   a. Alcohol

   b. Chronic hepatitis B or C

   c. Nonalcoholic fatty liver disease (NAFLD)

   d. Hemochromatosis

2. Less common causes

   a. Drugs and toxins (isoniazid, methotrexate, amiodarone)

   b. Autoimmune hepatitis

   c. Genetic metabolic diseases (Wilson disease, alpha-1-antitrypsin deficiency, glycogen storage diseases, porphyria)

   d. Infections (schistosomiasis, echinococcosis, brucellosis)

   e. Cardiac

   f. Primary or secondary biliary cirrhosis

The 2 most common causes of cirrhosis in the United States are alcoholic liver disease and chronic hepatitis C.

B. Pathophysiology

1. Advanced fibrosis, or cirrhosis, causes architectural distortion of the hepatic vasculature, leading to shunting of the blood coming into the liver via the portal vein directly to the hepatic vein outflow system, which causes

   a. Impaired hepatocyte function due to loss of normal sinusoids

   b. Increased intrahepatic resistance, or portal hypertension

   c. Increased risk of hepatocellular carcinoma related to regenerative activity and DNA damage

2. Consequences of cirrhosis and portal hypertension include

   a. Formation of portosystemic collaterals (ie, varices)

   b. Splanchnic vasodilation

   c. Renal vasoconstriction and hypoperfusion of the kidneys, causing salt and water retention

   d. Increased cardiac output

   e. Decreased production of albumin and clotting factors

   f. Increased capillary hydrostatic pressure

   g. Edema due to a combination of salt and water retention (increasing hydrostatic pressures) and hypoalbuminemia (decreasing intravascular oncotic pressure)

C. Prognosis

1. Median survival from time of diagnosis of compensated cirrhosis is 10–12 years.

2. Up to 60% of patients progress to decompensated cirrhosis, defined as worsening portal hypertension and decreased hepatic reserve, at 10 years after diagnosis.

3. Rates of progression are quite variable and are related to the etiology of the cirrhosis, presence of other liver disease, available treatment (such as for chronic hepatitis B and C), and avoidance of hepatic toxins (such as alcohol).

4. 5-year mortality approaches 85% after decompensation if transplantation is not performed.

   a. In patients with cirrhosis but no varices and no ascites, the 1-year mortality rate is 1%.

   b. In those with varices but no ascites, the 1-year mortality rate is 3.4%.

   c. In those with varices and ascites, the 1-year mortality rate is 20%; in those with variceal bleeding and ascites, the 1-year mortality is 57%.

5. The Childs-Pugh-Turcotte classification of cirrhosis severity predicts prognosis (see Chapter 19, GI Bleeding).

Evidence-Based Diagnosis

A. Cirrhosis is a pathologic diagnosis definitively made only by examining the entire liver at autopsy or after liver transplantation.

B. The traditional gold standard is percutaneous liver biopsy, although due to sampling error, the sensitivity has been reported to be as low as 70–80%.

C. The clinical presentation is variable, making clinical diagnosis difficult.

1. Patients may have physical findings suggestive of chronic liver disease (see below), constitutional symptoms, asymptomatic liver enzyme or radiologic abnormalities, manifestations of portal hypertension (see below), or no symptoms at all. Cirrhosis is sometimes diagnosed at autopsy in patients in whom the disease never manifested.

2. Physical findings may increase the likelihood that a patient with liver disease has cirrhosis, but rarely rule out cirrhosis (Table 17-2).

Table 17-2. Physical exam findings for the diagnosis of cirrhosis in patients with liver disease.

Physical Finding	LR+	LR−
Caput medusae	9.5	0.72
Gynecomastia	7	0.43
Ascites	6.6	0.8
Testicular atrophy	5.8	0.18
Spider angiomata	4.5	0.5
Palmar erythema	4.3	0.6
Jaundice	3.8	0.8
Peripheral edema	3	0.7
Splenomegaly	2.5–3.5	0.8
Hepatomegaly	2.3	0.6

3. Patients who show manifestations of portal hypertension (see below) are assumed to have cirrhosis.

D. Laboratory tests

1. A low platelet count in a patient with liver disease increases the probability of cirrhosis.

   a. Platelet count $< 110 \times 10^3$/mcL: LR+ = 9.8

   b. Platelet count $< 160 \times 10^3$/mcL: LR+ = 6.3; LR− = 0.29

2. Albumin < 3.5 g/dL (LR+ = 4.4) and a prolonged international normalized ratio (INR) (LR+ = 5.0) also increase the likelihood of cirrhosis.

3. The Bonacini cirrhosis discriminant score combines the alanine aminotransferase:aspartate aminotransferase (ALT:AST) ratio, the platelet count, and the INR into a score from 0–11; scores > 7 increase the likelihood of cirrhosis (LR+ = 9.4).

E. Several noninvasive models and techniques (FibroSURE, FibroScan) have been developed to predict cirrhosis *in patients with chronic hepatitis C*, although they are not currently used in place of biopsy.

1. FibroSURE includes the biomarkers alpha-2 macroglobulin, haptoglobin, gamma-glutamyl transpeptidase, apolipoprotein A_1, ALT, and total bilirubin.

   a. Correlates well with liver biopsy

   b. Useful for distinguishing mild fibrosis from cirrhosis, but less accurate in identifying moderate fibrosis.

2. FibroScan is an imaging method that measures liver stiffness, which correlates with cirrhosis.

   a. For predicting cirrhosis, the sensitivity is 86% and specificity 93% (LR+, 12.2; LR−, 0.15).

   b. Less accurate in identifying moderate fibrosis (sensitivity 64%, specificity 87%; LR+, 4.9; LR−, 0.41)

F. Test characteristics of ultrasound to diagnose cirrhosis are variable (LR+, 2.5–11.6; LR−, 0.13–0.73).

G. MRI has sensitivity and specificity as high as 93% and 82%, respectively.

Treatment

Once it has been determined that the patient probably or definitively has cirrhosis, it is important to determine the specific cause of the cirrhosis (see Chapter 26, Jaundice & Abnormal Liver Enzymes) and to determine whether the patient has manifestations of portal hypertension: variceal bleeding, ascites, hepatic encephalopathy, and hypersplenism. The treatment of cirrhosis depends on the underlying cause. Treatments for selected causes of cirrhosis are discussed in Chapter 26, Jaundice & Abnormal Liver Enzymes.

Manifestations of Portal Hypertension

1. Variceal Bleeding

See Chapter 19, GI Bleeding.

2. Ascites

Textbook Presentation

The patient complains of an inability to fasten her pants due to increasing abdominal girth, sometimes accompanied by dyspnea and edema.

Disease Highlights

A. Epidemiology

1. Over 10 years, ascites develops in 50% of patients with cirrhosis.

2. 1-year survival rates drop significantly once ascites develops.

B. Pathophysiology: Portal hypertension → arterial vasodilation of the splanchnic circulation → reduction in systemic vascular resistance → underfilling of arterial circulation → sodium and free water retention by the kidneys; also reduced glomerular filtration rate (GFR) → increased capillary permeability and lymph formation in the splanchnic organs.

C. Complications of ascites

1. Respiratory compromise due to compression of lung volumes

2. Hepatorenal syndrome (HRS): a syndrome of acute kidney injury associated with cirrhosis and a poor prognosis. The acute kidney injury may be acute (type 1) or subacute (type 2).

 a. Diagnostic criteria

 (1) Cirrhosis with ascites

 (2) Serum creatinine > 1.5 mg/dL

 (3) Serum creatinine stays above 1.5 mg/dL after at least 2 days of diuretic withdrawal and volume expansion with albumin.

 (4) Absence of shock

 (5) No current or recent treatment with nephrotoxic drugs

 (6) Absence of parenchymal kidney disease (< 500 mg/day of proteinuria, < 50 RBC/hpf, abnormalities on renal ultrasound)

 b. Clinical phases (Table 17-3).

 c. Incidence in patients with cirrhosis and ascites is 18% at 1 year and 39% at 5 years.

 d. The prognosis is poor: 6-month mortality is about 50% for patients with type 2 HRS and 100% for those with type 1.

 e. Precipitants of type 1 HRS include bacterial infections (especially spontaneous bacterial peritonitis), GI bleeding, acute hepatitis, over-diuresis, and large volume paracentesis.

Table 17-3. Clinical phases of hepatorenal syndrome (HRS).

Phase	Pathophysiology	Clinical Manifestations
1	Impaired sodium metabolism with normal renal perfusion, GFR, free water clearance	None; ascites or edema may develop with rapid infusion of IV saline
2	Renal sodium excretion further reduced	Ascites develops when oral sodium intake > renal excretion
3	Urinary sodium < 10 mEq/d; plasma renin/aldosterone increase to maintain plasma volume, cardiac output, and peripheral vascular resistance; renal perfusion normal or slightly reduced	Ascites and edema develop
4	High renin/aldosterone levels; arterial vasoconstriction; reduced renal perfusion/GFR; reduced free water clearance	Type 2 HRS: steady decrease in creatinine over weeks to months; hyponatremia; refractory ascites
5	Systemic hypotension → decreased renal perfusion and renal ischemia	Type 1 HRS: doubling of serum creatinine to > 2.5 mg/dL in < 2 weeks

GFR, glomerular filtration rate.

 f. Treatment of HRS

 (1) Liver transplantation is the definitive treatment for both types of HRS.

 (2) There are limited data regarding the use of transvenous intrahepatic portosystemic shunts (TIPS) and vasopressin derivatives to treat type 1 HRS.

3. Spontaneous bacterial peritonitis (SBP)

 a. Prevalence of 10–30% in hospitalized cirrhotic patients, with 1-year recurrence rate of 70% and mortality rate of about 20%; 96% of patients with SBP have a Childs-Pugh-Turcotte grade of B or C

 b. Overgrowth of intestinal bacterial and increased intestinal permeability lead to movement of bacteria into mesenteric lymph nodes; the bacteria can then enter the systemic circulation and colonize the ascitic fluid.

 c. The 3 most common isolates are *Escherichia coli, Klebsiella pneumoniae,* and pneumococci.

 d. Symptoms include fever (50–75% of patients), abdominal pain (27–72%), chills (16–29%), nausea/vomiting (8–21%), mental status changes (up to 50%), and decreased renal function (33%); about 13% of patients are asymptomatic.

 e. Risk factors for SBP include ascitic fluid total protein level ≤ 1 g/dL, upper GI bleeding, a prior episode of SBP.

 f. Diagnosis of SBP

 (1) Criteria for performing a diagnostic paracentesis in patients with cirrhosis and ascites:

 (a) Admission to the hospital for any reason

 (b) Change in clinical status (fever, abdominal pain, mental status changes, ileus, septic shock)

(c) Development of leukocytosis, acidosis, or acute kidney injury

(d) Active GI bleeding

(2) Always inoculate blood culture tubes with ascitic fluid at the bedside to maximize yield of fluid cultures.

(3) Interpretation of ascitic fluid cell counts and cultures (Table 17-4)

Consider secondary peritonitis if more than 1 organism is cultured from the ascitic fluid.

(4) Other ascitic fluid findings that increase the likelihood of SBP include WBC count > 1000 cells/mcL (LR+ = 9.1), pH < 7.35 (LR+ = 9.0), and blood-ascitic fluid pH gradient ≥ 0.1 (LR+ = 11).

g. Treatment of SBP

(1) Empiric treatment should be started prior to return of culture results.

(2) IV cefotaxime is the best-studied antibiotic for SBP; oral ofloxacin can be used in outpatients without signs of sepsis or hepatic encephalopathy.

(3) IV albumin has been shown to reduce mortality and development of renal impairment, particularly in patients with a total bilirubin > 4 mg/dL, BUN > 30 mg/dL, or creatinine > 1 mg/dL.

(4) All patients who recover from SBP should receive secondary prophylaxis with oral norfloxacin, and all patients with acute GI bleeding should receive prophylaxis; other primary prophylaxis is controversial.

(5) Since 2-year survival after SBP is only about 30%, liver transplantation should be considered in patients who recover from SBP.

Evidence-Based Diagnosis

A. Physical exam: See Chapter 26, Jaundice & Abnormal Liver Enzymes

B. Peritoneal fluid analysis should be done in all patients with new ascites.

1. Initial tests should include cell count, albumin, total protein, and culture.

Table 17-4. Interpretation of ascitic fluid results.

Condition	Polymorphonuclear Count (cells/mcL)	Culture Results
Spontaneous bacterial peritonitis	≥ 250	Single organism
Culture-negative neutrophilic ascites	≥ 250	Negative
Monomicrobial nonneutrocytic bacterascites	< 250	Single organism
Secondary bacterial peritonitis	≥ 250	Polymicrobial
Polymicrobial bacterascites	< 250	Polymicrobial

2. Serum-ascites albumin gradient is used to distinguish ascites due to portal hypertension from ascites due to other causes.

a. In portal hypertension, ascites occurs due to transudation, without changes in permeability that would allow albumin to leak into the ascitic fluid.

b. Therefore, the albumin content of ascitic fluid is low relative to serum.

c. This is in contrast to exudative types of ascites, such as ascites from infection or malignancy, in which albumin can leak into the ascitic fluid.

d. A serum ascites-albumin gradient (serum albumin-ascitic fluid albumin) of ≥ 1.1 mg/dL has a LR+ of 4.6 for the diagnosis of ascites due to portal hypertension; a serum ascites-albumin gradient of < 1.1 mg/dL has a LR– of 0.06 for the diagnosis of portal hypertension.

Treatment

A. Sodium restriction (sodium intake < 2 g/day) is commonly recommended, but there are no clinical trials showing that it leads to improved outcomes; fluid restriction of 1000–1500 mL/day is recommended if the serum sodium is < 130 mEq/L.

B. Spironolactone is the diuretic of choice to treat the aldosterone driven salt and water retention seen in cirrhosis.

1. 75% of patients respond

2. Furosemide or other loop diuretics can be added in patients who do not respond to spironolactone alone; 90% of patients respond to sodium-restricted diets, spironolactone, and loop diuretics.

3. Hydrochlorothiazide and metolazone are not recommended.

4. In order to avoid hypovolemia and renal impairment, the rate of weight loss should not exceed 0.5 kg/day in the absence of peripheral edema or 1 kg/day in the presence of edema.

Aspirin and NSAIDs blunt the natriuretic effect of diuretics and should not be used in patients with ascites.

C. Large volume paracentesis with volume expansion (dextran or albumin) is done in patients unresponsive to diuretics.

D. TIPS

1. Creates a shunt between the high-pressure portal vein and the low-pressure hepatic vein, leading to improved hemodynamics and a decrease in ascites.

2. Complications include bleeding, shunt stenosis or thrombosis, right-sided HF, and encephalopathy in 30% of patients.

3. Used as a bridge to transplant

E. Liver transplantation

F. When should ascites be treated with measures beyond sodium restriction?

1. Not in grade 1 ascites (detectable only by ultrasound)

2. Grade 2 (moderate) and grade 3 (severe) ascites are generally treated due to patient discomfort and respiratory compromise.

a. Grade 2 should be treated with diuretics.

b. Grade 3 should be treated with paracentesis followed by diuretics.

3. Refractory ascites (ascites not responsive to maximal tolerated medical therapy) should be treated with repeated paracentesis or TIPS, or both.

3. Hepatic Encephalopathy

Textbook Presentation

The classic presentation of hepatic encephalopathy is a patient with known cirrhosis who has mental status changes or is in a coma.

Disease Highlights

A. A spectrum of reversible neuropsychiatric abnormalities seen in patients with cirrhosis

B. Must exclude other neurologic or metabolic causes prior to diagnosing hepatic encephalopathy

C. Overt hepatic encephalopathy (Table 17-5, grades 1–4) is found in 30–45% of patients with cirrhosis.

D. Minimal hepatic encephalopathy (deficits manifested only on neuropsychological testing) is found in 60% of patients with cirrhosis.

E. Patients with severe hepatic encephalopathy requiring hospitalization have a 1-year survival rate of < 50%.

F. Can be precipitated by a wide variety of insults including

  1. Increased ammonia production due to

    a. Excess dietary protein

    b. Constipation

    c. GI bleeding

    d. Infection

    e. Azotemia

    f. Hypokalemia

    g. Systemic alkalosis

  2. Reduced metabolism of toxins because of hepatic hypoxia due to

    a. Dehydration

    b. Arterial hypotension

    c. Anemia

  3. Increased central nervous depressant effect with use of benzodiazepines or other psychoactive drugs

  4. Reduced metabolism of toxins because diversion of portal blood, due to surgical or intrahepatic shunts

Always look for the underlying cause of worsening hepatic encephalopathy.

Evidence-Based Diagnosis

A. There is some correlation between the degree of elevation of ammonia (either arterial or venous) and the severity of the encephalopathy, but the *ammonia level cannot be used to determine the presence or absence of hepatic encephalopathy.*

B. Diagnosis is based on history and exclusion of other causes of encephalopathy in a patient with significant liver dysfunction.

Treatment

A. Identify and treat precipitating causes

B. Patients with an episode of overt hepatic encephalopathy should be treated indefinitely; the approach to minimal hepatic encephalopathy is evolving.

C. Treatment focuses on reduction of intestinal accumulation of ammonia.

D. Lactulose removes both dietary and endogenous sources of ammonia through its cathartic action; it also lowers pH, which reduces the population of urease-producing bacteria, and traps ammonia as ammonium ions in the gut lumen.

  1. Frequently used in clinical practice, although most studies showing an improvement in encephalopathy are of poor quality.

  2. Daily dose should be titrated to result in 2–4 soft stools/day.

  3. Complications include hypovolemia and hypernatremia.

E. Antibiotics reduce the population of urease-producing bacteria.

  1. Rifaximin may be superior to lactulose for overt hepatic encephalopathy and has been shown to improve cognitive status in patients with minimal hepatic encephalopathy.

  2. Neomycin is equivalent to lactulose but has the potential to cause ototoxicity and nephrotoxicity with long-term use.

F. Consideration of liver transplantation is indicated in patients with hepatic encephalopathy.

4. Hypersplenism

Textbook Presentation

Cytopenias are found on routine blood testing in a patient with cirrhosis.

Table 17-5. West Haven Criteria for hepatic encephalopathy.

Grade	Level of Consciousness	Clinical Symptoms	Neurologic Signs	EEG Abnormalities
0	Normal	None	None	None
Minimal hepatic encephalopathy	Normal	Normal	Abnormal neuropsychological testing	None
1	Sleep-wake reversal, restlessness	Forgetfulness, agitation, irritability, mild confusion	Tremor, apraxia, incoordination	Present
2	Lethargy, slow responses	Disorientation, amnesia, inappropriate behavior	Asterixis, dysarthria, ataxia, hypoactive reflexes	Present
3	Somnolence, confusion	Disorientation, aggressive behavior	Asterixis, hyperactive reflexes, positive Babinski sign, muscle rigidity	Present
4	Coma	Unresponsive	Decerebration	Present

Disease Highlights

A. Splenomegaly is found in 36–92% of patients with cirrhosis; 11–55% have the clinical syndrome of hypersplenism, defined as the presence of leukopenia or thrombocytopenia (or both) with splenomegaly.

B. There is a rough correlation between spleen size and degree of decrease in blood cells.

C. Blood cell abnormalities in liver disease
   1. Thrombocytopenia is due to platelet sequestration in the spleen, impaired bone marrow production, and decreased platelet survival.
   2. Leukopenia is due to sequestration in the spleen and is rare compared with thrombocytopenia (1 series found 64% of cirrhotic patients had thrombocytopenia, but only 5% had leukopenia).
   3. Although not part of the syndrome of hypersplenism, anemia often occurs in patients with cirrhosis and is due to increased destruction in the spleen as well as iron or folate deficiency; there is also reduced erythropoietin production.

Evidence-Based Diagnosis

A. Hypersplenism is a clinical syndrome without a specific set of diagnostic criteria.

B. Hypersplenism is manifested by splenomegaly and a significant reduction in 1 or more cellular elements of the blood, in the presence of normal or hypercellular bone marrow.

Treatment

A. Treatment is usually not necessary.

B. Splenectomy or partial splenic embolization is sometimes done for severe thrombocytopenia with bleeding complications.

C. Granulocyte-macrophage colony-stimulating factor and erythropoietin are rarely used.

D. TIPS does not correct thrombocytopenia.

MAKING A DIAGNOSIS

Initial laboratory test results follow: WBC, 9700/mcL; Hgb, 10.5 g/dL; HCT, 31%; MCV, 86 mcm³; platelet, 123,000/mcL; electrolytes normal; BUN, 8 mg/dL; creatinine, 0.4 mg/dL; glucose, 97 mg/dL; albumin, 2.1 g/dL; alkaline phosphatase, 95 units/L; total bilirubin, 1.2 mg/dL; ALT, 102 units/L; AST, 66 units/L; PT/PTT normal; urinalysis, 2+ protein with no cells or casts.

Have you crossed a diagnostic threshold for the leading hypothesis, cirrhosis and portal hypertension? Have you ruled out the active alternatives? Do other tests need to be done to exclude the alternative diagnoses?

The physical exam findings of splenomegaly and ascites, along with the laboratory abnormalities of thrombocytopenia, elevated transaminases, and hypoalbuminemia, are all consistent with chronic liver disease. The absence of pulmonary crackles and elevation of the jugular venous pressure makes HF unlikely. However, the findings of proteinuria and hypoalbuminemia are also consistent with nephrotic syndrome.

Alternative Diagnosis: Nephrotic Syndrome

Textbook Presentation

Patients with nephrotic syndrome classically have edema (often periorbital), hypertension, hypoalbuminemia, hyperlipidemia, and at least 3.5 g/24 hour of proteinuria.

Disease Highlights

A. Etiology
   1. Primary glomerular diseases
      a. Etiology uncertain but probably immune mediated
      b. Most common pathologies found in adults are membranous and focal segmental glomerulosclerosis (33% each), with membranous being more common in white patients and focal segmental glomerulosclerosis more common in black patients.
      c. Less common pathologies found in adults are minimal change disease (15%) and membranoproliferative glomerular disease (including IgA nephropathy) (14%).
      d. In patients over age 65 who undergo kidney biopsy (recognizing that many patients with presumed diabetic nephropathy do not have a biopsy), approximately 15% have minimal change disease, 30–40% have membranous, and 10–12% have amyloidosis.
   2. Secondary glomerular disease
      a. Diabetes is the most common cause in the United States.
      b. Systemic lupus erythematosus (SLE) generally causes an inflammatory nephritis, but sometimes causes a noninflammatory, membranous pathology.
      c. Amyloidosis and multiple myeloma should be considered in patients over age 40.
      d. Infections commonly associated with nephrotic syndrome include HIV, hepatitis B, hepatitis C, syphilis, and malaria.
      e. Malignancies, especially lung, breast, prostate, and colon cancer, and Hodgkin lymphoma are associated with nephrotic syndrome.
         (1) 5–25% of patients with membranous nephropathy have a malignancy, with the association being strongest for patients over 60 years old.
         (2) The cancer may be diagnosed at the same time as the kidney disease but often is found later.
      f. Many drugs, including NSAIDs, captopril, tamoxifen, lithium, and heroin, can cause nephrotic syndrome.

B. Clinical consequences
   1. Primary sodium retention by the kidney, related to low effective circulating volume, causes edema and hypertension.
   2. Albumin excretion leads to hypoalbuminemia, which also contributes to edema formation.
   3. Alterations in lipoprotein production and catabolism lead to elevations of low-density lipoprotein and sometimes triglycerides.
   4. Immunoglobulin excretion and depression of T cell function causes increased susceptibility to infection.
   5. Thromboembolic complications
      a. Due to increased procoagulatory factors and fibrinogen, altered fibrinolytic system, urinary loss of antithrombin III, and increased platelet activity
      b. Relative risk of DVT is 1.7 with an annual incidence of 1.5%; the annual incidence of renal vein thrombosis is 0.5%.

c. Relative risk of pulmonary embolism is 1.4 but is 6.8 for patients aged 18–39 years.

d. Risk factors for venous thromboembolism include serum albumin < 2.0–2.5 mg/dL, protein excretion > 8 g/24 h, being within 6 months of diagnosis

e. The role of prophylactic anticoagulation is unclear but should be considered in high-risk patients.

f. Arterial thrombosis is rare.

Evidence-Based Diagnosis

A. Nephrotic syndrome is defined by the presence of urinary protein excretion of at least 3.5 g/24 hours, measured with either a 24-hour specimen or a spot albumin/creatinine ratio > 3000–3500 mcg/mg.

B. Laboratory evaluation should include

  1. CBC

  2. Comprehensive metabolic panel (kidney and liver function, including serum albumin)

  3. Fasting glucose and HgbA$_{1c}$

  4. Antinuclear antibody

  5. HIV

  6. Hepatitis B serology (surface antigen, core antibody)

  7. Hepatitis C antibody

  8. Serum and urine protein electrophoresis

C. Renal ultrasound should be done.

D. Renal biopsy is often necessary.

Treatment

A. All patients with nephrotic syndrome should be referred to a nephrologist.

B. Loop diuretics are used to treat the edema; high doses are often needed due to the primary sodium retention by the kidney.

C. Angiotensin-converting enzyme inhibitors reduce proteinuria in both hypertensive and normotensive patients.

  1. The antiproteinuric effect becomes maximal in 28 days.

  2. The effect can be increased by a low-salt diet, diuretic treatment, or both.

D. Corticosteroids and other immunosuppressives are used in selected patients.

CASE RESOLUTION

Mrs. V's hepatitis C antibody is positive, with negative hepatitis B serologies. Her total cholesterol is 145 mg/dL, and her 24-hour urinary protein excretion is 1.4 g. An abdominal CT scan demonstrates a small, nodular liver; splenomegaly; and ascites. You schedule an esophagogastroduodenoscopy to screen for varices, start spironolactone because of the discomfort she is having from the edema, and refer her to a hepatologist.

CHIEF COMPLAINT

PATIENT 2

Mrs. E is a 62-year-old woman with a long history of hypertension that is well controlled with hydrochlorothiazide, metoprolol, and amlodipine. She comes in today with a new complaint of swelling in her legs and feet for several weeks. It is generally most noticeable late in the day and is often absent when she first gets up in the morning. She has no history of liver or kidney disease or alcohol use. She has no chest pain and no shortness of breath, although notes she finds it tiring to climb stairs or walk more than a few blocks. She smoked a few cigarettes a day for 20 years, but quit 20 years ago.

Her physical exam is notable for a BMI of 38, clear lungs, an S$_4$ with no S$_3$ or murmurs, and a normal abdomen. Her legs show 1+ edema to the knees bilaterally. She has a long-standing goiter that is unchanged from previous exams. It is difficult to identify her jugular venous pressure due to the shape of her neck.

At this point, what is the leading hypothesis, what are the active alternatives, and is there a must not miss diagnosis? Given this differential diagnosis, what tests should be ordered?

RANKING THE DIFFERENTIAL DIAGNOSIS

Once again, given the pivotal finding of bilateral edema, the first step is to look for systemic causes, focusing first on cardiac, hepatic, and renal causes. Mrs. E's long-standing history of hypertension raises the possibility of diastolic dysfunction, and the lack of physical exam findings does not rule this out. There are no clinical clues to suggest liver or kidney disease, but these are easy to test for and should always be ruled out. Amlodipine commonly causes edema, but she has taken it for years without symptoms. "Dependent edema," edema that is worsened by standing and improves or resolves with leg elevation, is consistent with, but not specific for, venous insufficiency. A final consideration would be pulmonary hypertension. Patients with pulmonary hypertension commonly complain of dyspnea in addition to edema, and the tired feeling she experiences with exertion could represent dyspnea. Additionally, she is overweight, putting her at risk for obstructive sleep apnea and consequent pulmonary hypertension. Table 17-6 lists the differential diagnosis.

Initial laboratory test results include BUN, 15 mg/dL; creatinine, 0.9 mg/dL; albumin/creatinine ratio, 5 mcg/mg; normal liver enzymes, albumin, and prothrombin time.

(continued)

Table 17-6. Diagnostic hypotheses for Mrs. E.

Diagnostic Hypotheses	Demographics, Risk Factors, Symptoms and Signs	Important Tests
Leading Hypothesis		
Diastolic dysfunction	History of hypertension Dyspnea Orthopnea, PND Edema Elevated JVP S$_3$ or S$_4$	Echocardiogram BNP
Active Alternatives—Most Common		
Venous insufficiency	Dependent edema Varicose veins Typical skin changes (see text for description)	Physical exam Duplex ultrasound
Active Alternatives—Must Not Miss		
Renal and liver disease	See Table 17-1	See Table 17-1
Other Hypotheses		
Pulmonary hypertension	Dyspnea, often long-standing Obesity Edema Syncope	Echocardiogram Right heart catheterization

BNP, B-type natriuretic peptide; JVP, jugular venous pressure; PND, paroxysmal nocturnal dyspnea.

Table 17-7. Classification and etiology of pulmonary hypertension (PH).

Classification	Etiology
Group 1: Pulmonary arterial hypertension	Idiopathic Heritable Drug/toxin induced Associated with connective tissue disease,[1] HIV, portal hypertension, congenital heart disease, chronic hemolytic anemia, schistosomiasis
Group 2: Pulmonary venous hypertension due to left heart disease	Systolic heart failure Diastolic heart failure Valvular disease
Group 3: PH due to hypoxia	Chronic obstructive pulmonary disease Interstitial lung disease Sleep disordered breathing Alveolar hypoventilation Chronic exposure to high altitude
Group 4: PH due to chronic thromboembolic disease	Chronic thromboembolic disease
Group 5: PH due to miscellaneous causes	Myeloproliferative disorders Sarcoid Glycogen storage diseases Fibrosing mediastinitis

[1]Most commonly seen with scleroderma, mixed connective tissue disease, and systemic lupus erythematosus.

The ECG and chest radiograph are normal. An echocardiogram shows normal left ventricle size and function, elevated pulmonary pressures consistent with moderate pulmonary hypertension (estimated mean PAP 30 mm Hg), mild tricuspid regurgitation, and normal right ventricular size and function.

 Is the clinical information sufficient to make a diagnosis? If not, what other information do you need?

There is no evidence of kidney disease, liver disease, or diastolic dysfunction. However, the echocardiogram shows the somewhat unexpected finding of pulmonary hypertension (PH). This necessitates revising the original set of diagnostic hypotheses: the leading hypothesis is now PH, and venous insufficiency is the remaining active alternative.

Leading Hypothesis: Pulmonary Hypertension

Textbook Presentation

Patients commonly complain of long-standing dyspnea that progresses over months or years. Syncope, exertional chest pain, and edema occur with more severe PH and impaired right heart function.

Disease Highlights

A. Definition

1. The normal mean pulmonary artery pressure (PAP) is 12 mm Hg.

2. The clinical classification was revised in 2008 (Table 17-7).

3. PH is defined as a mean PAP ≥ 25 mm Hg and a pulmonary capillary wedge pressure (PCWP) ≤ 15 mm Hg; however, in Group 2 PH related to left heart disease (see Table 17-7), the PCWP is > 15 mm Hg.

B. Epidemiology

1. The prevalence of Group 1 PAH is 6 cases/million (about 3% of patients with PH); approximately one-half of these are idiopathic (including heritable and drug related), 15–30% are related to connective tissue disease, 10–24% to congenital heart disease, 1–6% to HIV, and 7–10% to portal hypertension.

2. Left heart disease is the etiology of PH in about 65% of cases; up to 83% of patients with diastolic HF have PH.

3. Over 50% of patients with advanced chronic obstructive pulmonary disease have PH, as do 32–39% of patients with interstitial lung disease.

4. Chronic thromboembolic disease is the etiology in 0.5–2% of patients with PH.

Evidence-Based Diagnosis

A. History

1. In 1 series of patients with PAH, initial symptoms included dyspnea (60%), fatigue (19%), chest pain (7%), syncope (8%), edema (3%).

2. At the time these patients were given the diagnosis of PAH and were enrolled in the study, 98% had dyspnea, 73% fatigue, 47% chest pain, 36% syncope, 37% edema, and 33% palpitations.

B. Physical exam

　1. Characteristic findings include the following:

　　a. An accentuated pulmonary component of S_2

　　b. A sustained left lower parasternal movement

　　c. Increased jugular a and v waves

　　d. A tricuspid regurgitation murmur

　　e. Hepatojugular reflux

　　f. A pulsatile liver

　　g. Elevated jugular venous pressure

　　h. Edema

　2. Sustained left lower parasternal movement for detecting severe PH with a mean PAP > 50 mm Hg: sensitivity, 71%; specificity, 80%; LR+, 3.6; LR−, 0.4

　3. A palpable P_2 for detecting severe PH with a mean PAP > 50 mm Hg (studied in patients with mitral stenosis): sensitivity, 96%; specificity, 73%; LR+, 3.6; LR−, 0.05

C. ECG

　1. Expected findings include right axis deviation, right ventricular hypertrophy, and P-pulmonale pattern (right atrial enlargement).

　2. Not sensitive or specific enough to diagnosis PH (sensitivity, 51%; specificity, 86%; LR+, 3.6; LR−, 0.56)

D. Chest film

　1. Expected findings include enlargement of pulmonary arteries and right ventricular enlargement.

　2. Not sensitive or specific enough to diagnose PH (sensitivity, 46%; specificity, 63%; LR+, 1.24; LR−, 0.85)

E. Transthoracic echocardiogram is the best first screening test.

　1. Echocardiogram estimates often correlate fairly well with invasively determined PAPs, but differences of 10–20 mm Hg are common.

　2. Sensitivity ranges from 79% to 100%.

　3. Specificity ranges from 80% to 98%; the specificity may be lower than 50% in patients with mildly elevated PAP on an echocardiogram.

F. Right heart catheterization is the gold standard for diagnosing PH, and most patients with suspected PH need a right heart catheterization to confirm the diagnosis.

Treatment

A. Depends on underlying etiology

B. Correct underlying cause when possible

　1. For obstructive sleep apnea, administer continuous positive airway pressure.

　2. For chronic thromboembolism, begin anticoagulation and consider thromboendarterectomy.

　3. For valvular disease, replace the valve.

　4. For congenital heart disease, repair surgically.

　5. For left ventricular dysfunction, optimize medical regimen.

C. Oxygen therapy for patients with hypoxemia (PO_2 < 55 mm Hg at rest, oxygen saturation < 85% with exercise)

D. Most patients require loop diuretics.

E. Most treatment studies have been performed in patients with PAH.

MAKING A DIAGNOSIS

Mrs. E has a normal physical exam, ECG, and chest radiograph, normal right ventricular function on echocardiogram, and the isolated finding of moderately elevated PAP seen on an echocardiogram. The echocardiogram estimate of PAP alone is not specific enough to make the diagnosis of PH, and Mrs. E has no other findings supporting the diagnosis of PH. Furthermore, Mrs. E's dyspnea is minimal, suggesting that she has neither significant PH nor pulmonary disease.

You explain the puzzling finding to Mrs. E. She does not want to undergo a right heart catheterization to verify the PAP. She reports that she is able to walk a mile every morning without shortness of breath, and that her edema is most noticeable when she has been on her feet for a long time.

Have you crossed a diagnostic threshold for the leading hypothesis, pulmonary hypertension? Have you ruled out the active alternatives? Do other tests need to be done to exclude the alternative diagnoses?

Alternative Diagnosis: Venous Insufficiency

Textbook Presentation

Venous insufficiency can be asymptomatic or manifested just by small visible, but nonpalpable veins. In more severe cases, the patient has large varicose veins and skin changes ranging from edema to fibrosing panniculitis to ulceration. Symptoms include leg fullness or heaviness, aching leg pain, and nocturnal leg cramps. Symptoms are often worse at the end of the day and in heat, and are sometimes relieved by elevation.

Disease Highlights

A. Anatomy (Figure 17-3)

　1. The superficial saphenous veins join the deep system at the knee (popliteal vein) and the groin (femoral vein).

　2. Perforating veins directly connect the saphenous veins and the deep veins at various points along their parallel courses.

　3. Valves within the veins prevent reflux back toward the feet.

B. Pathophysiology and epidemiology

　1. Chronic venous disease is due to venous hypertension caused by reflux through incompetent valves, venous outflow obstruction, or lack of calf muscle pumping due to obesity or immobility.

　　a. Reflux occurs in the superficial system in about 45% of patients, both the superficial and deep systems in about 40%, and in the deep system only in the remainder of patients.

　　b. Prolonged standing leads to marked increases in venous pressure in all people; while those with competent valves quickly lower the venous pressure with walking, individuals with incompetent valves have only slight decreases in pressure with walking.

　2. Varicose veins are found in 25–33% of women and 10–20% of men.

　3. Prevalence of skin changes is 3–11%; prevalence of skin ulcers is 0.3–1%.

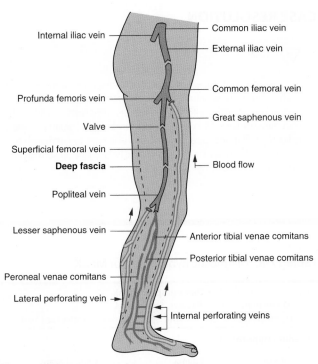

Figure 17-3. Anatomy of the superficial venous system.

4. Risk factors for venous insufficiency include female sex, advancing age, obesity, a history of phlebitis or venous thrombosis, serious leg trauma, pregnancy, prolonged standing, and greater height.

5. Postthrombotic syndrome (venous insufficiency after a DVT) occurs in 35–69% of patients at 3 years and in 49–100% of patients at 5–10 years; incidence is reduced to 8% if patients are treated with adequate anticoagulation, early mobilization, and long-term use of compression stockings.

C. Classification

1. Class 1: telangiectasias or reticular veins (nonpalpable subdermal veins up to 4 mm in diameter)

2. Class 2: varicose veins (palpable, subcutaneous veins > 4 mm in diameter)

3. Class 3: edema without skin changes

    a. Initially present just at the end of day but can become persistent and massive

    b. Can be unilateral initially

    c. Often begins around medial malleolus

4. Class 4: skin changes

    a. Pigmentation due to breakdown of extravasated RBCs

    b. Stasis dermatitis: itching, weeping, scaling, erosions, and crusting

    c. Lipodermatosclerosis or fibrosing panniculitis

       (1) Induration initially at medial ankle, spreading circumferentially round the entire leg, up to mid calf

       (2) The skin is heavily pigmented and fixed to subcutaneous tissues, with brawny edema above the fibrosis and in the foot below

       (3) High risk for cellulitis

5. Classes 5 and 6: healed or nonhealed ulcers

    a. Usually low on the medial ankle or along the path of the long or short saphenous vein

b. Never above the knee or on the forefoot

c. Chronic and recurrent, often lasting for months or even years

Evidence-Based Diagnosis

A. Diagnosis is often made based on the appearance of the leg.

B. Venography is the gold standard.

C. Duplex ultrasonography is the best noninvasive test.

1. Should be done if the diagnosis is in doubt (especially to rule out DVT), in patients with atypical symptoms or presentations, or if surgery is being considered

2. For diagnosing valvular incompetence, the sensitivity is 84%, specificity is 88%, LR+ = 7, and LR– = 0.18.

3. For diagnosing severe venous insufficiency, the sensitivity is 77%, specificity is 85%, LR+ = 5.1, and LR– = 0.26.

D. Because many patients have both arterial and venous insufficiency, concurrent arterial disease must be ruled out with the ankle-brachial index.

Treatment

A. Compression stockings are the most important treatment modality.

1. Have been shown to reduce the risk of postthrombotic syndrome, to accelerate ulcer healing, and to prevent recurrent ulceration

2. Classified into several grades, based on degree of compression at the ankle

    a. 20–30 mm Hg: for patients with varicose veins, edema, leg fatigue (Classes 2 and 3)

    b. 30–40 mm Hg: for patients with severe varicosities or moderate disease (Classes 4–6)

    c. 40–50 mm Hg: for patients with recurrent ulceration

3. Knee high stockings are better tolerated than thigh high stockings.

4. Compliance often poor due to skin irritation, discomfort, and difficulty putting on the stockings.

 Compression stockings should not be used in patients with peripheral arterial disease or with invasive infection at an ulcer site.

5. Alternative ways to provide compression include elastic wraps and intermittent pneumatic compression pumps.

6. Ulcers should be covered with a dressing before putting on the compression device.

B. Diuretics are ineffective for the edema unless given with compression therapy.

C. Treatment of venous insufficiency ulcers

1. Occlusive dressing

2. Leg elevation and compression

3. Aspirin, 325 mg daily, might accelerate healing.

4. Pentoxifylline might accelerate healing.

5. Topical antibiotics have no role.

6. Systemic antibiotics indicated only if cellulitis or other invasive infection is present.

D. Interventional therapies

1. Sclerotherapy for spider veins, venous lakes, varicose veins 1–4 mm in diameter

2. Endovenous radiofrequency ablation and laser: alternative to vein stripping for great saphenous vein reflux

3. Iliac vein stenting for venous outflow abnormalities

4. Vein stripping and ligation

    a. Usually involves removing the saphenous vein with high ligation of the saphenofemoral junction

    b. Shown to result in significant improvement in symptoms in patients with Class 2–6 disease

    c. Surgery plus compression is better than compression alone for preventing ulcer recurrence (12% combined therapy vs. 28% compression alone).

CASE RESOLUTION

You decide that Mrs. E's symptoms are more consistent with venous insufficiency than with PH. Duplex ultrasonographic scans confirm valvular incompetence, and you recommend that Mrs. E wear compression stockings. She returns in 3 months reporting that she has no edema when she wears the stockings, and that she continues to walk 1 mile daily without any dyspnea.

CHIEF COMPLAINT

PATIENT ▽3

Mrs. K is a 64-year-old woman who had a right mastectomy 2 years ago for breast cancer. She was treated with adjuvant radiation therapy and has been taking tamoxifen since completing the radiation. She has had no evidence of recurrent disease but has had some right arm swelling for at least 18 months. She comes to see you now because 2 days ago the swelling of her right arm worsened, with associated pain and redness. This morning her temperature was 37.9°C.

 At this point, what is the leading hypothesis, what are the active alternatives, and is there a must not miss diagnosis? Given this differential diagnosis, what tests should be ordered?

RANKING THE DIFFERENTIAL DIAGNOSIS

Mrs. K has unilateral limb edema, a key pivotal point limiting the differential. Exploring her history, it is notable that she has chronic lymphedema due to disruption of lymphatic drainage by her previous surgery and radiation therapy. This is an important clinical clue, since patients with lymphatic disruption and lymphedema are at high risk for skin and subcutaneous infections. Pathophysiologically, the edema found in cellulitis is due to a localized increase in capillary permeability due to inflammation; however, patients with underlying limb abnormalities will often present with more diffuse edema. The other primary consideration in *any* patient with unilateral limb swelling is DVT. Mrs. K has several risk factors for this, including history of cancer, possible venous scarring secondary to radiation, and use of tamoxifen (a drug associated with a relative risk for DVT of about 3). Table 17-8 lists the differential diagnosis.

 Always think about DVT in a patient with unilateral limb swelling.

▽3

On physical exam, Mrs. K is clearly uncomfortable. Her temperature is 38.3°C, pulse 102 bpm, RR 16 breaths

(continued)

Table 17-8. Diagnostic hypotheses for Mrs. K.

Diagnostic Hypotheses	Demographics, Risk Factors, Symptoms and Signs	Important Tests
Leading Hypothesis		
Cellulitis or erysipelas	Edema Erythema Pain Fever Entry site for infection Underlying venous insufficiency or lymphedema	Clinical exam
Active Alternative—Must Not Miss		
Upper extremity DVT	Unilateral arm/neck swelling Feeling of fullness or heaviness DVT risk factors (especially indwelling intravenous catheter)	Duplex ultrasound CT MRA Venography

DVT, deep venous thrombosis; MRA, magnetic resonance angiography.

per minute, and BP 125/80 mm Hg. Her right upper arm and chest are bright red, hot, and tender. The border of the erythema is sharply demarcated, and the area of erythema feels indurated. She has eczema of all of her fingers, with multiple areas of cracked skin.

 Is the clinical information sufficient to make a diagnosis? If not, what other information do you need?

Leading Hypothesis: Cellulitis & Erysipelas

Textbook Presentation

A painful, red, hot, and swollen limb develops acutely in a patient with underlying venous or lymphatic disease.

Disease Highlights

A. Definitions

　1. Cellulitis is an infection of the dermis and subcutaneous tissue.

　2. Erysipelas is a superficial cellulitis with prominent lymphatic involvement.

B. Cellulitis highlights

　1. Risk factors

　　a. Edema

　　b. Venous insufficiency

　　c. Obesity

　　d. Diabetes mellitus

　　e. History of cellulitis

　　f. Injection drug use

　　g. Breast cancer treatment

　　　(1) Cellulitis of the ipsilateral arm is seen in women in whom lymphedema of the arm develops after mastectomy.

　　　(2) Cellulitis of the ipsilateral breast is seen in women in whom localized lymphedema develops after lumpectomy, axillary node dissection, and radiation therapy.

　2. Often an entry site for infection can be identified (leg ulcer, trauma, tinea pedis, eczema, subcutaneous abscess)

　3. Clinical presentation

　　a. Presence of systemic symptoms (eg, fever, chills, myalgias) is unusual and suggests concomitant bacteremia or a more serious infection such as necrotizing fasciitis.

　　b. Physical findings

　　　(1) Nonpalpable, confluent erythema with indistinct margins

　　　(2) Generalized swelling

　　　(3) Warmth and tenderness of involved skin

　　　(4) Tender regional adenopathy sometimes found

　　　(5) Lymphangitis and abscess formation sometimes seen

　　　(6) In women who have been treated for breast cancer and have arm lymphedema, the humeral area of the ipsilateral extremity is most often involved, with extension to the shoulder and forearm.

　　　(7) In breast cellulitis, the infection starts at the lumpectomy site and can extend to the remainder of the breast, the anterior shoulder, back, and ipsilateral upper extremity.

　4. Microbiology

　　a. Beta-hemolytic streptococci and *Staphylococcus aureus* are the most common organisms; *S aureus* is the more likely cause if there is an abscess or drainage, and streptococci are more likely if there is no abscess or drainage.

　　　(1) Community-acquired methicillin-resistant *S aureus* (CA-MRSA), usually the USA300 genotype, is increasingly common; it is now the most common pathogen cultured from skin and soft tissue infections in urban emergency departments.

　　　(2) Risk factors for MRSA

　　　　(a) Recent antibiotic use or hospitalization

　　　　(b) Recurrent needle sticks (injection drug use, hemodialysis, insulin use)

　　　　(c) Homelessness, incarceration

　　　　(d) Contact sports

　　　　(e) Patients with a previous CA-MRSA infection or colonization

　　　(3) Many patients with CA-MRSA have none of these risk factors

　　　(4) Skin abscesses, often with central necrosis, are a very common manifestation of CA-MRSA; patients often think they have been bitten by a spider or other insect.

　　　(5) Other manifestations include cellulitis, necrotizing pneumonia, pleural empyema, necrotizing fasciitis, septic thrombophlebitis, myositis, and severe sepsis.

　　b. A variety of other organisms may be seen with specific exposures or sites of infection (Table 17-9).

C. Erysipelas highlights

　1. Risk factors for development of erysipelas

　　a. Similar to those for cellulitis

　　b. Lymphedema and an identified portal of entry (primarily tinea pedis) are the 2 strongest risk factors in 1 study.

 Always treat tinea pedis in a patient with cellulitis, erysipelas, or risk factors for developing those infections.

Table 17-9. Microbiology of cellulitis.

Cellulitis Syndrome	Location/Key Point	Likely Organisms
Periorbital	Periorbital	*Staphylococcus aureus*, pneumococcus, group A streptococcus (GAS)
Orbital	Emergent because of potential to affect oculomotor function and visual acuity	Staphylococcus, streptococcus
Perianal	Evaluate for underlying abscess	GAS
Breast cancer treatment	See text	Non-group A hemolytic streptococcus
Saphenous vein harvest	Ipsilateral leg	GAS or non-group A streptococcus
Injection drug use	Extremities, neck	Staphylococcus, streptococcus (groups A, C, F, G), gram-negative organisms, anaerobes
Crepitant cellulitis	Trunk, extremities; consider necrotizing fasciitis	GAS, anaerobes, *Clostridia*
Salt water exposure	Exposed body part	*Vibrio vulnificus*
Fresh water exposure	Exposed body part	*Aeromonas hydrophilia*
Hot tub exposure	Bathing suit distribution	*Pseudomonas aeruginosa*

2. Clinical presentation
   a. Sudden onset of fever (85% of patients), erythema, edema, and pain
   b. Physical findings
      (1) Palpable plaque of erythema that extends by 2–10 cm/day
      (2) Sharply demarcated border
      (3) Leg is the most common site (90%), then the arm (5%), and then the face (2.5%).
      (4) Regional adenopathy and lymphangitis sometimes seen
   c. Recurrence rate of 10% at 6 months and 30% at 3 years is usually due to untreated local factors.
   d. Patients should respond to antibiotic therapy in 24–72 hours.
3. Microbiology
   a. Streptococci are the causative organisms in 90% of cases (group A in about 58–67% of cases caused by streptococci, group B in 3–9%, and group C or G in 14–25%).
   b. *S aureus* is also found in 10% of cases, although it is unclear whether it is contributing to the infection or just colonizing.

 Consider necrotizing fasciitis in patients with a rapid increase in the size of the infected area, evolution of violaceous bullae, a reddish-purple discoloration of the skin, woody induration of the infected area, disproportionally severe pain or tenderness, severe systemic toxicity.

Evidence-Based Diagnosis

A. Both cellulitis and erysipelas are clinical diagnoses.
B. Blood cultures are positive in 2–5% of patients.
C. Skin biopsy cultures are positive in 5–40% of patients but are rarely necessary.
D. Aspiration of the leading edge of erythema is sometimes done, but the yield is low.
E. Toe web cultures are sometimes helpful in patients with tinea pedis.
F. If there is a skin abscess associated with the cellulitis, it should be drained and the fluid cultured.
G. CT or MRI should be done if necrotizing fasciitis is suspected; MRI is more sensitive, but CT is more specific.

 Cultures are rarely helpful in cellulitis or erysipelas without an associated abscess.

Treatment

A. Cellulitis (2011 Infectious Disease Society of American Guidelines)
   1. Outpatients with purulent cellulitis (associated with purulent drainage or exudate but no drainable abscess): empiric treatment for CA-MRSA with clindamycin, trimethoprim-sulfamethoxazole (TMP-SMX), doxycycline, or linezolid for 5–10 days

2. Outpatients with nonpurulent cellulitis (no exudate or drainage; no abscess): empiric treatment for beta-hemolytic streptococci with a beta-lactam (cephalexin, amoxicillin, or similar drugs) for 5–10 days
   a. Patients who do not respond should be treated for CA-MRSA.
   b. To treat for both CA-MRSA and beta-hemolytic streptococci, use clindamycin, TMP-SMX (or doxycycline) *and* a beta-lactam, or linezolid.
3. 10–20% of MRSA isolates that are sensitive to clindamycin, but resistant to erythromycin, develop inducible clindamycin resistance due to the presence of the *erm* gene.
4. Clindamycin sensitive/erythromycin resistant isolates should undergo the "D-Zone Test" to look for inducible resistance (Figure 17-4).

B. Erysipelas
   1. Penicillin G or amoxicillin is effective in > 80% of patients with erysipelas.
   2. Other drugs that have been studied include macrolides and fluoroquinolones.
   3. Should treat for 10–20 days

C. Uncomplicated, slowly progressive infection in a well-appearing patient can be treated with oral antibiotics if
   1. The patient has no GI upset
   2. The limb can be elevated
   3. Serial exams are feasible

D. Patients who appear ill, who have rapidly progressive infection, are immunocompromised, or who might not be able to follow treatment instructions should be admitted for

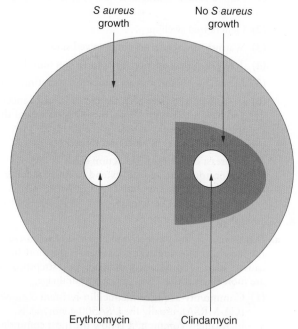

When there is inducible clindamycin resistance, the zone of clindamycin inhibition is blunted on the side next to the erythromycin disk, resulting in a "D" shaped area of no growth surrounding the clindamycin disk. If there is no inducible resistance, the no growth area around the clindamycin disk will be a more symmetric circle

Figure 17-4. D-Zone test

IV antibiotics, generally including either vancomycin, clindamycin, linezolid, or daptomycin.

E. Obtain infectious disease and surgical consultations for patients with rapidly progressive infections, especially if progression occurs while they are receiving appropriate antibiotics and those in whom necrotizing fasciitis is suspected.

MAKING A DIAGNOSIS

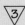

Initial laboratory tests include the following: WBC 11,700/mcL, 83% PMNs, 10% basophils, 7% lymphocytes; Hgb, 13.5 g/dL; glucose, 88 mg/dL; creatinine, 0.8 mg/dL.

Have you crossed a diagnostic threshold for the leading hypothesis, cellulitis or erysipelas? Have you ruled out the active alternatives? Do other tests need to be done to exclude the alternative diagnoses?

Alternative Diagnosis: Upper Extremity DVT (UEDVT)

Textbook Presentation

Patients can be asymptomatic, but generally arm, shoulder, or neck discomfort or fullness as well as arm swelling are the presenting symptoms.

Disease Highlights

A. Classification
1. Primary UEDVT (20% of cases)
   a. Idiopathic
   b. Effort thrombosis, also known as Paget-Schroetter syndrome
      (1) Occurs in young men after strenuous exercise, which causes microtrauma to the veins
      (2) Narrowing of the thoracic outlet at the level of the first rib and clavicle leads to compression of the subclavian vein
2. Secondary UEDVT (80% of cases) (Table 17-10)
   a. Indwelling central venous catheter–associated UEDVT (up to 70% of cases)
      (1) UEDVT occurs more often with large catheters than with smaller ones.
      (2) Risk increases with duration of catheter use, being negligible within 6 days and increasing significantly after 2 weeks.
      (3) Risk is higher with polyvinyl chloride-coated catheters than with silicone ones.
      (4) One study found that the risk is about 2.5 times higher with peripherally inserted central catheters than with other central venous catheters.
   b. Malignancy (> 40% of cases): patients with cancer and an indwelling catheter are at especially high risk.
   c. Hypercoagulable states
   d. Other miscellaneous causes (surgery, infection, immobility, concurrent lower extremity DVT)

Table 17-10. Risk factors for upper extremity deep venous thrombosis.

Risk Factor	Adjust Odds Ratio (95% CI)
Cancer plus central venous catheter (CVC)	43.6 (25.5–74.6)
CVC plus inherited coagulation disorder	~30
Cancer	18.1 (9.4–35.1)
Oral contraceptives plus factor V Leiden or prothrombin G20210A mutation	13.6 (2.7–67.3)
Upper extremity surgery	13.1 (2.1–80.6)
Metastatic vs. localized cancer	11.5 (1.6–80.2)
Indwelling (CVC)	9.7 (7.8–12.2)
Upper extremity plaster cast	7.0 (1.7–29.5)

B. Sites
1. Subclavian in 18–69% of cases
2. Axillary in 5–42% of cases
3. Internal jugular in 8–29% of cases
4. Brachial in 4–13% of cases
5. Multiple veins are often involved, but bilateral UEDVT is rare.

C. Clinical features
1. Pain is present in ~40% of patients.
2. Edema is present ~80% of patients in some series, but patients with catheter-related UEDVT often do not have edema.
3. Patients may note numbness, heaviness, paresthesias, pruritus, and coldness.
4. Dilated cutaneous veins sometimes visible.

D. Complications
1. Pulmonary embolism has been reported to occur in up to 36% of cases and is more often seen with secondary UEDVT, especially catheter-related; however, more recent studies have found a much lower rate of pulmonary embolism.

 UEDVT can cause pulmonary embolism.

2. Recurrent thrombosis occurs in up to 10% of patients.
3. Postthrombotic syndrome is seen in up to 4–34% of patients in different series.

Evidence-Based Diagnosis

A. Venography is the gold standard.
B. Duplex ultrasonography is the most commonly used noninvasive test.
1. Disadvantages include a blind spot caused by the clavicle, inability to determine compressibility in veins located in the thoracic cavity, and difficulties interpreting the study if there are collateral veins.
2. Test characteristics come from two small, low quality studies: sensitivity 97%; specificity 94%; LR+, 16.2; LR–, 0.03
C. The test characteristics of D-dimer for the diagnosis of UEDVT are not known.

D. Magnetic resonance and CT venography are sometimes done; sensitivity and specificity are unknown.

E. The American College of Chest Physicians 2012 Guidelines recommend the following diagnostic approach:

1. Initial evaluation with duplex ultrasound

2. Follow up testing with a highly sensitive D-dimer or venography (CT, MR, or conventional) in patients with a normal ultrasound and a high clinical suspicion.

3. No further testing in patients with negative follow up testing

Treatment

A. Anticoagulation with heparin, followed by at least 3 months of warfarin; patients with cancer or chronic indwelling central venous catheters should receive anticoagulation therapy indefinitely.

B. Thrombolysis with or without stent placement is sometimes done, especially in patients who require permanent indwelling catheters.

CASE RESOLUTION

Mrs. K's presentation of a sharply demarcated, erythematous plaque, fever, and leukocytosis is diagnostic of erysipelas. The portal of entry is the eczematous, cracked skin on her hands. Although she has some risk factors for UEDVT, it is not necessary to test for it at this point. Because of the extent of infection, Mrs. K is admitted to the hospital and treated with IV cefazolin. One of 2 blood cultures grows group A beta-hemolytic streptococci. She improves rapidly, is switched to oral penicillin and is discharged.

REFERENCES

Angeli P, Merkel C. Pathogenesis and management of hepatorenal syndrome in patients with cirrhosis. J Hepatol. 2008;28:S93–S103.

Baarslad HJ, van Beek EJR, Koopman MMW, Reekers JA. Prospective study of color duplex ultrasonography compared with contrast venography in patients suspected of having deep venous thrombosis of the upper extremities. Ann Intern Med. 2002;136:865–72.

Bates SM, Jaeschke R, Stevens SM et al. Diagnosis of DVT. Antithrombotic Therapy and Prevention of Thrombosis, 9th ed:American College of Chest Physicians Evidence-Based Clinical Practice Guidelines. Chest. 2012;141(2)(Suppl):e351S–e418S.

Bergan JJ, Schmid-Schonbein GW, Smith PD, Nicolaides AN, Boisseau MR, Eklof B. Chronic venous disease. N Engl J Med. 2006;355:488–98.

Bernardi E, Pesavento R, Prandoni P. Upper extremity deep venous thrombosis. Semin Thromb Hemost. 2006;32:729–36.

Bonnetblanc JM, Bedane C. Erysipelas. Am J Clin Dermatol. 2003;4:157–63.

Chin KM, Rubin LJ. Pulmonary arterial hypertension. J Am Coll Cardiol. 2008;51:1527–38.

Eberhardt RT, Raffetto JD. Chronic venous insufficiency. Circulation. 2005;111:2398–2409.

Eron LL. In the Clinic: Cellulitis and soft-tissue infections. Ann Intern Med. 2009;150:ITC1-1.

Glassock RJ. Attending rounds: an older patient with nephrotic syndrome. Clin J Am Soc Nephrol. 2012;7:665–70.

Gordon FD. Ascites. Clin Liver Dis. 2012;16:285–99.

Hoeper MM. Definition, classification, and epidemiology of pulmonary arterial hypertension. Semin Respir Crit Care Med. 2009;30:369–75.

Hull RP, Goldsmith DJA. Nephrotic syndrome in adults. BMJ. 2008;336:1185–9.

Khungar V, Poordad F. Hepatic encephalopathy. Clin Liver Dis. 2012;16:301–20.

Kodner C. Nephrotic syndrome in adults: diagnosis and management. Am Fam Physician. 2009;80:1129–34.

Jou JH, Muir AJ. In the Clinic: Hepatitis C. Ann Intern Med. 2012;157:ITC6-1–ITC6-16.

Liu C, Bayer A, Cosgrove SE et al. Clinical practice guidelines by the Infectious Diseases Society of America for the treatment of methicillin-resistant *Staphylococcus aureus* infections in adults and children. Clin Infect Dis. 2011;52:e18–55.

McGee S. Evidence based physical diagnosis. W.B. Saunders; 2012.

McGoon M, Gutterman D, Steen V et al; American College of Chest Physicians. Screening, early detection, and diagnosis of pulmonary hypertension: ACCP evidence-based clinical practice guidelines. Chest. 2004;126:14S–34S.

Schuppan D, Afdhal NH. Liver cirrhosis. Lancet. 2008;371:838–51.

Shah SJ. Pulmonary hypertension. JAMA. 2012;308:1366–74.

Udell JA, Wang CS, Tinmouth J et al. Original article: does this patient with liver disease have cirrhosis? In: Simel DL, Rennie D, eds. *The Rational Clinical Examination: Evidence-Based Clinical Diagnosis.* New York, NY: McGraw-Hill; 2013. http://www.jamaevidence.com/content/3502402. Accessed 9/25/2013

Wong CL, Holroyd-Leduc J, Thorpe KE, Straus SE. Does this patient have bacterial peritonitis or portal hypertension? How do I perform a paracentesis and analyze the results? JAMA. 2008;299:1166–78.

I have a patient with fatigue. How do I determine the cause?

CHIEF COMPLAINT

PATIENT 1

Mrs. M is a 42-year-old woman who has had fatigue for the past 6 months.

What is the differential diagnosis of fatigue? How would you frame the differential?

CONSTRUCTING A DIFFERENTIAL DIAGNOSIS

Before considering the differential diagnosis, it is important to understand what the patient means by fatigue, which is conventionally defined as a sensation of exhaustion after usual activities, or a feeling of insufficient energy to begin usual activities. Most people consider the terms fatigue, tiredness, and lack of energy synonymous. However, patients sometimes use these terms when they are actually experiencing other symptoms, especially excessive sleepiness, weakness, or dyspnea on exertion.

Always ask patients what they mean when they report fatigue. Always ask directly about weakness, excessive sleepiness, and dyspnea.

Acute fatigue is common in conjunction with a variety of acute illnesses, ranging from uncomplicated viral infections to exacerbations of heart failure (HF). Fatigue is also a prominent symptom in some chronic diseases, such as multiple sclerosis and cancer. This chapter will not discuss fatigue in such patients but will focus on evaluating the symptom of fatigue lasting weeks to months in patients without already diagnosed conditions known to cause fatigue.

The differential diagnosis of fatigue is extremely broad and best organized with an organ/system approach.

A. Psychiatric
  1. Depression
  2. Anxiety
  3. Somatization disorder
  4. Substance abuse

B. Sleep disorders
  1. Insomnia
  2. Obstructive sleep apnea (OSA)
  3. Periodic leg movements
  4. Narcolepsy

C. Endocrine
  1. Thyroid disease
  2. Diabetes mellitus
  3. Hypoadrenalism

D. Medications (Table 18-1)

E. Hematologic or oncologic
  1. Anemia
  2. Cancer

F. Renal: chronic kidney disease

G. Liver disease

H. Cardiovascular: chronic heart disease

I. Pulmonary: chronic lung disease

J. Neuromuscular: myositis, multiple sclerosis

K. Infectious: chronic infections

L. Rheumatologic: autoimmune diseases

M. Fatigue of unknown etiology
  1. Chronic fatigue syndrome
  2. Idiopathic chronic fatigue: fatigue for which no medical, psychiatric, or sleep pattern explanation can be found.

Figure 18-1 outlines the diagnostic approach to fatigue.

The most common causes of fatigue are psychiatric disorders, sleep disorders, and medication side effects.

1

Mrs. M reports that she is tired all the time, beginning first thing in the morning and lasting all day. She also reports frontal headaches several mornings per week, intermittent lower abdominal pain relieved by bowel movements, and low back pain. She does not complain of any trouble sleeping.

Her past medical history is notable for menorrhagia and iron deficiency anemia when she was in her 20s and is otherwise unremarkable. Currently, her menses occur every 30 days, with bleeding for 3–4 days. Her family history is notable for thyroid disease in her mother and breast cancer in her paternal grandmother.

She takes no medications, does not smoke, and does not drink alcohol. She has never used illicit drugs. She works as a teacher, and her husband is a security guard. They have 2 children, ages 9 and 12. She does not report any recent changes at home or work.

At this point, what is the leading hypothesis, what are the active alternatives, and is there a must not miss diagnosis? Given this differential diagnosis, what tests should be ordered?

Table 18-1. Medications that affect sleep.

Medications that cause insomnia	Antidepressants: Bupropion, venlafaxine, fluoxetine, sertraline
	Anticholinergics: Ipratropium
	CNS stimulants: Methylphenidate, modafinil
	Hormones: Oral contraceptives, thyroid hormone, corticosteroids, progesterone
	Sympathomimetic amines: Albuterol, theophylline, phenylpropanolamine, pseudoephedrine
	Antineoplastics: Leuprolide, goserelin, pentostatin, interferon alfa
	Miscellaneous: Phenytoin, nicotine, levodopa, quinidine, caffeine, alcohol
Medications that cause drowsiness	Tricyclic antidepressants: Amitriptyline, imipramine, nortriptyline
	Other antidepressants: Mirtazapine, trazodone, paroxetine
	Opioids
	Benzodiazepines
	Nonsteroidal antiinflammatory drugs
	Neuropathic pain agents: Gabapentin, pregabalin
	Alcohol
	Antihistamines: Diphenhydramine, hydroxyzine, meclizine
	Atypical antipsychotics

RANKING THE DIFFERENTIAL DIAGNOSIS

A specific causative medical disease (other than psychiatric disease and sleep disorders) that explains fatigue is found in less than 10% of patients who seek medical attention from their primary care physician. Up to 75% of patients with fatigue have psychiatric symptoms. Sleep disorders, especially OSA and insomnia syndromes, are also common in patients with fatigue, and in one referral clinic, 80% of patients with fatigue had sleep disorders. Because the differential diagnosis of fatigue is broad and difficult to limit during the initial assessment, it is necessary to explore for symptoms and signs of many possible etiologies in most patients, even those with pivotal psychiatric or sleep disorder symptoms. Patients with several somatic complaints, such as Mrs. M, are particularly likely to have psychiatric causes for fatigue, as are patients who feel tired constantly. Because sleep disorders are so common, either in association with psychiatric disorders or alone, they are always an active alternative in patients with fatigue. Patients often do not spontaneously describe sleep disturbances and psychiatric symptoms, so it is important to ask about them directly.

 All patients with fatigue need a detailed psychosocial and sleep history.

Although most patients with fatigue do *not* have anemia, hypothyroidism, or diabetes mellitus, these conditions are important and treatable, and so are generally considered "must not miss" diagnoses. Anemia and hypothyroidism are somewhat likely in Mrs. M because of her previous history of anemia and her family history of

thyroid disease. Finally, on occasion, fatigue may be the presenting symptom in patients with undiagnosed cardiac, pulmonary, renal, liver, rheumatologic, or chronic infectious disease. Table 18-2 lists the differential diagnosis.

 Despite the rarity of positive results, most patients with fatigue need basic laboratory testing consisting of a blood count, chemistry panel (including glucose, electrolytes, BUN, creatinine, calcium, and liver function tests), and a TSH.

Mrs. M does not lack interest in her usual activities or feel depressed. She has not lost or gained weight. She worries about money and her family but has never had a panic attack and does not consider herself excessively nervous or anxious.

On physical exam, she appears healthy and her affect is normal. Her BMI is 35. HEENT exam is normal. There is no thyromegaly or adenopathy. Lungs are clear. There are no breast masses. Cardiac and abdominal exams are normal, and there is no edema. Her CBC, glucose, electrolytes, BUN, creatinine, liver function tests, and TSH are all normal.

 Is the clinical information sufficient to make a diagnosis? If not, what other information do you need?

Leading Hypotheses: Depression & Anxiety

See Chapter 32, Unintentional Weight Loss.

Mrs. M does not meet DSM criteria for anxiety or depression. It is therefore necessary to consider the alternative diagnoses.

Mrs. M works as a teacher, rising at 6 AM, leaving her house at 7 AM, and returning home about 5 PM. She then prepares dinner for her family, helps her 2 children with their homework, and grades papers until 9:30 PM. She watches a little television, and then goes to sleep about 10:00 PM. Her husband works from 3 PM to 11 PM, and she often wakes up when he gets home at midnight. He needs some time to "wind down" before he goes to sleep, so they often talk and watch TV in bed for an hour or so. After her husband dozes off, she often cannot fall back asleep, and will sit in bed "surfing" the Internet on her laptop for an hour or two. She also comments that she feels tired even when she sleeps straight through the night on the weekends, and her husband complains about her snoring.

 Is the clinical information sufficient to make a diagnosis? If not, what other information do you need?

Mrs. M's sleep history clearly uncovers several sleep hygiene issues. However, she is also obese, a risk factor for OSA. Re-exploring her symptoms, it is notable that she has some morning headaches, feels fatigued even when she sleeps all night, and snores.

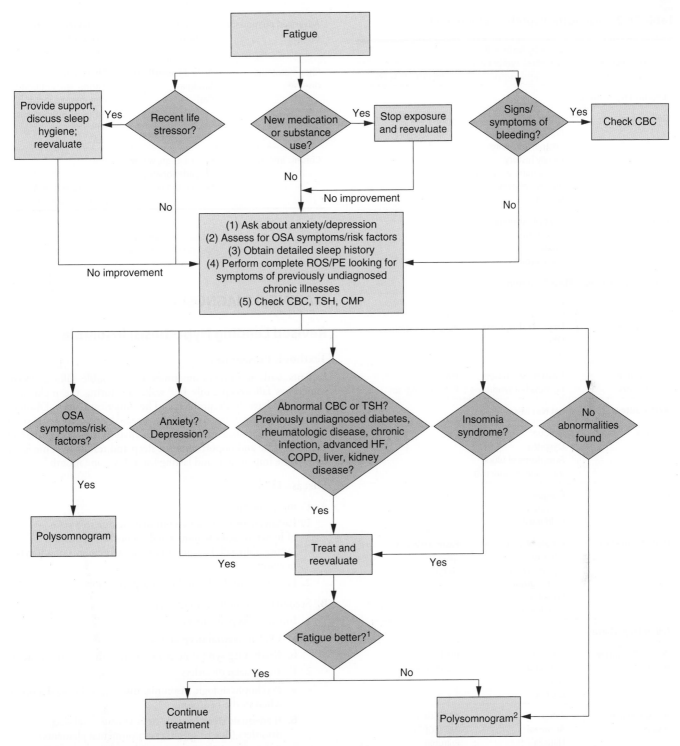

[1]Symptoms of depression and anxiety are common in patients with OSA. A polysomnogram should be considered even in patients who respond to treatment for depression or anxiety.
[2]Not all patients with OSA have identifiable risk factors. Additionally, periodic leg movement disorder is frequently not reported by patients and is detected during polysomnography. Therefore, all patients with persistent fatigue that does not respond to treatment should have a polysomnogram.

CBC, complete blood cell; CMP, complete metabolic profile; COPD, chronic obstructive pulmonary disease; HF, heart failure; OSA, obstructive sleep apnea; ROS/PE, review of systems/physical exam; TSH, thyroid-stimulating hormone.

Figure 18-1. Diagnostic approach: fatigue.

Table 18-2. Diagnostic hypotheses for Mrs. M.

Diagnostic Hypotheses	Demographics, Risk Factors, Symptoms and Signs	Important Tests
Leading Hypotheses		
Depression	History of loss Prior depression Postpartum state Family history > 6 somatic symptoms Positive depression screen	History
Anxiety	Multiple somatic symptoms Anxiety Panic attacks	History
Active Alternatives—Most Common		
Insomnia	Fatigue	History
Sleep apnea	Daytime sleepiness Obesity Hypertension	Polysomnogram
Periodic limb movements	Daytime sleepiness Restless leg syndrome	History Polysomnogram
Active Alternatives—Must Not Miss		
Anemia	Fatigue Dyspnea Symptoms of blood loss, pale conjunctiva	CBC
Hypothyroidism	Fatigue Constipation Cold intolerance	TSH
Diabetes mellitus	Family history Obesity Hypertension Ethnic group Polyuria Polydipsia	Fasting plasma glucose HgbA$_{1c}$
Other Hypotheses		
Advanced kidney disease	Fatigue Anorexia Nausea Edema	BUN Creatinine
Advanced liver disease	Fatigue Anorexia Nausea Edema History of alcohol abuse or chronic hepatitis	AST (SGOT) ALT (SGPT) Bilirubin Alkaline phosphatase
Advanced cardiac disease	Dyspnea Orthopnea Paroxysmal nocturnal dyspnea Edema Jugular venous distention, S$_3$ gallop	ECG Echocardiography Stress test
Advanced pulmonary disease	Dyspnea Cachexia	Pulmonary exam Pulmonary function tests
Rheumatologic disease	Arthralgias/arthritis Myalgias Rash	Chest radiograph Antinuclear antibody Rheumatoid factor Anti-CCP antibody ESR/CRP CBC
Chronic infection	Fever, cough, weight loss, adenopathy, heart murmur	HIV CBC Chest radiograph Echocardiography

ALT, alanine aminotransferase; AST, aspartate aminotransferase; BUN, blood urea nitrogen; anti-CCP, anti-cyclic citrullinated peptide; ESR/CRP, erythrocyte sedimentation rate/C-reactive protein; TSH, thyroid-stimulating hormone.

MAKING A DIAGNOSIS

Revised Leading Hypothesis: Insomnia

Textbook Presentation

Patients with insomnia sometimes have trouble falling asleep, sometimes fall asleep easily but wake up during the night, and sometimes have both problems. The American Sleep Disorder Association defines insomnia as "a repeated difficulty with sleep initiation, duration, consolidation, or quality that occurs despite adequate time and opportunity for sleep and results in some form of daytime impairment and lasting for at least one month."

Disease Highlights

A. Primary insomnia

1. Pathogenesis is unknown but may be due to a state of hyperarousal (demonstrated on positron emission tomography (PET) scans and by measurements of adrenal hormones).

2. Prevalence of 2–4% in the adult population

B. Secondary (comorbid) insomnia

1. Intrinsic sleep disorders

   a. OSA or central sleep apnea

   b. Restless leg syndrome/periodic limb movement disorder

2. Extrinsic sleep disorders

   a. Psychophysiologic insomnia: due to conditioned arousal when in the bedroom

   b. Inadequate sleep hygiene or environmental sleep disorders (due to specific environmental elements)

   c. Related to alcohol or other substance use (stimulants, withdrawal from hypnotic drugs)

3. Circadian rhythm sleep disorders

   a. Shift work disorder

   b. Delayed or advanced sleep phase syndrome (major sleep phase late or early compared to clock time)

   c. Time zone change syndrome (jet lag)

4. Related to medical conditions (chronic pain; nocturia; uncontrolled HF, chronic obstructive pulmonary disease/asthma, gastroesophageal reflux disease)

C. 35–50% of adults have insomnia symptoms; 12–20% have insomnia disorders

D. Risk factors for insomnia include depression, female sex, older age, lower socioeconomic status, concurrent medical and mental disorders, marital status (divorced/separated > married), race (African-American > white)

Evidence-Based Diagnosis

A. Obtaining a thorough history helps establish the diagnosis of insomnia. Ask about predisposing, precipitating and perpetuating factors. Initial screening questions include the following:

1. Difficulty initiating sleep, staying asleep, or both?

2. Early awakening?

3. Nonrestorative sleep?

4. Daytime consequences? (Lack of daytime fatigue or sleepiness suggests the insomnia is not clinically significant.)

5. Frequency and duration?

B. Follow-up questions

1. Precipitating events, progression, ameliorating or exacerbating factors?

2. Sleep-wake schedule?

3. Cognitive attitude toward sleep?

   a. Negative expectations regarding the ability to sleep and distortions about the effects of insomnia lead to perpetuation of the insomnia.

   b. Attitudes toward previous treatments are also important.

4. Psychiatric disorder present?

5. Substance misuse or medication use?

6. Medical illness with nocturnal symptoms?

7. Symptoms of sleep apnea, restless legs? (See discussion below.)

Treatment

A. Behavioral therapy

1. Stimulus control therapy

   a. Also known as sleep hygiene

   b. Based on premise that insomnia is a conditioned response to temporal and environmental cues

   c. Has been shown to be effective for sleep onset and maintenance

   d. Principles of sleep hygiene

      (1) Go to bed only when sleepy.

      (2) Use the bedroom only for sleep and sex, not reading, watching television, eating, working, or using a computer

      (3) If unable to sleep after 20 minutes in bed, get out of bed, go into another room, read or listen to quiet music, and then return to bed when sleepy.

      (4) Maintain a consistent sleep-wake schedule; go to bed and get up at the same time each day.

      (5) Avoid daytime napping; if napping is necessary, limit the nap to less than 30 minutes and take the nap no later than the early afternoon.

      (6) Avoid caffeine, alcohol, and other stimulants (such as decongestants).

      (7) Exercise regularly, but not in the late evening.

2. Relaxation therapy

   a. Methods include progressive muscle relaxation, biofeedback to reduce somatic arousal, imagery training, and meditation.

   b. Useful for both sleep onset and maintenance

   c. Often requires practice with a trained professional

3. Sleep restriction therapy

   a. Decreases the amount of time spent in bed in order to increase the percentage of time in bed spent sleeping

   b. Usually keep waking time constant and make bedtime later, with progressive moving up of bedtime as sleep improves

   c. Effective for sleep onset and maintenance

B. Cognitive therapy involves identifying dysfunctional beliefs about sleep and then substituting more functional attitudes that can reduce anxiety.

C. Combination therapy: combining cognitive and behavioral therapy has been shown to be superior to relaxation therapy alone.

D. Pharmacotherapy

1. Most studies of pharmacologic agents are short (12 days to 6 months), so data about long-term effects are lacking.

2. Basic principles for using pharmacotherapy to treat chronic insomnia

   a. Use agents with shorter half-lives to minimize daytime sedation.

   b. Use the lowest effective dose.

   c. Try to dose intermittently, such as 2–4 times per week, rather than daily.

   d. Try to limit daily use to a maximum of 3–4 weeks.

   e. Discontinue medication gradually.

   f. Monitor for rebound insomnia when medications are stopped.

   g. Side effects, including delirium, are more likely to occur in elderly patients.

   h. Commonly used sleep aids are summarized in Table 18-3.

E. Pharmacologic therapy versus cognitive behavioral therapy

1. Data comparing pharmacotherapy with behavioral and cognitive therapy are limited.

   a. Overall, treatment effects are similar.

   b. Perhaps more rapid improvement with pharmacotherapy

   c. Perhaps more sustained improvement with behavioral therapy

2. Studies of combined cognitive behavioral and pharmacologic therapy versus cognitive behavioral therapy alone show that the cognitive behavioral therapy alone group maintained results at 10–24 months, but the combined group did not.

Alternative Diagnosis: Obstructive Sleep Apnea

Textbook Presentation

Patients with OSA often complain of daytime sleepiness or fatigue. Bed partners often note snoring or actual apneic episodes. Most patients are obese.

Disease Highlights

A. Characterized by repetitive episodes of complete or partial upper airway obstruction during sleep

1. An obstructive **apnea** is at least 10 seconds of cessation of ventilation accompanied by respiratory efforts.

Table 18-3. Medications used to treat insomnia.

Medication	Dose Range (mg)	Half-life of Drug and Active Metabolites (hrs)	Benefits	Side Effects
Benzodiazepines				
Triazolam[1]	0.125–0.25	2–5	Faster sleep initiation; better sleep maintenance	Daytime sedation, amnesia, falls, rebound insomnia
Temazepam[1]	7.5–30	8–15		
Estazolam[1]	0.5–2	10–24		
Lorazepam	0.5–4	8–24		
Clonazepam	0.5–2	19–60		
Benzodiazepine receptor agonists (BZRAs)				
Zaleplon[1]	5–20	1	Faster sleep initiation; better sleep maintenance	Daytime sedation, amnesia, falls, rebound insomnia; all generally less than with benzodiazepines
Zolpidem[1]	5–10	3		
Eszopiclone[1]	1–3	5–7		
Antidepressants				
Tricyclics	25–50	8–24	Faster sleep initiation; better sleep maintenance	Sedation, amnesia, rebound insomnia, anticholinergic effects, falls
Trazodone	25–100	5–9	Faster sleep initiation; better sleep maintenance	Priapism, syncope
Antihistamines				
Diphenhydramine	25–50	2.4–9.3	Faster sleep initiation; better sleep maintenance	Anticholinergic effects, dizziness, sedation

[1]Approved by the US Food and Drug Administration for treatment of insomnia.

2. A **hypopnea** is at least a 30% reduction in air flow for 10 seconds or longer with at least a 4% reduction in oxygen saturation.

3. A **respiratory effort related arousal (RERA)** is an occurrence of disordered breathing that does not meet criteria for apnea or hypopnea but does cause arousal.

4. The apnea-hypopnea index (AHI) is the total number of apneas plus hypopneas per hour; the respiratory disturbance index (RDI) includes apneas, hypopneas, and RERAs.

   a. OSA is defined as an AHI or RDI ≥ 5 with daytime somnolence, or an AHI or RDI ≥ 15 regardless of symptoms.

   b. Mild OSA is an AHI or RDI of 5–14; moderate is an AHI or RDI of 15–30, and severe is an AHI or RDI > 30.

B. Prevalence of OSA

1. When OSA is defined as an AHI ≥ 5, the prevalence in the community ranges from 9% to 17%, with higher rates in men.

2. Using a threshold of ≥ 15, the prevalence is 6%.

3. The prevalence is 50% in referral populations.

C. Pathophysiology

1. There are normal decreases in tonic pharyngeal muscle tone and compensatory reflex dilators during sleep.

2. Patients with OSA have smaller upper airways due to increased parapharyngeal fat, tongue prominence, elongated palate, or thickened lateral pharyngeal walls, and are unable to maintain airway stability.

3. During inspiration, the negative upper airway pressures close these narrowed airways, resulting in apneas or hypopneas.

D. Risk factors

1. Obesity

   a. The strongest risk factor for OSA

   b. There is a 6-fold increase in the risk of OSA with a 10% weight gain.

   c. Neck circumference, a measurement of upper body obesity, is a predictor of OSA.

2. Gender: OSA is 2–3 times more common in men than women.

3. Menopausal status: 4-fold increase in risk in postmenopausal compare to premenopausal women

4. Craniofacial morphology, especially mandibular length, may explain presence of OSA in otherwise low-risk patients.

E. Consequences of OSA

1. Increased rate of motor vehicle accidents (relative risk = 2.5–5)

2. Hypertension (relative risk = 2.89)

3. HF (relative risk = 2.38)

4. Higher rates of mortality and adverse cardiac events in patients with coronary artery disease and untreated OSA.

5. An association with impaired glucose tolerance has been observed.

6. Long-standing, severe OSA can lead to cor pulmonale.

Evidence-Based Diagnosis

A. History and physical exam

1. Excessive daytime sleepiness is reported by about 35–40% of patients with OSA and by about 18% of patients without sleep disordered breathing

2. Lack of energy, tiredness, or fatigue is reported by about 50% of patients with OSA.

3. Depressive symptoms occur in up to 50% of OSA patients.

4. Cognitive impairment, especially in motor coordination, executive function, and some memory functions, can occur.

5. Individual clinical symptoms are not very useful in identifying patients with OSA.

   a. Nocturnal choking/gasping has the best LR+ (3.3), with morning headache having an LR+ of 2.6.

   b. The symptoms reported apnea, excessive daytime sleepiness, and snoring all have LR+ of < 1.5.

   c. The absence of snoring has an LR– ranging from 0.2 to 0.45; all other individual symptoms have an LR– near 1.

6. Several clinical decision rules have been developed to identify patients at high risk for OSA, but none is recommended for widespread use due to suboptimal or inconsistent test characteristics.

   a. The Berlin, STOP-Bang, and Snoring Severity Scale are somewhat useful in reducing the likelihood a patient has OSA; none of them significantly increases the likelihood a patient has OSA.

   b. Berlin Questionnaire (10 questions about snoring, observed apneas, sleepiness, BP, body mass index [BMI])

     (1) For AHI > 5: LR+, 1.4; LR–, 0.43

     (2) For AHI > 15: LR+, 1.5; LR–, 0.28

   c. STOP-Bang (snoring, tiredness, observed apnea, BP, BMI, age, neck circumference, gender)

     (1) For AHI > 5: LR+, 1.8; LR–, 0.23

     (2) For AHI > 15: LR+, 1.4; LR–, 0.20

   d. Snoring Severity Scale (0–3 points each to frequency of nights with snoring, duration of snoring, and loudness of snoring)

     (1) In patients with a BMI > 26 and a positive score, defined as ≥ 4

     (2) LR+, ; LR–, 0.07

B. Polysomnography

1. Records electroencephalogram, electromyelogram, ECG, heart rate, respiratory effort, airflow, and oxygen saturation during sleep

2. Gold standard for diagnosis of OSA

3. One study found sensitivity of 66% for the first night study in patients who underwent 2 consecutive night studies; the sensitivity increased by 25% after the second night.

4. The more severe the OSA, the less variability in the night-to-night polysomnogram results.

Treatment

A. Risk factor modification

1. Weight loss, smoking cessation, avoiding alcohol or hypnotics before bedtime

2. A 10% weight loss leads to a 25–30% reduction in the AHI.

B. Nasal therapies (external dilator strips, internal nasal dilators, lubricants): limited data, generally not sufficient treatment

C. Continuous positive airway pressure (CPAP)

1. Pneumatically splints the upper airway throughout the respiratory cycle

2. The pressure must be determined during polysomnography (a "CPAP titration") and is set to eliminate, or at least reduce, apneas and hypopneas.

3. CPAP has been shown to reduce symptoms of sleepiness/fatigue and slightly lower BP; observational studies suggest better cardiovascular outcomes in treated patients compared to untreated patients. There is minimal evidence of benefit in patients without daytime sleepiness.

D. Oral appliances

1. Designed to advance the mandible, pulling the tongue forward and opening the pharyngeal airway

2. Less effective than CPAP

3. Indicated in patients with mild to moderate OSA who prefer an oral appliance or do not respond to positive airway pressure therapy

E. Surgery

1. Considered second-line therapy unless there are specific, correctible anatomic abnormalities

2. Data on outcomes limited; maxillary and mandibular advancement procedures can result in improvement similar to that seen with CPAP.

3. Tracheostomy is reserved for patients with life-threatening disease who do not respond to other treatments.

CASE RESOLUTION

1

Mrs. M is reassured that her laboratory tests are normal. A polysomnogram shows an AHI of 2 when she sleeps on her side, and an AHI of 15 when she is on her back. After listening to you explain the principles of sleep hygiene, she decides to talk with her husband about ways they could spend time together without interrupting her sleep so often. Since she has an elevated AHI only when she is supine, you recommend that she wear a backpack or use special pillows to help her stay on her side during sleep.

When she returns 6 months later, she reports that she is still tired because she values the time she spends with her husband at night. However, she now asks him to sleep in the guest room when she feels exceptionally fatigued, so she can have a few nights of uninterrupted sleep. She is successfully using a body pillow to stay on her side at night. She has also found that a 15-minute nap at lunchtime helps.

REVIEW OF OTHER IMPORTANT DISEASES

Periodic Limb Movement Disorder (PLMD)

Textbook Presentation

The patient complains of daytime sleepiness or fatigue, and the bed partner complains that the patient is very restless, even kicking the bed partner.

Disease Highlights

A. Periodic episodes of repetitive and stereotyped limb movements occurring during non-REM sleep, generally consisting of big toe extension in combination with partial flexion of the ankle, knee, and hip.

B. The movements recur at regular intervals of 20–40 seconds and cause arousal, although the patient is usually unaware.

C. Rare in persons younger than 30 years; found in 5% of persons aged 30–50, 33% in persons aged 50–65, and in 44% of persons older than 65 years.

D. Primary cause of insomnia in 17% of patients

E. Can be unmasked after successful treatment of OSA

F. Accompanied by restless leg syndrome (RLS) in 25% of patients

   1. Diagnostic criteria for RLS

      a. The urge to move the legs, accompanied by uncomfortable or unpleasant sensations, often described as "creeping" or "crawling"

      b. Worsening of symptoms when inactive

      c. Partial symptom relief with movement

      d. Presence of symptoms only in the evening or at night, or worsening of daytime symptoms in the evening

   2. Found in 2–15% of the general population, and 10–35% of patients over 65

   3. Accompanied by PLMD in 85% of cases

   4. Can be primary or secondary to iron deficiency anemia, chronic kidney disease, or peripheral neuropathy; possibly related to celiac disease; all patients with PLMD should have iron studies done

Evidence-Based Diagnosis

A. PLMD is confirmed by polysomnography

B. RLS is a clinical diagnosis

Treatment of PLMD

Effective medications include dopamine agonists (pramipexole or ropinirole) and anti-epileptics (such as gabapentin, pregabalin, or carbamazepine).

Hypothyroidism

Textbook Presentation

Patients with hypothyroidism commonly complain of fatigue, constipation, or cold intolerance.

Disease Highlights

This discussion focuses on primary hypothyroidism in nonpregnant adults.

A. Epidemiology

   1. Prevalence of overt hypothyroidism (elevated TSH with low free T4) is 0.1% in men and 1–2% in women (see below for a discussion of subclinical hypothyroidism)

   2. Prevalence increases with age

   3. 10 times more common in women than men

B. Etiology

   1. Primary hypothyroidism: failure of the thyroid gland to produce adequate thyroid hormone

      a. Most common cause in iodine sufficient areas is chronic autoimmune (Hashimoto) thyroiditis

         (1) Both cell-mediated and antibody-mediated destruction of the thyroid gland

         (2) Autoantibodies against thyroid peroxidase, thyroglobulin, and TSH receptor

         (3) Patients may or may not have a goiter on presentation

      b. Iodine deficiency is a common cause worldwide; patients have large goiters

      c. Thyroidectomy or radioactive iodine therapy both cause hypothyroidism

         (1) Patients with partial thyroidectomy may not need replacement but should be monitored annually.

         (2) Postablative hypothyroidism develops several weeks after the radioactive iodine therapy.

      d. Can develop years later in patients who have undergone external neck radiation

      e. Amiodarone and lithium commonly cause hypothyroidism

      f. Less common etiologies include infiltrative diseases, such as sarcoidosis, and thyroid agenesis

   2. Central hypothyroidism: reduction in TSH due to pituitary or hypothalamic disorder

      a. Pituitary adenoma is the most common cause; also can occur post neurosurgery or brain radiation or as a complication of postpartum hemorrhage

      b. Granulomatous diseases, especially sarcoidosis, can infiltrate the hypothalamus.

C. Clinical manifestations

   1. Metabolic: Decreased metabolism that can lead to weight gain, cold intolerance, and increased total and LDL cholesterol (due to decreased clearance)

   2. Cardiac: Reduction in myocardial contractility and heart rate

   3. Skin: Nonpitting edema, due to accumulation of glycosaminoglycans; dry skin; coarse, brittle hair

   4. CNS: fatigue, delayed relaxation phase of the deep tendon reflexes

   5. Pulmonary: hypoventilation seen with severe hypothyroidism

   6. GI: reduced intestinal motility causing constipation

   7. Reproductive: menstrual abnormals, reduced fertility, increased risk of miscarriage.

Evidence-Based Diagnosis

A. The signs and symptoms of hypothyroidism all lack sensitivity and specificity.

B. The TSH is the best screening test both primary hypothyroidism and hyperthyroidism; it is necessary to measure thyroid hormone levels initially un central hypothyroidism is suspected.

C. If the TSH is normal, no further ng is necessary (LR− for hypothyroidism is < 0.01)

D. If the TSH is elevated (LR+ for hypothyroidism is > 99), the free T_4 should be ordered next.

   1. Most of T_4 is bound to thyroxine-binding globulin and albumin.

   2. The levels of these binding proteins are affected by a variety of medical conditions, thus altering the level of total T_4.

   3. Free T_4 better reflects the patient's thyroid function than total T_4.

 To assess thyroid function, order a TSH followed by a measurement of free T_4; do not order a total T_4 (TT_4). It is not necessary to order a T_3 when evaluating patients for hypothyroidism.

E. If the TSH is elevated, and the free T_4 is decreased, the patient has overt hypothyroidism and should be treated.

F. If the TSH is elevated and the free T_4 is normal, the patient may have subclinical hypothyroidism.

   1. The TSH and free T_4 should be repeated to confirm the diagnosis.

   2. The most common cause is chronic autoimmune (Hashimoto) thyroiditis.

   3. The overall prevalence is 4–8% but is up to 20% in women over 60.

   4. The progression rate to overt hypothyroidism is 4–18%/year; patients with higher levels of TSH and positive thyroid antibodies are more likely to progress.

   5. A recent study found an increased risk of coronary heart disease events (relative risk 1.89) and coronary heart disease mortality (relative risk 1.58) in patients with subclinical hypothyroidism and a TSH ≥ 10; whether treatment lowers this risk is not known.

   6. Other causes of an elevated TSH with a normal T_4 include recovery from non-thyroidal illness and the recovery phase of subacute thyroiditis.

Treatment

A. Overt hypothyroidism

   1. All patients should be treated with levothyroxine (T_4).

   2. The full replacement dose is 1.6 mcg/kg/day, but in older patients or those with underlying coronary disease, it is preferable to start with a lower of dose of 25–50 mcg/day.

   3. Levothyroxine is best absorbed on an empty stomach, with a 40% reduction in absorption if taken with food; calcium, iron, antacids, proton pump inhibitors, and anticonvulsants also interfere with absorption.

   4. The half-life of levothyroxine is 7 days, so steady state concentration is reached in about 6 weeks.

   5. The TSH level should be checked 6 weeks after every dose adjustment, with the goal of increasing the dose until the TSH is within the normal range.

   6. Once the dose is stable, it is sufficient to check the TSH annually.

B. Subclinical hypothyroidism

   1. Experts agree that patients with a TSH > 10 mcU/mL should be treated; many experts would also treat patients with TSH levels of 5–10, and elevated LDL, symptoms, or positive thyroid antibodies.

   2. Patients may report improved symptoms with treatment; effects on LDL and cardiovascular outcomes are inconclusive.

REFERENCES

Buysse DJ. Insomnia. JAMA. 2013;309:706–16.

Doghramji K. The evaluation and management of insomnia. Clin Chest Med. 2010;31:327–39.

Falloon K, Arroll B, Elley CR, Fernando A 3rd. The assessment and management of insomnia in primary care. BMJ. 2011;342:d2899.

McDermott MT. In the Clinic. Hypothyroidism. Ann Intern Med. 2009;151:ITC61.

Lurie A. Obstructive sleep apnea in adults: epidemiology, clinical presentation, and treatment options. Adv Cardiol. 2011;46:1–42.

Myers KA, Mrkobrada M, Simel DL. Does this patient have obstructive sleep apnea? JAMA. 2013;310:731–41.

Neubauer DN. Insomnia. Prim Care. 2005;32:375–88.

Ramachandran SK, Josephs LA. A meta-analysis of clinical screening tests for obstructive sleep apnea. Anesthesiology. 2009;110:928–39.

Rondondi N, den Elzen WP, Bauer DC et al. Subclinical hypothyroidism and the risk of coronary heart disease and mortality. JAMA. 2010;304:1365–74.

Sateia MJ, Nowell PD. Insomnia. Lancet. 2004;364:1959–73.

Silber MH. Chronic insomnia. N Engl J Med. 2005;353:803–10.

Wilson JF. In the Clinic. Insomnia. Ann Intern Med. 2008;148: ITC13-1–ITC13–16.

I have a patient with GI bleeding.
How do I determine the cause?

CHIEF COMPLAINT

PATIENT 1

Mr. T is a 66-year-old man who arrives at the emergency department with bloody stools and dizziness. His symptoms started 2 hours ago.

What is the differential diagnosis of GI bleeding? How would you frame the differential?

CONSTRUCTING A DIFFERENTIAL DIAGNOSIS

The approach to GI bleeding is similar to the approach to other potentially life-threatening illnesses. Patient stabilization, specifically, hemodynamic stabilization is the first step in management. In a patient with GI bleeding, management precedes diagnosis, usually made by colonoscopy or esophagogastroduodenoscopy (EGD).

Initial management follows a regimented course. The patient must be hemodynamically stabilized, preparation must be made in case of further bleeding, and initial diagnostic tests must be completed.

A. Hemodynamic stabilization
   1. Clinically assess volume status.
      a. Signs of shock may be seen with 30–40% volume depletion.
      b. Orthostasis can be seen with 20–25% volume depletion.
      c. Tachycardia may be present with 15% volume depletion.
   2. Calculate necessary replacement (weight in kg × 0.6 (lean body weight made up of water) × % volume depletion).
   3. Replace fluid losses initially with normal saline or Ringer solution.
   4. Consider the need for blood transfusion.
      a. In patients who are not bleeding, withholding transfusions until the hemoglobin reaches 7–8 g/dL is a conservative approach supported by recent data.
      b. There has, until recently been general agreement on the following recommendations for transfusion in actively bleeding patients.
         (1) Patients should receive a blood transfusion when there has been 30% loss of blood volume (manifested by tachycardia, hypotension, tachypnea, decreased urinary output, or CNS symptoms [eg, anxiety/confusion]).

(2) Alternatively, if 2 L of crystalloid have been given without successful resuscitation, blood should be transfused.
         (3) If a hemoglobin level is available, actively bleeding patients should receive a transfusion when the level falls below 10 g/dL.
         (4) If large amounts of blood are needed (> 4 units of packed red blood cells), fresh frozen plasma and platelets should also be given.
      c. A recent randomized trial of patients with upper GI bleeding compared a restrictive strategy of transfusion (threshold for transfusion of hemoglobin < 7 g/dL) with a liberal strategy (threshold of hemoglobin < 9 g/dL).
         (1) This study demonstrated a mortality benefit with the restrictive strategy.
         (2) Exclusion criteria in this study were massive exsanguinating bleeding, an acute coronary syndrome, symptomatic peripheral vasculopathy, stroke, or transient ischemic attack.
         (3) All patients had endoscopy within 6 hours of presentation.
         (4) Patients in this study also received blood if symptoms of anemia or massive bleeding developed or if they required surgery.
      d. It is important to remember that patients may initially have a normal hemoglobin level when they present with an acute hemorrhage. It will only fall after fluid resuscitation.

Even after a large hemorrhage, patients may initially have a normal hemoglobin level. The level will only fall after fluid resuscitation.

B. Preparation for further bleeding
   1. All patients should have their blood typed and be cross-matched for at least 2 units of packed red blood cells.
   2. Two large bore IVs
      a. IVs should be 16 gauge or greater.
      b. Flow = ΔP ($\pi r^4/8\mu L$) where ΔP is the pressure differential, r is the radius of the IV, μ is the viscosity of the fluid, and L is the length of the IV.
      c. Flow can therefore be maximized by
         (1) Increasing the pressure behind the fluid being infused (squeezing the bag).
         (2) Decreasing the length of the IV.

(3) Increasing the gauge of the IV (the most effective as the flow goes up by the fourth power of any increase).

d. Large gauge IVs (16 and larger) are much more effective than central lines for volume resuscitation.

 Always make sure your patient has 2 usable large bore IVs, so you do not have to worry about IV access should life-threatening bleeding develop.

e. In the setting of severe hemorrhage, a urinary catheter, with regular monitoring of urinary output, helps monitor the adequacy of volume resuscitation.

C. Initial diagnostic tests

1. CBC and platelet count

2. Basic metabolic panel (chem-7)

3. Liver function tests (LFTs) (Abnormal LFTs raise the risk of underlying severe liver disease and thus coagulopathy and varices.)

4. Prothrombin time and partial thromboplastin time

5. Upright chest radiograph

a. Most important if there is abdominal tenderness to assess for free air in the abdomen arising from a perforated viscus

b. Patients taking immunosuppressants (including corticosteroids) may have free air in the abdomen with only mild abdominal symptoms.

c. Radiographs may, infrequently, provide other diagnostic clues.

6. Nasogastric (NG) tube placement, which was once considered standard, is now more controversial.

a. An NG tube is a minimally invasive way to assess the acuity of bleeding and to help localize its source.

b. Blood or coffee grounds in an NG aspirate is indicative of an upper GI bleed (LR+, 9.6).

c. On the other hand, a negative lavage does not exclude an upper GI source.

d. A recent study strongly suggested that NG tube placement does not change patient outcomes (mortality, length of stay, volume of transfused blood, need for surgery).

The differential diagnosis of GI bleeding is based on an anatomic framework. Upper GI bleeds originate proximal to the ligament of Treitz, while lower GI bleeds originate from areas distal to the ligament and are primarily colonic. The pivotal points in a patient's evaluation are therefore characteristics that argue for an upper or lower GI source. Among others, these include history of previous upper or lower bleeding episodes, epigastric pain, melena, and blood in an NG lavage, all of which suggest an UGI bleed. The causes of upper and lower GI bleeding are arranged below in the approximate order of frequency. Bleeding from a small bowel source is less common. The last category is anorectal bleeding. These are generally smaller bleeds with limited potential to cause hemodynamic instability.

A. Upper GI bleeds

1. Common

a. Peptic ulcer disease

b. Esophageal or gastric varices

c. Mallory-Weiss tear

2. Less common

a. Angiodysplasia

b. Gastritis

c. Malignancy

d. Esophagitis

e. Dieulafoy lesion

B. Lower GI bleeds

1. Common

a. Diverticulosis

b. Malignancy or polyp

c. Colitis

(1) Inflammatory

(2) Infectious

(3) Ischemic

d. Angiodysplasia

2. Less common small bowel sources

a. Angiodysplasia

b. Ulcers

c. Malignancy

d. Crohn disease

e. Meckel diverticulum

C. Anorectal bleeding

1. Hemorrhoids

2. Anal fissures

 Mr. T was well until this morning. Abdominal cramping developed while he was eating breakfast. He did not have nausea. He went to the bathroom and passed a large bowel movement of stool mixed with blood. Afterward, he felt better and went to lie down. About 30 minutes later, he had the same sensation and this time passed what he described as "about a pint" of bright red blood. While getting up from the toilet, he became dizzy and had to sit on the bathroom floor for 15 minutes before he could crawl to the phone to dial 911.

 At this point, what is the leading hypothesis, what are the active alternatives, and is there a must not miss diagnosis? Given this differential diagnosis, what tests should be ordered?

RANKING THE DIFFERENTIAL DIAGNOSIS

The lack of nausea, vomiting, or abdominal pain, and the presence of bright red blood per rectum are pivotal points in this case and make a lower GI source most likely. Cramping is often seen with GI bleeds, caused by blood passing through the bowel. The acuity and volume of blood makes bleeding from diverticuli, colitis, malignancy, or angiodysplasia the most likely diagnoses. Whether he has had a recent change in bowel habits, weight loss, or previous bloody stools are unknown; all these factors would heighten suspicion for colitis or malignancy. The amount of blood loss makes hemorrhoids or fissures unlikely. Upper sources of bleeding must also be considered. A brisk bleed from an upper source can present with bright red blood per rectum. Assuming there is no history of liver disease, peptic ulcer disease would be the most likely upper source. Table 19-1 lists the differential diagnosis.

Table 19-1. Diagnostic hypotheses for Mr. T.

Diagnostic Hypotheses	Demographics, Risk Factors, Symptoms and Signs	Important Tests
Leading Hypothesis		
Diverticular bleed	Brisk self-limited bleeds History of diverticuli	Colonoscopy
Active Alternative		
Angiodysplasia	Diverse presentations but brisk lower GI bleeds are common More common with end-stage renal disease	Colonoscopy or small bowel endoscopy
Other Alternative		
Peptic ulcer disease	Often asymptomatic May present with epigastric pain or weight loss History of NSAID use (including ASA)	Esophagogastroduodenoscopy
Active Alternative—Must Not Miss		
Colon cancer	History of anemia or changing bowel habits	Colonoscopy

ASA, aspirin; NSAID, nonsteroidal antiinflammatory drug.

 Blood is a cathartic. A brisk bleed from an upper source can present with bright red blood per rectum.

 Mr. T reports no recent illness or change in bowel habits. He reports no family history of colon cancer, and he has never had a colonoscopy. He has a fifty-pack year smoking history and quit about 6 years ago. He reports drinking 2–4 beers each night.

On physical exam, Mr. T looks anxious but is otherwise well. While sitting, his BP is 120/92 mm Hg and his pulse is 100 bpm. While standing, his BP is 100/80 mm Hg and his pulse is 122 bpm. His temperature is 37.0°C and his RR is 16 breaths per minute. There is no conjunctival pallor. Lungs and heart exams are normal. There are hyperactive bowel sounds but the abdomen is soft, nontender, and with no organomegaly. Rectal exam reveals bright red blood.

 Is the clinical information sufficient to make a diagnosis? If not, what other information do you need?

Leading Hypothesis: Diverticular Bleed

Textbook Presentation

The typical presentation is an episode of bright red blood per rectum in an older patient. There may be abdominal cramping but no real pain. A history of previously diagnosed diverticuli (on a screening colonoscopy, for instance) and possibly a previous, self-limited hemorrhage may be present.

Disease Highlights

A. Most common cause of lower GI bleeding

1. The prevalence of the various causes of GI bleeding varies from study to study.

2. One large review gave the following data:

   a. Diverticulosis: 35%

   b. Inflammatory bowel disease (IBD) or other colitis: 14%

   c. Colonic malignancy or polyp: 7%

   d. Angiodysplasia: 3%

   e. Anorectal cause: 12%

B. The risk of diverticular hemorrhage in a patient with diverticuli is not known but is estimated to be 3–15%.

C. Data from case control studies suggest that nonsteroidal antiinflammatory drug (NSAID) use and hypertension are risk factors for diverticular hemorrhage.

D. Although diverticuli are most commonly left sided, right-sided lesions are responsible for the majority of bleeding episodes.

E. Bleeding occurs as a vessel is stretched over the dome of a diverticulum. Luminal trauma likely leads to bleeding from the weakened vessel.

F. Spontaneous cessation and only moderate blood loss is the rule, but recurrence is common.

1. ≈ 75% of patients experience spontaneous cessation of hemorrhage.

2. Nearly all patients require < 4 units of packed red blood cells.

3. ≈ 40% of patients have recurrent bleeding.

G. Diverticular hemorrhage carries a poor short-term prognosis.

1. In general, lower GI bleeding carries a better overall prognosis than upper GI bleeding with about half the mortality rate.

2. Mortality rates for diverticular hemorrhage are higher (11% at 1 year and 20% at 4 years) although the cause of death is rarely related to the GI hemorrhage.

 Although diverticular hemorrhage seldom causes death, it is a marker for a relatively poor, short-term prognosis.

Evidence-Based Diagnosis

The first step in making the diagnosis of any GI bleed is to determine whether the source of the bleeding is the upper or lower tract.

A. History and physical exam

1. Certain historical features may point to a specific diagnosis (Table 19-2).

   a. These features should be sought in every patient with GI bleeding.

   b. They are, however, only suggestive and by no means diagnostic.

Table 19-2. Historical features in the diagnosis of GI bleeding.

Historical Feature	Suggested Diagnosis
NSAID use	Peptic ulcer disease
Severe vascular disease	Ischemic colitis
Pelvic radiation	Radiation colitis
Febrile illness	Infectious colitis
Aortic graft	Aortoenteric fistula (duodenal most common)
Liver disease or alcohol history	Esophageal varices
Retching preceding hematemesis	Mallory-Weiss tear
Recent colonic polypectomy	Post polypectomy bleeding
Severe constipation	Stercoral ulcer

NSAID, nonsteroidal antiinflammatory drug.

2. Other than frank hematemesis, only a few features are strongly predictive in localizing the site of bleeding to the upper or lower tract. These are outlined in Table 19-3.

   a. Patients who are volume depleted, orthostatic, or hypotensive are about twice as likely to have an upper GI bleed than a lower GI bleed.

   b. A BUN/creatinine ratio > 30 suggests an upper GI source (sensitivity, 39%; specificity, 94%; LR+ = 6.5, LR− = 0.64)

Table 19-3. Test characteristics of clinical findings for upper vs lower GI bleeding.

Clinical Finding	Sensitivity	Specificity	LR+	LR−
Upper GI Bleeds				
Melenic stools on exam	49%	98%	25	0.52
Blood or coffee grounds in an NG aspirate	44%	95%	9.6	0.58
Prior history of upper GI bleed	22%	96%	6.2	0.81
History of black stool	77–95%	81–87%	5.1–5.9	0.06–0.27
Age < 50	27%	92%	3.5	0.80
Cirrhosis	5%	99%	3.1	0.93
Lower GI Bleeds				
Presence of blood clots in stool	14%	99%	14	0.87
History of lower GI bleed	36%	94%	6	0.68
Physician seeing bright red blood	46%	90%	4.6	0.6

c. Although hematochezia generally suggests a lower GI source of bleeding, 10–15% of patients with hematochezia have an upper GI source. These patients are more likely to be older and to have duodenal ulcers.

 10–15% of patients with hematochezia have an upper GI source of bleeding.

B. Endoscopy

1. In a patient with GI bleeding, EGD is usually recommended as the first procedure unless the suspicion for a lower GI bleed is very high (based on history and a negative NG tube aspirate). This recommendation is based partly on the higher potential for severe blood loss from upper GI bleeds.

2. Colonoscopy

   a. The diagnosis of diverticular hemorrhage is usually made on colonoscopy.

   b. It is important to realize that this diagnosis is usually presumptive (87% of the time in some studies) based on seeing diverticuli and blood in the same region of the colon.

   c. Less commonly, a definitive diagnosis is made when active bleeding or stigmata of recent bleeding in a diverticulum is seen.

C. Radionuclide scintigraphy

1. Uses either radio labeled sulfur colloid or labeled red blood cells.

2. Can detect bleeds as slow as 0.05 mL/min.

3. Utility

   a. Most commonly used for detecting the source of bleeding in patients with persistent bleeding and normal upper and lower endoscopies.

   b. Also used to localize bleeding prior to resection or angiography.

4. The test characteristics are not well defined, varying from study to study.

   a. In a representative study, only 39% of patients had positive scans (sensitivity = 39%).

   b. In this study of patients who had further evaluation of their bleeding, 48% were found to have bleeding at the sight of the positive scan and 10% were found to have bleeding at a different site.

   c. Scans in patients who recently required transfusion are most likely to be positive; scans that turn positive quickly are best at localizing bleeding (≈ 95% accurate).

D. Angiography

1. Requires bleeding at a rate of about 0.5 mL/min to detect active bleeding.

2. Sensitivity is about 50% (though that number depends greatly on selection of patients).

3. Like radionuclide scintigraphy, angiography can be useful for localizing the site of bleeding before surgery and is considered far more reliable.

4. Also has therapeutic potential.

Treatment

A. Management of blood loss

1. As discussed above, all GI bleeds call for similar treatment of a patient who has lost, or has the potential to lose, a significant amount of blood.

2. Patients need to be closely monitored for signs of bleeding (increasing tachycardia, orthostasis, oliguria, declining Hgb).

3. Typically, patients have a CBC checked every 6 hours until stability has been achieved but the intensity of monitoring varies with risk of rebleeding.

B. Management of diverticular hemorrhage

1. Because most diverticular hemorrhages stop spontaneously, specific treatment is often not necessary.

2. Endoscopic treatment is primarily clipping, although thermocoagulation and sclerotherapy are occasionally used.

3. Angiographic intervention, with vasoconstrictor agents or embolization, can also be used. Occasionally, local vasopressin infusion may be a temporizing measure.

C. Colectomy

1. Curative therapy for diverticular bleeding is removal of the portion of the colon containing the diverticuli.

2. Recommended for either persistent, large bleeds (over 4 units in 24 hours or 10 units during the course of a single bleed) or for frequent recurrences.

The diagnosis of diverticular hemorrhage is often presumptive. Localization of the bleeding site before surgery must be as definitive as possible.

MAKING A DIAGNOSIS

Mr. T was given 1 L of normal saline. While in the emergency department, he again passed a large amount of bright red blood.

Initial laboratory tests are normal. Important values are BUN, 12 mg/dL; creatinine, 1.1 mg/dL; Hgb, 13.9 g/dL. NG tube lavage did not reveal any blood. The patient was admitted to the medical ICU.

Have you crossed a diagnostic threshold for the leading hypothesis, diverticular bleed? Have you ruled out the active alternatives? Do other tests need to be done to exclude the alternative diagnoses?

Mr. T weighs 75 kg and his orthostasis suggests 20% volume depletion. His fluid deficit is about 9 L (75 kg × 20% volume depletion × 60%). Assuming this deficit is all from the GI bleed, it is very likely that his Hgb will fall once he is hydrated.

His hematochezia, normal BUN/creatinine ratio, and clear NG tube lavage are suggestive of a lower GI bleed. The patient was admitted to an ICU bed because, although he is relatively young and without comorbidities, he is orthostatic and has shown evidence of active bleeding. Following stabilization, initial endoscopy with either colonoscopy or EGD would be reasonable.

Alternative Diagnosis: Angiodysplasia

Textbook Presentation

Bleeding from angiodysplasia can look like any other cause of lower GI bleeding. It is seen almost exclusively in older adults and can present with anything from hematochezia to occult blood loss. In general, hemorrhage from angiodysplasia tends to be less brisk than bleeding from diverticuli.

Disease Highlights

A. Angiodysplasias, also called arteriovenous malformations, are dilated submucosal veins that are most commonly seen in the right colon of adults over age 60.

B. Present in < 5% of patients over age 60.

C. Most patients with angiodysplasias do not bleed and those that do tend to have occult blood loss rather than brisk, overt, hemorrhage.

D. Angiodysplasia has historically been associated with various diseases (eg, aortic stenosis, cirrhosis) but only a relationship to end-stage renal disease seems definite.

Evidence-Based Diagnosis

A. Similar to the diagnosis of diverticular hemorrhage, colonoscopy, tagged red blood cell scan, and angiography are all used.

B. Colonoscopy is the most common tool. It allows good visualization of the cecum, which is the site of most angiodysplasias.

C. Angiography can provide evidence of a diagnosis even without active bleeding if suspicious vascular patterns are seen.

D. As in diverticular hemorrhage, the diagnosis is often presumptive, made on the basis of visualizing nonbleeding angiodysplasia in a patient with GI bleeding.

Treatment

A. Both acute and chronic bleeding is generally treated endoscopically with thermal or laser ablation. This method can be repeated for recurrent bleeding.

B. Angiographic intervention, with vasoconstrictor agents or embolization, is rarely used.

C. Surgical management (right hemicolectomy) is sometimes required for frequent, recurrent bleeding.

D. Hormonal therapy with estrogen has been used to prevent recurrent bleeding in angiodysplasia, but recent studies suggest that this is not very effective.

E. Whenever possible, long-term antiplatelet therapy should be discontinued.

Alternative Diagnosis: Colon Cancer

Colon cancer is discussed in Chapter 2, Screening & Health Maintenance.

CASE RESOLUTION

Six hours and 3 L of normal saline after his initial Hgb of 13.9 g/dL, a repeat Hgb was 10.3 g/dL. Given the clinical suspicion of a lower GI bleed, colonoscopy was done about 6 hours after admission. There were multiple left-sided diverticuli and a right-sided diverticulum with a nonbleeding visible vessel. A diagnosis of a diverticular hemorrhage was made.

Mr. T remained clinically euvolemic and his Hgb stabilized around 10.0 g/dL. He remained in the hospital for about 48 hours during which there was no recurrent bleeding and his Hgb remained stable. No further treatment (eg, surgery) was necessary.

CHIEF COMPLAINT

PATIENT ▽2

Mr. M is a 39-year-old man who arrives at the emergency department after vomiting blood. He reports waking the morning of admission with an "upset stomach." He initially attributed this to a hangover. After about an hour he vomited "a gallon of blood" with no other stomach contents. Almost immediately afterward, he had a second episode of hematemesis and called 911.

At this point, what is the leading hypothesis, what are the active alternatives, and is there a must not miss diagnosis? Given this differential diagnosis, what tests should be ordered?

RANKING THE DIFFERENTIAL DIAGNOSIS

Mr. M is having an upper GI bleed. The hematemesis is a pivotal point in this case and localizes the source of the bleeding to above the ligament of Treitz. Peptic ulcer disease and gastritis are the most common causes of upper GI bleeding. Although not always present, preceding symptoms of abdominal distress are common with peptic ulcer disease and gastritis. Esophageal varices should be considered in the differential diagnosis given the patient's history of alcohol use. The details of the patient's alcohol use are still unknown, so his risk of portal hypertension cannot be predicted. A Mallory-Weiss tear is also possible, but the patient would report vomiting before the onset of bleeding. Table 19-4 lists the differential diagnosis.

Table 19-4. Diagnostic hypotheses for Mr. M.

Diagnostic Hypotheses	Demographics, Risk Factors, Symptoms and Signs	Important Tests
Leading Hypothesis		
Peptic ulcer disease	Abdominal pain NSAID use Relation of pain to eating	Esophagogastroduodenoscopy (EGD) Tests for *Helicobacter pylori*
Active Alternative		
Gastritis	Often asymptomatic prior to hemorrhage	EGD
Active Alternative—Must Not Miss		
Esophageal varices	History of portal hypertension, usually due to cirrhosis Stigmata of chronic liver disease Alcohol use	EGD Liver function tests
Other Alternative		
Mallory-Weiss tear	Hematemesis preceded by vomiting, especially with retching	EGD

On further history, the patient reports no previous episodes of GI bleeding. He reports occasional stomach upset, usually following drinking binges. He denies NSAID use. Mr. M says that he has been drinking heavily since his late teens. He drinks at least a fifth of hard liquor and a 6-pack of beer daily for the last 20 years. He reports that he has not seen a doctor since his pediatrician.

On physical exam, Mr. M is anxious and appears tired. He smells of alcohol. While sitting, his BP is 140/80 mm Hg and his pulse is 100 bpm. While standing, his BP is 100/80 mm Hg and his pulse is 130 bpm. His temperature is 37.0°C and RR is 16 breaths per minute. Sclera are slightly icteric. Lungs are clear and heart is tachycardic but regular. Abdomen is soft without hepatomegaly. There is no ascites but the spleen is palpable about 2 cm below the costal margin.

Given the alcohol history, scleral icterus, and splenomegaly, a hemorrhage from esophageal varices needs to move above peptic ulcer disease on the differential diagnosis.

Is the clinical information sufficient to make a diagnosis? If not, what other information do you need?

Leading Hypothesis: Esophageal Variceal Hemorrhage

Textbook Presentation

A patient with known cirrhosis presents with heavy upper GI bleeding (hematemesis or melena). There are stigmata of chronic liver disease and frequently a history of previous hemorrhages. Laboratory data demonstrate LFTs consistent with cirrhosis and thrombocytopenia.

Disease Highlights

A. Esophageal varices are portosystemic collaterals that dilate when portal pressures exceed 12 mm Hg.

B. Although varices are the second most common cause of upper GI bleeding, they account for 80–90% of GI bleeds in patients with cirrhosis.

C. Gastroesophageal varices are present in about 50% of patients with cirrhosis.

D. The prevalence of varices depends on the severity of the cirrhosis.

E. The Child-Turcotte-Pugh system classifies patients based on the severity of their cirrhosis.

  1. The system takes into account the presence of encephalopathy, ascites, hyperbilirubinemia, hypoalbuminemia, and clotting deficiencies (Table 19-5).

  2. 40% of patients with Child-Turcotte-Pugh grade A disease have varices, while 85% of patients with grade C disease have varices.

F. Approximately 33% of patients with varices experience hemorrhage.

G. Varices may develop from cirrhosis of any cause.

H. Of all GI bleeds, those from varices carry the worst prognosis.

  1. Nearly 33% of patients die at the time of their first variceal hemorrhage.

Table 19-5. Child-Turcotte-Pugh classification.

Parameter	1 point	2 points	3 points
Ascites	Absent	Slight	Moderate
Bilirubin mg/dL	≤ 2	2–3	> 3
Albumin, g/dL	> 3.5	2.8–3.5	< 2.8
International normalized ratio	< 1.7	1.8–2.3	> 2.3
Encephalopathy	None	Grade 1–2	Grade 3–4

Grade A (well-compensated disease, 2-year survival 85%): 5–6 points
Grade B (significant functional compromise, 2-year survival 60%): 7–9 points
Grade C (decompensated disease, 2-year survival 35%): 10–15 points

2. Up to 70% of survivors have recurrent bleeding in the first year.

3. A variceal bleed carries a 32–80% 1-year mortality.

Esophageal varices are by far the most lethal type of GI bleeding.

Evidence-Based Diagnosis

A. Esophageal varices are diagnosed with endoscopy.

B. Screening for varices

1. Because variceal bleeding carries such a high mortality, the goal is to detect varices before they bleed so that prophylactic treatment can be initiated.

2. All patients with cirrhosis should undergo screening endoscopy every other year.

3. Patients with cirrhosis but without splenomegaly or thrombocytopenia are at the lowest risk for having varices (≈ 4%). Endoscopy may be delayed in these patients.

C. Of all causes of GI bleeding, varices are probably the easiest to predict. One study has the sensitivity and specificity of physicians predicting variceal hemorrhage at 82% and 96%, respectively.

Treatment

A. Primary prophylaxis (patients with varices but no previous bleeding)

1. Beta-blockers (usually propranolol or nadolol) effectively decrease portal pressures.

2. Patients at higher risk for bleeding should also undergo band ligation of the varices.

B. Secondary prophylaxis (patients who have had a previous variceal hemorrhage)

1. Portosystemic shunt procedures, either surgical or transjugular, should be considered.

2. Liver transplantation is the definitive therapy.

C. Treatment of acute hemorrhage

1. Even more than other GI bleeds, achievement of hemodynamic stability in variceal bleeds is of primary importance because the hemorrhage is potentially massive.

2. Patients with variceal bleeding are at high risk for bacterial infections, especially spontaneous bacterial peritonitis. Administration of antibiotics (ceftriaxone or norfloxacin), given prior to endoscopy, have been shown to decrease both the rate of bacterial infections and mortality.

3. Attention should be paid to the patient's coagulation status. Given the prevalence of liver disease in these patients there is often coagulopathy related to factor deficiency or thrombocytopenia.

4. Somatostatin or octreotide should be given as soon as variceal hemorrhage is suspected. These drugs decrease portal pressure and decrease bleeding.

5. Endoscopic banding or sclerotherapy are done initially and if bleeding recurs.

6. Balloon tamponade may be used as a temporizing measure prior to endoscopic therapy.

7. Transvenous intrahepatic portosystemic shunting (TIPS) is an option for patients who continue to bleed despite intervention.

8. Surgical intervention is seldom called for as the mortality is extremely high.

MAKING A DIAGNOSIS

NG tube lavage in the emergency department revealed bright red blood that did not clear with flushing. The patient was admitted to the ICU and received 1 L of normal saline and 2 units of O– packed RBCs. A Foley catheter was placed to assist monitoring his volume status. After another large episode of hematemesis, Mr. M was intubated for airway protection. IV octreotide was begun, and the GI service was called to perform urgent endoscopy.

Have you crossed a diagnostic threshold for the leading hypothesis, variceal hemorrhage? Have you ruled out the active alternatives? Do other tests need to be done to exclude the alternative diagnoses?

The patient is having a large upper GI bleed and is clearly actively bleeding. Initial management is aimed at hemodynamic stabilization. The decision to place the patient in the ICU was based on his hemodynamic instability, active bleeding, and need for close monitoring. Given the alcohol history, the volume of the bleed, and the lack of previous abdominal symptoms, bleeding from esophageal varices is highest on the differential diagnosis, and empiric therapy is begun with octreotide and antibiotics. Peptic ulcer disease is the most common cause of upper GI bleeding, and we do not yet know whether this patient has cirrhosis.

Alternative Diagnosis: Peptic Ulcer Disease

The details of peptic ulcer disease are discussed in Chapter 32, Unintentional Weight Loss. This section will only deal with hemorrhage from peptic ulcers.

Textbook Presentation

The classic presentation is a middle-aged person with chronic dyspepsia; long-term use of NSAIDs (including aspirin); or *Helicobacter pylori* infection who has an episode of hematemesis, melena, or both.

Disease Highlights

A. Most common cause of GI bleeds.

1. Upper GI bleeds are 4–8 times more common than lower GI bleeds.

2. Peptic ulcer disease accounts for at least 50% of upper GI bleeds.

B. Bleeding occurs when an ulcer erodes into a vessel in the stomach or duodenal wall.

C. About 50% of patients with bleeding or perforation have had no previous symptoms.

D. Causative factors are long-term use of NSAIDs, *H pylori* infection, or stress from critical illness.

E. Similar to diverticuli, most cases are self-limited ($\approx$ 80%).

Evidence-Based Diagnosis

A. Except in rare cases, all patients with GI bleeding in whom an ulcer is suspected undergo endoscopy. Endoscopy is useful from diagnostic, prognostic, and therapeutic standpoints.

B. Endoscopy has a 92% sensitivity for ulcers. Biopsy during endoscopy allows for exclusion of malignancy and *H pylori* infection as a cause of the ulcer.

C. Endoscopy is also useful because it gives information about a patient's risk of recurrent bleeding and thus enables discharge planning. Table 19-6 gives approximate rates for recurrent bleeding by endoscopic finding.

D. Other endoscopic findings associated with high risk are ulcer size > 2 cm and arterial bleeding.

E. Clinical factors such as transfusion requirements, age, comorbid conditions, and hemodynamic stability must also be taken into account.

Treatment

A. Hemodynamic stabilization

B. Endoscopy

  1. Early endoscopy achieves hemostasis in > 94% of patients and decreases length of hospital stay.

  2. For patients with a high-risk lesion, endoscopic intervention such as clipping, thermocoagulation, or sclerotherapy is warranted.

  3. Repeat endoscopy is effective in the 15–20% of patients who have a recurrence of bleeding.

C. Medication

  1. IV H_2-blockers are no longer recommended for acutely bleeding ulcers.

  2. Proton pump inhibitors

    a. IV proton pump inhibitors should be given to patients admitted with suspected bleeding ulcers.

    b. Patients found to be at high risk for rebleeding (Table 19-6) on endoscopy should continue this therapy for 72 hours.

    c. Patients at low risk can be switched to oral proton pump inhibitors.

    d. All patients who are discharged should be taking proton pump inhibitors (as well as *H pylori* therapy, if warranted) to ensure ulcer healing.

D. Patients who have rebleeding that cannot be controlled endoscopically can either undergo embolization or surgical therapy.

Alternative Diagnosis: Mallory-Weiss Tear

Textbook Presentation

Mallory-Weiss tear is typically seen in patients with vomiting of any cause in whom hematemesis develops acutely.

Disease Highlights

A. Mallory-Weiss tears are mucosal tears at the gastroesophageal junction.

B. It is a common misconception that Mallory-Weiss tears always follow retching. In fact, a history of retching preceding hematemesis is present in about 33% of cases.

Evidence-Based Diagnosis

Diagnosis is routinely made on upper endoscopy.

Treatment

Mallory-Weiss tears seldom require specific treatment. Rebleeding is quite rare.

CASE RESOLUTION

Emergency endoscopy was performed in the ICU. Mr. M was found to have large esophageal and gastric varices. A clear bleeding source was found and treated with banding. Although there was no clinically significant rebleeding, other complications developed. He remained intubated for 5 days for presumed aspiration pneumonia, experienced alcohol withdrawal symptoms, and developed mild encephalopathy.

During the hospitalization he was found to have Child-Turcotte-Pugh grade B cirrhosis. At the time of discharge, he was taking propranolol and lactulose. Follow-up in an outpatient alcohol program and the hepatology practice was scheduled. He did not come to any follow-up visits.

Mr. M's emergent endoscopy was indicated by the severity of the bleeding. His bleeding was controlled with a combination of medical and endoscopic management. The complicated hospital course is not surprising given the comorbid conditions frequently present in patients with varices. Mr. M had advanced cirrhosis and alcohol dependence.

Table 19-6. Approximate rates for recurrent bleeding by endoscopic finding.

Lesion	Rebleeding Rate
Actively oozing vessel	55%
Nonbleeding visible vessel	45%
Adherent clot	15–35%
Clean based ulcer	5%

CHIEF COMPLAINT

PATIENT 3

Ms. S is a 35-year-old woman who comes to the out-patient clinic for an initial visit. She is well and is without complaints. On review of systems, she notes that she occasionally passes bright red blood per rectum. This has happened about 4 times over the past 5 years. It is never associated with pain. She sometimes sees the blood on the toilet paper and sometimes in the bowl.

At this point, what is the leading hypothesis, what are the active alternatives, and is there a must not miss diagnosis? Given this differential diagnosis, what tests should be ordered?

RANKING THE DIFFERENTIAL DIAGNOSIS

Ms. S has recurrent, lower GI bleeding that has occurred inter-mittently over a number of years without obvious negative health effects. This type of bleeding can be categorized as benign sound-ing anorectal bleeding. It is bleeding in a young patient without "red flags" for serious disease such as anemia, change in bowel hab-its, weight loss, or diarrhea. Between 10% and 20% of the popula-tion will have this type of bleeding. The goal is to diagnose these patients appropriately without missing occasional serious lesions and without subjecting excessive numbers of patients to unpleasant evaluation. The pivotal points in this case are the patient's young age, the small volume of blood loss, and the absence of "red flags."

The differential diagnosis includes hemorrhoidal bleeding and bleeding from anal fissures. Anal fissures are usually painful so hem-orrhoids are the more likely diagnosis in this case. IBD, especially ulcerative colitis, could cause similar symptoms, but the intermit-tent nature of symptoms makes IBD less likely. We need to know more about the patient's bowel habits. Diverticuli and colonic angiodysplasia could account for the patient's symptoms but would be very unusual in a patient this age. Colon or rectal cancer is also rare in this age group but should be considered. Table 19-7 lists the differential diagnosis.

3

On further history Ms. S reports no recent change in bowel habits, no weight loss, and says she feels well. She does report that although the bleeding has never been associ-ated with pain, it is sometimes associated with constipa-tion. She has never used any treatment.

Is the clinical information sufficient to make a diagnosis? If not, what other information do you need?

Leading Hypothesis: Hemorrhoidal Bleeding

Textbook Presentation

Hemorrhoidal bleeding typically presents with severe rectal pain and bleeding. The pain is worst with bowel movements, straining, or sit-ting. Occasionally, hemorrhoids can present with painless bleeding.

Table 19-7. Diagnostic hypothesis for Ms. S.

Diagnostic Hypotheses	Demographics, Risk Factors, Symptoms and Signs	Important Tests
Leading Hypothesis		
Hemorrhoids	Painful or painless bright red blood per rectum	Anoscopy CBC
Active Alternative—Most Common		
Anal fissures	Bright red blood per rectum, often associated with severe pain	External inspection and anoscopy
Active Alternative—Must Not Miss		
Ulcerative colitis	Usually associated with diarrhea	Colonoscopy
Colon cancer	History of anemia or changing bowel habits Family history of colon cancer	Colonoscopy

Disease Highlights

C. Hemorrhoids are generally classified as internal or external.
   1. External hemorrhoids
      a. Occur below the dentate line.
      b. Present either as painless bleeding or with engorged, painful, swollen perianal tissue; or with thrombosis. Thrombosed hemorrhoids are purple, extremely painful, and may bleed.
   2. Internal hemorrhoids
      a. Occur above the dentate line.
      b. Symptoms can be a feeling of internal fullness, painless bleeding, or prolapse. Prolapse is usually painful and sometimes associated with bleeding.
   3. Both internal and external hemorrhoids will be most symptomatic with sitting, straining, and constipation.

A clinician should always verify a patient's self-diagnosis of hemorrhoids. Many patients refer to all perianal symptoms as hemorrhoids.

Evidence-Based Diagnosis

A. Hemorrhoidal bleeding is diagnosed by direct observation.
   1. This may be accomplished visually in patients with external hemorrhoids.
   2. Patients with internal hemorrhoids require anoscopy to see hemorrhoids.

B. An important question is "When does benign sounding ano-rectal bleeding need a more extensive evaluation than an anal exam with or without anoscopy?"
   1. One study looked at 201 patients whose review of symptoms revealed rectal bleeding.
      a. 24% of these patients were found to have serious disease. The diseases were polyps in 13%, colon cancer in 6.5%, and IBD in 4% of patients.

b. Factors associated with risk of serious disease were age, short duration of bleeding, and blood mixed with stool.

c. No cancers were found in patients younger than 50.

d. 6 of the 37 patients who had a clear source of anorectal bleeding (fissures or hemorrhoids) also had polyps or cancer.

2. Another study found only 10 polyps among 314 patients under 40 with rectal bleeding compared with 27 polyps and 1 case of cancer among 256 patients between the ages of 40 and 50.

C. In general, if a young patient (under age 40) with rectal bleeding does not have a clear anorectal source or if the bleeding continues despite treatment of the anorectal source, a more complete evaluation (with colonoscopy) should be done. Patients over 40 should always be evaluated.

 Although serious disease is rare among young people with rectal bleeding, it does occur.

Treatment

A. Most hemorrhoids and anal fissures can be treated conservatively with general recommendations for perianal well being.

1. Sitz baths to relax anal sphincter.

2. Analgesia with acetaminophen, topical creams, or short-term topical corticosteroids. A doughnut cushion is sometimes helpful for prolonged sitting.

3. Soften stool with increased fluid intake, a high-fiber diet, and docusate sodium or mineral oil.

4. Avoid anything that may lead to constipation.

5. Avoid prolonged sitting, especially on the toilet.

B. Internal hemorrhoids that prolapse or continue to bleed usually require surgical removal.

C. Thrombosed, irreducible internal hemorrhoids and thrombosed external hemorrhoids require rapid surgical treatment.

MAKING A DIAGNOSIS

 Ms. S has a normal general physical exam. External anal exam and digital rectal exam are normal. Anoscopy reveals 1 large, nonbleeding internal hemorrhoid. A CBC is normal.

 Have you crossed a diagnostic threshold for the leading hypothesis, hemorrhoidal bleeding? Have you ruled out the active alternatives? Do other tests need to be done to exclude the alternative diagnoses?

The patient has an internal hemorrhoid on exam. This is almost certainly, but not definitely, the cause of her bleeding. Because she is currently asymptomatic, it would be reasonable to postpone further work-up for now.

Alternative Diagnosis: Anal Fissures

Textbook Presentation

Patients typically have severe rectal pain with bowel movements and bright red blood on the toilet paper. On physical exam, a fissure can be found at the midline, posterior to the anal opening.

Disease Highlights

A. Anal fissures occur secondary to trauma to the mucosa of the anal canal, most commonly by hard stool.

B. Fissures usually present as acute onset, painful defecation, usually with bleeding.

C. Fissures can become chronic.

1. Pain causes anal sphincter spasm that, in turn, causes recurrent trauma.

2. Chronic fissures can be associated with sentinel piles (essentially a thickening of the skin at the end of a fissure).

D. Fissures are present at the midline.

1. Fissures are usually posterior in men and can be posterior or anterior in women.

2. Other diagnoses, such as Crohn disease or sexually transmitted diseases, should be considered when fissures are lateral to the anal opening.

Evidence-Based Diagnosis

A. Fissures are diagnosed by direct observation.

B. Physical exam is sometimes difficult since patients are often in pain.

Treatment

A. In most cases, general supportive recommendations outlined above for the treatment of hemorrhoids will bring relief of symptoms in days to weeks.

B. More chronic fissures often need therapy to relax the anal sphincter.

1. Topical nitrates and injected botulinum toxin are effective.

2. Surgical sphincterotomy is almost always effective but carries a small risk of permanent fecal incontinence.

CASE RESOLUTION

 One year later Ms. S returns to the clinic with recurrent bleeding. Anoscopy revealed a bleeding internal hemorrhoid. Symptoms resolve with supportive care, but bleeding recurs 1 month later. Colonoscopy is performed and reveals only internal hemorrhoids. The patient declines definitive therapy and continues to experience rare episodes of hemorrhoidal bleeding.

The patient's history of recurrent bleeding is quite common. Many patients with hemorrhoids will have occasional flares. The decision to perform colonoscopy was a difficult one. Although her young age and presence of an abnormality on anoscopy makes serious disease unlikely, evaluation of any patient with recurrent rectal bleeding is appropriate.

REVIEW OF OTHER IMPORTANT DISEASES

Occult GI Bleeding

Textbook Presentation

Occult GI bleeding presents in 1 of 2 ways: either in a patient with newly discovered iron deficiency anemia or in a patient with positive fecal occult blood tests.

Disease Highlights

A. Generally a disease of older patients; average age in most studies is the early 60s.

B. Upper GI lesions cause occult GI bleeding slightly more commonly than lower GI lesions.

C. The common causes of upper and lower GI bleeding account for most causes of occult GI bleeding.

D. Long-term aspirin, NSAID, or alcohol use is found in about 40% of patients with an upper GI tract lesion.

E. A small percentage of patients, ≈ 5%, have lesions of both the upper and lower GI tract.

Evidence-Based Diagnosis

A. All patients with occult GI bleeding need evaluation of the GI tract.

B. All patients with iron deficiency anemia need to have the cause of the iron deficiency identified (see Chapter 6, Anemia).

   1. Iron deficiency is usually due to chronic blood loss. Rarely, it is due to poor iron intake or iron malabsorption.

   2. Menstrual and GI blood loss are the most common sources.

   3. All men, all women without menorrhagia, and all women over 50 (even those with menorrhagia) need to have an evaluation of the GI tract.

   4. Women under age 40 with menorrhagia do not necessarily need further GI evaluation unless they have GI symptoms or a family history of early colon cancer.

   5. Women between 40 and 50 years of age with menorrhagia need to be managed carefully. They should be asked about minimal GI symptoms (celiac sprue causes iron deficiency through malabsorption and the symptoms can be easily attributed to irritable bowel syndrome). There should be a low threshold for recommending colonoscopy in this subset of patients.

 Always determine the source of blood loss in occult GI bleeding and iron deficiency anemia.

C. Evaluation of the GI tract in patients with occult GI bleeding should be done as follows:

   1. Colonoscopy alone is sufficient in patients with only a positive fecal occult blood test and no iron deficiency.

   2. Evaluation of entire GI tract is recommended by most experts for those patients with iron deficiency anemia or iron deficiency anemia and positive fecal occult blood testing.

   3. Video capsule endoscopy should be used in patients in whom EGD and colonoscopy are inconclusive.

Obscure GI Bleeding

Textbook Presentation

Obscure GI bleeding refers to GI bleeding with normal upper and lower endoscopy and small bowel evaluation by a radiographic procedure. As the evaluation of occult GI bleeding comes to include capsule endoscopy, this diagnosis should become less common.

Disease Highlights

A. Included in the diagnosis of obscure GI bleeding are patients with occult bleeding, as discussed above, who have had a normal evaluation but persistent bleeding and those patients with acute GI bleeding and an unrevealing initial evaluation.

B. About 25% of the patients with obscure GI bleeding have an upper or colonic source. Peptic ulcer disease or ulcers within hiatal hernias are common.

C. The small bowel, a rare source of blood loss in patients with GI bleeding, is the most likely origin of obscure GI bleeding.

   1. Angiodysplasia is the most common small bowel source.

   2. Ulcers, malignancy (accounting for about 10% of small bowel bleeding), Crohn disease, and Meckel diverticula are also represented in most series.

Evidence-Based Diagnosis

A. A directed history may provide clues to the source of obscure GI bleeding. Ask about use of medications that can cause mucosal damage (eg, NSAIDs, bisphosphonates) as well as a history of diseases that predispose patients to GI bleeding (HIV, neurofibromatosis).

B. Repeat endoscopy, looking for lesions that were missed on the initial evaluation, is the initial step in the diagnosis.

C. If repeated upper and lower endoscopies are negative, capsule endoscopy should be used to image the small bowel.

D. Other means of endoscopically visualizing the small bowel include:

   1. Enteroscopy, in which a long endoscope (often a colonoscope) is passed orally.

   a. Visualization of 40–60 cm of jejunum is common.

   b. Diagnostic yields of 40–75% have been reported.

   2. Double balloon enteroscopy can allow visualization of the entire small bowel.

   3. Intraoperative endoscopy.

E. Meckel diverticulum scan uses a nuclear tracer that binds to parietal cells.

   1. Sensitivity for detecting a Meckel diverticulum is between 75% and 100%.

   2. Diagnosis only really considered when obscure bleeding occurs in a patient younger than 30.

Treatment

The treatment of obscure bleeding varies by the cause of bleeding.

REFERENCES

Barkun AN, Bardou M, Kuipers EJ; International Consensus Upper Gastrointestinal Bleeding Conference Group. International consensus recommendations on the management of patients with nonvariceal upper gastrointestinal bleeding. Ann Intern Med. 2010;152(2):101–13.

Cuellar RE, Gavaler JS, Alexander JA et al. Gastrointestinal tract hemorrhage. The value of a nasogastric aspirate. Arch Intern Med. 1990;150(7):1381–4.

Helfand M, Marton KI, Zimmer-Gembeck MJ, Sox HC Jr. History of visible rectal bleeding in a primary care population. Initial assessment and 10-year follow-up. JAMA. 1997;277(1):44–8.

Huang ES, Karsan S, Kanwal F, Singh I, Makhani M, Spiegel BM. Impact of nasogastric lavage on outcomes in acute GI bleeding. Gastrointest Endosc. 2011;74(5):971–80.

Lewis JD, Shih CE, Blecker D. Endoscopy for hematochezia in patients under 50 years of age. Dig Dis Sci. 2001;46(12):2660–5.

Madhotra R, Mulcahy HE, Willner I, Reuben A. Prediction of esophageal varices in patients with cirrhosis. J Clin Gastroenterol. 2002;34(1):81–5.

McGuire HH Jr. Bleeding colonic diverticula. A reappraisal of natural history and management. Ann Surg. 1994;220(5):653–6.

Ohmann C, Thon K, Stoltzing H, Yang Q, Lorenz W. Upper gastrointestinal tract bleeding: assessing the diagnostic contributions of the history and clinical findings. Med Decis Making. 1986;6(4):208–15.

Olds GD, Cooper GS, Chak A, Sivak MV Jr, Chitale AA, Wong RC. The yield of bleeding scans in acute lower gastrointestinal hemorrhage. J Clin Gastroenterol. 2005;39(4):273–7.

Pickhardt PJ, Choi JR, Hwang I et al. Computed tomographic virtual colonoscopy to screen for colorectal neoplasia in asymptomatic adults. N Engl J Med. 2003;349(23):2191–200.

Raju GS, Gerson L, Das A, Lewis B; American Gastroenterological Association. American Gastroenterological Association (AGA) Institute technical review on obscure gastrointestinal bleeding. Gastroenterology. 2007;133(5):1697–717.

Sharara AI, Rockey DC. Gastroesophageal variceal hemorrhage. N Engl J Med. 2001;345(9):669–81.

Srygley FD, Gerardo CJ, Tran T, Fisher DA. Does this patient have a severe upper gastrointestinal bleed? JAMA. 2012;307(10):1072–9.

Strate LL. Lower GI bleeding: epidemiology and diagnosis. Gastroenterol Clin North Am. 2005;34(4):643–64.

Villanueva C, Colomo A, Bosch A et al. Transfusion strategies for acute upper gastrointestinal bleeding. N Engl J Med. 2013;368(1):11–21.

Witting MD, Magder L, Heins AE, Mattu A, Granja CA, Baumgarten M. ED predictors of upper gastrointestinal tract bleeding in patients without hematemesis. Am J Emerg Med. 2006;24(3):280–5.

I have a patient with headache. How do I determine the cause?

CHIEF COMPLAINT

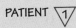

PATIENT 1

Mr. M is a 34-year-old man who comes to an outpatient practice complaining of intermittent headaches.

What is the differential diagnosis of headache? How would you frame the differential?

CONSTRUCTING A DIFFERENTIAL DIAGNOSIS

Headache is one of the most common physical complaints. Because less than 1% of all headaches are life-threatening, the challenge is to reassure and appropriately treat patients with benign headaches while finding the rare, life-threatening headache without excessive evaluation.

Headaches are classified as primary or secondary. Primary headaches are syndromes unto themselves rather than signs of other diseases. Although potentially disabling, they are reliably not life-threatening. Secondary headaches are symptoms of other illnesses. Unlike primary headaches, secondary headaches are potentially dangerous.

The distinction of primary and secondary headaches is useful diagnostically. Primary headaches, such as tension headaches, are diagnosed clinically, sometimes using diagnostic criteria (the most commonly used are published by the International Headache Society, IHS). Traditional diagnostic studies (laboratory studies, radiology, pathology) cannot verify the diagnosis. Secondary headaches, such as headaches caused by central nervous system (CNS) tumors, often can be definitively diagnosed by identifying the underlying disease.

Clinically, primary and secondary headaches can be difficult to distinguish. The single most important question when developing a differential diagnosis for a headache is, "Is this headache new or old?" Chronic headaches tend to be primary, while new-onset headaches are usually secondary. This is the first and most important pivotal point in diagnosing headaches. This distinction is not perfect. There are some chronic headaches that are secondary headaches (headaches caused by cervical degenerative joint disease for example) and even classic, primary headaches (such as migraines) can present as a new headache. The differentiation of old versus new also depends on how rapidly a patient brings his or her symptoms to medical attention. This being said, the classification of headaches as primary vs secondary and new vs old provides not only a memorable framework for the differential diagnosis but also a clinically useful structure by which the differential can be organized by pivotal points. The differential diagnosis appears below.

Figure 20-1 shows the potential diagnoses in a more algorithmic form as they are often considered clinically.

A. Old headaches
  1. Primary
     a. Tension headaches
     b. Migraine headaches
     c. Cluster headaches
  2. Secondary
     a. Cervical degenerative joint disease
     b. Temporomandibular joint syndrome
     c. Headaches associated with substances or their withdrawal
        (1) Caffeine
        (2) Nitrates
        (3) Analgesics (often presenting as chronic daily headaches)
        (4) Ergotamine

B. New headaches
  1. Primary
     a. Benign cough headache
     b. Benign exertional headache
     c. Headache associated with sexual activity
     d. Benign thunderclap headache
     e. Idiopathic intracranial hypertension (pseudotumor cerebri)
  2. Secondary
     a. Infectious
        (1) Upper respiratory tract infection
        (2) Sinusitis
        (3) Meningitis
     b. Vascular
        (1) Temporal arteritis
        (2) Subarachnoid hemorrhage (SAH)
        (3) Parenchymal hemorrhage
        (4) Malignant hypertension
        (5) Cavernous sinus thrombosis
     c. Space-occupying lesions
        (1) Brain tumors
        (2) Subdural hematoma
     d. Medical morning headaches
        (1) Sleep disturbance
        (2) Night-time hypoglycemia

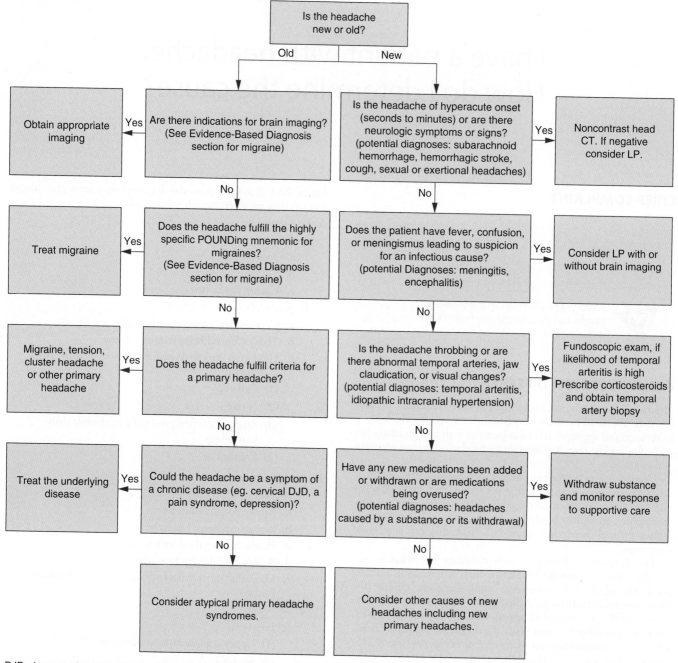

DJD, degenerative joint disease; LP, lumbar puncture.

Figure 20-1. Diagnostic approach: headache.

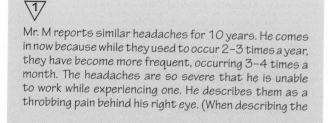

Mr. M reports similar headaches for 10 years. He comes in now because while they used to occur 2–3 times a year, they have become more frequent, occurring 3–4 times a month. The headaches are so severe that he is unable to work while experiencing one. He describes them as a throbbing pain behind his right eye. (When describing the

(continued)

headache, he places the base of his hand over his eye with his fingers wrapping over his forehead.) The headaches are often associated with nausea and, in the last few months, he has occasionally vomited with them.

At this point, what is the leading hypothesis, what are the active alternatives, and is there a must not miss diagnosis? Given this differential diagnosis, what tests should be ordered?

RANKING THE DIFFERENTIAL DIAGNOSIS

The severity and chronicity of the headaches are pivotal points in this case that enable us to limit the differential. Although Mr. M's headaches are severe, they have to be classified as old headaches since they have been occurring for years. This fact is reassuring, meaning that his headaches are most likely a primary headache syndrome. In a young healthy person with chronic headaches, migraine, tension, and cluster headaches are most likely. Given the severity of the headaches, migraines are more likely than tension headaches. Given the severe, throbbing nature of the headaches, a vascular cause should at least be considered. An intracranial aneurysm could cause similar symptoms, but the chronicity makes this less likely. Table 20-1 ranks the differential diagnosis considering the demographic information, risk factors, symptoms and signs available to us at this point.

Severity is less important than quality in distinguishing a new headache from an old headache. A severe headache that is identical in quality to chronic headaches is less worrisome than a mild headache that is dissimilar to any previous headache.

Mr. M has used ibuprofen in the past with good response, but this is no longer working well. His past history is remarkable only for car-sickness as a child.

Is the clinical information sufficient to make a diagnosis? If not what other information do you need?

Table 20-1. Diagnostic hypotheses for Mr. M.

Diagnostic Hypotheses	Demographics, Risk Factors, Symptoms and Signs	Important Tests
Leading Hypothesis		
Migraine headache	Moderate to severe unilateral throbbing headache, sometimes associated with aura	Diagnostic criteria and exclusion of secondary headaches
Active Alternatives—Most Common		
Tension headache	Chronic, pressure-type headache of mild to moderate intensity	Diagnostic criteria and exclusion of secondary headaches
Cluster headaches	Unilateral headache, worst around the orbit or temporal area, associated with conjunctival injection, lacrimation, or nasal congestion	Diagnostic criteria and exclusion of secondary headaches
Active Alternative—Must Not Miss		
Intracranial aneurysm	Acute or subacute headache Headache features are nonspecific	CT angiography, MR angiography, or traditional angiography

Leading Hypothesis: Migraine Headaches

Textbook Presentation

Migraines most often first present in women in their teens or 20s. The headaches are unilateral and throbbing and are severe enough to make it impossible to do work during an attack. They are occasionally preceded by about 20 minutes of flickering lights in a visual field (aura). Patients often find it necessary to lie in a dark, quiet room.

Disease Highlights

A. The description of migraine headaches adopted by the IHS is, "Recurring headache disorder manifesting in attacks lasting 4–72 hours. Typical characteristics of headache are unilateral location, pulsating quality, moderate or severe intensity, aggravation by routine physical activity and association with nausea, and/or photophobia and phonophobia."

B. Migraine headaches are a chronic headache syndrome caused by a neurovascular disorder. Neural events lead to intracranial vasodilatation.

C. They may begin at any age but most commonly begin during adolescence.

D. They are more common (2–3 times) and more severe in women than men.

E. Auras frequently accompany migraines.

   1. Somewhere between 33% and 75% of patients with migraines have auras. Of all people with migraine,

      a. 18% always have auras

      b. 13% sometimes have auras

      c. 8% have auras without headaches.

   2. Auras are usually visual, precede the headache, and last for about 20 minutes.

   3. Descriptions of auras

      a. Frequently, patients will initially describe a blind spot.

      b. Auras usually involve 1 portion of the visual field.

      c. Auras may vary. The frequency of some types of aura is given in Table 20-2.

Table 20-2. Qualities of migraine auras.

Types of aura	Prevalence
Zigzags	56%
Stars or flashes	83%
Scotoma	40%
Hemianopsia	7%
Sensory aura	20%
Aphasia	11%
Motor aura	4%
Duration of aura	**Prevalence**
< 30 minutes	70%
30–60 minutes	18%
> 60 minutes	7%

Adapted, with permission, from Smetana GW. The diagnostic value of historical features in primary headache syndromes: a comprehensive review. Arch Intern Med. 2000;160:2729–37. Copyrighted © 2000 American Medical Association. All rights Reserved.

d. Scintillating scotoma often occur. These are often described as flashing lights, spots of light, zigzag lines, or squiggles.

Migraine auras are stereotypical. Listening closely to patients with migraines describe their aura will make it easy to recognize auras in other patients.

Evidence-Based Diagnosis

A. Migraine headaches are among the most severe of all the recurrent headache syndromes. (Cluster headache is the other primary headache that causes severe pain.)

1. They should be considered in any patient with headaches severe enough to be the chief complaint at a doctor visit.

2. Of initial visits for headaches in the primary care setting, 90% meet criteria for migraines.

The diagnosis of migraine headache should be seriously considered in any patient who has recurrent headaches that cause disability.

B. As with other primary headaches, diagnosis is guided by the IHS's diagnostic criteria rather than by diagnostic tests.

C. The criteria for migraines are divided into migraines with and without aura.

1. Migraine without aura

a. A patient must have at least 5 attacks that last 4–72 hours.

b. The headache must have 2 of the following qualities:

(1) Unilateral pain

(2) Pulsating pain

(3) Moderate to severe (must limit activity)

(4) Aggravated by routine physical activity

c. And have 1 of the following associated symptoms:

(1) Nausea and/or vomiting

(2) Photophobia or phonophobia

2. Migraine with aura

a. Definition: "Recurring disorder manifesting in attacks of reversible focal neurological symptoms that usually develop gradually over 5–20 minutes and lasting less than 60 minutes." A migraine-type headache usually follows the aura symptoms. Less commonly, auras can be followed by a headache that lacks migrainous features or auras can occur with no subsequent headache.

b. A patient must have at least 2 attacks.

D. It is important to remember that diagnostic criteria, although helpful, need to be used carefully when applied to an individual patient. A patient who clearly has the disease in question may not perfectly fit the criteria. Consider these data about some of classic migraine symptoms:

1. 50% of patients with migraines have nonpulsatile headaches.

2. 40% have bilateral headaches.

Diagnostic criteria are more helpful for research than patient care. They should be used cautiously with individual patients.

E. There are other less common types of migraine.

1. These include headaches with aura lasting longer than 60 minutes and migraine aura without a headache.

2. These syndromes are difficult to diagnose and require exclusion of other diseases (such as cerebrovascular accident, transient ischemic attack, or retinal detachment) that could cause similar symptoms.

F. Besides the diagnostic criteria, there are many other aspects of the history that are suggestive of migraine headaches.

1. A systematic review suggested the mnemonic POUNDing as a diagnostic test for migraines.

a. Is the headache **p**ulsatile?

b. Does it last between 4 and 72 h**o**urs without medications?

c. Is it **u**nilateral?

d. Is there **n**ausea?

e. Is it **d**isabling?

 2. If 4 or 5 questions are answered with "Yes," the LR+ is 24, which rules in the diagnosis of migraine headache.

3. Another review provided test characteristics for various headache qualities in distinguishing migraines from tension headaches. Table 20-3 shows those characteristics that have at least a moderate effect on posttest probability.

 4. When differentiating migraines from tension headaches, nausea is an important clue to migraines.

5. Interestingly, some commonly considered characteristics, such as headache duration and relationship of headache to stress, weather, menses, fatigue, and odors, were not helpful in differentiating migraines from tension headaches.

6. Presence of a family history was helpful in making the diagnosis with a LR+ of 5.0.

7. Patients with migraines are also more likely to have had vomiting attacks as children and to have suffered from motion sickness.

G. Given the severity of migraine, a common issue that comes up is whether a patient with a probable migraine undergos neuroimaging. The following are predictors of abnormal neuroimaging in patients with headaches and are generally agreed upon indications.

Table 20-3. Test characteristics for symptoms of migraine.

Criteria	Sensitivity	Specificity	LR+	LR−
Nausea	82%	96%	23.2	0.19
Photophobia	79%	87%	6.0	0.24
Phonophobia	67%	87%	5.2	0.38
Exacerbated by physical activity	81%	78%	3.7	0.24
Unilateral	66%	78%	3.1	0.43
Throbbing	76%	77%	3.3	0.32
Precipitated by chocolate	22%	95%	4.6	0.82
Precipitated by cheese	38%	92%	4.9	0.68

1. Abnormal neurologic exam or symptoms that are atypical for aura, especially dizziness, lack of coordination, numbness or tingling, or worsening of headache with the Valsalva maneuver

2. Increasing frequency of headaches or a change in headache quality or pattern

3. Headaches that awaken patients from sleep

4. New headaches in patients over 50

5. First headache, worst headache, or abrupt-onset headache

6. New headache in patients with cancer, immunosuppression, or pregnancy

7. Headache associated with loss of consciousness

8. Headache triggered by exertion

9. Special consideration should be given to a person who is receiving warfarin therapy.

Treatment

A. Treatment of migraines is either abortive or prophylactic.

B. Abortive therapy

1. Abortive therapy should be used at the very first sign of a migraine. Patients should be advised not to wait until they "are sure it is a migraine."

2. Effective drugs are outlined in Table 20-4 with the individual considerations mainly from the consensus comments from the US Headache Consortium.

Table 20-4. Recommended abortive treatments for migraine.

Drug	Considerations
NSAIDs	First-line therapy May be used with antiemetics
Acetaminophen plus aspirin plus caffeine	First-line therapy May also be used with antiemetics
Triptans (SQ, PO, IN)	For moderate to severe migraines Combination with NSAIDS probably more effective that monotherapy
Dihydroergotamine (SQ, IV, IM, IN)	For moderate to severe migraines Maybe used with antiemetics
Antiemetics (prochlorperazine maleate or metoclopramide)	Used as adjunctive therapy
Opioids	For moderate to severe migraine Use should be limited because of the risk of rebound and medication overuse
Corticosteroids	Rescue therapy for intractable migraines
Butalbital plus aspirin plus caffeine	Occasional use for moderate and severe migraines
Acetaminophen, dichloralphenazone, and isometheptene	Occasional use for mild to moderate migraines

IM, intramuscular; IN, intranasal; IV, intravenous; NSAIDs, nonsteroidal antiinflammatory drugs; PO, oral; SQ, subcutaneous.

C. Prophylactic therapy

1. Prophylactic therapy is instituted when patient and doctor agree that the migraines are frequent enough, severe enough, or persistent enough to warrant regular medications.

2. Prophylactic therapy does not need to be used every day. It can be used only around the times that migraines predictably occur (such as perimenstrually).

3. There are many effective medications in multiple classes. Some of the most effective and commonly used are:

a. Beta-blockers
(1) Propranolol
(2) Metopolol
(3) Timolol

b. Antidepressants
(1) Amitriptyline
(2) Venlafaxine

c. Anticonvulsants
(1) Valproic acid
(2) Topiramate

MAKING A DIAGNOSIS

Mr. M's physical exam, including a detailed neurologic exam, is completely normal.

Mr. M's headaches fulfill the criteria for migraine headaches. They are pulsatile, unilateral, disabling, and associated with nausea, thus fulfilling 4 of the POUNDing criteria. The history of motion sickness provides another clue. The increasing frequency and severity of the headaches is somewhat worrisome, and neurologic imaging would be reasonable but not entirely necessary given the high positive likelihood of the POUNDing criteria.

Have you crossed a diagnostic threshold for the leading hypothesis, migraine headaches? Have you ruled out the active alternatives? Do other tests need to be done to exclude the alternative diagnoses?

Alternative Diagnosis: Tension Headaches

Textbook Presentation

Tension headaches are the most common type of headache. They generally occur a few times each month and are described as bilateral and squeezing. They are usually relieved with over-the-counter analgesics and are seldom severe enough to cause real disability.

Disease Highlights

A. The IHS definition of episodic tension-type headache is, "Recurrent episodes of H/A lasting minutes to days. The pain is typically pressing/tightening in quality, of mild or moderate intensity, bilateral in location and does not worsen with routine physical activity. Nausea is absent, but photophobia or phonophobia may be present."

B. Most common type of headache; the 1-year prevalence of tension headaches is 63% in men and 86% in women.

C. The IHS criteria divide tension headaches into multiple subtypes: episodic, chronic, with or without associated tenderness of pericranial muscles.

D. The pathophysiology of tension headaches is still a topic of debate.

1. Episodic tension headaches are likely related to tenderness and spasm in the pericranial muscles while chronic tension headaches are related to changes in the CNS caused by the chronic pain of tension headaches.

2. There is evidence to suggest that people who suffer from more frequent tension headaches have higher levels of perceived stress and lower pain thresholds than those without headaches.

E. Tension headaches can be troublesome but are seldom disabling.

Evidence-Based Diagnosis

A. Because tension headaches are the most common form of headaches, they are the default diagnosis in almost every patient with a mild to moderate headache syndrome.

B. A detailed history and physical exam is required to exclude other headache syndromes that require specific treatment.

C. Special attention should be given to excluding migraines.

D. The IHS diagnostic criteria for episodic tension headaches are:

1. At least 10 previous headaches

2. Duration of 30 minutes to 7 days

3. 3 of the following:

   a. Pressing or tightening (nonpulsating) quality

   b. Mild to moderate in severity (inhibits but does not prevent activity)

   c. Bilateral

   d. Not aggravated by routine activity

4. No nausea or vomiting

5. Photophobia or phonophobia may be present, but not both

E. Chronic tension-type headaches often develop from the more common episodic headaches. These are similar in quality but occur at least 15 days of the month.

1. Chronic tension-type headaches are commonly referred to chronic daily headaches.

2. Chronic tension-type headaches may often be caused by overuse of analgesic drugs used to treat headaches.

Treatment

A. Episodic tension headaches

1. Usually treated by patients without the input of a physician.

2. Simple analgesics (acetaminophen or nonsteroidal antiinflammatory drugs [NSAIDs]) are the basis of most treatment.

3. For more severe headaches, combinations that include caffeine or codeine can be used.

4. In patients with frequent, but still episodic tension headaches, efforts at stress reduction are helpful.

B. Chronic tension headaches

1. These are often quite difficult to treat especially if they have been caused by medication overuse.

2. One of the first interventions in treating chronic tension headaches should almost always be "detoxification" from the patient's regimen of pain medications.

   a. Long-term use of many headache medications has the potential to cause or exacerbate chronic tension headaches.

   b. The most common culprit medications are ergotamine, NSAIDs, caffeine, and opioids.

   c. Detoxification can be difficult and occasionally requires hospitalization.

3. While all previous medications are being withdrawn, the addition of tricyclic antidepressants (TCAs) and stress management, either alone or in combination, are effective.

   a. TCAs work faster than stress management.

   b. Even a combination of both TCAs and stress management only reduce headache frequency and severity by about 50%.

Alternative Diagnosis: Cluster Headaches

Textbook Presentation

Cluster headaches are severe headaches that occur in young men, often beginning in their 20s. The headache is unilateral, usually occurring around the eye or temporal region and is associated with ipsilateral conjunctival injection, lacrimation, nasal congestion, or rhinorrhea. Sufferers are often restless during attacks.

Disease Highlights

A. The prevalence of cluster headaches is about 0.1%. They occur more commonly in men (4:1).

B. The headaches are unilateral, severe, and are associated with autonomic findings related to both parasympathetic overactivity and sympathetic underactivity.

C. Cluster headaches are generally brief, lasting from 15 minutes for 3 hours.

D. The headaches occur in clusters with frequent headaches occurring for 6–12 weeks before a headache-free period.

Evidence-Based Diagnosis

A. Classic cluster headaches present in a memorable, stereotypical way.

B. The IHS criteria for a cluster headache are:

1. The patient must have at least 5 attacks.

2. The headache must last 15–180 minutes; be severe; and be characterized by unilateral pain that is orbital, supraorbital, or temporal.

3. The headache is accompanied by at least 1 of the following:

   a. Ipsilateral conjunctival injection and/or lacrimation

   b. Ipsilateral nasal congestion and/or rhinorrhea

   c. Ipsilateral eyelid edema

   d. Ipsilateral forehead and facial sweating

   e. Ipsilateral miosis and/or ptosis

   f. A sense of restlessness or agitation

4. Attacks occur anywhere from every other day to 8/day during a cluster.

Treatment

A. Treatment for cluster headaches is similar to the treatment for migraines in that one may use either acute abortive therapies or prophylactic therapies.

B. Abortive therapy

1. High-flow oxygen is the treatment with the least side effects and best evidence base.

2. Triptans, similar to those used in the treatment of migraines, are also effective.

C. Prophylactic therapy

1. Verapamil is usually considered the first-line therapy for preventing cluster headaches.

2. Corticosteroids and topiramate have also been used successfully.

Alternative Diagnosis: Headache due to Unruptured CNS Aneurysm

Textbook Presentation

The classic presentation of a headache caused by a CNS aneurysm is a unilateral and throbbing headache that is new in a middle-aged patient.

Disease Highlights

A. CNS aneurysm may present in 3 ways.

1. Asymptomatic detection: This commonly occurs when a patient has a ruptured aneurysm and another, nonruptured aneurysm is found during the evaluation.

2. Acute rupture or expansion (discussed later in the chapter)

3. Chronic headache

B. The studies of the chronic headaches caused by unruptured aneurysms are, by their nature, somewhat flawed since they must be retrospective.

Evidence-Based Diagnosis

A. The headaches of unruptured aneurysms are nonspecific.

1. One study looked retrospectively at the symptoms of 111 patients referred for therapy of unruptured aneurysms; 54 of the patients had symptoms referable to the aneurysm at the time of diagnosis.

2. Of the 54 patients with symptoms, 35 (65%) had chronic symptoms.

3. In 18 of these 35 patients, the chronic symptom was headache without other neurologic signs.

4. Patient's headaches were divided equally between unilateral and bilateral.

B. Neuroimaging

1. CT angiography and magnetic resonance angiography are very sensitive means of detecting CNS aneurysms.

   a. Sensitivity for aneurysms > 1 cm in diameter is probably 100%.

   b. Sensitivity for all aneurysms is lower (62% for CT and 45% for MRI).

      (1) Aneurysms < 1 cm can, rarely, cause symptoms. These symptoms may include chronic headaches.

      (2) Repair of aneurysms < 1 cm in a patient who has not had a previous rupture is generally not recommended since the rupture rates are so low.

2. Traditional angiography

   a. Considered the gold standard for diagnosis

   b. Usually required prior to repair

   c. There are case reports of small aneurysms being missed on traditional angiography and being seen on CT and magnetic resonance angiography.

Treatment

A. The treatment of CNS aneurysms can be accomplished with neurosurgical or endovascular procedures.

B. Management decisions are difficult in a patient with a small aneurysm and a suspicious headache because there is no definitive way to know whether the aneurysm is causing the headache prior to surgery.

Because the quality of Mr. M's headaches had not changed at all, the decision was made not to image his brain. He was given long-acting propranolol at 80 mg/day as a prophylactic medication and prescribed oral sumatriptan to be used as needed as abortive therapy. At a 1-month follow-up, the patient reported only a single mild headache for which he used ibuprofen.

CASE RESOLUTION

The decision to forgo imaging was difficult. Although the likelihood of finding another cause of headaches was small, the frequency of the patient's headaches had changed. His complete response to migraine prophylaxis is diagnostic.

CHIEF COMPLAINT

PATIENT 2

Mrs. L is a 65-year-old woman who comes to an outpatient clinic complaining of headaches. She reports waking up almost every morning with a moderate to severe, bitemporal headache. She reports never having headaches of any consequence in the past but has been quite troubled for the last 2 months.

At this point, what is the leading hypothesis, what are the active alternatives, and is there a must not miss diagnosis? Given this differential diagnosis, what tests should be ordered?

RANKING THE DIFFERENTIAL DIAGNOSIS

Mrs. L's headaches are of concern because she is older and the headaches are new. Her age and the acuity of the headaches are pivotal features that limit the differential diagnosis. Both these features raise the likelihood that the headaches are secondary and, therefore, potentially dangerous. Morning headaches are classically associated with brain tumors. Edema forms around the CNS lesion while the patient is supine at night leading to headaches from increased intracranial pressure in the morning. Further history is needed, as brain tumors are most likely in patients with other types of cancer.

Morning headaches are also a fairly common symptom of many habits, diseases, and exposures. Headaches associated with substances or their withdrawals are a common cause of morning headaches. Alcohol, caffeine, and carbon monoxide are probably the most common. Morning headaches are frequently the symptoms of diseases that are active at night or that disturb sleep. Nighttime hypoglycemia and obstructive sleep apnea (OSA) are common causes of headaches in this category. Tension headaches should always be in the differential of headaches and may, on occasion, cause morning headaches.

The presence of a new, bitemporal headache in an older patient should raise the possibility of temporal arteritis. Although these headaches are not classically morning headaches, they should still be considered. Temporal arteritis will be discussed later in the chapter. Table 20-5 lists the differential diagnosis.

 Even more than with most headaches, a careful history is necessary in a patient with morning headaches.

Table 20-5. Diagnostic hypotheses for Mrs. L.

Diagnostic Hypotheses	Demographics, Risk Factors, Symptoms and Signs	Important Tests
Leading Hypothesis		
Brain tumor	History of malignancy Focal neurologic deficit	CNS imaging
Active Alternatives		
Substance exposure or withdrawal	*Caffeine:* Worst when sleeping late, often worst on vacations or weekends	Response to caffeine
	Alcohol: Occurs following intoxication	Relation to alcohol use
	Carbon monoxide poisoning: Headache that occurs in an exposed cohort and resolves upon leaving site of exposure	Carboxyhemoglobin levels
Morning headaches as symptoms of other diseases	*Nighttime hypoglycemia:* Most common in diabetics with recent medication or diet changes	2 AM glucose level
	Obstructive sleep apnea: Obesity and daytime somnolence	Polysomnogram
Tension headaches	Chronic, pressure-type headache of mild to moderate intensity	Diagnostic criteria and exclusion of secondary headaches
Temporal arteritis	Throbbing headache Symptoms of polymyalgia rheumatica Temporal artery abnormalities (such as prominence, tenderness, beading)	Erythrocyte sedimentation rate Temporal artery biopsy

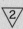

Mrs. L reports otherwise feeling well. She says the headaches occur nearly every morning, irrespective of day of the week or whether she has slept at home or at her weekend house. She denies neurologic symptoms such as focal numbness, weakness, or visual disturbances. She denies snoring or excessive daytime somnolence. She read on an Internet site that new-onset, morning headaches are classic for brain tumors and she is very nervous.

Her medical history is notable only for noninsulin-dependent diabetes mellitus, which has always been under good control. She reports no recent change in her diet, weight, or medication.

Medications are 325 mg/day of aspirin, 10 mg/day orally of atorvastatin, and 5 mg of oral glyburide taken twice daily.

 Is the clinical information sufficient to make a diagnosis? If not, what other information do you need?

Many patients seeking care for a headache believe they have a brain tumor. It is important to recognize this—a little definitive reassurance can go a long way.

Leading Hypothesis: Intracranial Neoplasms

Textbook Presentation

Brain tumors classically present with progressive morning headaches associated with focal neurologic deficits.

Disease Highlights

A. Brain tumors are classified as metastatic, primary extra-axial, and primary intra-axial.

B. The relative frequency of types of tumors within each type are listed below:
1. Metastatic
   a. Lung, 37%
   b. Breast, 19%
   c. Melanoma, 16%
2. Primary extra-axial
   a. Meningioma, 80%
   b. Acoustic neuroma, 10%
   c. Pituitary adenoma, 7%
3. Primary intra-axial
   a. Glioblastoma, 47%
   b. Astrocytoma, 39%

C. Metastatic tumors are about 7 times more common than primary tumors. Thus, a patient with known malignancy and new headaches should undergo imaging.

D. Intracranial neoplasms generally present with seizure, focal neurologic signs, or signs of increased intracranial pressure such as headache.

E. Although the presenting symptoms vary with type of tumor, the most common symptoms are:
1. Headache (about 50% of the time)
2. Seizure

3. Hemiparesis

4. Change in mental status

Evidence-Based Diagnosis

A. History

1. The history of a patient's headache is not particularly helpful in making a diagnosis of intracranial neoplasms.

2. One very good report retrospectively studied 111 patients with brain tumors. The symptoms were nonspecific.

   a. Only 48% of patients had headaches.

   b. Only 17% had classic brain tumor headache (defined as severe, worse in the morning and associated with nausea and vomiting).

   c. 77% of patients met the criteria for tension headaches.

   d. 9% of patients had migraine-like headaches.

   e. The most common qualities were

      (1) Intermittent, 62%

      (2) Frontal, 68%

      (3) Bilateral, 72%

Brain tumor headaches are nonspecific. A patient with a new headache and a preexisting cancer that could potentially metastasize to the CNS should undergo imaging.

B. Neuroimaging

1. Contrast-enhanced CT

   a. A reasonable choice for screening patients in whom there is a low suspicion.

   b. The sensitivity of a contrast-enhanced CT for intracranial neoplasm is around 90%.

2. MRI with contrast is the procedure of choice for imaging brain tumors. The sensitivity of MRI is nearly 100%, and the detail provided often suggests a likely pathology.

Treatment

A. The treatment of brain tumors depends on the pathology.

B. Importantly, patients with signs of increased intracranial pressure or seizure should be hospitalized immediately enabling both rapid diagnosis and treatment.

MAKING A DIAGNOSIS

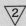

Mrs. L's physical exam, including a detailed neurologic exam, is normal. Laboratory tests done on the day of the visit revealed a normal CBC, normal chem-7, and a glycosylated Hgb of 5.9% (down from 7% 3 months earlier). A noncontrast head CT done on the day of the visit was normal. The patient was asked to set her alarm and check a finger-stick glucose at 2 AM. Her reading was 42 mg/dL.

Have you crossed a diagnostic threshold for the leading hypothesis, intracranial neoplasms? Have you ruled out the active alternatives? Do other tests need to be done to exclude the alternative diagnoses?

Given that intracranial neoplasms are rare in patients without preexisting cancers and the presence of morning headaches is a nonspecific finding, it is unlikely that the patient has a brain tumor. The noncontrast head CT was probably a reasonable test to do. Although it is not as sensitive as a contrast-enhanced study, with the low pretest probability it effectively rules out a tumor and, given the patient's concern, it was an effective method of calming her.

After the normal CT and unrevealing laboratory test results, attention must be turned to possible exposures or the "medical morning headaches." The patient's marked drop in her glycosylated Hgb and early morning hypoglycemia are suggestive of a diagnosis.

Alternative Diagnosis: Morning Headaches as Symptoms of Other Diseases

Textbook Presentation

Various diseases can cause headaches that occur predominantly in the morning. The headaches are generally worst upon awakening and then improve as the day progresses. Classically, the more common symptoms of the underlying disease (daytime hypoglycemia with overly controlled diabetes mellitus or daytime somnolence with OSA) are present.

Disease Highlights

A. The most rigorously defined morning headaches are those caused by disturbed sleep. The sleep disturbance can be of almost any etiology.

1. Primary sleep disturbance

   a. OSA

   b. Periodic leg movement of sleep (PLMS)

2. Abnormal sleep duration

   a. Excessive sleep

   b. Interrupted sleep

   c. Sleep deprivation

3. Secondary to another disease

   a. Chronic pain

   b. Depression

B. Hypoglycemia that occurs while asleep or awake can cause headaches.

Evidence-Based Diagnosis

A. The attribution of morning headaches to another disease depends on recognition of the underlying disease, its treatment, and the response of the presenting headache.

B. Recognition of the OSA and nighttime hypoglycemia can be difficult since clinical clues are nonspecific.

1. Nighttime hypoglycemia should be considered in any patient treated for diabetes with morning headaches. Abnormal nocturnal glucose readings and resolution of headaches with achievement of euglycemia are diagnostic.

2. Clinical predictors of OSA are poor (See Chapter 18, Fatigue). Polysomnography is diagnostic and will also provide information about PLMS and, sometimes, insomnia related to chronic pain.

A sleep study is a reasonable diagnostic test in a patient with morning headaches and no readily apparent cause.

Treatment

The treatment of medical morning headaches depends on the cause.

A. Nighttime hypoglycemia: improved management of diabetes mellitus

B. OSA: Continuous positive airway pressure

C. PLMS: Carbidopa and levodopa

D. Pain syndromes: Improved pain control

Alternative Diagnosis: Headaches Associated with Substances or Their Withdrawal

Textbook Presentation

These are headaches that occur in close temporal relation to substance exposure or substance withdrawal. They resolve when the culprit substance is no longer used.

Disease Highlights

A. Many substances can cause headaches acutely, with long-term use, or after their withdrawal.

   1. Acute exposure

      a. Nitrites ("hot dog headache")

      b. MSG ("Chinese restaurant syndrome")

      c. Carbon monoxide

   2. Long-term exposure (analgesics)

   3. Withdrawal from acute exposure (alcohol)

   4. Withdrawal from chronic exposure

      a. Caffeine

      b. Opioids

      c. Multiple other medications including estrogen, corticosteroids, TCAs, selective serotonin reuptake inhibitors, and NSAIDs.

B. Of these headaches, caffeine withdrawal, hangovers, and carbon monoxide poisoning are probably the most common or important causes of morning headaches.

Evidence-Based Diagnosis

A. Caffeine withdrawal headaches

   1. The IHS criteria require that:

      a. Patients have a headache that is bilateral or pulsating or both.

      b. Patients drink ≥ 200 mg of caffeine daily for > 2 weeks.

      c. The headaches occur within 24 hours of the last caffeine intake and are relieved within 1 hour by 100 mg of caffeine.

      d. That the headache resolves within 7 days of total caffeine withdrawal.

   2. An average cup of coffee contains about 100 mg of caffeine.

   3. Premium coffees may contain significantly more. A 12-oz coffee at Starbucks contains 260 mg of caffeine.

   4. The average adult American ingests approximately 280 mg of caffeine each day.

   5. Caffeine withdrawal should be suspected if headaches seem to occur when coffee intake changes, such as on weekends and during vacations.

 Caffeine withdrawal should be considered when headaches occur when patients sleep later than usual or occur mainly on weekends or vacations.

B. Carbon monoxide poisoning

   1. Presentation runs the spectrum from mild headache to headache with nausea, vomiting, and anxiety to coma and cardiovascular collapse.

   2. Historical features that increase the suspicion of this diagnosis.

      a. A patient's headache only occurs in a single location and resolves when the patient is removed from this setting.

      b. Multiple family members or roommates have similar symptoms.

      c. Carbon monoxide poisoning is most common in the winter.

   3. An elevated carboxyhemoglobin level makes the diagnosis. Routine arterial blood gas measurements and pulse oximetry do not detect carbon monoxide poisoning.

 Because carbon monoxide poisoning is potentially life-threatening, the diagnosis should be considered whenever a patient has a potentially consistent history.

Treatment

A. Treatment of headaches associated with substances or their withdrawal depends on the substance.

B. Patients with headaches from carbon monoxide poisoning should be removed from their house while the source is repaired.

C. Patients with caffeine withdrawal headaches should either be weaned off caffeine or counseled on the need to continue regular use (an option generally preferred by medical students).

CASE RESOLUTION

A tentative diagnosis of morning headaches due to nocturnal hypoglycemia was made. The patient was advised not to take the evening dose of glyburide; her headaches resolved the next day. At her next visit, the patient's medications were inspected. The label on the bottle was correct, but inspection of the pills revealed that 10-mg pills had been mistakenly dispensed, doubling her dose.

Adverse effects of medications are common. Although most commonly intrinsic to the medication, they can also be related to inappropriate prescribing or incorrect dispensing.

CHIEF COMPLAINT

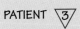

PATIENT

Mr. J is a 27-year-old man who arrives at his primary care physician's office complaining of a headache. He has a long history of mild tension-type headaches managed with acetaminophen. Three days ago, a severe headache suddenly developed while he was weight lifting. He describes this headache as the "worst headache of his life." The headache slowly resolved over about 2 hours. He is now feeling completely well. He has been afraid to exercise since this headache.

At this point, what is the leading hypothesis, what are the active alternatives, and is there a must not miss diagnosis? Given this differential diagnosis, what tests should be ordered?

RANKING THE DIFFERENTIAL DIAGNOSIS

Both the acuity and severity of this headache are worrisome and pivotal. The onset during exercise is also concerning. This type of headache, one that begins at its peak intensity, is referred to as a thunderclap headache.

Limiting the differential based on the pivotal points of the headache being new and of hyperacute onset, SAH is the leading hypothesis and must not miss diagnosis. His designation of the headache as the "worst headache of his life" is classic for SAH, although the resolution of the pain is not typical. Other headaches can present in similar fashion. Benign thunderclap headache is a rare headache syndrome that is clinically indistinguishable from SAH. Headaches due to cough, exertion, and sexual activity are primary headache syndromes that may mimic SAH. A parenchymal hemorrhage is possible but unlikely given the patient's age and absence of a history of hypertension.

There are some rare diseases that can occasionally present with a thunderclap headache; these include cerebral venous sinus thrombosis, pituitary apoplexy, carotid dissection, and spontaneous intracranial hypotension from cerebrospinal fluid (CSF) leaks. Table 20-6 lists the differential diagnosis.

Table 20-6. Diagnostic hypotheses for Mr. J.

Diagnostic Hypotheses	Demographics, Risk Factors, Symptoms and Signs	Important Tests
Leading Hypothesis		
Subarachnoid hemorrhage (SAH)	"Worst headache of life" Acute onset	Noncontrast head CT scan Lumbar puncture
Active Alternatives		
Cough, exertional, and sexual headaches	Acute headaches associated with cough, exertion, or sexual activity	History CNS imaging
Benign thunderclap headaches	Indistinguishable from SAH	Noncontrast head CT scan Lumbar puncture
Intracerebral hemorrhage	Headache with focal neurologic signs	Noncontrast head CT scan

 A headache that starts abruptly and is reaches its maximal severity within seconds (a thunderclap headache) should be assumed to be caused by a SAH until proven otherwise.

Mr. J's past medical history is notable only for mild asthma for which he uses albuterol as needed.

On physical exam, he appears well and not in any distress. His vital signs are temperature, 36.9°C; pulse, 82 bpm; BP, 112/82 mm Hg; RR, 14 breaths per minute. His neck is supple and detailed neurologic exam is also normal.

 Is the clinical information sufficient to make a diagnosis? If not, what other information do you need?

Leading Hypothesis: SAH

Textbook Presentation

A middle-aged patient experiences "the worst headache of his life." Soon after the headache begins, the patient vomits and develops neck pain and stiffness. Patients may also lose consciousness. If the patient is alert at the time of medical assessment, focal neurologic signs and meningismus may be present on the physical exam.

Disease Highlights

A. SAH is primarily caused by rupture of a saccular aneurysm in or near the circle of Willis (≈ 85%).

B. Aneurysms are present in about 7% of the population.

C. Large aneurysms (> 1 cm) rupture at a rate of about 0.5%/year.

D. The vast majority of ruptures occur in persons 40–65 years old.

E. SAH carries a mortality of about 50%.

F. It is generally accepted that anywhere from 10% to 50% of patients will have a warning or sentinel headache in the weeks preceding the SAH.

1. Likely caused by the expansion of, or a small leak from, an aneurysm.

2. This headache is usually the same sort of abrupt onset (thunderclap) headache as SAH but resolves within 24 hours.

3. About 50% of patients with warning headaches actually seek medical care at the time of the headache.

Evidence-Based Diagnosis

A. Pretest probability

1. SAH accounts for 1–4% of headaches presenting to the emergency department.

2. Among headaches presenting to the emergency department, SAH accounts for

a. 12% of patients with the "worst headache of my life"

b. 25% of patients with the "worst headache of my life" and neurologic findings

3. The following findings are common in patients in whom SAH is ultimately diagnosed. (Prevalence figures are estimates from 2 large studies.)

a. Headache, 90%

b. In patients presenting with headache, 82.4% report a thunderclap headache, and 99.2% reported the worst headache of their life.

    c. Stiff neck, 75%

    d. Change in mental status, 60%

    e. Stupor or coma, 27%

B. Diagnostic tests

  1. The initial diagnostic test is a noncontrast head CT. The sensitivity of this test varies with the time since the onset of symptoms.

    a. First 12 hours, 97%

    b. 12–24 hours, 93%

    c. Falls to as low as 80% after 2 weeks.

  2. Next to angiography, CSF examination for RBCs and xanthochromia (the result of first oxyhemoglobin and later bilirubin from deteriorating RBCs) is the most accurate diagnostic method.

    a. RBCs are seen immediately in the CSF in 100% of patients. The specificity, however, can be limited by traumatic lumbar punctures.

    b. Sensitivity of RBCs begins to fall after about 24 hours.

    c. Spectrophotometric detection of xanthochromia is 100% specific for SAH.

    d. Most experts suggest delaying the lumbar puncture for 6–12 hours after the onset of a headache (if clinically safe) in a patient with a suspicious headache and normal CT scan since it takes 12–24 hours for the sensitivity to reach nearly 100%.

    e. The sensitivity of xanthochromia remains at 100% for over 1 week.

  3. In all patients with documented SAH, angiography is performed to assist in surgical planning. Angiography might also be done for patients in whom the diagnosis is unclear even after lumbar puncture.

  4. There is less data for the use of MRI in the diagnosis of SAH. MRI maybe as sensitive as CT early in the course of disease and probably remains sensitive for longer.

  5. A recently derived decision rule suggests that SAH may be excluded in patients who arrive at the emergency department with acute nontraumatic headache that reached maximal intensity within 1 hour and who had normal neurologic exam findings if they lack the following findings:

    a. Age over 40 years

    b. Neck pain or stiffness or limited neck flexion on exam

    c. Witnessed loss of consciousness

    d. Onset during exercise

    e. Thunderclap headache

C. Importance of correct diagnosis

  1. About 25% of patients with SAH are initially misdiagnosed.

  2. Patients with less severe clinical presentations are most commonly misdiagnosed.

  3. Patients who are initially misdiagnosed are only about half as likely to have a good or excellent outcome.

 All patients in whom SAH is suspected should undergo a noncontrast head CT. If the CT is normal, a lumbar puncture should be performed in any patient with more than a minimal pretest probability.

Treatment

A. Prevention of rebleeding

  1. The primary treatment of a SAH is to occlude the culprit aneurysm to prevent rebleeding.

  2. This is usually accomplished by deploying platinum coils via arterial catheters within the aneurysm to cause occlusion.

  3. Neurosurgical clipping of aneurysms is now second-line therapy.

B. Prevention of cerebral vasospasm and resulting ischemia

  1. The cause of cerebral vasospasm is poorly understood but is predicted by size of the hemorrhage and loss of consciousness at the time of hemorrhage.

  2. Calcium antagonists, primarily nimodipine, decrease the risk of vasospasm.

C. Management of hydrocephalus

MAKING A DIAGNOSIS

The patient had a thunderclap headache that he describes as the worst headache of his life, which mandates urgent evaluation.

Mr. J is referred from clinic for a noncontrast head CT. The results are normal.

 Have you crossed a diagnostic threshold for the leading hypothesis, SAH? Have you ruled out the active alternatives? Do other tests need to be done to exclude the alternative diagnoses?

Alternative Diagnoses: Primary Cough Headache, Primary Exertional Headache, & Headache Associated with Sexual Activity

Textbook Presentation

These headaches are primary headaches precipitated by cough, exertion (usually involving the Valsalva maneuver), and sexual activity. They may mimic SAH.

Disease Highlights

A. Cough headaches

  1. Most common in men (≈ 3:1)

  2. More common in older patients (mean age, 67)

  3. Last < 1 minute

B. Exertional headaches

  1. Most common in men (≈ 90%)

  2. Occurs in young people (mean age, 24)

  3. Often bilateral and throbbing

  4. Sometimes related to migraines (some patients may induce migraines with physical activity)

  5. Lasts from 5 minutes to 24 hours

C. Sexual headaches

  1. Also most common in men (≈ 85%)

  2. Mean age, 41

3. Lasts < 3 hours

4. Can occur as 3 types

   a. Dull type: dull headache worsening with sexual excitement

   b. Explosive type: SAH-like headache occurring at orgasm

   c. Postural type: postural headache developing after coitus

Evidence-Based Diagnosis

A. Although these headaches may be indistinguishable from more concerning headaches, the clinical presentation can sometimes help identify the diagnosis.

B. They should be considered when the headache starts with cough, sexual activity, or exercise.

C. One review suggested other distinguishing features.

1. Cough headaches

   a. Either represented the primary headache syndrome or symptoms of an Arnold-Chiari type I malformation in which the cerebellar tonsils protrude out of the base of the skull

   b. Those headaches lasting > 30 minutes were usually secondary to a Chiari type I malformation.

   c. Patients with Chiari type I malformations were younger than those with primary cough headaches (mean age, 39 vs 67).

2. Sexual headaches

   a. Almost always (93%) benign

   b. In this study, only 1 sexual headache was found to symptomatic of another disease. This headache was caused by a SAH.

   c. Patients with benign sexual headaches tended to have multiple episodes of the headache.

3. Exertional headaches

   a. Represent either the primary headache syndrome or secondary headaches (causes included SAH and brain tumor).

   b. The primary and secondary headaches were generally indistinguishable.

 Because exertional headaches are clinically indistinguishable from SAH, a patient presenting with such a headache must be carefully evaluated to rule out the latter.

Treatment

A. Cough headaches are effectively treated with cough suppression and NSAIDs.

B. Exertional headaches are treated by avoiding strenuous activity (especially in hot weather or at high altitudes) or by using preexertion ergotamine, beta-blockers, or NSAIDs.

C. Sexual headaches are effectively treated with prophylactic beta-blockers.

Alternative Diagnosis: Benign Thunderclap Headache

Textbook Presentation

The presentation of benign thunderclap headaches is indistinguishable from SAH. The diagnosis is made after normal results are obtained on CT scan and lumbar puncture. These headaches occasionally recur in an unpredictable way.

Disease Highlights

A. Primary headache syndrome

B. Clinically indistinguishable from SAH but lacks any associated neurologic symptoms or signs.

C. Headaches frequently recur over 1–2 weeks and then intermittently over years.

D. In the best study of these headaches:

1. SAH developed in none of the 71 patients studied.

2. Headaches generally lasted from 8 to 72 hours.

3. 51 (72%) of the patients had their headaches unrelated to cough, sexual activity, or exertion.

4. 17% of the patients had recurrent, similar headaches.

Evidence-Based Diagnosis

A. Benign thunderclap headaches are diagnosed when there is a suspicious clinical presentation and SAH is ruled out.

B. Given the poor prognosis of SAH, CT scan and lumbar puncture should be performed in all patients prior to making this diagnosis.

 Because benign thunderclap headaches are clinically indistinguishable from SAH, they can only be diagnosed after SAH has been ruled out.

Treatment

A. Treatment is challenging because these headaches are short-lived and very intermittent.

B. As-needed analgesics are probably the only reasonable therapy.

Alternative Diagnosis: Intracerebral Hemorrhage

Textbook Presentation

Intracerebral hemorrhage (hemorrhagic stroke) generally presents in older, hypertensive patients with acute-onset headache and focal neurologic symptoms and signs.

Disease Highlights

A. Intracerebral hemorrhage accounts for about 10% of strokes, being less common than embolic and thrombotic strokes.

B. Hypertension is the most common cause, followed by amyloid angiopathy, saccular aneurysm rupture, and arteriovenous malformation rupture.

C. Among patients with hypertension, Asians and blacks have the highest risk of hemorrhagic cerebrovascular accidents.

D. The incidence of hypertension-related intracerebral hemorrhage has declined over the last 3 decades with better control of hypertension.

E. In young patients without hypertension, diseases such as arteriovenous malformation, aneurysm rupture, and drug use should be considered.

F. Arteriovenous malformations are present in 0.01% to 0.05% of the population and usually present in persons between the ages of 20 and 40 years.

1. Presentation may be with hemorrhage, seizure, or headache.

2. About 50% of patients with arteriovenous malformation present with a hemorrhagic event. Patients with hypertension or a previous hemorrhage have the highest rate of bleeding.

Evidence-Based Diagnosis

A. Patients with intracerebral hemorrhage usually have headache and focal neurologic signs.

B. A thunderclap-type headache is the presenting sign in nearly 60% of patients.

C. Vomiting is present in about 50% of patients, and seizures are present in about 10%.

D. Noncontrast CT and MRI are equally accurate in making this diagnosis with sensitivities of nearly 100%. MRI may be better at detecting hemorrhagic transformation of ischemic strokes.

Treatment

See the Treatment section under Cerebellar Hemorrhage in Chapter 14, Dizziness.

CASE RESOLUTION

> Given the acute-onset during exercise, the normal neurologic exam, and the lack of symptoms during the intervening
>
> *(continued)*

3 days, the patient was thought to have primary exertional headache. A sentinel headache, preceding a SAH, however, was a must not miss alternative. Given this, the patient underwent lumbar puncture that revealed no RBCs and no xanthochromia. He subsequently experienced a similar headache 2 weeks later with exercise. He was then treated with preexercise propranolol with good response.

This patient received the appropriate evaluation. Although he was feeling well at the time of the visit, the test threshold for SAH needs to be very low given the severity of disease. SAH tends to be misdiagnosed in patients with the mildest symptoms. This is because the physician's suspicion is lowest in these patients and probably because the CT scan may be less sensitive in people with presumably small hemorrhages. Accurate diagnosis of these patients is highly desirable as they potentially have the best outcomes.

With a normal CT scan and lumbar puncture, the diagnosis becomes either benign thunderclap headache or benign exertional headache. The difference is likely semantic, but the headache's onset and recurrence during exercise makes benign exertional headache the diagnosis. Intracerebral bleed from an arteriovenous malformation was a possibility but was ruled out with the normal CT scan.

CHIEF COMPLAINT

> **PATIENT 4**
>
> Mrs. T is an 80-year-old woman who comes to your office complaining of headaches for the past 3 months. She reports always having had mild headaches that never troubled her enough to see a doctor. This headache has been persistent, bilateral, band-like, and throbbing.
>
> At her present visit, she reports no visual changes, no recent head trauma, and no neurologic deficits. She does report fatigue and says that she has lost about 15 lbs over the last month. She denies jaw symptoms.
>
> Her past medical history is notable for hypertension for which she takes losartan, morbid obesity, and a breast mass noted 2 years before. The mass was thought to be low suspicion for malignancy and the patient declined work-up.

At this point, what is the leading hypothesis, what are the active alternatives, and is there a must not miss diagnosis? Given this differential diagnosis, what tests should be ordered?

RANKING THE DIFFERENTIAL DIAGNOSIS

This presentation is of concern because the patient is elderly, she has a new headache, and she has experienced weight loss. The differential diagnosis must take into account these pivotal points of age, subacute onset, and constitutional symptoms. The persistence of the headache probably excludes diagnoses such as intracerebral hemorrhage or infections. As we explore the limited differential diagnosis for this patient, the patient's gender and obesity are important.

Temporal arteritis and malignancy are both possible given the patient's age and subacute presentation. The throbbing nature of the pain and weight loss could certainly be consistent with either of these types of headache. The history of a breast mass has to make metastatic disease a real consideration. Subdural hematoma is possible, but the lack of a history of head trauma or use of anticoagulation medications makes this less likely. Although a diagnosis of tension headaches should be given with extreme caution in an elderly person with new headaches, the persistent band-like description raises this possibility. A new headache in a woman with obesity also raises the possibility of idiopathic intracranial hypertension. This disease is more commonly seen in young women. Table 20-7 lists the differential diagnosis.

> **4**
>
> Soon after the headache began (3 months prior to her current presentation), she went to an emergency department and cervical osteoarthritis was diagnosed. She was given ibuprofen, muscle relaxants, and a referral to a rheumatologist. She saw the rheumatologist about 2 weeks later. An ESR done at that visit was 56 mm/h.

Is the clinical information sufficient to make a diagnosis? If not, what other information do you need?

Table 20-7. Diagnostic hypotheses for Mrs. T.

Diagnostic Hypotheses	Demographics, Risk Factors, Symptoms and Signs	Important Tests
Leading Hypothesis		
Temporal arteritis	Throbbing headache Symptoms of polymyalgia rheumatica Temporal artery abnormalities (such as prominence, tenderness, beading)	Erythrocyte sedimentation rate Temporal artery biopsy
Active Alternative—Most Common		
Tension headache	Chronic, pressure-type headache of mild to moderate intensity	Diagnostic criteria and exclusion of secondary headaches
Active Alternatives		
Brain tumor	History of malignancy Focal neurologic deficit	CNS imaging
Idiopathic intracranial hypertension	Severe headache Female gender Obesity	Papilledema Exclusion of secondary causes of intracranial hypertension
Other Alternative		
Subdural hematoma	Elderly patients with a history of falls or anticoagulation	Noncontrast head CT scan

Leading Hypothesis: Temporal Arteritis

Textbook Presentation

Temporal arteritis classically presents in white women over age 50 as a bilateral, throbbing headache. Jaw pain and fatigue with chewing (jaw claudication) may be present. There may be a history of polymyalgia rheumatica or consistent symptoms (shoulder and hip girdle pain) and the physical exam can reveal beading and tenderness of the temporal arteries. The erythrocyte sedimentation rate (ESR) is usually elevated.

Disease Highlights

A. Temporal (or giant cell) arteritis is a corticosteroid-responsive vasculitis of large arteries.

B. Primarily involves the vessels of the aortic arch, particularly the external carotid.

C. Affects people over age 50, women more commonly than men.

D. D. Although the most common presentation is a new headache, temporal arteritis can present with nonspecific manifestations of a chronic inflammatory disorder.

1. Fever

2. Anemia

3. Fatigue

4. Weight loss

5. Elevated ESR or C-reactive protein

Temporal arteritis is in the differential diagnosis for older people presenting with nonspecific inflammatory conditions.

E. It can also present with specific complications of the disease.

1. Jaw claudication

2. Blindness (secondary to ophthalmic artery vasculitis)

F. Related to polymyalgia rheumatica

1. 15% of patients with polymyalgia rheumatica have temporal arteritis.

2. As many as 40% of patients with temporal arteritis have polymyalgia rheumatica.

G. Rapid diagnosis and treatment are critical to prevent vasculitis-associated thrombosis in the effected vessels.

Evidence-Based Diagnosis

A. Clinical findings

1. The clinical signs and symptoms of temporal arteritis are not highly predictive.

2. Two systematic reviews presented test characteristics for many of the commonly cited findings. These are outlined in Table 20-8.

3. A few combinations of signs and symptoms have been found to have very high positive LRs.

a. Headache and jaw claudication: LR+ 8.0

b. Scalp tenderness and jaw claudication: LR+ 17.0

4. Reflecting the poor performance of clinical predictors, only 30–40% of patients referred for temporal artery biopsy have the disease.

Because the clinical signs and symptoms of temporal arteritis are not highly predictive, temporal artery biopsy should be used in any patient in whom the clinical suspicion is even moderate.

B. B. ESR has been used to "rule out" temporal arteritis.

1. The sensitivity of an abnormal ESR is 96–99%.

2. The test characteristics of the ESR at various cut points are shown below. (A normal ESR is usually considered to be < age/2 in men and (age + 10)/2 in women.)

a. Abnormal: LR+, 1.1–1.2; LR–, 0.025–0.2

b. ESR > 50 mm/h: LR+, 1.2; LR–, 0.35

c. ESR > 100 mm/h: LR+, 1.9; LR–, 0.8

Table 20-8. Positive LRs for signs and symptoms of temporal arteritis.

Symptom or Sign	LR+
Jaw claudication	4.2–6.7
Diplopia	3.4–3.5
Beaded temporal artery	4.6
Enlarged temporal artery	4.3
Scalp tenderness	3.0
Temporal artery tenderness	2.6
Any temporal artery abnormality	2.0

C. Temporal artery ultrasound
1. Ultrasound has been used as a diagnostic tool.
2. Inflamed arteries have a hypoechoic halo around the lumen.
3. Most studies have found this finding to be insensitive and not specific enough to avoid biopsy.

D. Temporal artery biopsy
1. Considered the gold standard for diagnosing temporal arteritis.
2. Given the difficulty of clinically diagnosing temporal arteritis and the common side effects of the treatment, temporal artery biopsy is always recommended to establish the diagnosis of temporal arteritis.
3. Although biopsy should be done as quickly as possible once the disease is suspected, a short delay after beginning treatment (≈ 7 days) probably does not affect the results.

 Treatment of temporal arteritis should not be delayed to perform a biopsy in a patient in whom temporal arteritis is suspected.

4. Biopsy of a palpably abnormal artery is the most accurate. If the artery is palpably normal, longer and bilateral biopsies are useful.
5. There are cases of biopsy-negative temporal arteritis. One much quoted study gave the following test characteristics for temporal artery biopsy:
   a. Sensitivity, 85%; specificity, 100%
   b. LR+, ∞ LR–, 0.15

 Even in the setting of a negative temporal artery biopsy, a patient with very high suspicion for temporal arteritis should be monitored closely or treated.

Treatment

A. The treatment of temporal arteritis is corticosteroids.
1. Should be started immediately in a patient in whom temporal arteritis is suspected.
2. Can be tapered slowly once there has been clinical remission as long as the inflammatory markers (ESR, C-reactive protein) remain depressed.

B. Methotrexate might be an option in patients who have recurrent disease upon withdrawal of corticosteroids.

MAKING A DIAGNOSIS

Physical exam is notable for vital signs of temperature, 37.1°C; BP, 130/82 mm Hg; pulse, 72 bpm; RR, 10 breaths per minute. Head and neck exam revealed prominence of the temporal arteries. Cataracts limited the fundoscopic examination. Heart, lung, and abdominal exams were normal. Breast exam revealed a 2 × 3 cm mass in the left breast that was soft and freely mobile, which seemed unchanged from a description in the patient's chart from 2 years earlier. Extremity exam was notable for bruises over her left elbow and shoulder from a fall. Neurologic exam is fully intact.

 Have you crossed a diagnostic threshold for the leading hypothesis, temporal arteritis? Have you ruled out the active alternatives? Do other tests need to be done to exclude the alternative diagnoses?

Temporal arteritis certainly remains high on the differential diagnosis. Her headache and physical exam are both suspicious. Assuming a pretest probability of 40% (the usual percentage of positive biopsies among people in whom temporal arteritis is suspected), the prominence of her temporal arteries (LR+ = 2) increases the likelihood of the diagnosis to 57%.

Alternative Diagnosis: Subdural Hematoma

Textbook Presentation

Subdural hematoma is usually seen in older patients with a history of falls and neurologic deterioration. The classic triad of symptoms of chronic subdural hematoma is headache, somnolence, and change in mental status.

Disease Highlights

A. Subdural hematomas may be acute (within 24 hours of injury), subacute (1–14 days after injury), or chronic.

B. Acute and subacute subdural hematomas generally pose little diagnostic problem. They usually produce evolving, focal neurologic deficits.

C. Chronic subdural hematomas can present with subtle symptoms, weeks to months after trauma and can pose a real diagnostic challenge.

D. Chronic subdural hematoma is a disease seen in the elderly and others with cerebral atrophy. Cerebral atrophy allows accommodation of a slowly expanding collection of blood in the subdural space.

E. Risk factors for subdural hematomas are frequent falls, alcoholic dependence, and use of anticoagulant medications such as warfarin or aspirin.

Evidence-Based Diagnosis

A. History and physical exam
1. Diagnosis requires a high index of suspicion because the presenting symptoms are often subtle.
2. The mean age at diagnosis is around 70 years in most studies.
3. The most common presenting symptoms are falls and progressive neurologic deficit.
4. Head trauma, transient neurologic deficit, seizure, and headache are not uncommon modes of presentation.
5. The absence of a trauma history should not be particularly reassuring as this history is often hard to establish.

 The most common presenting symptom of chronic subdural hematoma is a history of falls. A high index of suspicion should be present for subdural hematoma in any elderly patient with a history of falls and subacute neurologic deficits.

B. Neuroimaging
1. CT scan and MRI are both effective means of diagnosing acute subdural hematoma.
2. Caution should be used with noncontrast head CT scan because the blood in a chronic subdural hematoma can sometimes be isodense with cortical tissue.

Treatment

Chronic subdural hematomas are treated with surgical drainage unless they are small and asymptomatic.

Alternative Diagnosis: Idiopathic Intracranial Hypertension

Textbook Presentation

Patients tend to be young women who are obese. Headaches caused by idiopathic intracranial hypertension are severe, occur daily, and may awaken the patient from sleep. These types of headaches are associated with transient visual disturbances.

Disease Highlights

A. Idiopathic intracranial hypertension is frequently referred to as pseudotumor cerebri.

B. The characteristics of idiopathic intracranial hypertension were well described from a series of patients in the early 1990s.

   1. The disease tends to effect young (mean age around 30) woman (> 90%)

   2. Sufferers are overwhelmingly obese (94%).

   3. The headaches are usually severe, pulsatile, and often awaken people from sleep.

   4. Visual disturbances (usually lasting only seconds) and pulsatile tinnitus are also common.

C. The presence of papilledema is a very important finding in idiopathic intracranial hypertension. It is present in the overwhelming majority of cases.

D. Idiopathic intracranial hypertension carries the risk of permanent visual loss and must be diagnosed and treated.

Evidence-Based Diagnosis

A. The diagnosis of idiopathic intracranial hypertension is based on recognition of the headache syndrome, diagnosis of increased intracranial pressure, and exclusion of other causes of increased pressure.

B. The headache in idiopathic intracranial hypertension must occur daily, be diffuse and/or constant, or be aggravated by coughing.

C. Intracranial hypertension

   1. Generally first detected on a physical exam by the presence of papilledema, an enlarged blind spot, a visual field defect, or a sixth cranial nerve palsy.

   2. To make the diagnosed, intracranial hypertension must be demonstrated on lumbar puncture (> 200 mm H_2O in nonobese patients, > 250 mm H_2O in obese patients).

   3. Other causes of intracranial hypertension must be excluded.

      a. Neuroimaging (usually an MRI) must be done before the lumbar puncture.

      b. CSF studies must be normal.

      c. Other diseases that can cause intracranial hypertension with a normal MRI need to be excluded (use of growth hormone, tetracyclines, or hypervitaminosis A).

D. The headache must improve after lumbar puncture (with a postprocedure pressure of 120–170 mm H_2O) and resolve after treatment of idiopathic intracranial hypertension.

Treatment

A. Weight loss and carbonic anhydrase inhibitors, which reduce the rate of CSF production) are the mainstay of therapy.

B. Loop diuretics may be use as an adjunctive therapy.

C. Surgical procedures (CSF shunting procedures and optic nerve sheath fenestration) are rarely used for people with refractory disease.

Laboratory tests are done, and the patient is sent for a precontrast head CT to look for hemorrhage and a postcontrast study to increase the sensitivity for parenchymal lesions. The patient's test results follow: Hgb, 9.0 g/dL (11.7 g/dL 1 month earlier); HCT, 28.1% (36.6% 1 month earlier); ESR, 125 mm/h. The head CT was normal other than cerebral atrophy expected for the patient's age.

Mrs. T was given 60 mg of prednisone daily and referred for a temporal artery biopsy. This was done 3 days later and was diagnostic for temporal arteritis. Her headache improved after 1 week of therapy. Over the next 2 years, multiple attempts at weaning corticosteroids failed, and the patient continues to take 15 mg of prednisone. While taking prednisone, a spinal compression fracture, acne, diabetes mellitus, and difficult-to-control hypertension develop.

CASE RESOLUTION

The elevated ESR made the diagnosis of temporal arteritis likely but by no means certain. Taking the pretest probability of 57%, as it stood after the physical exam, an ESR > 100 mm/h raises the probability to 72%. This is probably not high enough to accept the side effects of long-term prednisone therapy without a more definitive diagnosis.

REVIEW OF OTHER IMPORTANT DISEASES

Meningitis

Textbook Presentation

Classically, meningitis presents with the acute onset of the triad of headache, fever, and a stiff neck. Meningitis may occur in the setting of a cluster of cases.

Disease Highlights

A. A. The presentation of fever and headache is common and can be worrisome, potentially caused by anything from influenza to meningitis. The differential includes:

   1. Viral infections and almost any other febrile illness

   2. Meningitis (bacterial, fungal, viral, or parasitic)

   3. Encephalitis

   4. Sinusitis

   5. CNS abscess

   6. Septic cavernous sinus thrombosis

B. Although certainly not the most common cause of fever and headache, meningitis is a relatively common, potentially life-threatening illness.

C. Viral causes are 3–4 times more common than bacterial causes and have a generally favorable prognosis.

D. Bacterial meningitis must be treated as a medical emergency.

E. Mortality rates vary by organism but community-acquired bacterial meningitis has a mortality rate of about 25%.

F. Mortality rates are higher for hospital-acquired infections.

G. The most common organisms are listed in Table 20-9.

Evidence-Based Diagnosis

A. A review studied patients in Holland in whom community-acquired bacterial meningitis was diagnosed over a 3 1/2 year time period; the prevalence of various exam features follow:

  1. 95% of patients had at least 2 of the findings of headache, fever, stiff neck, or mental status changes

    a. 87% had a headache

    b. 83% had stiff neck

    c. 77% had temperature > 38.0°C

    d. 69% had a change in mental status

  2. 33% had focal neurologic findings

  3. 34% of those who had imaging done had an abnormal CT scan

B. Patients with suppressed immune systems and the elderly are less likely to have a stiff neck.

  1. Two of the most commonly used meningeal signs are Kernig (the inability to extend the knee with a flexed hip) and Brudzinski (the demonstration of flexion of both the knees and hips upon forced flexion of the neck).

  2. These signs are present in only about 60% of patients with meningitis.

C. Lumbar puncture

  1. Lumbar puncture is the only means of making a definitive diagnosis.

  2. The CSF in acute bacterial meningitis will demonstrate WBCs with neutrophil predominance, low glucose, and high protein.

D. Patients with contraindications to lumbar puncture

  1. Frequently, the question of contraindication to lumbar puncture is raised.

  2. Performing a lumbar puncture in a patient with a CNS mass, elevated intracranial pressure, or a bleeding diathesis places the patient at risk for complications such as herniation, paraspinal hemorrhage, and death.

  3. CNS imaging should be performed before lumbar puncture in any patient in whom there is a suspicion of increased intracranial pressure.

  4. Findings associated with mass effect on CT scan are

    a. Age > 60 years

    b. Immunocompromise

    c. Preexisting CNS disease

    d. Seizure within the previous week

    e. Abnormal level of consciousness

    f. Inability to answer 2 consecutive questions or follow 2 consecutive commands correctly

    g. Gaze palsy, abnormal visual fields, facial palsy, arm or leg drift, aphasia

 Patients with an abnormal neurologic exam should undergo CNS imaging prior to lumbar puncture.

  5. If CNS imaging is required, a patient with suspected meningitis should have blood cultures drawn and then receive empiric antibiotics immediately, undergo a CT scan, and then have the lumbar puncture.

Treatment

A. As with all infectious diseases, the specific treatment depends on the pathogen.

B. Because of the severity of meningeal infections, empiric therapy is recommended while waiting for Gram stain and culture results.

C. Antibiotic treatment should be ordered when the diagnosis of meningitis is suspected and given immediately after CSF begins to be collected.

D. In adult patients with suspected community-acquired meningitis, the current recommendations are to treat empirically with a third-generation cephalosporin and vancomycin.

E. If *Listeria monocytogenes* is suspected, ampicillin is also added.

F. Corticosteroids should be added to the regimen in patients with a Glasgow coma scale ≥ 8. (Table 20-10).

Headaches Associated with Head Trauma

Textbook Presentation

A common presentation of a posttraumatic headache would be a middle-aged person who recently suffered head trauma, usually without detectable cranial or neurologic injury, with a headache similar in quality to tension headaches. The headaches are often associated with symptoms such as irritability or anxiety.

Disease Highlights

A. Head trauma can cause serious cranial or neurologic injury including subdural, epidural or parenchymal hematoma, SAH, cerebral contusion, or depressed skull fracture.

B. More commonly, head trauma can cause new headaches or worsen preexisting headache syndromes.

Table 20-9. Common causes of meningitis in adults.

Organism	Characteristics
Viruses	Enteroviruses (echovirus and coxsackievirus) most common More common in children than adults Summer and Fall predominance
Streptococcus pneumoniae	Most common bacterial meningitis in adults of all ages May occur de novo or by contiguous spread (sinuses, ears) Mortality rates ≈ 30%
Neisseria meningitidis	Second most common cause overall May occur in epidemics Most commonly seen in young adults Mortality rates ≈ 10%
Listeria monocytogenes	Disease of older adults (older than 60 years) and immunosuppressed (including patients with diabetes and alcohol abuse)
Haemophilus influenzae	Previously very common cause of meningitis in children; now rare because of vaccination

Table 20-10. The Glasgow Coma Scale.

	1	2	3	4	5	6
Eyes	Does not open eyes	Opens eyes in response to painful stimuli	Opens eyes in response to voice	Opens eyes spontaneously		
Verbal	Makes no sounds	Incomprehensible sounds	Utters inappropriate words	Confused, disoriented	Oriented, converses normally	
Motor	Makes no movements	Extension to painful stimuli (decerebrate response)	Abnormal flexion to painful stimuli (decorticate response)	Flexion/ withdrawal to painful stimuli	Localizes painful stimuli	Obeys commands

C. Trauma-related headaches might occur after minor or major trauma. The IHS requires 2 of the following to qualify as major trauma:

1. Loss of consciousness > 30 minutes
2. 45 minutes of posttraumatic amnesia
3. Objective measures of cranial or neurologic trauma

D. There appears to be a significant amount of psychiatric distress and disability associated with posttraumatic headaches.

Evidence-Based Diagnosis

A. Acute evaluation of head trauma

1. In a patient with head trauma or a headache seemingly associated with head trauma, the first goal is to identify important and potentially treatable injury.

2. The initial test is usually a head CT scan. A difficult question is who can be clinically cleared without a CT scan.

   a. Two clinical decision rules (The Canadian Head CT Rule and the Nexus II).

   b. Nexus II says that if none of the following signs are present, the patient does not need a head CT: Evidence of significant skull fracture, scalp hematoma, neurologic deficit, altered level of alertness, abnormal behavior, coagulopathy, persistent vomiting, age > 65.

   c. The Canadian Head CT Rule is referenced at the end of the chapter.

   d. Both rules have nearly 100% sensitivity for clinically important brain injuries and injuries requiring neurosurgical intervention.

B. Diagnosis of posttraumatic headaches

1. The next step is to diagnose ongoing headaches as posttraumatic.

2. The IHS classifies these headaches into headaches following minor or major trauma (see above) and into acute (occurs within 7 days of the injury and resolves within 3 months) or chronic (occurs within 7 days of the injury and does not resolve within 3 months).

3. Headache develops in about 25% of patients following minor trauma.

   a. These headaches are most likely to be chronic.

   b. They are also most likely to meet criteria for tension-type headaches.

Treatment

A. The treatment of posttraumatic headaches is generally similar to the treatment of clinically similar headaches.

B. It does appear that associated psychological treatment, such as biofeedback and treatment of associated posttraumatic stress syndrome, might be beneficial.

REFERENCES

Detsky ME, McDonald DR, Baerlocher MO, Tomlinson GA, McCrory DC, Booth CM. Does this patient with headache have a migraine or need neuroimaging? JAMA. 2006;296(10):1274–83.

Edlow JA, Caplan LR. Avoiding pitfalls in the diagnosis of subarachnoid hemorrhage. N Engl J Med. 2000;342(1):29–36.

Forsyth PA, Posner JB. Headaches in patients with brain tumors: a study of 111 patients. Neurology. 1993;43(9):1678–83.

Holroyd KA, O'Donnell FJ, Stensland M, Lipchik GL, Cordingley GE, Carlson BW. Management of chronic tension-type headache with tricyclic antidepressant medication, stress management therapy, and their combination: a randomized controlled trial. JAMA. 2001;285(17):2208–15.

Li MH, Chen SW, Li YD et al. Prevalence of unruptured cerebral aneurysms in Chinese adults aged 35 to 75 years: a cross-sectional study. Ann Intern Med. 2013;159:514–21.

Mower WR, Hoffman JR, Herbert M et al. Developing a decision instrument to guide computed tomographic imaging of blunt head injury patients. J Trauma. 2005;59(4):954–9.

Pascual J, Iglesias F, Oterino A, Vazquez-Barquero A, Berciano J. Cough, exertional, and sexual headaches: an analysis of 72 benign and symptomatic cases. Neurology. 1996;46(6):1520–4.

Perry JJ, Stiell IG, Sivlotti ML et al. Clinical decision rules to rule out subarachnoid hemorrhage for acute headache. JAMA. 2013;310(12):1248–55.

Raps EC, Rogers JD, Galetta SL et al. The clinical spectrum of unruptured intracranial aneurysms. Arch Neurol. 1993;50(3):265–8.

Smetana GW. The diagnostic value of historical features in primary headache syndromes: a comprehensive review. Arch Intern Med. 2000;160(18): 2729–37.

Smetana GW, Shmerling RH. Does this patient have temporal arteritis? JAMA. 2002;287(1):92–101.

Snow V, Weiss K, Wall EM, Mottur-Pilson C. Pharmacologic management of acute attacks of migraine and prevention of migraine headache. Ann Intern Med. 2002;137(10):840–9.

Stiell IG, Clement CM, Rowe BH et al. Comparison of the Canadian CT Head Rule and the New Orleans Criteria in patients with minor head injury. JAMA. 2005;294(12):1511–8.

The International Classification of Headache Disorders: 2nd edition. Cephalalgia. 2004;24 Suppl 1:9–160.

van de Beek D, de Gans J, Spanjaard L, Weisfelt M, Reitsma JB, Vermeulen M. Clinical features and prognostic factors in adults with bacterial meningitis. N Engl J Med. 2004;351(18):1849–59.

van Gijn J, Kerr RS, Rinkel GJ. Subarachnoid haemorrhage. Lancet. 2007;369(9558): 306–18.

Wall M. The headache profile of idiopathic intracranial hypertension. Cephalalgia. 1990;10(6):331–5.

Weir B. Headaches from aneurysms. Cephalalgia. 1994;14(2):79–87.

Wijdicks EF, Kerkhoff H, van Gijn J. Long-term follow-up of 71 patients with thunderclap headache mimicking subarachnoid haemorrhage. Lancet. 1988;2(8602): 68–70.

Younge BR, Cook BE Jr, Bartley GB, Hodge DO, Hunder GG. Initiation of glucocorticoid therapy: before or after temporal artery biopsy? Mayo Clin Proc. 2004;79(4):483–91.

I have a patient with hematuria.
How do I determine the cause?

CHIEF COMPLAINT

PATIENT

Mr. Y is a 56-year-old man who has had several episodes of red urine in the past few days.

What is the differential diagnosis of hematuria? How would you frame the differential?

CONSTRUCTING A DIFFERENTIAL DIAGNOSIS

Red urine is not always caused by hematuria. A variety of medications, food dyes, and metabolites can cause heme-negative red urine, or pigmenturia (Table 21-1). Furthermore, not all dipstick tests positive for blood are due to hematuria. In addition to detecting heme in intact red blood cells (RBCs), urine dipsticks detect free hemoglobin and myoglobin, hence leading to false-positive tests for hematuria.

Whenever the urine dipstick is positive for blood, and the microscopic exam of the urine does not show RBCs, myoglobinuria and hemoglobinuria should be considered.

True macroscopic (visible) hematuria is always pathologic. Microscopic (nonvisible) hematuria may be transient, spurious, or persistent. Transient causes of microscopic hematuria include urinary tract infections (UTIs) (which sometimes also cause macroscopic hematuria) and strenuous exercise; hematuria due to these causes would be expected to resolve on repeat testing after 48 hours of treatment or after discontinuing exercise for 72 hours. Spurious causes include urinary contamination from menstruation and sexual intercourse in women. This chapter will focus on persistent, true hematuria.

All patients with hematuria should have a urine culture performed, regardless of the likelihood of infection.

The differential diagnosis of hematuria is often divided into microscopic hematuria or macroscopic hematuria. Microscopic hematuria is present when microscopic inspection of at least 2 properly collected urine specimens show > 3 RBCs per high-powered field (hpf). Macroscopic hematuria is red or brown urine, sometimes with blood clots. However, there is considerable overlap in the causes of microscopic and macroscopic hematuria, and it may be more practical to first consider whether the hematuria is glomerular in origin. Pivotal points that help distinguish glomerular hematuria from nonglomerular hematuria include dysmorphic RBCs (acanthocytes),

red cell casts, new or acutely worsening hypertension or proteinuria, and increased creatinine. While these abnormalities may also be seen in some of the interstitial and vascular causes of hematuria, they will not be found when hematuria is caused by a renal structural abnormality or an abnormality distal to the kidneys. Visible blood clots, which are never due to a glomerular cause, are another pivotal point, indicating a lower urinary tract source of the hematuria.

A. Renal
  1. Glomerular
    a. IgA nephropathy
    b. Alport disease and thin basement membrane nephropathy (TBMN)
    c. Other primary and secondary glomerulonephritides
      (1) Postinfectious or infection-related
      (2) Systemic lupus erythematosus
      (3) Goodpasture syndrome
      (4) Henoch-Schünlein purpura (HSP) and other small or medium vessel vasculitides
      (5) Hemolytic uremic syndrome (HUS)
  2. Nonglomerular
    a. Neoplastic
      (1) Renal cell or transitional cell carcinoma
      (2) Benign renal mass
    b. Tubulointerstitial
      (1) Nephrolithiasis
      (2) Polycystic kidney disease or medullary sponge kidney
      (3) Pyelonephritis
      (4) Acute interstitial nephritis
      (5) Papillary necrosis
    c. Vascular
      (1) Arterial embolus or thrombosis
      (2) Arteriovenous malformation or arteriovenous fistula
      (3) Renal vein thrombosis
      (4) Nutcracker syndrome (compression of left renal vein)
      (5) Malignant hypertension
    d. Metabolic (hypercalciuria, hyperuricosuria)
B. Extrarenal
  1. Ureter
    a. Mass: benign polyp or malignancy
    b. Stone
    c. Stricture

Table 21-1. Causes of heme-negative red urine (pigmenturia).

Causes	Examples
Medications	Azathioprine
	Chloroquine
	Deferoxamine
	Doxorubicin
	Ibuprofen
	Iron sorbitol
	Laxatives
	Nitrofurantoin
	Phenazopyridine
	Phenytoin
	Riboflavin
	Rifampin
Food dyes	Beets
	Blackberries
	Food coloring
Metabolites	Bilirubin
	Melanin
	Methemoglobin
	Porphyrin
	Tyrosinosis
	Urates

2. Bladder

   a. Transitional cell or squamous cell carcinoma

   b. Noninfectious cystitis (radiation or medication [cyclophosphamide])

   c. Infectious cystitis

   d. Stone

3. Urethra

   a. Urethritis

   b. Urethral diverticulum

   c. Traumatic catheterization

   d. Urethral stricture

4. Prostate

   a. Benign prostatic hypertrophy (BPH)

   b. Prostate cancer

   c. Post prostatic procedure

   d. Prostatitis

Figures 21-1 and 21-2 reorganize the differential diagnosis using pivotal points and outline the diagnostic approach to hematuria.

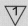

Mr. A reports several episodes of painless visible hematuria over the last several days, along with occasional mild lower abdominal discomfort. He is feeling well otherwise and has no other complaints. His medical history is significant for chronic kidney disease (CKD) stage 3, hypertension treated with hydrochlorothiazide and enalapril, and a remote appendectomy. He has no family history of kidney stones, but his father did have prostate cancer. He has smoked 1 pack per day of cigarettes for 35 years. He is a philosophy professor, and has no known toxin exposures. Initial urinalysis shows many nondysmorphic RBCs, with no WBCs, bacteria, casts, or proteinuria.

At this point, what is the leading hypothesis, what are the active alternatives, and is there a must not miss diagnosis? Given this differential diagnosis, what tests should be ordered?

RANKING THE DIFFERENTIAL DIAGNOSIS

Mr. A does not have the pivotal urinalysis findings that suggest a glomerular source of the hematuria. Therefore, nonglomerular causes should be considered first. Given the patient's sex (male), age (>40), and 35 pack year smoking history, all risk factors for malignancy, bleeding from a urothelial bladder cancer needs to move to the top of the differential diagnosis. Although he does not have abdominal or flank pain suggestive of renal colic, stone disease is common and should be considered. Prostate cancer, BPH, and prostatitis are also common, and men with prostatitis may have vague abdominal discomfort, as Mr. A does. Renal cell carcinoma (RCC) is rare but must always be considered in a patient with hematuria. The otherwise bland urinalysis makes interstitial causes and UTI unlikely. He has no history of radiation or chemotherapy to suggest an associated cystitis. Table 21-2 lists the differential diagnosis.

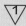

Mr. A's physical exam is normal, with no abdominal masses or tenderness. External genitalia are normal, and digital rectal exam shows a symmetric, nontender prostate without nodules. Serum creatinine is 1.8 mg/dL, unchanged from previous values.

   Urine culture is negative.

Is the clinical information sufficient to make a diagnosis? If not, what other information do you need?

Leading Hypothesis: Bladder Cancer

Textbook Presentation

Bladder cancer classically presents as painless visible hematuria in an older male smoker. Microscopic hematuria occurs in nearly all patients with bladder cancer. Other symptoms include dysuria or obstructive symptoms.

Disease Highlights

A. Accounts for 90% of urothelial cancers

B. Visible painless hematuria, often intermittent, occurs in 85% of patients

C. Risk factors for bladder cancer

   1. Male sex and white race: white males are 3–4 times more likely to develop bladder cancer than African American males or white females

   2. Smoking: accounts for 60% of bladder cancers in males and 30% in females

   3. Age > 40: median age at diagnosis is 70

   4. Preexisting urothelial cancer (RCC, ureteral, prostate)

   5. History of pelvic radiation

   6. Chronic UTI

   7. Schistosomiasis (in Africa and the Middle East)

   8. Industrial chemical/toxin exposure

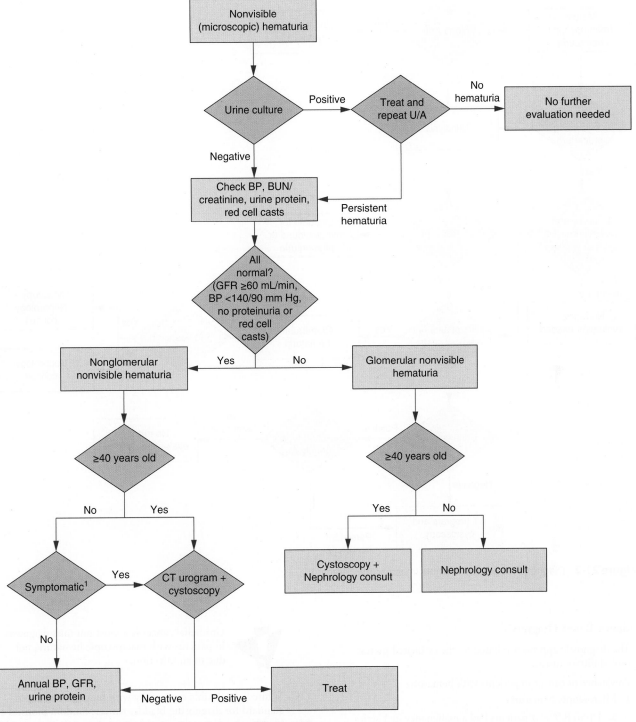

[1]Symptoms include dysuria, flank pain, abdominal pain, difficulty voiding.

BP, blood pressure; BUN, blood urea nitrogen; GFR, glomerular filtration rate; U/A, urinalysis.

Figure 21-1. Diagnostic approach to nonvisible (microscopic) hematuria.

a. Kidneys filter and concentrate metabolic toxins into the urine which pool in the bladder, promoting oncogenesis
b. Accounts for about 20% of bladder cancers
c. 10- to 20-year latency period between exposure and disease
d. Compounds associated with bladder cancer include aromatic amines, aniline dyes, nitrates, nitrites, coal, and arsenic

e. Occupations associated with a higher risk of bladder cancer include miners, bus drivers, rubber workers, motor mechanics, leather workers, blacksmiths, machine setters, hairdressers, and mechanics.

D. Prognosis: 10-year survival for muscle-invasive cancer still confined to the bladder is 65–72%.

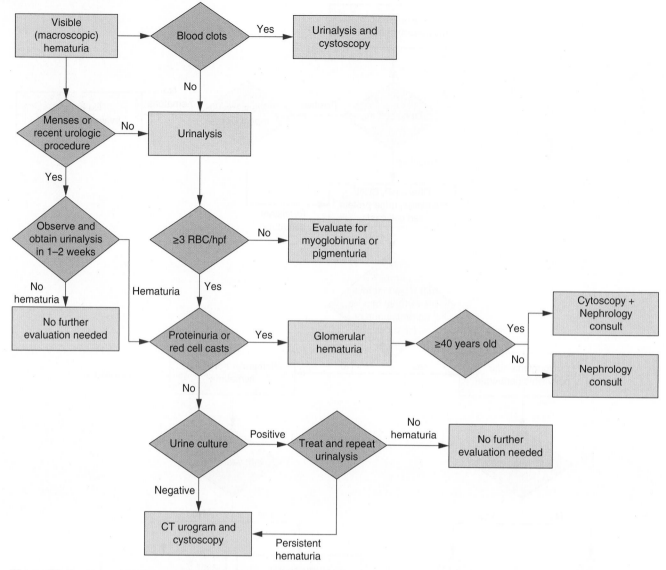

Figure 21-2. Diagnostic approach to visible (macroscopic) hematuria.

Evidence-Based Diagnosis

A. The diagnostic approach is based on the estimated pretest probability of disease.

B. Prevalence of cancer in patients with hematuria

1. Microscopic hematuria

   a. Up to 8.9% of patients had a malignancy in 1 series

   b. Another cohort found bladder cancer in 3.7%, RCC in 1%, and ureteral cancer in 0.2%.

   c. Malignancy was extremely rare in patients under the age of 40 with microscopic hematuria.

2. Macroscopic hematuria: studies generally included older patients who presented to "hematuria clinics"

   a. Up to 30% had a malignancy

   b. 20–25% had bladder cancer

   c. 1.3–10% had prostate cancer

   d. 0.6–2% had RCC

   e. 21% had stones

   f. 12–13% had BPH

 Urothelial cancer is a must not miss diagnosis in patients with macroscopic hematuria not due to an infection.

C. White light flexible cystoscopy with biopsies is the gold standard for diagnosing bladder cancer; random biopsies of bladder tissue are taken to detect carcinoma in situ not visible to the naked eye.

D. Hexaminolevulinate fluorescence cystoscopy is also useful for detection of carcinoma in situ.

E. Multiphasic CT urography is done with and without contrast and includes imaging in the excretory phase.

1. Has largely replaced other imaging modalities such as IV pyelogram, ultrasound, conventional CT, and retrograde pyelography to evaluate unexplained hematuria

2. Comparatively higher sensitivity (92–100%) and specificity (94–97%) for the detection of renal masses, urinary tract stones, and genitourinary transitional cell carcinomas

3. May improve the sensitivity of cystoscopy if done first

Table 21-2. Diagnostic hypotheses for Mr. A.

Diagnostic Hypotheses	Demographics, Risk Factors, Symptoms and Signs	Important Tests
Leading Hypothesis		
Bladder cancer	Painless hematuria sometimes with blood clots Smoking history Male sex Toxin exposure Age over 40	Cystoscopy Urine cytology CT urogram
Active Alternatives—Most Common		
Stone disease	**Bladder:** hematuria, bladder pain	Noncontrast CT Cystoscopy
	Ureter or kidney: hematuria, flank/abdominal pain, renal colic	Noncontrast CT
BPH	Urgency frequency, nocturia, urge incontinence, stress incontinence, hesitancy, poor flow, straining, dysuria	Rectal exam
Prostatitis	Abdominal pain, recent/concurrent urinary tract infection, fever, chills, urinary retention, recent prostate biopsy	Rectal exam, urinalysis, urine culture
Active Alternatives—Must Not Miss		
Prostate cancer	Hematuria	Rectal exam Prostate-specific antigen
Renal cell carcinoma	Hematuria Flank pain Abdominal mass	CT scan

4. Delivers a relatively high radiation dose; therefore, some guidelines recommend avoiding in low-risk patients

F. Ultrasound
   1. The sensitivity of ultrasound for bladder cancer is 63% and the specificity 99%.
   2. Ultrasound is less sensitive than CT for detecting renal tumors < 3 cm.

G. Urine cytology and biomarkers
   1. None of the many urine biomarkers investigated has adequate test characteristics.
   2. Urine cytology sensitivity is 7–17% for low-grade and 53–90% for high-grade cancers; specificity is 90–98%.

 Patients ≥ 40 years old, or with visible urinary blood clots, require cystoscopy even if the bleeding is glomerular.

Treatment

A. Superficial or minimally invasive tumors are treated with transurethral resection for both diagnostic confirmation and cure.

B. Intravesicular chemotherapy (most often with BCG) is given immediately after the operation.

C. Muscle-invasive tumors are treated with radical cystectomy and cisplatin-based chemotherapy.

MAKING A DIAGNOSIS

 Although you are concerned about malignancy, because of his CKD you order an ultrasound rather than a CT scan. It shows a 1 mm stone in the right renal pelvis, and a 2 cm cyst in the left kidney. You order a PSA and refer him to urology for a cystoscopy.

 Have you crossed a diagnostic threshold for the leading hypothesis, bladder cancer? Have you ruled out the active alternatives? Do other tests need to be done to exclude the alternative diagnoses?

Alternative Diagnosis: Nephrolithiasis

See Chapter 3, Abdominal Pain.

Alternative Diagnosis: Prostate Cancer

See Chapter 2, Screening & Health Maintenance.

Alternative Diagnosis: BPH

See Chapter 28, Acute Kidney Injury.

Alternative Diagnosis: Prostatitis

See Chapter 16, Dysuria.

Alternative Diagnosis: Renal Cell Carcinoma

Textbook Presentation

RCC classically presents with the triad of hematuria, flank pain, and a palpable abdominal mass but now is far more commonly detected incidentally as a renal mass seen on a radiographic examination done for other reasons.

Disease Highlights

A. Epidemiology
   1. Arises from the renal epithelium and accounts for over 80% of renal cancers, with a 1.6:1 male predominance and peak incidence between the sixth and eighth decades of life
   2. About 2% of cases are associated with inherited syndromes like von Hippel-Lindau disease
   3. Risk factors
      a. Smoking
      b. Obesity
      c. Hypertension
      d. Toxic exposures
      e. Acquired cystic kidney disease associated with end-stage renal disease (ESRD)

B. Etiology

1. The most common histologic form is clear cell, which accounts for 75–85% of cases.

2. Other histologies are papillary (10–15%) and chromophobe (5–10%).

3. The pathogenesis is incompletely understood, but the von Hippel-Lindau (*VHL*) tumor suppressor gene is mutated in most sporadic cases of RCC.

C. Presentation

1. Many patients with RCC are asymptomatic until the disease is advanced, with roughly 25% having distant metastases or locally advanced disease at time of presentation.

2. Hematuria occurs with tumor invasion of the renal collecting system, ranging from microscopic to visible blood clots.

3. An abdominal or flank mass, generally only palpable in thin individuals, is usually firm, homogenous, and nontender, moving with respiration.

4. Nonspecific symptoms such as fatigue, weight loss, and anemia, are common.

D. Prognosis

1. Stage I: 5-year survival > 90%

2. Stage II: 75–95%

3. Stage III who undergo nephrectomy: 59–70% 5-year survival

4. Stage IV: median survival of 16–20 months; < 10% 5-year survival rate for patients with distant metastases

Evidence-Based Diagnosis

A. RCC appears as a solid renal lesion on abdominal imaging.

1. On ultrasound, the mass does not meet criteria for a simple cyst.

2. On CT, features of RCC include thickened irregular walls or septa and enhancement with IV contrast.

B. RCC can remain localized, invade surrounding fascia and adjacent organs, and/or metastasize.

1. CT scan is used for staging.

   a. 78% sensitive and 96% specific for the detection of renal vein invasion

   b. 83% sensitive and 88% specific for the detection of metastatic adenopathy

   c. 46% sensitive and 98% specific for the detection of perinephric invasion

   d. 100% specific for detecting adjacent organ invasion

2. Bone scan, CT chest, MRI, or PET scanning are used to detect distant metastases.

Treatment

A. For patients with isolated, solid renal masses, resection with either partial or complete nephrectomy is preferred to biopsy since it is both diagnostic and therapeutic; consultation with urology is essential to determine whether surgery or surveillance is indicated.

B. Deciding whether to perform a partial or complete (radical) nephrectomy depends on

1. Stage and location of the tumor

2. Baseline renal function

3. Functional status

4. Presence of other comorbidities

C. A reasonable alternative for individuals at high risk for complications from surgery is thermal ablation (eg, cryotherapy or radiofrequency ablation)

D. Consultation with oncology is indicated for patients with locally advanced or metastatic RCC.

CASE RESOLUTION

Mr. A's cystoscopy detects a small papillary tumor localized to the uroepithelium of his bladder. Hexaminolevulinate fluorescence cystoscopy does not detect any carcinomas in situ. CT urography does not demonstrate any masses elsewhere in the upper urinary tract or kidneys. His bladder cancer is classified as superficial and he is treated with transurethral resection followed by BCG therapy. At a follow-up visit 1 year later he is cancer free and feeling well.

CHIEF COMPLAINT

Mr. S is a 24-year-old white man who comes to your office after being told there was 'some blood detected' on a screening urinalysis 2 weeks ago prior to enlistment in the Army. He has not seen any blood in his urine, is anxious to start basic training, and 'doesn't understand what all the fuss is about.' He denies any dysuria, abdominal pain, fevers, or urethral discharge. Exam is notable for a fit, well-developed young man in no acute distress. His vital signs were temperature 37.2°C; pulse of 68 bpm; BP 126/78 mm Hg; RR 16 breaths per minute. His exam is completely normal with a notable absence of abdominal pain, costovertebral angle tenderness, urethral discharge or testicular pain, and lower extremity edema.

His screening and in-office urinalyses both show 2+ protein, 2+ blood, and 5–10 RBCs/hpf. The dipstick is otherwise negative, and there are no WBCs or bacteria. Microscopic analysis of the urine in the office also reveals occasional dysmorphic RBCs but no RBC casts.

 At this point, what is the leading hypothesis, what are the active alternatives, and is there a must not miss diagnosis? Given this differential diagnosis, what tests should be ordered?

RANKING THE DIFFERENTIAL DIAGNOSIS

Mr. S is asymptomatic with nonvisible (or microscopic) hematuria. Based on the 2 separate urinalyses, it is persistent. In young patients (under age 40) without risk factors, cancer is an uncommon cause

Table 21-3. Diagnostic hypotheses for Mr. S.

Diagnostic Hypothesis	Demographics, Risk Factors, Symptoms and Signs	Important Tests
Leading Hypothesis		
IgA nephropathy	Episodes of macroscopic hematuria (tea-colored urine) that coincide with respiratory infections	Urinalysis with microscopy Serum creatinine Renal biopsy
Active Alternative		
Thin basement membrane nephropathy	Family history of hematuria without history of chronic kidney disease	Urinalysis with microscopy Serum creatinine Renal biopsy
Active Alternative		
Infection-related glomerulonephritis	Antecedent group A streptococcal pharyngitis 1–3 weeks prior to episode of gross hematuria, often with high BP and edema	Urinalysis with microscopy Serum creatinine Antibodies to streptococcal antigens Serum complement levels
Other Alternative		
Alport syndrome	Hematuria with strong family history of progressive renal disease and sensorineural hearing loss	Urinalysis with microscopy Serum creatinine Family history Renal biopsy

of asymptomatic nonvisible hematuria; in the absence of lower urinary symptoms, a urologic cause is rare. Notably, the concomitant proteinuria and the dysmorphic RBCs are pivotal points for a glomerular source. The most common glomerular causes are IgA nephropathy and TBMN. Table 21-3 lists the differential diagnosis.

The patient reports no prior medical or surgical history; he has not seen a physician since his last pediatrician visit at age 18. No one in his family has any known history of hematuria or kidney problems. He has been in a stable, monogamous relationship with his girlfriend for over a year and is not taking any medications or supplements. On more detailed questioning, he does recall "3 or 4" previous episodes of his urine changing color for a few days, which he associated with colds or minor respiratory infections. Basic metabolic profile is normal, with a creatinine of 0.9 mg/dL and BUN of 12 mg/dL.

Is the clinical information sufficient to make a diagnosis? If not, what other information do you need?

Leading Hypothesis: IgA Nephropathy

Textbook Presentation

IgA nephropathy (IgAN) most commonly presents with visible hematuria within 12–72 hours of a mucosal (typically an upper respiratory) infection. It can also be discovered upon detection of asymptomatic, nonvisible hematuria with or without proteinuria during routine medical screening.

Disease Highlights

A. The most common cause of primary glomerulonephritis worldwide.
   1. Peak incidence of IgAN is between the second and fourth decades of life, though it can present at any age.
   2. Occurs with greatest frequency in Asians and whites.

B. An important cause of progressive CKD, with up to 50% of patients developing ESRD within 25 years of diagnosis.

C. Etiology of IgAN
   1. Caused by glomerular deposition of A1 isotype of IgA in the mesangium.
   2. No evidence of a role for any specific antigen despite the relation between mucosal infections and episodes of visible hematuria.
   3. Most cases of IgAN are sporadic, although familial cases do occur and appear to be transmitted as an autosomal dominant trait with incomplete penetrance.

D. Clinical manifestations of IgAN
   1. One or more episodes of visible hematuria, usually associated with upper respiratory infection (often called **synpharyngitic hematuria**) and sometimes accompanied by flank pain and low-grade fever (present in 40–50% of patients).
   2. Nonvisible hematuria and typically mild proteinuria, detected incidentally on routine screening (present in 30–40% of patients).
   3. Advanced, progressive CKD, hypertension, and heavy proteinuria, in addition to hematuria (seen in small proportion of patients); nephrotic range proteinuria (present in ~5% of patients).
   4. IgAN rarely occurs secondary to other conditions like cirrhosis, celiac disease, and HIV infection, all of which are associated with a high frequency of IgA deposition.

Evidence-Based Diagnosis

A. Urine dipstick with microscopy and culture should be used to rule out infection, confirm the findings of hematuria, and evaluate for proteinuria.

B. A definitive diagnosis can only be made by renal biopsy with immunofluorescence or immunoperoxidase studies for IgA deposits.
   1. In the absence of proteinuria, hypertension, or decreased glomerular filtration rate (GFR), the clinical course (at least short-term) of patients with IgAN is generally benign and renal biopsy is usually not indicated; periodic monitoring is recommended in these cases.
   2. Proteinuria (> 500–1000 mg/day), elevated serum creatinine, or hypertension suggests more severe or progressive disease and are indications for renal biopsy to establish the diagnosis.

C. The pathognomonic biopsy finding of IgAN is prominent, globular deposits of IgA in the mesangium on immunofluorescence microscopy.

Treatment

A. Patients with isolated hematuria, normal GFR, and no significant proteinuria should be monitored every 6–12 months for signs of progression (worsening proteinuria, BP, and GFR).

B. Clinical predictors of progression of IgAN, including proteinuria > 500–1000 mg/day, decreased GFR, and hypertension often signal the need for treatment.

C. Treatment is primarily aimed at reducing proteinuria and optimizing BP to minimize risk of progression.

D. Treatment of progressive IgAN

1. Angiotensin-converting enzyme (ACE) inhibitor or angiotensin-receptor blocker (ARB) therapy slows progression by optimizing BP control and reducing proteinuria.

2. Fish oil has also been used in IgAN patients with > 1000 mg/day of proteinuria despite 3–6 months of ACE inhibitor or ARB therapy.

3. Some patients with IgAN with signs of more severe inflammatory disease on biopsy may require immunosuppressive therapy.

4. Renal transplantation is an option for patients with IgAN who have had progression to ESRD, but recurrence is common.

MAKING A DIAGNOSIS

A spot urine total protein to creatinine ratio, to quantify the amount of protein in the urine, is found to be 1100 mg/day. He now remembers that he did have a sore throat prior to the first urine sample.

Have you crossed a diagnostic threshold for the leading hypothesis, IgA nephropathy? Have you ruled out the active alternatives? Do other tests need to be done to exclude the alternative diagnoses?

Alternative Diagnosis: Thin Basement Membrane Nephropathy

Textbook Presentation

Most individuals with TBMN have isolated hematuria with normal renal function, no or minimal proteinuria, and a uniformly thinned glomerular basement membrane (GBM) on electron microscopy analysis of biopsy specimen.

Disease Highlights

A. The most common cause of persistent hematuria in children and adults

1. Occurs in at least 1% of the general population and is often familial

2. A family history of hematuria is present in 30–50% of TBMN cases.

B. Characteristically presents with persistent or intermittent hematuria incidentally discovered on routine urinalysis.

1. Most patients have isolated hematuria, which can present at virtually any age, without proteinuria or renal impairment.

2. Dysmorphic RBCs are commonly seen, and RBC casts may occur.

3. Episodes of visible hematuria may occur in a small percentage of individuals with TBMN (12%) but are far more common in Alport syndrome (33%) and IgA nephropathy (88%).

4. Proteinuria is rarely seen in children with TBMN, but mild proteinuria (up to 1 g/day) may be seen in a minority of adult patients.

C. TBMN is caused by defects in type IV collagen genes, which leads to a diffuse thinning of the GBM seen on electron microscopy.

D. The long-term prognosis in most patients with true TBMN is excellent.

Evidence-Based Diagnosis

A. The only way to definitively diagnose TBMN is by renal biopsy and electron microscopy.

1. Renal biopsy is usually not performed in patients with isolated hematuria, normal renal function, and no or minimal proteinuria. The diagnosis is often inferred in these patients with positive family history of hematuria and negative family history of CKD.

2. Renal biopsy is more commonly performed in patients with suspected TBMN who also have proteinuria (> 200–300 mg/day).

B. Biopsy reveals diffuse, uniform thinning of the GBM on electron microscopy, and the absence of other significant glomerular pathology.

C. Immunohistochemical evaluation of the type IV collagen alpha-3 to alpha-5 chains is useful in helping distinguish between TBMN and early Alport syndrome (with microscopic hematuria and thin GBM), as these chains are usually absent or abnormally distributed in Alport syndrome.

Treatment

A. Progressive CKD with TBMN is rare, but regular follow-up and monitoring is important.

B. While there are no proven therapies for TBMN, a goal BP of < 130/80 mm Hg and ACE inhibition is recommended for patients with TBMN and proteinuria > 1 g/day.

Alternative Diagnosis: Infection-Related Glomerulonephritis

Textbook Presentation

The classic presentation of infection-related glomerulonephritis (IRGN) is new onset of hematuria, proteinuria, and edema, often with hypertension and mild acute kidney injury, following or concurrent with an infection.

Disease Highlights

A. Epidemiology

1. In the developing world, IRGN (especially poststreptococcal glomerulonephritis [GN]) occurs primarily in children (ages 6–10) and young adults, with a male predominance (2–3:1).

2. In the developed world, IRGN affects mostly adults, especially those with immunocompromising comorbidities such as diabetes mellitus and alcoholism.

B. Etiology

1. Upper respiratory and skin infections are the 2 most common sites of infection leading to IRGN, although multiple other sites have also been implicated.

2. Historically, most cases have been attributed to group A streptococci, specifically *Streptococcus pyogenes.*

3. More recently, it has become clear that other strains of streptococci (groups C and G), staphylococci, gram-negative bacilli, mycobacteria, parasites, fungi, and viruses can also cause IRGN.

4. One-third to one-half of cases of IRGN in developed countries are associated with infections of gram-negative bacilli.

C. Clinical manifestations

1. Acute nephritic syndrome (poststreptococcal GN is the prototypical form)

   a. Presents with hematuria, proteinuria, and edema, often accompanied by hypertension and mild acute kidney injury

   b. Urinary output usually improves after 5–7 days, followed rapidly by resolution of edema and normalization of BP

2. Rapidly progressive nephritic syndrome

   a. Rarely, acute postinfectious GN (usually poststreptococcal) is complicated by rapidly worsening GFR

   b. Crescent formation often present on biopsy but tends to be limited

3. Subclinical or asymptomatic GN

   a. Present in many patients with mild, self-limited streptococcal infections

   b. Characterized by low-grade proteinuria (< 1 g/day), pyuria, and nonvisible (microscopic) hematuria; often goes undetected

Evidence-Based Diagnosis

A. In children, nephritis typically follows pharyngitis by 1–2 weeks and skin infection by 2–4 weeks.

1. During this time asymptomatic nonvisible (microscopic) hematuria and proteinuria is often present.

2. Upon symptomatic presentation (eyelid and diffuse edema, smoky colored urine), a urinalysis shows proteinuria (mild to nephrotic range), pyuria (97%), and often hematuria (30–37%) with RBC casts.

3. Acute kidney injury and hypertension are also common (60–80%).

4. Hypocomplementemia is present in 90% of children with poststreptococcal GN and 35–80% of adults with IRGN.

   a. C3 is typically low while C4 is normal.

   b. One-third of patients with IRGN will have both low C3 and low C4.

5. Serologies for recent streptococcal infection (ASO, DNase B, streptokinase, hyaluronidase, anti-NAD) are often positive, even when patients do not report recent respiratory or skin infection.

   a. The streptozyme test measures all 5 of these streptococcal antibodies and performs better than any individual antibody measurement alone.

   b. It has a sensitivity of 95% in patients with recent group A streptococcal pharyngitis and 80% in those with streptococcal skin infections.

6. Biopsy is usually not recommended in children.

B. In a significant proportion (45%) of adults, the precipitating infection is still present and only discovered at the time IRGN is diagnosed.

1. Adults present with gross hematuria and diffuse edema; proteinuria can lead to foamy urine and hypertension can cause headaches.

2. Exam may reveal signs of infection, such as pharyngitis, pneumonia, cellulitis/abscess, endocarditis, or urethral/vaginal discharge.

3. Older adults (25%) may have additional signs of volume overload (increased jugular venous pressure, S_3 gallop, pulmonary crackles, lower extremity edema) stemming from acute volume overload precipitated by the acute kidney injury.

4. Urinalysis shows at least nonvisible (microscopic) hematuria, although gross hematuria is often already present.

5. Proteinuria (mild to nephrotic range) is usually present, and RBC casts may be seen on microscopy.

6. Biopsy is usually recommended in adults to confirm diagnosis and rule out glomerulonephritides that require immediate immunosuppressive therapy.

Treatment

A. Children should be treated with supportive therapy.

B. Adults

1. Treat underlying infection, which is often ongoing at the time of diagnosis.

2. Manage complications of nephritis.

   a. Antihypertensives, specifically ACE inhibitor if moderate to heavy proteinuria

   b. Diuretics and sodium restriction

3. Immunosuppressive therapy is not recommended.

C. Prognosis

1. Complete recovery occurs in almost all children, although potentially with increased likelihood of CKD and hypertension later in life.

2. Adults with IRGN have a poorer prognosis.

   a. Up to 50% have persistent renal dysfunction, and up to 33% progress to ESRD.

   b. Elderly and diabetic patients have the highest risk of persistent CKD and ESRD.

CASE RESOLUTION

In the absence of any family history of hematuria or CKD, IgA nephropathy is the most likely diagnosis. Mr. S has normal BP and renal function but needs a biopsy because of the proteinuria. The results show classic IgA nephropathy. Given his significant proteinuria, which is a risk factor for more rapid decline in renal function, Mr. S was started on an ACE inhibitor with close BP monitoring for a target < 125/75 mm Hg. After 1 month, repeat testing demonstrated persistent nonvisible hematuria, stable renal function, and that the proteinuria had decreased to 250 mg/day. Although he was disqualified from military service, he continued with regular follow-up every 6–12 months and has done well without significant progression of his disease.

REFERENCES

Chou R, Dana T. Screening adults for bladder cancer: a review of the evidence for the US preventive services task force. Ann Intern Med.2010;153(7):461–8.

Cohen HT, McGovern FJ. Renal-cell carcinoma. N Engl J Med. 2005 Dec 8;353(23):2477–90.

Cohen RA, Brown RS. Clinical practice. Microscopic hematuria. N Engl J Med. 2003 Jun 5;348(23):2330–8.

Davis R, Jones JS, Barocas DA et al. Diagnosis, evaluation and follow-up of asymptomatic microhematuria (AMH) in adults: AUA guideline. J Urol. 2012 Dec;188(6 Suppl):2473–81.

Hudson BG, Tryggvason K, Sundaramoorthy M, Neilson EG. Alport's syndrome, Goodpasture's syndrome, and type IV collagen. N Engl J Med. 2003 Jun 19;348(25):2543–56.

Kanjanabuch T, Kittikowit W, Eiam-Ong S. An update on acute postinfectious glomerulonephritis worldwide. Nat Rev Nephrol. 2009 May;5(5):259–69.

Kaufman DS, Shipley WU, Feldman AS. Bladder cancer. Lancet. 2009 Jul 18;374(9685):239–49.

O'Connor OJ, McSweeney SE, Maher MM. Imaging of hematuria. Radiol Clin North Am. 2008;46:113.

Wyatt RJ, Julian BA. IgA Nephropathy. N Engl J Med. 2013;368(25):2402–14.

I have a patient with hypercalcemia.
How do I determine the cause?

CHIEF COMPLAINT

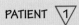

PATIENT

Mrs. D is a 60-year-old, African American woman who complains of long-standing constipation. Initial laboratory evaluation reveals a normal TSH, normal electrolytes, and a calcium level of 10.8 mg/dL (nl 8.4–10.2).

What is the differential diagnosis of hypercalcemia? How would you frame the differential?

CONSTRUCTING A DIFFERENTIAL DIAGNOSIS

In general, hypercalcemia is detected in 1 of 3 clinical circumstances. First, hypercalcemia may be discovered during routine laboratory work-ups in patients with no symptoms. These patients may or may not have a risk factor for hypercalcemia, such as malignancy. Most cases of hypercalcemia are diagnosed in these asymptomatic people. Second, hypercalcemia may be found during evaluation of patients with symptoms or findings that can be related to hypercalcemia, such as constipation, weakness, fatigue, depression, nephrolithiasis, or osteopenia. Third, severe hypercalcemia may present as altered mental status.

Although most cases of hypercalcemia are due to only a handful of conditions (primary hyperparathyroidism, hypercalcemia of malignancy, chronic kidney disease (CKD), and the milk-alkali syndrome), the complete differential diagnosis is extensive. The most commonly used framework for the differential is organized by pathophysiology. What follows is a somewhat abbreviated list organized by etiology.

A. Parathyroid hormone (PTH)–related

  1. Primary hyperparathyroidism

  2. Secondary hyperparathyroidism (with calcium supplementation)

  3. Tertiary hyperparathyroidism

  4. Lithium therapy (causes hypercalcemia in about 10% of patients)

  5. Familial hypocalciuric hypercalcemia

B. Hypercalcemia of malignancy

  1. Secretion of parathyroid hormone–related protein (PTHrP)

    a. Squamous cell carcinomas

    b. Adenocarcinoma of lung, pancreas, kidney, and others

  2. Osteolytic metastasis

    a. Breast cancer

    b. Multiple myeloma

  3. Production of calcitriol (Hodgkin disease)

C. Vitamin D–related

  1. Hypervitaminosis D

  2. Granulomatous diseases

D. Other relatively common causes of hypercalcemia

  1. Milk-alkali syndrome (mainly seen in patients with CKD who are taking calcium carbonate)

  2. Hyperthyroidism

  3. Thiazide diuretics

  4. Falsely elevated serum calcium (secondary to increased serum binding protein)

    a. Hyperalbuminemia

    b. Hypergammaglobulinemia

Clinically, the differential diagnosis is most commonly organized by the pivotal findings of whether or not the PTH is elevated and whether the patient has a known malignancy. A useful clinical algorithm is presented in Figure 22-1.

Before returning to the case, it is worthwhile to briefly review the basics of calcium metabolism. Calcium levels are dictated by the actions of PTH, calcitonin, and calcitriol (1,25-dihydroxyvitamin D). PTH levels rise and fall in response to serum calcium levels. High levels of PTH stimulate a rise in serum calcium by increasing both renal tubular calcium reabsorption and bone resorption. PTH also stimulates the conversion of calcidiol to calcitriol in the kidneys. Calcitriol leads to a further increase in serum calcium via increased absorption of calcium in the small intestine. Phosphate metabolism is also controlled by PTH and calcitriol; PTH generally lowers phosphate levels through its effects on the kidney, while calcitriol generally raises phosphate levels through its effects on the intestine and inhibitory effects on PTH levels. Calcitonin lowers calcium by suppressing calcium release from bones by inhibiting the function of osteoclasts.

Mrs. D comes to your office for an initial visit. Her constipation has been long-standing and severe enough to lead to physician visits over the past 5 years. Evaluation with colonoscopy had been normal. Results of laboratory tests, drawn over the last few years by previous physicians, show normal results (including kidney function and TSH), with the exception of calcium levels in the range of 11 mg/dL. Despite use of stool softeners and high-fiber supplements, she often needs laxatives to move her bowels more than once a week.

In addition to constipation, the patient's other medical problems are hypertension and tobacco use. She feels well.

(continued)

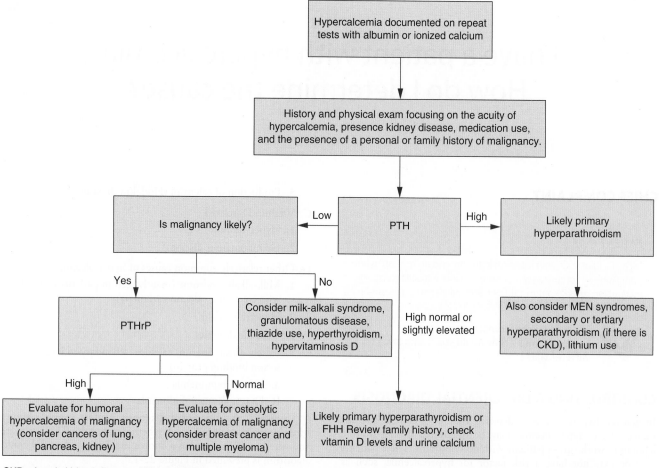

CKD, chronic kidney disease; FHH, familial hypocalciuric hypercalcemia; MEN, multiple endocrine neoplasia; PTH, parathyroid hormone; PTHrP, parathyroid hormone-related protein.

Figure 22-1. Diagnostic approach: hypercalcemia.

Her medications are atenolol and hydrochlorothiazide. Family history is notable only for hypertension in both parents. She is up-to-date on routine healthcare maintenance (mammography, colonoscopy, Pap smears) and her physical exam is unremarkable.

Following the laboratory results, she was told to stop taking the diuretic and return in 1 week to have her calcium level and BP rechecked.

 At this point, what is the leading hypothesis, what are the active alternatives, and is there a must not miss diagnosis? Given this differential diagnosis, what tests should be ordered?

RANKING THE DIFFERENTIAL DIAGNOSIS

In healthy ambulatory patients with hypercalcemia, primary hyperparathyroidism is, by far, the most common diagnosis. This disease is often asymptomatic or minimally symptomatic. The chronicity of this patient's hypercalcemia, as well as her relatively good health, are pivotal points that make this diagnosis even more likely. Hypercalcemia related to thiazide use is also possible. Although thiazide diuretics generally cause chronic hypercalcemia in patients with other abnormalities in calcium metabolism, they occasionally do cause mild hypercalcemia in patients with no other cause. Familial hypocalciuric hypercalcemia (FHH) is another cause of chronic, usually asymptomatic hypercalcemia. Although it is usually diagnosed early in life, it can present similarly to primary hyperparathyroidism. Most patients with hypercalcemia due to a malignancy have a known malignancy when presenting with hypercalcemia. Sarcoidosis is not a common cause of hypercalcemia but should probably be considered, given the patient's race, if another diagnosis is not made. Table 22-1 lists an appropriately limited differential diagnosis for this patient.

 After the thiazide diuretic is discontinued, the calcium level is remeasured and remains unchanged. A PTH level is drawn.

 Is the clinical information sufficient to make a diagnosis? If not, what other information do you need?

Leading Hypothesis: Primary Hyperparathyroidism

Textbook Presentation

Primary hyperparathyroidism usually presents with hypercalcemia found during routine laboratory screening. Occasionally, it is

Table 22-1. Diagnostic hypotheses for Mrs. D.

Diagnostic Hypotheses	Demographics, Risk Factors, Symptoms and Signs	Important Tests
Leading Hypothesis		
Primary hyperparathyroidism	Elevated calcium without evident underlying disease	PTH level
Active Alternatives		
Familial hypocalciuric hypercalcemia	Chronic asymptomatic hypercalcemia	PTH level Family history Urine calcium excretion
Thiazide diuretic use	Transient hypercalcemia or exacerbation of hypercalcemia in patient with underlying disease	Resolution with cessation of drug
Active Alternative—Must Not Miss		
Hypercalcemia of malignancy	Usually presents in patients with known malignancy	Diagnosis of malignancy Demonstration of PTHrP or skeletal metastasis
Other Alternative		
Sarcoidosis	Pulmonary disease with hilar lymphadenopathy or interstitial lung disease	Demonstration of noncaseating granulomas and exclusion of other causes of granulomatous disease

PTH, parathyroid hormone; PTHrP, parathyroid hormone–related protein.

detected during the evaluation of nonspecific symptoms, such as fatigue or constipation.

Disease Highlights

A. Primary hyperparathyroidism most commonly presents with a modestly elevated calcium and few (if any) symptoms rather than the classic presentation of "stones, bones, groans, and psychiatric overtones."

Primary hyperparathyroidism accounts for more than 90% of cases of hypercalcemia in otherwise healthy ambulatory patients.

B. Etiology of primary hyperparathyroidism
1. 85% of the cases of primary hyperparathyroidism are due to solitary parathyroid adenomas.
2. Parathyroid hyperplasia, multiple adenomas, and the rare carcinoma, cause the other 15% of cases.
   a. Parathyroid hyperplasia can be sporadic or inherited.
   b. Inherited syndromes of parathyroid hyperplasia include the multiple endocrine neoplasia (MEN) type I and IIA syndromes. Patients with other relevant diagnoses

such as pituitary tumors, islet cell tumors, medullary thyroid carcinomas, and pheochromocytomas should be evaluated for these syndromes.

C. Clinical manifestations of primary hyperparathyroidism
1. Nonspecific symptoms such as fatigue, irritability, and weakness are more common among patients with primary hyperparathyroidism.
2. Decreased bone density is common in patients with primary hyperparathyroidism while classic osteitis fibrosis cystica is exceedingly rare today.
3. Nephrolithiasis is present in 15–20% of patients with primary hyperparathyroidism.
4. Other symptoms of primary hyperparathyroidism probably include increased frequency of hypertension, gout, and calcium pyrophosphate deposition disease.

Evidence-Based Diagnosis

A. Hypercalcemia should be confirmed before evaluating a patient for primary hyperparathyroidism.
1. The calcium level should be remeasured.
2. Ideally, the ionized calcium should be measured. Alternatively, a corrected calcium can be calculated to account for the plasma protein binding of calcium. The corrected calcium = Total calcium (mg/dL) + 0.8(4-albumin [g/dL]).

B. Other effects of elevated PTH levels (hypercalciuria, hypophosphatemia, hyperphosphaturia) are seldom useful in differentiating primary hyperparathyroidism from hypercalcemia of malignancy—the second most common cause of hypercalcemia.

C. The diagnosis of primary hyperparathyroidism is usually straightforward.
1. The diagnosis is extremely likely in an otherwise healthy patient with chronic hypercalcemia.
2. An elevated PTH level is confirmatory, distinguishing primary hyperparathyroidism from hypercalcemia of malignancy which has low serum PTH levels.
3. About 10% of patients with primary hyperparathyroidism have normal PTH levels (a finding that is in fact inappropriate given the hypercalcemia). In these patients, FHH must be excluded.

Treatment

A. Definitive treatment for primary hyperparathyroidism is surgical parathyroidectomy.

B. Who needs surgery?
1. Because of the generally benign course of primary hyperparathyroidism, not everyone needs surgery.
2. Recommendations from consensus panels are based on who is most likely to progress to symptomatic disease and who would benefit most from surgery.
3. Indications for surgery
   a. Symptoms of hypercalcemia
   b. Elevated serum calcium > 1 mg/dL above normal
   c. Creatinine clearance < 60 mL/min
   d. Osteoporosis (bone density with T score < 2.5 at any site) or fragility fracture
   e. Age younger than 50
   f. Patient preference or patient inability to comply with long-term monitoring

C. This approach to deciding which patients undergo surgery appears to be effective. A recent study observing 52 asymptomatic people for up to 10 years demonstrated the disease is usually not progressive.

   1. 38 (73%) had no progression of disease

   2. Patients who required surgery did so for the following reasons:

      a. Hypercalcemia worsened in 2 patients

      b. Hypercalciuria developed in 8 patients

      c. Low bone density developed in 6 patients

D. Parathyroidectomy

   1. Parathyroidectomy is markedly effective at inducing normocalcemia (95–98%), improving bone density (100%), and improving symptoms (82%).

   2. Preoperative nuclear imaging of the parathyroid glands is very helpful in identifying abnormal glands, thus decreasing the need for detailed neck exploration. The data below is for the identification of abnormal glands.

      a. Sensitivity, 69%; specificity, 98%

      b. LR+, 34.5; LR–, 0.32

   3. Intraoperative PTH assays also serve to improve the surgical success rates.

E. Monitoring (for patients not undergoing surgery)

   1. Assessment of symptoms, calcium level, and kidney function yearly.

   2. Biyearly bone density screening of the hip, spine, and wrist.

   3. Initial screening for nephrolithiasis with radiographs or CT scans.

F. If surgery is indicated but the patient declines or is unfit for surgery, medical therapy is indicated.

   1. Patients should be encouraged to remain active, stay well hydrated, and maintain moderate calcium and vitamin D intake in order to retain bone health and reduce the risk of kidney stones.

   2. Thiazide diuretics and lithium carbonate, both of which can exacerbate hypercalcemia, should be avoided.

   3. Bisphosphonates are often used to maintain bone density.

   4. Cinacalcet is probably a good option for patients with primary hyperparathyroidism who cannot or will not undergo surgery.

MAKING A DIAGNOSIS

Final laboratory test results for Mrs. D follow:

Calcium: 10.9 mg/dL
Inorganic phosphate: 3.3 mg/dL (nl 2.5–4.4)
Ionized calcium: 6.20 mg/dL (nl 4.60–5.40)
PTH: 166 pg/mL (nl < 60 pg/mL)

A diagnosis of primary hyperparathyroidism was made.

 Have you crossed a diagnostic threshold for the leading hypothesis, primary hyperparathyroidism? Have you ruled out the active alternatives? Do other tests need to be done to exclude the alternative diagnoses?

Other than primary hyperparathyroidism, the differential diagnosis of hypercalcemia in a patient with an elevated PTH is lithium use, MEN syndromes, secondary or tertiary hyperparathyroidism, or familial hypocalciuric hypercalcemia. Given the patient's medications, normal kidney function, age at presentation, and lack of a family history of hypercalcemia, primary hyperparathyroidism is clearly the most likely diagnosis. FHH would remain a possibility if not for the markedly elevated PTH level. Thiazide diuretic use does not cause hypercalcemia via hyperparathyroidism and thus does not explain the patient's hypercalcemia. It could have been a contributing factor in the initial presentation.

Alternative Diagnosis: Familial Hypocalciuric Hypercalcemia

Textbook Presentation

The diagnosis of FHH is usually made in childhood during evaluation of asymptomatic hypercalcemia or during screening because of a positive family history. The condition may also present during adulthood as hypercalcemia with a normal to slightly elevated PTH.

Disease Highlights

A. The mutation in FHH makes the calcium sensing receptor, found on various tissues throughout the body, less sensitive to calcium. In the parathyroid glands, this means that higher serum calcium levels are needed to suppress PTH release. The defect leads to:

   1. Secretion of PTH inappropriate to calcium levels

   2. Renal absorption of calcium inappropriate to calcium levels

B. Most patients with FHH are asymptomatic at the time of presentation.

Evidence-Based Diagnosis

A. FHH is usually easily distinguished from primary hyperparathyroidism as the former usually has mildly elevated calcium levels and a normal PTH level while the latter has an elevated PTH level.

B. Differentiation can be difficult because patients with FHH sometimes have a mildly elevated PTH, and patients with primary hyperparathyroidism often have mild hypercalcemia and have a normal PTH 10% of the time.

C. Three important distinguishing features are:

   1. Patients with FHH usually have family members with FHH. The genetic defect is inherited in an autosomal dominant manner.

   2. Urinary calcium excretion is reduced (> 99% reabsorption vs < 99% in primary hyperparathyroidism).

      a. A urinary calcium < 200 mg/day suggests FHH.

      b. A fractional excretion of calcium < 0.01 is nearly diagnostic of FHH. Patients with primary hyperparathyroidism usually have results > 0.02. (Fractional excretion of calcium = (urine calcium × serum creatinine)/(serum calcium × urine creatinine)

   3. Serum magnesium is often increased in FHH.

   4. Genetic testing is available when the diagnosis is difficult to make.

Treatment

Treatment for FHH is not necessary because the hypercalcemia is mild and only very rarely leads to complications.

Alternative Diagnosis: Thiazide-Induced Hypercalcemia

Textbook Presentation

Thiazide-induced hypercalcemia usually occurs transiently after starting a thiazide diuretic. It is generally mild and is not associated with hyperparathyroidism.

Disease Highlights

A. Thiazide diuretics cause hypocalciuria.

1. Sodium depletion causes increased sodium and calcium retention in the proximal tubule.

2. Thiazides probably also augment the effect of PTH.

B. Hypercalcemia is generally mild and short lived because reduced PTH secretion will normalize calcium levels.

C. Some patients may have persistently, although still only mildly, elevated calcium levels.

D. Patients with underlying hyperparathyroidism, or other causes of increased bone turnover, are more likely to have persistent and more pronounced degrees of hypercalcemia.

Evidence-Based Diagnosis

A. The diagnosis of thiazide-induced hypercalcemia depends on documenting hypercalcemia temporally related to beginning a diuretic.

B. Resolution of the abnormality with cessation of the drug is diagnostic.

C. Patients taking a thiazide who have persistent elevations of calcium of > 0.5 mg/dL above normal should be evaluated for other causes of hypercalcemia.

Treatment

Because the hypercalcemia is almost always mild and short lived, no treatment is necessary.

CASE RESOLUTION

The combination of hypercalcemia and an elevated PTH confirms the diagnosis of primary hyperparathyroidism. Based on the patient's severe constipation, without another cause, the decision was made to treat her hyperparathyroidism. She underwent nuclear scanning of the parathyroid glands and then parathyroidectomy. A 3 × 3 cm, 4-g parathyroid adenoma was found and surgically removed without complication.

On follow-up, after close monitoring of her calcium postoperatively (when hypocalcemia can occur) the patient had rapid normalization of her calcium levels. Her constipation, however, persisted. In the end, the constipation was considered to be functional and unrelated to the hypercalcemia.

As discussed above, the patient's symptoms are an indication for surgery. However, since the patient's symptoms were nonspecific, there was no guarantee that they were related to the hyperparathyroidism.

CHIEF COMPLAINT

Mrs. W is an 80-year-old woman who is admitted to the hospital because of lethargy, abdominal pain, and hypercalcemia. She reports 1 year of epigastric pain that was initially mild but has become severe and persistent over the last 6 weeks. Her daughter, who found her somewhat confused at their weekly lunch, brought her to the office.

On evaluation she is found to be lethargic but oriented to person and place. Vital signs: temperature, 36.9° C; pulse, 94 bpm; BP, 110/90 mm Hg; RR, 14 breaths per minute. She is orthostatic. Her exam is remarkable for cachexia and hepatomegaly.

Initial laboratory test results in the physician's office were:

Sodium: 134 mEq/L
Potassium: 3.9 mEq/L
Chloride: 99 mEq/L
CO2: 26 mEq/L
BUN: 24 mg/dL
Creatinine: 0.8 mg/dL
Glucose: 117 mg/dL
Calcium: 15.0 mg/dL
Albumin: 3.9 g/dL
Total bilirubin: 0.9 g/dL
Conjugated bilirubin: 0.6 g/dL
Alkaline phosphatase: 800 units/L
AST (SGOT): 124 units/L
ALT (SGPT): 86 units/L
Phosphate: 1.4 mg/dL

At this point, what is the leading hypothesis, what are the active alternatives, and is there a must not miss diagnosis? Given this differential diagnosis, what tests should be ordered?

RANKING THE DIFFERENTIAL DIAGNOSIS

This is an elderly woman with abdominal pain and marked hypercalcemia. Although primary hyperparathyroidism is a possibility, there are multiple pivotal points that suggest other diagnoses. These include the degree of hypercalcemia and the abnormalities found on physical exam and laboratory studies. Hypercalcemia of malignancy needs to be considered given the patient's age and hepatomegaly. Most patients with hypercalcemia of malignancy have a previously diagnosed cancer, but it is possible for symptoms of cancer and hypercalcemia to present simultaneously or for symptoms of hypercalcemia to be the presenting symptoms of the malignancy. Malignancy usually leads to hypercalcemia through the elaboration of PTHrP or through osseous metastasis.

The milk-alkali syndrome should be considered. This syndrome is often caused by ingestion of large amounts of calcium carbonate in an effort to treat dyspepsia. This syndrome typically presents with hypercalcemia, metabolic alkalosis, and acute kidney injury. The presence of only 1 of the syndrome's 3 features

Table 22-2. Diagnostic hypotheses for Mrs. W.

Diagnostic Hypotheses	Demographics, Risk Factors, Symptoms and Signs	Important Tests
Leading Hypothesis		
Humoral hypercalcemia of malignancy	Presence of malignancy, usually previously diagnosed Squamous cell carcinomas and adenocarcinomas of the lung, pancreas, and kidney most common	PTHrP
Active Alternatives		
Local osteolytic hypercalcemia of malignancy	Presence of malignancy, usually previously diagnosed Multiple myeloma and breast cancer most common	Demonstration of bony metastases
Primary hyperparathyroidism	Elevated calcium without evident underlying disease	PTH level
Other Alternative		
Milk-alkali syndrome	Hypercalcemia, metabolic alkalosis, and acute kidney injury	Normal PTH level and history of calcium and absorbable alkali ingestion

PTH, parathyroid hormone; PTHrP parathyroid hormone–related protein.

(hypercalcemia) makes this diagnosis less likely. The presence of other illnesses or medication use may suggest less common causes of hypercalcemia, such as granulomatous disease. Table 22-2 lists the differential diagnosis for this patient.

The patient reports no significant prior medical history but she has not seen a physician in over 5 years. She has been using calcium carbonate (Tums) for her abdominal pain but reports only intermittent use and none for the last few days. She is not taking any other medications. Review of systems is unremarkable other than the previously noted fatigue and abdominal pain.

An abdominal ultrasound reveals multiple hepatic masses.

Is the clinical information sufficient to make a diagnosis? If not, what other information do you need?

Leading Hypothesis: Humoral Hypercalcemia of Malignancy

Textbook Presentation

Hypercalcemia of malignancy is most commonly detected in patients with previously diagnosed cancers. It is uncommon for

symptomatic hypercalcemia to be the presenting symptom of a malignancy. Hypercalcemia of malignancy carries a horrendous prognosis with 50% 30-day mortality.

Disease Highlights

A. Hypercalcemia of malignancy is a heterogeneous process.

   1. The most common pathophysiology behind hypercalcemia in malignancy is elaboration of PTHrP by tumor cells. This is referred to as humoral hypercalcemia of malignancy (HHM).

   2. Tumors metastatic to bone may also cause hypercalcemia through local osteolytic effects on the bones, sometimes via local elaboration of PTHrP. This syndrome is discussed below.

   3. It is likely there is a great deal of overlap between these first 2 causes.

   4. Rarely, tumors can cause hypercalcemia by elaborating vitamin D (seen most commonly with lymphoma).

B. The malignancies that commonly cause hypercalcemia are (in approximate order of frequency):

   1. Lung

   2. Breast

   3. Multiple myeloma

   4. Lymphoma

   5. Head and neck

   6. Renal

   7. Prostate

C. PTHrP is a normal, physiologic, protein that is produced by many non-neoplastic tissues.

   1. The protein shares considerable sequence homology to PTH and binds to the same receptor.

   2. PTH and PTHrP affect the bones and kidneys in the same way.

   3. Certain malignancies elaborate the protein in relatively large amounts.

      a. PTHrP is detectable in 80% of patients with hypercalcemia and malignancy.

      b. The most common tumors that produce PTHrP are squamous cell carcinomas and adenocarcinomas of the lung, pancreas, and kidney.

   4. In hypercalcemia of malignancy secondary to PTHrP, hypercalcemia commonly precedes bony metastasis.

Evidence-Based Diagnosis

A. Similar to primary hyperparathyroidism, hypercalcemia of malignancy seldom presents significant diagnostic confusion.

B. In patients with a known malignancy, the diagnosis is made by detecting high PTHrP and low PTH levels.

Treatment

A. Patients with hypercalcemia of malignancy benefit from treatment of the underlying disease.

B. Beyond treatment of the malignancy, treatment aimed directly at hypercalcemia depends on its severity.

C. The mainstays of treatment for moderate and severe elevations of calcium are the bisphosphonates.

   1. Bisphosphonates work by inhibiting osteoclast activity.

   2. Pamidronate and zoledronic acid are both approved for the treatment of hypercalcemia of malignancy in the United States.

D. For patients with severe, symptomatic hypercalcemia, therapy must be more rapidly effective than treatment of the underlying disease or bisphosphonate therapy (which takes about 48 hours to reach full effectiveness).

  1. Saline hydration treats the dehydration that frequently accompanies hypercalcemia and decreases reabsorption of calcium in the proximal tubule of dehydrated, hypercalcemic patients.

  2. Once hydration is attained, a loop diuretic can further assist in achieving calciuresis.

  3. While calcitonin rapidly decreases hypercalcemia, it also decreases bone resorption.

  4. While immediate therapy for hypercalcemia is instituted, a bisphosphonate should be given and long-term treatment of the malignancy should be planned.

E. In all patients being treated for hypercalcemia of malignancy, care should be taken to institute other measures known to decrease serum calcium. Calcium supplements should be stopped, drugs that lead to hypercalcemia (lithium, thiazides) should be held, hypophosphatemia should be treated and weight-bearing exercise should be encouraged.

Given the results of the patient's ultrasound, it is highly likely that she has a malignancy that is causing the hypercalcemia. The next step is to make a definitive diagnosis of the malignancy so that specific treatment can be instituted. Determining how the malignancy is causing hypercalcemia will be part of this evaluation; is the hypercalcemia a result of osseous metastasis or of PTHrP?

The patient was given normal saline for hydration and furosemide for diuresis when mild peripheral edema developed. Her calcium dropped over the first 3 days in the hospital to 11.2 mg/dL, where it remained stable.

As a follow-up to the ultrasound, a chest/abdomen/pelvis CT was ordered. This revealed a large lung mass and multiple liver masses. CT-guided biopsy of the liver was consistent with metastatic squamous cell carcinoma, likely of pulmonary origin.

Have you crossed a diagnostic threshold for the leading hypothesis, hypercalcemia of malignancy (elaboration of PTHrP)? Have you ruled out the active alternatives? Do other tests need to be done to exclude the alternative diagnoses?

MAKING A DIAGNOSIS

Alternative Diagnosis: Local Osteolytic Hypercalcemia of Malignancy

Textbook Presentation

Similar to hypercalcemia of malignancy caused by PTHrP, hypercalcemia due to malignancies metastatic to bone generally presents in patients with previously diagnosed cancer. Breast cancer and multiple myeloma (discussed in detail here) are the most common causes.

Multiple myeloma commonly presents with bone pain (often back pain), anemia, hypercalcemia, or acute kidney disease in patients in their 60s. Plain radiographs commonly demonstrate

osteolytic lesions and the diagnosis is made by the demonstration of paraproteinemia and increased plasma cells on bone marrow exam.

Disease Highlights

A. Multiple myeloma (and breast cancer) only cause hypercalcemia after metastasizing to bone.

B. The hypercalcemia is caused by local osteolytic effects on bone.

C. Multiple myeloma is caused by a malignant proliferation of plasma cells. The plasma cells usually secrete a single immunoglobulin, or fragment of immunoglobulin, called the M component (monoclonal component).

D. Multiple myeloma most commonly affects patients in the seventh decade of life. Blacks are affected at twice the rate as whites.

E. Symptoms are varied and result from the effect of plasma cell proliferation on multiple systems.

  1. Anemia: Secondary to plasma cell infiltration of the bone marrow.

  2. Infections: When the M component is excluded, patients with myeloma usually have hypogammaglobulinemia.

  3. Bone pain and hypercalcemia: Proliferation of plasma cells in the bone cause osteolytic lesions.

  4. Kidney disease: Multiple myeloma can cause kidney disease in multiple ways:

    a. Light chains may injure the kidney via toxicity to the renal tubules or through obstruction secondary to the heavy burden of filtered protein.

    b. Hypercalcemia

    c. Amyloid deposition in the kidney

    d. Urate nephropathy

  5. Serum hyperviscosity may occur from hypergammaglobulinemia; the most common symptoms are headache and visual disturbances.

F. Symptoms at presentation as reported in 1 study of over 1000 patients:

  1. Anemia was present in 73% of patients. The anemia was usually mild, normochromic, normocytic.

  2. 58% of patients had bone pain at presentation and 67% had lytic bone lesions on radiographs.

  3. 19% had renal disease

  4. 13% had hypercalcemia > 11 mg/dL

  5. M component

    a. 82% of patients had an abnormal serum protein electrophoresis. Of the 18% with a normal serum electrophoresis, 97% had an abnormal urine protein electrophoresis.

    b. The M component most commonly appears in the gamma range and is most commonly IgG.

    c. 16% have only free light chains.

  6. A sizable minority (36%) had a history of or presence of another plasma cell abnormality present at the time of diagnosis (monoclonal gammopathy of unknown significance, plasmacytoma, amyloidosis).

G. Monoclonal gammopathy of unknown significance (MGUS)

  1. Commonly seen in older patients (≈ 3% of patient > 50)

  2. MGUS is diagnosed when there is M component present on serum protein electrophoresis but the patient does not fulfill criteria for myeloma (listed below).

3. The M component is generally small, < 3 g/dL

4. Patients with MGUS have an elevated risk of developing multiple myeloma (≈ 1%/year)

Evidence-Based Diagnosis

A. The diagnosis of multiple myeloma is based on the identification of:

1. Marrow plasmacytosis (> 10%)

2. Lytic bone lesions

3. M component detected on serum or urine electrophoresis.

B. Clues to the diagnosis are the presence of normocytic anemia, bone pain, and elevated immunoglobulins.

C. There are a few important issues that may confuse the diagnosis.

1. Filtered light chains are not detected on traditional urine dipsticks. A patient with light chain only myeloma may have normal amounts of serum protein, a normal serum protein electrophoresis and, apparently, no proteinuria. The presence of a monoclonal gammopathy will be detected only by urine protein electrophoresis.

2. The bone lesions of multiple myeloma are almost exclusively osteolytic. They will usually be missed on bone scans but are seen on radiographs.

Treatment

The treatment of hypercalcemia of malignancy due to local osteolytic metastases is the same as that for HHM discussed above.

Alternative Diagnosis: Milk-Alkali Syndrome

Textbook Presentation

There can be many presentations of the milk-alkali syndrome. Acute cases often present as hypercalcemia in women who use calcium carbonate for dyspepsia or osteoporosis.

Disease Highlights

A. The milk-alkali syndrome is a syndrome of hypercalcemia, metabolic alkalosis, and acute kidney injury caused by the ingestion of calcium and an absorbable alkali.

B. The syndrome was first described as a complication of a proposed ulcer therapy that included high doses of magnesium carbonate, sodium bicarbonate, bismuth subcarbonate, and about 1 liter of a milk/cream mixture daily.

C. The pathogenesis likely involves hypercalcemia secondary to the ingestion followed by a resultant decrease in glomerular filtration rate. The combination of acute kidney injury, hypercalcemia, and alkali ingestion then causes the metabolic alkalosis.

D. The modern presentation of the milk-alkali syndrome includes a wide range of calcium values, low to normal phosphate levels, moderate acute kidney injury (average creatinine 4.2 mg/dL in a review of modern, published cases), and calcium carbonate as the source of calcium and absorbable alkali.

E. The milk-alkali syndrome is a distant third among the leading causes of hypercalcemia in hospitalized patients, after malignancy and primary hyperparathyroidism.

Evidence-Based Diagnosis

The diagnosis of milk-alkali syndrome is based on history with supporting laboratory test results (hypercalcemia, metabolic alkalosis, and normal to low PTH).

Treatment

A. Cessation of calcium carbonate intake and hydration is usually sufficient treatment of milk-alkali syndrome.

B. Caution should be taken when treating patients with severe milk-alkali syndrome with fluid and loop diuretics. These patients appear to be at particular risk for subsequent, transient, hypocalcemia.

C. A subset of patients, possibly those with more prolonged or severe disease complicated by hypovolemia, may never recover normal renal function.

CASE RESOLUTION

The patient's laboratory test results follow:

PTHrP: 3.3 pmol/L (nl 0–1.9 pmol/L)
PTH: 13 pg/mL (nl < 60 pg/mL)

Mrs. W's hypercalcemia was diagnosed as humoral hypercalcemia of malignancy. She was treated with zoledronic acid and hydration. The patient opted to be treated with palliative chemotherapy. Her condition declined markedly over the next 12 weeks. Chemotherapy was discontinued, and she was transferred to a hospice center where she died 4 weeks later.

Because the patient had metastatic squamous cell lung cancer, her rapid decline was expected. The average life expectancy of patients with squamous cell carcinoma and extensive disease is a little less than 1 year and, as mentioned above, the presence of hypercalcemia worsens the prognosis of a malignancy.

REVIEW OF OTHER IMPORTANT DISEASES

Secondary & Tertiary Hyperparathyroidism

Disease Highlights

A. Secondary and tertiary hyperparathyroidism occur in patients with CKD.

B. Secondary hyperparathyroidism is usually associated with hypocalcemia. It is most commonly caused by the chronic hypocalcemia of CKD leading to parathyroid hyperplasia. Therapy for the hyperphosphatemia associated with secondary hyperparathyroidism, however, can lead to hypercalcemia.

1. Hyperphosphatemia develops in patients with CKD as the renal clearance of phosphate falls.

2. Early in the course of CKD, hypocalcemia, hypovitaminosis D, and hyperphosphatemia lead to (secondary) hyperparathyroidism. The elevated PTH is adaptive, increasing calcium release from bones and enhancing renal phosphate excretion.

3. As CKD worsens, hyperparathyroidism becomes counterproductive as the kidneys no longer respond to PTH by excreting phosphate while phosphate continues to be released, with calcium, from the bones.

4. Treatment of hyperphosphatemia in CKD

   a. Calcium carbonate and calcium acetate have been the traditional first-line therapy for hyperphosphatemia in CKD.

(1) Calcium carbonate and calcium acetate are effective phosphate binders, decreasing the GI absorption of phosphate.

(2) Calcium-based phosphate binders rarely bring phosphate into the normal range and may cause hypercalcemia.

(3) This hypercalcemia (and hyperphosphatemia) may be exacerbated by exogenous calcitriol, also used to treat secondary hyperparathyroidism.

(4) High levels of calcium and phosphate have deleterious cardiovascular effects.

b. Newer therapies offer alternatives for lowering phosphate more effectively without leading to hypercalcemia.

(1) Sevelamer is a synthetic phosphate-binding polymer.

(2) The calcium mimetic cinacalcet targets the calcium-sensing receptor in the parathyroid glands, lowering PTH levels.

(3) Newer vitamin D analogues may be able to lower PTH levels with less of a tendency to cause hypercalcemia and hyperphosphatemia.

c. It is important to realize that we do not yet have robust clinical data supporting the use of these new medications over the more traditional phosphate binders.

d. Tertiary hyperparathyroidism occurs when the parathyroid hyperplasia of secondary hyperparathyroidism becomes so severe that PTH production becomes autonomous, causing hypercalcemia beyond that expected by calcium and calcitriol therapy.

Evidence-Based Diagnosis

A. In patients with CKD, an elevated calcium level, in the setting of calcium carbonate use and an elevated PTH, is diagnostic of secondary hyperparathyroidism.

B. Tertiary hyperparathyroidism is diagnosed when PTH reaches higher levels and does not respond to calcium supplementation and vitamin D.

Treatment

A. The treatment of secondary hyperparathyroidism is very complicated and is predicated on treating the factors that stimulate PTH secretion in CKD: hypocalcemia, hypovitaminosis D, and hyperphosphatemia.

B. Treatment involves phosphate binders, calcium and/or calcimimetics, and vitamin D analogues all used in an effort to control the levels of PTH, calcium, and phosphate.

C. If tertiary hyperparathyroidism occurs and is symptomatic (based on hypercalcemia, bone disease, metastatic calcifications) parathyroidectomy is often required.

REFERENCES

Beall DP, Scofield RH. Milk-alkali syndrome associated with calcium carbonate consumption. Report of 7 patients with parathyroid hormone levels and an estimate of prevalence among patients hospitalized with hypercalcemia. Medicine (Baltimore). 1995;74:89–96.

Bilezikian JP, Potts JT Jr, Fuleihan Gel H et al. Summary statement from a workshop on asymptomatic primary hyperparathyroidism: a perspective for the 21st century. J Clin Endocrinol Metab. 2002;87:5353–61.

Block GA, Martin KJ, de Francisco AL et al. Cinacalcet for secondary hyperparathyroidism in patients receiving hemodialysis. N Engl J Med. 2004;350:1516–25.

Fraser WD. Hyperparathyroidism. Lancet. 2009 Jul 11; 374(9684):145–58.

Irvin GL 3rd, Carneiro DM. Management changes in primary hyperparathyroidism. JAMA. 2000;284:934–6.

Kyle RA, Gertz MA, Witzig TE et al. Review of 1027 patients with newly diagnosed multiple myeloma. Mayo Clin Proc. 2003;78:21–33.

Lundgren E, Ljunghall S, Akerstrom G, Hetta J, Mallmin H, Rastad J. Case-control study on symptoms and signs of "asymptomatic" primary hyperparathyroidism. Surgery. 1998;124:980–5.

Marcocci C, Cetani F. Primary hyperparathyroidism. N Engl J Med. 2011;365:2389–97.

Marx SJ. Hyperparathyroid and hypoparathyroid disorders. N Engl J Med. 2000;343:1863–75.

Pattou F, Torres G, Mondragon-Sanchez A et al. Correlation of parathyroid scanning and anatomy in 261 unselected patients with sporadic primary hyperparathyroidism. Surgery. 1999;126:1123–31.

Peacock M, Bilezikian JP, Bolognese MA et al. Cinacalcet HCl reduces hypercalcemia in primary hyperparathyroidism across a wide spectrum of disease severity. J Clin Endocrinol Metab. 2011 Jan; 96(1):E9–18.

Tonelli M, Pannu N, Manns B. Oral phosphate binders in patients with kidney failure. N Engl J Med. 2010;362:1312–24.

Silverberg SJ, Shane E, Jacobs TP, Siris E, Bilezikian JP. A 10-year prospective study of primary hyperparathyroidism with or without parathyroid surgery. N Engl J Med. 1999;341:1249–55.

Sippy B. Gastric and duodenal ulcer: Medical cure by an efficient removal of gastric juice corrosion. JAMA. 1915;64:1625.

Stewart AF. Clinical practice. Hypercalcemia associated with cancer. N Engl J Med. 2005;352:373–9.

I have a patient with hypertension. How do I determine the cause?

CHIEF COMPLAINT

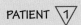

PATIENT

Mr. U is a 48-year-old man with a BP of 165/90 mm Hg.

What is the differential diagnosis of hypertension? How would you frame the differential?

CONSTRUCTING A DIFFERENTIAL DIAGNOSIS

First, what is normal BP, and when is a patient hypertensive? The first step is accurately measuring the BP. Table 23-1 summarizes guidelines for obtaining valid BP measurements.

Consensus guidelines classify BP as follows, based on the mean of 2 seated BP measurements on each of 2 or more office visits:

A. Optimal: systolic BP (SBP) < 120 mm Hg **and** diastolic BP (DBP) < 80 mm Hg

B. Normal: SBP 120–129 mm Hg **and** DBP 80–84 mm Hg

C. High normal: SBP 130–139 mm Hg **or** DBP 85–89 mm Hg

D. Grade 1 hypertension: SBP 140–159 mm Hg **or** DBP 90–99 mm Hg

E. Grade 2 hypertension: SBP 160–179 mm Hg **or** DBP 100–109 mm Hg

F. Grade 3 hypertension: SBP ≥ 180 mm Hg **or** DBP ≥ 110 mm Hg

G. Isolated systolic hypertension: SBP ≥ 140 mm Hg **and** DBP < 90 mm Hg

Hypertension is either primary (essential) or secondary (resulting from a specific identifiable cause). Causes of secondary hypertension can be organized using an organ/system framework:

A. Primary (essential) hypertension

B. Secondary hypertension

  1. Endocrine

    a. Primary aldosteronism

    b. Pheochromocytoma

    c. Thyroid disease

    d. Hyperparathyroidism

    e. Cushing syndrome

  2. Renal

    a. Chronic kidney disease (CKD)

    b. Acute kidney injury

  3. Vascular

    a. Renovascular disease

    b. Coarctation of the aorta

  4. Pulmonary: sleep apnea

  5. GI: obesity

  6. Drug-induced or drug-related

    a. Prolonged corticosteroid therapy

    b. Nonselective nonsteroidal antiinflammatory drugs (NSAIDs)

    c. Cyclooxygenase (COX)-2 inhibitors

    d. Cocaine

    e. Alcohol

    f. Sympathomimetics (decongestants, anorectics)

    g. Oral contraceptives

    h. Cyclosporine and tacrolimus

    i. Erythropoietin

    j. Stimulants (modafinil, amphetamines)

Mr. U's BP is high. He has wanted to avoid taking medication and has been trying to watch his diet and lose weight. Both of his parents and several of his siblings have hypertension. His medical history is notable only for smoking 1 pack/day for 30 years; he does not use alcohol and takes no medications.

At this point, what is the leading hypothesis, what are the active alternatives, and is there a must not miss diagnosis? Given this differential diagnosis, what tests should be ordered?

RANKING THE DIFFERENTIAL DIAGNOSIS

Ninety-five to 99% of patients with hypertension have essential hypertension. A family history of hypertension increases the pretest probability of essential hypertension and is a pivotal clue in Mr. U's history. Patients between the ages of 20 and 50 have about twice the risk of developing hypertension if they have 1 first-degree relative with hypertension; the relative risk is 3–4 if 2 first-degree relatives have hypertension. Common conditions that can contribute to or cause hypertension include obesity, hyperthyroidism or hypothyroidism, acute kidney injury or CKD, excessive alcohol use, sleep apnea, and the use of drugs listed previously. Other secondary causes are quite rare in *unselected* populations, with estimated prevalences of 0.18–4.4% for renovascular hypertension, 0.04–0.2%

Table 23-1. Guidelines for measuring BP.

- The patient should sit for several minutes in a quiet room before BP measurements are taken. Pain, stress, a full urinary bladder, a recent meal, and talking or active listening during measurement affect BP. Having smoked a cigarette within 15–20 minutes can elevate the BP by 5–20 mm Hg.
- Take at least 2 measurements spaced by 1–2 minutes and additional measurements if the first 2 are quite different.
- Using a bladder that is too narrow yields false high readings. Instead of the standard cuff (12–13 cm long, 35 cm wide) use an appropriate larger cuff in patients with increased arm circumference.
- Use phase I (first tapping sound) and V (disappearance) Korotkoff sounds to identify systolic and diastolic BP values, respectively.
- Do not deflate the cuff too rapidly, otherwise individual Korotkoff sounds are missed and too low a value is measured; start with a deflation rate of 2 mm/s.
- Measure the heart rate by palpation and watch out for arrhythmia, which mandates repeated BP measurements.
- At the first visit, measure BP in both arms and take the higher value as the reference; measure BP at 1 minute and 5 minutes after standing upright if the patient has a disorder that frequently causes orthostatic hypotension.

Adapted, with permission, from Messerli FH, Williams B, Ritz E. Essential hypertension. Lancet. 2007;370:591–603.

for pheochromocytoma, 0.01–0.4% for primary hyperaldosteronism, and 0.3% for Cushing syndrome. These conditions are more prevalent in populations of patients with *resistant* hypertension. Table 23-2 lists the differential diagnosis.

Mr. U's review of symptoms is negative for chest pain, shortness of breath, claudication, headache, dizziness, palpitations, weight change, constipation, daytime sleepiness, and snoring. On physical exam, BP is 165/90 mm Hg in both arms; pulse, 84 bpm; RR, 16 breaths per minute. He weighs 220 pounds, with a body mass index (BMI) of 30 kg/m². Fundoscopic exam shows some arteriolar narrowing with no hemorrhages or exudates. Jugular venous pressure is normal. Lungs are clear, and cardiac exam shows an S_4 but no S_3 or murmurs. There are no abdominal bruits; carotid, radial, femoral, posterior tibialis, and dorsalis pedis pulses are normal. There is no peripheral edema. Neurologic exam is normal.

Is the clinical information sufficient to make a diagnosis? If not, what other information do you need?

Leading Hypothesis: Essential Hypertension

Textbook Presentation

Essential hypertension generally presents as the gradual onset of elevated BP, most often in middle-aged people with positive family histories. Coexisting diabetes or obesity is common.

Disease Highlights

A. Patients who are normotensive at age 55 have a 90% lifetime risk of developing hypertension.

B. Across the BP range of 115/75 mm Hg to 185/115 mm Hg, each increment of 20 mm Hg systolic BP or 10 mm Hg diastolic BP doubles the risk of cardiovascular disease.

Table 23-2. Diagnostic hypotheses for Mr. U.

Diagnostic Hypotheses	Demographics, Risk Factors, Symptoms and Signs	Important Tests
Leading Hypothesis		
Essential hypertension	Family history Obesity Coexistent diabetes	HgbA$_{1c}$
Active Alternatives—Most Common		
Chronic kidney disease	Often none Sometimes edema, malaise	Serum creatinine Estimated GFR Urinalysis
Sleep apnea	Obesity Neck circumference > 17 in Frequent snoring Daytime somnolence Witnessed apnea	Polysomnogram
Thyroid disease	*Hyperthyroidism:* Weight loss Loose stools Palpitations Sweating *Hypothyroidism:* Weight gain Constipation Fatigue	TSH
Alcohol	Alcohol history	Alcohol history CAGE questionnaire
Drug/medication use	Medication/drug history	Medication/drug history
Other Hypotheses		
Renal artery stenosis	Abrupt onset or accelerated hypertension Azotemia after use of ACE inhibitor Hypertension refractory to ≥ 3 medications Abdominal or flank bruit Other vascular disease (coronary, carotid, or peripheral) Smoking Severe retinopathy	Duplex ultrasonography MRA with gadolinium CT angiography
Hyperaldosteronism	Resistant hypertension Hypokalemia	Aldosterone/renin ratio
Pheochromocytoma	Labile BP/paroxysmal hypertension Headache Sweating Orthostasis Tachycardia	Plasma metanephrine

ACE, angiotensin-converting enzyme; GFR, glomerular filtration rate; MRA, magnetic resonance angiography; TSH, thyroid-stimulating hormone.

Evidence-Based Diagnosis

The evaluation of patients with hypertension focuses primarily on assessing other cardiovascular risk factors and assessing the presence or absence of target organ damage (TOD). Extensive testing for secondary causes is generally not done unless the patient has specific symptoms strongly suggestive of a specific secondary cause or if BP control cannot be achieved. Therefore, there are 3 objectives of testing in patients with hypertension:

A. **Objective 1: Assess presence or absence of TOD** (Table 23-3).

B. **Objective 2: Assess presence or absence of other cardiovascular risk factors**.

  1. Smoking

  2. Obesity (BMI > 30 kg/m²)

  3. Physical inactivity

  4. Dyslipidemia

  5. Diabetes

  6. Microalbuminuria or estimated glomerular filtration rate (GFR) < 60 mL/min

  7. Age (> 55 for men, > 65 for women)

  8. Family history of premature cardiovascular disease (men < 55, women < 65)

  9. Calculate a global risk score such as the Framingham Risk Score (see Chapter 2, Screening & Health Maintenance)

C. **Objective 3: Identify secondary hypertension**.

  1. In the absence of any of the clinical clues listed previously, it is unlikely that the patient has renal artery stenosis, hyperaldosteronism, or pheochromocytoma.

Table 23-3. Assessing target organ damage in patients with hypertension.

Target organ	Clinical Manifestations	Important Tests
Heart	Left ventricular hypertrophy	Physical exam, ECG, Echocardiography in selected patients
	Coronary artery disease (angina, myocardial infarction)	History, ECG, Stress test in selected patients
	Heart failure	History, Physical exam, Echocardiography
Brain	Stroke, transient ischemic attack	History, Physical exam
Kidneys	Proteinuria, Chronic kidney disease	Albumin/creatinine ratio, Serum creatinine, urinalysis
Eyes	Retinopathy	Fundoscopic or ophthalmologic exam
Peripheral vasculature	Peripheral vascular disease	History and physical exam, ABI measurements in selected patients

ABI, ankle-brachial index; ECG, electrocardiogram.

  2. Testing should focus on screening for more common causes or contributors to hypertension, such as kidney or thyroid disease, that are easily diagnosed with simple blood tests.

 Initial testing in a patient with hypertension and no clinical clues should include an ECG, electrolytes, BUN, creatinine, calcium, TSH, urine albumin–creatinine ratio, fasting glucose, and fasting lipid panel (total cholesterol, high-density lipoprotein [HDL], triglycerides, low-density lipoprotein [LDL]).

Treatment

A. **Goal 1**: reduce BP to recommended target (2013 European Society of Hypertension guidelines)

  1. The SBP goal is < 140 mm Hg in all patients, including those with diabetes and CKD, except

    a. In patients 65–80 years of age, a SBP of 140–150 mm Hg is acceptable; a target of < 140 mm Hg should be considered in patients with high functional status and the ability to tolerate additional medication.

    b. In patients over 80 years of age, the target SBP is 140–150 mm Hg.

     (1) All of the studies of hypertension treatment in the elderly included only patients with SBP ≥ 160 mm Hg.

     (2) Decisions regarding whether to treat hypertension and target SBP in the elderly should be adapted based on the patient's functional status, comorbid conditions, and medication side effects.

  2. The DBP goal is < 90 mm Hg in all patients except

    a. In patients with diabetes, the DBP target is < 85 mm Hg.

    b. The American Diabetes Association recommends a DBP target of < 80 mm Hg.

  3. Lifestyle changes (Tables 23-4 and 23-5) should be initiated in all patients with any grade of hypertension, and in patients with high normal BP plus additional cardiovascular risk factors, CKD, diabetes mellitus, or TOD.

    a. Low-risk patients (grade 1 hypertension, no other cardiovascular risk factors, no TOD) should be given several months to achieve their target BP with lifestyle changes.

    b. Moderate-risk patients (grade 1–2 hypertension with < 3 other risk factors) should start taking medication if goal BP is not achieved after several weeks of lifestyle changes.

Table 23-4. Effects of lifestyle changes on BP.

Intervention	Approximate Reduction in Systolic BP
Weight reduction	5–20 mm Hg/10 kg weight loss
DASH diet (see Table 23-5)	8–14 mm Hg
Reduced sodium diet (< 2.4 g sodium/day)	2–8 mm Hg
Aerobic exercise, 30 minutes/day, several days/week	4–9 mm Hg
Limitation of alcohol consumption to ≤ 2 drinks/day for men and ≤ 1 drink/day for women	2–4 mm Hg

Table 23-5. DASH diet.

Food group	Number of Servings
Grains/grain products	7–8/day
Vegetables	4–5/day
Fruits	4–5/day
Low-fat dairy products	2–3/day
Meats, poultry, fish	2–3/day
Fats, oils	2–3/day
Sweets	5/week
Nuts, seeds, dried beans	4–5/week

Many clinicians would start medication simultaneously with the initiation of lifestyle changes.

  c. High-risk patients (grade 3 hypertension, lower grade hypertension with multiple risk factors, TOD, CKD stage 3, or diabetes mellitus) should start taking medication simultaneously with the initiation of lifestyle changes.

4. Selecting antihypertensive medication: general principles

  a. Monotherapy is successful in a limited number of patients.

  b. Combining 2 agents from any 2 classes reduces BP more than increasing the dose of a single agent.

  (1) Low-risk and many moderate-risk patients can be given 1 medication initially.

  (2) Patients with grade 3 hypertension or high cardiovascular risk may be given 2 medications initially.

  c. Current randomized trial evidence does not demonstrate major differences in clinical cardiovascular outcomes for different antihypertensive classes.

  d. Some patients have specific conditions that guide medication selection.

  e. Diuretics (thiazides, chlorthalidone, and indapamide), beta-blockers, dihydropyridine calcium antagonists, angiotensin-converting enzyme (ACE) inhibitors, and angiotensin receptor blockers (ARBs) can all be used as initial monotherapy in patients with no indications for specific agents; beta-blockers are possibly somewhat less effective in preventing cardiovascular outcomes than the other classes.

  f. Preferred 2 drug combinations include diuretics plus dihydropyridine calcium antagonists, diuretics plus ACE inhibitors **or** ARBs, and dihydropyridine calcium antagonists plus ACE inhibitors **or** ARBs

  g. ACE inhibitors and ARBs should not be used together since the combination has been shown to accelerate CKD.

  h. If target BP is not achieved using 1 of the preferred 2 drug combinations, add the class not already being used (diuretic, ACE inhibitor **or** ARB, or dihydropyridine calcium antagonist).

  i. If target BP is not achieved using the 3 preferred drug classes, the next class added is usually beta-blockers, followed by spironolactone, direct vasodilators (such as hydralazine), or alpha-adrenergic blockers.

  j. Antihypertensive therapy for patients with specific indications

  (1) Left ventricular hypertrophy: ACE inhibitors/ARBs, dihydropyridine calcium antagonists

  (2) Heart failure: loop diuretics, ACE inhibitors/ARBs, beta-blockers, spironolactone (see Chapter 15, Dyspnea, for a more detailed discussion of the treatment of heart failure)

  (3) Ischemic heart disease

  (a) Stable angina: beta-blockers
  (b) Acute coronary syndromes: use beta-blockers and ACE inhibitors
  (c) Postmyocardial infarction: use beta-blockers, ACE inhibitors **or** ARBs

  (4) Diabetes mellitus: ACE inhibitors/ARBs

  (5) CKD or microalbuminuria: ACE inhibitors/ARBs

B. Goal 2: Optimize other cardiovascular risk factors

1. Lipid lowering: The American College of Cardiology/American Heart Association (ACC/AHA) issued updated cholesterol treatment guidelines in 2013, based on the following findings:

  a. Statin therapy has been shown to reduce atherosclerotic cardiovascular disease (ASCVD) events in both primary and secondary prevention populations.

  (1) The relative risk reduction is about the same in all populations.

  (2) However, the number of events avoided per 1000 patients treated is smaller in lower risk populations (Figure 23-1).

  b. There was no randomized controlled trial evidence to support titrating drug therapy to a certain target LDL or to support the use of non-statin therapy in patients who can tolerate statins.

  c. High intensity statins lower LDL by ≥ 50% (Table 23-6).

  d. Moderate intensity statins lower LDL by 30–50% (Table 23-6).

  e. Low intensity statins lower LDL by < 30%.

  f. The guidelines are found in Table 23-7.

  g. There are no recommendations for patients with NYHA class II–IV ischemic systolic heart failure or patients receiving maintenance hemodialysis, since these patients were not included in the clinical trials; it is possible they would also benefit.

2. All patients should be counseled regarding exercise and diet.

3. Smoking cessation

4. Antiplatelet therapy (aspirin 81 mg daily, or clopidogrel in aspirin-allergic patients) if the Framingham Risk Score is > 10%

MAKING A DIAGNOSIS

Mr. U's initial test results are as follows:

ECG: Left ventricular hypertrophy by voltage, otherwise normal
TSH, 1.0 microunit/mL
Urine albumin–creatinine ratio: normal

(continued)

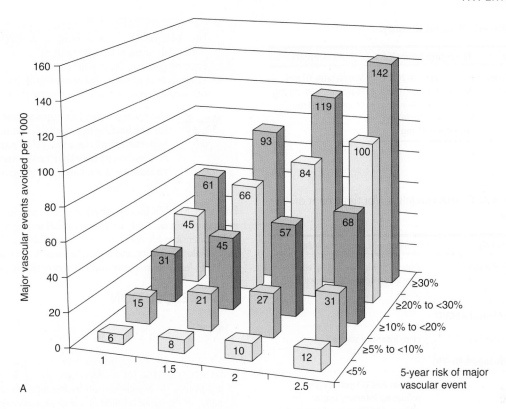

A

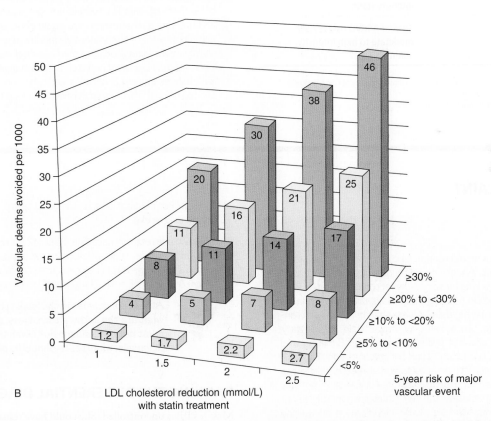

B

Figure 23-1. Predicted 5-year benefits of LDL cholesterol reductions with statin treatment at different levels of risk. (A) Major vascular events, and (B) vascular deaths. Lifetable estimates using major vascular event risk or vascular death risk in the respective risk categories and overall treatment effects per 1.0 mmol/L reduction in LDL cholesterol with statin (1 mmol/L = 38 mg/dL). Reproduced, with permission from Cholesterol Treatment Trialists' (CTT) Collaborators, Mihaylova B, Emberson J, Blackwell L et al. The effects of lowering LDL cholesterol with statin therapy in people at low risk of vascular disease: meta-analysis of individual data from 27 randomised trials. Lancet. 2012 Aug 11;380(9841):581–90.

Table 23-6. Intensity of statin therapy.

High Intensity	Moderate Intensity	Low Intensity
Atorvastatin 40–80 mg	Atorvastatin 10–20 mg	Simvastatin 10 mg
Rosuvastatin 20 mg	Rosuvastatin 5–10 mg	Pravastatin 10–20 mg
	Simvastatin 20–40 mg	Lovastatin 20 mg
	Pravastatin 40–80 mg	
	Lovastatin 40 mg	

Table 23-7. 2013 ACC/AHA guidelines for treatment of high cholesterol.

Clinical Group	Treatment Recommendation
Patients with clinical ASCVD	Age ≤ 75: high intensity statin Age > 75: moderate intensity statin
Patients without clinical ASCVD	
LDL ≥ 190 mg/dL (aged 20–75)	High intensity statin
LDL 70–189 mg/dL (aged 40–79)	
With diabetes	10-year ASCVD risk[1] < 7.5%: moderate intensity statin 10-year ASCVD risk[1] ≥ 7.5%: high intensity statin
Without diabetes	10-year ASCVD risk[1] ≥ 7.5%: moderate to high intensity statin

[1]10-year ASCVD risk based on Pooled Cohort Equations assessment (see Chapter 2, Screening & Health Maintenance).
ASCVD, atherosclerotic cardiovascular disease.

Na, 145 mEq/L; K, 4.2 mEq/L; Cl, 100 mEq/L; BUN, 11 mg/dL; creatinine, 0.5 mg/dL
Fasting glucose, 90 mg/dL
Fasting lipid panel: total cholesterol, 240 mg/dL; HDL, 40 mg/dL; triglycerides, 100 mg/dL; LDL, 180 mg/dL

 Have you crossed a diagnostic threshold for the leading hypothesis, essential hypertension? Have you ruled out the active alternatives? Do other tests need to be done to exclude the alternative diagnoses?

Based on Mr. U's history, physical exam, and initial laboratory test results, it is not necessary to do any further testing for secondary causes of hypertension. He does have other modifiable cardiovascular risk factors (smoking, obesity, and hypercholesterolemia), and some evidence for TOD (early retinopathy and left ventricular hypertrophy).

CASE RESOLUTION

Mr. U is counseled regarding smoking cessation and referred to a nutritionist for guidance regarding diet and exercise programs. He is started on hydrochlorothiazide, 12.5 mg daily, for his hypertension and atorvastatin, 40 mg daily, for his hypercholesterolemia (Table 23-6). One month later, his BP is 145/85 mm Hg. He has not yet started to exercise and has not quit smoking. You again counsel him regarding the importance of these lifestyle modifications and the possibility of avoiding a second medication if he exercises and loses weight. Six months later, after changing his diet and faithfully exercising 3 times a week, he has lost 5 pounds, and his BP is 135/82 mm Hg. He continues to smoke.

CHIEF COMPLAINT

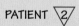
PATIENT 2

Mrs. X is a 58-year-old woman who comes to see you for a new patient visit. According to records from her previous doctor, she has a long history of hypertension treated with hydrochlorothiazide (25 mg daily), lisinopril (40 mg daily), and amlodipine (10 mg daily). Other than her antihypertensive medications, she takes only pravastatin 10 mg daily. Her BP, when last checked 1 year ago, was 138/88 mm Hg, and her BMI was 30. She last took her medications 1 month ago. She feels fine, with no headache, chest pain, shortness of breath, or edema. Her medical history is also notable for smoking 1 pack/day for 40 years, peripheral vascular disease manifested by stable claudication on walking 6 blocks, and CKD, with a serum creatinine of 1.7 mg/dL. In your office, her BP is 170/98 mm Hg and her BMI is 35. Physical exam is notable for clear lungs, an S₄ without an S₃ or murmurs, and decreased posterior tibial and dorsalis pedis pulses. Abdominal exam is normal. There is no peripheral edema, and there are no femoral or abdominal bruits.

You refill her medications, order blood tests, and ask her to return in 6 weeks.

When she returns, her BP is 150/92 mm Hg. She reports that she takes all of her medications every day and that her home BP readings have been similar to those obtained in the office. A repeat BP with a larger cuff is the same.

 At this point, what is the leading hypothesis, what are the active alternatives, and is there a must not miss diagnosis? Given this differential diagnosis, what tests should be ordered?

RANKING THE DIFFERENTIAL DIAGNOSIS

Mrs. X's BP is uncontrolled. She could have resistant hypertension, which is defined as a failure to reach a BP goal despite the use of 3 optimally dosed antihypertensive medications of different classes, ideally including a diuretic. Alternatively, she could have "pseudoresistance," meaning that her BP is uncontrolled due to poor BP measurement technique, poor adherence, white-coat effect, or an inadequate treatment regimen. The first steps in assessing patients with uncontrolled BP include repeating the BP measurement with

Table 23-8. Causes of resistant hypertension.

Lifestyle factors	Dietary salt Alcohol consumption Obesity
Drugs/medications	NSAIDs Sympathomimetic agents (decongestants, cocaine) Stimulants (methylphenidate, modafinil) Oral contraceptives Corticosteroids Erythropoietin Tricyclic antidepressants
Common secondary causes	Primary hyperaldosteronism Renal artery stenosis Chronic kidney disease Obstructive sleep apnea
Rare secondary causes	Pheochromocytoma Cushing disease Coarctation of aorta Intracranial tumor Carcinoid syndrome Hyperparathyroidism Hypothyroidism or hyperthyroidism

NSAIDs, nonsteroidal antiinflammatory drugs.

a properly sized cuff (if the cuff is too small, the systolic BP can be elevated as much as 15 mm Hg), reviewing medication adherence, obtaining home BP measurements, and reviewing the medication regimen itself. Mrs. X is adherent to her medications, is taking optimal doses of 3 medications from different classes including a diuretic, and has consistent BP readings at home and in the office. Thus, she meets the criteria for resistant hypertension.

After establishing that a patient has resistant hypertension, the next step is to consider the many potential causes (Table 23-8). Lifestyle factors are common contributors to resistant hypertension. Elderly patients, African-American patients, and those with CKD tend to be particularly salt sensitive. About 12–14% of people consuming more than 2 drinks/day are hypertensive. For every 10% increase in body weight, systolic BP increases by 6.5 mm Hg. Secondary causes of hypertension are more common in patients with resistant hypertension referred to hypertension specialty clinics, with about 20% having an identifiable secondary cause.

The clinical clues in Mrs. X's presentation include her vascular risk factors, suggesting she is at risk for renal artery stenosis. In addition, she does have preexisting CKD, a common cause of resistant hypertension. Her obesity is a risk factor for obstructive sleep apnea, another common cause. Hyperaldosteronism should be considered since it is found in 15–20% of patients with resistant hypertension. She has no symptoms to suggest a rare cause of secondary hypertension, pheochromocytoma (0.1–0.6% of patients). Table 23-9 lists the differential diagnosis.

She never adds salt to her food and reads food labels carefully. She does not drink alcohol and is afraid to use over-the-counter medications. She attributes her weight gain to being somewhat less active due to symptomatic

Table 23-9. Diagnostic hypotheses for Mrs. X.

Diagnostic Hypotheses	Demographics, Risk Factors, Symptoms and Signs	Important Tests
Leading Hypothesis		
Renal artery stenosis	Abrupt onset or accelerated hypertension Azotemia after use of ACE inhibitor Hypertension refractory to ≥ 3 medications Abdominal or flank bruit Other vascular disease (coronary, carotid, or peripheral) Smoking Severe retinopathy	Duplex ultrasonography MRA with gadolinium CT angiography
Active Alternatives—Most Common		
Worsening CKD	None Sometimes edema, malaise	Serum creatinine Estimated GFR
Lifestyle factors	History	History
Use of medications/drugs that increase BP	History	History
Obstructive sleep apnea	Obesity Neck circumference > 17 inches Frequent snoring Daytime somnolence	Polysomnogram
Other Hypotheses		
Hyperaldosteronism	Resistant hypertension Hypokalemia	Aldosterone/renin ratio

ACE, angiotensin-converting enzyme; CKD, chronic kidney disease; GFR, glomerular filtration rate; MRA, magnetic resonance angiography.

knee osteoarthritis. A recent polysomnogram was normal. Laboratory tests include the following: Na, 140 mEq/L; K, 3.4 mEq/L; Cl, 100 mEq/L; HCO_2, 26 mEq/L; BUN, 35 mg/dL; creatinine, 1.8 mg/dL; TSH, 3.2 microunit/mL.

Is the clinical information sufficient to make a diagnosis? If not, what other information do you need?

Leading Hypothesis: Atherosclerotic Renal Artery Stenosis

Textbook Presentation

Patients generally have either very abrupt hypertension, hypertension that worsens over 6 months, or hypertension refractory to treatment with 3 drugs. The classic patient with atherosclerotic renal artery stenosis has other vascular disease (cerebrovascular disease, coronary artery disease, peripheral arterial disease) or risk factors such as smoking or diabetes.

Disease Highlights

A. Must distinguish renovascular disease from renovascular hypertension

1. Renovascular disease means significant stenosis of 1 or both renal arteries.

   a. Can be due to fibromuscular dysplasia (most commonly in young women) or atherosclerosis (90% of cases)

      (1) Atherosclerotic renal artery stenosis (ARAS) is present in 1–6% of unselected patients with hypertension.

      (2) ARAS is found in more than 30% of patients undergoing cardiac catheterization.

   b. Does not necessarily cause hypertension and can exist in patients with essential hypertension.

2. Renovascular hypertension means hypertension caused by renal hypoperfusion as a result of renal artery stenosis.

   a. Stenosis leads to renal ischemia, activating the renin–angiotensin system, which leads to release of renin and production of angiotensin II.

   b. Although plasma renin levels are high initially, they decrease over time.

   c. Aldosterone secretion and vasoconstriction then occur, leading to hypertension.

   d. Aldosterone secretion also causes salt and water retention and hypokalemia.

   e. Ischemic nephropathy occurs when renal blood flow is so reduced that GFR decreases and there is loss of renal function.

   f. Some patients with bilateral renal artery stenosis present with episodic, unexplained pulmonary edema ("flash pulmonary edema"); echocardiograms in such patients show normal systolic function.

B. About 50% of patients with renal artery stenosis have renovascular hypertension.

Evidence-Based Diagnosis

A. Clinical clues to identify patients with high risk of having ARAS

1. Onset of hypertension before age 30, or severe hypertension after age 55

2. Accelerated, resistant, or malignant hypertension

3. New azotemia or worsening renal function after use of an ACE inhibitor or ARB

   a. A reversible increase in serum creatinine can develop in some patients with **bilateral** renal artery stenosis (or unilateral stenosis in patients with only 1 functioning kidney) when starting ACE inhibitor therapy.

      (1) The peak creatinine occurs somewhere between 4 days and 2 months.

      (2) Creatinine returns to baseline within 1 week of stopping the ACE inhibitor.

   b. One study reported that, in a population of high-risk patients, a 20% increase in creatinine had 100% sensitivity and 70% specificity for the diagnosis of renal artery stenosis (defined as > 50% **bilateral** stenosis).

4. Unexplained atrophic kidney or size discrepancy of > 1.5 cm between the kidneys

5. Sudden, unexplained pulmonary edema; unexplained heart failure; refractory angina

6. Multivessel coronary artery disease or peripheral arterial disease

7. Unexplained renal dysfunction

B. Abdominal bruits may be present.

1. Should listen over all 4 abdominal quadrants and also spine and flanks between T12 and L2

2. Must differentiate between systolic bruits and continuous (systolic and diastolic) bruits

   a. Systolic bruits occur in 4–20% of healthy persons, more commonly in people under 40 years of age.

      (1) May originate from the celiac artery

      (2) Modestly increase the likelihood of renal artery stenosis: LR+, 5.6; LR–, 0.6

   b. Continuous systolic-diastolic bruits often radiate to the side and strongly increase the likelihood of renal artery stenosis: LR+, 38.9; LR–, 0.6.

C. Family history of hypertension is often absent.

D. Hypokalemia is often seen as a result of stimulation of aldosterone release; metabolic alkalosis is also often seen.

E. Imaging studies

1. Intra-arterial digital subtraction angiography is the gold standard.

   a. Can also be therapeutic through performance of angioplasty or placement of stent in the rare cases this is indicated

   b. Complications include bleeding, dissection, embolization, and contrast nephropathy.

2. Duplex ultrasonography (2-dimensional ultrasound imaging combined with Doppler flow measurements)

   a. Results can vary depending on the level of experience of the technician and the body habitus of the patient.

   b. Accuracy ranges from 60% to 90%

   c. In optimal circumstances, sensitivity is 85% and specificity, 92% (LR+, 10; LR–, 0.16)

3. Magnetic resonance angiography with gadolinium

   a. The largest single study found that for ARAS the sensitivity was 78% and specificity was 88% (LR+ = 6.5, LR– = 0.25); for fibromuscular dysplasia, the sensitivity was only 22% but the specificity was 96%.

   b. Smaller studies report sensitivities and specificities over 90%.

4. CT angiography

   a. Preferable to avoid in patients with CKD due to the necessary IV contrast (see Chapter 28, Acute Kidney Injury)

   b. In the large study noted above, for ARAS, the sensitivity was 77% and specificity was 94% (LR+ = 12.8, LR– = 0.24); for fibromuscular dysplasia, the sensitivity was 28% and specificity was 99%.

   c. Smaller studies report sensitivities and specificities over 90%.

Treatment

A. All patients with ARAS should have optimal medical therapy with ACE inhibitors or ARBs, statins, and aspirin.

B. Most patients require multiple antihypertensive medications to reach BP goals.

C. Patients should stop smoking, and diabetes should be optimally controlled.

D. The role of renal artery revascularization is limited.

    1. Randomized, controlled trials have not shown that stenting is better than medical therapy with regard to preventing progression of renal disease or cardiovascular events.

    2. ACC/AHA guidelines recommend considering revascularization in patients with hemodynamically significant bilateral ARAS (or unilateral in patients with 1 kidney) and recurrent, unexplained heart failure or pulmonary edema. Other potential indications include progressive CKD, resistant or accelerated hypertension, and unstable angina.

MAKING A DIAGNOSIS

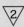

After you explain that most patients with ARAS are treated with aspirin, statins, and good BP control, Mrs. X declines any imaging studies.

 Have you crossed a diagnostic threshold for the leading hypothesis, renovascular hypertension? Have you ruled out the active alternatives? Do other tests need to be done to exclude the alternative diagnoses?

Worsening CKD, lifestyle factors, and medications/drugs have been ruled out by the history and unchanged serum creatinine. Primary aldosteronism needs to be considered in patients with resistant hypertension, especially those with hypokalemia.

Alternative Diagnosis: Primary Hyperaldosteronism

Textbook Presentation

Primary hyperaldosteronism is usually diagnosed when a patient with hypertension has unexplained hypokalemia or when a patient has resistant hypertension.

Disease Highlights

A. Etiology

    1. Results from a unilateral aldosterone-producing adenoma in 30–35% of cases (Conn syndrome)

    2. Results from idiopathic bilateral adrenal hyperplasia in most other patients (60–70%)

    3. Rarer causes include microadenomas, unilateral adrenal hyperplasia, and adrenal carcinoma.

B. The overall prevalence, based on community cohorts, is about 11%.

    1. Prevalence of 8–15.5% in patients with grade 2 hypertension (160–179/100–109 mm Hg) and of 13–19% in patients with grade 3 hypertension (≥ 180/≥ 110 mm Hg)

    2. Found in 17–23% of patients with resistant hypertension

    3. Prevalence uncertain in patients with hypertension and unprovoked hypokalemia; 1 study reported a prevalence of 50%

C. Pathophysiology

    1. High aldosterone levels lead to salt and water retention and potassium wasting.

    2. Because aldosterone is being produced autonomously, it is not suppressed by volume expansion, as it is normally.

    3. Volume expansion suppresses plasma renin levels.

D. Most patients have a normal potassium level; 48% of those with aldosterone-producing adenomas and 17% of those with bilateral adrenal hyperplasia are hypokalemic.

 A normal potassium level does not rule out hyperaldosteronism.

Evidence-Based Diagnosis

A. The Endocrine Society recommends screening for primary hyperaldosteronism in *hypertensive* patients with moderate-severe hypertension (BP > 160/100 mm Hg), resistant hypertension, unprovoked (by diuretics) hypokalemia associated with renal potassium wasting, an adrenal incidentaloma, diuretic-associated hypokalemia (especially in treatment resistant patients or when hypokalemia persists when potassium-sparing diuretics, ACE inhibitors, or ARBs are used), a family history of early onset hypertension, or cerebrovascular accident at < 40 years of age.

B. There are 3 steps in the diagnosis of primary hyperaldosteronism: screening, confirmatory testing, and determining the subtype.

    1. The plasma aldosterone concentration/plasma renin activity ratio (ARR) is the most commonly used screening test; since patients with primary hyperaldosteronism have elevated levels of aldosterone and suppressed renin levels, the ratio should be elevated.

        a. The ARR can be affected by potassium status, dietary sodium, medications, and age.

        b. Ideally, prior to measurement, the patient should have a normal potassium level and liberal sodium intake.

        c. Medications that minimally affect aldosterone levels include verapamil, hydralazine, and alpha-adrenergic blockers; other antihypertensive medications and NSAIDs should be stopped for 2–4 weeks when possible.

        d. The optimal cut point is unclear; a ratio > 20–30 is generally considered a positive test.

        e. Sensitivity ranges from 73% to 87%, with a specificity of about 75%.

    2. If the ARR is abnormal, the patient should be referred to an endocrinologist for confirmatory testing (oral sodium loading, saline infusion, fludrocortisone suppression, or captopril challenge).

    3. Patients with abnormal confirmatory testing should undergo adrenal CT, possibly followed by adrenal vein sampling.

Treatment

A. Laparoscopic adrenalectomy should be considered when lateralized aldosterone excess is demonstrated by adrenal vein sampling.

B. Otherwise, treat with the aldosterone antagonist spironolactone.

CASE RESOLUTION

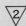

Mrs. X has an elevated ARR; however, confirmatory testing by the endocrinologist is negative. You stop the hydrochlorothiazide, substituting chlorthalidone, a longer acting diuretic. Her BP improves slightly, and she requires the addition of labetolol to achieve her BP goal.

CHIEF COMPLAINT

PATIENT 3

Mr. J is 45-year-old man with a 10-year history of hypertension. When you last saw him 1 year ago, his BP was 160/95 mm Hg. He ran out of his medications 6 months ago and was unable to obtain refills because of financial problems. Today, he has stopped by to see your nurse for new prescriptions. Because he is complaining of a headache, she checks his BP and then runs to find you because it is 220/112 mm Hg.

At this point, what is the leading hypothesis, what are the active alternatives, and is there a must not miss diagnosis? Given this differential diagnosis, what tests should be ordered?

RANKING THE DIFFERENTIAL DIAGNOSIS

Mr. J's BP clearly needs to be lowered, and the primary question is how quickly this needs to be accomplished. In other words, is this a **hypertensive emergency** or **hypertensive urgency**? These syndromes are defined by the degree of BP elevation and whether there is acute end organ damage.

A hypertensive emergency exists when there is severe BP elevation and acute target organ involvement: acute neurologic syndromes (encephalopathy, cerebrovascular accident, intracerebral or subarachnoid hemorrhage), acute aortic dissection, acute coronary syndrome, acute pulmonary edema, acute kidney injury, severe preeclampsia/eclampsia, microangiopathic hemolytic anemia, or acute postoperative hypertension.

In hypertensive urgency, there is severe BP elevation without any acute TOD. The exact definition of "severe BP elevation" has not been established, but many experts use a cutoff of > 180/110–120 mm Hg. Common causes of hypertensive urgency and emergency include medication nonadherence, abrupt cessation of clonidine, CKD, renovascular disease, drugs (cocaine, PCP), systemic lupus erythematosus, eclampsia, and postoperative state; Cushing disease and pheochromocytoma are less common causes.

A hypertensive emergency is defined by the presence of TOD, not by the degree of BP elevation.

To some extent, the degree of the acute TOD in patients with very elevated BP depends on the time course of the BP elevation. For example, normotensive women in whom acute hypertension develops from eclampsia can have significant TOD at pressures of 160/100 mm Hg, whereas patients with chronic hypertension can be asymptomatic at much higher pressures. So, despite his very elevated BP, it is quite likely that Mr. J falls into the "hypertensive urgency" rather than the "hypertensive emergency" category. Nevertheless, hypertensive emergency is always the "must not miss" diagnosis in such patients (Table 23-10).

3

You tell the nurse to put Mr. J in an exam room. On further history, he has no shortness of breath, chest pain, edema, abdominal pain, feelings of confusion, vomiting, or focal weakness or numbness. He generally appears well and

is clearly happy to have a new job. Physical exam confirms BP of 220/112 mm Hg, pulse of 84 bpm, and RR of 16 breaths per minute. There is no papilledema. Lungs are clear, jugular venous pressure is not elevated, there is an S_4 and a 2/6 systolic ejection murmur without an S_3, abdomen is nontender, there is no peripheral edema, and neurologic exam is normal.

Is the clinical information sufficient to make a diagnosis? If not, what other information do you need?

Leading Hypothesis: Hypertensive Urgency

Textbook Presentation

A patient with chronic hypertension has extremely high BP; by definition, patients have no symptoms or signs of acute TOD.

Disease Highlights

A. Hypertensive urgency or emergency occurs in about 1% of adults with hypertension; with urgency occurring in three-quarters of these patients.

B. The most common presenting symptoms are headache (22%), epistaxis (17%), faintness (10%), psychomotor agitation (10%), chest pain (9%), and dyspnea (9%).

Table 23-10. Diagnostic hypotheses for Mr. J.

Diagnostic Hypotheses	Demographics, Risk Factors, Symptoms and Signs	Important Tests
Leading Hypothesis		
Hypertensive urgency	Absence of hypertensive emergency syndromes	
Active Alternative—Must Not Miss		
Hypertensive emergencies Acute coronary syndrome	Chest pain	ECG Cardiac enzymes
Aortic dissection	Chest, back pain Diastolic murmur Absent pulses	Chest radiograph Transesophageal echocardiogram Chest CT
Pulmonary edema	Dyspnea Crackles S_3	Chest radiograph
Hypertensive encephalopathy	Headache Nausea/vomiting Delirium Seizures Coma Papilledema	MRI
Acute kidney injury	Nausea Fatigue	Serum creatinine

Evidence-Based Diagnosis

A. Must rule out acute TOD through history, physical, and selected laboratory tests.

B. BP should be measured in both arms, and pulses palpated in both the upper and lower extremities; all patients should have a complete cardiovascular and neurologic exam, including fundoscopic exam.

C. All patients should have a serum creatinine and urinalysis performed.

D. Patients with symptoms suggestive of myocardial ischemia or pulmonary edema should have an ECG, chest radiograph, and cardiac enzymes.

E. Patients with neurologic signs or symptoms need a head CT scan and sometimes a brain MRI.

Treatment

A. In stable outpatients with chronically elevated BP, there is NOT an urgent need to reduce the BP, and it is fine if it takes several days for the BP to be reduced.

B. There are several ways to approach treatment, depending on the overall condition of the patient, whether the patient has been treated previously, and the ability of the patient to return for follow-up.

   1. In patients who have stopped their medications, it is usually sufficient just to restart them.

   2. In previously untreated patients, options include

      a. Starting 2 long-acting agents, such as a diuretic and either a calcium channel blocker or ACE inhibitor

      b. Beginning treatment with more rapid-acting agents, such as oral labetalol or clonidine, and then transitioning to longer acting agents; patients can be observed for several hours to assess their response to the short-acting agents.

C. Too rapid reduction of BP can lead to hypotension and cerebral hypoperfusion with stroke.

D. IV and sublingual medications can have unpredictable effects on BP and should be avoided in asymptomatic patients.

   1. IV hydralazine causes a progressive and sometimes precipitous fall in BP 5–15 minutes after administration.

   2. Although the circulating half-life of hydralazine is only 3 hours, the half time of its effect on BP is 10 hours.

   3. Sublingual nifedipine causes completely unpredictable lowering of BP and should never be used.

 Do not be in a hurry to normalize BP in patients without acute TOD!

MAKING A DIAGNOSIS

 Mr. J's serum creatinine is 1.4 mg/dL, unchanged from 1 year ago. His urinalysis is normal. Mr. J wants to know if he can have a couple of acetaminophen tablets for his headache, get his prescriptions, and leave; he has to pick up his son at school.

 Have you crossed a diagnostic threshold for the leading hypothesis, hypertensive urgency? Have you ruled out the active alternatives? Do other tests need to be done to exclude the alternative diagnoses?

Alternative Diagnosis: Hypertensive Emergencies

Patients with hypertensive emergencies frequently present with chest pain (27%), dyspnea (22%), and neurologic deficits (21%). Cerebral infarction is found in about 24% of patients, with about 22% having pulmonary edema, 16% hypertensive encephalopathy, and 12% heart failure.

Acute coronary syndromes, aortic dissection, subarachnoid hemorrhage, and pulmonary edema are discussed in other chapters. This section focuses on hypertensive encephalopathy.

Textbook Presentation

Patients present with the acute or subacute development of lethargy, confusion, headache, and visual disturbances, sometimes followed by seizures (focal or generalized) and coma. The syndrome can occur with or without proteinuria and retinopathy.

Disease Highlights

A. Cerebral blood flow is autoregulated within specific limits.

   1. In normotensive people, cerebral blood flow is unchanged between mean arterial pressures (MAP) of 60–120 mm Hg (MAP = [(2 × diastolic) + systolic]/3)

      a. Cerebral vasoconstriction limits hyperperfusion up to a MAP of 180 mm Hg.

      b. Above a MAP of 180 mm Hg, autoregulation is overwhelmed.

   2. In hypertensive patients, cerebral blood flow can be maintained at MAPs of up to 200 mm Hg.

      a. Thought to be due to arteriolar thickening

      b. Such patients also need higher MAPs to maintain adequate cerebral blood flow (ie, abrupt lowering of the BP to a MAP of < 100–110 mm Hg can potentially lead to cerebral ischemia).

B. Failure of autoregulation leads to cerebral vasodilation, endothelial dysfunction, and cerebral edema.

C. The classic MRI finding in hypertensive encephalopathy is subcortical vasogenic edema.

   1. Also called reversible posterior leukoencephalopathy syndrome (RPLS)

   2. Generally in the posterior regions of the brain due to relatively sparse sympathetic innervation of the vertebrobasilar territory leading to more disruption of autoregulatory mechanisms, increased perfusion, and edema

   3. Can also see changes in the brainstem and anterior brain

   4. In 1 series, 92% of patients with RPLS presented with encephalopathy, 39% with visual symptoms, and 53% with headache; 87% of patients had seizures.

   5. Also seen with eclampsia and use of some immunosuppressive agents and cytotoxic drugs; in 1 series, 68% of patients with RPLS had hypertension, 11% eclampsia, 11% immunosuppressive use, and 11% other causes

6. Reversible with treatment of hypertension or removal of inciting agent, with MRI findings resolving in days to weeks; long-term antiepileptic therapy is not necessary.

Evidence-Based Diagnosis

A. Hypertensive encephalopathy is primarily a clinical diagnosis.

B. A head CT should be done to exclude intracranial hemorrhage (intracerebral or subarachnoid bleeding).

C. An MRI should be done to exclude acute ischemic stroke and to look for RPLS.

 MRI is much more sensitive than CT (83% vs 16% sensitivity; specificity of both > 95%) for the diagnosis of acute ischemic stroke.

Treatment

A. Hypertensive encephalopathy and other hypertensive emergencies should be treated in the ICU with parenteral, titratable antihypertensive agents.

B. There is little evidence to guide the choice of agents; commonly used medications include labetalol, esmolol, fenoldopam, clevidipine, nitroprusside, and nicardipine.

C. Generally, the BP should be reduced by about 10% in the first hour, and by another 15% in the next 2–3 hours; patients can often be transitioned to oral agents within 12–24 hours.

1. The BP should be reduced more quickly in acute aortic dissection, with a goal of < 120/80 mm Hg within 20 minutes.

2. Neurology consultation should be obtained for guidance regarding BP lowering in the setting of acute stroke.

CASE RESOLUTION

Mr. J has no signs or symptoms of stroke, intracranial hemorrhage, pulmonary edema, myocardial ischemia, or aortic dissection. He has a headache, but he does not have other symptoms, such as lethargy or confusion, to suggest hypertensive encephalopathy. His renal function is stable and his urinalysis is normal. There is no need to perform any further testing at this point.

Mr. J's previous regimen was hydrochlorothiazide, 25 mg; lisinopril 40 mg; and amlodipine, 10 mg. You instruct him to fill his prescriptions after he picks up his son at school, to take the amlodipine tonight, and then to take all 3 medications in the morning. When he returns in 2 days, his BP is 160/100 mm Hg; 3 weeks later it is 145/90 mm Hg.

REVIEW OF OTHER IMPORTANT DISEASES

Pheochromocytoma

Textbook Presentation

The classic presentation is a patient with attacks of paroxysmal hypertension, headache, palpitations, and sweating occurring several times daily, weekly, or every few months. Patients generally have orthostatic hypotension on physical exam.

Disease Highlights

A. 95% of patients have headache, sweating, or palpitations.

B. 10% of pheochromocytomas are malignant and tend to have a less typical presentation.

C. 10–15% are familial (multiple endocrine neoplasia type 2, von Hippel-Lindau disease, neurofibromatosis); these are more often asymptomatic (and normotensive) than sporadic cases.

D. Table 23-11 lists symptoms, taken from a series of patients with pheochromocytoma, about half of whom presented with paroxysmal hypertension and about half of whom had persistent hypertension.

Evidence-Based Diagnosis

A. Pretest probability of 0.5% in hypertensive patients who have suggestive symptoms, and of 0.2% in unselected hypertensive patients

B. Pretest probability of 4% in patients with incidentally discovered adrenal masses

C. Plasma free metanephrine is the single best test to rule out pheochromocytoma (Table 23-12).

1. Patients should fast overnight and be supine for 20 minutes prior to the blood draw.

2. Because caffeine and acetaminophen interfere with the assay, patients should avoid caffeine for 12 hours and acetaminophen for 5 days prior to testing.

3. The standard upper limit of normal for plasma metanephrines is 61 ng/L.

a. The overall (sporadic and hereditary cases) sensitivity at this cut off is 99% with a specificity of 89%.

b. A plasma metanephrine > 236 ng/L is 100% specific for the diagnosis of pheochromocytoma.

D. Patients with positive biochemical testing should undergo adrenal imaging.

1. CT: sensitivity of 93–100% for detecting adrenal pheochromocytomas, 90% for extra-adrenal tumors; specificity 50–70%

2. MRI: sensitivity 90%; specificity also 50–70%; better than CT for identifying vascular invasion

Table 23-11. Symptoms of pheochromocytoma.

Symptom	Patients with Pheochromocytoma and Paroxysmal Hypertension	Patients with Pheochromocytoma and Persistent Hypertension
Severe headaches	92%	72%
Sweating	65%	69%
Palpitations and/or tachycardia	73%	51%
Anxiety/panic	60%	28%
Tremulousness	51%	26%
Chest or abdominal pain	48%	28%
Nausea ± vomiting	43%	26%

Table 23-12. Diagnostic tests for sporadic pheochromocytoma.[1]

Test	Sensitivity	Specificity	LR+	LR−
Plasma free metanephrines	99%	82%	5.5	0.012
Plasma catecholamines	92%	72%	2.9	0.11
24-hour urine fractionated metanephrines	97%	45%	1.76	0.06
24-hour urine catecholamines	91%	75%	3.64	0.12
24-hour urine total metanephrines	88%	89%	8	0.13
24-hour urine vanillylmandelic acid level	77%	86%	5.5	0.26

[1]Test characteristics for the diagnosis in patients with hereditary pheochromocytoma are different and can be found in (Data from Lenders JWM. JAMA. 2002;287:1427–34.)

3. ^{131}I-MIBG or positron emission tomography scanning is sometimes used when the biochemistry is positive and both CT and MRI are negative.

Treatment

A. Surgery is the definitive treatment.

B. Must give both alpha- and beta-blocking agents preoperatively

1. The alpha-blocker opposes catecholamine-induced vasoconstriction.

2. The beta-blocker opposes the reflex tachycardia that occurs with alpha-blockade.

3. Unopposed beta-blockade causes inhibition of epinephrine-induced vasodilation, leading to increased BP, left heart strain, and possibly heart failure.

4. Should be done in consultation with an endocrinologist because of the complexities of ensuring adequate alpha-blockade

 Never give a patient with a pheochromocytoma a beta-blocker without first giving an alpha-blocker.

C. 27–38% of patients have residual hypertension.

D. Patients with familial pheochromocytoma often have multiple, bilateral tumors; the optimal approach to therapy is not clear.

REFERENCES

Calhoun DA, Jones D, Textor S et al. Resistant hypertension: diagnosis, evaluation and treatment. A Scientific Statement from the American Heart Association Professional Education Committee of the Council for High Blood Pressure Research. Hypertension. 2008;51:1403–19.

Dworkin LD, Cooper CJ. Renal artery stenosis. N Engl J Med. 2009;361:1972–8.

Funder JW, Carey RM, Fardella C et al; Endocrine Society. Case detection, diagnosis, and treatment of patients with primary aldosteronism: an endocrine society clinical practice guideline. J Clin Endocrinol Metab. 2008;93:3266–81.

Jellinger PS, Smith DA, Mehta AE et al; AACE Task Force for Management of Dyslipidemia and Prevention of Atherosclerosis. American Association of Clinical Endocrinologists' Guidelines for Management of Dyslipidemia and Prevention of Atherosclerosis. Endocrine Pract. 2012;18 (Suppl 1):1–78.

Lao D, Parasher PS, Cho KC, Yeghiazarians Y. Atherosclerotic renal artery stenosis—diagnosis and treatment. Mayo Clin Proceedings. 2011;86:649–57.

Lee VH, Wijdicks EFM, Manno EM, Rabinstein AA. Clinical spectrum of reversible posterior leukoencephalopathy syndrome. Arch Neurol. 2008;65:205–10.

Lenders JWM, Pacak K, Walther MM et al. Biochemical diagnosis of pheochromocytoma. Which test is best? JAMA. 2002;287:1427–34.

Manger WM, Gifford RW. Pheochromocytoma. J Clin Hypertension. 2002;4:62–72.

Mittendorf EA, Evans DB, Lee JE, Perrier ND. Pheochromocytoma: advances in genetics, diagnosis, localization, and treatment. Hematol Oncol Clin N Am. 2007;21:509–25.

Pisoni R, Ahmed MI, Calhoun DA. Characterization and treatment of resistant hypertension. Curr Cardiol Rep. 2009;11:407–13.

Rodriguez MA, Kumar SK, De Caro M. Hypertensive crisis. Cardiol Rev. 2010;18:102–7.

Rossi GP. A comprehensive review of the clinical aspects of primary aldosteronism. Nat Rev Endocrinol. 2011;7:485–95.

Schwartz GL. Screening for adrenal-endocrine hypertension: overview of accuracy and cost-effectiveness. Endocrinol Metab Clin N Am. 2011;40:279–94.

Smith SC Jr, Benjamin EJ, Bonow RO et al. AHA/ACCF secondary prevention and risk reduction therapy for patients with coronary and other atherosclerotic vascular disease: 2011 update: a guideline from the American Heart Association and American College of Cardiology Foundation endorsed by the World Heart Federation and the Preventive Cardiovascular Nurses Association. J Am Coll Cardiol. 2011;58:2432–46.

The Task Force for the management of arterial hypertension of the European Society of Hypertension (ESH) and of the European Society of Cardiology (ESC). 2013 ESH/ESC Guidelines for the management of arterial hypertension. Eur Heart J. doi:10.1093/eurheartj/eht151

Turnbull JM. Is listening for abdominal bruits useful in the evaluation of hypertension? JAMA. 1995;274:1299–1301.

Van de Ven PJG, Beutler JJ, Kaatee R et al. Angiotensin converting enzyme inhibitor induced renal dysfunction in atherosclerotic renovascular disease. Kidney Int. 1998;53:986–93.

Vasbinder G, Nelemans PJ, Kessels A et al. Accuracy of computed tomographic angiography and magnetic resonance angiography for diagnosing renal artery stenosis. Ann Intern Med. 2004;141:674–82.

C. 25–30% of patients have residual hypertension.

D. Patients with familial pheochromocytoma often have multiple tumors; therefore, the optimal approach to therapy is not clear.

REFERENCES

Table 23-12. Diagnostic tests for sporadic pheochromocytoma.

Test	Sensitivity	Specificity
Plasma free metanephrines		
Plasma catecholamines		
24-hour urine fractionated metanephrines		
24-hour urine catecholamines		
24-hour urine total metanephrines		
24-hour urine vanillylmandelic acid level		

3. [123I]MIBG or positron emission tomography scanning is sometimes used when the biochemistry is positive and both CT and MRI are negative.

Treatment

A. **Surgery** is the definitive treatment.

B. Must give both alpha- and beta-blocking agents preoperatively.

1. Alpha-blocker opposes catecholamine-induced vasoconstriction.

2. This helps to approach the volume makes that usually deficit with alpha-blockade.

3. Unopposed beta-blockade causes inhibition of epinephrine-induced vasodilation, leading to increased left ventricular strain and possibly heart failure.

4. Should be done in consultation with an endocrinologist because of the complexities of ensuring adequate alpha-blockade.

Never give a patient with a pheochromocytoma a beta-blocker without first giving an alpha-blocker.

I have a patient with hyponatremia. I have a patient with hypernatremia. How do I determine the cause?

HYPONATREMIA

CHIEF COMPLAINT

PATIENT 1

Mr. D is a 42-year-old man who is brought to the emergency department by the police department. He is disoriented and confused. Initial labs reveal a serum sodium concentration of 118 mEq/L.

What is the differential diagnosis of hyponatremia? How would you frame the differential?

CONSTRUCTING A DIFFERENTIAL DIAGNOSIS

As noted in Chapter 1, the first task when evaluating patients is to identify their problem(s). Mr. D's problems clearly include delirium and marked hyponatremia. While other causes of delirium should be considered, (see Chapter 11 Delirium & Dementia) the hyponatremia clearly requires evaluation because it is severe and thus likely to be causing the delirium.

Hyponatremia is defined as serum sodium concentration < 135 mEq/L and is significant when the concentration is < 130 mEq/L. The differential diagnosis for hyponatremia is long but the diagnostic approach can be easily framed in a few simple steps. These pivotal steps include (1) a quick search for rapid diagnostic clues; (2) a clinical assessment of the patients volume status to limit the differential; (3) in clinically euvolemic patients, a review of the patients urine sodium and response to a saline challenge to unmask subtle hypovolemia (4) in euvolemic patient further tests to distinguish the syndrome of inappropriate antidiuretic hormone (SIADH) from other less common causes of euvolemic hyponatremia; and finally (5) an exploration for the risk factors, associated symptoms, and signs for the diagnoses within each subgroup. Each of these steps is discussed below.

The first step recognizes that a few key clinical and laboratory features occasionally point to very specific diagnoses. Examples of these include thiazide use (suggesting diuretic-induced hyponatremia), recent participation in marathon events (suggesting exercise-associated hyponatremia [EAH]), hyperkalemia (suggesting kidney disease or primary adrenal insufficiency), very low urine osmolality (suggesting psychogenic polydipsia, Ecstasy use, or beer potomania) or markedly elevated blood glucose, or a normal serum osmolality (suggesting hyperglycemia-induced hyponatremia and pseudohyponatremia, respectively). Thus, the first pivotal step in approaching hyponatremia systematically reviews these few variables to search for clues (Figure 24-1).

For many patients, the previously mentioned clues are absent and the second pivotal step evaluates the patient's *clinical* volume status in order to determine whether they are clinically hypervolemic, clinically euvolemic, or clinically hypovolemic. This allows the differential diagnosis to be narrowed to that appropriate subset of diagnoses (Figure 24-2). Correct classification of the patient's volume status requires a review of the history, physical exam findings, and laboratory results. The clinical recognition of *hypervolemic patients* is very accurate because hyponatremia typically develops in patients with advanced heart failure (HF), cirrhosis, nephrotic syndrome, and chronic kidney disease when the disease is easily recognized. Similarly marked hypovolemia is often readily apparent when hypotension or orthostasis is present. However, *hypovolemia* may also be subtle. Hypovolemic patients may appear clinically euvolemic. Therefore, the differential diagnosis of patients that appear *clinically* euvolemic includes both euvolemic and hypovolemic etiologies.

The third pivotal step analyzes the clinically euvolemic group to unmask subtle hypovolemia by analyzing (1) the urine Na^+ or $FeNa^+$ and (2) the response to a small saline challenge (Figure 24-3).

A. Spot urine sodium and Fe_{Na+}

1. Since hypovolemia promotes avid sodium reabsorption, hypovolemia is usually associated with a low urinary sodium concentration (< 20–30 mEq/L) and low $FeNa^+$(< 0.5%). On the other hand, euvolemic patients do not have a stimulus to reabsorb urine sodium and usually have a higher urinary sodium (> 20–30 mEq/L) and Fe_{Na+}.

2. Average urinary sodium in hypovolemic patients: 18.4 mEq/L, compared with 72 mEq/L in euvolemic patients

3. Urine Na^+ < 30 mEq/L: 63–80% sensitive for hypovolemia, 72–100% specific, LR+ 2.2–∞, LR– 0.2–0.5

4. Fe_{Na+} may be more sensitive.
   a. $FE_{Na+} = (U_{Na+} \times P_{Cr})/(P_{Na+} \times U_{Cr})$
   b. Compares fraction of sodium excreted to fraction of sodium filtered. In hypovolemic states, the fraction excreted should be low (< 0.5%).
   c. One study reported $FeNa^+$ < 0.5% 100% sensitive for hypovolemia, 72% specific, LR+ 3.5, LR- 0

5. False-negative results (elevated urine sodium or $FeNa^+$ in hypovolemic patients) may be seen in hypovolemia secondary to:
   a. Diuretics
   b. Primary adrenal insufficiency in which the hypoaldosteronism directly leads to urinary sodium wasting.
   c. Vomiting with accompanying metabolic alkalosis. The metabolic alkalosis causes an obligatory urinary HCO_3^- loss, which is accompanied by sodium. Urine chloride may be low and diagnostic in such cases.

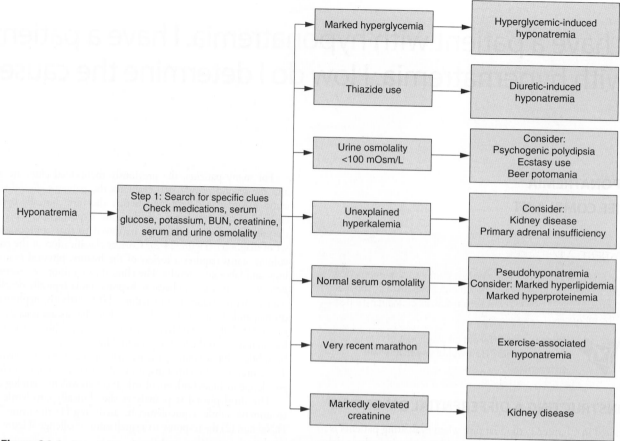

Figure 24-1. Step 1: Searching for pivotal clues in patients with hyponatremia.

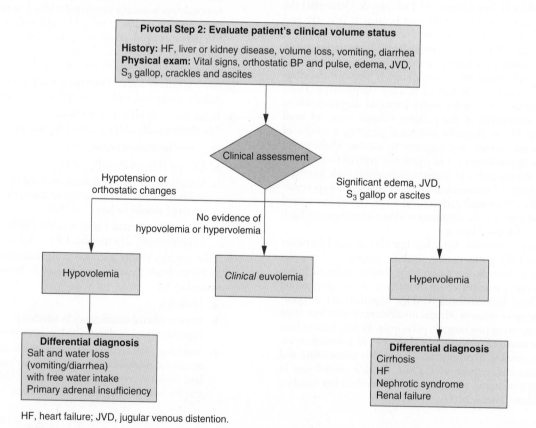

HF, heart failure; JVD, jugular venous distention.

Figure 24-2. Step 2: Organizing patients into subsets based on clinical volume status.

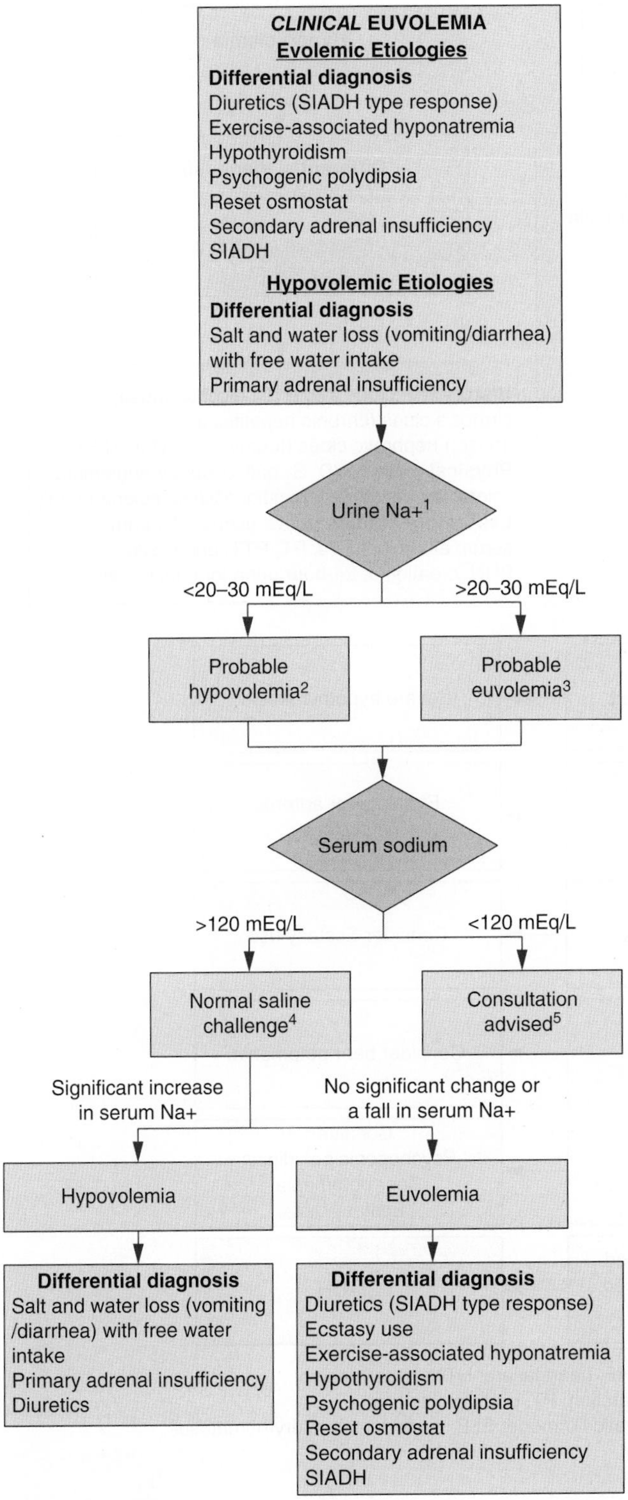

CLINICAL EUVOLEMIA
Evolemic Etiologies
Differential diagnosis
Diuretics (SIADH type response)
Exercise-associated hyponatremia
Hypothyroidism
Psychogenic polydipsia
Reset osmostat
Secondary adrenal insufficiency
SIADH

Hypovolemic Etiologies
Differential diagnosis
Salt and water loss (vomiting/diarrhea)
with free water intake
Primary adrenal insufficiency

Urine Na+[1]

<20–30 mEq/L → Probable hypovolemia[2]

>20–30 mEq/L → Probable euvolemia[3]

Serum sodium

>120 mEq/L → Normal saline challenge[4]

<120 mEq/L → Consultation advised[5]

Significant increase in serum Na+ → Hypovolemia

No significant change or a fall in serum Na+ → Euvolemia

Hypovolemia
Differential diagnosis
Salt and water loss (vomiting /diarrhea) with free water intake
Primary adrenal insufficiency
Diuretics

Euvolemia
Differential diagnosis
Diuretics (SIADH type response)
Ecstasy use
Exercise-associated hyponatremia
Hypothyroidism
Psychogenic polydipsia
Reset osmostat
Secondary adrenal insufficiency
SIADH

[1]Not reliable in patients taking diuretics.
[2]Exceptions include occasional patients with SIADH in whom a low salt intake leads to decreased urinary Na+ loss, and patients with psychogenic polydipsia.
[3]Exceptions include patients with a metabolic alkalosis in whom bicarbonaturia promotes sodium loss and those with primary adrenal insufficiency in which the hypoaldosteronism creates natriuresis.
[4]The saline challenge is expected to raise the serum sodium in patients with hypovolemia but may lower the serum sodium in patients with SIADH. In patients with serum sodium >120 mEq/L, 1 L of normal saline can be administered over 10 hours while the serum sodium is monitored. Since normal saline may decrease the serum sodium in patients with SIADH, this may not be safe in patients with an initial serum sodium of <120 mEq/L.
[5]Saline challenges may cause the serum sodium to fall and should be administered cautiously in patients with severe hyponatremia. Renal consultation is advised.

SIADH, syndrome of inappropriate antidiuretic hormone.

Figure 24-3. Step 3: Limiting the differential diagnosis in clinically euvolemic patients.

6. False-positive results (low urine sodium in euvolemic patients) may be seen in certain euvolemic patients.

   a. Psychogenic polydipsia. These patients are euvolemic but usually have low urine sodium *concentration* due to dilution of the excreted sodium in vast quantities of water.

   b. Some patients with SIADH *ingest* little sodium causing decreased urinary sodium output.

B. Finally the urine Na+ and the Fe_{Na+} should *not* be measured in clinically *hypervolemic* patients. Hypervolemia in such patients is usually associated with *ineffective circulating volume*, which promotes avid sodium reabsorption. Obtaining urine sodium measurements in such patients may mislead clinicians into classifying these patients as hypovolemic.

C. The response to a small saline challenge can also be diagnostically useful. In hypovolemic hyponatremia patients, antidiuretic hormone (ADH) is triggered by the hypovolemia and suppressed by volume resuscitation. Therefore, saline challenges can suppress ADH, promote a water diuresis, and cause a rise in the serum sodium. On the other hand, in euvolemic patients ADH is not volume dependent and persists despite the saline challenge. The persistent ADH results in retention of the water contained in the saline whereas the sodium is excreted resulting in a paradoxical *fall* in the serum sodium with a normal saline challenge.

D. Together the urinary sodium and saline challenge can usually accurately categorize euvolemic and hypovolemic patients (see Figure 24-3). Because normal saline can *decrease* the serum sodium in patients with SIADH, normal saline should *not* be used in patients with an initial serum sodium < 120 mEq/L. Consultation is advised.

In euvolemic patients a fourth step is required to distinguish SIADH from less common causes of euvolemic hyponatremia (Figure 24-4). Attending "raves" may suggest Ecstasy use. Maximally dilute urine suggests beer potomania, psychogenic polydipsia, or Ecstasy use and a high thyroid-stimulating hormone (TSH) or low cortisol can suggest hypothyroidism or adrenal insufficiency, respectively. Euvolemic patients without any of the aforementioned diagnoses likely have SIADH.

The final step reviews the diagnoses within the appropriate subset, searching for risk factors and associated symptoms or signs that suggest one of those diseases.

The differential diagnosis of hyponatremia classified by volume status is listed below.

Differential Diagnosis of Hyponatremia

A. Hypervolemia

  1. HF

  2. Cirrhosis

  3. Nephrotic syndrome

  4. Renal failure (glomerular filtration rate [GFR] < 5 mL/min)

B. Euvolemia

  1. Thiazide diuretics

  2. SIADH

    a. Cancers (eg, pancreas, lung)

    b. CNS disease (eg, cerebrovascular accident, trauma, infection, hemorrhage, mass)

    c. Pulmonary diseases (eg, infections, respiratory failure)

    d. Drugs

      (1) ADH analogues (vasopressin, desmopressin acetate [DDAVP], oxytocin)

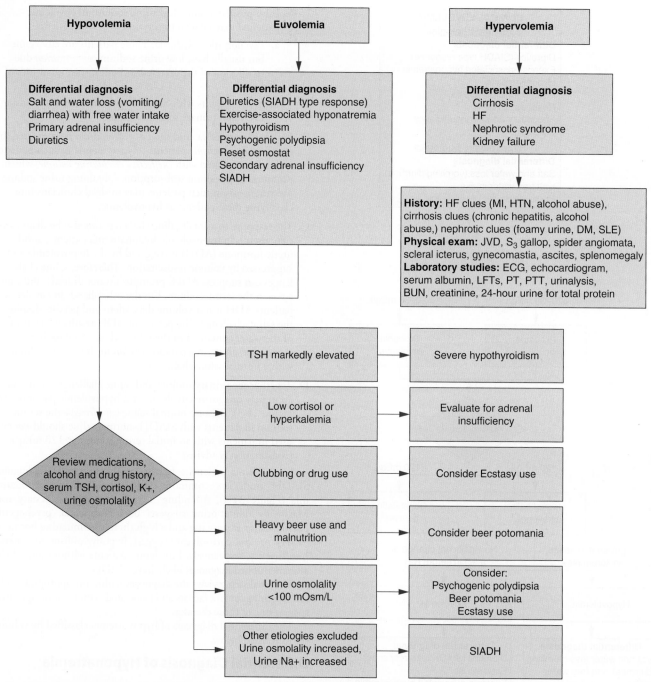

BUN, blood urea nitrogen; DM, diabetes mellitus; ECG, electrocardiogram; HF, heart failure; HTN, hypertension; JVD, jugular venous distention; LFTs, liver function tests; MI, myocardial infarction; PT, prothrombin time; PTT, partial thromboplastin time; SIADH, syndrome of inappropriate antidiuretic hormone; SLE, systemic lupus erythematosus; TSH, thyroid-stimulating hormone.

Figure 24-4. Evaluation of patients with euvolemic hyponatremia.

(2) Chlorpropamide (6–7% of treated patients)

(3) Carbamazepine

(4) Antidepressants (tricyclics and selective serotonin reuptake inhibitors) and antipsychotics

(5) Nonsteroidal antiinflammatory drugs (NSAIDs)

(6) Ecstasy (MDMA)

(7) Others (cyclophosphamide, vincristine, nicotine, opioids, clofibrate)

3. Hypothyroidism, severe

4. Psychogenic polydipsia

5. Secondary adrenal insufficiency

6. EAH

7. Beer potomania

C. Hypovolemia

1. Thiazide diuretics

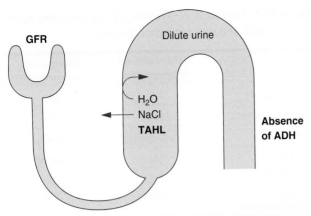

Figure 24-5. Pathophysiology of free water excretion. Free water diuresis requires (1) an adequate glomerular filtration rate (GFR), (2) functioning thick ascending limb of the loop of Henle (TAHL), and (3) absence of antidiuretic hormone (ADH).

2. Salt and water loss with free water replacement (ie, vomiting or diarrhea)

3. Primary adrenal insufficiency

Before proceeding, it is useful to briefly review the pathophysiology of hyponatremia. Hyponatremia develops when patients do not excrete their daily ingested excess (or free) water. Free water excretion requires 3 distinct mechanisms: glomerular filtration, a functioning thick ascending loop of Henle (to separate water from solute), and low levels of ADH, which prevent water reabsorption from the tubules into the interstitium. Interference with these 3 mechanisms contributes to hyponatremia (Figure 24-5).

Symptoms of Hyponatremia

The adverse effects and manifestations of hyponatremia depend on its severity and rapidity of development. Acute hyponatremia leaves the serum hypotonic relative to the brain. This osmotic gradient drives water into the brain, resulting in cerebral edema and CNS symptoms. *Severe acute* hyponatremia may cause brain damage, brainstem herniation, respiratory arrest, and death. Rhabdomyolysis may occur. On the other hand, in chronic hyponatremia (most cases) CNS adaptations occur. Neurons decrease their intracellular osmolality, decreasing the osmotic flux of water into the brain in turn causing less cerebral edema. Although minor symptoms are common in chronic hyponatremia, seizures and herniation are much less frequent. Typically, patients with serum sodium levels > 130 mEq/L are asymptomatic; those with levels from 120 mEq/L to 130 mEq/L may have nausea, vomiting, abdominal symptoms, mild cognitive and gait disturbances. Headache, agitation, and confusion may develop in patients with levels < 125 mEq/L. Levels below 120 mEq/L have been associated with seizures and coma.

Due to his confusion, Mr. D cannot give a medical history. His chart is requested. Physical exam reveals a disheveled man appearing older than 42. He smells of alcohol. His vital signs are BP, 90/50 mm Hg; pulse, 90 bpm; temperature, 36.0°C; RR, 18 breaths per minute. His lungs are clear to auscultation. Neck veins are flat. Cardiac exam reveals a regular rate and rhythm. There is no jugular venous distention (JVD), S₃ gallop, or murmur. His abdomen is distended, and his flanks are bulging. Extremity exam reveals 3+ pitting edema extending all the way up his thighs.

Laboratory studies reveal a glucose of 100 mg/dL, K+ 3.8 mEq/L, a BUN of 28 mg/dL, creatinine 1.0 mg/dL, and a serum osmolality of 252 mOsm/L. Urine osmolality is 480 mOsm/L.

At this point, what is the leading hypothesis, what are the active alternatives, and is there a must not miss diagnosis? Given this differential diagnosis, what tests should be ordered?

RANKING THE DIFFERENTIAL DIAGNOSIS

The first step in evaluating the patient with hyponatremia is to review the history and physical exam for highly specific results that point to a particular diagnosis (see Figure 24-1). Mr. D's serum glucose and potassium are normal, ruling out hyponatremia from marked hyperglycemia, and decreasing the likelihood of primary adrenal insufficiency. The urine osmolality is high enough to effectively rule out psychogenic polydipsia, beer potomania, or Ecstasy use (see below). The low serum osmolality confirms true hypo-osmolar hyponatremia ruling out pseudohyponatremia. His serum creatinine is also normal ruling out chronic renal failure. The second key pivotal point in the evaluation of hyponatremia is to ascertain whether Mr. D is clinically hypervolemic, euvolemic, or hypovolemic. Mr. D's marked peripheral edema clearly indicates that he is *hypervolemic*. Since he is clinically hypervolemic there is no need to check urinary Na+ or Fe$_{Na+}$. The final step in clinically hypervolemic patients explores the differential diagnosis looking for risk factors, associated symptoms and signs of possible diagnoses: HF, nephrotic syndrome, cirrhosis, and renal failure. Of these, cirrhosis seems most likely. The smell of alcohol raises the suspicion of alcohol abuse and liver disease, and the bulging flanks suggest ascites due to cirrhosis. HF is also possible although Mr. D has neither an S₃ gallop nor JVD. Nonetheless, HF should still be considered since neither finding is sensitive enough to rule out HF. Renal failure is effectively ruled out by his normal creatinine. Nephrotic syndrome remains a possibility since we do not have any information yet about proteinuria or the serum albumin level. Table 24-1 lists the differential diagnosis.

Review of Mr. D's past medical record reveals that he has a long history of alcohol-related complications. Six months ago he was hospitalized for bleeding esophageal varices.

Is the clinical information sufficient to make a diagnosis of cirrhosis? If not, what other information do you need?

Leading Hypothesis: Cirrhosis

Textbook Presentation

See Chapter 17, Edema for a full discussion. Patients with cirrhosis may have ascites, variceal hemorrhage, encephalopathy, jaundice, hypoalbuminemia, coagulopathy, and elevated transaminases.

Disease Highlights

A. Hyponatremia is a marker of advanced cirrhosis found in 3% of patients with Child-Pugh class A, 16% in those with class B, and 31% of those with class C.

Table 24-1. Diagnostic hypotheses for Mr. D.

Diagnostic Hypothesis	Demographics, Risk Factors, Symptoms and Signs	Important Tests
Leading Hypothesis		
Cirrhosis	*History:* Heavy alcohol use, hepatitis C or chronic hepatitis B, esophageal varices *Physical exam:* Scleral icterus, spider angiomata, gynecomastia, ascites (bulging flanks, shifting dullness), splenomegaly	Serum albumin, ALT, AST, bilirubin, GGT, alkaline phosphatase, PT, PTT, hepatitis B surface antigen, hepatitis C antibody, liver ultrasound and Doppler
Active Alternatives—Most Common and Must Not Miss		
Heart failure	History of myocardial infarction or poorly controlled hypertension, S_3 gallop, JVD, crackles on lung exam, peripheral edema	Echocardiogram, ECG
Active Alternatives		
Nephrotic syndrome	History of foamy urine, diabetes, SLE	Serum albumin, urinalysis, spot protein-creatinine ratio, BUN, creatinine

ALT, alanine aminotransferase; AST, aspartate aminotransferase; BUN, blood urea nitrogen; GGT, gamma glutamyl transferase ; JVD, jugular venous distention; PT, prothrombin time; PTT, partial thromboplastin time; SLE, systemic lupus erythematosus.

B. Hyponatremia is associated with a higher frequency of adverse outcomes (including hepatorenal syndrome, hepatic encephalopathy, spontaneous bacterial peritonitis, and death), especially if there is no clear precipitant.

1. One study of hospitalized patients reported a 25% mortality among cirrhotic patients without hyponatremia compared with 93% among those with hyponatremia.

2. Furthermore, greater degrees of hyponatremia are associated with an increasing risk of the hepatorenal syndrome and hepatic encephalopathy (Table 24-2).

C. Among patients with cirrhosis and ascites, 22% have sodium ≤ 130 mEq/L.

D. Pathogenesis of hyponatremia in cirrhosis

1. Hypoalbuminemia and splanchnic dilatation decrease effective circulating volume and decrease systemic vascular resistance respectively, leading to decreased mean arterial pressure, resulting in:

   a. Elevated ADH (particularly important)

   b. Decreased GFR

   c. Increased proximal reabsorption of solute causing decreased solute delivery to loop of Henle

   d. The combination of increased ADH, decreased GFR, and decreased solute delivery to the loop of Henle result in free water retention.

Table 24-2. Comparison of findings in patients who have cirrhosis with and without hyponatremia.

	Patients without Hyponatremia	Patients with Hyponatremia
Small liver size	25%	85%
Child-Pugh class C	31%	60%
BP	112/59 mm Hg	99/54 mm Hg
Hepatorenal syndrome	5%	17–85%[1]
Hepatic encephalopathy	15%	38%

[1]The wide variation between the incidence of hepatorenal syndrome in patients with hyponatremia and cirrhosis reflects the incidence in different patient populations. The rate of 85% was reported in patients hospitalized for an acute complication.

2. NSAIDs may worsen edema by reducing GFR and worsen hyponatremia. NSAIDs also lower renal PGE_2, which normally antagonizes ADH.

E. Hyponatremia may act synergistically with hyperammonemia to increase cerebral edema and encephalopathy.

Evidence-Based Diagnosis

A. No clinical finding is terribly sensitive for cirrhosis, but some are fairly specific.

1. Jaundice: 28% sensitive, 93% specific; LR+ 4.0, LR– 0.8

2. Variceal bleeding: 50% sensitive

3. Ascites: 35% sensitive, 95% specific, LR+ 7, LR– 0.7

4. Encephalopathy: 16% sensitive, 98% specific, LR+ 8, LR– 0.9

5. Splenomegaly: 34% sensitive, 90% specific, LR+ 3.4, LR– 0.7

B. However, certain physical exam findings are common in cirrhotic patients *with* hyponatremia.

1. Ascites present in 100%

 Ascites is a very sensitive sign of cirrhosis in hyponatremic patients. Its absence effectively rules out cirrhosis in these patients.

2. Peripheral edema seen in 59%

C. Laboratory studies:

1. Mean urine sodium 4 mEq/L (measurements made after diuretics have been stopped for 5 days). (Decreased effective circulating volume causes increased renal reabsorption of sodium.)

2. Patients with HF also occasionally have ascites, which can erroneously suggest cirrhosis. One study found that a serum NT-proBNP distinguished patients with ascites due to HF from patients with ascites due to cirrhosis. 98% of patients with cirrhosis had levels < 1000 pg/mL whereas all HF patients had levels over 1000 pg/mL. Patients with levels over 1000 pg/mL could have both HF and cirrhosis.

Treatment

A. Since the hyponatremia develops gradually, severe symptoms due to the hyponatremia are uncommon. Nonetheless patients with severe neurologic symptoms (coma or seizures) and severe

Table 24-3. Hyponatremia: approach to treatment.

	Severely symptomatic or acute hyponatremia[1]	Chronic hyponatremia: (> 48 h duration)	
Monitor serum Na+ every 4–6 h until Na+ > 125 mEq/L		Low risk of ODS	High risk of ODS[2]
Goal increase in serum Na+[3]	Urgent 4–6 mEq/L increase	4–8 mEq/L /d	4–6 mEq/L /d
Maximal increase in serum Na+	Symptom improvement	≤ 13 mEq/L /d and ≤ 18 mEq/L /2d	≤ 8 mEq/L /d
Intervention	100 mL 3% NaCl over 10 min. May repeat × 2 if needed[4] For mild-moderate symptoms: 0.5 – 2 mL/kg/h	Depends on etiology. See text	Depends on etiology. See text
Indications to reverse therapy to prevent ODS	Not usually necessary	Exceed maximal rate of correction. Options include • Administer 2–4 mcg of desmopressin every 8 h with • 3mL/kg IV D5W over 1 hour. • Repeat D5W until serum sodium within limit range • Stop vaptan • Follow serum sodium hourly	

[1]Severely symptomatic patients include those with coma or seizures. Acute hyponatremia is likely in patients with hyponatremia due to Ecstasy use, recent marathon participation (within hours), acute water intoxication or those in whom it has been documented to be new in the last 24–48 hours. Therapy should be discontinued when life-threatening symptoms abate or serum sodium exceeds 120 mEq/L.
[2]Patients with any of the following are at an increased risk for ODS. Hypovolemic hyponatremia, diuretic-associated hyponatremia, treated cortisol deficiency, Na+ < 105 mEq/L, hypokalemia, alcohol abuse, malnutrition, advanced liver disease.
[3]Once goal met for that 24 hour period, IV therapy should be stopped (as well as vaptans if used) and ongoing urinary water losses should be replaced with D5W or water by mouth. Alternatively DDAVP may be used to prevent further free water urinary losses (but may be ineffective in patients treated with vaptans).
[4]Stop 3% normal saline if life-threatening symptoms abate or the serum sodium exceeds 120 mEq/L.
ODS, osmotic demyelination syndrome.

hypernatremia should be treated emergently with hypertonic (3%) normal saline (Table 24-3).

B. Similar to all patients with chronic hyponatremia, careful and frequent sodium measurement should be performed to ensure the hyponatremia is not corrected too rapidly to ensure that osmotic demyelination syndrome does not develop (see below).

C. Therapy has not been shown to improve survival and is not recommended in asymptomatic patients with serum sodium levels ≥ 120 mEq/L.

D. Fluid restriction is recommended particularly in symptomatic patients and those with severe hyponatremia (< 120 mEq/L).

E. Vaptans: The FDA has recommended vaptans *not* be used in patients with cirrhosis.

MAKING A DIAGNOSIS

Lab studies reveal an albumin of 2.1 g/dL, bilirubin 6.2 mg/dL, AST (SGOT) 85 units/L, ALT (SGPT) 45 units/L, INR of 1.8. An abdominal ultrasound reveals moderate ascites and a small liver with coarse architecture suggestive of cirrhosis.

Have you crossed a diagnostic threshold for the leading hypothesis, cirrhosis? Have you ruled out the active alternatives? Do other tests need to be done to exclude the alternative diagnoses?

Mr. D's findings point fairly conclusively to hypervolemic hyponatremia secondary to cirrhosis. The prior history of varices and ascites point to portal hypertension while the jaundice, hypoalbuminemia, and increased INR suggest synthetic failure by the liver. HF secondary to an alcoholic cardiomyopathy is still possible. Other causes of hypervolemia hyponatremia, such as nephrotic syndrome, are less likely but possible. Finally, there is no history of thiazide use to suggest diuretic-induced hyponatremia.

Alternative Diagnosis: HF & Hyponatremia

Textbook Presentation

Typically, patients with HF complain of shortness of breath, dyspnea on exertion, fatigue, and orthopnea. (See Chapter 15, Dyspnea for a complete discussion of HF.)

Disease Highlights

A. Patients with HF and hyponatremia have marked *increases* in both total body sodium and water retention producing edema and volume overload.

B. In hyponatremic HF patients, free water clearance is impaired and water retention *exceeds* sodium retention (causing the hyponatremia).

C. Free water clearance is impaired in large part secondary to elevated ADH levels. The fall in cardiac output triggers carotid baroreceptors that in turn stimulate ADH release. Free water excretion is also impaired by decreased renal perfusion (which decreases the GFR) and an increase in proximal sodium reabsorption (which limits delivery to the thick ascending limb of the loop of Henle).

D. Hyponatremia is observed in patients with severe HF and is associated with an increased risk of death.

E. Diuretic therapy (particularly thiazides) can worsen the hyponatremia.

Evidence-Based Diagnosis

See HF discussion in Chapter 15, Dyspnea.

Treatment

A. Treatment of underlying HF

1. Similar to other patients with HF (see Chapter 15, Dyspnea).

2. Angiotensin-converting enzyme (ACE) inhibitors

   a. Can help restore sodium levels to normal. ACE inhibitors improve cardiac output, decrease ADH secretion, and facilitate free water excretion. They also directly antagonize the effect of ADH on the collecting tubules.

   b. Hyponatremic HF patients usually have activation of the renin angiotensin system and are susceptible to ACE inhibitor–induced hypotension. Therefore, therapy with ACE inhibitors should be initiated at *low* doses.

3. Avoid NSAID use, which can decrease prostaglandin-dependent renal blood flow and worsen renal function.

B. Treatment of hyponatremia

1. Patients with severe symptomatic hyponatremia (comas, seizures) should receive 3% normal saline (see Table 24-3). Furosemide should be given concurrently to prevent volume overload.

2. Asymptomatic or mildly symptomatic patients

   a. Consider excessive diuresis accompanied by increased thirst and ingestion of excessive free water.

   b. Restrict water intake < 1000 mL/d and add furosemide to volume overloaded patients to facilitate natriuresis and augment free water loss (furosemide decreases renal medullary gradients which augments free water loss).

   c. Vaptans can also be added if free water restriction and furosemide are inadequate (Table 24-4).

   d. The rate of rise of serum sodium should be carefully monitored. Recent recommendations guide the goal and maximal rate of rise for the serum sodium (Table 24-3). Correction that exceeds these limits should be countered with therapy to reduce the serum sodium (Table 24-3).

   e. Discontinue thiazide diuretics.

Alternative Diagnosis: Nephrotic Syndrome

Textbook Presentation

See Chapter 17, Edema for full discussion. Patients typically complain of edema.

Disease Highlights

A. Lesions may be primary and idiopathic (eg, minimal change lesion) or secondary to systemic disease (eg, diabetes mellitus, malignancy).

B. Glomerular lesion leads to albuminuria and hypoalbuminemia.

1. Hypoalbuminemia decreases oncotic pressures decreasing effective circulating volume.

2. Decreased effective circulating volume triggers sodium retention (which may be aggravated by renal insufficiency).

3. The combination of sodium retention and hypoalbuminemia cause edema and hypervolemia.

4. The ineffective circulating volume can also trigger ADH release, reduce free water clearance, and promote hyponatremia.

5. Pseudohyponatremia may be seen secondary to marked hypertriglyceridemia.

Evidence-Based Diagnosis

A. Nephrotic syndrome is characterized by urine protein excretion ≥ 3.5 g/d, edema, hypoalbuminemia, and hyperlipidemia.

B. Renal biopsy can help identify certain underlying disease states.

Treatment

A. Free water restriction.

B. Vaptans may be effective in patients with a GFR > 50 mL/min in patients who do not respond adequately to water restriction (see Table 24-4).

CASE RESOLUTION

An echocardiogram reveals normal left ventricular function and a urinalysis reveals only 1+ proteinuria not suggestive of nephrotic syndrome. A paracentesis is performed to rule out spontaneous bacterial peritonitis and is normal.

Mr. D's history, physical exam, and laboratory findings clearly point to severe cirrhosis. HF and nephrotic syndrome are effectively ruled out by the echocardiogram and urinalysis. The key therapeutic decision is the rate at which to increase his serum sodium. Several features suggest

Table 24-4. Vaptan treatment of hyponatremia.

Available agents	Tolvaptan (oral V2 selective) Conivaptan (IV nonselective)
Side effects	Thirst Transaminase elevations Decreased renal function (conivaptan) Potential for over rapid correction of hyponatremia and osmotic demyelination syndrome (ODS)
Recommendations to minimize the risk of ODS in patients receiving vaptans	Hospitalize patients when initiated Measure serum sodium every 6–8 h for the first 24–48 h Do not use with or immediately after other therapies that raise the serum sodium (eg, fluid restriction or 3% normal saline) Discontinued if patients unable to ingest fluid (confusion, nothing by mouth, etc.)
FDA guidelines[1]	The FDA advises limiting use to 30 days

[1]Approved for euvolemic and hypervolemic hyponatremia. Not indicated in hypovolemic hyponatremia. Not approved in patients with cirrhosis or liver disease. Not recommended for patients with severe symptomatic hyponatremia < 120 mEq/L.

great care should be given to avoid overcorrection. First, he does not have severe neurologic symptoms (coma or seizures) that would mandate acute and rapid correction. Second, the hyponatremia is likely chronic. Both the chronicity and his liver disease increase his risk for osmotic demyelination syndrome, a potentially fatal neurologic complication that may develop when chronic hyponatremia is corrected too rapidly (Table 24-5). An important aspect of his care is to ensure a safe and gradual return of his serum sodium to normal.

Mr. D's mild hyponatremia is corrected slowly. He is begun on free water restriction and his sodium gradually improves to 128 mEq/L. His mental status returns to normal.

Table 24-5. Osmotic demyelination syndrome (ODS).

1. ODS is a complication of overly rapid correction of severe *chronic* hyponatremia (< 120 mEq/L for 2 or more days)
2. Rapid correction of chronic hyponatremia makes the serum hypertonic compared to the brain causing osmotic demyelination
3. Develops 2–6 days after correction.
4. Spastic quadriparesis and pseudobulbar palsy, coma, ataxia, behavioral disorders, and death may occur.
5. Pons most commonly affected but other areas of white matter may also be affected.
6. Increased risk in patients with hypovolemic hyponatremia, diuretic-associated hyponatremia, treated cortisol deficiency, Na+ < 105 mEq/L, hypokalemia, alcohol abuse, malnutrition, or advanced liver disease.
7. Lesions may not be apparent on MRI for up to 4 weeks after symptoms develop.

CHIEF COMPLAINT

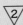

PATIENT 2

Mrs. L is a 60-year-old woman who comes to see you for a follow-up of her hypertension. She only complains of mild fatigue. On physical exam, her BP is well controlled at 126/84 mm Hg. Routine chemistries reveal a serum sodium of 128 mEq/L. Her potassium and other electrolytes and creatinine are normal. Her glucose is 108 mg/dL and BUN is 28 mg/dL. Urine specific gravity is 1.025. Serum osmolality is 278 mOsm/L.

At this point, what is the leading hypothesis, what are the active alternatives, and is there a must not miss diagnosis? Given this differential diagnosis, what tests should be ordered?

RANKING THE DIFFERENTIAL DIAGNOSIS

Again, the first step in evaluating the patient with hyponatremia is to review the history, physical exam, and initial lab findings for highly specific clues that point to a particular diagnosis (ie, a history of thiazide use, recent marathon, marked hyperglycemia, unexplained hyperkalemia, a maximally dilute urine or normal serum osmolality) (see Figure 24-1). She reports that her hypertension is treated with amlodipine (a calcium channel blocker) and her blood glucose and potassium are normal, ruling out marked hyperglycemic hyponatremia and making the diagnosis of primary adrenal insufficiency less likely. Although her urine osmolality is not reported, her urine specific gravity is *not* very low and not suggestive of psychogenic polydipsia. Finally, the serum osmolality is low, confirming true hypo-osmolar hyponatremia and ruling out pseudohyponatremia. The second key pivotal point is to classify Mrs. L's clinical volume status as hypervolemic, euvolemic, or hypovolemic (see Figure 24-2). A careful exam should search for signs of hypervolemia (edema, JVD, S_3 gallop, crackles, or ascites) and for signs of hypovolemia (hypotension, tachycardia, or orthostatic hypotension).

Mrs. L denies any history that suggests volume loss (vomiting, diarrhea, or excessive perspiration). She denies symptoms suggestive of hypervolemia such as edema, dyspnea on exertion, or orthopnea. Furthermore, she has

no history of any diseases associated with hypervolemic states (HF, cirrhosis, renal failure, or nephrotic syndrome). On physical exam, BP is normal with no significant change going from lying to standing. There is no pretibial or pedal edema. Cardiovascular exam reveals no JVD or S_3 gallop. She has no crackles on lung exam and there are no signs of ascites (bulging flanks, shifting dullness).

Mrs. L's history and exam suggest neither hypervolemia or hypovolemia. Therefore, she is classified as *clinically* euvolemic.

The third key pivotal step reviews her urine sodium and response to a saline challenge to determine if she is truly euvolemic or has subtle hypovolemia (see Figure 24-3).

Mrs. L's urine sodium concentration is 60 mEq/L.

The elevated urine sodium argues against hypovolemia and is consistent with the clinical impression that Mrs. L is euvolemic. As noted in the introduction, 1 L normal saline challenge can also be diagnostically useful, since it may distinguish subtle hypovolemia (which may improve with a normal saline challenge) from euvolemia, which may worsen (see above).

Following a 1 L normal saline challenge, Mrs. L's urinary output does not rise significantly. A repeat serum sodium 4 hours later is 126 mEq/L.

Mrs. L's lab studies and lack of response to saline confirms euvolemic hyponatremia (see Figure 24-3). The final step explores the differential diagnosis for euvolemic hyponatremia (see Figure 24-4). Causes include SIADH (most common), adverse effect of medication, secondary adrenal insufficiency, severe hypothyroidism (TSH > 50 milli-international units/mL), Ecstasy use, psychogenic polydipsia, and beer potomania. Psychogenic polydipsia and beer potomania are ruled out by the high urine osmolality. At this point the leading hypothesis is SIADH. Table 24-6 lists the differential diagnosis. Further history and laboratory studies may help rank the differential diagnosis.

Table 24-6. Diagnostic hypotheses for Mrs. L.

Diagnostic Hypotheses	Demographics, Risk Factors, Symptoms and Signs	Important Tests
Leading Hypothesis		
SIADH	History of cancer (or cancer risks) Unusual cough Hemoptysis or lymphadenopathy Neurologic or pulmonary disease HIV	Urine Na+ > 20-30 mEq/L Urine osmolality usually > 300 mOsm/L Exclusion of hypothyroidism and adrenal insufficiency
Active Alternative—Most Common		
Medication	Medication history	Response to discontinuation of medication
Hypothyroidism	Fatigue, cold intolerance	TSH
Active Alternative—Must Not Miss		
Adrenal insufficiency	Long-term corticosteroid therapy, pituitary disease, HIV, sarcoidosis	Serum cortisol Corticotropin stimulation test

SIADH, syndrome of inappropriate antidiuretic hormone; TSH, thyroid-stimulating hormone.

Past medical history: Hypertension treated with amlodipine. Social history: 40-pack-year history of smoking. Alcohol use is minimal. Mrs. L denies any drug use. Review of systems positive only for a cough that has been present over the last 1–2 months. Her TSH is 2.3 milli-international units/L (normal < 4.0 milli-international units/L).

Mrs. L's history is not particularly diagnostic. Her normal TSH essentially rules out primary hypothyroidism. Her recent cough and tobacco history raises the possibility of SIADH from a lung cancer. Adrenal insufficiency is a potentially life-threatening cause of hyponatremia and should be considered a "must not miss" diagnosis. Although hyperkalemia suggests adrenal insufficiency, a normal potassium does not rule it out.

 Is the clinical information sufficient to make a diagnosis? If not, what other information do you need?

Leading Hypothesis: SIADH

Textbook Presentation

Patients are often (although not always) elderly, with a chief complaint of falls, weakness, or confusion. Alternatively, mild hyponatremia may be discovered incidentally on serum chemistries.

Disease Highlights

A. Most common cause of hyponatremia

B. Secondary to inappropriate ADH release despite hypotonicity and euvolemia.

C. Patients are clinically euvolemic. Clinically unapparent volume expansion due to water retention leads to urinary sodium loss.

D. Etiologies

1. Cancer, 15%: Ectopic production by small cell carcinoma of the lung is the most common malignancy but many other cancers can cause SIADH.

2. Neurologic disease (eg, stroke, hemorrhage, meningitis, tumors or trauma)

3. Intrathoracic disease (eg, pneumonia, tuberculosis, acute respiratory failure)

4. Drugs: Carbamazepine (20–30% of patients), Ecstasy, ADH analogues (vasopressin, DDAVP, oxytocin [5% of patients]), chlorpropamide, NSAIDs, antidepressants (tricyclics and selective serotonin reuptake inhibitors), antipsychotics, cyclophosphamide, vincristine, nicotine, opioids, clofibrate, and many other medications

5. AIDS

   a. SIADH may be secondary to *Pneumocystis* pneumonia, CNS infections, or cancer.

   b. Hyponatremia may also develop secondary to HIV-related adrenal insufficiency or diarrhea (with free water ingestion).

 Evaluate patients with HIV and hyponatremia for adrenal insufficiency.

6. Temporal arteritis

7. Idiopathic

E. Reset osmostat

1. A variant of SIADH in which ADH control is modulated to maintain serum sodium levels at a lower range than normal. Patients retain ability to excrete water load at a new equilibrium point.

2. Therefore, hyponatremia is not progressive.

3. Patients typically have serum sodium levels between 125 mEq/L and 135 mEq/L.

4. Very dilute urine osmolality may be seen following water load (< 100 mOsm/L).

5. Etiology is similar to SIADH.

6. Treatment is directed at the underlying disorder.

Evidence-Based Diagnosis

A. Standard criteria

1. Effective plasma osmolality < 275 mOsm/L; can be calculated using the following equation: Effective osmolality = $(2 \times Na^+) + (Glucose/18)$

2. Urine sodium is typically > 20-30 mEq/L.

3. Urine osmolality not maximally dilute due to active ADH (urine osmolality > 100 mOsm/L, usually > 300 mOsm/L).

4. Patients clinically euvolemic and other causes of euvolemic hyponatremia must be excluded (hypothyroidism, psychogenic polydipsia, secondary adrenal insufficiency).

5. Patients are not using diuretics.

B. Urine sodium

1. Patients with SIADH are euvolemic.

2. Since there is no volume stimulus for sodium retention, sodium is usually > 20–30 mEq/L.

3. However, 13–42% of patients have low urine sodium and low FE_{Na} due to low sodium intake.

Treatment

A. Determine and treat underlying etiology.

1. Review medications; consider CT scan of the chest and head.

2. SIADH often resolves with treatment of the underlying disorder (eg, cancer, infection). When due to cancer, recurrent SIADH suggests cancer recurrence.

B. It is important to note that *isotonic saline* without furosemide may *worsen* hyponatremia because the ADH stimulus promotes water retention while the sodium is excreted. Therapeutic options include fluid restriction < 800 mL/d, salt tablets, salt tablets with furosemide, hypertonic 3% saline, and ADH receptor antagonists.

 Normal saline may worsen hyponatremia in patients with SIADH.

1. Discontinue any medications that may cause SIADH.

2. Fluid restriction is often used. Of note, it is unlikely to be successful as the sole measure if urinary osmolality is > 500 mOsm/L.

3. Salt tablets can increase urinary osmolality and facilitate increased water loss.

4. Furosemide may be a useful adjunct to salt supplementation because it decreases the concentration of solute in the renal medulla, which impairs water retention and thereby facilitates water excretion.

5. Hypertonic saline (3%) augments water elimination and is effective.

   a. Recommended for patients with severe neurologic symptoms (coma, seizures; Table 24-3)

   b. May be useful for patients with severe hyponatremia who have less severe neurologic symptoms (confusion, lethargy), but care must be used not to exceed recommended rates of correction (Table 24-3) and avoid subsequent osmotic demyelination syndrome (Table 24-5).

      (1) Careful calculations (Table 24-7) and frequent sodium monitoring should guide therapy.

      (2) Hypertonic saline may be used with or without furosemide.

6. ADH receptor antagonists can be used (see Table 24-4).

Table 24-7. Predicted response to normal or hypertonic saline.

The impact of 1 liter of fluid can be predicted as follows:

Δ Serum $[Na^+] = ($Infusate $[Na^+] -$ serum $[Na^+])/($TBW $+ 1)$

In men, TBW = 0.6 X weight(kg)

In women, TBW = 0.5 X weight(kg)

Infusate $[Na^+]$: Normal saline $[Na^+]$ = 154 mEq/L; 3% normal saline $[Na^+]$ = 513 mEq/L

Example: 70-kg man with serum sodium of 110 mEq/L given 1 L of normal saline

TBW = 70 * 0.6 = 42L

Predicted Δ Serum $[Na^+] = (154 - 110)/(42 + 1) = 1$ mEq/L increase in serum sodium for every liter of normal saline administered.

TBW, total body water.

7. Demeclocycline diminishes renal sensitivity to ADH but may cause nephrotoxicity and photosensitivity and is rarely used.

MAKING A DIAGNOSIS

The urine osmolality is 480 mOsm/L. The serum osmolality is 266 mOsm/L.

Have you crossed a diagnostic threshold for the leading hypothesis, SIADH? Have you ruled out the other active alternatives that cause euvolemic hyponatremia? Do other tests need to be done to exclude the alternative diagnoses?

Mrs. L's elevated urine osmolality is consistent with SIADH. It is important to consider the alternative diagnosis before concluding that she in fact has SIADH. If SIADH is confirmed, a search for the underlying cause is appropriate.

Alternative Diagnosis: Adrenal Insufficiency

Textbook Presentation

Patients may have chronic symptoms of fatigue, weight loss, nausea, vomiting, orthostasis, and abdominal pain or acute symptoms, such as a clinical constellation that suggests septic shock (hypotension and fever). Adrenal insufficiency may also cause hypoglycemia. Both primary and secondary adrenal insufficiency may cause hyponatremia.

Disease Highlights

A. Pathophysiology

1. Adrenal insufficiency may be primary or secondary.

   a. Primary adrenal insufficiency occurs when damage to the adrenal gland results in inadequate cortisol production. ACTH increases because the hypothalamic pituitary axis attempts to compensate for the hypocortisolism.

   b. Secondary adrenal insufficiency develops when damage to the hypothalamic pituitary system results in inadequate corticotropin (ACTH) production thereby producing inadequate adrenal stimulation and hypocortisolism.

2. Cortisol normally suppresses ADH release. Decreased cortisol causes increased ADH levels and promotes hyponatremia.

3. Primary adrenal insufficiency

   a. May decrease the synthesis of other adrenal hormones

      (1) Aldosterone, DHEA, and catecholamine synthesis may be impaired.

      (2) Aldosterone deficiency results in salt losses and clinical hypovolemia. The hypovolemia may further stimulate ADH release. Finally, the aldosterone deficiency may also cause hyperkalemia.

 Suspect primary adrenal insufficiency in hyponatremic patients with hyperkalemia.

      (3) DHEA deficiency affects women (but not men due to testicular androgen synthesis). Findings may

include decreased libido, decreased axillary and pubic hair, and amenorrhea.

   (4) Catecholamine synthesis is also usually impaired (except in autoimmune adrenal disease).

4. Secondary adrenal insufficiency (hypothalamic-pituitary insufficiency)

   a. Results in *isolated* cortisol deficiency which, in turn, causes elevated ADH levels and hyponatremia.

   b. Aldosterone is primarily under control of the renin angiotensin system and is unaffected so that patients are often euvolemic and do not suffer from hyperkalemia.

   c. Hyponatremia may be precipitated by inter-current illness, leading to inadequate cortisol response; 43% of patients with secondary adrenal insufficiency had superimposed infection when presenting with hyponatremia.

B. Etiology

1. Etiologies of primary adrenal insufficiency

   a. Autoimmune adrenalitis (80–90% of cases in developed nations)

   b. HIV infection: Up to 20% of patients with HIV have adrenal insufficiency.

   c. Tuberculosis (most common cause in developing nations)

   d. Less common etiologies: Fungal or cytomegalovirus infections, bilateral adrenal hemorrhage (seen in septic shock, meningococcemia, postoperative patients, and in patients taking anticoagulants), infiltration (cancer), inherited disorders and certain drugs (ketoconazole, rifampin, phenytoin, and others)

2. Etiologies of secondary adrenal insufficiency (hypothalamic-pituitary insufficiency)

   a. Iatrogenic due to corticosteroid therapy

      (1) Up to 50% of patients taking long-term corticosteroid therapy (ie, > 7.5 mg/d prednisone for > 3 weeks) have adrenal insufficiency

      (2) Recovery of hypothalamic-pituitary-adrenal axis may take 9–12 months.

   b. Sepsis

   c. Pituitary tumors (30% of patients with a pituitary macroadenoma exhibit adrenal insufficiency)

   d. Less common etiologies: Pituitary infarction, irradiation, autoimmune hypophysitis, traumatic brain injury, HIV, sarcoidosis, hemorrhage, hemochromatosis, empty sella syndrome

 Suspect hypopituitarism as the cause of hyponatremia in any patient with a history of pituitary disease (eg, macroadenoma, infarction, empty sella syndrome).

C. Adrenal crisis

1. 3% of patients per year

2. Often secondary to insufficient increases in glucocorticoid during times of stress

Evidence-Based Diagnosis

A. History and physical exam

1. Acute adrenal insufficiency (adrenal crisis)

   a. Often presents similarly to septic shock with hypotension (90%), abdominal pain (with rigidity or rebound in 22%), vomiting (47%), confusion (42%) and unexplained fever (66%). Patients may also have unexplained hypoglycemia, hyponatremia, and hyperkalemia.

   b. Often precipitated by inter-current stress (myocardial infarction or infection). May occur in patients without known adrenal insufficiency or in those with diagnosed disease who fail to increase glucocorticoid therapy during infection or stress.

   c. Rare in patients with secondary adrenal insufficiency because aldosterone secretion is preserved in such patients.

2. Chronic adrenal insufficiency

   a. May present with a variety of nonspecific symptoms (eg, fatigue, weakness, weight loss, musculoskeletal pains).

   b. The frequency of presenting symptoms may be overestimated in the literature dominated by very old case series that discovered advanced disease.

   c. Hypotension and hyperpigmentation are seen only in primary adrenal insufficiency.

      (1) Hypotension occurs due to concomitant aldosterone deficiency and occurs in ≡ 90% of patients with primary adrenal insufficiency.

      (2) Hyperpigmentation

         (a) Develops secondary to a compensatory increase in the release of proopiomelanocortin (POMC), the precursor hormone that contains both ACTH and melanocyte-stimulating hormone.

         (b) Typically develops in exposed areas such as the face, dorsum of hands and knuckles, as well as the palmer creases of interphalangeal joints. There may also be a blue black hyperpigmentation of the buccal mucosa. Patients often appear "tanned."

         (c) Older reports suggest hyperpigmentation was invariable in primary adrenal insufficiency. A more recent report found hyperpigmentation in only 18% of such patients.

   d. Other findings in chronic adrenal insufficiency

      (1) Weakness, tiredness, fatigue: 100%

      (2) Weight loss and anorexia: 100%

      (3) Musculoskeletal complaints 94%

         (a) Myalgia 71%

         (b) Flexion contractures 55%

         (c) Back pain 33%

         (d) Arthralgia 22%

      (4) Gastrointestinal symptoms

         (a) Nausea: 86%

         (b) Vomiting: 75%

         (c) Diarrhea: 16%

      (5) Amenorrhea: 25% of women

      (6) Postural dizziness: 12%

      (7) Psychiatric manifestations (memory impairment, delirium, depression, and psychosis): 5–50%

      (8) Vitiligo: 10–20% (another autoimmune phenomenon)

      (9) Salt craving: 16%

      (10) Visual field defects may occur in secondary adrenal insufficiency when pituitary tumors compress the optic tracts.

B. Laboratory tests (Figure 24-6)

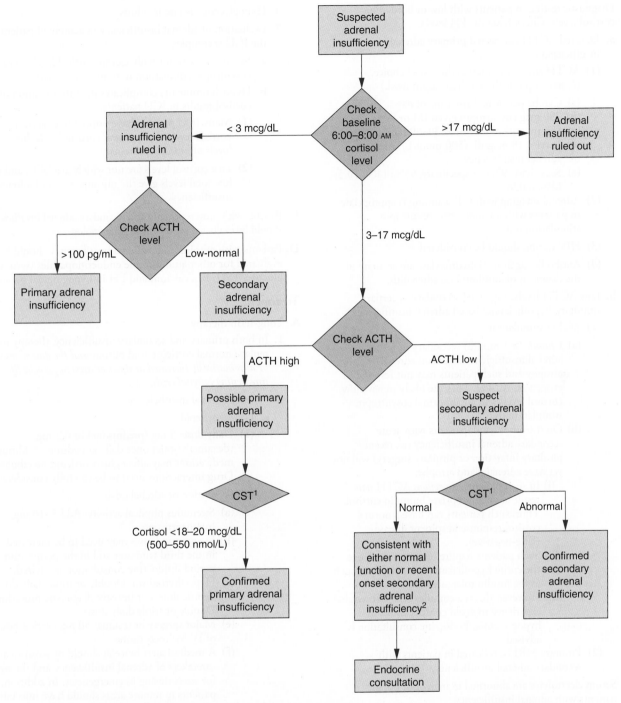

^{1}ACTH cosyntropin stimulation test (CST): Administer 250 mcg as IV bolus and check cortisol level in 30–60 minutes.
  (Normal response: cortisol >18 mcg/dL)
^{2}Recent secondary adrenal insufficiency should be suspected in patients with recent pituitary surgery or infarction.

Figure 24-6. Evaluation of suspected adrenal insufficiency.

1. Morning cortisol levels
   a. Cortisol secretion demonstrates a marked diurnal variation.
   b. Early morning cortisol levels can help establish or refute adrenal insufficiency.
      (1) Morning levels > 17 mcg/dL rule out adrenal insufficiency.
      (2) Morning levels between 3 mcg/dL and 17 mcg/dL are nondiagnostic.

   (3) Morning levels < 3 mcg/dL establish adrenal insufficiency.
      (a) In such patients, 8 AM ACTH measurements differentiate primary from secondary adrenal insufficiency.
      (b) ACTH is elevated in primary adrenal insufficiency.
      (c) ACTH is low in adrenal insufficiency secondary to hypothalamic-pituitary dysfunction.

2. Diagnostic testing in patients with low or borderline cortisol levels. Check 8 AM ACTH levels.

    a. Elevated ACTH (suspected primary adrenal insufficiency)

        (1) ACTH stimulation test is the test of choice. (Cosyntropin is the synthetic agent used.)

            (a) Can be performed any time of day

            (b) 250 mcg cosyntropin given IM or IV

            (c) Serum cortisol measured 30–60 minutes later

            (d) Level < 18 mcg/dL (500 nmol/L) rules in adrenal insufficiency

            (e) Sensitivity, 97.5%; specificity, 95%; LR+, 19.5; LR−, 0.026

        (2) Adrenal imaging with CT scanning is appropriate in patients with an abnormal cosyntropin stimulation test.

        (3) HIV testing should be considered.

        (4) Antibodies against 21-hydroxylase are accurate in the diagnosis of autoimmune adrenalitis.

    b. Low ACTH levels: suspected secondary or tertiary (pituitary-hypothalamic) based adrenal insufficiency

        (1) ACTH stimulation

            (a) *Chronic* (> 1 month) secondary or tertiary adrenal insufficiency results in adrenal atrophy and such patients may not respond to exogenous ACTH. They are likely to have low cortisol levels and an abnormal cosyntropin stimulation test.

            (b) On the other hand, patients with acute secondary adrenal insufficiency (ie, recent pituitary infarction or pituitary surgery) will not yet have adrenal gland atrophy.

                (i) In such patients, *exogenous* ACTH *will* result in an appropriate bump in cortisol. Thus, such patients can have a normal cortisol response in spite of disease (false-negative).

                (ii) Such patients require tests that challenge the entire hypothalamic-pituitary axis, such as the insulin tolerance test.

                (iii) However, this is a complex test that requires experience to avoid complications of hypoglycemia. Endocrine consultation is advised.

        (2) Pituitary MRI is indicated in patients with secondary adrenal insufficiency.

3. Serum electrolytes are abnormal in many but not all patients with adrenal insufficiency.

    a. Hyponatremia develops in 88% of patients with primary or secondary adrenal insufficiency due to increased ADH levels.

    b. Hyperkalemia develops in 50% of patients with primary adrenal insufficiency due to aldosterone deficiency. It is not seen in patients with isolated glucocorticoid deficiency (secondary adrenal insufficiency).

4. Urine electrolytes in hyponatremic patients with adrenal insufficiency: Decreased cortisol causes lack of suppression of ADH, leading to increased ADH and laboratory values similar to SIADH (average urinary sodium, 110 mmol/L; average urine osmolality, 399 mOsm/L)

5. Eosinophilia has been reported in 17% of patients.

6. Hypoglycemia is rare in adults.

7. Evaluation of adrenal insufficiency in acutely ill patients in the ICU is complex.

    a. Severe stressors normally elevate cortisol levels so that cosyntropin stimulation tests are unnecessary.

    b. Hypoalbuminemia complicates the interpretation of cortisol results in ICU patients.

        (1) Many ICU patients have normal free (active) cortisol levels but low *total* cortisol levels due to low levels of binding proteins.

        (2) Free cortisol levels are not widely available, and the low total levels give the misimpression of adrenal insufficiency.

C. Patients with proven primary and secondary adrenal insufficiency should be evaluated for the underlying etiology.

D. Patients with autoimmune adrenal insufficiency should be evaluated for other autoimmune endocrinopathies (serum glucose, TSH, B_{12}, calcium and LH in hypogonadal patients).

Treatment

A. Long-term therapy

  1. In both primary and secondary insufficiency, therapy must replace normal corticosteroid output *and the dosage must be automatically increased at times of stress to prevent life-threatening adrenal crisis.*

  2. Primary adrenal insufficiency

    a. Glucocorticoid

        (1) Daily dose: 5 mg (prednisone) or 0.5 mg (dexamethasone) once daily at bedtime. Additional medications may affect glucocorticoid metabolism. Drug interactions need to be carefully considered.

        (2) Prevention of adrenal crisis

            (a) Strenuous physical activity: Add 5–10 mg hydrocortisone

            (b) Pregnancy: Doses may need to be increased in the third trimester and in the peripartum period. Endocrine consultation is advised.

            (c) Hyperthyroidism: Double or triple daily dose

            (d) Febrile illness or invasive diagnostic procedures: Double or triple daily dose

            (e) Major surgery or trauma: 50 mg every 8 hours of IV hydrocortisone

            (f) A medical alert bracelet should be worn to alert caretakers of adrenal insufficiency and the need for stress dosing in emergencies. In addition, patients in remote areas should have injectable glucocorticoids for emergency situations.

    b. Mineralocorticoid

        (1) 0.05–0.2 mg/d of fludrocortisone

        (2) Monitor potassium levels as well as BP

    c. DHEA (50 mg/d) can be considered for women with impaired sense of well being despite glucocorticoid and mineralocorticoid replacement.

  3. Secondary adrenal insufficiency: Glucocorticoids as for primary adrenal insufficiency

B. Treatment of adrenal crisis

  1. Hydrocortisone 100 mg IV and then 100 mg IV every 6–8 hours. For patients who are still being evaluated for adrenal insufficiency, dexamethasone is substituted for hydrocortisone because it is not detected by the cortisol assays.

2. Normal saline (often up to 1 L/h)

3. Patients should be monitored closely to ensure that over rapid correction of hyponatremia does not develop with steroid therapy. Both glucocorticoids and fluid resuscitation suppresses ADH, promotes a water diuresis and may result in overcorrection.

4. Patients with fever should be evaluated for infectious etiologies and treated appropriately. It should *not* be assumed that fever is secondary to adrenal insufficiency.

5. Endocrinology consultation is advised.

 When adrenal crisis is suspected, blood tests should be drawn for cortisol and ACTH. Treatment should commence immediately and not await laboratory results.

C. In patients with concomitant hypothyroidism, adrenal insufficiency should be corrected prior to the initiation of thyroid replacement (which can worsen symptoms).

CASE RESOLUTION

The serum cortisol level following 250 mcg of corticotropin is 800 nmol/L.

Her corticotropin stimulation tests are normal ruling out adrenal insufficiency and as previously noted her TSH was normal ruling out primary hypothyroidism. (Secondary adrenal insufficiency of recent onset is still theoretically possible, but nothing in the history suggests the patient is at risk for pituitary disease.) Therefore, Mrs. L has SIADH. The final step will be to determine the etiology of the SIADH. As noted above, SIADH can result from a variety of pulmonary, neurologic, or malignant causes. Following clinical clues is important. Her recent cough and long history of tobacco use suggests an underlying pulmonary etiology.

A chest film reveals a 5-cm pulmonary mass adjacent to the right hilum. Bronchoscopy and biopsy confirms small cell carcinoma of the lung. Mrs. L is referred to medical oncology. Her hyponatremia is controlled with free water restriction.

REVIEW OF OTHER IMPORTANT DISEASES

Alternative Diagnosis: Diuretic-Induced Hyponatremia

Textbook Presentation
The most common clinical situation is a small elderly woman taking a thiazide diuretic for hypertension. Patients may be asymptomatic or complain of weakness, lethargy, or occasionally confusion due to hyponatremia.

Disease Highlights

A. One of the most common causes of hyponatremia

B. Often associated with more severe hyponatremia than frequently seen due to other etiologies (mean serum sodium, 116 mEq/L)

C. Most commonly seen with thiazide diuretics; rarely seen with loop diuretics

D. More common in patients over 70 years (OR 3.9)

E. 70% of patients are women

F. Hyponatremia can be multifactorial; pathogenesis may vary in different patients.

G. Pathophysiology

1. Thiazide diuretics interfere with NaCl transport in cortical diluting segments, causing natriuresis and interfering with the generation of free water within the tubule. This limits free water excretion.

2. The natriuresis results in hypovolemia.

3. Hypovolemia may increase ADH levels, and interfere with free water clearance.

4. Hypovolemia also reduces the GFR, which increases proximal sodium reabsorption leading to reduced distal sodium delivery and reduced free water clearance.

5. In some patients, hyponatremia develops due to a combination of increased water intake coupled with ADH independent water retention. Such patients appear clinically euvolemic.

H. NSAID use may increase the risk of thiazide-induced hyponatremia.

I. Hyponatremia may persist for 1 month after discontinuation of thiazide.

Evidence-Based Diagnosis

A. Clinical dehydration is evident in only 24% of patients.

B. Symptoms included lethargy 49%, dizziness 47%, vomiting 35%, confusion 17%, and seizures 0.9%.

C. Despite volume depletion, urine sodium concentration may be elevated if diuretic action is still present.

Treatment

A. Symptomatic hyponatremia: See Table 24-3

B. Asymptomatic hyponatremia: Stopping the diuretic is usually adequate. Thiazides should *not* be reinitiated later. Rapid and dangerous hyponatremia often recurs.

C. Hypovolemic patients

1. Consider *careful* volume resuscitation with normal saline.

2. Unlike euvolemic or hypervolemic patients, fluid resuscitation in a hypovolemic patient may suppress ADH. This may result in rapid water losses and an overly rapid and dangerous correction of the serum sodium concentration resulting in osmotic demyelination syndrome (Table 24-5). Serum sodium levels should be monitored closely and electrolyte replacement may need to be terminated (and free water administered) if serum sodium levels or urinary output rise abruptly (see Table 24-3).

Hypothyroidism

Hypothyroidism is reviewed in detail in Chapter 18, Fatigue. This section will focus on hyponatremia in hypothyroidism.

A. Hyponatremia may occur in 10% of patients with hypothyroidism but is rarely symptomatic.

B. Hyponatremia arises in part secondary to ADH release triggered by a decrease in cardiac output.

C. Hyponatremia only typically develops in severe hypothyroidism (TSH > 50 milli-international units/mL). Patients with mild hypothyroidism and hyponatremia should be evaluated for other causes.

Hypovolemic Hyponatremic Syndromes

Textbook Presentation

Hyponatremia may develop in volume-depleted patients if sodium losses (resulting from vomiting, diarrhea, or excessive perspiration) are replaced with free water. Patients may have orthostatic hypotension or dry mucous membranes.

Disease Highlights

A. The primary controller of ADH release is serum osmolality. Hypo-osmolality normally inhibits ADH release leading to free water diuresis.

B. *Significant* hypovolemia can stimulate ADH release independent of serum osmolality.

C. Free water ingestion in face of elevated ADH levels causes hyponatremia.

D. Typical urine findings include

1. Decreased urine sodium concentration (< 30 mEq/L)

2. Decreased FE_{Na} (< 0.5%)

3. Increased urine osmolality (> 450 mOsm/L)

4. Prerenal azotemia (BUN/Cr > 20)

5. Elevated uric acid

Treatment

A. For mildly symptomatic patients, normal saline can be used (see calculations above).

B. For severely symptomatic patients with coma or seizures, 3% normal saline can be used (Table 24-3).

C. These patients are at particularly high risk for osmotic demyelination syndrome (Table 24-5) because fluid resuscitation will suppress ADH, promote a water diuresis, and cause the serum sodium to rise faster than formulas predict.

D. Frequent monitoring of serum sodium is mandatory and a lowering of the serum sodium may be necessary if the correction rate exceeds recommended limits (Table 24-3).

Exercise-Associated Hyponatremia

Textbook Presentation

Exercise-associated hyponatremia (EAH) usually presents in patients during or within hours of completing an endurance event (marathon). Symptoms range from weakness and nausea to coma, seizures, and death.

Disease Highlights

A. Typically follows prolonged workout and developed in 6-30% of athletes completing marathons, was severe (< 130 mEq/L) in 2%, and critical (< 120 mEq/L) in 0.6%

B. Secondary to a combination of both excessive fluid intake combined in some patients with inappropriate ADH release.

1. The leading risk factor is weight gain during the event. Hyponatremia developed in 17% of runners who gained > 2 kg during the race, compared with < 2% of runners who gained < 2 kg.

   a. Ingestion of excessive water or carbohydrate sports drinks can both produce EAH. (Carbohydrate sports drinks are still markedly hypotonic compared with plasma.)

   b. Some studies have also reported an increased risk in women, NSAID users, and long race times.

2. Hyponatremia should suppress ADH. The finding that 44% of runners with EAH did not have maximally dilute urine suggests that SIADH contributes to hyponatremia in some patients.

C. Rapid onset of hyponatremia renders the plasma hypotonic relative to the brain, leading to cerebral edema.

D. Hyponatremia and cerebral edema cause neurologic symptoms, including confusion, headaches, seizures, coma, and death.

E. Noncardiogenic pulmonary edema has been reported in patients with EAH.

Treatment

A. Prevention

1. Athletes should be advised to weigh themselves before and after exercise, and counseled to avoid excessive weight gain (> 2 kg).

2. Thirst should be used as a guide to drinking during marathon events rather than fixed, regular, fluid intake.

3. Sporadic weight checks during endurance events could also detect athletes with significant weight gain at risk for EAH.

B. Treatment

1. Individuals who collapse or have neurologic symptoms during or following endurance events should be immediately evaluated for EAH (as well as hypernatremia, hyperthermia, hypoglycemia, and myocardial infarction).

2. Unlike chronic hyponatremia, EAH develops rapidly and does not allow the brain time to adapt to the hypo-osmolarity.

3. Therefore, brain edema is more likely (and osmotic demyelination syndrome unlikely). A more aggressive treatment approach is therefore safer and recommended to correct the acute hyponatremia in patients with symptomatic EAH.

4. 3% normal saline is recommended in patients with hyponatremia (≤ 125 mEq/L) and severe symptoms (confusion, seizures, coma). An initial bolus of 100 mL (of 3% normal saline) is recommended. This may be repeated twice if necessary. Hypertonic saline is optional for patients with a serum sodium of 126–130 mEq/L.

5. Isotonic saline should *not* be administered because it may worsen the hyponatremia in patients who have elevated ADH levels.

6. The osmotic demyelination syndrome from over rapid correction of the serum sodium in patients with EAH has *not* been reported.

Psychogenic Polydipsia

Textbook Presentation

Psychogenic polydipsia typically occurs in patients with a psychiatric history and unexplained hyponatremia. Patients are unaware of or do not usually admit to excessive water intake. (SIADH may also be seen in psychiatric patients.)

Disease Highlights

A. Increased water intake suppresses ADH, which increases free water excretion and the formation of a dilute urine.

B. Water ingestion is triggered by excessive thirst.

C. Hyponatremia develops only when massive water ingestion is sufficient to overcome maximal urinary free water excretion (usually requires > 8–10 L/d fluid intake).

D. Urine osmolality is maximally dilute ($\approx$ 40-100 mOsm/L).

E. Reported in 6–20% of chronically ill, hospitalized psychiatric patients

F. Since volume status is normal, renal excretion of sodium is usually normal. However, spot urine sodium *concentration* is low due to dilution by massive water intake. The FENa is usually > 1%.

G. Complications are secondary to both hyponatremia and marked polyuria (incontinence, hypocalcemia, hydronephrosis (from massive urinary output), and HF.

H. Surprisingly, not all patients with psychogenic polydipsia have a maximally dilute urine. Several problems can aggravate the hyponatremia in psychogenic polydipsia and complicate the diagnosis.

 1. Psychotic episodes may cause a transient release of ADH or an increased renal responsiveness to ADH.

 2. In addition, psychiatric medications can induce concomitant SIADH (including selective serotonin reuptake inhibitors and phenothiazines). This accentuates the hyponatremia and can produce a higher than expected urine osmolality.

Evidence-Based Diagnosis

A. Water restriction test can prove the diagnosis by demonstrating rapid resolution of hyponatremia.

B. Mean urine sodium concentration is 18 mEq/L.

C. FE_{Na} > 0.5% in 66%

D. Mean urine osmolality 144 $\pm$ 23 mOsm/L vs 500 mOsm/L in SIADH and 539 mOsm/L in hypovolemic patients.

E. CNS tumors may trigger polydipsia and cause hyponatremia. CNS imaging is recommended before making the diagnosis of psychogenic polydipsia.

Treatment

A. For severe neurologic symptoms (eg, seizures, coma), hypertonic saline can be used.

B. Careful free water restriction allows gradual restoration of serum sodium concentration. Over rapid correction should be avoided (see Table 24-3).

Ecstasy (MDMA) Intoxication

Textbook Presentation

Patients are typically college students, attending clubs (raves), who often present on the weekend with anxiety, restlessness, delirium, or seizures.

Disease Highlights

A. MDMA is a synthetic sympathomimetic amphetamine that stimulates the release of norepinephrine, dopamine, and serotonin, and blocks their reuptake.

B. Frequent drug of abuse (up to 5–10% of high school seniors and 39% of US college students have reported use). Its use has been reported in 60–76% of rave participants.

C. Symptoms and signs among emergency department MDMA visits include agitation (38%), anxiety (29%), disorientation (25%), shaking (23%), hypertension (21%), headache (19%), mood changes (19%), psychotic disturbances (17%), loss of consciousness (13%), tachycardia (10%), dilated pupils (10%), hyperthermia (6%).

D. Serious complications among MDMA emergency department visits have included hypoglycemia, hyponatremia, hyperthermia, malignant hypertension, stroke, coma, seizures, myocardial infarction, arrhythmias, nontraumatic rhabdomyolysis, acute kidney injury, liver failure, disseminated intravascular coagulation, and death (even in first time users).

E. Commonly ingested with other drugs

F. Hyponatremia

 1. Discovered in 6% of MDMA-related emergency department visits.

 2. Hyponatremia may be severe and cause cerebral edema, seizures, coma, and death. The mortality in patients with MDMA-induced hyponatremia is 50%.

 3. Secondary to ADH secretion (SIADH) *and* water intoxication. The water intoxication is prompted by hyperthermia, diaphoresis, and increased thirst. It is further aggravated by "recommendations" to drink large amounts of water.

 4. Unlike other MDMA complications, women are more susceptible to MDMA-induced hyponatremia than men. (85% of the case reports of MDMA-induced hyponatremia have been in women.)

 5. Hyponatremia can occur after just a single dose.

Evidence-Based Diagnosis

A. MDMA is excreted in the urine and can be detected by specific tests.

B. Numerous congeners of MDMA exist.

C. Urine studies may not detect various congeners and the diagnosis is often made clinically.

Treatment

A. The treatment of MDMA intoxication is beyond the scope of this text. Treatment will focus on the hyponatremia.

B. ICU monitoring is usually required.

C. For asymptomatic patients with mild hyponatremia, fluid restriction is usually adequate.

D. For marked symptoms (coma, seizures) in patients with severe hyponatremia (< 120 mEq/L), see Table 24-3.

Pseudohyponatremia

Textbook Presentation

Certain rare conditions interfere with the accurate measurement of sodium and cause the sodium concentration to appear *spuriously* low. These conditions are referred to as **pseudohyponatremia**. Causes include *marked* hyperlipidemia and *marked* hyperproteinemia. In these conditions, the serum sodium in the plasma phase is actually normal and the measured serum osmolality is normal. However, the measured serum sodium is low because the plasma phase within any aliquot is smaller than normal due to the marked increase in lipid or proteins causing the instrument to calculate a low serum sodium level. These conditions may be suspected in patients with marked hyperproteinemia (ie, patients with multiple myeloma or following immunoglobulin infusions), or marked hyperlipidemia or when there is a significant difference between the measured and calculated serum osmolality. Since the *calculated* osmolality uses the measured serum sodium level (which is spuriously low), the calculated osmolality is also spuriously low whereas the measured serum osmolality is correct. The difference between the two (the *osmolar gap*) is elevated. The osmolar gap can be calculated by the following equations:

Osmolar gap = Measured serum osmolality – calculated serum osmolality (normal < 10). Calculated serum osmolality = 2 × sodium + glucose/18 + BUN/2.8

Marked hyperglycemia works somewhat differently. Marked hyperglycemia draws water into the intravascular space and thereby produces hyponatremia. In this situation, the hyperglycemia makes the serum hyperosmolar. This discussion will be limited to patients with hyponatremia secondary to marked hyperglycemia.

Disease Highlights

A. In poorly controlled diabetes, intravascular glucose acts as an osmotic agent drawing water from the cells into the plasma resulting in hyponatremia.

B. Serum osmolality is elevated (due to the marked hyperglycemia).

C. The elevated serum osmolality stimulates ADH release further accentuating hyponatremia. (Hypernatremia may also occur if water intake is limited. See below.)

D. Correction factors can help predict the serum sodium concentration after the hyperglycemia is treated (and the intravascular water relocates to the intracellular space). The optimal correction factor is controversial.

E. Experiments suggest that the sodium concentration will increase by 2.4 mEq/L for every 100 mg/dL that glucose falls with treatment. A sodium of 129 mEq/L in a patient with a serum glucose of 1000 mg/dL would correct as follows:

  1. Serum glucose will fall 900 mg/dL with treatment (to about 100 mg/dL).

  2. Correct sodium concentration by 2.4 per 100 mg/dL fall in glucose.

  3. 9 × 2.4 = 21.6

  4. Corrected sodium = 129 + 21.6 = 150.6

HYPERNATREMIA

CHIEF COMPLAINT

PATIENT 3

Mr. R is an 80-year-old nursing home resident with a history of severe dementia brought to the emergency department with lethargy and confusion. Serum chemistries reveal a sodium level of 168 mEq/L.

As noted in Chapter 1, the first task when evaluating patients is to identify their problem(s). Like hyponatremic patients, hypernatremic patients often suffer from an altered sensorium and serum chemistries reveal hypernatremia. In addition to evaluating other possible causes of confusion, the cause of the hypernatremia should be determined and treatment initiated since the hypernatremia may be contributing to the delirium.

What is the differential diagnosis of hypernatremia? How would you frame the differential?

CONSTRUCTING A DIFFERENTIAL DIAGNOSIS

Hypernatremia is almost always secondary to a free water deficit. The differential diagnosis of hypernatremia is markedly simpler than that of hyponatremia and usually develops in 1 of 3 situations: (1) impaired water intake, (2) hyperglycemic hyperosmolar state, or rarely (3) diabetes insipidus.

Hypernatremia and hyperosmolality are potent stimulators of thirst, which promotes drinking and protects against hypernatremia. Therefore, hypernatremia occurs almost exclusively in patients who are either unaware of their thirst or physically unable to get to water. The most common clinical scenarios involve infants or debilitated elderly patients with severe dementia. In such patients, normal insensible water losses or increased water loss (ie, from diarrhea) are not matched by oral intake and hypernatremia develops. Normal kidneys respond by maximizing water reabsorption

resulting in a high urine osmolality (> 600 mOsm/L). In over 50% of elderly patients, a superimposed process (ie, pneumonia, urinary tract infection, or cerebrovascular accident) is present. The 30-day mortality in elderly hypernatremic patients has been reported at 41.5%.

Clinicians should search for an underlying cause in patients discovered to have hypernatremia.

Hypernatremia may also develop in patients with marked hyperglycemia. The osmotic diuresis results in a free water loss and may result in hypernatremia if free water intake is impaired due to an altered sensorium. This may not be obvious on initial laboratory results because the hyperglycemia draws water from the intracellular compartment into the extracellular compartment diluting the sodium concentration. With treatment of the hyperglycemia, water moves back to the intracellular space and the hypernatremia worsens.

Other causes of hypernatremia are rare and will be touched upon here only briefly. Hypernatremia may develop in patients who have an impairment in renal *water conservation* (ie, diabetes insipidus). Even in these patients, increased thirst normally prompts increased water intake and allows such patients to compensate and maintain normal sodium levels. (These patients complain of polydipsia and polyuria.) Hypernatremia may develop when a superimposed process limits water intake. The urine osmolality in such patients is inappropriately low (< 600 mOsm/L). Diabetes insipidus can result from pituitary processes that decrease ADH production or renal processes, which cause resistance to ADH. Finally, very rare causes of hypernatremia include hypothalamic lesions, which render patients unaware of thirst despite a normal sensorium, or increased salt intake (ie, infusion of hypertonic saline or salt water ingestion).

In summary the approach to hypernatremia focuses on a thorough history and physical exam with particular emphasis on the assessment of vital signs, orthostasis, and dehydration. A urine osmolality, serum electrolytes, BUN, creatinine, and glucose are often adequate to determine the etiology. Figure 24-7 outlines the approach to hypernatremia.

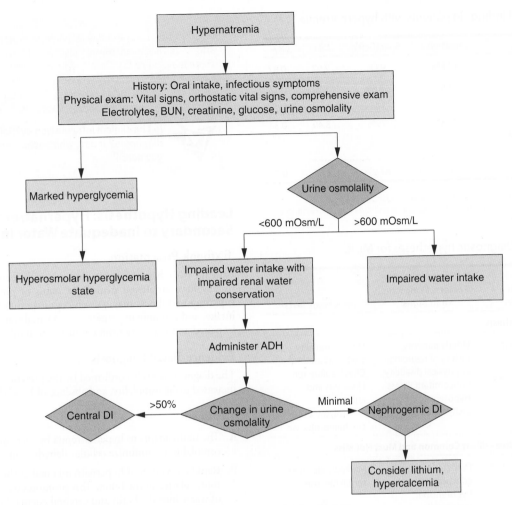

ADH, antidiuretic hormone; BUN, blood urea nitrogen; DI, diabetes insipidus.

Figure 24-7. Approach to hypernatremia.

Differential Diagnosis of Hypernatremia

A. Impaired water intake: urine osmolality > 600 mOsm/L
   1. Neurologic disease (eg, dementia, delirium, coma, stroke)
   2. Water unavailable (ie, desert conditions)

B. Osmotic diuresis with impaired water intake
   1. Hyperosmolar hyperglycemia
   2. Postobstructive diuresis

C. Rare etiologies
   1. Diabetes insipidus (if associated with decreased water intake)
      a. Neurogenic diabetes insipidus (decreased ADH production)
      b. Nephrogenic diabetes insipidus (ADH resistance)
         (1) Long-term lithium ingestion
         (2) Hypercalcemia
   2. Hypothalamic lesions causing decreased thirst
   3. Increased salt intake
      a. Salt water ingestion
      b. Hypertonic saline
      c. Isotonic saline replacement of hypotonic saline loss

 How reliable is the history and physical exam for detecting hypernatremia?

Signs and symptoms develop due to dehydration (tachycardia, orthostatic hypotension, dry mucous membranes and axilla) and due to the hypernatremia (depressed sensorium, coma, focal deficits, and seizures). Hypernatremia-induced brain shrinkage can also result in rupture of cerebral veins and subarachnoid hemorrhage. Symptoms are more severe when hypernatremia develops rapidly. The clinical findings in patients with hypernatremia are summarized in Table 24-8. No finding was highly sensitive for hypernatremia.

RANKING THE DIFFERENTIAL DIAGNOSIS

The patient's underlying dementia put him at increased risk for hypernatremia due to inadequate water intake, particularly if a superimposed illness has resulted in delirium. This is the leading hypothesis. Marked hyperglycemia should always be considered a "must not miss" alternative. Inadequate water conservation due to diabetes insipidus is possible but far less common. Table 24-9 lists the differential diagnosis.

Table 24-8. Findings in patients with hypernatremia.

Finding	Sensitivity	Specificity	LR+	LR−
Tachycardia	17.8%	94%	2.97	0.87
Orthostatic hypotension	61.5%	50.6%	1.24	0.76
Abnormal subclavicular skin turgor[1]	73.3%	79%	3.49	0.34
Dry oral mucosa[2]	49%	87.8%	4.02	0.58

[1]Defined as lasting ≥ 3 seconds after 3 seconds of pinching.
[2]Defined as placing the finger inside the cheek and assessing whether it is wet or dry.

Table 24-9. Diagnostic hypotheses for Mr. R.

Diagnostic Hypotheses	Demographics, Risk Factors, Symptoms and Signs	Important Tests
Leading Hypothesis		
Inadequate water consumption	Elderly patients, history of neurologic or physical disability Concomitant illness Hypotension, tachycardia	Urine osmolality > 600 mOsm/L Chest radiograph Urinalysis and culture Electrolytes, BUN, creatinine, glucose
Active Alternative—Most Common and Must Not Miss		
Hyperglycemia	Diabetes mellitus, concurrent illness, hypotension, tachycardia	Markedly elevated serum glucose
Active Alternative		
Diabetes insipidus	Complaints of polydipsia, polyuria	Urine osmolality < 600 mOsm/L
Central diabetes insipidus	History of CNS trauma, surgery, CVA, sarcoidosis	ADH levels low Administration of exogenous ADH markedly increases urine osmolality
Nephrogenic diabetes insipidus	Lithium ingestion	ADH levels elevated Exogenous ADH minimally elevates urine osmolality

ADH, antidiuretic hormone; BUN, blood urea nitrogen; CNS, central nervous system; CVA, cerebrovascular accident.

The nursing home reports that Mr. R has had a cough for the last 3 days with low-grade fever. Over the last 48 hours, he has become progressively less responsive and his oral intake and urinary output have dropped dramatically.

Mr. R is minimally responsive to stimuli. Vital signs are BP, 110/70 mm Hg; pulse, 110 bpm; temperature, 38.1°C; RR, 20 breaths per minute. His oral mucosa is parched and

his axilla dry. Lung exam is difficult to evaluate due to poor effort. Cardiac exam reveals tachycardia; neck veins are flat. There is no S_3 or S_4. Chest radiograph reveals a right lower lobe infiltrate. Laboratory findings: Na, 168 mEq/L; K, 4.2 mEq/L; HCO_3^-, 24 mEq/L; chloride, 134 mEq/L; BUN, 45 mg/dL; creatinine, 1 mg/dL. Serum glucose is 150 mg/dL.

Is the clinical information sufficient to make a diagnosis? If not, what other information do you need?

Leading Hypothesis: Hypernatremia Secondary to Inadequate Water Intake

Textbook Presentation

Patients with hypernatremia due to inadequate water ingestion usually have an altered neurologic status or physical disability. A superimposed illness may worsen cognitive function, decrease oral intake, and promote hypernatremia. Mental status is almost always impaired and may vary from confusion to frank coma.

Evidence-Based Diagnosis

The diagnosis is easily confirmed by the presence of hypernatremia, increased urine osmolality, and absence of hyperglycemia.

Treatment

A. The brain adapts to hypernatremia by increasing intracellular osmolality to minimize cellular dehydration.

B. Rapid correction of hypernatremia makes the serum hypotonic relative to the brain. This promotes osmotic movement of water into the brain and cerebral edema. Seizures and death can occur if correction is too rapid.

C. Hypernatremia should be corrected slowly ≅ 0.5 mEq/L/h (≤ 12 mEq/L/d). A reasonable target is 10 mEq/L/d.

D. Calculating infusion rates

1. Calculate free water deficit = TBW * {(Na_s/140) − 1}.
    a. Na_s is the patient's serum sodium.
    b. TBW = total body water.
        (1) In hypernatremic men TBW = 0.5 × weight (kg)
        (2) In hypernatremic women TBW = 0.4 × weight (kg)
2. Calculate correction time (days) = (Na_s − 140)/10. Assuming a serum sodium of 160 mEq/L and target sodium of 140, and a reduction rate of 10 mEq/L per day, the correction time (days) = (160 − 140)/10 = 2 days (48 hours)
3. Calculate infusion rate = free water deficit/correction time
4. Example: A 70-kg man with a serum sodium of 165 mEq/L
    a. Free water deficit = 35{(165/140)-1} = 6.25 liters
    b. Correction time: (Na_s - 140)/10 = (165 − 140)/10 = 2.5 days or 60 hours
    c. Infusion rate (per hour) of D5W = 6.25L/60 hours = 104 mL/h of D5W
    d. Note that if D5.45NS is used, each liter provides 500 mL of free water. To deliver 6.25 L of free water would require 12.5 L of D5 0.45 NS over 60 hours = 208 mL/h of D5 0.45 NS
    e. Insensible losses should be added, which can be estimated at 30–40 mL/h of D5W. In addition,

any other observed ongoing losses (ie, from diarrhea) must be matched.

f. Online utilities can help with calculations http://www.mdcalc.com/free-water-deficit-in-hypernatremia/

g. Careful, frequent monitoring of the serum sodium (initially every 4-6h) is required to ensure that correction occurs at a safe rate.

5. Many such patients are markedly hypovolemic on presentation. Patients who are hypotensive should initially receive normal saline to normalize BP, orthostasis, and urinary output and then be switched to D5W at the appropriate rate to correct the free water deficit.

MAKING A DIAGNOSIS

An elevated urine osmolality can confirm urinary concentrating ability and establish inadequate fluid intake (versus inadequate conservation) as the etiology. An evaluation of the underlying precipitant is also important.

> Mr. R's urine osmolality is 850 mOsm/L. Blood cultures grow *Streptococcus pneumoniae*.

As in the overwhelming majority of cases of hypernatremia, the diagnosis is straightforward. The history, exam, and elevated urine osmolality all confirm hypernatremia due to decreased intake. Urine concentrating ability is intact. Serum glucose is normal. Further diagnostic testing is not required.

CASE RESOLUTION

Mr. R is given D5W. His body weight is measured at 140 lbs (63 kg). The rate of free water administration must be determined. He is given piperacillin-tazobactam to treat his aspiration pneumonia.

Three days after D5W is started, his electrolytes are normal. He gradually returns to his baseline neurologic function and is discharged after 6 days of therapy to continue his oral antibiotics at the nursing home.

REVIEW OF OTHER IMPORTANT DISEASES

Hyperosmolar Hyperglycemic State

See Chapter 12, Diabetes.

REFERENCES

Almond CS, Shin AY, Fortescue EB et al. Hyponatremia among runners in the Boston Marathon. N Engl J Med. 2005;352(15):1550–6.

Angeli P, Wong F, Watson H, Gines P, Investigators C. Hyponatremia in cirrhosis: Results of a patient population survey. Hepatology. 2006;44(6):1535–42.

Bunnag S, Pattanasombatsakul K. N-terminal-pro-brain natriuretic peptide for the differential diagnosis of hypovolemia vs. euvolemia in hyponatremic patients. J Med Assoc Thai. 2012;95(Suppl 3):S69-74.

Chassagne P, Druesne L, Capet C, Menard JF, Bercoff E. Clinical presentation of hypernatremia in elderly patients: a case-control study. J Am Geriatr Soc. 2006;54(8):1225–30.

Chow KM, Kwan BC, Szeto CC. Clinical studies of thiazide-induced hyponatremia. J Ntl Med Assoc. 2004;96(10):1305–8.

Chung HM, Kluge R, Schrier RW, Anderson RJ. Clinical assessment of extracellular fluid volume in hyponatremia. Am J Med. 1987;83(5):905–8.

Dunlop D. Eighty-six cases of Addison's disease. BMJ. 1963;2(5362):887–91.

Musch W, Decaux G. Utility and limitations of biochemical parameters in the evaluation of hyponatremia in the elderly. Int Urol Nephrol. 2001;32(3):475–93.

Musch W, Thimpont J, Vandervelde D, Verhaeverbeke I, Berghmans T, Decaux G. Combined fractional excretion of sodium and urea better predicts response to saline in hyponatremia than do usual clinical and biochemical parameters. Am J Med. 1995;99(4):348–55.

Musch W, Verfaillie L, Decaux G. Age-related increase in plasma urea level and decrease in fractional urea excretion: clinical application in the syndrome of inappropriate secretion of antidiuretic hormone. Clin J Am Soc Nephrol. 2006;1:909-14.

Nerup J. Addison's disease–clinical studies. A report of 108 cases. Acta Endocrinologica. 1974;76(1):127–41.

Porcel A, Diaz F, Rendon P, Macias M, Martin-Herrera L, Giron-Gonzalez JA. Dilutional hyponatremia in patients with cirrhosis and ascites. Arch Intern Med. 2002;162(3):323–8.

Ruf AE, Kremers WK, Chavez LL, Descalzi VI, Podesta LG, Villamil FG. Addition of serum sodium into the MELD score predicts waiting list mortality better than MELD alone. Liver Transplant. 2005;11(3):336–43.

Sanghvi SR, Kellerman PS, Nanovic L. Beer potomania: an unusual cause of hyponatremia at high risk of complications from rapid correction. Am J Kidney Dis. 2007;50(4):673–80.

Sheer TA, Joo E, Runyon BA et al. Usefulness of serum N-terminal-ProBNP in distinguishing ascites due to cirrhosis from ascites due to heart failure. J Clin Gastroenterol. 2010;44:e23-e26.

Siegel AJ, Verbalis JG, Clement S et al. Hyponatremia in marathon runners due to inappropriate arginine vasopressin secretion. Am J Med. 2007;120(5):461 e11–7.

Udell JA, Want CS, Tinmouth J et al. Does this patient with liver disease have cirrhosis? JAMA. 2012;307(8):832-42.

Verbalis JG, Goldsmith SR, Greenberg A et al. Diagnosis, evaluation, and treatment of hyponatremia: expert panel recommendations. Am J Med. 2013;126:S1-S42.

I have a patient with hypotension. How do I determine the cause?

CHIEF COMPLAINT

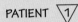

PATIENT 1

Ms. P is a 75-year-old woman with weakness and hypotension.

 What is the differential diagnosis of hypotension? How would you frame the differential?

CONSTRUCTING A DIFFERENTIAL DIAGNOSIS

When a patient presents with hypotension, the important question is whether or not the patient is in shock. Shock is present if there is evidence of multisystem organ hypoperfusion. This may manifest itself as tachycardia, tachypnea, diaphoresis, poorly perfused skin and extremities, altered mental status, or decreased urinary output. In addition, it is not necessary for a patient to have overt hypotension to be in shock since a marked reduction in a patient's usual BP may cause shock (but still be in the low-normal range in previously hypertensive patients). Given the life-threatening nature of shock, hemodynamic stabilization must be prompt and cannot wait for a long series of investigations to be completed.

Therefore, a rational, rapid approach to hypotension is necessary. The 3 main etiologies of shock include **distributive** (low total peripheral resistance, usually septic), **cardiogenic** (low cardiac output despite adequate intravascular volume), and **hypovolemic** (low cardiac output due to low intravascular volume). In terms of epidemiology, septic shock is by far and away the most common. In a trial of over 1600 patients with shock, 62% had septic shock, 16% had hypovolemic shock, and 16% had cardiogenic shock.

Differential Diagnosis of Shock

A. Distributive shock
   1. Septic shock
   2. Hepatic failure
   3. Pancreatitis
   4. Anaphylactic shock
   5. Adrenal insufficiency
   6. Neurogenic shock
   7. Arteriovenous shunts

B. Hypovolemic shock
   1. Hemorrhage
      a. Trauma
      b. Gastrointestinal hemorrhage
      c. Postsurgical, postprocedural bleeding
      d. Intra-abdominal (eg, abdominal aortic aneurysm, ruptured ectopic pregnancy)
   2. Volume depletion
      a. Vomiting
      b. Diarrhea
      c. Excessive diuresis (from diuretics or uncontrolled diabetes)

C. Cardiogenic shock
   1. Poor contractility
      a. Left ventricular (LV) failure
         (1) Myocardial infarction (MI)
         (2) Myocarditis
         (3) Metabolic derangements (eg, profound acidosis, hypophosphatemia, hypocalcemia)
         (4) Depressant drugs (beta-blockers, calcium-channel blockers)
         (5) Miscellaneous causes of heart failure (HF) (eg, alcoholic cardiomyopathy, adriamycin-related cardiomyopathy, dilated cardiomyopathy)
      b. Right ventricular (RV) failure
         (1) MI
         (2) Pulmonary vascular disease
         (3) Hypoxic pulmonary vasoconstriction
   2. Outflow obstruction
      a. Aortic stenosis
      b. Hypertrophic cardiomyopathy
      c. Malignant hypertension
      d. Pulmonary embolism (PE)
   3. Arrhythmogenic
      a. Significant bradycardia
      b. Significant tachycardia
   4. Backflow
      a. Acute mitral regurgitation – papillary muscle rupture or dysfunction
      b. Rupture septum or free wall
      c. Acute aortic regurgitation
   5. Reduced filling
      a. Constrictive pericarditis
      b. Tension pneumothorax
      c. Mitral stenosis

PATIENT

Ms. P has a past medical history of coronary artery disease (CAD), hypertension and diabetes. She complains of weakness, anorexia, nausea and vomiting. Her initial vitals signs demonstrate a pulse of 110 bpm and BP of 85/55 mm Hg. She is having difficulty staying awake during the interview.

At this point, what is the leading hypothesis, and what are the active alternatives? What other tests should be ordered?

RANKING THE DIFFERENTIAL DIAGNOSIS

The first step in approaching patients with hypotension and shock is recognition. Is there evidence of decreased perfusion? This may be manifest by any 1 or more of the following:

A. Significantly decreased BP
   1. Typically systolic BP < 90 mm Hg
   2. A patient may be in shock with a "normal" BP; comparison to prior BPs is necessary.
   3. BP should be measured with a manual cuff. BPs measured with automatic BP cuffs may be inaccurate at lower BPs, especially the pulse pressure.
   4. The pulse pressure should be calculated: pulse pressure = systolic BP – diastolic BP. Wide pulse pressures suggest high cardiac output, whereas narrow pulse pressures suggest low cardiac output.

B. Tachycardia

C. Increased respiratory rate

D. Alteration of mental status

E. Decreased urinary output

F. Decreased arterial pH

The first diagnostic pivotal step utilizes a combination of the history, physical exam, and laboratory studies to determine if the shock is clearly due to sepsis, hypovolemia or cardiogenic. Hypovolemic shock is often obvious due to a history of hemorrhage or dehydration and patients usually have a history of melena, bright red blood per rectum, vomiting, diarrhea, or poor oral intake. In addition, it is typically associated with signs of low cardiac output including a narrow pulse pressure, cold extremities and poor capillary refill. Anemia or acute kidney injury may be evident on laboratory exam. Distributive shock is most frequently due to sepsis, which is often apparent due to a history of fever, rigors, other infectious symptoms (cough, rash, abdominal pain, urinary urgency, or dysuria) and signs of high cardiac output (warm extremities, bounding pulses, a wide pulse pressure, and brisk capillary refill). However, some patients with advanced sepsis have a poor cardiac output. Laboratory evidence of sepsis often suggests underlying infection, including a leukocytosis, an infiltrate on chest film, pyuria on urinalysis, or diagnostic findings on abdominal CT in patients with abdominal pain. Finally, patients with cardiogenic shock often have a history of CAD or HF or symptoms of acute MI. Their physical exam suggests low cardiac output (poor capillary refill, narrow pulse pressure, and cold extremities) and may also reveal evidence of high filling pressures (jugular venous distention [JVD] or an S_3 gallop). The physical exam, ECG, and echocardiogram can determine whether cardiogenic shock is secondary to poor contractility, outflow obstruction, an arrhythmia, reduced filling, or backflow from valve failure.

The final pivotal step addresses patients in whom the initial evaluation does not delineate a likely etiology of shock. Patients with evidence of a high cardiac output (wide pulse pressure, brisk capillary refill, warm extremities) without an obvious source of sepsis, should be evaluated for unusual causes of systemic inflammatory response syndrome (SIRS) (eg, pancreatitis), occult infections, and other causes of distributive shock (hepatic failure, anaphylaxis, adrenal insufficiency). Patients with evidence of a low cardiac output of unclear etiology (narrow pulse pressure, sluggish capillary refill, cold extremities) should be evaluated for occult massive hemorrhage (eg, intra-abdominal) and less common causes of cardiogenic shock such as PE and pericardial tamponade. Such patients should also be evaluated for septic shock. An echocardiogram can be useful in such patients by revealing unsuspected cardiac etiologies (eg, pericardial tamponade, acute aortic regurgitation due to dissection or right HF suggesting PE).

Finally, it is important to realize that overlapping etiologies are common, especially septic and cardiogenic shock. Figure 25-1 illustrates the diagnostic approach to shock.

Ms. P is clearly hypotensive and the combination of her hypotension, tachycardia, and difficulty staying awake clearly suggest inadequate tissue perfusion and shock. The next pivotal step considers the 3 most common categories of shock: hypovolemic, septic and cardiogenic.

 1

Ms. P has vomited once this morning, but she ate and drank fluids normally the day before. She denies diarrhea, melena, or bright red blood per rectum. She denies any chest pain or pressure. She admits to urinary frequency over the last few days and chills and fever that began the previous night. On physical exam her temperature is 38.4°C. Her hands are cool but pulses are full with adequate capillary refill. Her neck veins are flat and lungs are clear. There is no JVD or S_3 gallop. She has costovertebral angle tenderness. Laboratory exam reveals a WBC of 15,000/mcL and her lactate was 3 mmol/L.

At this point, what is the leading hypothesis, what are the active alternatives, and is there a must not miss diagnosis? Given this differential diagnosis, what tests should be ordered?

Ms. P clearly has several features suggesting septic shock. Her urinary tract symptoms, fever, and costovertebral angle tenderness point to a possible urinary tract infection. Her leukocytosis is also suggestive. Septic shock is therefore the leading and must not miss hypothesis. Her episode of vomiting suggests some hypovolemia but her hypotension is out of proportion to her 1 episode of emesis. Another possible diagnosis would be hypovolemia due to an osmotic diuresis from severe diabetic hyperosmolar state. Finally, given her diabetes mellitus and prior CAD, cardiogenic shock from an acute MI needs to be considered. Table 25-1 lists the differential diagnosis.

Leading Hypothesis: Septic Shock

Textbook Presentation

Patients with septic shock typically have fever, tachypnea, tachycardia, and hypotension. Whereas patients with cardiogenic or hemorrhagic shock often have cold extremities, patients with septic shock often have warm extremities and bounding pulses after fluid resuscitation. (Pulses are bounding due to a widened pulse pressure.) Mentation may be impaired and urinary output decreased.

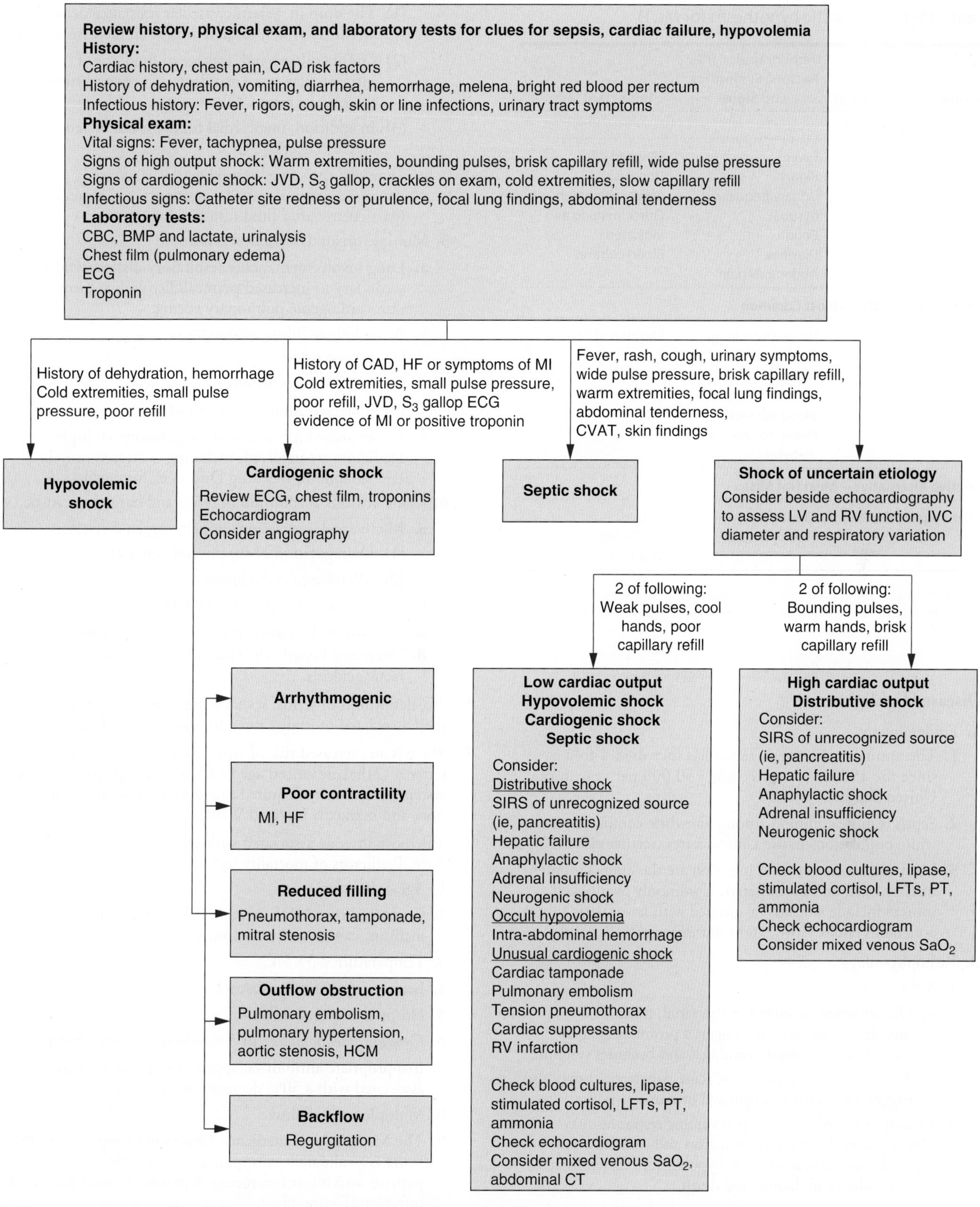

Review history, physical exam, and laboratory tests for clues for sepsis, cardiac failure, hypovolemia
History:
Cardiac history, chest pain, CAD risk factors
History of dehydration, vomiting, diarrhea, hemorrhage, melena, bright red blood per rectum
Infectious history: Fever, rigors, cough, skin or line infections, urinary tract symptoms
Physical exam:
Vital signs: Fever, tachypnea, pulse pressure
Signs of high output shock: Warm extremities, bounding pulses, brisk capillary refill, wide pulse pressure
Signs of cardiogenic shock: JVD, S_3 gallop, crackles on exam, cold extremities, slow capillary refill
Infectious signs: Catheter site redness or purulence, focal lung findings, abdominal tenderness
Laboratory tests:
CBC, BMP and lactate, urinalysis
Chest film (pulmonary edema)
ECG
Troponin

History of dehydration, hemorrhage
Cold extremities, small pulse pressure, poor refill

History of CAD, HF or symptoms of MI
Cold extremities, small pulse pressure, poor refill, JVD, S_3 gallop ECG evidence of MI or positive troponin

Fever, rash, cough, urinary symptoms, wide pulse pressure, brisk capillary refill, warm extremities, focal lung findings, abdominal tenderness, CVAT, skin findings

Hypovolemic shock

Cardiogenic shock
Review ECG, chest film, troponins
Echocardiogram
Consider angiography

Septic shock

Shock of uncertain etiology
Consider beside echocardiography to assess LV and RV function, IVC diameter and respiratory variation

2 of following:
Weak pulses, cool hands, poor capillary refill

2 of following:
Bounding pulses, warm hands, brisk capillary refill

Arrhythmogenic

Poor contractility
MI, HF

Reduced filling
Pneumothorax, tamponade, mitral stenosis

Outflow obstruction
Pulmonary embolism, pulmonary hypertension, aortic stenosis, HCM

Backflow
Regurgitation

Low cardiac output
Hypovolemic shock
Cardiogenic shock
Septic shock

Consider:
Distributive shock
SIRS of unrecognized source (ie, pancreatitis)
Hepatic failure
Anaphylactic shock
Adrenal insufficiency
Neurogenic shock
Occult hypovolemia
Intra-abdominal hemorrhage
Unusual cardiogenic shock
Cardiac tamponade
Pulmonary embolism
Tension pneumothorax
Cardiac suppressants
RV infarction

Check blood cultures, lipase, stimulated cortisol, LFTs, PT, ammonia
Check echocardiogram
Consider mixed venous SaO_2, abdominal CT

High cardiac output
Distributive shock
Consider:
SIRS of unrecognized source (ie, pancreatitis)
Hepatic failure
Anaphylactic shock
Adrenal insufficiency
Neurogenic shock

Check blood cultures, lipase, stimulated cortisol, LFTs, PT, ammonia
Check echocardiogram
Consider mixed venous SaO_2

BMP, basic metabolic profile; CAD, coronary artery disease; CBC, complete blood count; CVAT, costovertebral angle tenderness; ECG, electrocardiogram; HCM, hypertrophic cardiomyopathy; HF, heart failure; IVC, inferior vena cava; JVD, jugular venous distention; LFTs, liver function tests; LV, left ventricle; MI, myocardial infarction; PT, prothrombin time; RV, right ventricle; SIRS, systemic inflammatory response syndrome.

Figure 25-1. Diagnostic approach: shock.

Table 25-1. Diagnostic hypotheses for Ms. P.

Diagnostic Hypothesis	Demographics, Risk Factors, Symptoms and Signs	Important Tests
Leading Hypothesis		
Septic shock	Fever Rigors Urinary frequency/ dysuria Cough Diarrhea Abdominal pain	Elevated WBC Urinalysis Chest radiograph Other imaging as indicated Blood cultures
Active Alternative—Most Common		
Hypovolemic shock	Nausea/vomiting Decreased oral intake Melena, bright red blood per rectum Poorly controlled diabetes	Elevated BUN, creatinine Urinalysis Low Fe_{Na} CBC Glucose
Active Alternative—Must Not Miss		
Cardiogenic shock	Chest pain History of CAD	ECG CK/CK-MB Troponin

BUN, blood urea nitrogen; CAD, coronary artery disease; CBC, complete blood count; CK, creatine kinase; ECG, electrocardiogram; Fe_{Na}, fraction excretion of sodium; WBC, white blood cell.

Disease Highlights

A. Epidemiology
  1. The annual incidence of sepsis has increased 4-fold since the 1970s, now exceeding 750,000 per year in the United States.
  2. Sepsis is more common among nonwhite compared with white populations in the United States (relative risk 1.90).
  3. Most common sources of infection are the lung, abdomen, urinary tract, and IV catheters. Commonly overlooked sources include sinusitis (associated with nasogastric tubes), acalculous cholecystitis, and *Clostridium difficile* colitis.

B. Pathophysiology
  1. Sepsis
    a. Occurs when an infection (bacterial, fungal, mycobacterial, or viral) triggers a proinflammatory reaction that is poorly regulated and becomes systemic.
    b. A noninfectious process (eg, acute pancreatitis) may also trigger a similarly dysregulated immune response.
  2. In early stages of sepsis, hyperimmune responses may play a role in the organ dysfunction and cause multiple organ dysfunction syndrome, hypotension, disseminated intravascular coagulation, and death.
  3. In later stages of sepsis, patients may be hypoimmune. Hypoimmunity may also contribute to infection and death.
  4. Mechanisms of hypotension include
    a. Vasodilation (decreased systemic vascular resistance) mediated by elevated nitrous oxide levels, increased prostacyclin levels, and low vasopressin levels, lowers BP.
    b. Cardiac output can be increased or decreased in sepsis.

  (1) The drop in systemic vascular resistance decreases afterload, which often results in an increase in CO.
  (2) On the other hand, leakage of fluid out of intravascular space can decrease venous return and thereby decrease CO.
  (3) In addition, myocardial function can be reduced and also decrease CO.
    c. Typically, the *initial* hemodynamic response is decreased systemic vascular resistance and increased CO (particularly after fluid resuscitation).
  5. Multiple organ dysfunction syndrome
    a. Lung involvement: acute respiratory distress syndrome secondary to increased permeability with subsequent non-cardiogenic pulmonary edema.
    b. Acute kidney injury secondary to
      (1) Hypotension
      (2) Renal vasoconstriction
      (3) Increased tumor necrosis factor
    c. Disseminated intravascular coagulation: Multiple mediators are involved, including decreased protein C (see Chapter 8, Bleeding Disorders, for details).
  6. Lactic acidosis is common in sepsis and has many causes.
    a. Microcirculatory lesions impair oxygen delivery.
      (1) Dysregulation of supply and demand
      (2) Microvascular occlusion
    b. Hypotension impairs oxygen delivery.
    c. Mitochondrial injury impairs oxygen utilization.
    d. Decreased hepatic clearance of lactate contributes to lactic acidosis.

C. The definitions of sepsis, severe sepsis, and septic shock and their associated mortality rates are shown in Table 25-2.

D. There is an increased risk of septic shock in patients with bacteremia (21%), advanced age ($\geq$ 65 years), impaired immune system, community-acquired pneumonia, abdominal infection, and markedly elevated WBC.

E. The mortality rate associated with sepsis ranges from 20% to 50%. Predictors of mortality include
  1. Age > 40 years
  2. Comorbidities: AIDS, hepatic failure, HF, diabetes mellitus, cancer, or immunosuppression.
  3. Temperature < 35.5°C
  4. Leukopenia < 4000 cells/mcL
  5. Hospital-acquired infection
  6. *Candida, Pseudomonas,* or *Staphylococcus aureus* infection.
  7. Inappropriate antibiotics: appropriate antibiotics are associated with a 50% decrease in mortality.
  8. Multiple organ failure
  9. The Mortality in Emergency Department Sepsis (MEDS) Score is a validated scoring index that predicts mortality in patients arriving at emergency departments with suspected infection (Figure 25-2).

Evidence-Based Diagnosis

A. Predictors of bacteremia (Table 25-3)
  1. Fever
    a. In emergency department patients, fever was higher among bacteremic patients (38.8°C) than

Table 25-2. Definitions of stages of sepsis.

Category	Definition	Mortality
Sepsis	Infection and ≥ 2 of following: Temperature > 38.5°C or < 35.0°C Pulse > 90 bpm Respiratory rate > 20/min or $PaCO_2$ < 32 mm Hg WBC > 12,000/mcL or < 4000/mcL or > 10% bands	16%
Severe sepsis	Sepsis and at least 1 of the following signs of inadequate tissue perfusion: Altered mental status Oliguria Lactic acidosis Platelet count < 100,000/mcL ALI/ARDS	20%
Septic shock	Severe sepsis with mean BP < 60 mm Hg (or < 80 mm Hg if the patient has baseline hypertension) after fluid resuscitation or the need for vasopressors	46%

ALI/ARDS, acute lung injury/acute respiratory distress syndrome.

Table 25-3. Predictors of bacteremia.

Finding	Sensitivity	Specificity	LR+	LR-
Shaking chills	45%	90%	4.7	0.61
Injection drug use	7%	98%	2.9	0.95
Central venous catheter	23%	90%	2.4	0.85
Acute abdomen	20%	91%	2.2	0.9
WBC > 15,000/mcL	28%	87%	2.2	0.8
WBC < 1000/mcL	14%	94%	2.3	0.9
Bandemia ≥ 1500/mcL	44%	69%	1.4	0.8
Chills (any type)	88%	52%	1.7	0.23
Comorbidity	86%	37%	1.4	0.14

nonbacteremic patients (38.1°C). However, 5% of bacteremic patients are normothermic (temperature < 37.6°C) and 13% of patients were hypothermic.

 b. The absence of fever was associated with increased mortality.

2. Chills

 a. Chills can vary from mild to moderate to shaking chills (ie, teeth chattering, bed shaking chills).

 b. Chills of some kind (mild, moderate, or severe) are common in bacteremic patients (sensitivity 88%).

 c. Shaking chills (rigors) are less sensitive but more specific for bacteremia (sensitivity, 45%; specificity, 90%; LR+, 4.7, LR-, 0.61).

 Providers should consider bacteremia in older patients with significant fever or rigors. Patients presenting with rigors should have blood cultures drawn and antibiotics administered.

3. Rashes: Certain life-threatening infections may produce characteristic rashes (ie, meningococcemia, Rocky Mountain spotted fever, or staphylococcal toxic shock syndrome).

 Patients with fever and a rash should be immediately evaluated for life-threatening diseases including toxic shock syndrome, meningococcemia, or Rocky Mountain spotted fever.

Mortality in Emergency Department Sepsis (MEDS) Score	Points
Age >65 years	3
Nursing home resident	2
Rapidly terminal comorbid illness	6
Lower respiratory infection	2
Bands >5%	3
Tachypnea or hypoxemia	3
Shock	3
Platelet count <150,000/mm³	3
Altered mental status	2

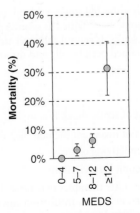

Figure 25-2. Mortality in Emergency Department Sepsis (MEDS) Score observed versus mortality (error bars are 95% confidence intervals). Reproduced with permission from Howell MD, Donnino MW, Talmor D, Clardy P, Ngo L, Shapiro NI. Performance of severity of illness scoring systems in emergency department patients with infection. Acad Emerg Med. 2007;14(8):709–14.

4. Patients with severe sepsis or septic shock have a high incidence of bacteremia (38% and 69%, respectively)

5. WBC > 15,000/mcL is only 28% sensitive for bacteremia.

 A normal WBC does not rule out bacteremia.

6. Catheter site infections

a. Signs of inflammation at the insertion site are *uncommon* in patients with central venous catheter infections (sensitivity 27%). Erythema is present in only 3% of patients with catheter-related bloodstream infections.

 Consider central catheter line infection in septic patients even in the absence of erythema or pus.

b. Certain findings are highly specific for catheter infection, including gross pus at the catheter site.

7. Injection drug use or an acute abdomen (or both) also increase the risk of bacteremia.

8. Incidence of bacteremia is low (2%) in patients without *any* of the following risk factors:

a. Temperature > 38.3°C

b. Shaking chills

c. Injection drug use

d. Acute abdomen on exam

e. Major comorbidity

9. Procalcitonin is an emerging marker of bacterial infection.

a. Polypeptide upregulated during *bacterial* infection in a manner that mirrors the severity of the infection.

b. Procalcitonin's release is attenuated by cytokines released during viral infections, particularly interferon-gamma.

c. Elevated levels suggest bacterial infections whereas normal levels in sepsis suggest a systemic inflammatory response without bacterial infection.

d. The accuracy is limited (sensitivity, 77%; specificity, 79%; LR+, 3.7; LR−, 0.29) and results must be viewed in context of all of the clinical data.

10. A lactic acidosis can suggest sepsis. Serum lactate levels are more sensitive for detecting a lactic acidosis from any cause than an increase in the anion gap. An elevated anion gap is only 44-67% sensitive.

B. Cultures from suspected sources (blood, urine, sputum, fluid collection) should be obtained as soon as possible in patients evaluated for sepsis. If central catheters are in place, blood should be obtained peripherally and through the central catheter.

Treatment

A. The treatment of septic shock is complex.

B. The principles of treatment include the following:

1. Treat the underlying cause.

2. Prompt volume resuscitation

3. A variety of other therapies may be critical including vasopressors, inotropes, intubation and mechanical ventilation, blood products and others.

4. Recommendations evolve frequently. Readers are referred to specialized text for details.

MAKING A DIAGNOSIS

Ms. P has several features that suggest sepsis, including her fever, urinary symptoms, and leukocytosis. An ECG shows no acute changes and a serum troponin level is undetectable. Her blood glucose is 150 mg/dL.

 Have you crossed a diagnostic threshold for the leading hypothesis, septic shock? Have you ruled out the active alternatives? Do other tests need to be done to exclude the alternative diagnoses?

Alternative Diagnosis: Hypovolemic Shock

Typically, a patient with hypovolemic shock will have an obvious source of bleeding, a drop in hematocrit, or recognizable gastrointestinal fluid or renal losses.

Disease Highlights

A. Patients who are hypovolemic have 1 of 2 clinical conditions:

1. Volume depletion due to vomiting, diarrhea, inadequate oral intake, or excessive diuresis (from diuretics or uncontrolled diabetes)

2. Hemorrhage (due to trauma, gastrointestinal or intra-abdominal hemorrhage)

B. Hospitalizations related to gastrointestinal hemorrhage are common, 150/100,000 population per year, and have a case fatality rate of 3-10%.

C. Degree of bleeding is often difficult to assess.

1. Melena can occur with massive hemorrhage or as little as 100 mL of blood loss.

2. Admission hematocrit correlates poorly with degree of blood loss and mortality.

 Massive hemorrhage may be present in patients despite a normal hematocrit.

D. Hypovolemia secondary to dehydration sufficiently severe to cause hypovolemic shock disproportionately affects the elderly. Common risk factors include:

1. Female sex

2. Age > 85

3. Greater than 4 chronic medical conditions

4. Taking 4 or more medications

5. Being confined to bed

Evidence-Based Diagnosis

A. In a review of physical exam findings in hypovolemia, abnormal vital signs are relatively specific but not sensitive (Table 25-4).

1. Orthostatic vital signs, particularly an increase in pulse are more sensitive than supine vital signs.

a. When measuring orthostatic vital signs, wait 2 minutes before measuring supine vitals and wait 1 minute after patient stands to measure upright vitals.

b. Helpful physical findings include:

(1) Severe postural dizziness (unable to measure upright vital signs due to dizziness).

Table 25-4. Operating characteristics of vital signs in detecting hypovolemia.

Physical Examination Finding	Sensitivity	Specificity	LR+ (95% CI)	LR– (95% CI)
Large blood loss				
Postural pulse increment > 30 bpm	97%	98%	48.5	0.03
Supine hypotension	33%	97%	11.0	0.7
Moderate blood loss				
Postural pulse increment > 30 bpm	22%	98%	11.0	0.8
Supine hypotension	13%	97%	4.3	0.9
Dehydration				
Postural pulse increment > 30 bpm	43%	75%	1.7 (0.7-4.0)	0.8 (0.5-1.3)
Mucus membranes dry	85%	58%	2.0 (1.0-4.0)	0.3 (0.1-0.6)
Sunken eyes	62%	82%	3.4 (1.0-12.2)	0.5 (0.3-0.7)

Data from Sinert R, Spektor M. Clinical assessment of hypovolemia. Ann Emerg Med. 2005;45:327-9. McGee S, Abernethy WB, Simel DL. Is this patient hypovolemic? JAMA. 1999;281:1022-9.
Supine hypotension = Systolic blood pressure < 95 mm Hg

    (2) Postural pulse increment of 30 beats/min or more.
2. Dry axilla supports hypovolemia in the elderly (sensitivity, 50%; specificity, 82%; LR+ 2.8, LR– 0.61).
3. Poor skin turgor has no proven diagnostic value in adults.
B. Laboratory evidence is often more revealing.
  1. Hematocrit
    a. Decreased in hemorrhage if bleeding has been ongoing
    b. However, in acute bleeding, isovolemic blood loss prior to hemodilution (from IV or oral fluid repletion) may result in a normal hematocrit.

 A normal hematocrit does not rule out life-threatening acute hemorrhage.

    c. The hematocrit is often elevated in patients with nonhemorrhagic hypovolemia.
  2. Other laboratory findings typically seen in hypovolemic patients include:
    a. An elevated BUN/Cr ratio > 20 (see Chapter 28, Acute Kidney Injury)
    b. A low urine sodium concentration < 30 mEq/L and a $Fe_{Na} < 1\%$
    c. In patients taking diuretics, the $Fe_{urea} < 35\%$ may be more accurate (see Chapter 28, Acute Kidney Injury)
C. A brisk BP response to a 500 mL bolus given over 10 minutes supports hypovolemia (but may also be seen in sepsis).

Treatment

A. The treatment of hypovolemia is the restoration of an adequate mean pressure by fluid resuscitation.
B. In the case of hemorrhagic hypovolemia, the source of bleeding must be identified and stopped.
C. Vasopressors are not indicated. They can increase BP; however, they may have a detrimental effect on cardiac output and perfusion of vascular beds.

CASE RESOLUTION

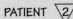

After a 2 L fluid resuscitation, Ms. P's BP increases to 100/50 mm Hg, her skin is warmer, and her pulses are bounding. Antibiotics were started for empiric treatment of urosepsis. After initial stabilization, hypotension recurred and urinary output dropped. She was transferred to the ICU. Four hours later her oxygenation deteriorated and a chest film revealed a diffuse infiltrate consistent with acute respiratory distress syndrome. She was intubated, cultures were drawn, and she was given IV fluids, norepinephrine, antibiotics, and mechanical ventilation. Her blood and urine cultures grew *Escherichia coli*. Over the next 24 hours, her BP stabilized. Seventy-two hours later she was extubated. She eventually made a full recovery.

CHIEF COMPLAINT

PATIENT

Mr. A is a 71-year old man who arrives at the emergency department feeling weak. He has a history of CAD and mitral valve regurgitation. One week ago, he underwent a 2-vessel coronary artery bypass grafting (CABG) and mitral valve replacement with a mechanical valve. He denies any recent nausea, vomiting, melena, or bright red blood per rectum. He has not had a cough, dysuria, urinary frequency, abdominal pain, or fever. On physical exam his pulse is 115 bpm and BP is 85/65 mm Hg. His neck veins are visible to the angle of his jaw and his skin is cool.

 At this point, what is the leading hypothesis, what are the active alternatives, and is there a must not miss diagnosis? Given this differential diagnosis, what tests should be ordered?

RANKING THE DIFFERENTIAL DIAGNOSIS

The first step in the evaluation is to recognize shock. Mr. A's BP is exceptionally low for a 71-year-old man. His BP, combined with his complaint of weakness and cool extremities, makes shock likely. The next pivotal diagnostic step is to evaluate the history, physical exam, and laboratory data to determine if this is likely hypovolemic, septic, or cardiogenic shock. There are no signs or symptoms of sepsis, nor any history to suggest hypovolemia. His cool extremities are consistent with a low cardiac output state (which is often seen in hypovolemic or cardiogenic shock) and his JVD suggests that the low cardiac output is due to cardiogenic, not hypovolemic, shock. Furthermore, his past medical history increases the probability of cardiogenic shock. Possible etiologies of cardiogenic shock include poor contractility (potentially from LV or RV MI or preexistent HF), outflow obstruction (due to, for example, aortic stenosis or PE), backflow (from acute aortic regurgitation or a failed regurgitant mitral valve), or reduced filling (from tamponade or a failed stenotic mitral valve). Given the patient's history, you consider MI to be most likely. Active alternatives include mitral valve failure or tamponade (given recent cardiac surgery). Table 25-5 lists the differential diagnosis.

Leading Hypothesis: Cardiogenic Shock

Textbook Presentation

Typically, cardiogenic shock presents during or immediately after an MI. The patient presents with chest pain, cool extremities, low BP, and ST elevation myocardial infarction (STEMI).

Disease Highlights

A. Cardiogenic shock is defined as persistent hypotension (systolic BP < 90 mm Hg) or mean arterial pressure 30 mm Hg lower than baseline with severe reduction in cardiac index (< 1.8 L/min/m^2) and adequate or elevated filling pressure (LV end-diastolic pressure > 18 mm Hg or RV end-diastolic pressure > 10-15 mm Hg).

Table 25-5. Diagnostic hypotheses for Mr. A.

Diagnostic Hypothesis	Demographics, Risk Factors, Symptoms and Signs	Important Tests
Leading Hypothesis		
Cardiogenic shock: MI	History of CAD Chest pain	ECG Troponin CK/CK-MB
Active Alternatives—Must Not Miss		
Cardiogenic shock: Mitral valve failure	Discontinued anticoagulation therapy New murmur Lung crackles	Echocardiogram
Cardiogenic shock: Cardiac tamponade	Recent cardiac surgery Dyspnea Pulses paradox JVD	Chest film ECG Echocardiogram
Cardiogenic shock: Pulmonary embolism	PE risk factors (immobilization, surgery, cancer, prior VTE) Dyspnea, chest pain, leg swelling	CTA

CAD, coronary artery disease; CK, creatine kinase; CTA, computed tomography angiography; ECG, electrocardiogram; JVD, jugular venous distention; MI, myocardial infarction; PE, pulmonary embolism; VTE, venous thromboembolism.

B. The majority of cardiogenic shock cases are related to MI.

  1. The incidence of cardiogenic shock appears to be decreasing with increasing use of percutaneous intervention for acute MI.

  2. However, cardiogenic shock still complicates 5-8% of STEMI and 2.5% of non-STEMI.

    a. This translates to 40,000 to 50,000 cases per year in the United States.

    b. Infarction location was anterior in 55% of cases and in multiple locations in 50%.

    c. In the SHOCK trial registry, 53.4% of patients have 3-vessel disease and 15.5% have significant left main disease.

  3. Risk factors for cardiogenic shock include older age, anterior MI, hypertension, diabetes mellitus, multivessel CAD, prior MI or angina, prior diagnosis of HF, STEMI, and left bundle branch block.

  4. The magnitude of LV ejection fraction reduction does not need to be profound for shock to develop. In a large registry of cardiogenic shock, the mean LV ejection fraction was 30%.

  5. Mechanical complications of MI (rupture of the ventricular septum, free wall or papillary muscles) cause 12% of cardiogenic shock cases.

    a. Ventricular septal rupture has a mortality of 87%.

    b. Women and elderly are at increased risk for these complications, particularly elderly individuals who undergo thrombolysis.

C. Any cause of severe RV or LV dysfunction can lead to cardiogenic shock. Other typical etiologies include:

  1. Acute myocarditis

    a. Cardiogenic shock complicates 10-15% of cases.

    b. Patients are younger than those with MI and often present with dyspnea rather than chest pain.

  2. Takotsubo cardiomyopathy

    a. Stress-induced condition that leads to apical ballooning after emotional or respiratory distress.

    b. Leads to cardiogenic shock in 4.2% of cases.

  3. Acute valvular regurgitation

  4. Aortic dissection causing either acute, severe aortic insufficiency or extension of dissection to coronary arteries leading to infarction.

  5. Acute stress in the setting of mitral or aortic stenosis

  6. Cardiac tamponade

  7. PE

  8. Arrhythmia

D. Pathophysiology

  1. In MI effecting the LV, decreased coronary perfusion lowers cardiac output, which further decreases coronary perfusion.

  2. Hypoperfusion causes catecholamine release and activation of the renin-angiotensin system increasing contractility and peripheral blood flow but also increasing myocardial oxygen demand and promotes arrhythmia.

  3. This leads to further ischemia and greater reduction in cardiac output.

  4. Activation of the neurohormonal cascade also leads to salt and water retention and exacerbates pulmonary edema.

  5. Treatment relies on breaking this cycle.

Evidence-Based Diagnosis

The diagnosis of the individual etiologies of cardiogenic shock (eg, MI, PE, etc) is covered elsewhere. The focus of this section will be on the diagnosis of cardiogenic shock itself.

A. Diagnosing cardiogenic shock relies on recognizing signs of decreased cardiac output despite an adequate or elevated filling pressure. However, signs and symptoms have limited accuracy in detecting elevated filling pressures.

1. JVP ≥ 12 cm H_2O sensitivity, 65%; specificity, 64%; LR+ 1.8; LR– 0.55

2. In a single-center study, elevation of the *external* jugular vein correlated with catheter-measured central venous pressure

   a. External JVP < 5 cm H_2O predicted a low central venous pressure

      (1) Senior students and interns: sensitivity, 47%; specificity, 100%; LR+ ∞; LR– 0.5

      (2) Junior and senior residents: sensitivity, 78%; specificity 92%; LR+ 9.8; LR– 0.2

   b. External JVP > 10 cm H_2O predicted a high central venous pressure

      (1) Senior students and interns: sensitivity, 61%; specificity, 75%; LR+ 2.4; LR– 0.5

      (2) Junior and senior residents: sensitivity, 78%; specificity, 93%; LR+ 11.1; LR– 0.2

3. 2 pillow orthopnea (86% sensitive, 25% specific, LR+ 1.1, LR– 0.56)

4. Cold extremities 20% sensitive, 88% specific (LR+ 1.7, LR– 0.9)

5. The proportional pulse pressure can suggest cardiogenic shock.

   a. Typically, the pulse pressure increases as the systolic BP increases.

   b. A relatively low pulse pressure compared to the systolic BP suggests a low stroke volume.

   c. Proportional pulse pressure (PPP = (systolic BP – diastolic BP) / systolic BP)

   d. A PPP < 25% is 10% sensitive, 96% specific (LR+ 2.5, LR– 0.94) for cardiac index < 2.3 L / (min-m²). This must be measured with manual BP cuff.

B. Once the diagnosis of cardiogenic shock is considered and the need for immediate catheterization for treatment of acute MI (the most common cause) is assessed, echocardiography should be performed early.

C. Bedside portable ultrasound is becoming more prevalent and has been shown to be useful in assessing the cause of cardiogenic shock as well as in undifferentiated shock.

1. It is especially useful to

   a. Assess for pericardial effusion

   b. Determine global cardiac systolic function

   c. Identify marked LV or RV enlargement

   d. Gauge intravascular volume status by assessing inferior vena cava diameter and respiratory variation.

2. Preliminary data suggests hand held devices are accurate in residents with limited training (3 hours of didactic training and 5 hours of hands-on training)

   a. LV dysfunction: 88% sensitive, 89% specific, LR+ 8, LR– 0.13

   b. Pericardial effusion: 83% sensitive, 96% specific, LR+ 20.8, LR– 0.18

Treatment

Complete discussion of the treatment of cardiogenic shock is beyond the scope of this chapter. However, when cardiogenic shock is a result of myocardial ischemic, early revascularization (percutaneous coronary intervention or CABG) results in a significant survival benefit and is clearly indicated.

MAKING A DIAGNOSIS

An ECG showed no evidence of MI and troponins were normal. Chest film revealed an enlarged cardiac silhouette. Measurement of pulsus paradoxus demonstrated a pulsus of 12 mm Hg.

The patient's clinical picture suggests cardiogenic shock but the etiology remains obscure. Neither the ECG nor troponins suggest an acute MI. You consider the shock is due to one of the less common causes of cardiogenic shock (tamponade, valve failure).

Leading Hypothesis: Cardiac Tamponade

Textbook Presentation

Weakness, hypotension, and tachycardia are typically present. Other classic findings include an elevated jugular venous pressure and muffled heart sounds. However, the signs and symptoms associated with tamponade are quite nonspecific.

Disease Highlights

A. Cardiac tamponade results when fluid accumulation in the pericardial space compresses the heart and causes a reduction in cardiac output. This occurs as a result of pericardial effusion or hemorrhage.

B. As the signs and symptoms associated with it are nonspecific, diagnosing cardiac tamponade relies on understanding the conditions that can lead to pericardial effusion and careful assessment.

C. The incidence of cardiac tamponade and pericardial effusions are not well documented, and there is little data regarding how often pericardial effusions progress to tamponade. However, pericardial effusions are not uncommon; therefore, identifying clinically significant effusions is of great importance.

1. Common etiologies of pericardial effusions that may lead to tamponade include

   a. Idiopathic pericarditis (20-30%)

   b. Malignancy (13-36%)

   c. Iatrogenic (16%)

   d. Infection (5-21%)

   e. Acute MI (8%)

   f. Collagen vascular disease (5%)

2. Of these, effusions due to infection (bacterial, fungal, HIV-associated infections) and neoplasm have the greatest incidence of progression to tamponade.

3. Cardiac tamponade occurs in 1-2% of patients following cardiac surgery and commonly occurs as late as 7 days postoperatively.

4. Cardiac tamponade was found in almost 19% of patients with a type A aortic dissection. These patients had significantly higher mortality.

D. Tamponade has a wide range of presentations depending on pericardial fluid volume, accumulation rate, and degree of compression. It is typically grouped into 2 main types:

1. Acute tamponade
   a. Occurs following traumatic injury, rupture of the heart or aorta, or an invasive diagnostic or therapeutic procedure.
   b. Presents with cardiogenic shock (cool extremities, altered mental status, peripheral cyanosis, and JVD)

2. Subacute tamponade
   a. Occurs in the setting of inflammatory disease or malignancy.
   b. Symptoms often mimic HF (fatigue, dyspnea, chest fullness).
   c. Pericardial effusion may reach as much 2 L before tamponade physiology occurs.

E. Physiology: Tamponade occurs as increasing intrapericardial pressure compresses the cardiac chambers. The key components that determine when tamponade occurs are the rate of fluid accumulation relative to pericardial stretch.

1. True filling pressure of the heart is the transmural pressure, which is calculated as follows: intracardiac pressure – pericardial pressure.

2. Rising pericardial pressure offsets intracardiac pressure at some point and leads to competition for the chambers to fill:
   a. During systole, reduced ventricular volume leads to decreased pericardial pressure and atrial filling is preserved.
   b. During diastole, increased ventricular volume leads to increased pericardial pressure, decreased atrial transmural pressure and as tamponade approaches, late diastolic atrial collapse.
   c. As the pericardial effusion continues to increase and pericardial pressure rises, the ventricles compete for limited space. This stress more easily affects the RV and can lead to early diastolic collapse of the RV.

3. During inspiration, decreased pleural pressure is transmitted to the pericardium and causes increased transmural pressure and increased venous return and right heart filling. In tamponade this RV expansion compresses the LV and results in shift of the interventricular septum and decreased pulmonary venous return and reduced stroke volume.

4. As cardiac output drops, increases in heart rate, contractility, and peripheral arterial vasoconstriction defend circulation until circulatory collapse occurs.

Evidence-Based Diagnosis

A. Signs and symptoms
   1. Tachypnea and dyspnea nearly always present with cardiac tamponade (87-88%).
   2. Other common findings in patients with cardiac tamponade are tachycardia, elevated jugular venous pressure and pulsus paradoxus with pooled sensitivities of 76-82%.
   3. Chest pain, cough, fever, lethargy, and palpitations are present in 25% or less of patients.
   4. ECG findings associated with tamponade are insensitive with low voltage QRS and electrical alterans having estimated sensitivities of 43% and 16-21%, respectively.
   5. Cardiomegaly on chest film is common with a pooled sensitivity of 89% in 4 studies of 165 patients.
   6. Hypotension and diminished heart sounds are insensitive (28% and 26%, respectively).

B. Pulsus paradoxus
   1. Defined as an exaggerated decrease in BP with the normal inspiration

2. The paradox comes from decreased systolic BP despite increased venous return during inspiration.

3. In tamponade, when inspiration increases RV filling, the expansion of the RV within the confined pericardial space pushes the interventricular septum to the left and diminishes left heart filling.

4. Additionally, inspiratory expansion of the lungs leads to pulmonary venous pooling and even further reduced LV filling.

5. When the LV diastolic pressures are elevated as in end-stage renal disease, cardiac tamponade does not result in pulsus paradoxus.

6. Making an accurate measurement of pulsus paradoxus requires a manual sphygmomanometer, a quiet location, and patience.
   a. The sphygmomanometer is fully inflated and slowly deflated, in 1-2 mm Hg steps as the likely pressure is approached listening for the first Korotkoff sounds (which will be heard only with exhalation). Record this pressure.
   b. The cuff is deflated further in 1-2 mm Hg steps until the Korotkoff sounds are heard with inspiration and expiration.
   c. The difference between these pressures is the pulsus paradoxus; a difference > 10 mm Hg suggests cardiac tamponade but may also be seen in severe respiratory distress, massive PE, and other forms of severe hypertension.

C. When cardiac tamponade is suspected, transthoracic echocardiography is the primary diagnostic test to confirm the diagnosis.

D. The main findings on the transthoracic echocardiography include a pericardial effusion associated with the following:
   1. Late diastolic collapse of the right atria
   2. Early to mid diastolic collapse of the RV
   3. Septal shift toward the left during inspiration and toward the right with expiration
   4. Suppression of deep inspiratory collapse of the inferior vena cava

Treatment

A. Once cardiac tamponade is diagnosed, pericardial drainage is required unless tamponade is due to aortic dissection or free wall rupture.

B. Symptomatic management may be used if the patient is hemodynamically stable or in a "pre-tamponade" state. This consists primarily of volume resuscitation with isotonic fluids and supplemental oxygen until drainage can be performed.

C. Pericardiocentesis can be accomplished under ultrasound guidance at the bedside in the ICU if needed emergently. Alternatively, this can be performed under ultrasound or fluoroscopic guidance in the catheterization laboratory.

D. If the effusion is loculated, there is a need for pericardial window, or if the effusion is due to acute traumatic hemopericardium, surgical pericardiotomy is required.

CASE RESOLUTION

Echocardiography revealed a large pericardial effusion with late diastolic collapse of the right atrium. The patient was taken to the catheterization laboratory urgently and underwent pericardiocentesis; 500 mL of blood was removed. The patient felt better immediately. His pulse dropped to 75 bpm and BP increased to 110/70 mm Hg.

CHIEF COMPLAINT

PATIENT 3

Ms. M is a 70 year-old woman who arrives at the emergency department complaining of shortness of breath and dizziness. On physical exam, her pulse is 105 bpm, BP 75/45 mm Hg, and her skin exam is notable for hives. She is warm and has bounding pulses. The patient recently underwent surgery to have a mechanical mitral valve placed and took amoxicillin for the first time as prophylaxis for an upcoming dental procedure.

As noted above, the first step in the evaluation of the hypotensive patient is the recognition of shock. The patient's profound hypotension, particularly at this age, and dizziness suggest symptomatic hypotension and inadequate cerebral perfusion diagnostic of shock. The first pivotal diagnostic step is to consider whether the history and physical exam suggest 1 of 3 leading causes of shock: septic shock, hypovolemic shock, or cardiogenic shock. Her bounding pulses and warm extremities suggest distributive shock, a high output form of shock. As mentioned above, the most common form of distributive shock is septic shock, a must not miss hypothesis. However, her hives and recent use of amoxicillin is a pivotal clue that suggests another cause of distributive shock, anaphylactic shock. This is both the leading and must not miss hypothesis. Table 25-6 lists the differential diagnosis.

Leading Hypothesis: Anaphylactic Shock

Textbook Presentation

Anaphylaxis is an acute systemic reaction caused by IgE-mediated immunologic release of mediators from mast cells and basophils to allergenic triggers like food, insect venom, or medications. Typically, the reaction may affect the patient's skin, the cardiovascular system, or respiratory system. Anaphylactoid reactions produce the same clinical picture; however, they are not immune-mediated.

Disease Highlights

A. Triggers and mechanisms
   1. Foods are most common triggers in infants, children, and teenagers.

Table 25-6. Diagnostic hypotheses for Ms. M.

Diagnostic Hypothesis	Demographics, Risk Factors, Symptoms and Signs	Important Tests
Leading Hypothesis		
Anaphylactic shock	Recent new medication, nut or shellfish ingestion, bee sting Hives, itching, wheezing, angioedema	
Septic shock	Fever Rigors Urinary frequency/ dysuria Cough Diarrhea Abdominal pain	Elevated WBC Urinalysis Chest radiograph Other imaging as indicated Blood cultures

a. As much as 2% of the US population may have food allergies.
   (1) Peanut allergies are most common in children.
   (2) Shellfish allergies are most common in adults.
b. Each year in the United States there are as many as 100 deaths due to anaphylactic reactions to food.
2. When the cause of anaphylaxis is identified in adults, the most common culprits are antibiotics or nonsteroidal antiinflammatory drugs, with penicillins responsible for 75% of fatal cases.

B. The patient history is the most important tool to determine whether a patient has had anaphylaxis and the cause of the episode.
   1. Respiratory symptoms may include nasal stuffiness or itching; difficulty in breathing; retrosternal tightness; or pharyngeal, epiglottic, or glottis edema.
   2. Cardiovascular symptoms include dizziness, chest tightness, or overt hypotension.
   3. Skin complaints include itching, warmth, minor swelling, or characteristic urticaria.
   4. Severity, onset, and symptom patterns may vary considerably and results in discrepancies in diagnosis.

C. The estimated lifetime prevalence of anaphylaxis is 0.05-2%. However, even the high-end estimate may be too low as significant evidence points toward underreporting of anaphylaxis.
   1. In Australia, anaphylaxis admissions doubled from 1995 to 2005 to over 10:100,000 population. The increase in incidence is likely more pronounced among young patients, with food the most common trigger.
   2. Deaths related to medicine-induced anaphylaxis have increased 300%. Medicines account for 57% of anaphylaxis-related deaths.

D. Physiology
   1. Interaction of antigen with mast cell IgE or direct drug actions (by histamine, leukotrienes, kinins, prostaglandins or platelet activating factor) cause mast cells to release the mediators of anaphylaxis or anaphylactoid reactions.
   2. These mediators cause vasodilation and the leakage of fluid from capillaries and the post-capillary venules resulting in hypotension.
   3. Several of these substances, in particular leukotrienes, cause respiratory symptoms related to bronchoconstriction and increased mucus production.
   4. When untreated, death may result from hypoxemia due to upper airway angioedema, bronchospasm and mucus plugging and/or shock resulting in multi-organ system failure.

Evidence-Based Diagnosis

A. The sudden onset of skin, cardiovascular, and respiratory symptoms should point toward a diagnosis of anaphylaxis.
   1. However, even if just 2 of these organ systems are involved, or hypotension alone, anaphylaxis should be considered.
   2. Often, these reactions may be self-limited; however, failure to make a diagnosis puts the patient at risk for future life-threatening allergen exposure.

B. Clinical criteria for the diagnosis of anaphylaxis. Essential questions to be asked:
   1. Were there cutaneous manifestations, specifically pruritus, flushing, urticaria, and angioedema?

2. Was there any sign of airway obstruction involving either the upper airway or the lower airway?

3. Were syncope or presyncopal symptoms present?

C. According to the National Institute of Allergy and Infectious Disease, the diagnosis of anaphylaxis is highly likely if *any* the following criteria are met:

1. Sudden onset of an illness (within minutes to several hours) with involvement of the skin, mucosal tissue, or both **and**

    a. Respiratory compromise (dyspnea, wheeze-bronchospasm, hypoxemia), **or**

    b. Reduced BP or associated symptoms of end-organ dysfunction (hypotonia, syncope, or incontinence).

2. Sudden onset of 2 or more of the following symptoms after exposure to a *likely* allergen or other trigger for that patient:

    a. Skin or mucosal symptoms (hives, itch-flushing, swollen lips-tongue-uvula)

    b. Respiratory compromise

    c. Reduced BP or associated symptoms

    d. Persistent gastrointestinal symptoms

3. Reduced BP (systolic BP < 90 mm Hg or greater than 30% decrease from baseline) after exposure to a *known* allergen for that patient (minutes to hours)

4. The test characteristics for the criteria are sensitivity, 96.7%; specificity, 82.4%; LR+, 5.5; LR–, 0.04.

D. The sensitivity of individual findings:

1. Skin/mucosa: 100% skin or mucosal tissue findings, 60.5% generalized hives, 42% pruritus, 44% angioedema, and 30% flushing/diaphoresis.

2. Respiratory: respiratory compromise 90%, dyspnea 72%, wheezing 24%

3. Reduced BP or associated end-organ dysfunction, 24%

E. Mature tryptase is released from mast cells when activated. Therefore, measurement of tryptase can be useful to confirm a diagnosis of anaphylaxis.

1. An increase > 2.0 mcg/L between arrival, 1 hour later and just before discharge was 75% sensitive for severe anaphylaxis.

2. This test does not have benefit at the time of presentation; however, it may be beneficial to ensure that a diagnosis of anaphylaxis is made when appropriate and minimize the risk for recurrence.

Treatment

A. Initial management of suspected anaphylaxis relies on quick recognition and appropriate supportive care.

1. Assess patient's circulation, airway, breathing, mental status, skin, and body weight.

2. Inject intramuscular epinephrine in the mid-anterolateral aspect of the thigh, 0.01 mg/kg of a 1:1000 (1 mg/mL), maximum 0.5 mg (adult) or 0.3 mg (child). Repeat in 5-15 minutes if needed.

3. H_1- and H_2- antihistamines as well as corticosteroids are considered second-line agents and are not considered essential medications for the treatment of anaphylaxis. If given, antihistamines may decrease itching, flushing, urticarial, and nasal symptoms but have no effect on airway obstruction or hypotension.

4. Corticosteroids do not affect the initial symptoms of anaphylaxis but may reduce the likelihood and severity of protracted symptoms. There is no consensus regarding the type of corticosteroid, the route, or the dose that may be beneficial.

5. Place the patient on their back and elevate lower extremities.

6. If indicated, provide respiratory support; this may range from supplemental oxygen via nasal cannula to mechanical ventilation.

7. Establish IV access with wide-bore cannula (16 gauge if possible) and bolus 1-2 L of 0.9 normal saline.

B. Once the patient recovers from the acute episode, steps must be taken to prevent a recurrence.

1. Provide self-injectable epinephrine from an auto-injector.

2. Establish an anaphylaxis emergency plan and medical identification of the patient's allergy (bracelet, wallet card).

3. Referral to an allergy/immunology specialist to confirm sensitivity to a specific allergen and to discuss long-term risk reduction strategies including immune modulation.

CASE RESOLUTION

Anaphylactic shock was quickly recognized, and Ms. M promptly received an IM injection of epinephrine as well as fluids. Her BP and shortness of breath quickly improved.

REFERENCES

Agarwal R, Schwartz DH. Procalcitonin to guide duration of antimicrobial therapy in intensive care units: a systematic review. Clin Infect Dis. 2011;53:379-87.

Angus DC, van der Poll T. Severe sepsis and septic shock. N Engl J Med. 2013;369(9):840-51.

Biais M, Carrie C, Delauney F, Morel N, Revel P, Janvier G. Evaluation of a new pocket echoscopic device for focused cardiac ultrasonography in an emergency setting. Crit Care. 2012;16:R82.

Bodson L, Bouferrache K, Vieillard- Baron. Cardiac tamponade. Curr Opin Crit Care. 2011;17:416-24.

Bonow RO, Mann DL, Zipes DP, Libby P (2012). *Braunwald's Heart Disease: A Textbook of Cardiovascular Medicine*, 9th ed. Philadelphia, PA: Saunders.

Butman SM, Ewy GA, Standen JR, Kern KB, Hahn E. Bedside cardiovascular examination in patients with severe chronic heart failure: importance of rest or inducible jugular venous distension. J Am Coll Cardiol. 1993;22:968-74.

Coburn B, Morris AM, Tomlinson GT, Detsky AS. Does this adult patient with suspected bacteremia require blood cultures? JAMA. 2012;308(5):502-11.

Drazner MH, Hellkamp AS, Leier CV et al. Value of clinician assessment of hemodynamics in advanced heart failure: the ESCAPE trial. Circ Heart Fail. 2008;1:170-7.

Gelincik A, Demirturk M, Yilmaz E et al. Anaphylaxis in a tertiary adult allergy clinic: a retrospective review of 516 patients. Ann Allergy Asthma Immunol. 2013;110:96-100.

Hall JB, Schmidt GA, Wood LDH. *Principles of Critical Care*, 3rd ed. New York, NY: McGraw-Hill Professional, 2005.

Jacob S, Sebastian JC, Cherian PK, Abraham A, John SK. Pericardial effusion impending tamponade: a look beyond Beck's triad. Am J Emerg Med. 2009;27:216-9.

Khunnawat C, Mukerji S, Havlichek D, Touma R, Abela GS. Cardiovascular manifestations in human immunodeficiency virus-infected patients. Am J Cardiol. 2008;102:635-42.

Kirkbright SJ, Brown SGA. Anaphylaxis: recognition and management. Aust Fam Phys. 2012;41:366-70.

Kobal SL, Trento L, Baharami S et al. Comparison of effectiveness of hand-carried ultrasound to bedside cardiovascular physical examination. Am J Cardiol. 2005;96:1002-6.

Koplin JJ, Martin PE, Allen KJ. An update on epidemiology of anaphylaxis in children and adults. Curr Opin Allergy Clin Immunol. 2011;11:492-6.

Labovitz AJ, Noble VE, Bierig M et al. Focused cardiac ultrasound in the emergent setting: a consensus statement of the American Society of Echocardiography and American College of Emergency Physicians. J Am Soc Echocardiogr. 2010;23:1225-30.

Lieberman P, Camargo CA, Bohlke K et al. Epidemiology of anaphylaxis: findings of the American College of Allergy, Asthma and Immunology epidemiology of anaphylaxis working group. Ann Allergy Asthma Immunol. 2006;97:596-602.

Lieberman P, Kemp SF, Oppenheimer J et al. The diagnosis and management of anaphylaxis: an updated practice parameter. J Allergy Clin Immunol. 2005;115:S483-523.

Lighthall G. Use of physiologic reasoning to diagnose and manage shock states. Crit Care Res Practice. 2011; Article ID 105348.

Manasia AR, Nagaraj HM, Kodali RB et al. Feasibility and potential clinical utility of goal-directed transthoracic echocardiography performed by noncardiologist intensivists using a small hand-carried device in critically ill patients. J Cardiothor Vasc An. 2005;19:155-9.

McGee S, Abernethy WB, Simel DL. Is this patient hypovolemic? JAMA. 1999;281:1022-9.

Meurin P, Tabet JY, Thabut G et al. Nonsteroidal anti-inflammatory drug treatment for postoperative pericardial effusion. Ann Intern Med. 2010;152:137-43.

Mjolstad OC, Andersen GN, Dalen H et al. Feasibility and reliability of point-of-care pocket-size echocardiography performed by medical residents. Eur Heart J Cardiovasc Imaging. 2013 Dec;14(12):1195-202.

Patel AK, Hollenberg SM. Cardiovascular failure and cardiogenic shock. Semin Respir Crit Care Med. 2011;32:598-606.

Rame JE, Dries DL, Drazner MH. The prognostic value of the physical examination in patients with chronic heart failure. Congest Heart Fail. 2003;9:170-5.

Reddy PS, Curtiss EI, O'Toole JD, Shaver JA. Cardiac tamponade: hemodynamic observations in man. Circulation. 1978;58:265-72.

Reynolds HR, Hochman JS. Cardiogenic shock, current concepts and improving outcomes. Circulation. 2008;117:686-97.

Roy CL, Minor MA, Brookhart MA, Choudhry NK. Does this patient with a pericardial effusion have cardiac tamponade? JAMA. 2007;297:1810-8.

Sagrista-Sauleda J, Merce J, Permanyer-Miralda G, Soler-Soler J. Clinical clues to the causes of large pericardial effusions. Am J Med. 2009;109:95-101.

Simons FER, Ardusso LRF, Bilo MB et al. 2012 update: World Allergy Organization guidelines for the assessment and management of anaphylaxis. Curr Opin Allergy Clin Immunol. 2012;12:389-99.

Sinert R, Spektor M. Clinical assessment of hypovolemia. Ann Emerg Med. 2005;45:327-9.

Soni NJ, Samson DJ, Galaydick JL, Vats V, Pitrak DL, Aronson N. Procalcitonin-guided antibiotic therapy: comparative effectiveness review no. 78 AHRQ Publication No. 12(13)-EHC124-EF. Rockville, MD: Agency for Healthcare Research and Quality. October 2012.

Spodick DH. Acute cardiac tamponade. N Engl J Med. 2003;349:684-90.

Topalian S, Ginsberg F, Parrillo JE. Cardiogenic shock. Crit Care Med. 2008;36(Suppl):S66-S74.

Vazquez R, Gheorghe C, Kaufman D, Manthous CA. Accuracy of bedside physical examination in distinguishing categories of shock. J Hosp Med. 2010;5:471-4.

Vignon P, Dugard A, Abraham J et al. Focused training for goal-oriented hand-held echocardiography performed by noncardiologist residents in the intensive care unit. Intensive Care Med. 2007;33:1795-9.

Vinayak AG, Levitt J, Gehlbach B, Pohlman AS, Hall JB, Kress JP. Usefulness of the external jugular vein examination in detecting abnormal central venous pressure in critically ill patients. Arch Intern Med. 2006;166:2132-7.

Vincent JL, De Backer D. Circulatory Shock. N Engl J Med. 2013;369:1726-34.

Wacker C, Prkno A, Brunkhorst FM, Schlattmann P. Procalcitonin as a diagnostic marker for sepsis: a systematic review and meta-analysis. Lancet ID. 2013;13:426-35.

I have a patient with jaundice or abnormal liver enzymes. How do I determine the cause?

CHIEF COMPLAINT

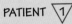

PATIENT 1

Ms. B is a 56-year-old woman who comes to your office because her skin and eyes have been yellow for the past 2 weeks.

What is the differential diagnosis of jaundice? How would you frame the differential?

CONSTRUCTING A DIFFERENTIAL DIAGNOSIS

The differential diagnosis of jaundice, or hyperbilirubinemia, is often organized pathophysiologically. It is helpful to review some basic physiology first.

A. Oxidation of the heme moiety of Hgb generates biliverdin, which is metabolized into **unconjugated bilirubin,** and then bound to albumin.

B. There are 3 steps in bilirubin metabolism in the liver:

1. **Uptake:** The unconjugated bilirubin-albumin complex reaches the hepatocyte; bilirubin dissociates from albumin and then enters the hepatocyte.

2. **Conjugation:** Unconjugated bilirubin and glucuronic acid combine to make **conjugated bilirubin.**

3. **Excretion:** The hepatocyte excretes conjugated bilirubin into the bile.

   a. The rate-limiting step of bilirubin metabolism in the liver

   b. If excretion is impaired, conjugated bilirubin enters the hepatic sinusoids and then into the bloodstream.

C. Conjugated bilirubin in the bile is transported through the biliary ducts into the duodenum; it is not reabsorbed by the intestine.

1. Can be excreted unchanged in the stool

2. Can be converted to **urobilinogen** by colonic bacteria

   a. Urobilinogen can be reabsorbed, entering the portal circulation.

   b. Some is taken up by the liver and re-excreted into the bile.

   c. Some bypasses the liver and is excreted by the kidney, thus appearing in the urine in small amounts.

   d. Can be converted in the bowel to stercobilin rendering the stool brown.

D. **Unconjugated bilirubin is not found in the urine** because it is bound to albumin and cannot be filtered by the glomeruli.

E. **Conjugated bilirubin is filtered and excreted in the urine** when there is conjugated hyperbilirubinemia.

The first pivotal point in the differential diagnosis of hyperbilirubinemia is determining which kind of bilirubin is elevated.

Dark, tea-colored urine means the patient has conjugated hyperbilirubinemia.

Light stools, often described as "clay colored," occur when extrahepatic obstruction prevents bilirubin from entering the intestine.

If the patient has unconjugated hyperbilirubinemia (> 50% of the bilirubin is unconjugated), use a pathophysiologic framework:

A. Increased bilirubin production

1. Hemolysis

2. Dyserythropoiesis

3. Extravasation of blood into tissues

B. Impaired hepatic bilirubin uptake

1. Heart failure

2. Sepsis

3. Drugs (rifampin, probenecid, chloramphenicol)

4. Fasting

5. Portosystemic shunts

C. Impaired bilirubin conjugation (decreased hepatic glucuronosyltransferase activity)

1. Hereditary

   a. Gilbert syndrome

   b. Crigler-Najjar syndrome

2. Acquired

   a. Neonates

   b. Hyperthyroidism

   c. Ethinyl estradiol

   d. Liver disease (causes mixed hyperbilirubinemia; usually predominantly conjugated)

   e. Sepsis

Most patients with unconjugated hyperbilirubinemia have hemolysis, Gilbert syndrome, heart failure, sepsis, or very advanced cirrhosis.

Although many sources organize the differential diagnosis for conjugated hyperbilirubinemia (when > 50% is conjugated) using a pathophysiologic framework, a more practical, clinical approach uses the results of other liver function tests:

A. Normal liver enzymes (ALT [SGPT], AST [SGOT])

 1. Sepsis or systemic infection

 2. Rotor syndrome

 3. Dubin-Johnson syndrome

B. Elevated liver enzymes

 1. **Hepatocellular** pattern: transaminases more elevated than alkaline phosphatase

 a. Marked transaminase elevations (> 1000 units/L)

 (1) Acute viral hepatitis

 (2) Ischemic hepatitis

 (3) Medication- or toxin-induced hepatitis

 (4) Autoimmune hepatitis

 (5) Acute bile duct obstruction

 (6) Acute Budd-Chiari syndrome

 b. Mild to moderate elevations (mild elevation: defined as < 5 times the upper limit of normal [approximately < 175–200 units/L])

 (1) Alcoholic liver disease

 (2) Medications/toxins

 (3) Chronic hepatitis B or C

 (4) Nonalcoholic fatty liver disease (NAFLD)

 (5) Autoimmune hepatitis

 (6) Hemochromatosis

 (7) Wilson disease (in patients < 40 years old)

 (8) Alpha-1-antitrypsin deficiency

 2. **Cholestatic** pattern: alkaline phosphatase more elevated than transaminases

 a. Extrahepatic cholestasis (bile duct obstruction)

 (1) Common bile duct stone

 (2) Benign stricture

 (3) Benign polyp

 (4) Malignancy (pancreatic cancer, cholangiocarcinoma, ampullary cancer)

 (5) Periportal adenopathy

 b. Intrahepatic cholestasis (primarily due to impaired excretion)

 (1) Hepatitis (viral, alcoholic)

 (2) Intrahepatic cholestasis of pregnancy

 (3) Cirrhosis

 (4) Medications and toxins

 (5) Sepsis

 (6) Total parenteral nutrition

 (7) Postoperative jaundice

 (8) Infiltrative diseases (amyloidosis, lymphoma, sarcoidosis, tuberculosis)

 (9) Primary sclerosing cholangitis

 (10) Primary biliary cirrhosis

Regardless of how you organize this differential, the first step is to determine whether the hyperbilirubinemia is primarily unconjugated or conjugated. The differential of unconjugated hyperbilirubinemia is relatively limited. If the hyperbilirubinemia is conjugated,

the second step is to determine whether there is extrahepatic obstruction or intrinsic liver dysfunction due to 1 of many possible etiologies. Although other liver function tests can serve as a guide, it is clear from the way the above differentials overlap that these tests are not very specific. Table 26-1 summarizes the commonly used liver tests. Figure 26-1 outlines the diagnostic approach to hyperbilirubinemia.

Ms. B also tells you she has dark urine, light-colored stools, anorexia, and fatigue. She has no nausea, vomiting, abdominal pain, or fever. Ms. B's physical exam shows scleral icterus and jaundice as well as hepatomegaly, with her liver edge palpable 7 cm below the costal margin. The liver extends across the midline, and the spleen tip is palpable. There is no abdominal tenderness or distention. There is no peripheral edema, and the rest of her exam is normal.

How reliable is the physical exam for detecting signs of liver disease?

A. Jaundice

 1. Detectable on physical exam when total bilirubin is > 2.5–3.0 mg/dL.

Scleral icterus is detectable before jaundice of the skin.

 2. For bilirubin > 3.0 mg/dL, sensitivity of physical exam is 78.4% and specificity is 68.8% (LR+ = 2.5, LR− = 0.31).

Table 26-1. Biochemical markers used to evaluate the liver.

Test	Aspect of Liver Assessed	Origins
Aspartate aminotransferase (AST [SGOT])	Hepatocyte integrity	Liver Heart Skeletal muscle Kidney Brain RBC
Alanine aminotransferase (ALT [SGPT])	Hepatocyte integrity	Liver
Alkaline phosphatase (AP)	Cholestasis	Liver Bone Intestine Placenta
Gamma-glutamyl transpeptidase (GGTP)	When elevated with AP, indicates liver origin of AP	Liver
Bilirubin (conjugated)	Cholestasis	Liver
Serum albumin	Reflects synthetic capacity of liver	Liver or diet
Prothrombin time	Reflects synthetic capacity of liver	Vitamin K dependent clotting factors synthesized by liver

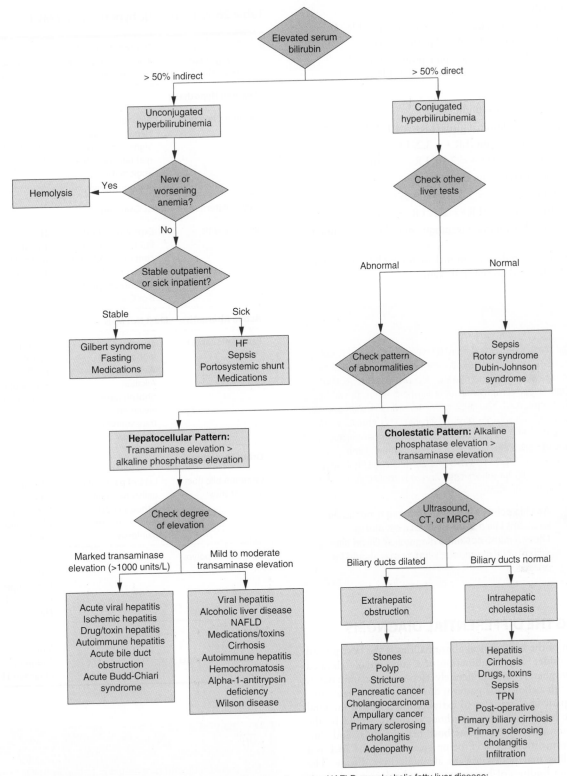

HF, heart failure; MRCP, magnetic resonance cholangiopancreatography; NAFLD, nonalcoholic fatty liver disease; TPN, total parenteral nutrition.

Figure 26-1. Diagnostic approach to hyperbilirubinemia.

3. For bilirubin > 15.0 mg/dL, sensitivity of physical exam is 96.4%.

B. Hepatomegaly

1. On ultrasound, the upper limit of normal for the cephalocaudad dimension of the liver is 13 cm.

2. While examiners are always correct when they report palpating the liver edge (LR+ = 233), a palpable liver edge is not a reliable sign of hepatomegaly (sensitivity, 39–71%; specificity, 56–85%; LR+, 1.9; LR–, 0.6) since the liver may be pushed caudally by enlarged lungs.

C. Splenomegaly

1. Percussion methods have inadequate negative LRs (all around 0.45) and minimal positive LRs.

 2. Palpation of a spleen in a supine position is highly predictive of splenomegaly: LR+ = 8.5, LR– = 0.41.

D. Ascites

1. The best 3 historical findings are

   a. Increased abdominal girth (LR+ = 4.1, LR– = 0.17)

   b. Recent weight gain (LR + = 3.2, LR– = 0.42)

   c. Ankle swelling (LR+ = 2.80, LR– = 0.10)

2. The best physical exam findings are

   a. Fluid wave (LR+ = 5.3, LR– = 0.57)

   b. Shifting dullness (LR+ = 2.1, LR– = 0.4)

   c. Proper physical exam technique must be used to obtain these LRs.

3. Ultrasound can detect minimal ascites, far less than could ever be detected on physical exam.

Given the pivotal historical points (dark urine and light colored stools) and the physical exam findings of jaundice, hepatomegaly, and splenomegaly, you are confident that Ms. B has hyperbilirubinemia and suspect that it will be primarily conjugated. You obtain the following initial tests: total bilirubin, 13 mg/dL; direct bilirubin, 9.6 mg/dL; AST, 250 units/L; ALT, 113 units/L; alkaline phosphatase, 503 units/L; albumin, 2.8 g/dL; prothrombin time (PT), 15.4 s (control 11.1 s); WBC = 22,000 cells/mcL with 80% PMNs, 16% lymphocytes, and 4% monocytes. The platelet count is normal.

 At this point, what is the leading hypothesis, what are the active alternatives, and is there a must not miss diagnosis? Given this differential diagnosis, what tests should be ordered?

RANKING THE DIFFERENTIAL DIAGNOSIS

The pattern of the biochemical abnormalities is the next pivotal point to consider. The combination of a substantially elevated alkaline phosphatase and moderately elevated transaminases is consistent with a cholestatic pattern, due either to a disease causing intrahepatic cholestasis or to extrahepatic obstruction. Viral or alcoholic hepatitis, with or without cirrhosis, would be the most common diseases that cause both hepatocellular and cholestatic abnormalities; the AST being greater than the ALT is a pivotal finding that points toward alcoholic liver disease. The physical exam findings of hepatomegaly and splenomegaly both modestly increase the likelihood of chronic liver disease (LR+, 2.3 for hepatomegaly; 2.9 for splenomegaly). Extrahepatic obstruction must be considered also, since she could have an obstruction in addition to chronic liver disease. Cancer and stricture are more likely causes of painless jaundice than common bile duct stones. Pancreatic cancer is the most common malignancy that causes extrahepatic obstruction; cholangiocarcinoma and ampullary carcinoma are 2 other possibilities. Occasionally, obstruction is due to benign polyps in the biliary tree. Table 26-2 lists the differential diagnosis.

Table 26-2. Diagnostic hypotheses for Ms. B.

Diagnostic Hypotheses	Demographics, Risk Factors, Symptoms and Signs	Important Tests
Leading Hypothesis		
Alcoholic hepatitis	Alcohol history Hepatomegaly Signs of cirrhosis (palmar erythema, angiomata, splenomegaly)	CT scan Liver biopsy AST > ALT
Active Alternative—Most Common		
Viral hepatitis	Exposure to body fluids, needles, or contaminated food Signs of cirrhosis if chronic hepatitis B or C	Hepatitis A antibody Hepatitis B antigen and antibodies Hepatitis C antibody
Active Alternative—Must Not Miss		
Pancreatic cancer	Jaundice (with or without pain) Weight loss Alkaline phosphatase elevation > transaminase elevation	CT scan MRCP ERCP Endoscopic ultrasound
Other Hypotheses		
Common bile duct (CBD) stones	Lack of pain makes gallstones unlikely, although CBD stones can present painlessly	CT scan MRCP Endoscopic ultrasound ERCP
Strictures or polyps	Painless jaundice	CT scan MRCP Endoscopic ultrasound ERCP
Ampullary carcinoma or cholangiocarcinoma	Painless jaundice	CT scan MRCP Endoscopic ultrasound ERCP

Ms. B had a blood transfusion in Latvia in 1996. She has no history of injection drug use, tattoos, or smoking, but she has consumed between 2 glasses and 1 bottle of wine daily for years. Her past medical history is notable only for *Helicobacter pylori*–positive gastric and duodenal ulcers 6 years ago, treated with eradication therapy. She is taking no medications.

 Is the clinical information sufficient to make a diagnosis? If not, what other information do you need?

Leading Hypothesis: Alcoholic Liver Disease (ALD)

Textbook Presentation

Patients may be asymptomatic, have incidentally discovered hepatomegaly or transaminase elevation, have symptoms of acute alcoholic hepatitis, or have manifestations of cirrhosis. Some or all of these symptoms may develop in an individual patient during the course of the disease.

Disease Highlights

A. Alcohol ingestion is the most important risk factor for ALD.

1. Beer and spirits are more associated with ALD than wine.

2. Drinking outside of meal time and binge drinking increase the risk.

B. Other risk factors include female sex, African-American and Hispanic ethnicity, obesity, and genetic factors.

C. ALD is more frequent and worse in patients with other chronic liver diseases, especially hepatitis C.

D. There are 3 histologic stages: steatosis, alcoholic steatohepatitis, and chronic hepatitis with fibrosis or cirrhosis.

1. Hepatic steatosis is generally asymptomatic.

   a. 70% of patients have hepatomegaly

   b. Occurs in up to 90% of patients who consistently consume > 6 drinks (60 g) per day

   c. Potentiates liver damage from other insults, such as viral hepatitis or acetaminophen toxicity, and promotes obesity-related liver disease.

   d. Usually completely reversible with abstinence from alcohol for 4–6 weeks

      (1) Despite abstinence, cirrhosis will develop in 5–15% of patients with steatosis.

      (2) Cirrhosis develops in 30% of those who continue to drink.

2. Alcoholic steatohepatitis occurs in 15–30% of patients with ALD.

   a. Often presents acutely in the context of chronic liver disease

   b. Symptoms often include fever, hepatomegaly, ascites, encephalopathy, AST:ALT ratio > 1.5, and leukocytosis, all in the context of heavy alcohol use.

   c. Malnutrition is seen in 90% of patients.

   d. Concomitant cirrhosis is found in > 50% of patients with alcoholic hepatitis.

   e. 3-month mortality between 15% (mild alcoholic hepatitis) and 55% (severe alcoholic hepatitis)

   f. Several tools have been developed to risk stratify patients with alcoholic hepatitis.

      (1) The Modified Discriminant Function (mDF) = 4.6 × (patient PT − control PT) + serum bilirubin level: patients with a score ≥ 32 have a poor prognosis

      (2) The Mayo End-stage Liver Disease (MELD) score incorporates the total bilirubin, international normalized ratio (INR), and serum creatinine (http://www.mayoclinic.org/meld/mayomodel7.html).

         (a) A MELD score > 11 is similar to an mDF ≥ 32 in predicting mortality.

         (b) A MELD score > 20 1 week after admission had a sensitivity of 91% and specificity 85% for identifying patients who will die within 30 days.

      (3) The Glasgow Alcoholic Hepatitis Score (GAHS) includes age, WBC count, BUN, PT/INR, and total bilirubin (http://www.mdcalc.com/glasgow-alcoholic-hepatitis-score/): a score ≥ 9 is associated with a poor prognosis and has an accuracy of 81% in predicting 28-day mortality

3. Cirrhosis (also see Chapter 17, Edema)

   a. Increased risk in men who consume > 60–80 g/day and women who consume > 20 g/day of alcohol for ≥ 10 years

      (1) Only 6–41% of such individuals develop cirrhosis

      (2) Fibrosis develops in 40–60% of people who consume > 40–80 g/day for 25 years

   b. In patients without any other chronic liver disease, 21 drinks/week in men and 7–14/week in women probably will not lead to ALD.

   c. The prognosis of alcoholic cirrhosis varies, depending on whether the patient stops consuming alcohol.

      (1) 5-year survival of 90% if patient becomes abstinent

      (2) 5-year survival of 70% if patient continues to consume alcohol

      (3) 5-year survival of 30–50% once complications of cirrhosis appear

Evidence-Based Diagnosis

A. ALD is diagnosed by documenting alcohol excess in the presence of liver disease.

B. Biomarkers such as GGT, AST, and ALT are not sensitive or specific enough to diagnose ALD; macrocytosis may be seen but is also insensitive

C. Alcoholic steatosis is diagnosed by seeing fatty infiltration on imaging in patients with excessive alcohol consumption.

D. Alcoholic hepatitis is a clinical diagnosis.

1. Criteria used in randomized trials of therapy include history of excessive alcohol consumption; serum bilirubin > 4.5 mg/dL; AST < 500 units/L; ALT < 300 units/L; exclusion of acute viral, autoimmune, obstructive, or malignant liver disease.

2. Transaminases are elevated but generally < 6–7 times the upper limit of normal.

   a. AST:ALT ratio > 2 in 70–80% of patients, with ratios > 3 being more specific

   b. Another study showed mean ratio of 2.6 for patients with alcoholic liver disease, compared with mean of 0.9 for patients with nonalcoholic steatohepatitis; however, there was some overlap.

3. GGTP (gamma-glutamyl transpeptidase) is often elevated, and the GGTP/alkaline phosphatase ratio is often > 2.5.

4. Imaging (with ultrasound or CT) is most helpful for ruling out other diagnoses; can variably see fatty infiltration, hepatomegaly, ascites, or cirrhosis.

5. Liver biopsy is the gold standard for diagnosis but is not always necessary.

E. Cirrhosis is diagnosed when portal hypertension is present or on biopsy (also see Chapter 17, Edema).

Treatment

A. Abstinence is the primary treatment for all forms of ALD.

B. Although the data are conflicting, current guidelines recommend that patients with severe alcoholic hepatitis, defined as an mDF score ≥ 32, should be treated with corticosteroids; pentoxifylline could be considered in patients intolerant of corticosteroids.

C. Patients with advanced disease or alcoholic hepatitis should be assessed for nutritional deficiencies and repleted as necessary.

MAKING A DIAGNOSIS

Ms. B's transaminases are consistent with, but not diagnostic of, ALD. An imaging study is necessary not to rule in ALD but rather to exclude alternative diagnoses. As discussed in Chapter 3, Abdominal Pain, ultrasound is the best first test to look for stones in the gallbladder, although the sensitivity is less for common bile duct stones. However, in this patient, pancreatic cancer or other malignancies are more likely causes of extrabiliary obstruction than stones; therefore, an abdominal CT scan or MRCP would be a better first test. Tests for hepatitis are necessary in all patients with liver disease and are especially important in Ms. B because of her history of a blood transfusion.

Ms. B has an abdominal CT scan, which shows an enlarged, nodular liver, moderate ascites, and a normal pancreas. Her ANA, hepatitis A IgM antibody, HBsAg hepatitis B IgM core antibody, and hepatitis C antibody are all negative.

 Have you crossed the diagnostic threshold for the leading hypothesis, alcoholic hepatitis? Have you ruled out the active alternatives? Do other tests need to be done to exclude the alternative diagnoses?

Alternative Diagnosis: Pancreatic Cancer

Textbook Presentation

Patients with pancreatic cancer often have vague abdominal pain for weeks or months, followed by weight loss and perhaps the abrupt onset of painless jaundice.

Disease Highlights

A. > 90% of cases are ductal carcinomas; 70–80% are in the pancreatic head and 20–25% in the body or tail

B. Risk Factors

1. Smoking (related to up to 20% of cases) and family history of pancreatic cancer (present in 7–10% of patients) are the most important risk factors.

2. Other risk factors include the following:
   a. Family history of chronic pancreatitis, older age, male sex, African-American ethnic origin
   b. Diabetes, obesity
   c. Non-O blood group
   d. Occupational exposures (chlorinated hydrocarbon solvents and nickel)
   e. High fat diet; high meat/low vegetable diet

C. Clinical presentation (Table 26-3)

1. Symptoms are insidious and often present for more than 2 months.

2. Abdominal pain is a presenting complaint, occurring in up to 80% of patients.
   a. Often described as gnawing, visceral pain, sometimes radiating from the epigastrium to the sides or back.

Table 26-3. Clinical presentation of pancreatic cancer.

Sign/Symptom	All cases	Cases by Anatomic Location		
		Head (79% of cases)	Body (13% of cases)	Tail (7% of cases)
Asthenia	86%	85%	89%	80%
Weight loss	85%	82%	95%	100%
Anorexia	83%	85%	89%	60%
Abdominal pain	79%	78%	95%	60%
Jaundice	56%	73%	10%	0
Nausea	51%	55%	58%	20%
Back pain	49%	48%	68%	63%
Diarrhea	44%	47%	26%	30%
Vomiting	33%	35%	42%	10%
Hepatomegaly	30%	32%	32%	10%
Steatorrhea	25%	28%	10%	0

   b. Sometimes improves with bending forward; worse at night or after eating.
   c. Back pain is prominent if splanchnic nerve or celiac plexus infiltration occurs.

3. Weight loss is common.

4. Jaundice
   a. In over 70% of patients with cancers in the head; more if mass is > 2 cm
   b. Can occur when the cancer is in the body but is then due to liver metastases
   c. Can be painless or associated with abdominal pain

5. Less common presentations include acute pancreatitis, malabsorption, migratory thrombophlebitis, and GI bleeding.

Evidence-Based Diagnosis

A. The first imaging study in most patients presenting with jaundice is an ultrasound.

1. The overall sensitivity for pancreatic cancer is 90%, with a lower sensitivity for tumors < 3 cm in size.

2. The sensitivity may be less in obese patients or with less experienced sonographers.

B. If the ultrasound shows a pancreatic mass, the next test should be a triphasic pancreatic-protocol multidetector CT.

1. Sensitivity = 86%; specificity = 90%

2. Sensitivity lower for cancers < 2 cm (77%) compared with those > 2 cm (89%)

3. Best test for determining potential resectability

C. If an initial ultrasound does not show a mass, pancreatic protocol CT, magnetic resonance cholangiopancreatography (MRCP), endoscopic ultrasound (EUS), or endoscopic retrograde cholangiopancreatography (ERCP) should be done.

1. MRCP is noninvasive and has sensitivity = 84%, specificity = 97% for detecting pancreatic cancer.

2. EUS requires endoscopy but does not lead to as many complications as ERCP; sensitivity = 89–92%; specificity = 96%.

3. ERCP is invasive and has a sensitivity of only 50–60% for detecting pancreatic cancer, with a specificity of 94%; complications include pancreatitis and hemorrhage.

D. CA 19–9

1. For levels above 37–40 units/mL: sensitivity = 76–90%, specificity = 68–98%

2. For levels above 100–120 units/mL, specificity = 87–100%

3. For levels > 1000 units/mL, specificity = 94–100%

E. There is no universally accepted standard algorithm to diagnose pancreatic cancer; one approach is outlined in Figure 26-2.

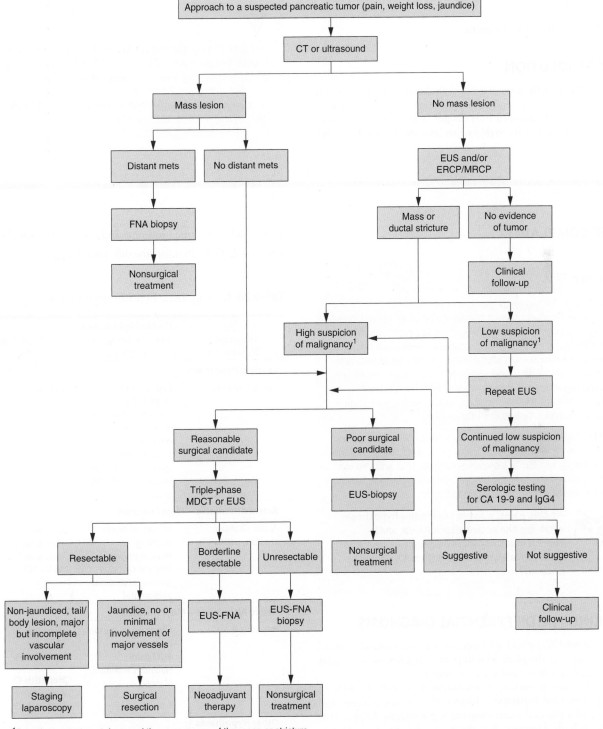

[1]Based on symptomatology and the appearance of the mass or stricture.

CA 19-9, cancer antigen 19-9; ERCP, endoscopic retrograde cholangiopancreatography; EUS, endoscopic ultrasound; FNA, fine-needle aspiration; mets, metastases; MDCT, multidetector row computed tomography; MRCP, magnetic resonance cholangiopancreatography.

Figure 26-2. Approach to diagnosing pancreatic cancer. (Reproduced with permission from Gress FG. Endoscopic ultrasound in the staging of exocrine pancreatic cancer. In: UpToDate [Accessed on 6/10/14] Copyright 2014.)

Treatment

A. Complete resection is possible in ~15% of patients; 5-year survival is still only 20–25%.

B. Palliative approach for patients with nonresectable cancer

1. Biliary diversion, either percutaneous or surgical

2. Radiation therapy for pain relief

3. Gemcitabine for improved quality of life but not increased survival

4. Median survival is 6 months.

CASE RESOLUTION

With an LR– of 0.16, a normal CT scan does not always rule out pancreatic cancer. However, in this patient, given that her CT scan shows evidence of advanced liver disease (a more likely diagnosis for her), it is not necessary to do further imaging studies. The other active alternative, chronic hepatitis, is ruled out by her negative serologies. These test results, combined with her alcohol intake history, makes alcoholic liver disease the most likely diagnosis. At this point, some clinicians would proceed with treatment for alcoholic hepatitis, while others would confirm the diagnosis and, for prognostic purposes, establish the presence or absence of cirrhosis with a liver biopsy.

Her liver biopsy showed acute alcoholic hepatitis with cirrhosis. Because her mDF was > 32, she was treated with prednisolone. She was also advised to abstain from alcohol. She completed the course of prednisolone and has remained abstinent. Several weeks later, her bilirubin was normal and she felt well.

CHIEF COMPLAINT

PATIENT

Mr. R is a 24-year-old graduate student with no past medical history who comes to see you because his girlfriend thought his eyes looked yellow yesterday. He has felt tired and a bit queasy for the last couple of weeks but thought he was just overworked and anxious. He has had some aching pain in the right upper quadrant and epigastrium, not related to eating or bowel movements. He has had no fevers, chills, or sweats. He has noticed dark urine for 1 or 2 days but attributed it to not drinking enough.

On physical exam, he appears tired. He has scleral icterus; his liver is palpable 2 cm below the costal margin and is mildly tender. The spleen is not palpable, and the rest of his abdomen is nontender and nondistended. He has no edema, and the rest of his exam is normal.

At this point, what is the leading hypothesis, what are the active alternatives, and is there a must not miss diagnosis? Given this differential diagnosis, what tests should be ordered?

RANKING THE DIFFERENTIAL DIAGNOSIS

The differential diagnosis for fatigue, nausea, and vague abdominal pain is broad, but the pivotal findings of scleral icterus and tender hepatomegaly point toward a hepatic source.

Mr. R's clinical picture is consistent with that of 90% of patients with viral hepatitis: a history of anorexia, malaise, and nausea, and a physical exam showing hepatomegaly, hepatic tenderness, or both. Hepatitis A is the most frequent cause of acute viral hepatitis; hepatitis C is the second most frequent but is usually asymptomatic acutely. Hepatitis B can also present acutely. By virtue of being common, alcoholic hepatitis is another active alternative diagnosis, and the presentation can mimic that of viral hepatitis. Biliary obstruction is always a consideration in patients with jaundice, but the prodrome and type of abdominal pain are not typical. Table 26-4 lists the differential diagnosis.

Table 26-4. Diagnostic hypotheses for Mr. R.

Diagnostic Hypotheses	Demographics, Risk Factors, Symptoms and Signs	Important Tests
Leading Hypothesis		
Acute hepatitis A	Exposure to potentially contaminated food Travel to developing nations Right upper quadrant (RUQ) pain Nausea ± vomiting Malaise	IgM anti-HAV
Active Alternative—Most Common		
Acute alcoholic steatohepatitis	History of binge drinking Hepatomegaly Signs of cirrhosis (palmar erythema, angiomata)	CT scan Liver biopsy Ultrasound AST > ALT
Active Alternative—Must Not Miss		
Hepatitis B or C	Exposure to needles/ body fluids RUQ pain Nausea ± vomiting Malaise	**Hepatitis B:** HBsAg IgM anti-HBc **Hepatitis C:** Anti-HCV HCV RNA
Other Hypotheses		
Epstein Barr virus (EBV) or cytomegalovirus (CMV) hepatitis	Adenopathy Pharyngitis	EBV, CMV IgM antibodies
Biliary obstruction	Biliary colic	Ultrasound

Acute viral hepatitis is unlikely in the absence of nausea, anorexia, malaise, hepatomegaly, or hepatic tenderness.

He has no past medical history and takes no medications; he does not smoke or use illicit drugs. He drinks 1–2 beers most weeks, and occasionally shares a bottle of wine with friends. He has never had a blood transfusion or a tattoo, and has had only 1 sexual partner. He enjoys trying different restaurants, and frequently eats sushi and ceviche. Initial laboratory tests include the following: total bilirubin, 6.5 mg/dL; conjugated bilirubin, 4 mg/dL; ALT, 1835 units/L; AST, 1522 units/L; alkaline phosphatase, 175 units/L; WBC, 9800 cells/mcL (normal differential); Hgb, 14.5 g/dL; HCT, 44%.

Is the clinical information sufficient to make a diagnosis? If not, what other information do you need?

Pivotal points in Mr. R's lab tests include the following: he has a conjugated hyperbilirubinemia with a hepatocellular pattern, marked elevation of the transaminases, and the ALT is greater than the AST. This pattern is consistent with viral hepatitis. Exploring his history, he does not have clear risk factors for hepatitis B or C, but does have potential exposure to contaminated food, suggesting possible hepatitis A.

Leading Hypothesis: Hepatitis A

Textbook Presentation

The classic presentation is the gradual onset of malaise, nausea, anorexia, and right upper quadrant pain, followed by jaundice.

Disease Highlights

A. Prevalence: Accounts for 20–40% of cases of viral hepatitis in the United States.

B. Clinical manifestations

1. Symptoms develop in 70–80% of adults, compared with < 30% of children under the age of 6.

2. Average incubation period is 25–30 days (range 15–49 days), followed by prodromal symptoms of fatigue, malaise, nausea, vomiting, anorexia, fever, and right upper pain; about 1 week later, jaundice appears.

3. 70% of patients have jaundice, and 80% have hepatomegaly.

4. Other physical findings include splenomegaly, cervical lymphadenopathy, rash, arthritis, and leukocytoclastic vasculitis.

5. Uncommon extrahepatic manifestations include optic neuritis, transverse myelitis, thrombocytopenia, and aplastic anemia.

C. Transmission

1. Fecal-oral transmission, either sporadically or in an epidemic form

   a. Contaminated water, shellfish, frozen strawberries, etc.

   b. Contamination from infected restaurant worker

   c. Exposure history not always clear

2. No maternal-fetal transmission

D. Clinical course

1. Generally self-limited, with rare cases of fulminant hepatic failure (0.015–0.5% of patients with hepatitis A)

   a. Fulminant course is more common in patients with underlying hepatitis C or other chronic liver diseases.

   b. 1.1% fatality rate in adults > age 40

2. 85% of patients fully recover in 3 months, and nearly 100% by 6 months

3. Transaminases normalize more rapidly than serum bilirubin.

E. Prevention

1. Vaccination is available for preexposure prophylaxis.

   a. Immunity develops within 4 weeks in 90% of patients and within 26 weeks in 100% of patients.

   b. A second dose given 6–12 months later provides persistent immunity.

2. Can use immune serum globulin with vaccination for postexposure prophylaxis.

   a. Immune globulin provides 3–5 months of protection against hepatitis A and can be used for preexposure prophylaxis in patients who need immediate coverage.

   b. Immune globulin is 69–89% effective in preventing symptomatic illness when used postexposure.

   c. A randomized trial comparing vaccination with immune globulin given within 14 days of exposure found that hepatitis A developed in 4.4% of vaccine recipients and 3.3% of immune globulin recipients (relative risk = 1.35 (95% confidence interval [CI], 0.70 to 2.67).

Evidence-Based Diagnosis

A. Liver function tests

1. ALT and AST are generally over 1000 units/L, and may be as high as 10,000 units/L; ALT is generally > AST.

2. Bilirubin is commonly > 10 mg/dL.

3. Alkaline phosphatase is usually modestly elevated.

B. Antibody tests (Figure 26-3)

1. Serum IgM anti-HAV detects acute illness, being positive even before the onset of symptoms and remaining positive for 4–6 months.

2. LR+ = 99, LR– = 0.01

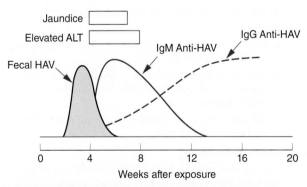

Figure 26-3. Natural history of hepatitis A symptoms and antibodies. ALT, alanine aminotransferase; HAV, hepatitis A virus. (Reproduced with permission from Frauci AS, Kasper DL, Braunwald E, Hauser SL, Longo DL, Jameson JL, Loscalzo J: Harrison's Principles of Internal Medicine, 18th Edition: http://www.accessmedicince.com. Copyright © The McGraw-Hill Companies, Inc. All rights reserved.)

3. Serum IgG anti-HAV appears in the convalescent phase of the disease and remains positive for decades.

Treatment

A. Supportive therapy: rest, oral hydration, and antiemetic medications as needed

B. Admit if INR is elevated or patient is unable to hydrate orally.

C. Liver transplant if fulminant hepatitis and liver failure occur

MAKING A DIAGNOSIS

Considering the hepatocellular pattern of Mr. R's liver test abnormalities, the acute onset of his symptoms, and his lack of signs of chronic liver disease, the pretest probability for some form of viral hepatitis is so high that it is not necessary to consider other diagnoses at this point. Although Mr. R's history of food exposure suggests hepatitis A, it is generally necessary to test for all 3 of the primary hepatitis viruses since the exposure history for both hepatitis B and C is often unclear.

His hepatitis A IgM antibody is positive, with negative HBsAg, IgM anti-HBc, and anti-HCV.

 Have you crossed a diagnostic threshold for the leading hypothesis, acute hepatitis A? Have you ruled out the active alternatives? Do other tests need to be done to exclude the alternative diagnoses?

Alternative Diagnosis: Acute Hepatitis B

Textbook Presentation

The classic presentation is the gradual onset of malaise, nausea, anorexia, right upper quadrant pain, followed by jaundice. Hepatitis B is often subclinical.

Disease Highlights

A. Prevalence of hepatitis B virus (HBV) carriers

1. About 5% worldwide, with substantial geographic variation

   a. 0.1–2% (low prevalence) in the United States, Canada, and Western Europe

   b. 2–8% (medium prevalence) in Mediterranean countries, Japan, central Asia, the Middle East, and Latin and South America

   c. 10–20% (high prevalence) in Southeast Asia, China, and sub-Saharan Africa

B. Clinical manifestations

1. 70% of adult patients have subclinical infection or are anicteric; 30% of patients have icteric hepatitis

2. Incubation period is 1–4 months.

3. Symptoms are similar to those of hepatitis A, but serum sickness–like syndrome can be part of the prodrome (fever, urticarial rash, arthralgias).

4. Fulminant hepatic failure occurs in 0.1–0.5% of patients, with a mortality rate of 70%.

C. Transmission

1. In high prevalence areas, transmission is primarily perinatal, occurring in 90% of babies born to HBeAg-positive mothers and in 10–20% born to HBeAg-negative mothers.

2. In medium prevalence areas, most infections occur from childhood exposure to contaminated household objects, via minor breaks in the skin or mucous membranes.

3. In low prevalence areas, transmission is most often sexual, via percutaneous inoculation (eg, injection drug use, accidental needlestick, tattooing, body piercing, acupuncture), or from contaminated blood transfusion or medical equipment (such as dialysis equipment).

D. Prevention of hepatitis B

1. Vaccination for preexposure prophylaxis

2. Vaccination *and* HB immune globulin within 12 hours for perinatal exposure and within 1 week for other postexposure prophylaxis (percutaneous, mucosal, or sexual)

3. Vaccinated individuals will have positive hepatitis B surface antibody (HBsAb) tests.

Evidence-Based Diagnosis

A. Liver function tests: similar to hepatitis A

1. Transaminases normalize in 1–4 months if acute infection resolves.

2. Elevation of ALT for > 6 months indicates progression to chronic hepatitis (see below).

B. Acute infection is diagnosed by the presence of hepatitis B surface antigen (HBsAg) and IgM hepatitis B core antibody (IgM anti-HBc).

1. HBsAg appears 1–6 weeks prior to symptoms or elevations of transaminases (Figure 26-4).

   a. Should be present in patients with acute symptoms

   b. Should clear in 4–6 months, although small amounts of viral DNA can be detected in serum and mononuclear cells for years after seroclearance

2. IgM anti-HBc appears 1–2 weeks after HBsAg.

   a. The only marker of acute infection detectable during the "window period," the several weeks to months

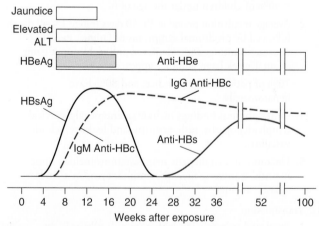

Figure 26-4. Natural history of acute hepatitis B infections. (Reproduced with permission from Frauci AS, Kasper DL, Braunwald E, Hauser SL, Longo DL, Jameson JL, Loscalzo J: Harrison's Principles of Internal Medicine, 18th Edition: http://www.accessmedicince.com. Copyright © The McGraw-Hill Companies, Inc. All rights reserved.)

between the disappearance of HBsAg and the appearance of HBsAb.

  b. Persists for up to 6 months *after HBsAg is cleared*

  c. LR+ = 27, LR– = 0.2

C. Previous infection is diagnosed by the presence of HBsAb and IgG anti-HBc.

  1. HBsAb appears weeks to months after disappearance of HBsAg

  2. HbsAb test characteristics: LR+ = 45, LR– = 0.1

Treatment

A. Supportive therapy: rest, oral hydration, and antiemetic medications as needed

B. Admit if INR is elevated or patient is unable to hydrate orally.

C. Antiviral therapy is used for chronic infection (see below) and antiviral therapy or liver transplant can be used for fulminant hepatitis.

Alternative Diagnosis: Chronic Hepatitis B

Textbook Presentation

Manifestations can range from asymptomatic, to isolated fatigue, to cirrhosis with portal hypertension. There is often no history of clinical acute hepatitis B.

Disease Highlights

A. Defined as presence of HBsAg for more than 6 months

B. Occurs when the hepatitis B specific CD4 and CD8 response is insufficient

C. Risk of progression from acute to chronic hepatitis B varies, depending on the host

  1. < 1% when the acute infection is acquired by an immunocompetent adult

  2. 90% when the infection is acquired perinatally

  3. 20% when the infection is acquired during childhood

D. 10–20% have extrahepatic findings (eg, polyarteritis nodosa, glomerular disease)

E. There are 4 phases of chronic HBV (Figure 26-5), categorized by the activity of the infection, as defined by levels of viral DNA, degree of transaminitis, and presence or absence of HBe antigen and antibody (HBe antigen is a secretory protein considered to be a marker of HBV replication and infectivity. The presence of HBeAg usually indicates high levels of viral DNA and rates of transmission.)

  1. The immune tolerant phase occurs when the infection is acquired perinatally.

  2. Infections acquired later in life begin in the immune active phase, characterized by intermittent flares in up to 25% of patients per year; 8–12% of patients per year seroconvert from HBeAg positive to HBeAg negative and become HBeAb positive.

  3. Most patients who seroconvert enter a lifelong inactive state; however, up to 20% revert to HBeAg positive or develop HBeAg negative chronic hepatitis.

F. Risk factors for progression from chronic hepatitis to cirrhosis include high viral DNA levels, longer duration of the immune active phase, male sex, increasing age, HBeAg positivity, genotype C, concurrent hepatitis C or HIV infection, severe inflammatory histology.

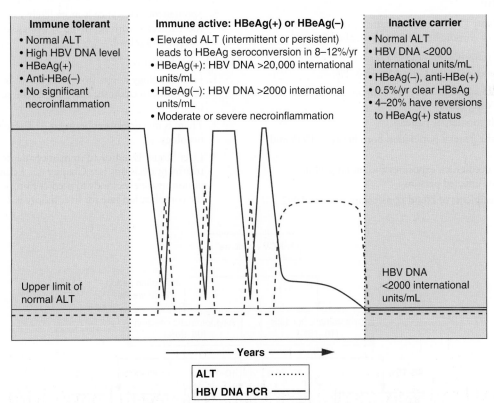

Figure 26-5. Phases of chronic hepatitis B infections. These states do not occur in all patients and transitions between states are dynamic and can be nonconsecutive. ALT, alanine aminotransferase; HBV, hepatitis B virus; PCR, polymerase chain reaction. (Modified, with permission, from Kuo A, Gish R. Chronic hepatitis B infection. Clin Liv Dis. 2012;16:347–69.)

G. Hepatitis B cirrhosis leads to hepatic decompensation in 15–20% of patients over 5 years.

    1. 5-year survival rate is 80–85% in patients with compensated cirrhosis and 30–50% in those with decompensated cirrhosis.

    2. Each year, hepatocellular carcinoma develops in 3–6% of patients.

Evidence-Based Diagnosis

A. HBsAg is always positive.

B. See Figure 26-5 for patterns of HBeAg, HBV DNA, and ALT in different phases.

Treatment

A. The goals of treatment include suppression of viral DNA levels, HBeAg seroconversion, stopping or reducing hepatic inflammation and necrosis, and preventing progression to cirrhosis.

B. Current treatment options include interferon alfa, pegylated interferon-alfa-2a; nucleoside analogues such as lamivudine, and nucleotide analogues such as adefovir.

Alternative Diagnosis: Hepatitis C

Textbook Presentation

Most patients are asymptomatic, with jaundice developing in < 25%. When present, symptoms are similar to those of other viral hepatitis and last 2–12 weeks.

Disease Highlights

A. Accounts for about 15% of cases of acute hepatitis; the most common cause of chronic hepatitis in the United States

B. Prevalence and transmission rates

    1. Overall prevalence in the United States is 2%.

        a. 45% in US adults aged 20–59 with any history of injection drug use

        b. 8.9% in hemodialysis patients

        c. 4.3% in the general population born between 1945 and 1965

        d. 1–5% in needlestick exposures and monogamous partners of infected persons

        e. 10% in recipients of blood transfusions prior to 1992

    2. Transmission

        a. Since 1992, rarely acquired from blood transfusion in developed countries but contaminated blood still common in undeveloped countries

        b. Now, hepatitis C is primarily transmitted through injection drug use, with occasional cases due to ear or body piercing, sex with an injection drug user, or accidental needlesticks.

        c. Household contacts are rarely infected.

        d. Transmission between monogamous partners is < 1%/year; risk of sexual transmission is higher if index carrier also has HIV or there are multiple partners.

        e. Perinatal transmission occurs in 4–7% of cases; risk for transmission increases 4- to 5-fold if the mother has both hepatitis C and HIV.

        f. 15–30% of patients report no risk factors

C. Clinical course (Figure 26-6)

    1. Jaundice develops in only 10–20% of symptomatic patients.

    2. Fulminant hepatitis is rare.

    3. Extrahepatic manifestations are common, being found in about 75% of patients.

        a. Fatigue, arthralgias, paresthesias, myalgias, pruritus, and sicca syndrome are found in > 10% of patients.

        b. Vasculitis secondary to cryoglobulinemia is found in 1% of patients, although cryoglobulinemia is present in about 40%.

        c. Depression and anxiety are more common than in uninfected persons.

    4. 74–86% of patients have detectable HCV RNA at 6 months and therefore have chronic hepatitis C.

    5. Spontaneous clearance is more likely to occur in females, those infected with genotype 3, whites, and those with a low peak viral load.

D. Chronic hepatitis C

    1. Liver histology ranges from no fibrosis, to varying degrees of fibrosis, to cirrhosis; there are several scoring systems in use.

    2. There is no correlation between ALT levels and liver histology.

    3. Liver biopsy is indicated in many patients to guide treatment decisions (see Chapter 17, Edema for discussion of noninvasive methods to predict fibrosis and cirrhosis); the complication rate for liver biopsy is 1–5%.

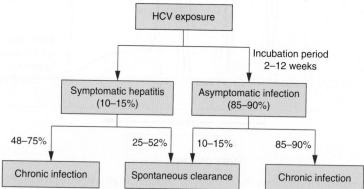

Figure 26-6. Clinical course of hepatitis C infection. (Reproduced, with permission, from Maheshwari A, Ray S, Thuluvath PJ. Acute hepatitis C. Lancet. 2008;372:321–32.)

4. Cirrhosis develops in 5–25% of patients after 20 years of infection.

    a. Rates are low in community cohorts and cohorts of blood donors (4–7%).

    b. Rates are higher in other populations (24%).

    c. Liver histology is the best predictor of progression to cirrhosis.

    d. Other predictors of progression to cirrhosis include

      (1) Age at infection (> 40 years of age → more progression)

      (2) Longer duration of infection

      (3) Consumption of alcohol > 50 g/d

      (4) HIV or HBV coinfection

      (5) Male sex

      (6) Higher ALT

      (7) Baseline fibrosis

      (8) Possibly steatosis

    e. Hepatocellular carcinoma develops in 1–3% of cirrhotic patients per year.

E. Prevention

    1. No vaccine available

    2. No role for immunoglobulin

F. Screening guidelines

    1. Centers of Disease Control and Prevention and US Preventive Services Task Force recommend 1 time screening for all persons born between 1945 and 1965 as well as risk factor–based screening

    2. Risk–factor based screening includes

      a. History injection drug use

      b. Receipt of blood products prior to 1992

      c. Long-term hemodialysis

      d. Exposure to known HCV-positive blood (needlestick or mucosal exposure in health care workers)

      e. HIV infection

      f. Child of a HCV-positive woman

      g. History of multiple sex partners or sexually transmitted infections

Evidence-Based Diagnosis

A. Anti-HCV antibody tests (enzyme immunoassays)

    1. HCV antibodies generally detectable within 8–12 weeks of acquiring the infection.

    2. Sensitivity, 94–100%; specificity, 97–98%; LR+, 31–49; LR–, 0.01–0.06

    3. False-positive results do occur in low prevalence screening populations, with positive predictive values as low as 39%.

    4. False-negative results can occur in immunocompromised patients, such as organ transplant recipients, HIV-infected patients, hemodialysis patients, or those with hypogammaglobulinemia.

B. Quantitative HCV RNA tests (polymerase chain reaction and transcription-mediated amplification)

    1. Lower limit of detection using current methods is 10–50 international units/mL.

    2. Sensitivity, 96%; specificity, 99%; LR+, 96; LR–, 0.04

    3. Levels do not correlate with liver injury, duration of infection, or disease severity.

C. Genotype testing

    1. Used for prediction of response to treatment and choice of treatment duration

    2. Genotypes do not change, so this test needs to be done only once.

    3. In the United States, 71.5% of cases are from genotype 1, 13.5% from genotype 2, 5.5% from genotype 3, and 1.1% from genotype 4.

D. Choosing and interpreting hepatitis C tests

    1. American Association for the Study of Liver Disease Guidelines for testing:

      a. First, test for anti-HCV antibodies in patients in whom acute or chronic hepatitis C is suspected.

      b. Test for HCV RNA in patients with (1) a positive antibody test; (2) unexplained liver disease whose antibody test is negative and who are immunocompromised or in whom acute HCV infection is suspected.

    2. Table 26-5 summarizes the interpretation of hepatitis C tests.

Treatment

A. Goals of treatment: Prevention of cirrhosis and its complications, reduction of extrahepatic manifestations, and reduction of transmission

B. A sustained virologic response is defined as nondetectable HCV RNA 6 months after completion of therapy.

C. Current therapy includes pegylated interferon and ribavirin; the treatment approach is continuously evolving.

CASE RESOLUTION

Mr. R clearly has acute hepatitis A, presumably from contaminated food. Although he is nauseated, he is able to drink adequate fluid. His INR is normal at 1.1. You recommend rest and oral hydration for Mr. R, and serum immune globulin and vaccination for his girlfriend. He feels much better when he returns 1 month later.

The best test of the liver's synthetic function is the PT. It is important to check the INR in all patients with hepatitis to look for signs of liver failure.

Table 26-5. Interpretation of HCV tests.

Anti-HCV antibody	HCV RNA	Interpretation
Positive	Positive	Acute or chronic infection, depending on the clinical context
Positive	Negative	Resolution of HCV, or acute HCV during period of low level viremia
Negative	Positive	Early acute infection, or chronic infection in an immunocompromised patient, or false positive test
Negative	Negative	No HCV infection

CHIEF COMPLAINT

PATIENT 3

Ms. H is a 40-year-old woman with unexpected transaminase abnormalities.

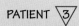 What is the differential diagnosis of mild asymptomatic transaminase elevations? How would you frame the differential?

CONSTRUCTING A DIFFERENTIAL DIAGNOSIS

Most patients with asymptomatic transaminase elevations have mild or moderate elevations; it is very unusual for patients with marked elevations to be asymptomatic. Therefore, the diagnostic thinking should focus on chronic diseases. The basic framework separates hepatic from nonhepatic causes.

A. Hepatic causes
   1. Marked elevations (> 1000 units/L)
      a. Acute viral hepatitis
      b. Ischemic hepatitis
      c. Medication- or toxin-induced hepatitis
      d. Autoimmune hepatitis
      e. Acute bile duct obstruction
      f. Acute Budd-Chiari syndrome
   2. Mild to moderate elevations
      a. ALD
      b. Medications/toxins
      c. Chronic hepatitis B or C
      d. NAFLD
      e. Autoimmune hepatitis
      f. Hemochromatosis
      g. Wilson disease (in patients < 40 years old)
      h. Alpha-1-antitrypsin deficiency
B. Nonhepatic causes
   1. Celiac disease
   2. Hyperthyroidism
   3. Inherited disorders of muscle metabolism or acquired muscle disease (AST elevation only)
   4. Strenuous exercise (AST elevation only)

Ms. H comes in for a routine new patient visit. She feels fine. Her past medical history is notable for type 2 diabetes mellitus and hypertension. Her medications include metformin, atorvastatin, hydrochlorothiazide, and lisinopril. She does not smoke, and has a glass of wine about twice per month. Her physical exam shows a BP of 125/80 mm Hg, pulse of 80 bpm, RR of 16 breaths per minute, weight 230 lbs, and height 5 ft 9 in (BMI = 34.0). Pulmonary, cardiac, and abdominal exams are all normal.

She shows you blood test results from a recent health fair at work: creatinine, 0.9 mg/dL; HgbA₁c, 6.8%; LDL, 95 mg/dL; platelet count, 272/mcL; bilirubin, 0.8 mg/dL; AST, 85 units/L; ALT, 92 units/L; albumin, 4.0 g/dL; and a normal

alkaline phosphatase. She reports she was told a few months ago that 1 of her liver tests was a little abnormal. No one in her family has had liver disease, but her mother has thyroid disease. She does recall taking several acetaminophen tablets in the days prior to the recent blood test.

 At this point, what is the leading hypothesis, what are the active alternatives, and is there a must not miss diagnosis? Given this differential diagnosis, what tests should be ordered?

RANKING THE DIFFERENTIAL DIAGNOSIS

In the absence of an obvious nonhepatic cause of liver enzyme elevations, the initial approach is to focus on the hepatic causes. The prevalence of the liver diseases in the differential diagnosis varies widely, depending on the population studied. For example, in a study of over 19,000 young, healthy military recruits, of whom 99 had enzyme elevations, only 11 were found to have any liver disease (4 had hepatitis B, 4 had hepatitis C, 2 had autoimmune hepatitis, 1 had cholelithiasis). A study of 100 blood donors with elevated enzymes found that 48% had alcoholic liver disease, 22% had NAFLD, and 17% had hepatitis C. In another study, patients with elevated enzymes in whom a diagnosis could not be made by history or blood tests underwent liver biopsy; NAFLD was found in over 50% of them.

Pivotal points in Ms. H's presentation include that the transaminase abnormalities are mild and probably chronic. The key findings in the history and physical exam are the patient's diabetes and elevated body mass index (BMI). NAFLD is extremely common in obese, diabetic patients, so Ms. H is at high risk for this disease. She has no specific risk factors for viral hepatitis, but often the exposure history is unclear and these diagnoses cannot be ruled out without further testing. Her alcohol intake is minimal, but sometimes even small amounts of alcohol can cause liver enzyme elevations. Additionally, other drug and toxin exposure always should be considered. Even therapeutic doses of acetaminophen can cause transaminitis; in 1 study, 50% of patients taking 4 g of acetaminophen daily developed transaminases > 2 times the upper limit of normal. Mild transaminase elevations are seen in 0.5–3% of patients taking statins (it is not necessary to stop the statin in such cases, and the FDA no longer recommends routine testing after obtaining a baseline at the start of therapy). Finally, her family history of thyroid disease, presumably autoimmune, increases the likelihood of autoimmune hepatitis or hyperthyroidism. Hemochromatosis, a fairly common gene mutation, can present with liver enzyme abnormalities and diabetes mellitus. Table 26-6 lists the differential diagnosis.

Ms. H abstains from alcohol and stops taking any acetaminophen and atorvastatin for 2 weeks. Repeat liver enzymes show AST = 90 units/L and ALT = 95 units/L. Her TSH is normal. Her grandparents emigrated from Northern Europe.

 Is the clinical information sufficient to make a diagnosis? If not, what other information do you need?

Table 26-6. Diagnostic hypotheses for Ms. H.

Diagnostic Hypotheses	Demographics, Risk Factors, Symptoms and Signs	Important Tests
Leading Hypothesis		
Nonalcoholic fatty liver disease	Obesity (BMI > 30) Diabetes	Ultrasound Liver biopsy
Active Alternatives—Most Common		
Hemochromatosis	Family history Diabetes	Serum iron/TIBC Ferritin
Alcohol	Intake history	Abstinence Liver biopsy AST > ALT
Medication	Medication history (prescription and nonprescription)	Stopping the medication
Active Alternatives—Must Not Miss		
Hepatitis B or C	Exposure to body fluids, needles	HBsAg Anti-HBc Anti-HCV
Other Hypotheses		
Autoimmune hepatitis	Other autoimmune disease	Serum protein electrophoresis Antinuclear antibody Anti-smooth muscle antibody Liver biopsy
Wilson disease	Age < 40 Neuropsychiatric symptoms	Ceruloplasmin
Alpha-1-antitrypsin deficiency	Emphysema	Alpha-1-Antitrypsin level and phenotype
Celiac disease	Diarrhea	IgA level Endomysial antibody
Hyperthyroidism	Weight loss Tachycardia Diarrhea	TSH

Leading Hypothesis: NAFLD

Textbook Presentation

Patients are often asymptomatic but sometimes complain of vague right upper quadrant discomfort. It is common to identify patients by finding hepatomegaly on exam or asymptomatic transaminase elevations.

Disease Highlights

A. The definition of NAFLD is evidence of excessive fat in the liver, either by imaging or biopsy, in the absence of causes of secondary hepatic fat accumulation.

B. Secondary causes of excessive fat in the liver include significant alcohol use (> 14 drinks/week for women, > 21 for men), Wilson disease, jejunoileal bypass, prolonged total parenteral nutrition, protein-calorie malnutrition, and drugs (methotrexate, amiodarone, estrogens, corticosteroids, aspirin, cocaine, antiretroviral agents)

C. Patients with NAFLD have steatosis, either with or without inflammation.

  1. In simple steatosis (nonalcoholic fatty liver [NAFL]), there is no liver injury and the risk of progression to cirrhosis is minimal.

  2. Steatosis plus inflammation, with or without fibrosis, is called nonalcoholic steatohepatitis (NASH).

    a. Up to 21% of patients have regression of fibrosis.

    b. Up to 40% progress to more advanced fibrosis or cirrhosis

    c. The strongest predictor of progression is the degree of inflammation on the first biopsy.

  3. Liver failure develops over 7–10 years in 38–45% of patients with cirrhosis

  4. The risk of hepatocellular carcinoma in patients with NAFLD cirrhosis is less than that of patients with hepatitis C cirrhosis.

D. NAFLD can coexist with other chronic liver diseases.

E. Epidemiology

  1. Risk factors include the metabolic syndrome, obesity, type 2 diabetes mellitus, insulin resistance, hyperlipidemia, and family history of NAFLD.

  2. Prevalence varies based on population studied.

    a. Worldwide prevalence ranges from 6.3% to 33%; NASH prevalence 3–5%

    b. One US study found an overall NAFLD prevalence of 46% (58% in Hispanics, 44% in whites, 35% in African Americans); 30% had NASH

    c. 91% in obese patients (BMI > 35 kg/m^2) undergoing bariatric surgery, with 37% having NASH

    d. Found in 69% of patients with type 2 diabetes mellitus, 50% of patients attending lipid clinics, 50% of morbidly obese patients

  3. Most common cause of abnormal liver test results in the United States.

Evidence-Based Diagnosis

A. Blood tests

  1. Transaminases elevation is usually < 400 units/L, with ALT > AST; in advanced fibrosis or cirrhosis, AST may be > ALT.

  2. Serum ferritin is elevated in 60% of patients but is rarely > 1000 mcg/L.

  3. Alkaline phosphatase is elevated in 30% of patients.

B. Imaging can detect steatosis when it replaces more than 30% of the liver volume; it cannot distinguish NAFL from NASH.

  1. Ultrasound: sensitivity, 60%; specificity, 93%; LR+, 8.6; LR–, 0.43

  2. CT scan: sensitivity, 82%; specificity, ~95%; LR+, 16.4; LR–, 0.19

  3. MRI: sensitivity, ~95%; specificity, ~95%; LR+, 19; LR–, 0.05

C. Liver biopsy is the gold standard for diagnosis and staging.

  1. NASH is missed in 27% of single biopsies.

  2. Test characteristics of a single biopsy for the diagnosis of NASH: sensitivity, 73%; specificity, 92%; LR+, 8.6; LR–, 0.3

  3. Advanced fibrosis is less often missed: LR+, 7.7; LR–, 0.16

D. Liver biopsy should be considered when it is necessary to exclude other causes of chronic liver disease and in patients with a high risk of having NASH and advanced fibrosis.

   1. The NAFLD Fibrosis Score is used to identify high risk patients.

      a. Need to know age, BMI, diabetes status, ALT, AST, albumin, and platelet count

      b. On line calculator: http://nafldscore.com/

      c. A low score (< –1.455) reduces the likelihood of advanced fibrosis: sensitivity, 90%; specificity, 60%; LR+, 2.25; LR–, 0.16

      d. A high score (> 0.676) significantly increases the likelihood of advanced fibrosis: sensitivity, 67%; specificity, 97%; LR+, 22; LR–, 0.34

      e. 20–58% of patients studied were between the two cut offs and could not be classified.

   2. Patients with the metabolic syndrome are also considered high risk.

 It is necessary to rule out other causes of liver disease listed in the above differential before diagnosing NAFLD.

Treatment

A. Weight loss can improve both steatosis and inflammation.

B. Exercise may improve steatosis independent of weight loss.

C. Diabetes and hyperlipidemia should be optimally treated.

D. Metformin has been studied and is not effective.

E. Vitamin E has been shown to improve histology in non-diabetic adults with biopsy proven NASH.

F. Pioglitazone is effective in reducing inflammation but not fibrosis; the long-term safety and efficacy are not established.

MAKING A DIAGNOSIS

You should take a stepwise approach to evaluating asymptomatic liver enzyme abnormalities. As was done with Ms. H, the first step is to stop alcohol and, if possible, potentially hepatotoxic medications, and then remeasure the liver enzymes. Although aspects of the history can increase the likelihood of a specific diagnosis, the history is not sensitive or specific enough to make a diagnosis, and it is necessary to test somewhat broadly. If liver enzyme abnormalities persist after stopping alcohol and potentially hepatotoxic medications, the American Gastroenterological Association recommends beginning with a PT; serum albumin; CBC; hepatitis A, B, and C serologies; and iron studies (serum iron, total iron-binding capacity [TIBC], ferritin).

IgM and IgG anti-HAV are both negative. HBsAg and IgM anti-HBc are negative; IgG anti-HBc and anti-HBs are positive. Anti-HCV is negative. The transferrin saturation is 35%, and the serum ferritin is 190 ng/mL.

 Have you crossed a diagnostic threshold for the leading hypothesis, NAFLD? Have you ruled out the active alternatives? Do other tests need to be done to exclude the alternative diagnoses?

Alternative Diagnosis: Hereditary Hemochromatosis

Textbook Presentation

Most patients are asymptomatic, but a few have extrahepatic manifestations of iron overload (see below). Some patients are identified by screening the family members of affected individuals.

Disease Highlights

A. An autosomal recessive disease causing deficiency of the iron regulatory hormone hepcidin, leading to increased intestinal iron absorption and accumulation in tissues

B. Iron deposition occurs throughout the reticuloendothelial system, leading to a broad range of potential manifestations.

   1. Liver manifestations range from hepatomegaly to fibrosis to cirrhosis; hepatocellular carcinoma risk is increased only in patients with cirrhosis.

   2. Any joint can be affected, but the second and third metacarpophalangeal joints are typical.

   3. Cardiac infiltration leads to cardiomyopathy.

   4. Other manifestations include secondary hypogonadism (pituitary infiltration), diabetes (pancreatic infiltration), and hypothyroidism (thyroid infiltration).

C. There are several possible gene mutations; the most common is the *HFE* C282Y mutation, thought to have initially occurred in a Viking or Celtic ancestor.

   1. In a meta-analysis of people of European ancestry with iron overload, 81% were homozygous for the *HFE* C282Y mutation.

   2. 5% were compound heterozygous for the C282Y/H63D mutation.

   3. In another study, nearly 100,000 primary care patients were screened for iron overload and *HFE* mutations; 299 homozygotes were found.

      a. The prevalence of homozygosity was 0.44% in whites, 0.11% in Native Americans, 0.027% in Hispanics, 0.014% in blacks, 0.012% in Pacific Islanders, and 0.000039% in Asians.

      b. The prevalence of heterozygosity for the mutation was 10% in whites, 5.7% in Native Americans, 2.9% in Hispanics, 2.3% in blacks, 2% in Pacific Islanders, and 0.12% in Asians.

D. The gene expression is quite variable, with the penetrance of iron overload in homozygotes (abnormal transferrin saturation or ferritin) ranging from 38% to 76%; clinical disease is found in only 2–38% of men and 1–10% of women.

E. 72% of patients with serum ferritin levels > 1000 mcg/L have cirrhosis, compared with 7.4% of those with ferritin levels < 1000 mcg/L.

F. Screening primary care populations for hemochromatosis is not recommended by the USPSTF or the American College of Physicians.

Evidence-Based Diagnosis

A. Liver biopsy with measurement of hepatic iron index is the gold standard.

B. Initial testing should be done with a transferrin saturation (serum iron/TIBC) and a serum ferritin (the test characteristics are for identifying homozygous patients).

   1. Transferrin saturation ≥ 50% in men

      a. Sensitivity, 82.4%; specificity, 92.5%

      b. LR+ = 10.9, LR– = 0.19

2. Transferrin saturation ≥ 45% in women

    a. Sensitivity, 73.8%; specificity, 93.1%

    b. LR+ = 10.8, LR– = 0.28

3. Ferritin ≥ 200 ng/mL in men

    a. Sensitivity, 78%; specificity, 76%

    b. LR+ = 3.25, LR– = 0.23

4. Ferritin ≥ 200 ng/mL in women

    a. Sensitivity, 54%; specificity, 95%

    b. LR+ = 11, LR– = 0.48

C. Patients who have a transferrin saturation ≥ 45% and an elevated ferritin should undergo *HFE* gene testing, looking for the hereditary hemochromatosis mutations.

 All first-degree relatives of patients with hereditary hemochromatosis should undergo gene testing, regardless of the results of the iron studies.

1. If C282Y/C282Y homozygous mutation is found

    a. If age is < 40 years, ferritin < 1000 ng/mL, and transaminases are normal, proceed to treatment.

    b. Otherwise, perform liver biopsy to determine severity.

2. If other mutations or no mutations are found, look for other causes of iron overload or perform liver biopsy for diagnosis.

Treatment

Periodic phlebotomy to reduce the iron overload has been shown to reduce the risk of progression to cirrhosis.

Alternative Diagnosis: Autoimmune Hepatitis

Textbook Presentation

The clinical presentation is variable, ranging from asymptomatic transaminase elevation to nonspecific constitutional symptoms, to advanced liver disease.

Disease Highlights

A. A chronic inflammatory disease of the liver

B. Annual incidence of 1.4 cases/100,000; 3–4 times more common in women than in men

C. 72% of cases diagnosed after the age of 40 years

D. 36% of patients have cirrhosis at presentation; of those without cirrhosis at presentation, 12% will develop it over 10 years

    1. Risk factors for progression include time to normalization of ALT and number of relapses.

    2. Risk of developing hepatocellular carcinoma is 1–1.9%/year, occurring at a mean age of 60–63 years.

E. 50% 5-year mortality rate in untreated patients

F. Drug-induced autoimmune hepatitis, reported with minocycline, nitrofurantoin, atorvastatin, and infliximab, has a more benign course that idiopathic autoimmune hepatitis.

Evidence-Based Diagnosis

G. Autoantibodies

    1. Antinuclear antibodies (ANA): sensitivity, 32%; specificity, 76%; LR+, 1.3; LR–, 0.89

    2. Antismooth muscle antibody (SMA): sensitivity, 16%; specificity, 96%; LR+, 4; LR–, 0.87

Table 26-7. Diagnostic criteria for autoimmune hepatitis.

Variable	Points[1]
ANA or SMA ≥1:40	1
ANA or SMA ≥1:80	2
OR Anti-LKM ≥ 1:40	
OR Anti-SLA positive	
IgG > upper limit of normal	1
IgG > 1.1 x ULN	2
Histology compatible with autoimmune hepatitis	1
Histology typical for autoimmune hepatitis	2
Absence of viral hepatitis	2
Interpretation: 6 points = probable autoimmune hepatitis; ≥ 7 points = definite autoimmune hepatitis	

[1]Maximal points for all autoantibodies = 2.
ANA, antinuclear antibodies; LKM, liver kidney microsome; SLA, soluble liver antigen; SMA, antismooth muscle antibody; ULN. upper limit of normal.

3. ANA and SMA: sensitivity, 43%; specificity, 99%; LR+, 43; LR–, 0.57

4. Diagnostic criteria have been developed (Table 26-7).

    a. For a diagnosis of probable autoimmune hepatitis (6 points): sensitivity, 88%; specificity, 97%; LR+, 29; LR–, 0.12

    b. For a diagnosis of definite autoimmune hepatitis (≥ 7 points): sensitivity, 81%; specificity, 99%; LR+, 81; LR–, 0.19

Treatment

A. Treatment is indicated for all patients with evidence of active inflammation, either by transaminase elevation or histology.

B. Prednisone alone, or prednisone and azathioprine are used to induce remission; 90% of patients respond within 2 weeks.

C. Many patients require maintenance therapy, most commonly with azathioprine.

D. Other immunosuppressives are used in patients who do not respond to or cannot tolerate the first-line treatments.

E. Liver transplant is often successful in patients with cirrhosis and decompensated end-stage liver disease, although autoimmune hepatitis can recur in the transplanted liver.

CASE RESOLUTION

Ms. H's transaminase levels remained elevated after abstaining from alcohol and discontinuing medications, making those etiologies unlikely. Her hepatitis A and C serologies are negative; her hepatitis B serologies are consistent with a previous infection and not chronic hepatitis B. Her transferrin saturation is normal, and the slightly elevated ferritin is not specific for any particular disease. You order an ANA, SMA, ceruloplasmin, and alpha-1-antitrypsin levels and phenotype, all of which are normal.

At this point, NAFLD is by far the most likely diagnosis. An ultrasound is not absolutely necessary, but it could confirm the presence of steatosis.

Ms. H has an ultrasound, which shows an enlarged liver with diffuse fatty infiltration. Her NAFLD Fibrosis Score is low, suggesting that NASH is unlikely. She begins to walk

20 minutes 4 times/week, and reduces her portion sizes. Her transaminases remain stable for the next several months. One year later, she has lost 20 pounds, and her transaminases have decreased to around 40.

REVIEW OF OTHER IMPORTANT DISEASES

Figure 26-7 outlines the diagnostic approach to a patient with an isolated elevation of the alkaline phosphatase.

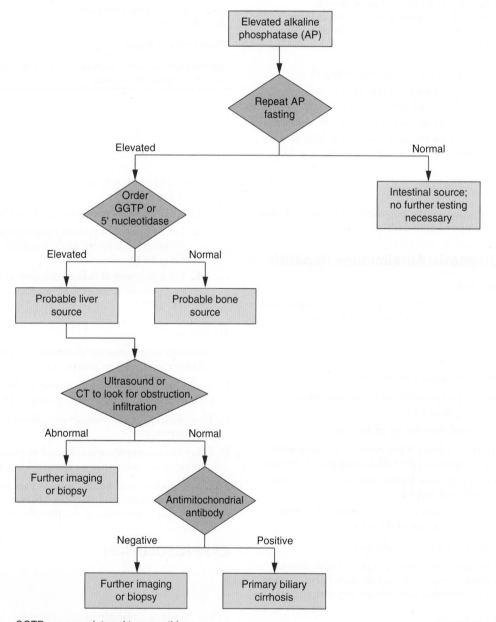

GGTP, gamma-glutamyl transpeptidase.

Figure 26-7. Diagnostic approach to elevated alkaline phosphatase.

REFERENCES

Adams PC, Barton JC. Hemochromatosis. Lancet. 2007;370:1855–60.

Adams PC, Reboussin DM, Barton JC et al. Hemochromatosis and iron overload screening in a racially diverse population (HEIRS study). N Engl J Med. 2005;352:1769–78.

Afdhal NH. Management of nonalcoholic fatty liver disease. JAMA. 2012;308:608–16.

American Gastroenterological Association. Evaluation of liver chemistry tests. Gastroenterology. 2002;123:1364–66.

Barkun AN, Grover SA, Muir A. Update: splenomegaly. In: Simel DL, Rennie D, eds. *The Rational Clinical Examination: Evidence-Based Clinical Diagnosis.* New York, NY: McGraw-Hill; 2009. http://www.jamaevidence.com/content/3487298. Accessed 10/8/2013

Brundage SC, Fitzpatrick AN. Hepatitis A. Am Fam Physician. 2006;73:2162–8.

Chalasani N, Younossi Z, Lavine JE et al. The diagnosis and management of non-alcoholic fatty liver disease: Practice guideline by the American Association for the Study of Liver Diseases, American College of Gastroenterology, and the American Gastroenterological Association. Hepatology. 2012;55:2005–23.

Forrest EH. The management of alcoholic hepatitis. Br J Hosp Med. 2009;70:680–4.

Ghany MG, Strader DB, Thomas DL, Seeff LB. Diagnosis, management and treatment of hepatitis C: an update. Hepatology. 2009;49:1335.

Giannini EG, Testa R, Savarino V. Liver enzyme alteration: a guide for clinicians. CMAJ. 2005;172:367–79.

Hennes EM, Zeniya M, Czaja AJ et al. Simplified criteria for the diagnosis of autoimmune hepatitis. Hepatology. 2008;48:169–76.

Hung OL, Kwon NS, Cole AE et al. Evaluation of the physician's ability to recognize the presence or absence of anemia, fever, and jaundice. Acad Emerg Med. 2000;7:146–56.

Kuo A, Gish R. Chronic hepatitis B infection. Clin Liv Dis. 2012;16:347–69.

Liaw YF, Chu CM. Hepatitis B infection. Lancet. 2009;373:582–92.

Maheshwari A, Ray S, Thuluvath PJ. Acute hepatitis C. Lancet. 2008;372:321–32.

McGee S. *Evidence-Based Physical Diagnosis,* 3rd edition. Saunders. 2012.

Musso G, Gambino R, Cassader M, Pagano G. Meta-analysis: natural history of nonalcoholic fatty liver disease and diagnostic accuracy on noninvasive tests for liver disease severity. Ann Med. 2011;43:617–49.

O'Shea RS, Dasarathy S, McCullough AJ. Alcoholic liver disease: ACG Practice Guidelines. Am J Gastroenterol. 2010;105:14–32.

Porta M, Fabregat X, Malats N et al. Exocrine pancreatic cancer: symptoms at presentation and their relation to tumour site and stage. Clin Transl Oncol. 2005;7:189–97.

Rosen HR. Chronic hepatitis C infection. N Engl J Med. 2011;364:2429–38.

Sass DA, Shaikh OS. Alcoholic hepatitis. Clin Liver Dis. 2006;10:219–37.

Schaefer E, Pratt DS. Autoimmune hepatitis: current challenges in diagnosis and management in a chronic progressive liver disease. Curr Opin Rheumatol. 2012;24:84–9.

Simel DL, Hatala R, Edelman D. Update: ascites. In: Simel DL, Rennie D, eds. *The Rational Clinical Examination: Evidence-Based Clinical Diagnosis.* New York, NY: McGraw-Hill; 2009. http://www.jamaevidence.com/content/3475877. Accessed 10/8/2013

Simel DL, D'Silva M. Update: hepatomegaly. In: Simel DL, Rennie D, eds. *The Rational Clinical Examination: Evidence-Based Clinical Diagnosis.* New York, NY: McGraw-Hill; 2009. http://www.jamaevidence.com/content/3480910. Accessed 10/8/2013

van Bokhoven MA, van Deursen C, Swinkels DW. Diagnosis and management of hereditary haemochromatosis. BMJ. 2011;342:c7251.

Vincent A, Herman J, Schulick R et al. Pancreatic cancer. Lancet. 2011;378:607–20.

Wilkins T, Malcolm J, Raina D, Schade RR. Hepatitis C: diagnosis and treatment. Am Fam Physician. 2010;81:1351–7.

REFERENCES

I have a patient with joint pain. How do I determine the cause?

CHIEF COMPLAINT

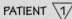

PATIENT 1

Mrs. K is a 75-year-old woman who complains of a painful left knee.

What is the differential diagnosis of joint pain? How would you frame the differential?

CONSTRUCTING A DIFFERENTIAL DIAGNOSIS

The causes of joint pain range from common to rare and from not particularly dangerous to joint and life-threatening. Even the most benign causes of joint pain can lead to serious disability. The evaluation of a patient with joint pain calls for a detailed history and physical exam (often focusing on extra-articular findings) and occasionally the sampling of joint fluid and possibly analyzing radiologic and serologic tests.

The differential diagnosis of joint pain can be framed with the use of 3 pivotal questions. First, is a single joint or are multiple joints involved (is the joint pain articular or polyarticular). If the pain involves just 1 joint, the next question is, is the pain articular or extra-articular? Although this distinction may seem obvious, abnormalities of periarticular structures can mimic articular disease. Finally, are the involved joints inflamed or not? Further down the differential, the acuity of the pain may also be important.

Figure 27-1 shows a useful algorithm organized according to these pivotal points. Because periarticular joint pain is almost always monoarticular, the first pivotal point differentiates monoarticular from polyarticular pain. Periarticular syndromes are discussed briefly at the end of the chapter.

The differential diagnosis below is organized by these 3 pivotal points as well. When considering both the algorithm and the differential diagnosis, it is important to recognize that all of the monoarticular arthritides can present in a polyarticular distribution, and classically polyarticular diseases may occasionally only affect a single joint. Thus, this organization is useful to organize your thinking but should never be used to exclude diagnoses from consideration.

A. Monoarticular arthritis
  1. Inflammatory
    a. Infectious
      (1) Nongonococcal septic arthritis
      (2) Gonococcal arthritis
      (3) Lyme disease
    b. Crystalline
      (1) Monosodium urate (gout)
      (2) Calcium pyrophosphate dihydrate deposition disease (CPPD or pseudogout)
  2. Noninflammatory
    a. Osteoarthritis (OA)
    b. Traumatic
    c. Avascular necrosis
B. Polyarticular arthritis
  1. Inflammatory
    a. Rheumatologic
      (1) Rheumatoid arthritis (RA)
      (2) Systemic lupus erythematosus (SLE)
      (3) Psoriatic arthritis
      (4) Other rheumatic diseases
    b. Infectious
      (1) Bacterial
        (a) Bacterial endocarditis
        (b) Lyme disease
        (c) Gonococcal arthritis
      (2) Viral
        (a) Rubella
        (b) Hepatitis B
        (c) HIV
        (d) Parvovirus
      (3) Postinfectious
        (a) Enteric
        (b) Urogenital
        (c) Rheumatic fever
  2. Noninflammatory: OA

1

Mrs. K's symptoms started after she stepped down from a bus with unusual force. The pain became intolerable within about 6 hours of onset and has been present for 3 days now. She otherwise feels well. She reports no fevers, chills, dietary changes, or sick contacts.

On physical exam she is in obvious pain, limping into the exam room on a cane. Her vital signs are temperature, 37.0°C; RR, 12 breaths per minute; BP, 110/70 mm Hg; pulse, 80 bpm. The only abnormality on exam is the right knee. It is red, warm to the touch, and tender to palpation. The range of motion is limited to only about 20 degrees.

At this point, what is the leading hypothesis, what are the active alternatives, and is there a must not miss diagnosis? Given this differential diagnosis, what tests should be ordered?

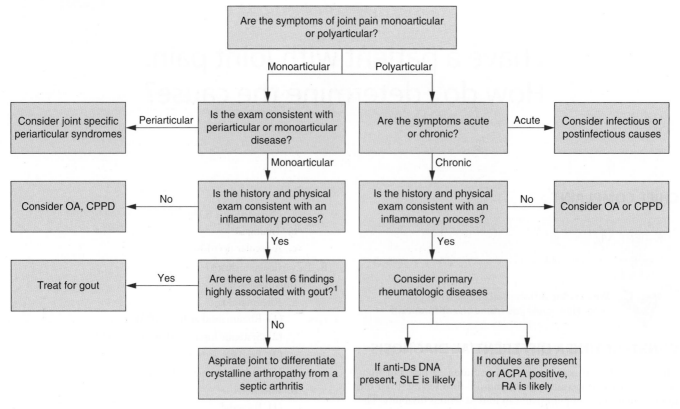

¹see text
ACPA, anti-citrullinated protein antibody; CPPD, calcium pyrophosphate deposition disease; OA, osteoarthritis;
SLE, systemic lupus erythematosus.

Figure 27-1. Diagnostic approach: joint pain.

RANKING THE DIFFERENTIAL DIAGNOSIS

The patient's symptoms and physical exam clearly localize to the problem to articular rather than periarticular structures as the exam reveals an inflamed joint with limited range of motion. Considering the pivotal points in this case, we can limit the differential diagnosis to those diseases that cause acute, monoarticular, inflammatory joint pain. These include septic arthritis, gout, and pseudogout. Traumatic injury to the knee, such as a meniscal injury or intra-articular fracture, are probably less likely given the mild nature of the injury and the inflammation of the joint.

Salient points of the patient's presentation are the rapid onset of the pain; the mild, antecedent trauma; and the lack of systemic symptoms, such as fever, fatigue, or weight loss.

Gout is the leading hypothesis given its high incidence, the patient's age, and the single inflamed joint. CPPD (also called pseudogout) is common in the knee of elderly patients, so this must also be high in the differential diagnosis. Traumatic injury to the knee, such as a meniscal injury or intra-articular fracture, are probably less likely given the mild nature of the injury and the inflammation of the joint.

An infectious arthritis is probably less likely, given the sudden onset and lack of systemic symptoms, but it is a must not miss diagnosis since it would be potentially disastrous if left untreated. Both gonococcal and nongonococcal septic arthritis are possibilities. Lyme disease can affect multiple joints but most commonly causes a monoarticular arthritis of the knee. Table 27-1 lists the differential diagnosis.

Mrs. K has never had a similar episode before. Her other medical problems include diabetes mellitus with diabetic nephropathy, hypertension, and hypercholesterolemia. Her medications are insulin, enalapril, atorvastatin, and hydrochlorothiazide. There is no history of alcohol or drug abuse.

 Is the clinical information sufficient to make a diagnosis? If not, what other information do you need?

Leading Hypothesis: Gout

Textbook Presentation

Gout most commonly presents in older patients with acute and severe pain of the first metatarsophalangeal (MTP) joint. The pain generally begins acutely and becomes unbearable within hours of onset. Classically, patients say that they are not even able to place a bed sheet over the toe. On physical exam, the first MTP joint is warm, swollen, and red.

Disease Highlights

A. Gout is the most common crystal-induced arthropathy.

Table 27-1. Diagnostic hypotheses for Mrs. K.

Diagnostic Hypotheses	Demographics, Risk Factors, Symptoms and Signs	Important Tests
Leading Hypothesis		
Gout	Men > women Previous episodes Rapid onset Involvement of first MTP joint	Classic presentation or demonstration of sodium urate crystals in synovial fluid
Active Alternative		
CPPD (pseudogout)	May present as chronic or acute arthritis	Demonstration of calcium pyrophosphate crystals in synovial fluid or classic radiographic findings
Active Alternative—Must Not Miss		
Bacterial arthritis (gonococcal or nongonococcal)	Fever with monoarticular or polyarticular arthritis	Positive synovial (or other body) fluid cultures
Lyme disease	Exposure to endemic area History of tick bite Rash	Clinical history Serologies Response to treatment
Other Alternative		
Traumatic injury	Usually history of severe trauma	Appropriate imaging (radiograph for fracture, MRI for cartilaginous injury)

CPPD, calcium pyrophosphate dihydrate deposition disease; MTP, metatarsophalangeal.

B. Gouty attacks occur when sodium urate crystallizes in synovial fluid inducing an inflammatory response and causing an abrupt, remarkably painful arthritis.

C. The primary risk factor for gout is hyperuricemia.

D. The prevalence of gout increases with age and is more common in men than women.

E. Location
1. The classic location for gout is the first MTP joint (podagra).
2. The joints of the lower extremities and the elbows are also common sites (though usually after an initial attack of podagra).

F. Gouty attacks often occur after abrupt changes in uric acid levels. Common causes are:
1. Large protein meals
2. Alcohol binges
3. Initiation of thiazide or loop diuretics
4. Initiation of urate-lowering therapy
5. Worsening kidney disease

G. Gouty attacks can also be induced by trauma, hospitalization, or surgery.

H. The initial attack nearly always involves a single joint, while later attacks may be polyarticular.

I. Forms of gout
1. Acute gouty arthritis is by far the most common type of gout.
2. Chronic arthritis can develop in patients who have untreated hyperuricemia.
3. Tophaceous gout occurs when there is macroscopic deposition of sodium urate crystals in and around joints.
4. The kidney can also be affected by gout. Sodium urate stones or a urate nephropathy can develop in patients.

J. Evaluation of a patient with gout
1. Patients with a new diagnosis of gout should be evaluated for alcoholism, chronic kidney disease, myeloproliferative disorders, and hypertension.
2. Patients in whom gout first occurs in their teens and twenties should be evaluated for disorders of purine metabolism.

Evidence-Based Diagnosis

A. Acute, inflammatory, monoarticular arthritis is an absolute indication for arthrocentesis.

B. Sampling synovial fluid will not only rule out potentially joint destroying septic arthritis but will also usually make a diagnosis.

 Every acute, inflammatory joint effusion should be aspirated.

C. Arthrocentesis
1. Joint fluid is routinely sent for cell count, Gram stain, culture, and crystal analysis.
2. Normal joint fluid is small in volume and clear with a very low cell count.
3. Characteristics of abnormal synovial fluid are shown in Table 27-2. These numbers should be used as estimates.
4. Joint fluid obtained during an acute flare of a crystal arthritis will be highly inflammatory in nature.
5. The only setting in which it is reasonable not to aspirate a monoarticular effusion is when a septic joint is extremely unlikely and there is truly no diagnostic question. This may be the case
   a. When a patient has recurrent inflammatory flares secondary to documented process (gout).
   b. When the diagnosis is clear (podagra for gout or joint trauma in a patient with a bleeding diathesis for hemarthrosis).

D. Clinical diagnosis
1. Despite the crucial role of arthrocentesis in the diagnosis of acute monoarticular arthritis, the diagnosis of gout can occasionally be made with some certainty without joint aspiration.
2. The following clinical points make a diagnosis of gout probable:
   a. More than 1 attack of acute arthritis
   b. Maximal inflammation in < 1 day
   c. Monoarthritis

Table 27-2. Characteristics of synovial fluid.

Characteristic	Normal	OA	RA or Similar Arthritides	Acute Crystal or Septic Arthritis
Color and clarity	Yellow and clear	Yellow and clear	Yellow green and cloudy	Yellow green and opaque
Volume	0–4 mL	1–10 mL	5–50 mL	15–50 mL
WBC/mcL	< 500	< 2000	1000–50,000	10,000–100,000
%PMN	< 25	< 50	> 50	> 75

OA, osteoarthritis; PMN, polymorphonuclear; RA, rheumatoid arthritis.

    d. Joint erythema

    e. First MTP involvement

    f. Unilateral MTP arthritis

    g. Unilateral tarsal acute arthritis

    h. Tophus

    i. Asymmetric joint swelling

    j. Hyperuricemia

    k. Bone cysts without erosion on radiograph

    l. Negative joint fluid culture

3. The predictive values for these findings are

    a. 6 or more of the clinical points: sensitivity, 87%; specificity, 96%; LR+, 22; LR–, 0.13

    b. 5 or more of the clinical points: sensitivity, 95%; specificity, 89%, LR+, 8.6; LR–, 0.05

    c. Serum uric acid > 7 mg/dL: sensitivity, 90%; specificity, 54%; LR+, 1.9; LR–, 0.19

 4. The presence of 6 findings highly consistent with gout rules in the diagnosis even without arthrocentesis.

5. Fever may accompany acute attacks.

    a. Present in 44% of patients

    b. 10% of patients have fevers > 39.0°C

6. Other findings that make gout more probable are

    a. Hypertension

    b. Use of thiazide or loop diuretics

    c. Obesity

    d. Alcohol use

Treatment

A. Therapy for gout is classified as either abortive (to treat an acute flare) or prophylactic (to prevent flares and the destructive effects on the joints and kidneys).

B. Abortive therapy is outlined in Table 27-3.

    1. All of the therapies are effective, and the choice is usually made by the potential adverse effects.

    2. Most frequently, patients are treated with a combination of a potent nonsteroidal antiinflammatory drug (NSAID) and colchicine.

C. Prophylactic therapy

    1. There are 5 basic indications for prophylactic therapy:

        a. Frequent attacks

        b. Disabling attacks

        c. Urate nephrolithiasis

        d. Urate nephropathy

        e. Tophaceous gout

Table 27-3. Immediate therapies for gout and their potential adverse effects.

Therapy	Potential Adverse Effects
Nonsteroidal antiinflammatory drugs	Nephrotoxicity GI toxicity
Colchicine	GI toxicity (diarrhea)
Oral corticosteroids	GI toxicity Hyperglycemia
Intra-articular corticosteroids	Complications of joint injection Hyperglycemia

    2. Prophylactic therapy should begin with nonpharmacologic interventions to decrease uric acid levels and decrease the risk of gouty flares.

        a. Abstinence from alcohol use

        b. Weight loss

        c. Discontinuation of medications that impair urate excretion (eg, aspirin, thiazide diuretics).

    3. Potential prophylactic treatments are listed below.

        a. NSAIDs

        b. Colchicine

        c. Allopurinol

        d. Probenecid

        e. Sulfinpyrazone

        f. Febuxostat

        g. Uricase agents (eg, pegloticase) are in the early stage for testing as prophylactic therapies.

    4. Colchicine should be used during the initiation of urate-lowering therapy to prevent recurrent gouty flares.

        a. NSAIDs may be added if necessary.

        b. Colchicine is usually continued for at least the first 6 months (longer in the case of patients with tophi) of urate-lowering therapy.

    5. Allopurinol is usually the first antihyperuricemic drug used, although it is relatively contraindicated in patients with chronic kidney disease or liver disease.

    6. If allopurinol is ineffective, uric acid excretion should be measured. Patients with low uric acid excretion (present in 80% of patients with gout) should be given a uricosuric agent, such as probenecid.

MAKING A DIAGNOSIS

The evaluation of this patient clearly requires joint aspiration. Septic arthritis is in the differential of any acutely inflamed joint. Mrs. K has 4 of the findings common for gout (maximal inflammation in < 1 day, monoarthritis, joint erythema, and asymmetric joint swelling), so although gout remains likely, especially given the presence of hypertension and her use of a thiazide, the diagnosis is not certain.

Radiographs of the knee demonstrate evidence of mild OA but no evidence of fracture. Joint fluid is aspirated from the patient's knee.

Have you crossed a diagnostic threshold for the leading hypothesis, gout? Have you ruled out the active alternatives? Do other tests need to be done to exclude the alternative diagnoses?

Alternative Diagnosis: Calcium Pyrophosphate Deposition Disease (CPPD)

Textbook Presentation

CPPD generally presents in older patients. It may present with an acute flare (pseudogout) or, more commonly, as a degenerative arthritis with suspicious radiographic findings that distinguish it from OA. Patients often have other diseases associated with CPPD, such as hyperparathyroidism.

Disease Highlights

A. CPPD is a crystal-induced arthropathy that can present in multiple different ways.
   1. CPPD is often asymptomatic, being diagnosed as an incidental radiographic finding of chondocalcinosis, the linear calcifications of articular cartilage.
   2. Pseudogout is an acute, inflammatory, usually monoarticular arthritis that can be clinically indistinguishable from gout, except for the presence of calcium pyrophosphate dihydrate crystals in the joint fluid.
   3. Pyrophosphate arthropathy is a chronic arthritis that is clinically similar to OA (sometimes referred to pseudo OA); distinguishing between the 2 conditions may be difficult. However, pyrophosphate arthropathy may affect joints less commonly affected by OA like the wrists, MCPs, and shoulders.
   4. A small percentage of patients with CPPD (≈5%) can have a chronic, inflammatory polyarthritis resembling RA (sometimes referred to as pseudo RA).
   5. Rarely, CPPD can present as pseudoneuropathic arthropathy, resembling a Charcot joint. In this presentation there is a destructive monoarthropathy,

B. There are many other similarities between pseudogout and gout.
   1. Both are caused by the inflammatory response to crystals in the synovial space.
   2. Both cause acute painful monoarticular attacks.
   3. Both can cause polyarticular flares.
   4. Flares can be induced by trauma or illness.

5. Both can potentially cause destructive arthropathy.
6. Incidence increases with age.

C. There are some aspects of the disease quite distinct from gout.
   1. Episodic "gout-like" flares only occur in a small percentage of patients.
   2. As above, CPPD commonly manifests as a degenerative arthritis, pyrophosphate arthropathy (in about 50% of patients).
   3. It has highly specific radiologic features.
   4. It most commonly affects the knee.

Although CPPD is commonly thought of as pseudogout, it more commonly presents as a chronic degenerative arthritis.

D. Pseudogout has been associated with a number of diseases, the most common of which are:
   1. Hyperparathyroidism
   2. Hemochromatosis
   3. Hypomagnesemia
   4. Hypophosphatasia

Evidence-Based Diagnosis

A. Definite diagnosis of CPPD arthritis requires demonstration of the calcium pyrophosphate crystals in synovial fluid.

B. Certain radiographic findings are quite suggestive. The classic findings are punctate and linear calcific densities, most commonly seen in the cartilage of the knees, hip, pelvis, and wrist.

C. The following characteristics should make a clinician consider the diagnosis of CPPD:
   1. Acute arthritis of a large joint, especially the knees, in the absence of hyperuricemia.
   2. Chronic arthritis with acute flares.
   3. Chronic arthritis involving joints that would be atypical for OA such as the wrists, metacarpophalangeal (MCP) joints, and shoulders.

D. Evaluation of a patient with pseudogout should include testing for related diseases. The evaluation generally includes measuring the levels of the following:
   1. Calcium
   2. Magnesium
   3. Phosphorus
   4. Iron, ferritin, and total iron-binding capacity (TIBC)
   5. In the right setting, markers of other rheumatologic diseases (uric acid, rheumatoid factor [RF], anti-cyclic citrullinated peptide [anti-CCP])

Treatment

A. Treat an associated underlying disease, when present.
B. Acute attacks can be managed with
   1. NSAIDs
   2. Joint aspiration with corticosteroid injection
   3. Colchicine
C. Chronic degenerative arthritis is difficult to treat. NSAIDs are usually used.

Alternative Diagnosis: Septic Arthritis

Textbook Presentation

Septic arthritis usually presents as subacute joint pain, the knee being most common, associated with low-grade fever and progressive pain and disability. Because the infection is usually caused by hematogenous spread, a risk factor for bacteremia (such as injection drug use) is sometimes present. Disseminated gonorrhea is discussed separately below.

Disease Highlights

A. Septic arthritis usually occurs via hematogenous spread of bacteria.

B. Joint distribution

    1. The knee is the most commonly affected joint.

    2. Monoarticular arthritis is the rule, with multiple joints involved in < 15% of patients.

    3. Infection is most common in previously abnormal joints, such as those affected by OA or RA.

C. *Staphylococcus aureus* is the most common organism followed by species of streptococcus.

Evidence-Based Diagnosis

A. Clinical findings

    1. Fever is present in most patients.

        a. One meta-analysis found that 57% of patients with septic arthritis had fever.

        b. Recognize that this means that over 40% of patients with septic arthritis are afebrile.

        c. Fever > 39.0°C is rare.

    2. Findings predictive of a septic arthritis causing joint pain are recent joint surgery (LR+ 6.9) and the presence of a prosthetic knee or hip in the presence of a skin infection (LR+ 15.0).

Fever cannot distinguish septic arthritis from other forms of monoarticular arthritis. Patients with gout may be febrile while those with septic joints may not be.

B. Laboratory findings

    1. WBC > 10,000/mcL is seen in only 50% of patients.

    2. Definitive diagnosis is made by Gram stain and culture.

        a. Gram stain of synovial fluid is positive in about 75% of patients with septic arthritis.

        b. The yield is highest with *S aureus*.

    3. Elevated synovial fluid WBC count is predictive.

        a. Synovial fluid WBC count > 100,000/mcL: LR+ 28, LR+ 0.71.

        b. Lower WBC cut offs are not predictive.

    4. Joint fluid culture is positive in about 90% of cases.

    5. Blood (and sputum, when appropriate) should also be cultured as this may help identify an organism if one is not isolated from the synovium. About 50% of patients will have positive blood cultures.

Because of the potential for septic arthritis to cause joint destruction, a single, acutely inflamed joint should be assumed infected until proved otherwise.

Treatment

A. Antibiotic therapy is directed by Gram stain findings.

B. Empiric therapy should cover *S aureus*.

C. The affected joint should also be drained, either with a needle, arthroscope, or arthrotomy (opening the joint in the operating room).

    1. Small joints can usually be drained and lavaged with serial arthrocentesis.

    2. Large joints usually require surgical drainage.

    3. The knee is an exception, a large joint that, in many cases can be treated with serial arthrocentesis.

D. Patients who receive treatment within 5 days of symptom onset have the best prognosis.

Alternative Diagnosis: Disseminated Gonorrhea

Textbook Presentation

Disseminated gonorrhea is classically seen in young, sexually active women who have fever and joint pain. The most common presentation is severe pain of the wrists, hands, and knees with warmth and erythema diffusely over the backs of the hands. A rash may sometimes be present.

Disease Highlights

A. Disseminated gonorrhea is a disease with rheumatologic manifestations that is seen in young, sexually active persons.

B. Women are 3 times more likely to have the disease than men.

Disseminated gonorrhea usually occurs in patients without a history of a recent sexually transmitted disease.

C. Disseminated gonorrhea presents in 1 of 2 ways (with a good deal of overlap): a classic septic arthritis or a triad of tenosynovitis, dermatitis, and arthralgia.

    1. The triad presentation reflects a high-grade bacteremia with reactive features.

    2. The tenosynovitis presents predominantly as a polyarthralgia of the hands and wrists.

    3. The rash is a scattered, papular, or vesicular rash.

    4. The more classic, monoarticular septic joint presentation occurs in about 40% of patients.

    5. Table 27-4 gives the frequency of various findings in these 2 types of presentation.

Evidence-Based Diagnosis

A. Diagnosis is based on isolating the organism.

B. Besides synovial fluid cultures, blood, pharyngeal, and genital cultures should be sent.

C. If all cultures are negative, the disease can still be diagnosed if there is a high clinical suspicion and a rapid response to appropriate antibiotics.

Negative cultures do not necessarily exclude the diagnosis of disseminated gonorrhea.

Treatment

A. Ceftriaxone 1 g IV or IM every 24 hours or cefotaxime 1 g IV every 8 hours.

Table 27-4. Physical signs and culture results in patients with disseminated gonorrhea.

Characteristic	Septic Arthritis	Triad
% Female	63%	77%
Tenosynovitis	21%	87%
Fever	32%	50%
Skin lesions	42%	90%
Positive blood cultures	0%	43%
"Tapable" joint effusion[1]	100%	0%

[1]Note that this is how the groups were distinguished.
Data from O'Brien JP, Goldenberg DL, Rice PA. Disseminated gonococcal infection: a prospective analysis of 49 patients and a review of pathophysiology and immune mechanisms. Medicine (Baltimore). 1983;62:395–406.

B. IV therapy is generally recommended for 24–48 hours after improvement.

Alternative Diagnosis: Lyme Disease

Textbook Presentation

Lyme disease presents in different ways at different stages of the disease. A classic presentation of the joint symptoms is a patient with acute, inflammatory knee pain who has been in an area where the disease is endemic. There may be a history of a previous tick bite, rash, or nonspecific febrile illness.

Disease Highlights

A. Lyme disease is caused by the spirochete *Borrelia burgdorferi*, transmitted by a number of species of *Ixodes* ticks.

B. The tick most commonly transmits the disease during its nymphal stage.

C. The disease is endemic in certain places.

    1. In the United States: along the northern Atlantic Coast, in Wisconsin and Minnesota, in California and Oregon

    2. In Europe: Germany, Austria, Slovenia, Sweden

D. The clinical picture differs somewhat between that in the United States and that in Europe and Asia. The presentation in the United States is discussed below.

E. Peak incidence is in June and July, with disease occurring from March through October.

F. The disease is generally divided into 3 stages.

    1. Early localized disease

        a. Skin findings are most common, usually a large area of localized erythema.

            (1) 80% of patients have an acute rash.

            (2) 50% of the rashes occur below the waist.

            (3) The mean diameter of the rash is 10 cm.

            (4) About 60% of the rashes are an area of homogeneous erythema.

            (5) About 30% of rashes are the more classic target lesion.

            (6) About 10% of the patients have multiple lesions.

Only about 30% of patients with Lyme disease have the classic target rash on presentation.

        b. Other symptoms include

            (1) Myalgias and arthralgias (59%)

            (2) Fever (31%)

            (3) Headache (28%)

    2. Early disseminated disease can involve the heart and the central nervous system (CNS).

        a. Atrioventricular (AV) node block is the most common cardiac manifestation.

        b. Headache is the most common CNS finding, while meningitis and cranial nerve palsies (especially CN7) also occur.

    3. Joint symptoms predominate late in the disease.

        a. Occur in about 60% of untreated patients months after infection.

        b. Monoarticular knee arthritis is the most common finding.

        c. Intermittent attacks or an oligoarticular arthritis may also occur.

        d. Arthritis can become chronic, even in treated patients, in about 10% of cases.

Evidence-Based Diagnosis

A. Definitive diagnosis of Lyme disease is based on clinical characteristics, exposure history, and antibody titers.

B. Antibodies may be negative early in the disease and are thus not helpful in the setting of acute infection.

C. Antibodies are nearly 100% sensitive in the setting of arthritis.

Treatment

A. There are multiple antibiotic regimens effective in the treatment of localized and disseminated Lyme disease.

B. Prophylactic treatment with a single dose of doxycycline given after a tick bite is effective at preventing Lyme disease but is generally not recommended given the low likelihood of being infected with Lyme disease after a tick bite, even in endemic areas.

C. Treatment of arthritis caused by Lyme disease is either 4 weeks of oral antibiotics or 2–4 weeks of IV antibiotics.

D. Chronic and debilitating symptoms from Lyme disease rarely develop after appropriate treatment and, when they do occur, the etiology of these symptoms is not clear.

CASE RESOLUTION

Mrs. K's synovial fluid aspiration yielded 25 mL of translucent, yellow fluid. The WBC was about 55,000/mcL with 56% PMNs. The Gram stain was negative, and crystal exam with polarized light microscopy demonstrates negatively birefringent crystals consistent with monosodium urate crystals, thus making the diagnosis of gout.

The inflammatory joint fluid is consistent with the exam. Acute gout is commonly associated with very inflamed joints, often with very high WBC counts. The positive crystal exam makes the diagnosis of gout.

The patient was treated with NSAIDs and colchicine with a good response. Because this was Mrs. K's first attack, prophylactic therapy was not instituted.

CHIEF COMPLAINT

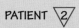

PATIENT 2

Mrs. C is a 50-year-old woman who comes to your office complaining of joint pain. She reports the pain has been present for about 2 years. The pain affects her hands and her wrists. She describes the pain as "a dull aching" and "a stiffness." It is worst in the morning and improves over 2 to 3 hours. She says that on particularly bad days she uses NSAIDs with moderate relief.

At this point, what is the leading hypothesis, what are the active alternatives, and is there a must not miss diagnosis? Given this differential diagnosis, what tests should be ordered?

RANKING THE DIFFERENTIAL DIAGNOSIS

Although morning stiffness is common with most types of arthritis, Mrs. C's prolonged symptoms are suggestive of an inflammatory arthritis. She does not seem to have other systemic symptoms, and she has no history of a recent infection. At this point the pivotal features in this case are the polyarticular and inflammatory nature of the joint pain and the chronicity of the symptoms.

Considering these points, as well as the fact that the patient is a middle aged woman, RA has to lead the differential. The chronicity, age at onset, and joint distribution all support this diagnosis. Psoriatic arthritis can be indistinguishable from RA, especially early in its course, and needs to be considered. SLE can also present as a chronic, inflammatory arthritis. The patient is older than the average age of onset for SLE, and we have not heard about other organ system involvement.

Degenerative arthropathies, such as OA and CPPD, should be considered, but the joint distribution and inflammatory nature of the arthritis makes these less likely. Table 27-5 lists the differential diagnosis.

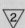

2

Mrs. C is otherwise well, except for a history of mild hypertension managed with an angiotensin-receptor blocker. She reports no other joint pains. She does not have a history of psoriasis.

Her vitals signs are temperature, 37.1°C; BP, 128/84 mm Hg; pulse, 84 bpm; RR, 14 breaths per minute. Her general physical exam is essentially normal. There is a 2/6 systolic ejection murmur. Joint exam reveals limited range of motion of the MCPs and wrists bilaterally. There is swelling of the third and fourth MCP on the right and the third on the left. There is pain at the extremes of motion and a boggy quality to the joints. A detailed skin exam is normal. The patient is wearing nail polish on the day of the visit.

Is the clinical information sufficient to make a diagnosis? If not, what other information do you need?

Leading Hypothesis: RA

Textbook Presentation

RA is most commonly seen in middle-aged patients with a symmetric polyarthritis manifesting itself with painful, stiff, and swollen

Table 27-5. Diagnostic hypotheses for Mrs. C.

Diagnostic Hypotheses	Demographics, Risk Factors, Symptoms and Signs	Important Tests
Leading Hypothesis		
Rheumatoid arthritis	Morning stiffness Symmetric polyarthritis Commonly involves the MCP joints	Clinical diagnosis Rheumatoid factor Anti-citrullinated protein antibody
Active Alternative		
Psoriatic arthritis	Psoriasis Dactylitis Spinal arthritis Often asymmetric Often involves the DIP joints	Clinical diagnosis
Systemic lupus erythematosus	Multisystem disease Most common in young, African American women	Clinical diagnosis aided by serologies and diagnostic criteria
Other Alternative		
Osteoarthritis	Chronic arthritis in weight-bearing joints In the hands, DIP and PIP involvement more common than MCP involvement	Radiograph of affected joints

DIP, distal interphalangeal; MCP, metatarsophalangeal; PIP, proximal interphalangeal.

hands. Morning stiffness is often a predominant symptom. Swollen and tender wrists, MCP, and proximal interphalangeal (PIP) joints are usually seen on exam. Laboratory evaluation may reveal an anemia of chronic inflammation and positive RF and anti-citrullinated protein antibody (ACPA, sometimes called anti-CCP).

Disease Highlights

A. RA is the paradigm for idiopathic inflammatory arthritides.

B. The sine qua non of RA is the presence of an inflammatory synovitis, most commonly involving the hands. This synovitis eventually forms a destructive pannus that injures articular and periarticular tissue.

C. RA is common, present in about 1% of the population, so the diagnosis should be considered in any adult patient presenting with joint symptoms and true findings of arthritis on exam.

RA should be considered in any adult with a chronic, symmetric polyarthritis.

D. Common findings in RA are:

1. Symmetric arthritis of the hands

2. Presence of serum RF and ACPA

3. Presence of radiographic changes typical of RA on hand and wrist radiographs.

4. Morning stiffness is a classic finding.

a. Although many people are stiff upon awakening, those with inflammatory arthritis can experience stiffness for an hour or more.

b. Morning stiffness improves with therapy.

Prolonged morning stiffness is a good clue to an inflammatory arthritis.

E. The joints most commonly involved are

1. Hand

   a. Wrists, MCP, and PIP joints are most commonly affected.

   b. Distal interphalangeal (DIP) joints are often spared.

   c. Ulnar deviation of the MCPs as well as swan neck and boutonnière deformities are classic findings.

   d. Figure 27-2 shows a hand with some of the classic findings of RA.

2. Elbow

3. Knee

4. Ankle

5. Cervical spine

   a. Usually presents as neck pain and stiffness.

   b. C1–C2 instability can occur secondary to associated tenosynovitis.

     (1) This can produce cervical myelopathy.

     (2) Advisable to radiographically image the cervical spines of patients with RA prior to elective endotracheal intubation.

F. Once RA is established, joint destruction begins to occur and can be seen on radiographs. The chronic synovitis causes erosions of bone and cartilage.

G. Long-standing RA can cause severe joint deformity through destruction of the joint and injury to the periarticular structures.

H. Nonarticular findings in RA

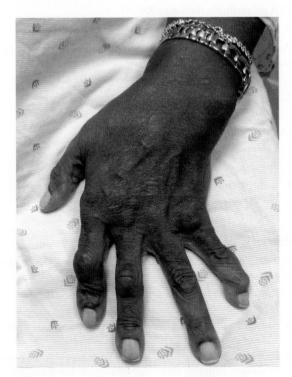

Figure 27-2. Rheumatoid arthritis of the hand.

1. Rheumatoid nodules, when present, are usually over extensor surfaces.

2. Dry eyes are common.

3. Pulmonary nodules or interstitial lung disease

4. Pericardial disease

   a. Asymptomatic pericardial effusion is most common.

   b. Restrictive pericarditis can occur.

5. Anemia of inflammation (see Chapter 6) is a typical finding in RA.

Evidence-Based Diagnosis

A. The diagnosis of RA can be difficult because it may resemble other causes of inflammatory arthritis around the time of onset.

B. Serologies

1. RF is a nonspecific test.

   a. It is occasionally positive in healthy people and in a number of inflammatory states such as infections, sarcoidosis, and periodontal disease.

   b. The test characteristics of RF vary in different studies but a meta-analysis found the following: sensitivity, 69%; specificity, 85%; LR+, 4.86; LR− 0.38.

2. ACPA is a newer test that is more predictive of RA than RF. The same meta-analysis found the following: sensitivity, 62%; specificity, 95%; LR+, 12.46; LR− 0.36.

A positive ACPA is very predictive of a diagnosis of RA.

3. In practice, RF and ACPA are used together. Patients are at high risk for RA when these tests are positive.

C. The American College of Rheumatology (ACR) has developed diagnostic criteria for RA (Table 27-6).

1. These criteria are meant to be used in patients who have clinical synovitis of at least 1 joint not explained by another disease.

2. A score of ≥ 6/10 fulfills the criteria.

3. Although meant to standardize research and not to be used as diagnostic criteria, they are helpful in highlighting the clinical characteristics of RA.

4. The test characteristics of the ACR criteria vary depending on when in the course of the illness they are evaluated and the end point used for the diagnosis of RA. Initial studies yield sensitivities and specificities of 62–84% and 60–78%, respectively.

D. Other very specific findings are the presence of rheumatoid nodules (LR+ > 30) and consistent radiographic changes (LR+ 11).

Treatment

A. The treatment for RA has changed rapidly in recent years and is now really the purview of the rheumatologist.

B. The treatments are often divided into those that treat the symptoms of the disease and those that modify the course of the disease.

C. The drugs used to treat the symptoms of the disease are:

1. NSAIDs

   a. Generally used early in the course of the disease for symptom relief while a diagnosis is being made.

   b. Rarely, patients with very mild disease can remain on these medications alone.

2. Corticosteroids

Table 27-6. 2010 American College of Rheumatology/
European League Against Rheumatism Classification
Criteria for RA.

Category	Criteria	Score
Joint involvement	1 large joint	0
	2–10 large joints	1
	1–3 small joints	2
	4–10 small joints	3
	> 10 joints (small or large)	5
Serology	Negative RF and negative ACPA	0
	Low-positive RF or low-positive ACPA	2
	High-positive RF or high-positive ACPA	3
Acute Phase Reactants	Normal CRP and normal ESR	0
	Abnormal CRP or abnormal ESR	1
Duration of symptoms	< 6 weeks	0
	≥6 weeks	1

RF, rheumatoid factor; ACPA, anti-citrullinated protein antibody; ESR, erythrocyte
sedimentation rate; CRP, C-reactive protein

   a. Generally provide excellent symptom control but due to
significant long-term side effects are used in the lowest
dose and for the least time possible.

   b. Their effect on slowing joint destruction from RA is
very controversial.

D. Disease-modifying antirheumatic drugs (DMARDs) include
sulfasalazine, hydroxychloroquine, methotrexate, leflunomide,
etanercept, and infliximab.

   1. Methotrexate is the most commonly used drug in this class.

   2. Patients with more severe disease also commonly receive
the TNF-alpha inhibitors etanercept or infliximab, or
leflunomide, a drug that impairs T-cell function.

   3. Newer therapies include rituximab, which depletes
B-lymphocytes, and abatacept, which blocks costimulation
of T-lymphocytes.

MAKING A DIAGNOSIS

The presentation of Mrs. C's symptoms is typical for RA. She
already fulfills 4 of the ACR criteria for RA. Further evaluation
should be directed toward gathering other information that might
suggest RA and make other diagnoses less likely.

A CBC with iron studies, RF, anti-CCP, and antinuclear antibodies (ANA) are done. Radiographs are ordered with fine
details of the hands.

Have you crossed a diagnostic threshold for
the leading hypothesis, RA? Have you ruled
out the active alternatives? Do other tests
need to be done to exclude the alternative
diagnoses?

Alternative Diagnosis: Psoriatic Arthritis

Textbook Presentation

Psoriatic arthritis most commonly presents as joint pain in middle-
aged patients with a history of psoriasis. There are signs and symptoms of an inflammatory arthritis often involving the wrists, MCP,
PIP, and DIP joints. Exam of the skin reveals psoriasis and psoriatic
nail changes.

Disease Highlights

A. Psoriasis is a very common skin disease that can be complicated by arthritis.

B. Psoriatic arthritis is one of the seronegative spondyloarthropathies.

   1. The seronegative spondyloarthropathies are diseases
characterized by inflammatory axial spine involvement,
asymmetric peripheral arthritis, enthesopathy, and
inflammatory eye diseases.

   2. Patients with these diseases classically have a negative ANA
and RF, giving the group the "seronegative" moniker.

   3. Other seronegative spondyloarthropathies are ankylosing
spondylitis, reactive arthritis, and the arthritis associated
with inflammatory bowel disease.

C. The distribution of the arthritis in psoriatic arthritis is quite
variable but follows 3 general presentations:

   1. Oligoarthritis often involving large joints and the hands.
Dactylitis, a swelling of the entire finger causing a "sausage
digit" secondary to both arthritis and tenosynovitis, is a
classic finding.

   2. A polyarthritis similar to RA

   3. A spinal arthritis

D. Psoriatic arthritis can be indistinguishable from RA, especially
early in the course of both diseases.

   1. Radiographs of the hands can show erosions.

   2. About 10% of patients with psoriatic arthritis have a
positive RF.

E. Distinguishing features include:

   1. Common involvement of DIP joints

   2. Spine involvement that is uncommon in RA

   3. Arthritis mutilans, a syndrome in which there is marked
boney destruction around joints causing "telescoping
digits."

Evidence-Based Diagnosis

A. The most diagnostic feature of psoriatic arthritis is the presence
of psoriasis.

   1. Psoriasis precedes the development of arthritis in about
70% of cases.

   2. Arthritis and psoriasis begin contemporaneously in about
15% of patients.

   3. In about 15% of patients, there is no psoriasis at the onset
of disease, although there may be a family history of the
skin disease.

B. A very careful skin exam should be done in all patients in whom the diagnosis is suspected.

C. Nail findings

1. Psoriasis can cause recognizable changes in the nails (eg, pitting, an oil stained appearance).

2. Nail changes occur in only about 20% of people with psoriasis but in about 80% of people with psoriasis and arthritis.

3. Nail changes are especially common in people with DIP arthritis.

 A detailed skin and nail exam is important when considering the diagnosis of psoriatic arthritis. Nail polish should be removed for the visit.

Treatment

The treatment of psoriatic arthritis is similar to the treatment of RA.

Alternative Diagnosis: SLE

Textbook Presentation

SLE classically presents in a young woman with fatigue and arthritis, commonly of the hands. There are often suspicious findings in the history such as an episode of pleuritis or undiagnosed anemia.

Disease Highlights

A. SLE is a truly systemic autoimmune disease primarily affecting women of childbearing age.

B. Various groups are more prone to disease.

1. Female:male ratio is about 9:1.

2. About 5% of patients reporting a first-degree relative with the disease.

3. Women of color are most commonly affected.

C. Almost every organ can be involved, although the joints, skin, serosa, and kidneys are most commonly affected.

D. The pathogenesis of the disease is related to the formation of autoantibodies to a number of nuclear antigens. The ANA is the most common.

E. The most common features of SLE, both at presentation and later in follow-up, are listed in Table 27-7.

Evidence-Based Diagnosis

A. The diagnosis of SLE, especially in people with mild disease, can be difficult.

B. The ACR has developed criteria to standardize the diagnosis for research purposes.

1. The criteria are:

   a. Malar rash

   b. Discoid rash

   c. Photosensitivity

   d. Oral ulcers

   e. Arthritis (nonerosive arthritis)

   f. Serositis (pleuritis or pericarditis)

   g. Renal disorder (proteinuria or cellular casts)

   h. Neurologic disorder (headache, seizures, or psychosis without other cause)

   i. Hematologic disorder (hemolytic anemia or any cytopenia)

Table 27-7. Clinical manifestations of SLE at onset and during disease.

Signs and Symptoms	Prevalence at Onset	Prevalence at any Time
Arthralgia	77%	85%
Rashes	53%	78%
Constitutional	53%	77%
Renal involvement	38%	74%
Arthritis	44%	63%
Raynaud phenomenon	33%	60%
CNS involvement (most commonly headache)	24%	54%
GI (most commonly abdominal pain)	18%	45%
Lymphadenopathy	16%	32%
Pleurisy	16%	30%
Pericarditis	13%	23%

SLE, systemic lupus erythematosus.

   j. Immunologic disorder (anti-DNA, anti-SM, or antiphospholipid antibodies)

   k. Positive ANA

2. The diagnosis of SLE requires the presence of 4 or more of these criteria.

3. Although the same reservations about using diagnostic criteria (that were developed for research purposes) clinically that were discussed above in the section of RA apply here, the SLE criteria are frequently used.

4. The test characteristics of these criteria are given in Table 27-8. Also included in this table are the test characteristics for the various individual criteria.

5. The presence of a malar rash, or satisfaction of the ACR criteria, is highly supportive of the diagnosis of SLE.

C. Autoantibodies

1. Measuring autoantibodies in SLE provides important diagnostic information.

2. ANA and anti-DsDNA

   a. ANA is the most sensitive test for SLE. It is very nonspecific.

   b. Anti-DsDNA is highly specific. It is also associated with the presence of lupus nephritis.

   c. ANA does not vary with disease activity while anti-DsDNA does.

   d. The predictive values of ANA and Anti-DsDNA are

      (1) ANA: sensitivity, 99%; specificity, 80%, LR+, 4.95; LR−, 0.0.1

      (2) DsDNA: sensitivity, 73%; specificity, 98%; LR+, 36.5; LR−, 0.28

 A negative ANA essentially rules out SLE. A positive anti-DsDNA essentially rules in SLE.

   e. Staining patterns are often reported with the ANA.

Table 27-8. Test characteristics for the ACR criteria (4 or more positive criteria) and individual criteria in the diagnosis of SLE.

Finding	Sensitivity	Specificity	LR+	LR−
ACR criteria	80%	98%	40	0.2
Discoid rash	18%	99%	18	0.83
Malar rash	57%	96%	14	0.45
Photosensitivity	43%	96%	11	0.59
Hematologic disorder	20%	98%	10	0.80
Renal disorder	51%	94%	8.5	0.52
Oral ulcers	27%	96%	6.8	0.76
Neurologic disorder	59%	89%	5.4	0.46
Serositis	56%	86%	4.0	0.51
Arthritis	86%	37%	1.4	0.38

ACR, American College of Rheumatology; SLE, systemic lupus erythematosus.
Data from Black ER. *Diagnostic strategies for common medical problems.* Philadelphia: American College of Physicians, 1999:421.

Table 27-9. Common serologies in rheumatologic diseases.

Antibody	Clinical Association
Anti-DsDNA	Nephritis in SLE
Anti–Smith	SLE
Anti-RNP	Raynaud phenomenon and myositis in SLE
Anti Ribosomal P	CNS disease in SLE
Anti SSA/Ro, Anti SSB/La	Sjögren syndrome and skin disease in SLE
Anti-histone antibodies	Drug-induced lupus
Anti-jo-1	Polymyositis/dermatomyositis
Anti-DNA topoisomerase I (Scl-70), anti-RNA polymerase I and III	Systemic sclerosis (scleroderma)
ANCA	Many vasculitic diseases including granulomatosis with polyangiitis, microscopic polyangiitis, and Churg-Strauss syndrome
Anti-U1 RNP antibodies	Mixed connective tissue disease
Anti-GBM	Anti-GBM antibody (Goodpasture disease)

(1) These patterns correlate, to some extent, with the other specific antibodies discussed below and their use has, to a great extent, been supplanted by these tests.

(2) In general, the meanings of the staining patterns are as follows:

  (a) Homogeneous: Seen in SLE, RA, and drug-induced lupus
  (b) Peripheral: Most specific pattern for SLE
  (c) Speckled: Least specific pattern. Commonly seen with low titer ANAs in people without rheumatic disease
  (d) Nucleolar: Common in patients with scleroderma and Raynaud phenomenon.

3. Other serologies are helpful because they tend to be associated with various subsets of disease.

  a. Anti-RNP: Associated with Raynaud phenomenon and myositis
  b. Anti-SSA/Ro and anti-SSB/La: Associated with Sjögren syndrome and photosensitivity
  c. Anti-ribosomal P: Associated with CNS manifestations of SLE

4. Table 27-9 outlines a variety of serologies that may be obtained in persons in whom rheumatologic disease is suspected.

D. Complement

1. Complement levels are helpful in tracking the activity of SLE but are nonspecific.

2. C3, C4, and CH50 levels tend to decline during episodes of lupus activity.

Treatment

A. Similar to RA, the treatment of SLE is complicated and to a great extent the purview of the rheumatologist.

B. In general, NSAIDs, corticosteroids, and immunosuppressants are the mainstay of therapy.

C. NSAIDs are generally used for symptomatic relief of inflammatory symptoms with careful monitoring because of their potential nephrotoxic effects.

D. Corticosteroids and hydroxychloroquine are commonly used in long-term therapy and high-dose corticosteroids are used for disease exacerbations.

E. Cyclophosphamide, mycophenolate mofetil, and azathioprine are the most commonly used immunosuppressants in SLE. They are used most widely for the treatment of lupus nephritis.

CASE RESOLUTION

Mrs. C's laboratory and radiology test results are as follows: Hgb, 10.5 g/dL; HCT, 31.0%; serum ferritin, 95 ng/mL (nl > 45 ng/mL); serum iron, 36 mcg/dL (nl 40–160 mcg/dL); TIBC, 200 mcg/dL (nl 230–430); RF, 253 international units/mL (nl < 10 international units/mL); anti-CCP 1000 units/mL (nl < 100 units/mL) ANA, 2560 titer (nl < 80); anti-DsDNA, < 10 titer (nl < 10); radiographs of hand, periarticular erosions of the 3 clinically involved MCP joints.

The diagnosis of RA is now fairly certain. The clinical picture, as well as the laboratory test showing an anemia of chronic inflammation, elevated RF and anti-CCP, and positive ANA all support the diagnosis. (About 40% of patients with RA have positive ANAs.) The first step in management is to control Mrs. C's symptoms. NSAIDs and prednisone are likely to accomplish this. There are already signs of joint destruction on the radiographs, so aggressive therapy with DMARDs is indicated.

CHIEF COMPLAINT

PATIENT ⬇3️⃣

Ms. T is a 21-year-old woman who comes to see you complaining of rash and joint pain for the past 2 days. She reports being well until 2 days ago when she awoke with severe pain in both knees and mild pain in both wrists. No other joints were involved. She also noted a nonpruritic rash on her distal arms and legs. She describes the rash as "splotchy." The joint pain has worsened over the last 2 days, and she reports that both her knees are swollen.

At this point, what is the leading hypothesis, what are the active alternatives, and is there a must not miss diagnosis? Given this differential diagnosis, what tests should be ordered?

RANKING THE DIFFERENTIAL DIAGNOSIS

Ms. T has acute onset polyarticular joint symptoms. From her history of knee swelling, it is likely that she has arthritis rather than arthralgias. The pivotal points are acute onset and polyarticular involvement. Considering these points, and limiting the differential diagnosis based on the patient's demographics and associated symptoms, we are able to come up with a fairly short list of probable etiologies.

Given the acuity of the illness, infectious arthritides need to be strongly considered. Many viral illnesses can cause arthritis. Parvovirus is probably the most common. Bacterial illnesses can cause polyarthritis in myriad ways. Septic arthritides, discussed above, can be polyarticular as can disseminated gonorrhea. Bacterial endocarditis can cause aseptic polyarthritis and can cause arthralgias. Acute rheumatic fever classically causes a migratory polyarthritis and rash. Lyme disease, discussed above, is most commonly monoarticular but can present in a polyarticular fashion. Reactive arthritis, occurring after enteric or urogenital infections, is also a possibility.

Although less likely, given the acute onset, primary rheumatologic diseases must also be considered. In a young woman with arthritis and a rash, SLE needs to be included on the differential diagnosis. As discussed above, rash, arthralgias, and arthritis are among the most common presenting symptoms in patients with SLE. Besides the acuity of the onset, the lack of other organ system involvement would be a little unusual for patients with SLE. RA would be less likely given the patient's age; however, Still disease, a variant of RA, may present acutely in young patients.

Given that the viral arthritides are more common than bacterial ones and, as far as we know, the patient has been previously well, viral arthritis is probably more likely than bacterial disease. Table 27-10 lists the differential diagnosis.

⬇3️⃣

On further history, Ms. T reports that 10 days before she came to see you she experienced 2 days of fatigue, myalgias, and fever to 39.4°C. There were no other symptoms. These symptoms resolved uneventfully.

She reports no travel outside Chicago, where she is in school, for the last year. She does not use recreational drugs. She is not sexually active.

Table 27-10. Diagnostic hypotheses for Ms. T.

Diagnostic Hypotheses	Demographics, Risk Factors, Symptoms and Signs	Important Tests
Leading Hypothesis		
Viral arthritis, parvovirus most common	Usually a history of preceding illness	Antibody titers and serology
Active Alternative		
Systemic lupus erythematosus	Multisystem disease Most common in young, African American women	Clinical diagnosis aided by serologies and diagnostic criteria
Active Alternative—Must Not Miss		
Rheumatic fever	Migratory polyarthritis Carditis Erythema marginatum	Jones criteria
Bacterial arthritis (gonococcal or nongonococcal)	Fever with monoarticular or polyarticular arthritis	Positive synovial (or other body) fluid cultures
Other Alternative		
Reactive arthritis	History of recent colonic or urogenital infection Presence of arthritis, urethritis, and iritis	Clinical diagnosis

On physical exam, she appears healthy. Her vital signs are temperature, 36.9°C; BP, 106/68 mm Hg; pulse, 84 bpm; RR, 14 breaths per minute. On extremity exam, her wrists have normal range of motion. There is pain with extremes of flexion and extension in the wrists and MCPs. There is mildly decreased range of motion and warmth in the knees as well as small effusions.

Skin exam reveals a diffuse erythematous rash with macules on the hands, feet, and distal extremities. Palms and soles are spared. The remainder of the exam was normal. There is no heart murmur.

The patient's history supports our initial hypothesis. The history of a recent febrile illness makes a viral or other postinfectious arthritis most likely. Lyme disease and bacterial endocarditis are very unlikely given her lack of suspicious exposure and the fact that she is otherwise presently well. SLE remains on the differential but is less likely.

In a patient with acute polyarthritis, a detailed history of recent illnesses must be taken.

Is the clinical information sufficient to make a diagnosis? If not, what other information do you need?

Leading Hypothesis: Parvovirus

Textbook Presentation

Parvovirus is commonly seen in young people who are in contact with children (mothers, teachers, daycare workers, and pediatricians).

Parvovirus often presents 10 days after a flu-like illness with a macular rash and moderately severe arthralgias of the joints of the upper extremities. There is no fever and symptoms improve over the course of weeks.

Disease Highlights

A. There are 5 major manifestations of parvovirus infection in humans.

1. Erythema infectiosum (fifth disease) in children

2. Acute arthropathy in adults

3. Transient aplastic crises in patients with chronic hemolytic diseases

4. Chronic anemia in immunocompromised persons

5. Fetal death complicating maternal infection prior to 20 weeks gestation.

B. In adults, the acute disease often proceeds in 2 phases with the arthritis following a systemic febrile infection.

1. Initial phase

   a. Nonspecific symptoms such as fever, malaise, headache, myalgia, diarrhea, and pruritus

   b. Generally resembles a nonspecific viral infection

2. Second phase

   a. Follows initial phase by 10 days with joint symptoms and rash dominating the clinical picture.

   b. Arthropathy accompanies about 50% of adult infections.

   c. The arthritis is a symmetric polyarthritis commonly involving the following joints:

      (1) Elbows

      (2) Wrists

      (3) Hands

      (4) Knees

      (5) Ankles

      (6) Feet

   d. The rash lasts 2–3 days.

      (1) It is usually a peripheral macular rash that occasionally spreads to the trunk.

      (2) Many different rashes have been described.

C. The incidence of parvovirus infection peaks between January and June.

D. Attack rates are 50–60%.

E. Contact with children is common among patients.

F. Other viruses cause arthritis less commonly. These are listed in Table 27-11.

Table 27-11. Common viral causes of arthritis.

Virus	Disease Characteristics
Rubella	Seen in about 50% of infections Occurs occasionally with vaccination Associated with rash
Hepatitis B	Arthritis usually precedes jaundice but is associated with transaminitis Rash may be present
HIV	May be symptom of seroconversion

Mumps, arboviruses, adenoviruses, coxsackieviruses, and echoviruses are all associated with arthritis

Evidence-Based Diagnosis

A. The diagnosis is made by identifying IgM to parvovirus in the serum of patients with a suspicious symptom complex.

B. The differential diagnosis of parvovirus includes SLE and the differentiation of these diseases can be challenging.

1. Both may present with arthritis, arthralgias, and rash.

2. Both are more common in women than men.

3. ANA can be transiently elevated in patients with parvovirus.

Treatment

A. The treatment of parvovirus is symptomatic.

B. NSAIDs generally provide good relief of symptoms.

C. Symptoms usually resolve within a couple of weeks, but as many as 10% of patients have symptoms that last longer.

MAKING A DIAGNOSIS

Ms. T was treated with NSAIDs and given a return appointment in 1 week. Laboratory tests were sent and revealed the following: Chem-7, normal; liver function tests, normal; WBC, 6800/mcL; Hgb, 12.9 g/dL; HCT, 37.9%; platelet, 182,000/mcL; ESR, 68 mm/h; rapid strep test, negative. ANA, streptococcal antibody titers, blood cultures, stool cultures, and parvovirus titer were pending when she left her first appointment.

Have you crossed a diagnostic threshold for the leading hypothesis, parvovirus? Have you ruled out the active alternatives? Do other tests need to be done to exclude the alternative diagnoses?

Parvovirus, or another viral arthritis, is highest on the differential diagnosis. Laboratory testing to rule in the most likely disease and rule out other possible diseases is essential. The normal liver function tests rule out hepatitis B as the cause of the patient's symptoms. Negative blood cultures will make endocarditis even less likely than it is based on the history alone. Lyme disease was thought so unlikely that serologies were not sent. Stool cultures were sent to evaluate the possibility of a reactive arthritis.

Alternative Diagnosis: Reactive Arthritis

Textbook Presentation

Reactive arthritis classically presents as a subacute, oligoarticular arthritis, often involving the knees, ankles, and back. Physical exam reveals arthritis. There may be a history of an antecedent infection and symptoms of urethritis and conjunctivitis.

Disease Highlights

A. Reactive arthritis is an acute arthritis complicating enteric and urogenital infections. This was formerly called Reiter syndrome.

B. Manifestations of the disease begin 1–4 weeks after the inciting infection, but more often than not, the inciting infection is asymptomatic.

Reactive arthritis often presents without an apparent antecedent infection.

Table 27-12. Features of reactive arthritis.

Feature	Prevalence
History of diarrhea	6%
Urethritis	46%
Conjunctivitis	31%
Location of arthritis	
Knees	68%
Ankles	49%
Feet	64%
Fever > 38.3°C	32%

Data from Arnett FC. Incomplete Reiter's syndrome: Clinical comparisons with classical triad. Ann Rheum Dis 1979;38(Suppl 1):suppl 73–78.

C. Reactive arthritis is typically an asymmetric oligoarthritis, usually involving the large joints of the lower extremities.

    a. Knees, ankles, and joints in the feet are the most common locations.

    b. Dactylitis, heel pain, and back pain also occur in 50–60% of patients.

D. The presentation of reactive arthritis often includes extra-articular manifestations such as enthesitis, tendinitis, bursitis, urethritis, or conjunctivitis.

    1. Urethritis is frequently the first finding followed by eye findings and then arthritis.

    2. Other associated findings include rash, nail changes, and oral ulcers.

    3. Table 27-12 shows the prevalence of various findings from an early study.

E. Reactive arthritis is 1 of the seronegative spondyloarthropathies.

    1. Early studies showed a high prevalence of HLA B-27 among affected patients.

    2. More recent studies have shown lower prevalences but have suggested that the presence of this antigen is associated with a more severe arthritis and predicts more protracted disease.

F. The bacteria commonly implicated in reactive arthritis are

    1. *Shigella*

    2. *Salmonella*

    3. *Yersinia*

    4. *Campylobacter*

    5. *Chlamydia*

G. The incidence of reactive arthritis varies by organism.

    1. Studies of outbreaks of GI infections have provided incidences of 0–29%.

    2. Population based studies, performed on people who had positive stool cultures for an enteric pathogen, have yielded incidence on the order of 1–3 cases/100,000.

H. GI infections are equally likely to be the inciting event in men and women. Arthritis complicating chlamydial infection is rare in women.

I. The age at diagnosis is generally in the 30s.

Evidence-Based Diagnosis

A. The diagnosis is a clinical one.

B. Although there are no agreed upon diagnostic criteria, proposed ones have included major criteria (asymmetric monoarticular or oligoarticular arthritis of the lower extremities and a preceding enteric or urogenital infection) and minor criteria (evidence of a triggering infection or persistent evidence of synovial inflammation).

C. A high clinical suspicion is warranted in a young patient with an asymmetric oligoarthritis.

Treatment

A. In most patients, symptoms resolve within 1 year.

B. NSAIDs are useful in treating the acute symptoms.

C. Culture-positive enteric or chlamydial infections should be treated.

D. A subset of patients experience relapse, development of a chronic arthritis, or development of ankylosing spondylitis.

E. There has been some recent suggestion that patients with a chronic arthritis, negative traditional cultures, but evidence of persistent chlamydial infection (positive synovial fluid or blood polymerase chain reaction [PCR]) be treated with antibiotics.

Alternative Diagnosis: Rheumatic Fever

Textbook Presentation

Rheumatic fever classically presents in a child in the weeks following streptococcal pharyngitis. The 5 cardinal manifestations are arthritis, carditis, rash, subcutaneous nodules, and chorea. The arthritis is typically migratory, involving the knees, ankles, and hands.

Disease Highlights

A. Rheumatic fever is an inflammatory disease that follows streptococcal pharyngitis by 2–4 weeks.

B. Unlike in children, clinical documentation of a previous streptococcal infection is rare in adults and the most pronounced symptoms are joint pain and stiffness.

C. The arthritis is classically a migratory polyarthritis.

    1. Individual joints are usually affected for less than a week.

    2. The joints in the legs are usually affected first.

    3. Subjective complaints are often more prominent than objective findings.

D. Carditis

    1. May involve any, or all, parts of the heart—pericarditis, myocarditis, endocarditis, or pancarditis.

    2. Endocarditis commonly causes valvular lesions that may progress over years to symptomatic valve disease, especially mitral stenosis.

Evidence-Based Diagnosis

A. The diagnosis of rheumatic fever is based on the Jones Criteria.

B. The criteria require evidence of an antecedent group A streptococcal infection (culture, antibody titer) with either 2 major criteria or 1 major and 2 minor criteria (Table 27-13).

Treatment

A. Anti-inflammatories

    1. Aspirin is the mainstay of therapy.

    2. Corticosteroids are given to patients with severe carditis.

Table 27-13. Jones criteria for the rheumatic fever.

Major Criteria	Minor Criteria
Polyarthritis	Fever
Carditis (pericarditis, myocarditis, endocarditis)	Arthralgia
Chorea	Inflammatory markers (eg, CRP, ESR)
Rash—Erythema marginatum, subcutaneous nodules	PR segment prolongation

CRP, C-reactive protein; ESR, erythrocyte sedimentation rate.

B. Antibiotics
   1. Penicillin for treatment of pharyngitis.
   2. Lifelong prophylactic therapy with penicillin is usually recommended after the initial therapy.

CASE RESOLUTION

Parvovirus clearly fits this patient's presentation. Reactive arthritis is possible although the patient's recent illness was not gastrointestinal or urogenital. Rheumatic fever seems less likely. Although she does have multiple Jones criteria (polyarthritis, arthralgia, elevated erythrocyte sedimentation rate [ESR]) and although the lack of a sore throat during the recent illness is not terribly helpful, the patient does not have a migratory arthritis or evidence of present streptococcal carriage.

Ms. T's blood work came back negative except for a positive ANA (titer 1:80) and a positive parvovirus IgM. She was treated with NSAIDs with good relief of her symptoms. Her rash resolved over 3–4 days, and joint pain was gone at a follow-up visit 2 weeks later.

CHIEF COMPLAINT

PATIENT 4

Mr. L is a 55-year-old man who comes to see you complaining of right hip pain. He reports suffering with the pain for about 2 years. The pain is worst in the morning and evening. In the morning, it is associated with stiffness. The stiffness lasts about 5 minutes and then improves. At the end of the day he routinely feels a dull ache that is worse if he has had a very active day. He recently noticed that he is unable to cross his legs (right over left) without significant discomfort.

At this point, what is the leading hypothesis, what are the active alternatives, and is there a must not miss diagnosis? Given this differential diagnosis, what tests should be ordered?

RANKING THE DIFFERENTIAL DIAGNOSIS

Mr. L is a middle-aged man with chronic, monoarticular symptoms. The time course, single joint involvement and noninflammatory nature of the process (we have not heard about warmth, erythema, or prolonged morning stiffness) are the pivotal points in this case.

Reviewing the initial differential diagnosis, the articular process that best fits the history is OA, a chronic, noninflammatory, often monoarticular arthritis. OA is so common in older adults that it becomes the diagnosis to disprove in all patients who have pain at all consistent with OA. The disease most commonly affects the fingers, knee, hip, and spine. CPPD, as was discussed previously, is another chronic degenerative arthritis that could produce similar symptoms and should be considered.

In patients with noninflammatory monoarticular symptoms, we also have to consider the specific periarticular symptoms that can affect the particular joint.

When considering the periarticular syndromes that cause hip pain, it is important to identify where exactly the patient feels the pain. Lumbar spine disease with radicular symptoms can cause pain in the buttocks or lateral hip. Trochanteric bursitis is

a common cause of lateral hip pain. Inguinal hernias may cause groin pain. Femoral stress fractures may cause groin or lateral hip pain. Although such stress fractures are rare and are most commonly seen in young women, they should not be missed. Use of bisphosphonates or corticosteroids should raise the possibility of other causes hip abnormalities, femoral shaft fractures and osteonecrosis, respectively. Table 27-14 lists the differential diagnosis.

"Hip pain" is a nonspecific complaint. It is important to identify the exact location of the pain.

4

When asked to pinpoint the location of his pain, Mr. L reports that he primarily feels it in the groin. Rest, acetaminophen, and heat all seem to help the pain. He comes in today because he is in more constant pain, and he has begun to limp on bad days. His past history is remarkable only for mild asthma. He denies any previous injury to the hip. He has never been hospitalized or taken corticosteroids. His only medication is albuterol.

Vital signs are temperature, 37.0°C; RR, 12 breaths per minute; BP, 132/70 mm Hg; pulse, 72 bpm. On physical exam, there is no warmth, erythema, or tenderness around the hip or over the trochanteric bursa. Testicular exam and hernia exam are normal. Flexion and extension of the right hip are nearly normal. There is decreased range of motion in hip rotation with about 10 degrees in internal rotation and 20 degrees in external rotation.

Is the clinical information sufficient to make a diagnosis? If not, what other information do you need?

Leading Hypothesis: OA

Textbook Presentation

OA most commonly presents in older patients as chronic joint pain and stiffness. Pain is usually worse with activity and improves with

Table 27-14. Diagnostic hypotheses for Mr. L.

Diagnostic Hypotheses	Demographics, Risk Factors, Symptoms and Signs	Important Tests
Leading Hypothesis		
Osteoarthritis	Chronic pain in weight-bearing joints	Radiograph of affected joints
Active Alternative		
CPPD	May present as chronic or acute arthritis	Demonstration of crystals in synovial fluid or classic radiographic findings
Active Alternatives—Nonarticular		
Inguinal hernia	Pain worse with straining	Physical exam
Trochanteric bursitis	Lateral hip pain Tenderness over the bursa	Physical exam Response to injection therapy
Lumbar nerve root compression	Positive straight leg raise	Physical exam MRI
Active Alternative—Must Not Miss		
Femoral stress fractures	Most common in young women involved in weight-bearing exercise	MRI Bone scan

rest. Knees, hips, and hands are most commonly affected. On examination of the joints, there is bony enlargement without significant effusions. Mild tenderness may be present along the joint lines. There is limited range of motion. Radiographs are diagnostic.

Disease Highlights

A. OA is a disease of aging, with peak prevalence in the eighth decade. However, as obesity is a risk factor, it may be seen in much younger people with severe obesity.

B. More common in women than men

C. Although often referred to as "wear and tear" arthritis, the pathophysiology is actually quite complicated.

D. Joint destruction manifests as a loss of cartilage with change to the underlying bone seen as bony sclerosis and osteophyte formation.

E. Joint distribution
  1. OA is most common in the knees, hips, hands, and spine.
  2. Nearly any joint can be affected.
  3. Non–weight-bearing joints other than the hand, such as the elbow, wrist, and shoulder, are less commonly affected by OA. The ankle is also not a common location.

F. Classic symptoms include
  1. Pain with activity
  2. Relief with rest
  3. Periarticular tenderness
  4. Occasional mildly inflammatory flares
  5. Gelling: Joint stiffness brought on by rest and rapidly resolving with activity.
  6. Late in the disease, constant pain with joint deformation and severe disability is common.

G. Physical exam findings
  1. Generally there is bony enlargement, crepitus, and decreased range of motion without signs of inflammation or synovial thickening.
  2. Knee
    a. Crepitus
    b. Tenderness on joint line
    c. Varus or valgus displacement of the lower leg related to asymmetric loss of the articular cartilage.
  3. Hip
    a. Marked decrease first in internal and then external rotation
    b. Groin pain with rotation of the hip
  4. Hand
    a. Tenderness and bony enlargement of the first carpometacarpal joint
    b. Joint involvement in decreasing order of prevalence is DIP, PIP, MCP.
    c. Heberden nodes (prominent osteophytes of the DIP joints)
    d. Bouchard nodes (prominent osteophytes of the PIP joints)
    e. Figure 27-3 shows a hand with some of the classic findings of OA.
  5. Spine
    a. Signs of spinal OA vary depending on location.
    b. Pain and limited range of motion are common.
    c. Radicular symptoms resulting from osteophyte impingement on nerve roots is seen.
    d. Spinal stenosis with associated symptoms (radiculopathy and pseudoclaudication) can result from bony hypertrophy (see Chapter 7, Back Pain).

Evidence-Based Diagnosis

A. The diagnosis of OA is clinical, based on a compatible history, physical exam, and radiologic findings.

B. Because of the high prevalence of OA, the diagnosis should lead the differential in any patient with suspicious symptoms.

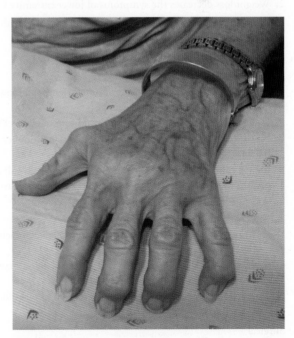

Figure 27-3. Osteoarthritis of the hand.

C. Diagnostic criteria have been established.

1. Hand

   a. Pain, aching, or stiffness

   b. 3 of the following

      (1) Hard tissue enlargement of at least 2 of the following joints:

         (a) Second and third DIP joints
         (b) Second and third PIP joints
         (c) First MCP joint

      (2) Hard tissue enlargement of 2 or more DIP joints

      (3) Fewer than 3 swollen MCP joints

      (4) Deformity of at least 1 of the joints listed in above entries a through c.

2. Hip

   a. Hip pain

   b. 2 of the following:

      (1) ESR < 20 mm/h

      (2) Osteophytes on radiograph

      (3) Joint-space narrowing on radiograph

3. Knee: There are multiple criteria, the easiest to remember is

   a. Knee pain

   b. Osteophytes on radiograph, and

   c. 1 of the following

      (1) Age older than 50 years

      (2) Stiffness < 30 minutes

      (3) Crepitus

D. The test characteristics for these criteria are shown in Table 27-15.

Treatment

A. Nonpharmacologic

1. Patient education and improved social support have been shown to improve pain and improve the efficacy of pharmacologic interventions.

2. Weight loss decreases the symptoms of lower extremity OA.

3. Physical and occupational therapy can help patients with functional impairment due to OA.

B. Pharmacologic

1. Acetaminophen

   a. Standard initial therapy given its effectiveness and low side-effect profile.

   b. Equally effective to NSAIDs for mild to moderate OA.

2. NSAIDs are probably more effective than acetaminophen for severe OA.

3. Oral combinations of glucosamine and chondroitan sulfate probably are modestly effective in some patients and have a very favorable side-effect profile.

4. Intra-articular medications

   a. Intra-articular corticosteroids are very effective for acute flares of OA.

   b. Hyaluronic acid given by intra-articular injection may provide a small benefit to some patients.

5. Tramadol and opioid analgesics are reasonable choices for patients with severe symptoms.

C. Surgical

1. Arthroscopic surgery for OA is probably ineffective.

Table 27-15. Test characteristics for the diagnostic criteria of OA.

Joint	Sensitivity	Specificity	LR+	LR−
Hand	94%	87%	7.2	0.07
Hip	89%	91%	9.9	0.12
Knee	91%	86%	6.5	0.1

OA, osteoarthritis.

2. Hip and knee replacement can have remarkable effects on decreasing pain and improving function in patients in whom conservative therapy has failed.

MAKING A DIAGNOSIS

Mr. L's history and physical exam are very suggestive of OA, but CPPD remains a possibility. Most of the periarticular syndromes that were considered initially have been made unlikely by the exam. Lumbar spine disease with radicular symptoms would not cause the limited range of motion that is seen on the patient's exam. The predominant symptom in patients with trochanteric bursitis is tenderness over the bursa. Mr. L does not have a hernia on exam. Femoral stress fractures may cause groin pain but should not really cause limited range of motion. That said, this is a diagnosis that must not be missed, so further consideration should be given.

The working diagnosis of OA was made and the patient was given 1000 mg of acetaminophen twice daily. A radiograph was ordered.

Have you crossed a diagnostic threshold for the leading hypothesis, OA? Have you ruled out the active alternatives? Do other tests need to be done to exclude the alternative diagnoses?

Alternative Diagnosis: Femoral Stress Fractures

Textbook Presentation

Femoral stress fractures are most commonly seen in young female athletes. Symptoms begin acutely with groin pain that persists and worsens as the day progresses. On physical exam, there is often mild tenderness over the proximal one-third of the femur. Range of motion of the hip is normal. Radiographs are usually normal.

Disease Highlights

A. Like other types of stress fractures, femoral stress fractures are most common in:

1. Athletes who have recently increased their level of training

2. Women

3. Persons with decreased bone density

B. The most common stress fractures are tibial and metatarsal.

C. Femoral stress fractures usually present with hip or groin pain with preserved range of motion of the hip.

Evidence-Based Diagnosis

A. Stress fractures in general and femoral stress fractures in particular are often not seen on initial radiographs.

B. MRI and bone scans are considered the diagnostic test of choice.

Treatment

A. Many stress fractures heal with reduced physical activity and short-term immobilization.

B. Femoral stress fractures may resolve with decreased weight bearing (crutches) or may require casting or internal fixation.

CASE RESOLUTION

The patient's hip radiograph showed changes consistent with OA.

The combination of a high clinical suspicion, pain, and consistent findings on a radiograph confirms the diagnosis.

REVIEW OF OTHER IMPORTANT DISEASES

Periarticular Syndromes

There are textbooks written about the numerous periarticular syndromes that commonly present to primary care physicians, orthopedists, and rheumatologists. Table 27-16 briefly outlines some of the most common.

Table 27-16. Some common periarticular pain syndromes.

Area of Pain	Diagnosis	History	Physical and Diagnostic Evaluation
Neck and shoulder	Sternocleidomastoid muscle spasm	Common cause of "stiff neck" in patient who is otherwise well Often noticed upon wakening	Neck pain with head tilt
	Cervical radiculopathy	Pain and stiffness of cervical spine, usually with radiation to upper back and arm Occasionally manifests solely as pain between spine and scapula	Radicular symptoms can be reproduced with manipulation of cervical spine MRI diagnostic
	Subacromial or rotator cuff disorder	Shoulder pain, often subacute onset, often worse at night	Positive painful arc test
	Rotator cuff tear	Pain similar to above Occurs after injury in younger patients Often spontaneous in older patients	Positive internal or external rotation lag test
Elbow	Lateral and medial epicondylitis	Pain over tendon insertion on medial and lateral epicondyle	Tenderness at site of pain Exacerbated with wrist flexion (medial) or extension (lateral)
	Olecranon bursitis	Pain over olecranon bursa	Tenderness and swelling over the olecranon bursa
Hand	DeQuervain tenosynovitis	Pain at the lateral base of the thumb	Worse with pincer grasp Positive Finkelstein maneuver (ulnar deviation of wrist with fingers curled over thumb)
Hip	Trochanteric bursitis	Pain over bursa	Tenderness over bursa
		Patient often notes pain when lying on area at night	Sometimes visualized on radiograph
	Meralgia paresthetica	Pain or numbness over lateral thigh Often after weight gain or loss	Neuropathic-type pain Abnormal sensation over lateral femoral cutaneous nerve distribution
Knee	Patellofemoral syndrome	Anterior knee pain, often worse climbing or descending stairs	Crepitus beneath patella
	Meniscal and ligamentous injuries	Ligament injuries tend to be traumatic Classically associated with the knee giving way Meniscal injuries may be traumatic or degenerative Knee locking is classic	Ligament injuries will manifest as laxity on exam Meniscal injuries as a click MRI is diagnostic
Foot and ankle	Achilles tendinitis	Pain over distal tendon Pain and stiffness worse after inactivity	Tenderness over insertion of tendon
	Plantar fasciitis	Pain anterior to heel Worse with first standing	History usually diagnostic Radiograph may show heel spur
	Morton neuroma	Pain between the second and third or third and fourth metatarsal heads	Tenderness at the area of pain
Polyperiarticular	Fibromyalgia	Diffuse pain syndrome Often nonrestorative sleep	Diagnosis depends on tenderness at 11 or more specific locations
	Polymyalgia rheumatica	Pain and disability of large muscles of shoulder and hips	Disease is often associated with signs of inflammatory disease (anemia, elevated CRP and ESR)

CRP, C-reactive protein; ESR, erythrocyte sedimentation rate.

REFERENCES

Aletaha D, Neogi T, Silman AJ et al. 2010 Rheumatoid Arthritis Classification Criteria: An American College of Rheumatology/European League Against Rheumatism Collaborative Initiative. Arthritis Rheum. 2010;62(9):2569–81.

Arnett FC. Incomplete Reiter's syndrome: clinical comparisons with classical triad. Ann Rheum Dis. 1979;38 Suppl 1:suppl 73–8.

Black ER. *Diagnostic strategies for common medical problems.* 2nd ed. Philadelphia: American College of Physicians; 1999.

Cader MZ. Performance of the 2010 ACR/EULAR criteria for rheumatoid arthritis: comparison with 1987 ACR criteria in a very early synovitis cohort. Ann Rheum Dis. 2011;70:949–55.

Hannu T. Reactive Arthritis. Best Pract Res Clin Rheumatol. 2011;5:347–57.

Margaretten ME, Kohlwes J, Moore D, Bent S. Does this adult patient have septic arthritis? JAMA. 2007;297(13):1478–88.

Neogi T. Gout. N Engl J Med. 2011;364:443–52.

Nishimura K, Sugiyama D, Kogata Y et al. Meta-analysis: diagnostic accuracy of anti-cyclic citrullinated peptide antibody and rheumatoid factor for rheumatoid arthritis. Ann Intern Med. 2007;146(11):797–808.

O'Brien JP, Goldenberg DL, Rice PA. Disseminated gonococcal infection: a prospective analysis of 49 patients and a review of pathophysiology and immune mechanisms. Medicine (Baltimore). 1983;62(6):395–406.

Primer on the rheumatic diseases. 13th ed. Atlanta, GA: Arthritis Foundation; 2008.

Richette P, Bardin T, Doherty M. An update on the epidemiology of calcium pyrophosphate dehydrate crystal deposition disease. Rheumatology (Oxford). 2009;48:711–15.

Shmerling RH. Origin and utility of measurement of rheumatoid factors. In: Rose B, ed. UpToDate, 2007.

Steere AC. Lyme disease. N Engl J Med. 2001;345(2):115–25.

van der Linden MP, Knevel R, Huizinga TW, van der Helm-van Mil AH. Comparison of the 1987 American College of Rheumatology Criteria and the 2010 American College of Rheumatology/European League Against Rheumatism Criteria. Arthritis Rheum. 2011;63(1):37–42.

28

I have a patient with acute kidney injury.
How do I determine the cause?

CHIEF COMPLAINT

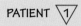

PATIENT 1

Mr. T is 77-year-old man with acute kidney injury (AKI).

What is the differential diagnosis of AKI? How would you frame the differential?

CONSTRUCTING A DIFFERENTIAL DIAGNOSIS

AKI is a syndrome defined as a reduction in kidney function that has occurred within the last 7 days. AKI can occur in patients with no known kidney disease but is more likely to develop in patients with preexisting kidney disease. Table 28-1 summarizes the current diagnostic criteria and staging for AKI, and acute and chronic kidney disease (CKD).

The framework for the differential diagnosis of AKI is a combination of anatomic and pathophysiologic:

A. Prerenal (due to renal hypoperfusion)

 1. Hypovolemia

  a. Gastrointestinal fluid loss

  b. Renal loss

  c. Hemorrhage

  d. Third spacing

 2. Decreased effective circulating volume (with or without hypotension)

  a. Heart failure (HF)

  b. Cirrhosis

 3. Hypotension

  a. Sepsis

  b. Cardiogenic shock

  c. Anaphylaxis

  d. Anesthesia- and medication-induced

  e. Relative hypotension below patient's autoregulatory level

 4. Changes in renal hemodynamics

  a. Nonsteroidal antiinflammatory drugs (NSAIDs) (including cyclooxygenase (COX)-2 inhibitors)

  b. Angiotensin-converting enzyme inhibitors/angiotensin receptor blockers

  c. Renal artery thrombosis or embolism

  d. Abdominal aortic aneurysm

B. Intrarenal

 1. Vascular

  a. Vasculitis

  b. Malignant hypertension

  c. Cholesterol emboli

  d. Thrombotic microangiopathies

   (1) Thrombotic thrombocytopenic purpura

   (2) Hemolytic uremic syndrome

   (3) Disseminated intravascular coagulopathy

 2. Glomerular

  a. Inflammatory

   (1) Postinfectious glomerulonephritis (GN)

   (2) Cryoglobulinemia

   (3) Henoch-Schönlein purpura

   (4) Systemic lupus erythematosus

   (5) Antineutrophil cytoplasmic antibody associated GN

   (6) Anti-glomerular basement membrane disease

  b. Thrombotic microangiopathies

 3. Tubular injury (acute tubular necrosis [ATN])

  a. Ischemic, due to prolonged renal hypoperfusion

  b. Toxin induced

   (1) Medications (such as aminoglycosides)

   (2) Radiocontrast media

   (3) Heavy metals (cisplatinum)

   (4) Intratubular pigments (myoglobin, hemoglobin), crystals (uric acid, oxalate), or proteins (myeloma)

 4. Interstitial

  a. Acute interstitial nephritis

  b. Bilateral pyelonephritis

  c. Infiltration (lymphoma, sarcoidosis)

C. Postrenal

 1. Mechanical

  a. Ureteral (must be bilateral obstruction to cause AKI)

   (1) Stones

   (2) Tumors

   (3) Hematoma

   (4) Retroperitoneal adenopathy or fibrosis

  b. Bladder neck

   (1) Benign prostatic hyperplasia (BPH) or prostate cancer

   (2) Tumors

   (3) Stones

  c. Urethral

Table 28-1. Diagnostic criteria and staging for kidney disease.

Syndrome	Serum Creatinine (Scr)/GFR Criteria	Evidence of Kidney Damage[1]	Staging		
			Stage[2]	Scr	Urinary Output
Acute kidney injury (AKI)	• Increase in serum creatinine by ≥ 0.3 mg/dL within 48 hours **or** • Increase to ≥ 1.5 times baseline within 7 days **or** • Urine volume < 0.5 mL/kg/h for 6 hours	Not required for diagnosis	1	↑ by ≥ 0.3 or 1.5–1.9 times baseline	< 0.5 mL/kg/h for 6–12 hours
			2	2–2.9 times baseline	< 0.5 mL/kg/h for ≥ 12 hours
			3	3 times baseline **or** ≥ 4 mg/dL **or** dialysis	< 0.3 mL/kg/h for ≥ 24 hours **or** anuria
Acute kidney disease (AKD)[3]	• AKI **or** • GFR < 60 mL/min for < 3 months **or** • Decrease in GFR by ≥ 35% **or** increase in serum creatinine > 1.5 times baseline for < 3 months	Present for < 3 months	No staging		
Chronic kidney disease (CKD)[3]	GFR < 60 mL/min for > 3 months	Present for > 3 months	**GFR stages**	**Albuminuria stages (ACR)**	
			G1 > 90 G2 60–89 G3a 45–59 G3b 30–44 G4 15–29 G5 < 15	A1 < 30 mcg/mg A2 30–299 mcg/mg A3 ≥ 300 mcg/mg	

[1] Kidney damage is defined as any of the following: urinalysis with casts (red cell, white cell, renal tubular epithelial, or granular), proteinuria [albumin/creatinine ratio (ACR) > 30 mg/g or protein/creatinine ratio (PCR) > 150 mg/g], abnormal histology, abnormalities on imaging (size abnormalities, hydronephrosis, cysts, stones), or presence of a transplanted kidney.
[2] Patients should be assigned the higher stage when Scr and urinary output criteria are discordant.
[3] Patients have AKD or CKD if they meet either the creatinine/GFR criteria **or** have evidence of kidney damage.
GFR, glomerular filtration rate.

(1) Strictures
(2) Tumors
(3) Obstructed indwelling catheters
2. Neurogenic bladder

Figure 28-1 outlines the diagnostic approach to AKI.

Measuring Kidney Function

A. Glomerular filtration rate (GFR)
  1. Best overall measure of kidney function
  2. Normal = 130 mL/min/1.73m^2 in young men (120 mL/min/1.73m^2 in women)
  3. Difficult to accurately measure in clinical practice

B. Serum creatinine
  1. Level varies with age, sex, race or ethnic group, muscle mass, diet, nutritional status
  2. The relationship between creatinine and GFR varies inversely and exponentially, so that early, small changes in serum creatinine may reflect clinically significant decreases in GFR.
    a. A 50-year-old white man with a baseline serum creatinine of 1.0 mg/dL has a GFR of 80 mL/min/1.73m^2; if his creatinine increases by 50% to 1.5 mg/dL, his GFR drops to 50 mL/min/1.73m^2.
    b. If his baseline serum creatinine is 4.0 mg/dL, his GFR is about 16 mL/min/1.73m^2; if his creatinine increases by 50% to 6.0 mg/dL, his GFR is about 10 mL/min/1.73m^2.

C. Cystatin C
  1. Freely filtered by glomerulus
  2. Less variable than creatinine
  3. Not yet in widespread use

D. Measured creatinine clearance
  1. Creatinine is filtered by glomeruli *and* secreted by the proximal tubule, so creatinine clearance overestimates GFR.
  2. Must be calculated with a 24-hour urine collection, which is inconvenient for patients and often incomplete.

E. Estimated GFR
  1. Cockcroft-Gault formula (multiply by 0.85 for women):

$$C_{cr} = \frac{[(140 - age) \times weight\ in\ kg]}{72 \times creatinine\ in\ mg/dL}$$

    a. Does not adjust for body surface area
    b. Does not accurately estimate renal function in those with normal GFRs, obese patients, or adults over 70 years.

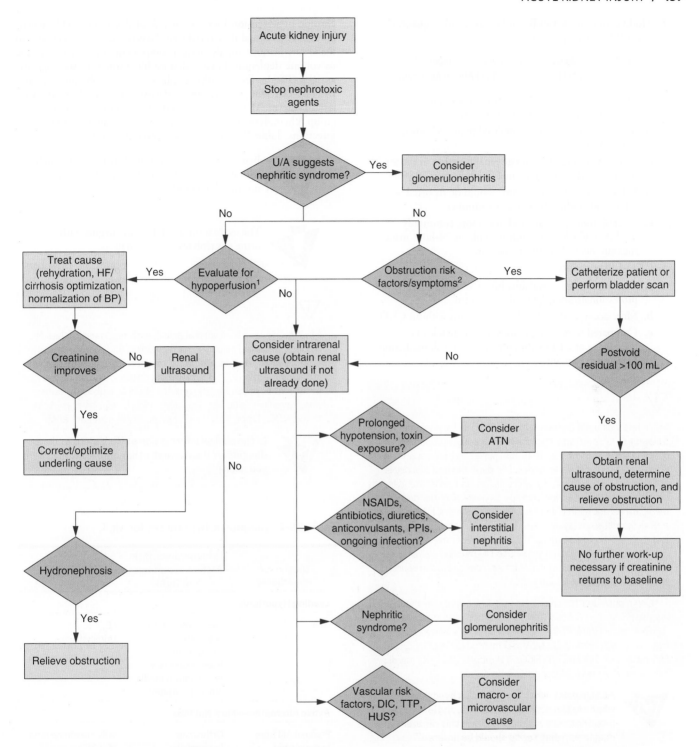

Figure 28-1. Diagnostic approach: acute kidney injury.

[1]History: symptoms related to hypovolemia (fever, nausea, vomiting, diarrhea, bleeding); heart failure (dyspnea, orthopnea, paroxysmal nocturnal dyspnea, edema), or cirrhosis (increased abdominal girth, edema)
Physical exam: hypotension, tachycardia, orthostasis, dry mucous membranes; signs of heart failure (pulmonary crackles, S3, elevated jugular venous pressure, edema) or cirrhosis (ascites, edema, spider angiomata)
Labs: specific gravity >1.020, FE_{Na} <1%, FE_{urea} < 35%
[2]Obstruction risk factors/symptoms: older age, male sex, anuria, anticholinergic medications, incontinence, dribbling.

ATN, acute tubular necrosis; DIC, disseminated intravascular coagulation; HF, heart failure; HUS, hemolytic uremic syndrome; NSAIDs, nonsteroidal anti-inflammatory drugs; PPIs, proton pump inhibitors; TTP, thrombotic thrombocytopenia; U/A, urinalysis.

2. Modification of Diet in Renal Disease Study Equation (MDRD) study equation:

$$GFR = 175 \times (standardized\ creatinine)^{-1.154} \times (age)^{-0.203}$$
$$\times 0.742\ (if\ female)\ or \times 1.212\ (if\ African\ American)$$

   a. Online calculator available: http://www.kidney.org/professionals/kdoqi/gfr_calculator.cfm

   b. Most accurate in nonhospitalized patients known to have CKD

   c. Does not accurately estimate renal function in those with normal GFRs, obese patients, or adults over 70 years

   d. Values > 60 mL/min/1.73m² should be reported as "above 60" rather than an exact number

   e. Overall, more accurate and now more commonly used than Cockcroft-Gault formula or 24-hour urine measurement of creatinine clearance.

3. CKD-EPI equation

   a. Online calculator available: http://www.kidney.org/professionals/kdoqi/gfr_calculator.cfm

   b. More accurate than MDRD in patients without CKD

   c. Compared to other equations, results in a lower prevalence of CKD with more accurate risk prediction for adverse outcomes.

Mr. T felt well until 3 days ago, when he had a shaking chill followed by a fever and the onset of a cough productive of rusty colored sputum. His fever has persisted, his cough has worsened, and he feels lethargic. His past medical history is notable for well-controlled hypertension and prostate cancer treated with radiation therapy 5 years ago. His current medications are hydrochlorothiazide and lisinopril. He smokes a few cigarettes a day and has 1 drink per week. His physical exam shows temperature, 38.6°C; BP, 90/60 mm Hg; pulse, 110 bpm; RR, 24 breaths per minute. His mucous membranes appear dry. Lung exam is notable for decreased breath sounds and crackles at the right lung base.

One month ago, his creatinine was 1.4 mg/dL. Six months ago, his PSA was 1.0. Laboratory test results now include WBC, 16,000/mcL (70% PMNs, 20% bands, 10% lymphocytes); Hgb, 10.2 g/dL; Hct, 32%; MCV, 88 mcm³; Na, 140 mEq/L; K, 5.4 mEq/L; Cl, 100 mEq/L; HCO₃, 19 mEq/L; BUN, 40 mg/dL; creatinine, 3.8 mg/dL; glucose, 102 mg/dL.

 At this point, what is the leading hypothesis, what are the active alternatives, and is there a must not miss diagnosis? Given this differential diagnosis, what tests should be ordered?

RANKING THE DIFFERENTIAL DIAGNOSIS

 Although 1 etiology may be more likely than the others based on the presentation, the initial testing is generally the same for every patient with AKI.

The pivotal point in this patient's presentation is the hypotension, due to hypovolemia, sepsis (presumably pneumococcal based on his classic presentation), or both. Transient hypovolemia or hypotension causes prerenal azotemia, but prolonged hypotension leads to renal ischemia. It is likely he has been hypotensive long enough for renal ischemia and consequent ATN to have developed. His history of CKD (baseline creatinine of 1.4 mg/dL), age, and

chronic hypertension increase his risk of developing ATN whenever his renal blood flow is reduced. Nevertheless, it is necessary to make sure he does not also have a component of prerenal AKI due to volume depletion. Finally, despite his normal prostate-specific antigen (PSA) a few months ago, he could have obstruction from BPH or recurrent prostate cancer. Post-streptococcal GN, an intrarenal cause of AKI, is not a consideration since that occurs after group A hemolytic streptococcal infections, not after pneumococcal infections. Table 28-2 lists the differential diagnosis.

 Because hypovolemia and obstruction are such treatable causes of AKI, they are always "must not miss" diagnoses.

 The evaluation of AKI always begins with urine electrolytes and a urinalysis.

Mr. T receives 1 L of normal saline, with no change in his BP. Urine is obtained prior to the fluid bolus and results include urine sodium, 40 mEq/h; urine chloride, 57 mEq/mL; urine creatinine, 45 mg/24 h, and urine urea nitrogen 250 g/24 h; urinalysis showed specific gravity, 1.010; leukocyte esterase, negative; glucose, negative; blood, negative; protein, trace; RBC, 1/hpf; WBC, 1–2/hpf; positive granular casts.

 Is the clinical information sufficient to make a diagnosis? If not, what other information do you need?

Table 28-2. Diagnostic hypotheses for Mr. T.

Diagnostic Hypotheses	Demographics, Risk Factors, Symptoms and Signs	Important Tests
Leading Hypothesis		
ATN	Hypotension from any cause Exposure to toxins (especially radiocontrast media, aminoglycosides)	FE_{Na} Urinalysis
Active Alternative—Must Not Miss		
Prerenal AKI from hypovolemia	Orthostatic hypotension Abnormal subclavicular skin turgor Dry axilla or mucous membranes History of vomiting or diarrhea Elderly	BUN/creatinine ratio FE_{Na}, FE_{urea} Specific gravity Response to fluid challenge
Obstruction	Incontinence Dribbling Pelvic discomfort Older man	Ultrasound Postvoid residual (by bladder scan or catheterization)

AKI, acute kidney injury; ATN, acute tubular necrosis; BUN, blood urea nitrogen; FE_{Na}, fractional excretion of sodium; FE_{urea}, fractional excretion of urea.

Leading Hypothesis: ATN

ATN is not synonymous with AKI; it is a cause of AKI.

Textbook Presentation

The presentation ranges from asymptomatic (with discovery of an increased creatinine on routine laboratory testing) to symptoms of uremia, such as lethargy, nausea, delirium, seizures, edema, and dyspnea.

Disease Highlights

A. Etiology

1. **Ischemia** due to renal hypoperfusion prolonged enough to cause tubular cell damage

   a. Due to autoregulation, patients with normal kidneys and normal renal arteries can maintain normal renal blood flow and GFR with mean arterial pressures (MAPs) as low as 80 mm Hg.

   b. When renal artery pressure decreases, there is a prostaglandin-mediated drop in afferent arteriolar resistance and an angiotensin II–mediated increase in efferent arteriolar resistance; these changes maintain glomerular capillary pressure and GFR.

   c. If renal artery pressure drops below the autoregulatory range, endogenous vasoconstrictors cause an increase in afferent arteriolar resistance, leading to reduced glomerular capillary pressure and GFR.

   d. Despite decreased perfusion, tubules remain intact initially; however, with prolonged ischemia, there is tubular injury and cell death.

   e. Patients with the conditions or exposures listed in Table 28-3, all of which impair autoregulation, are at higher risk for developing ATN.

2. **Toxin exposure** (radiocontrast media, aminoglycosides, amphotericin B, cisplatin, Hgb, myoglobin, crystals, myeloma proteins)

Table 28-3. Factors affecting autoregulation of glomerular pressure and glomerular filtration rate.

Inability to Decrease Afferent Arteriolar Resistance	Inability to Increase Efferent Arteriolar Resistance	Vascular Obstruction
Older age	ACE inhibitors	Renal artery stenosis
Atherosclerosis	Angiotensin receptor blockers	
Chronic hypertension		
Chronic kidney disease		
Malignant hypertension		
NSAIDs/COX-2 inhibitors		
Sepsis		
Hypercalcemia		
Cyclosporine/tacrolimus		
Renal artery stenosis		

ACE, angiotensin-converting enzyme; COX, cyclooxygenase; NSAIDs, nonsteroidal antiinflammatory drugs.

3. Contrast-induced nephropathy (CIN) is the most common toxin-induced ATN.

   a. Patient-related risk factors for CIN

      (1) Underlying CKD: patients with estimated GFR 45–60 mL/min have an intermediate risk of developing CIN; those with estimated GFR 30–45 mL/min have a high risk; those with estimated GFR < 30 mL/min have a very high risk.

      (2) Diabetes: patients with CKD and diabetes have especially high risk.

      (3) Intravascular volume depletion

      (4) HF

   b. Procedure-related risk factors for CIN

      (1) Volume of contrast used

      (2) Hyperosmolar contrast media

      (3) Intra-arterial contrast administration

   c. Serum creatinine levels peak at 3 days postexposure and usually return to baseline within 10 days.

B. Epidemiology and prognosis of ATN

1. ATN accounts for 55–60% of AKI in hospitalized patients and for 11% in outpatients.

2. Postoperative ATN and CIN are the most common causes.

3. Can be oliguric (urinary output < 400 mL/day) or nonoliguric.

4. Mortality in hospitalized patients with ATN is 15–30%; in ICU patients, mortality is about 40–60%.

5. Risk factors for increased mortality include

   a. Male sex

   b. Advanced age

   c. Comorbid illness

   d. Malignancy

   e. Oliguria

   f. Sepsis

   g. Mechanical ventilation

   h. Multiorgan failure

   i. Severity of illness

6. 60% of patients who survive recover renal function over 1–2 weeks; a "post ATN diuresis," during which urinary output transiently increases, may be seen.

7. CKD is more likely to develop in patients with normal kidneys who have recovered from ATN; those with preexisting CKD are more likely to need future dialysis.

Evidence-Based Diagnosis

Urine electrolytes, urinalysis, and serum BUN and creatinine are used to distinguish ATN from prerenal states; ultrasound is used to distinguish ATN from obstruction.

A. Urine chemistries

1. Hypoperfusion causes increased reabsorption of sodium, water, and urea by the tubules; if prolonged ischemia leads to tubular damage, the tubules can no longer increase reabsorption, leading to urinary sodium and urea loss.

2. Urea reabsorption is less affected by loop and thiazide diuretics than urine sodium.

3. There should be relatively little sodium and urea in the urine in prerenal AKI.

4. Fractional excretion of sodium (FE_{Na}) and fractional excretion of urea (FE_{urea}) are often used to distinguish prerenal AKI from ATN:

$$FE_{Na} = \frac{\text{urine Na} \times \text{plasma creatinine}}{\text{plasma Na} \times \text{urine creatinine}}$$

$$FE_{urea} = \frac{\text{urine urea nitrogen} \times \text{plasma creatinine}}{\text{blood urea nitrogen} \times \text{urine creatinine}}$$

5. The studies looking at the test characteristics of these calculations are limited by small numbers of patients, inconsistent definitions of the gold standard by which the cause of AKI was determined, and lack of generalizability.

   a. The sensitivity of FE_{urea} < 35–40% to detect prerenal AKI ranges from 68% to 98%, with specificities ranging from 48% to 98%.

   b. The sensitivity of FE_{Na} < 1% to detect prerenal AKI ranges from 58% to 96%, with specificities ranging from 75% to 95%.

   c. Some studies show that FE_{urea} is more sensitive that FE_{Na} in patients taking diuretics.

6. Table 28-4 lists situations in which the FE_{Na} result is the opposite of expected.

B. Urine microscopy

1. Granular casts and renal tubular epithelial cells are classic findings in ATN.

2. In 1 study, no patients with prerenal AKI had > 10 granular casts/hpf or > 6 renal tubular epithelial cells/hpf.

   a. Zero granular casts/hpf has a LR+ = 4.35 for the diagnosis of prerenal AKI.

   b. 6–10 granular casts/hpf has a LR+ = 9.68 for the diagnosis of ATN; >10 granular casts/hpf is 100% specific for ATN.

3. Hematuria suggests intrarenal or structural kidney disease and is not seen in prerenal AKI or ATN.

C. Other findings

1. Specific gravity > 1.020 and urine osmolality > 500 mOsm/kg are associated with prerenal states.

   a. Osmolality can be falsely low in prerenal states because of impairment of concentrating ability from underlying CKD, an osmotic diuresis, use of diuretics, or diabetes insipidus.

Table 28-4. Clinical scenarios with unexpected FE_{Na} results.

FE_{Na} < 1% Even Though the Patient Has ATN	FE_{Na} > 2% Even Though the Patient Has Prerenal AKI
AKI due to liver failure or HF	Use of diuretics
Sepsis associated AKI	Underlying CKD
Contrast induced nephropathy	FE_{Na} measured after IV fluids given
Non-oliguric ATN	Glucosuria
ATN due to myoglobinuria or hemoglobinuria	Bicarbonaturia
	Salt-wasting disorders

AKI, acute kidney injury; ATN, acute tubular necrosis; CKD, chronic kidney disease; FE_{Na}, fractional excretion of sodium; HF, heart failure; IV, intravenous.

b. Sensitivity and specificity of these findings are unknown.

2. The BUN/creatinine ratio is classically > 20:1 in prerenal states due to reabsorption of urea with sodium.

   a. Can also be elevated with gastrointestinal bleeding, use of corticosteroids, intake of a high-protein diet, or increased catabolism (postoperative or infection)

   b. Can be low in AKI secondary to rhabdomyolysis, or when production is decreased due to malnutrition or advanced liver disease.

D. Physical exam

1. See Chapter 31, Syncope, for a discussion of measuring orthostatic vital signs and their usefulness in assessing acute blood loss.

2. The ability of the physical exam to diagnosis hypovolemia is not well studied. Available data show:

   a. Orthostatic vital signs: pulse increment > 30 bpm and systolic BP decline > 20 mm Hg have moderate specificity (75% for pulse, 81% for BP) but poor sensitivity (43% for pulse, 29% for BP); LR+ and LR– are both ~1.

   b. Dry axilla (LR+ = 2.8), dry mucous membranes of the mouth and nose (LR+ = 3.1), and abnormal skin turgor in the subclavicular area (LR+ = 3.5) are the best predictors of hypovolemia.

   c. The absence of abnormal skin turgor in the subclavicular area and the absence of longitudinal furrows on the tongue reduce the likelihood of hypovolemia (LR– = 0.3 for both findings).

   d. One study suggests that a combination of findings (eg, confusion, nonfluent speech, dry mucous membranes, dry/furrowed tongue, extremity weakness, and sunken eyes) is highly predictive of hypovolemia.

 Patients can be hypovolemic in the absence of expected physical exam findings.

Treatment

A. Discontinue nephrotoxic agents.

B. Ensure volume status and perfusion pressure (MAP)

   1. MAP = 1/3 systolic BP + 2/3 diastolic BP

   2. General MAP goal is > 70 mm Hg; elderly patients may need MAP > 80–90 mm Hg

C. Obtain renal consultation within 48 hours.

D. Adjust doses of drugs for renal impairment as necessary.

E. Optimize nutritional support.

F. No evidence to support the use of loop diuretics, such as furosemide, or low-dose dopamine; both may actually be harmful.

G. Indications for acute dialysis

   1. Hyperkalemia

   2. Volume overload

   3. Metabolic acidosis refractory to medical therapy

   4. Uremic pericarditis or encephalopathy

H. Prevention of CIN

   1. Identify patients at risk

   2. Consider alternative imaging procedures

   3. Discontinue NSAIDs 1 day before and for 2–4 days following the procedure; hold metformin the day of the

procedure and for 2 days afterward to prevent metformin-induced lactic acidosis if CIN develops.

4. Optimize volume status prior to the procedure: there are good data to support the use of IV hydration in high-risk patients.

   a. Guidelines recommend 1 mL/kg/hour for 12 hours prior to and 12 hours following the procedure in inpatients; for outpatients and urgent procedures 3 mL/kg/hour for 1 hour prior to and 1–1.5 mL/kg/hour following the procedure

   b. There are conflicting data on the benefits of IV bicarbonate versus saline.

5. There are conflicting data on the benefits N-acetylcysteine; if used, give 1200 mg orally twice daily on the day prior to and the day of the procedure.

6. Use an iso-osmolar or low-osmolar contrast agent; administer the lowest possible dose of contrast.

7. Check serum creatinine 48–72 hours following the procedure.

MAKING A DIAGNOSIS

Mr. T's FE_{Na} is 2.41%, and his FE_{urea} is 53%. He is treated with IV antibiotics and fluids, with normalization of his BP. A repeat creatinine, done several hours later, is again 3.8 mg/dL.

 Have you crossed a diagnostic threshold for the leading hypothesis, ATN? Have you ruled out the active alternatives? Do other tests need to be done to exclude the alternative diagnoses?

The combination of sepsis, a $FE_{urea} > 50\%$, the finding of granular casts, lack of exposure to other toxins, and lack of response to IV fluids makes hypotension-induced ATN the most likely diagnosis and makes prerenal azotemia unlikely. However, it is not possible to rule out obstruction based on the information available so far, so it is necessary to do a renal ultrasound. (AKI due to obstruction will be discussed later in the chapter.)

 Exclude urinary tract obstruction in all patients with AKI.

CASE RESOLUTION

The ultrasound shows normal kidneys, with no hydronephrosis. Mr. T's BP remains stable, and at discharge 1 week later, his creatinine is 2.0 mg/dL. He returns to see you 2 weeks later, reporting that his osteoarthritis "flared" after so much time in bed, and he has been using celecoxib for relief. His creatinine is 2.5 mg/dL. You advise him to stop the celecoxib, and a repeat creatinine 2 weeks later is 1.5 mg/dL.

NSAIDs, even selective COX-2 inhibitors, can decrease renal perfusion due to prostaglandin inhibition, leading to prerenal AKI. Patients with abnormal renal function are at the highest risk for this complication, and such medications should be avoided. Renal function usually returns to baseline after stopping the drug.

CHIEF COMPLAINT

PATIENT

Mr. K is an 80-year-old man brought in by his family with the chief complaint of malaise, anorexia, and confusion for the past 3 days. He is generally healthy and independent, and he had been feeling fine, except for a cold several days ago. Over the last 3 days, his family noticed that he has seemed tired and a little confused. He has been drinking liquids but not eating much. They also report that he has had a couple of episodes of urinary incontinence, something he has never experienced before. His past medical history is notable only for osteoarthritis, for which he takes either acetaminophen or ibuprofen. On physical exam, he is alert and cooperative. His BP is 160/80 mm Hg, pulse is 88 bpm, RR is 16 breaths per minute, and he is afebrile. There is no adenopathy, lungs are clear, and cardiac exam is normal. Abdominal exam shows no masses or tenderness. His prostate is mildly enlarged, without nodules. There is no peripheral edema.

Initial laboratory test results include Na, 138 mEq/L; K, 4.8 mEq/L; Cl, 100 mEq/L; HCO_3, 20 mEq/L; BUN, 90 mg/dL; creatinine, 7.2 mg/dL.

 At this point, what is the leading hypothesis, what are the active alternatives, and is there a must not miss diagnosis? Given this differential diagnosis, what tests should be ordered?

RANKING THE DIFFERENTIAL DIAGNOSIS

All 3 etiologies of AKI need to be considered. His age, prostatic enlargement, and urinary incontinence are all pivotal points suggesting urinary tract obstruction. However, he also could have prerenal AKI from either NSAID use or intravascular volume depletion. He has no history suggesting a specific intrarenal cause, so intrarenal causes would be considered only if no postrenal or prerenal cause could be identified. Table 28-5 lists the differential diagnosis.

Mr. K's urine sodium is 20 mEq/h, with a FE_{Na} of 1%. He is given 500 mL of 0.9% saline intravenously. A couple of hours later, his creatinine is 7.0 mg/dL, and he reports lower abdominal pain. He has had several episodes of dribbling urine since receiving the IV fluids. A bladder scan shows

(continued)

Table 28-5. Diagnostic hypotheses for Mr. K.

Diagnostic Hypotheses	Demographics, Risk Factors, Symptoms and Signs	Important Tests
Leading Hypothesis		
Obstruction	Nocturia Incontinence Dribbling Slow stream Abdominal/pelvic discomfort Palpable bladder Older man	Catheterization or bladder scan Postvoid residual Ultrasound
Active Alternative—Most Common		
NSAID use	Medication history, including over-the-counter medications	FE_{Na} Stopping medication
Active Alternative—Must Not Miss		
Hypovolemia	Orthostatic hypotension Abnormal subclavicular skin turgor Dry axilla or mucous membranes History of vomiting or diarrhea Elderly	FE_{Na} BUN/creatinine ratio Response to fluid challenge

BUN, blood urea nitrogen; FE_{Na}, fractional excretion of sodium; NSAID, nonsteroidal anti-inflammatory drug.

a postvoid residual of several hundred milliliters. A Foley catheter is placed and 500 mL of urine quickly fills the bag.

Is the clinical information sufficient to make a diagnosis? If not, what other information do you need?

Leading Hypothesis: Urinary Tract Obstruction

Textbook Presentation

Symptoms vary with site, degree, and rapidity of onset of the obstruction. Obstruction may cause pain if acute or may be painless if chronic. Incontinence and dribbling are common if the obstruction is urethral.

Disease Highlights

A. Clinical manifestations

1. Upper ureteral or renal pelvic lesions can cause flank pain; lower obstruction can cause pelvic pain that sometimes radiates to the ipsilateral testicle or labium.

2. Obstruction must be bilateral to cause AKI; therefore, the most common cause of obstructive AKI is prostatic enlargement.

3. Urinary output

   a. Anuria, if obstruction is complete

      (1) Anuria is defined as < 100 mL of urine per day.

      (2) Also seen in shock, vascular lesions, severe ATN, or severe GN.

   b. Output can be normal or increased with partial obstruction.

   c. Increased output is due to tubular injury that impairs concentrating ability and sodium reabsorption.

   d. Incontinence, dribbling, decreased output, and hematuria may be present.

B. Obstruction accounts for 17% of cases of outpatient AKI, and for 2–5% of cases of inpatient AKI and is more commonly seen in men than women.

C. Obstruction can lead to a type 4 renal tubular acidosis with hyperkalemia due to tubular injury.

D. In patients with normal kidneys, unilateral obstruction often is undetected because the unobstructed kidney compensates enough to maintain normal renal function.

E. Prognosis

1. Complete or prolonged partial obstruction can lead to tubular atrophy and irreversible loss of renal function.

   a. Complete recovery of renal function occurs if total ureteral obstruction is relieved within 7 days; little or no recovery occurs if the total obstruction is present for 12 weeks.

   b. Obstruction is a rare cause of end-stage renal disease.

2. Prognosis of partial obstruction is unpredictable.

Evidence-Based Diagnosis

A. Urine electrolytes are not very helpful.

B. The postvoid residual will be increased (> 100 mL) if the obstruction is urethral; the postvoid residual will be normal if the obstruction is proximal to the bladder.

C. Renal ultrasound

1. The best first test to look for obstruction

2. Has a sensitivity of 90–98% and specificity of 65–84% for detecting urinary tract obstruction

3. There are 4 settings in which obstruction can occur without dilatation of the complete collecting system, leading to a false-negative ultrasound.

   a. With very early (< 8 hours) obstruction

   b. When the patient is also volume depleted; sometimes repeating an ultrasound after hydration will demonstrate the dilatation

   c. With retroperitoneal fibrosis, which can cause hydronephrosis without ureteral dilatation; the hydronephrosis and fibrosis are better seen on CT scan

   d. With obstruction so mild that there is no impairment in renal function

D. Noncontrast CT can detect sites of obstruction missed on ultrasound, and is superior to ultrasound for determining the site of ureteral obstruction.

Treatment

A. Relieve the obstruction immediately.

1. Modalities

   a. Foley catheter for bladder neck obstruction

Remember that indwelling catheters can be obstructed by clots.

b. Suprapubic catheter, if Foley is not possible

c. Percutaneous nephrostomy tubes for ureteral obstruction

2. Consequences

a. Rapid decompression of the bladder can rarely lead to hematuria and even hypotension

b. A postobstructive diuresis is common, with an initial urinary output of 500–1000 mL/hour

(1) Represents an attempt to excrete fluid retained during the period of obstruction but may also exceed this due to excretion of accumulated osmols

(2) Not necessary to replace entire urinary output; doing so will increase the diuresis

(3) Should treat with normal replacement fluids

(4) Should monitor electrolytes closely and replace as needed

B. Correct the underlying cause of the obstruction.

MAKING A DIAGNOSIS

A renal ultrasound shows bilateral ureteral dilatation and hydronephrosis, confirming the diagnosis of urinary tract obstruction. He is admitted to the hospital, and over several days, his creatinine returns to baseline of 1.5 mg/dL. The catheter is removed, and he urinates with his usual mild difficulty starting the stream. Several days after discharge, he arrives in the emergency department, reporting that he cannot urinate at all. As instructed, he has avoided all NSAID use but has been taking pseudoephedrine for cold symptoms.

 Have you crossed a diagnostic threshold for the leading hypothesis, urinary tract obstruction? Have you ruled out the active alternatives? Do other tests need to be done to exclude the alternative diagnoses?

No further tests are necessary to diagnose the cause of his AKI; however, it is important to determine the cause of the urinary tract obstruction, and that of his new, related problem, acute urinary retention.

Related Diagnoses: Acute Urinary Retention and BPH

1. Acute Urinary Retention

Acute urinary retention is most commonly seen in older men with prostatic hypertrophy causing bladder neck obstruction (seen in 10% of men in their 70s and up to 33% of men in their 80s). The risk is increased for older men, for those with moderate to severe lower urinary tract symptoms, for those with a flow rate < 12 mL/sec, and for those with a prostate volume > 30 mL by transrectal ultrasound.

In women, acute urinary retention is usually due to neurogenic bladder, and in younger patients, it is usually due to neurologic disease. Medications that commonly induce urinary retention in susceptible patients include antihistamines, anticholinergics, antispasmodics, tricyclic antidepressants, opioids, and alpha-adrenergic agonists.

2. BPH

Textbook Presentation

The classic presentation is an older man with urinary frequency, nocturia, reduced stream, and dribbling at the end of urination.

Disease Highlights

A. Defined as microscopic (histologic evidence of cellular proliferation), macroscopic (actual enlargement of the prostate), or clinical (symptoms resulting from macroscopic BPH)

B. Two-thirds of the adult prostate is glandular and one-third is fibromuscular.

1. Intraprostatic dihydrotestosterone, synthesized from testosterone by 5-alpha-reductase type 2, controls glandular growth.

2. The smooth muscle of the prostate, urethra, and bladder are under alpha-1-adrenergic control.

C. Prostatic enlargement causes symptoms due to compression of the periurethral area and of the bladder; the compression occurs because of the physical enlargement of the prostate and also because of increased muscle tone in the urethra, prostatic fibromuscular tissue, and bladder neck.

D. BPH is present in 80% of men in their seventies.

E. Risk factors for BPH include increasing age, African American race, obesity, diabetes mellitus, high alcohol consumption, and physical inactivity.

Evidence-Based Diagnosis

A. Symptoms can be categorized as

1. Storage symptoms (urgency frequency, nocturia, urge incontinence, stress incontinence)

2. Voiding symptoms (hesitancy, poor flow, straining, dysuria)

3. Postmicturition symptoms (dribbling, incomplete emptying)

B. Prostate size does not correlate with symptom severity.

C. Can use International Prostate Symptom Score (IPSS) to assess severity of symptoms and assess response to therapy.

1. There are 7 questions to be answered on a 0 to 5 scale, yielding a potential total of 35 points (Table 28-6).

2. 0–7 = mild BPH; 8–19 = moderate BPH; 20–35 = severe BPH

D. Digital rectal exam

1. Cannot ascertain anterior or posterior extension or feel entire posterior surface.

2. Therefore, prostate size is underestimated by 25–55% on digital rectal exam, compared with transrectal ultrasound; the underestimation increases the larger the prostate volume.

 The prostate is even bigger than you think it is on digital rectal exam.

E. Guidelines recommend all symptomatic patients have a digital rectal exam, urinalysis, and serum creatinine; other testing (urodynamics, imaging) is optional.

F. Although BPH can cause hematuria, other causes of hematuria should be considered (see Chapter 21, Hematuria).

G. PSA testing should be discussed (see Chapter 2, Screening & Health Maintenance).

Table 28-6. International Prostate Symptom Score.

	Not at All	< 1 Time in 5	< Than Half the Time	About Half the Time	> Half the Time	Almost Always
Over the past month, how often . . .						
have you had a sensation of not emptying your bladder completely after you finished urinating?	0	1	2	3	4	5
have you had to urinate again less than 2 hours after you finished urinating?	0	1	2	3	4	5
have you found you stopped and started again several times when you urinated?	0	1	2	3	4	5
have you found it difficult to postpone urination?	0	1	2	3	4	5
have you had a weak urinary stream?	0	1	2	3	4	5
have you had to push or strain to begin urination?	0	1	2	3	4	5
did you most typically get up to urinate from the time you went to bed at night until the time you got up in the morning?	0	1	2	3	4	5

Scoring Key: 0–7, mild; 8–19 moderate; 20–35, severe.
Modified, with permission, from Barry MJ et al. The American Urological Association symptoms index for benign prostatic hyperplasia. *J Urol.* 1992;148:1549.

H. Urinary flow rates, urodynamic measurements, and amount of postvoid residual do not correlate well with symptoms.

Treatment

A. Diuretics should be discontinued in order to minimize symptoms.

B. Men with mild symptoms (as defined by the IPSS) do not require treatment.

C. Men with moderate or severe symptoms (as defined by the IPSS) should be treated with pharmacotherapy.

   1. Alpha-blockers (terazosin and doxazosin) work on the alpha-adrenergic receptors of prostatic smooth muscle. Common side effects include orthostasis, hypotension, and fatigue. Selective alpha-blockers such as tamsulosin and alfuzosin will not effect blood pressure.

   2. 5-alpha reductase inhibitors (finasteride and dutasteride) prevent the conversion of testosterone to active dihydrotestosterone. Common side effects include decreased libido, erectile dysfunction, and gynecomastia.

   3. Phosphodiesterase inhibitors, such as tadalafil, are also effective.

   4. Combination therapy with an alpha-blocker and 5-alpha reductase inhibitor is more effective than monotherapy.

   5. Antimuscarinic agents may also help symptoms but have not been well established in clinical trials.

   6. The supplement saw palmetto is frequently used for BPH, but its efficacy has not been proven in clinical trials.

D. Surgical therapies, such as transurethral prostate resection (TURP) or microwave thermotherapy, are options for patients who do not respond to medical therapy, cannot tolerate medical therapy, or have acute urinary retention.

CASE RESOLUTION

Mr. K is catheterized, and 500 mL of urine is obtained. Because the urinary retention was precipitated by the use of an alpha-adrenergic agent (pseudoephedrine), he is given tamsulosin and the catheter is removed on a trial basis. He is again unable to urinate. He then undergoes transurethral resection of the prostate (TURP) with resolution of his urinary symptoms. His creatinine stays at 1.5 mg/dL throughout these events.

CHIEF COMPLAINT

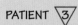

PATIENT

Mrs. F is a 63-year-old woman with a history of diastolic dysfunction, hypertension, and osteoarthritis. Her usual medications are atenolol, lisinopril, and acetaminophen, and her usual serum creatinine is 1.1 mg/dL. Four weeks ago, she came to see you reporting severe pain, erythema, and swelling of her right first metatarsophalangeal joint.

You diagnosed gout, and prescribed indomethacin 25 mg 3 times daily to use until the gout resolved. She returned for follow-up yesterday, reporting that the gout had resolved in a few days, but that she kept taking the indomethacin because it helped her arthritis so much. Despite your reservations, you agree to refill the prescription because she clearly feels so much better than usual. Today you receive the results of the blood tests you ordered during the visit:

(continued)

Na, 141 mEq/24 h; K, 5.0 mEq/24 h; Cl, 100 mEq/24 h; HCO₃, 20 mEq/L; BUN, 32 mg/dL; creatinine, 2.5 mg/dL.

 At this point, what is the leading hypothesis, what are the active alternatives, and is there a must not miss diagnosis? Given this differential diagnosis, what tests should be ordered?

RANKING THE DIFFERENTIAL DIAGNOSIS

At this point, the differential for her AKI is quite broad, but it is logical to focus on the pivotal point in this case, the recent use of indomethacin. Through prostaglandin inhibition, NSAIDs can cause decreased renal blood flow, leading to a prerenal state. NSAIDs are also 1 of the classes of drugs most commonly associated with an intrarenal disease, interstitial nephritis. Although obstruction must always be considered, she is having no urinary symptoms and has no risk factors. Table 28-7 lists the differential diagnosis.

 Mrs. F's urine sodium is 35 mEq/h, and the FE_{Na} is 1.5%. Urinalysis shows 1+ protein, 3 RBCs/hpf, 5–10 WBCs/hpf, and no casts. Renal ultrasound is normal.

 Is the clinical information sufficient to make a diagnosis? If not, what other information do you need?

Leading Diagnosis: NSAID-Induced Renal Hypoperfusion

Textbook Presentation

AKI caused by NSAIDs is usually asymptomatic and is most commonly detected by finding an increased serum creatinine.

Disease Highlights

A. Can occur with nonselective NSAIDs and COX-2 inhibitors.

B. Renal prostaglandins are particularly important in the autoregulation of glomerular pressure and GFR in patients with

Table 28-7. Diagnostic hypotheses for Mrs. F.

Diagnostic Hypotheses	Demographics, Risk Factors, Symptoms and Signs	Important Tests
Leading Hypothesis		
NSAID-induced renal hypoperfusion	Use of NSAIDs History of renal disease HF	FE_{Na} Stopping the medication
Active Alternative		
Interstitial nephritis	Exposure to NSAIDs, antibiotics Active infection	Stopping the medication Renal biopsy

FE_{Na}, fractional excretion of sodium; NSAIDs, nonsteroidal antiinflammatory drugs.

other causes of impaired autoregulation, such as CKD, hypertension, volume depletion, HF, and cirrhosis.

C. Prostaglandin inhibition in such patients can lead to significant decreases in renal blood flow, consequent reversible renal ischemia, and AKI.

D. Seen within 3–7 days of starting therapy.

E. Renal prostaglandins are not important regulators of blood flow in *normal* kidneys, and so AKI from NSAIDs does not develop in patients with *normal* renal function.

Evidence-Based Diagnosis

A. FE_{Na} should be < 1% since the mechanism is impaired perfusion. (Sensitivity and specificity are unknown.)

B. Reverses when the drug is stopped.

C. Not accompanied by hematuria or pyuria.

Treatment

Stop the exposure.

MAKING A DIAGNOSIS

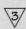 You call Mrs. F and tell her to stop taking the indomethacin. One week later, her creatinine is still 2.5 mg/dL. Urine eosinophils are negative.

 Have you crossed a diagnostic threshold for the leading hypothesis, NSAID-induced renal hypoperfusion? Have you ruled out the active alternatives? Do other tests need to be done to exclude the alternative diagnoses?

Mrs. F's FE_{Na} is higher than expected for NSAID-induced renal hypoperfusion. She has not used diuretics or received IV fluids, both of which can cause a falsely elevated urine sodium and FE_{Na}. In addition, her creatinine has not improved. Therefore, it is unlikely that prostaglandin inhibition is the reason for her kidney disease.

Alternative Diagnosis: Interstitial Nephritis

Textbook Presentation

Classic findings include AKI, hematuria, pyuria with WBC casts, fever, and eosinophilia. The full syndrome is rarely seen today since it occurs primarily with methicillin-induced acute interstitial nephritis.

Disease Highlights

A. Interstitial nephritis is found in 2–3% of all renal biopsies, and in 15–27% of patients who have a biopsy done for AKI.

B. Etiology
   1. Drug-induced
      a. Accounts for at least 2/3 of cases of acute interstitial nephritis; up to 90% of cases in some series
      b. Antimicrobial agents and NSAIDs cause the majority of cases; in 2 large series, NSAIDs caused 44% of the drug-induced cases.
      c. Also reported with allopurinol, acyclovir, famotidine, furosemide, omeprazole, phenytoin

2. Infection-related
   a. 15% of acute interstitial nephritis cases
   b. Can be caused by viral infections (eg, cytomegalovirus, Epstein-Barr virus, herpes simplex virus, HIV, mumps, and others), bacterial infections (staphylococci, streptococci, *Yersinia, Legionella,* and others), other infections such as mycobacteria, toxoplasmosis, syphilis
3. Idiopathic
   a. 5–10% of cases
   b. Includes tubulointerstitial nephritis and uveitis syndrome and anti-tubular basement membrane disease
4. Associated with systemic disease: sarcoidosis, systemic lupus erythematosus, Sjögren syndrome

C. Prognosis
   1. Most patients improve within 6–8 weeks and return to baseline renal function.
   2. Predictors of irreversible injury are diffuse infiltrates and frequent granulomas on biopsy, intake of the offending drug for longer than 1 month, delayed response to prednisone, and persistent kidney disease after 3 weeks.

Evidence-Based Diagnosis

A. Clinical findings
   1. Renal manifestations develop within 3 weeks of exposure in 80% of patients, with an average delay of 10 days (range 1 day to 18 months; longer delays often seen with NSAIDs).
   2. Symptoms develop more rapidly if the patient is rechallenged with the offending drug.
   3. The classic triad of fever, rash, and eosinophilia is seen in only 10–15% of patients.
   4. Table 28-8 summarizes the findings in 2 series reporting 121 cases of acute interstitial nephritis, 90% of which were drug-induced.

The absence of fever, rash, eosinophilia, or eosinophiluria does *not* rule out interstitial nephritis.

Table 28-8. Clinical features in acute interstitial nephritis.

Finding	% of Patients
Arthralgias	45
Fever	36
Rash	22
Non-nephrotic proteinuria	93
Pyuria	82
Microscopic hematuria	67
Eosinophilia[1]	35
Gross hematuria	5
Nephrotic range proteinuria	2.5
Complete nephrotic syndrome	0.8

[1]Less common in NSAID-related acute interstitial nephritis.

B. Urine eosinophils are less useful than early studies suggested: sensitivity, 40%; specificity, 72%; LR+ = 1.45, LR– = 0.83
C. FE_{Na} usually > 1%
D. Gallium scan
   1. Substantial renal uptake in acute interstitial nephritis, but uptake also seen in GN, pyelonephritis, and other conditions.
   2. Sensitivity and specificity are not well defined.
   3. No uptake with ATN, so possibly useful in distinguishing ATN from acute interstitial nephritis
E. Renal biopsy is the gold standard and is often necessary to establish the diagnosis.

Treatment

A. Stop exposure, if possible.
B. Corticosteroids are sometimes used, but there are no prospective randomized clinical trials.
   1. Consider in patients whose renal function does not improve within 1 week of stopping exposure, after biopsy confirms diagnosis.
   2. Consider empiric trial in patients who have worsening renal function and suspected acute interstitial nephritis, and who are poor candidates for biopsy.
   3. NSAID-induced acute interstitial nephritis is less responsive to corticosteroid therapy.
   4. Should see improvement in 2–3 weeks.

CASE RESOLUTION

Her urinalysis is consistent with interstitial nephritis, and the lack of urine eosinophils does not rule out the diagnosis. Renal biopsy is performed, which shows inflammatory infiltrates in the interstitium. Her renal function returns to baseline several weeks after the NSAIDs are discontinued. She is cautioned to never use NSAIDs in the future to avoid recurrent interstitial nephritis.

REVIEW OF OTHER IMPORTANT DISEASES

Acute Glomerulonephritis

Acute GN is caused by 1 of several disease processes, all of which involve immunologically mediated proliferative GN. The classic clinical "nephritic syndrome" consists of the *acute* onset of hematuria (with red cell casts), proteinuria, elevated creatinine, hypertension, and edema. See Table 28-9 for an overview of etiologies.

Rhabdomyolysis

Textbook Presentation

Patients may complain of muscle pain, weakness, and dark urine. Serum creatine kinase levels are elevated.

Disease Highlights

A. Direct trauma to the myocyte, or depletion of ATP within the cell, leads to increased intracellular calcium causing persistent contraction and eventual myocyte disintegration.

Table 28-9. Causes of acute glomerulonephritis (GN).

Type	Diseases	Serologic Markers	Highlights
Anti-GBM disease	Goodpasture syndrome	100% anti-GBM ab + 20% ANCA + C3 normal	Presents with abrupt onset of oliguria, hematuria, and renal failure Bimodal age distribution: young male smokers present with a pulmonary-renal syndrome, and women in their 50s to 60s present with kidney disease 30% develop ESRD
Pauci-immune GN	Microscopic polyangiitis	50-75% pANCA + Anti-GBM (-) C3 normal	Small- and medium-vessel vasculitis Renal involvement in 80%; pulmonary involvement in 20–55% Presents with constitutional symptoms, hematuria, and sometimes nephrotic range proteinuria 10–46% require dialysis
	Granulomatosis with polyangiitis	>90% cANCA + Anti-GBM (-) C3 normal	Upper and lower respiratory tract and GN Can be indolent prior to the onset of systemic vasculitis Seen primarily in white men and women in the fifth decade 1/3–1/2 have eye disease
	Churg-Strauss syndrome	65% pANCA + Anti-GBM (-) C3 normal IgE elevated	Asthma, eosinophilia, granulomatous vasculitis, and tissue eosinophilic infiltration Occurs in patients in their 30s and 40s Renal involvement typically mild
Immune –complex GN	SLE, poststreptococcal, membranoproliferative, endocarditis, visceral abscesses, shunt nephritis	Low C3 Anti-GBM (-) ANCA (-)	Post-streptococcal GN is the most common postinfectious GN, occurring 10–14 days after infection with a nephritogenic strain of group A beta-hemolytic streptococci Supportive treatment only; residual renal impairment rare
	Cryoglobulinemia	Low C4 Anti-GBM (-) ANCA (-)	Typically associated with chronic infection such as hepatitis C or hematologic malignancy Petechial rash, livedo reticularis, arthritis, systemic involvement
	IgA nephropathy, Henoch-Schönlein purpura (HSP), fibrillary GN	Normal C3, C4 Anti-GBM (-) ANCA (-)	IgA nephropathy is the most common cause of GN Purpura and GI symptoms seen in HSP

cANCA, cytoplasmic anti-neutrophilic cytoplasmic antibody; ESRD, end-stage renal disease; GBM, glomerular basement membrane; pANCA, perinuclear anti-neutrophilic cytoplasmic antibody; SLE, systemic lupus erythematosus.

B. Leakage of muscle cell contents (electrolytes, myoglobin, creatine kinase, other proteins) then occurs.

C. Causes of rhabdomyolysis include

1. Trauma (crush injury)

2. Exertion (strenuous exercise, seizures, alcohol withdrawal syndrome)

3. Muscle hypoxia (limb compression during prolonged immobilization, major artery occlusion)

4. Infections (influenza, coxsackievirus, Epstein-Barr virus, HIV, *Legionella*, *Streptococcus pyogenes*, *Staphylococcal aureus*, *Clostridium*, tick-borne infections)

5. Metabolic (hypokalemia, hypophosphatemia, hypocalcemia, diabetic ketoacidosis, nonketotic hyperosmotic conditions)

6. Drugs/toxins (fibrates, statins, alcohol, heroin, cocaine)

7. Body temperature changes (heat stroke, malignant hyperthermia, malignant neuroleptic syndrome, hypothermia)

8. Genetic defects

9. Idiopathic

D. AKI is the most serious complication of rhabdomyolysis.

    1. Rhabdomyolysis causes 7–10% of cases of AKI in the United States.

    2. Incidence of AKI is 13–50% and is higher in patients who use illicit drugs or alcohol, or who have multiple causes of rhabdomyolysis.

    3. Survival in patients with rhabdomyolysis and AKI is about 80%, with most patients recovering renal function.

    4. AKI occurs due to myoglobin-induced proximal tubule cytotoxicity, distal tubular obstruction from precipitation of myoglobin, and intrarenal vasoconstriction due to intravascular volume depletion and activation of renal vascular mediators.

Evidence-Based Diagnosis

A. Weak correlation between peak creatine kinase and development of AKI

    1. Risk of AKI is low when the admission creatine kinase is less than 15,000–20,000 units/liter.

    2. AKI may occur with creatine kinase levels as low as 5000 units/liter when coexisting conditions such as sepsis, dehydration, or acidosis are present.

B. Urine findings include

    1. Pigmented granular casts

    2. A reddish-brown supernatant

    3. Dipstick testing positive for blood with no red blood cells in the sediment (sensitivity of 80% for the detection of rhabdomyloysis)

C. BUN/creatinine ratio is often low.

D. Oliguria is frequent, with occasional anuria.

E. The FE_{Na} is < 1%, due to the contribution of vasoconstriction to the AKI.

F. Common electrolyte abnormalities include hyperkalemia, hyperphosphatemia, hyperuricemia, high anion gap metabolic acidosis, hypermagnesemia, and hypocalcemia.

Treatment

A. Aggressive fluid repletion is essential; some patients require up to 10 L/day.

B. Comparative studies show that early and high volume hydration is better than delayed hydration; there is no difference in outcomes regardless of which type of fluid is used (normal saline, lactated Ringer, sodium bicarbonate), and adding mannitol is not beneficial.

C. However, massive infusions of normal saline can cause metabolic acidosis, so experts recommend alternating 1 L of 0.45 normal saline + bicarbonate with each liter of normal saline if the urine pH is < 6.5.

Vascular Causes of AKI

Vascular events are serious, but rare, causes of AKI. There are 3 mechanisms of acute vascular compromise: renal artery thrombosis, thromboembolism of the renal arteries, and atheroembolism.

1. Renal Artery Thrombosis

Textbook Presentation

The classic presentation is severe flank pain, hematuria, nausea, vomiting, fever, and hypertension.

Disease Highlights

A. Blunt trauma is most common cause.

B. Nontraumatic causes include

    1. Dissecting aortic or renal artery aneurysms

    2. Vasculitis

    3. Cocaine abuse

    4. Antiphospholipid antibody syndrome

Evidence-Based Diagnosis

A. Angiogram is the gold standard.

B. Infused CT is often diagnostic.

Treatment

A. Nephrectomy, if renal infarction occurs

B. Revascularization or thrombolysis

C. Sometimes observation and medical management

2. Thromboembolism of the Renal Arteries

Textbook Presentation

Most patients have flank pain, often with hematuria or anuria.

Disease Highlights

A. Clinical features depend on severity and location of emboli.

B. Bilateral emboli or emboli to a solitary kidney more likely to produce AKI and anuria.

C. 75% of patients have abdominal or flank pain.

D. Variably see nausea, vomiting, hematuria

E. Fever and hypertension are common, but fever is often delayed until second or third day.

F. Sources of emboli

    1. Cardiac: atrial fibrillation, myocardial infarction, rheumatic valvular disease, prosthetic valves, subacute bacterial endocarditis

    2. Aortic or renal aneurysms

    3. Intra-arterial catheterization

Evidence-Based Diagnosis

A. Diagnosed at onset of symptoms in only 30% of patients

B. Usually have leukocytosis, increased lactate dehydrogenase (LD) and transaminases; the LD is increased more than the transaminases.

C. Alkaline phosphatase elevated in 30–50% of patients.

D. Angiography is gold standard for diagnosis; infused CT can be diagnostic.

Treatment

A. Unilateral embolism and normal contralateral kidney: streptokinase and/or angioplasty, followed by anticoagulation; no indication for surgery

B. Bilateral emboli, or embolus to solitary kidney: same as above, but try surgical reconstruction if cannot restore blood flow

3. Atheroembolism

Textbook Presentation

The classic presentation is a white man over age 60 with hypertension, smoking, and vascular disease in whom livedo reticularis and acute or subacute kidney injury develop after an inciting event.

Disease Highlights

A. Secondary to cholesterol crystal embolism from an atherosclerotic aorta

B. 3 syndromes: abrupt onset of kidney injury after an inciting event (such as angiography), subacute worsening of renal function a few weeks after an event, and chronic renal impairment

C. Risk factors include male sex, age > 60, hypertension, smoking, diabetes mellitus, and vascular disease.

D. Can occur spontaneously or after vascular surgery procedures, angiograms (especially coronary angiograms), and with anticoagulation

E. Incidence probably quite low (< 1–2%) but may be as high as 5–6% in high-risk patients.

F. Clinical manifestations (from 5 case series)

   1. Skin lesions (livedo reticularis) in 35–90%

   2. Gastrointestinal symptoms in 8–30%

   3. Eosinophilia in 22–73%

   4. CNS involvement in 4–23%

   5. Dialysis needed in 28–61%

Evidence-Based Diagnosis

A. Renal or skin biopsy

B. Can sometimes be diagnosed on fundoscopic exam

Treatment

A. Best approach beyond supportive therapy unknown

B. Avoid anticoagulation

C. Consider aggressive lipid management

REFERENCES

Bazari H, Guimaraes AR, Kushner YB. Case20-2012: A 77 year old man with leg edema, hematuria, and acute renal failure. N Engl J Med. 2012;366:2503–15.

Bosch X, Poch E, Grau JM. Rhabdomyolysis and acute kidney injury. N Engl J Med. 2009;361:62–72.

Goldfarb S, McCullough PA, McDermott J, Gay SB. Contrast-induced acute kidney injury: specialty specific protocols for interventional radiology, diagnostic computed tomography radiology, and interventional cardiology. Mayo Clin Proc. 2009;84:170–9.

Hilton R. Acute renal failure. BMJ. 2006;333:786–90.

KDIGO Clinical Practice Guideline for Acute Kidney Injury. Kidney International. 2012; volume 2, supplement 1.

Koyner JL. Assessment and diagnosis of renal dysfunction in the ICU. Chest. 2012;141:1584–94.

McGee S. *Evidence-Based Physical Diagnosis*, 3rd edition. Elsevier Saunders; 2012.

Perazella MA, Coca SG. Traditional urinary biomarkers in the assessment of hospital-acquired AKI. Clin J Am Soc Nephrol. 2012;7:167–74.

Praga M, Gonzalez E. Acute interstitial nephritis. Kidney Int. 2010;77:956–61.

Weisbord SD, Palevsky PM. Strategies for the prevention of contrast-induced acute kidney injury. Curr Opin Nephrol Hypertens. 2010;19:539–49.

I have a patient with a rash. How do I determine the cause?

CHIEF COMPLAINT

PATIENT

Ms. N is a 23-year-old woman who comes to see you complaining of a rash.

What is the differential diagnosis of a rash? How would you frame the differential?

CONSTRUCTING A DIFFERENTIAL DIAGNOSIS

In clinical practice, rashes are diagnosed through pattern recognition probably more than any other complaint. This is an effective way of making a diagnosis when the diagnosis is obvious or when the observer is very experienced. The risk with pattern recognition is that diagnostic hypotheses are heavily influenced by recent experience, rare diagnoses tend not to be recognized, and physicians often reach premature closure on an incorrect diagnosis.

The differential diagnosis of a rash should be based on the morphology of the lesion. To correctly categorize a lesion's morphology, the physician must first identify the primary lesion, the typical element of the eruption. This process can be complicated. Identifying the primary lesion may be difficult as it is often affected by secondary changes such as excoriation, erosion, crusting, or coalescence. The differential diagnosis of 1 lesion can also be extensive. Once the morphology of the primary lesion is identified, the next step in making the diagnosis is often to observe the distribution of lesions. Some eruptions will have characteristic distributions. What follows are some important definitions, followed by a differential diagnosis of some of the most common primary lesions.

1. Macule: lesion without elevation or depression, < 1 cm
2. Patch: lesion without elevation or depression, > 1 cm
3. Papule: any solid, elevated "bump" < 1 cm
4. Plaque: raised plateau-like lesion of variable size, often a confluence of papules
5. Nodule: solid lesion with palpable elevation, 1–5 cm
6. Tumor: solid growth, > 5 cm
7. Cyst: encapsulated lesion, filled with soft material
8. Vesicle: elevated, fluid-filled blister, < 1 cm
9. Bulla: elevated, fluid-filled blister, > 1 cm
10. Pustule: elevated, pus-filled blister, any size
11. Wheal: inflamed papule or plaque formed by transient and superficial local edema
12. Comedone: a plug of keratinous material and skin oils retained in a follicle; open is black, closed is white

Papulosquamous eruptions present with papules and plaques associated with superficial scaling. Folliculopapular eruptions begin as papules arising in a perifollicular distribution. Dermal reaction patterns result from infiltrative and inflammatory processes involving the dermal and subcutaneous tissues. Petechia and purpura occur when there is leakage of blood products into surrounding tissues from inflamed or damaged blood vessels. Blistering disorders present with vesicles and bullae. Figure 29-1 presents an algorithm of a possible approach to patients with rashes and skin lesions.

A. Papulosquamous eruptions (papules and plaques)
  1. Eczematous dermatitis
    a. Atopic dermatitis
    b. Allergic contact dermatitis
    c. Irritant contact dermatitis
  2. Pityriasis rosea
  3. Tinea infections
  4. Psoriasis
  5. Seborrheic dermatitis
B. Folliculopapular eruptions (perifollicular papules)
  1. Acne vulgaris
  2. Rosacea
  3. Folliculitis
  4. Perioral dermatitis
C. Dermal reaction patterns
  1. Urticaria
  2. Sarcoidosis
  3. Granuloma annulare
  4. Erythema nodosum
D. Purpura and petechiae
  1. Palpable purpura
    a. Leukocytoclastic vasculitis
      (1) Henoch-Schönlein purpura
      (2) Allergic vasculitis
    b. Infectious
      (1) Bacteremia
      (2) Rocky Mountain spotted fever
      (3) Meningococcemia
  2. Nonpalpable purpura
    a. Thrombocytopenia
    b. Medication-related
    c. Benign pigmented purpura
    d. Bacteremia
    e. Disseminated intravascular coagulation

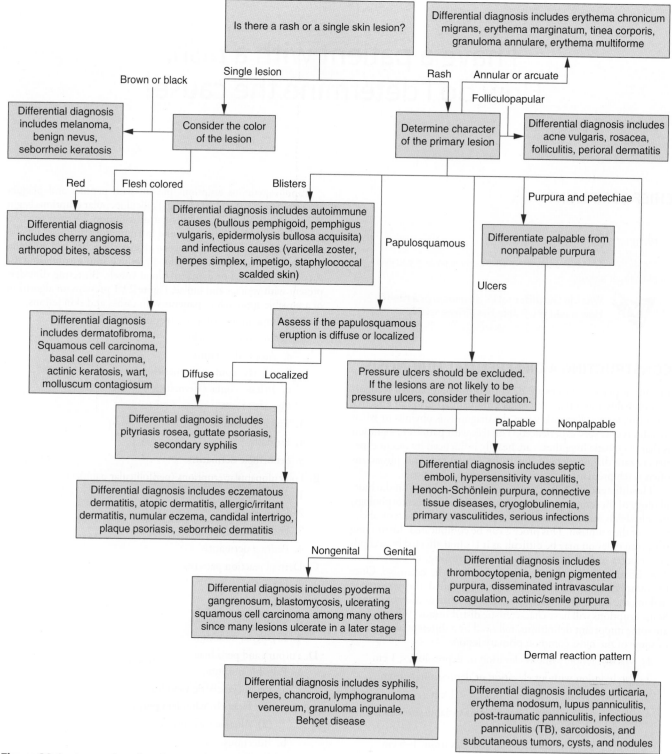

Figure 29-1. Approach to the patient with rash or skin lesion.

> f. Actinic/senile purpura
>
> g. Corticosteroid-associated
>
> h. Amyloidosis

E. Blistering disorders (vesicles, pustules, and bullae)

> 1. Autoimmune
>
>   a. Bullous pemphigoid
>
>   b. Pemphigus vulgaris
>
>   c. Epidermolysis bullosa acquisita

2. Infectious

> a. Varicella zoster
>
> b. Herpes simplex
>
> c. Impetigo
>
> d. Staphylococcal scalded skin

3. Hypersensitivity syndromes

> a. Stevens-Johnson syndrome
>
> b. Toxic epidermal necrolysis

Ms. N complains of frequent "breakouts" on her face for the last several years. She reports the use of many topical over-the-counter agents over the years. She complains of feeling greasy and the need to "squeeze pus" out of lesions on a regular basis.

On examination, over the forehead, cheeks, and chin there are many erythematous papules, occasional pustules, and open and closed comedones. There is a predominance of larger nodules along the jaw line. Similar erythematous papules involve the upper back and chest. There is neither significant background erythema nor scaling in the scalp, eyebrows, or nasolabial folds. Figure 29-2 shows her on her initial visit.

 At this point, what is the leading hypothesis, what are the active alternatives, and is there a must not miss diagnosis? Given this differential diagnosis, what tests should be ordered?

RANKING THE DIFFERENTIAL DIAGNOSIS

The pivotal clues in this case are the morphology of the lesion and its distribution. This patient has a folliculopapular eruption that predominantly affects the face, chest, and upper back. Primary lesions of inflammatory papules, pustules, and comedones place acne at the top of the differential. The history is typical for acne: a chronic course with intermittent flares.

Other folliculopapular conditions must be considered. The lack of background erythema and telangiectasias makes a diagnosis of rosacea less likely. Perioral dermatitis typically presents as monomorphic small papules and is closely associated with the use of topical corticosteroids and cosmetics. The mixture of lesion type, with comedones as well as papules and nodules, and the more diffuse distribution makes acne more likely than perioral dermatitis.

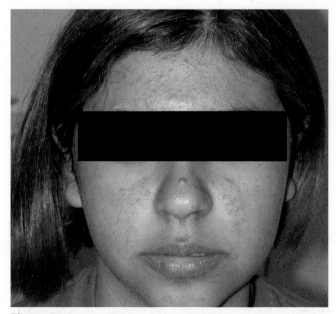

Figure 29-2. Ms. N on initial presentation.

An infectious folliculitis is possible, but the course of the disease makes this extremely unlikely (Table 29-1).

The patient is in good health and is not overweight. She is not taking any oral medications. She reports regular menstrual cycles and notes that the breakouts are worse around the time of her period. She does not report easy flushing or any increased hair growth on the face or chest. She has 1 healthy child.

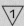 Is the clinical information sufficient to make a diagnosis? If not, what other information do you need?

Leading Hypothesis: Acne Vulgaris

Textbook Presentation

Typically, acne vulgaris presents in adolescence with chronic, waxing and waning lesions. A variety of lesions are present, including inflammatory papules, pustules, comedones, and nodulocysts over the face, chest, and back.

Disease Highlights

A. Description of lesion: inflammatory papules, pustules, comedones, and nodulocysts over the face, chest, and back (see Figure 29-2).

Table 29-1. Diagnostic hypotheses for Ms. N.

Diagnostic Hypotheses	Demographics, Risk Factors, Symptoms and Signs	Important Tests
Leading Hypothesis		
Acne vulgaris	Most common in adolescence and young adulthood Presence of comedones, papules, pustules, nodules Flares with menses Distribution over the face, chest and back	Clinical diagnosis
Active Alternative		
Rosacea	Most common in people with fair skin History of flushing Presence of telangiectasias and possibly inflammatory papules	Clinical diagnosis
Other Alternative		
Perioral dermatitis	Monomorphic eruption of fine erythematous papules clustered around mouth	Clinical diagnosis

B. Acne is a highly prevalent condition, most common during mid-to-late adolescence.

C. Acne may persist beyond adolescence, especially in women.

D. Acne is caused by the obstruction of sebaceous follicles on the face and trunk. Three factors are involved in the development of the lesions:

   1. Increased sebum is produced (androgen dependent) and accumulates in follicles.

   2. Desquamation of epithelial cells and keratin into sebum-rich follicles causes obstruction.

   3. Inflammation develops secondary to proliferation of the anaerobe *Propionibacterium acnes.*

E. Although the 3 factors discussed above are responsible for the overwhelming majority of acne, it is important to keep in mind other factors that may be contribute to the disease.

   1. Hyperandrogen states (eg, polycystic ovary syndrome [PCOS] or androgenic progestins in contraceptives).

   2. Exposure to topical comedogens (cocoa butter, mineral oil, lanolin, fatty acids).

   3. Numerous factors that lead to follicular obstruction (eg, habits or clothing that cause skin trauma or obstruct pores, and hot humid environments or heavy sweating leading to keratin over-hydration).

   4. Medications known to trigger or exacerbate acne (eg, corticosteroids, isoniazid, lithium, androgens).

Evidence-Based Diagnosis

A. The diagnosis is typically clinical.

B. Work-up for hyperandrogenism is appropriate when there are signs of polycystic ovary disease, virilization, or an atypical presentation (such as later in life).

Treatment

A. Establish that there are none of the acne precipitants discussed above.

B. Review general skin care techniques for acne-prone skin.

   1. Vigorous scrubbing can aggravate acne by promoting development of inflammatory lesions.

   2. Abrasive cleaners and mechanical devices also aggravate acne by promoting inflammation.

   3. Use of a mild cleanser with lukewarm water and one's hands is best.

   4. Use of moisturizers should be minimized and all cosmetics and lotions should be oil-free.

   5. Minimize contact of facial skin with hair gels and other styling products (pomade acne).

C. Medical therapy is aimed at the 3 factors involved in acne development.

   1. Decreasing sebum production

     a. No topical therapies are effective

     b. Estrogen

       (1) Most effective at doses of > 50 mcg of ethinyl estradiol

       (2) Common oral contraceptive pills containing ≤ 35 mcg ethinyl estradiol are still helpful.

     c. Antiandrogens (spironolactone)

     d. Isotretinoin (see later discussion)

   2. Alteration of epithelial turnover and cohesiveness

     a. Topical retinoids: tretinoin, tazarotene

     b. Adapalene: a naphthoic acid with retinoid activity

   3. *P acnes* proliferation and accompanying inflammation

     a. Topical antibiotics

       (1) Erythromycin

       (2) Clindamycin

       (3) Metronidazole

       (4) Benzoyl peroxide

     b. Systemic antibiotics

       (1) Tetracycline class

       (2) Erythromycin

       (3) Clindamycin

D. Guidelines for the use of these medications are as follows:

   1. Predominantly comedonal acne: retinoid or adapalene

   2. Mild inflammatory acne: topical antibiotic and benzoyl peroxide with or without retinoid or adapalene

   3. Moderate to severe but noncystic inflammatory acne: systemic antibiotic in combination with a topical retinoid

   4. Nodular cystic acne: isotretinoin

     a. Because of potential adverse effects with isotretinoin, it should only be prescribed by clinicians experienced in its use.

     b. Isotretinoin has the potential to cause hypertriglyceridemia and depression.

     c. Isotretinoin is a potent teratogen and effective contraception must be assured.

E. Additional considerations

   1. Oral contraceptives are useful in women with a strong hormonal component.

   2. Spironolactone can be useful in adult women with recalcitrant acne.

MAKING A DIAGNOSIS

A clinical diagnosis of acne is most likely. Although PCOS might by considered based on the older age of the patient and the distribution of lesions along the jaw line, the patient lacks the oligomenorrhea that, along with evidence of hyperandrogenism, is necessary for making the diagnosis.

A clinical diagnosis of acne is made, and discussion about the most appropriate therapy begins.

 Have you crossed a diagnostic threshold for the leading hypothesis acne vulgaris? Have you ruled out the active alternatives? Do other tests need to be done to exclude the alternative diagnoses?

Alternative Diagnosis: Rosacea

Textbook Presentation

Commonly presents in adults with a facial rash. There is gradual development of telangiectasias and persistent centrofacial erythema occasionally with inflammatory red papules and papulopustules. Comedones are absent. There is often a history of easy flushing. The rash may worsen with sun exposure, ingestion of spicy food and hot liquids, emotional stress, and exercise.

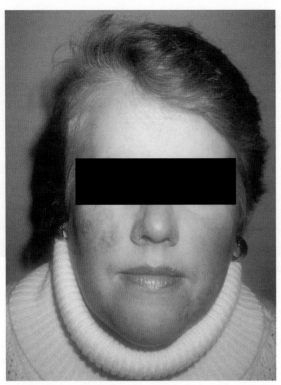

Figure 29-3. Rosacea. (Used with permission from Dr. Anne E. Laumann.)

Disease Highlights

A. Description of lesion: centrofacial persistent facial erythema, telangiectasias, and, occasionally, inflammatory papules and papulopustules (Figure 29-3).

B. Rosacea is most common in fair-skinned individuals of northern European descent but can be seen in people with darker skin as well.

C. Women are more commonly affected than men.

D. However, complicated disease with sebaceous gland hyperplasia and rhinophyma (sebaceous overgrowth causing deformity of the nose) develops more often in men.

E. Rosacea typically begins later than acne and reaches a peak in middle age. That said the 2 can overlap.

F. Sun exposure is thought to be a trigger and sun-damaged skin is frequently seen in patients with rosacea.

Evidence-Based Diagnosis

A. Diagnosis is by clinical presentation.

B. Histopathology, which is rarely necessary, varies according to the stage and variant of the disease and is often nonspecific.

Treatment

A. Sun protection

B. Avoidance of triggers of flushing
   1. Sun exposure
   2. Ingestion of spicy foods and hot liquids
   3. Emotional stressors
   4. Physical exertion: encourage frequent cool-downs

C. Topical agents: metronidazole decreases erythema and prevents papules and papulopustules.

D. Systemic agents: oral antibiotics of the tetracycline class control severe eruptions of inflammatory lesions.

E. Laser treatment
   1. Used to ablate telangiectasias and improve background erythema.
   2. May be helpful to reduce rhinophyma.

CASE RESOLUTION

A management plan was discussed with the patient, including an appropriate skin care regimen, appropriate product selection, and use of systemic and topical medications. At follow-up in 3 months, the patient had significantly fewer active lesions with evidence of dyspigmentation associated with resolving lesions.

CHIEF COMPLAINT

PATIENT 2

Mr. B is a 18-year-old man who was in good health until 1 week ago, when he noted that the left side of his chest was painful. One day before his visit, he noticed a rash on the left side of his chest, just lateral to his sternum. He describes the rash as small bumps, blisters, and red patches. He says that the skin is extremely sensitive to light touch. He otherwise feels well, without fever or constitutional symptoms.

At this point, what is the leading hypothesis, what are the active alternatives, and is there a must not miss diagnosis? Given this differential diagnosis, what tests should be ordered?

RANKING THE DIFFERENTIAL DIAGNOSIS

Several general etiologic categories need to be considered when presented with a patient with new-onset blisters or vesicles. Blisters can be a symptom of infection, autoimmune disease, or a reaction to an external stimulus. Infectious causes include varicella zoster virus (VZV), presenting either as chickenpox or herpes zoster (shingles), and bullous impetigo. Both are possible in this patient. The prodromal pain suggests VZV. Bullous impetigo can cause blisters in a young, healthy person, but these blisters often begin in intertriginous areas. Bullous impetigo is most common in children. Grouped blisters suggest VZV or herpes simplex virus (HSV), whereas other blistering diseases may demonstrate large distinct blisters or erosions.

Bullous arthropod bites can affect patients of any age. A history of exposure should be elicited. The numerous, small, clustered lesions in this case make arthropod bites a less likely diagnosis. Bullous pemphigoid and other autoimmune blistering disorders are rare but possible. Stevens-Johnson syndrome is unlikely given the subacute onset but is certainly a "must not miss" diagnosis (Table 29-2).

The patient reports no significant medical history. He recently finished a course of amoxicillin for pharyngitis. He does also frequently help his mother with gardening. The patient is afebrile with normal vital signs. The physical exam demonstrates clusters of small vesicles, filled with clear fluid, overlying erythematous skin. There is no lymphadenopathy. The rest of the skin exam is unremarkable (Figure 29-4).

 Is the clinical information sufficient to make a diagnosis? If not, what other information do you need?

Leading Hypothesis: Varicella Zoster Virus (Herpes Zoster/Shingles)

Textbook Presentation

This condition usually presents as a rash over a single, unilateral dermatome. The lesions begin as closely grouped vesicles on an

Table 29-2. Diagnostic hypotheses for Mr. B.

Diagnostic Hypotheses	Demographics, Risk Factors, Symptoms and Signs	Important Tests
Leading Hypothesis		
Varicella zoster virus	Prodromal pain symptoms Localized lesions in a dermatomal distribution	Usually diagnosed clinically Tzanck smear, PCR
Active Alternatives		
Bullous impetigo	Acute onset, intertriginous location Most common in children	Bacterial culture of lesion
Bullous arthropod bites	Pruritus Lack of constitutional symptoms Exposure history	Clinical
Bullous pemphigoid	May present with early urticarial lesions and pruritus Later intact blisters	Skin biopsy and direct immunofluorescence of skin
Active Alternative—Must Not Miss		
Stevens-Johnson syndrome	Rapidly progressive rash with associated mucosal lesions	Skin biopsy

PCR, polymerase chain reaction.

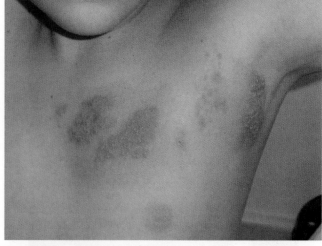

Figure 29-4. Mr. B. on initial presentation.

erythematous base. Over 2–3 days, the lesions become pustular and then crust over after 7–10 days. Pain and paresthesias along the involved dermatome often precede the rash by a few days.

Disease Highlights

A. Description of the lesion: small, tightly grouped vesicles on an erythematous base occurring in one dermatome (see Figure 29-4). Very early in the presentation, the lesions are large papules that then become vesicular, then pustular, and ultimately crusted.

B. Characteristics of the lesion

  1. The rash tends to occur in the region where the rash of primary VZV infection (chickenpox) was most severe.

    a. The most common dermatomes are trigeminal and T3–L2.

    b. It is not uncommon to have a few vesicles in contiguous dermatomes.

  2. New lesions may appear for several days, occasionally for up to 7 days.

C. Shingles is caused by reactivation of VZV in a dorsal root ganglion.

D. Complications

  1. Herpes zoster ophthalmicus

    a. Can occur when there is involvement of the first division of the trigeminal nerve.

    b. The tip of the nose is in this division so vesicles in this area should raise the possibility of herpes zoster ophthalmicus.

    c. Herpes zoster ophthalmicus carries high risk of corneal damage.

  2. Ramsay Hunt syndrome

    a. Reactivation of VZV within the geniculate ganglion

    b. Causes a Bell palsy (facial paralysis) and ear pain

    c. Vesicles can often be seen in the ear canal.

    d. Vestibular and hearing disturbances (vertigo and hearing loss or tinnitus) are frequently reported.

E. Disseminated varicella zoster may occur, most often in immunocompromised patients.

F. Shingles in the elderly

  1. Shingles can be associated with significant morbidity in elderly patients.

  2. The rash is more severe and generally lasts longer in the elderly.

  3. Postherpetic neuralgia, a potentially debilitating, long-term pain syndrome, is also most common in the elderly.

Evidence-Based Diagnosis

A. The diagnosis of shingles is usually made clinically without additional tests.

B. Viral polymerase chain reaction (PCR) done of the vesicle fluid is useful if the diagnosis is in doubt.

C. The bedside Tzanck smear of material scraped from a fresh vesicle can be supportive evidence but cannot distinguish between VZV and HSV.

Treatment

A. In the immunocompetent, the eruption is self-limited; supportive care with pain relievers may be all that is necessary.

B. Patients with any involvement of the eye should be evaluated by an ophthalmologist.

C. Antiviral agents (acyclovir, famciclovir, valacyclovir)

  1. When the rash is diagnosed within the first 72 hours, systemic antiviral medications are useful.

  2. They decrease the duration and severity of the disease.

  3. They prevent dissemination.

  4. Early treatment with antiviral agents may also prevent the development of postherpetic neuralgia.

 The use of antiviral drugs is not beneficial if the rash of herpes zoster has been present for more than 72 hours.

D. Symptomatic care: soaks and topical antipruritics might be useful.

E. Corticosteroids

  1. Corticosteroids have been used in conjunction with antiviral agents to reduce the duration of the rash and the acute pain syndrome.

  2. A recent meta-analysis showed that corticosteroids are probably ineffective in the treatment of shingles.

F. Infection control

  1. The vesicle fluid is infectious to individuals who have not had chickenpox or been vaccinated.

  2. Infection risk can, therefore, be reduced by preventing direct contact with the vesicle fluid.

G. Postherpetic neuralgia

  1. Most commonly complicates disease in the elderly

  2. Potentially severe neuropathic pain syndrome

  3. Can be treated with tricyclic antidepressants, gabapentin, or opioids

  4. Intrathecal methylprednisolone and lidocaine are effective for refractory disease.

H. Prevention

  1. The shingles vaccine is effective prevention.

  2. The original trial of this vaccine was conducted in a population over 60 years of age and demonstrated a 48.5% reduction in episodes of zoster (NNT = 63) and a 45% reduction in cases of postherpetic neuralgia (NNT = 434).

  3. The vaccine is recommended for patients over the age of 60.

    a. Patients should receive the vaccine regardless of whether there is a history of chickenpox.

    b. The vaccine should also probably be given 3–4 years after an episode of shingles.

  4. Because this is a live-virus vaccine, it is contraindicated in patients who are immunosuppressed, pregnant, or planning pregnancy.

MAKING A DIAGNOSIS

Given the patient's prodromal symptoms and classic dermatomal distribution, VZV is the leading diagnosis. Because the rash was thought to be somewhat atypical, a fresh vesicle was unroofed with a scalpel tip and the vesicle fluid was sent for PCR testing.

The diagnosis of varicella zoster is often clinical. The distribution and clinical appearance of lesions, as well as the associated prodromal symptoms, can make the diagnosis obvious. Impetigo, bullous arthropod bites, and autoimmune blistering diseases will typically demonstrate larger distinct blisters or erosions. Stevens-Johnson syndrome and other drug reactions must always be considered when medications are in use. This patient was taking amoxicillin. The clinical appearance of the lesions, their localized distribution, and the overall time course of the symptoms is not consistent with this eruption, so VZV must still lead the list.

 Have you crossed a diagnostic threshold for the leading hypothesis varicella zoster? Have you ruled out the active alternatives? Do other tests need to be done to exclude the alternative diagnoses?

Alternative Diagnosis: Bullous Impetigo

Textbook Presentation

Most commonly seen in children, bullous impetigo presents as flaccid, transparent bullae in the intertriginous areas. The blisters rupture easily and leave a rim of scale and a shallow moist erosion.

Disease Highlights

A. Description of the lesion: flaccid bullae on normal skin (Figure 29-5)

B. Location of the lesion

  1. Develops on grossly intact skin as a result of local toxin production.

  2. This is in contrast to nonbullous impetigo, shown in Figure 29-6, resulting from *Staphylococcus* or *Streptococcus* infection, which tends to affect previously traumatized skin.

  3. Lesions most commonly develop on moist, intertriginous skin.

C. Superficial skin infection that most commonly affects infants and young children

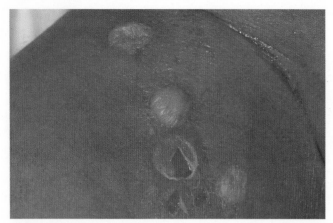

Figure 29-5. Bullous impetigo.

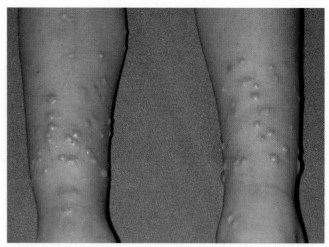

Figure 29-7. Bullous arthropod bites.

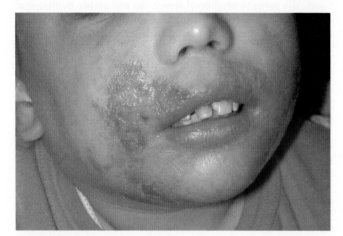

Figure 29-6. Impetigo.

D. Family members and close contacts may also be colonized and warrant investigation and treatment when appropriate. Environmental sources such as shared towels, athletic equipment and such should be considered.

Alternative Diagnosis: Bullous Arthropod Bites

Textbook Presentation

This condition commonly presents as a cluster of tense blisters on exposed skin. The blisters tend to be large (≥ 1 cm) and surrounding skin is normal.

Disease Highlights

A. Description of the lesion: large, often tense blisters on normal skin (Figure 29-7).

B. Character and location of the lesion
  1. The lesions tend to develop in exposed areas of the skin, such as the extremities.
  2. The patient will otherwise appear well.
  3. The lesions are typically extraordinarily pruritic.
  4. Although the blisters arise from otherwise normal skin, surrounding inflammatory changes from rubbing and scratching are often present.

C. Arthropod bite reactions are dermal hypersensitivity reactions to antigens in the saliva of insects.

D. Because bedbugs (as well as fleas) are a common culprit, this diagnosis has recently become more common.

Evidence-Based Diagnosis

A. Diagnosis is made by clinical presentation.

B. Histopathology, though rarely necessary, can be supportive, demonstrating edema, a subepidermal blister, and a dermal inflammatory infiltrate with numerous eosinophils.

Treatment

A. Avoidance of future bites with use of protective clothing and insect repellants.

B. Attention to eradicating the source of the biting insects, such as on pets, nests, etc.

D. The causative agent is *Staphylococcus aureus*.

E. The blistering is caused by the production of exfoliatin or epidermolytic toxins.

Evidence-Based Diagnosis

A. Diagnosis is by clinical presentation.

B. Culture of blister fluid or the moist edge of a crusted plaque may be diagnostic.

Treatment

A. Oral antibiotics active against *S aureus* should be prescribed for bullous impetigo. The possibility of methicillin-resistant *S aureus* (MRSA) must be considered.

B. Localized, nonbullous impetigo may be adequately treated with topical antibiotics (effective against gram-positive cocci) such as:
  1. Bacitracin
  2. Polymyxin
  3. Mupirocin

C. Recurrent infections may indicate staphylococcal carriage. Eradication measures including daily washing with chlorhexidine gluconate, intranasal mupirocin ointment, and oral rifampin and doxycycline have been modestly successful.

C. Supportive local care to prevent secondary infection and relieve pruritus.

Alternative Diagnosis: Bullous Pemphigoid

Textbook Presentation

Bullous pemphigoid is usually seen in elderly patients with the sudden onset of 1–2 cm tense blisters and bright red, urticarial plaques. Lesions often begin on the lower extremities and progress upward.

Disease Highlights

A. Description of the lesion: tense bullae arising on skin that may be normal, erythematous, or urticarial (Figure 29-8).

B. Bullous pemphigoid is an autoimmune disease primarily affecting the elderly.

C. Autoantibodies are targeted against components of the epidermal basement membrane zone, thus triggering separation and blistering.

D. The lesions heal without scarring.

E. Most cases occur sporadically without obvious precipitating factors.

F. Character and location of the lesion

  1. Predilection of blisters for the extremities

  2. Lesions range from asymptomatic to intensely pruritic.

  3. Mucosal surfaces are rarely involved.

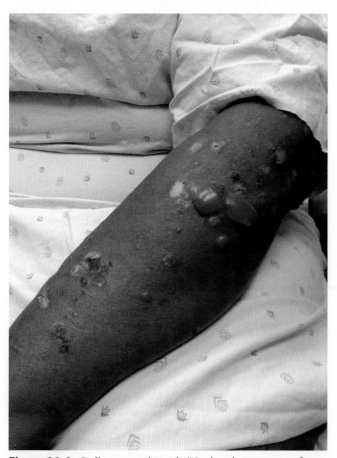

Figure 29-8. Bullous pemphigoid. (Used with permission from Dr. Duri Yun.)

G. Antibodies to several elements of the basements membrane zone have been isolated. These distinct antibodies cause other blistering syndromes, such as pemphigus vulgaris and epidermolysis bullosa acquisita.

Evidence-Based Diagnosis

A. Histopathology provides supportive information, demonstrating a subepidermal blister plane and accumulation of eosinophils.

B. Immunopathology confirms the diagnosis by demonstrating linear deposits of IgG and C3 at the dermal–epidermal junction.

C. In 70–80% of patients, circulating IgG that recognizes the identified antigens of the basement membrane zone can be found.

Treatment

A. Topical, potent corticosteroids can be effective.

B. Extensive disease can be treated with systemic corticosteroids.

C. Steroid-sparing immunosuppressives are used to limit the toxicities of systemic corticosteroids in chronic disease.

D. Alternative antiinflammatory regimens such as tetracycline and nicotinamide may be effective.

E. Remission is usually obtained within a few weeks; however, some degree of long-term therapy may be necessary.

F. Refractory cases may respond to plasmapheresis or intravenous gammaglobulin.

Alternative Diagnosis: Stevens-Johnson Syndrome

Textbook Presentation

Stevens-Johnson syndrome typically presents in a patient with fever, malaise, headache, and myalgias who is taking a potentially causative medication. After about 1 week of symptoms, a macular rash develops on the chest and face. These lesions subsequently blister and then rapidly erode. The skin is usually excruciatingly tender.

Disease Highlights

A. Description of the lesion: flaccid bullae and vesicles that develop centrally within preexisting target lesion. The bullae rapidly erode, leaving red and raw skin (Figure 29-9).

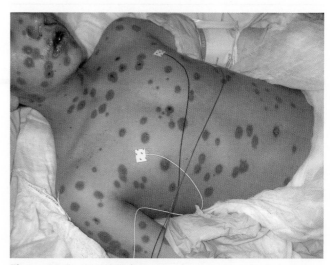

Figure 29-9. Stevens-Johnson syndrome.

B. Stevens-Johnson syndrome and toxic epidermal necrolysis are hypersensitivity reaction patterns involving the skin.

   1. These 2 conditions are often considered to be on a spectrum of severity. Stevens-Johnson syndrome involves less body surface area, whereas toxic epidermal necrolysis leads to considerable areas of full-thickness skin sloughing.

   2. Although the precise cause has not been found, drugs are involved in most cases.

C. More than 200 drugs have been implicated as causes of Stevens-Johnson syndrome and toxic epidermal necrolysis.

D. A well-done case-control trial identified the most likely culprits. These are listed in Table 29-3 with their associated ORs.

E. Disease course

   1. Prodromal symptoms, characterized by fever, malaise, headache, myalgias, as well as GI and respiratory complaints, occur over 1–2 weeks.

   2. The rash occurs initially on the face and central trunk as pink to red macules and papules.

Table 29-3. Medications most commonly implicated in Stevens-Johnson syndrome or toxic epidermal necrolysis.

Medications	OR
Short-term	
Sulfonamide antibiotics	172
Aminopenicillins	6.7
Quinolones	10
Cephalosporins	14
Long-term	
Carbamazepine	90
Phenobarbital	45
Phenytoin	53
Valproic acid	25
Piroxicam	12
Allopurinol	52
Corticosteroids	54

Data from Roujeau JC, Kelly JP, Naldi L et al. Medication use and the risk of Stevens-Johnson syndrome or toxic epidermal necrolysis. N Engl J Med. 1995; 333:1600–7. Massachusetts Medical Society.

   3. The rash may spread and evolve rapidly, with individual lesions becoming targetoid with dusky centers and ultimately coalescing into larger plaques.

   4. Flaccid bullae and vesicles may develop centrally within targets as the skin necroses.

   5. Blisters form and rapidly erode, leaving red and raw skin that becomes coated by a gray-white pseudomembrane.

   6. Mucous membranes

      a. Lesions on mucous membranes may accompany or precede the skin rash.

      b. The mucosal surfaces may be tender and burning.

      c. The lips are often swollen, cracked, bleeding, and crusted.

   7. The skin is extremely tender.

F. A hallmark of Stevens-Johnson syndrome and toxic epidermal necrolysis is the presence of exquisite skin tenderness.

Evidence-Based Diagnosis

A. Histopathology supports the clinical impression.

B. Pathology demonstrates epidermal necrosis with minimal evidence of epidermal and dermal inflammation.

Treatment

A. If an offending drug is present, it must be discontinued.

B. Some studies support the use of intravenous immunoglobulin in the early stages of the disease to abort progression.

C. Use of systemic corticosteroids is controversial. Studies have not proven that the benefit outweighs risk of immunosuppression.

D. Supportive care in a burn unit is recommended.

CASE RESOLUTION

PCR for VZV was positive, thus confirming the diagnosis of varicella zoster. The patient was prescribed valacyclovir for 7 days. He was instructed to keep the skin lesions covered to prevent contacts from being exposed to the infective vesicle fluid. He was counseled to avoid close contact with young infants and immunosuppressed individuals until all skin lesions are crusted.

CHIEF COMPLAINT

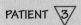

PATIENT 3

Ms. M is a 16-year-old girl who has many small red flaky spots. The rash developed first on her trunk and over the last 2 weeks is spreading to her extremities (Figure 29-10). She denies any history of similar eruptions. She states she is otherwise feeling well. This eruption is not particularly itchy. On examination, there are many 1–2 cm discrete, brightly erythematous plaques and papules with adherent white scale. The lesions are predominantly on the trunk but extend onto the extremities. Some lesions appear somewhat linear in configuration, whereas most are round to oval in shape. The scale is confluent over the surface of the lesions. The nails are normal and the palms and soles are clear. The oropharynx is injected with some tonsillar enlargement but without exudates. The tongue appears geographic. The rest of the physical exam is unremarkable.

(continued)

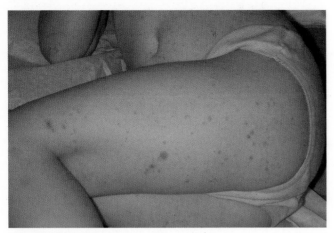

Figure 29-10. Ms. M on initial presentation.

At this point, what is the leading hypothesis, what are the active alternatives, and is there a must not miss diagnosis? Given this differential diagnosis, what tests should be ordered?

RANKING THE DIFFERENTIAL DIAGNOSIS

The appearance of the eruption suggests that this condition is papulosquamous in morphology (ie, it is composed primarily of papules and plaques with scale). Common causes of papulosquamous eruptions are psoriasis, pityriasis rosea, fungal infections, and nummular dermatitis.

The patient's age, acute onset of the rash, and the pattern of small papules and plaques are pivotal points suggesting either guttate psoriasis or pityriasis rosea. In addition, the finding of pharyngeal injection suggests that there may be an infectious component (as is common with guttate psoriasis). The configuration of the lesions and the scale can be very helpful in narrowing the differential diagnosis. This patient's scale is confluent over the surface of the lesions, consistent with guttate psoriasis. Tinea infections typically have scale at the border of the lesions (leading edge with advancing scale) and pityriasis rosea has scale at the center of the lesion (trailing scale). Nummular dermatitis is usually found on the extremities and is associated with significant pruritus, making it an unlikely diagnosis in this case. Secondary syphilis needs to be considered as a "must not miss" diagnosis. Syphilis can present with plaques, but they often involve the palms and soles and lack an adherent scale (Table 29-4).

On further questioning, the patient does recall a sore throat several weeks ago. Her medical history is unremarkable. Her family history is remarkable only for a father with psoriasis.

Is the clinical information sufficient to make a diagnosis? If not, what other information do you need?

Table 29-4. Diagnostic hypotheses for Ms. M.

Diagnostic Hypotheses	Demographics, Risk Factors, Symptoms and Signs	Important Tests
Leading Hypothesis		
Guttate psoriasis	Presents after acute pharyngitis Discrete small red papules and plaques with adherent silvery scale	Morphology and pattern of lesions and positive throat culture
Active Alternatives		
Pityriasis rosea	Classically starts with a single "herald patch" 1–2 weeks prior to disseminated eruption Primarily truncal distribution with "tree-like" appearance	Clinical diagnosis
Tinea corporis	Solitary or few lesions Annular lesions with a leading edge of scale Pruritic	Identification of fungus with KOH or culture
Nummular dermatitis	Well-defined plaques with crust and papulovesicles Pruritic Symmetric distribution on extremities	Clinical diagnosis
Secondary syphilis	Palms and soles involved Thinner plaques without adherent scale	RPR, FTA

FTA, fluorescent treponemal antibody; KOH, potassium hydroxide; RPR, rapid plasma reagin.

Leading Hypothesis: Guttate Psoriasis

Textbook Presentation

Guttate psoriasis generally presents with small, round, and slightly oval lesions on the back and trunk. The lesions often have somewhat silvery, adherent scales.

Disease Highlights

A. Description of lesion: small (0.5–1.5 cm), round or slightly oval lesions with characteristic overlying silvery scales (see Figure 29-10).

B. Character of the lesion

1. Lesions tend to occur over the upper trunk and proximal extremities.

2. Face, ears, and scalp may also be involved.

3. The lesions may localize to sites of minor skin trauma, such as scrapes (Koebner phenomenon).

4. Eruption generally persists for 3–4 months and then remits spontaneously.

C. Most commonly seen in young adults, frequently preceded by a streptococcal throat infection.

D. Affected patients are at increased risk for development of psoriasis vulgaris in the next 3–5 years.

E. There is an increased incidence of psoriasis in families.

Evidence-Based Diagnosis

A. The diagnosis is often made based on the clinical presentation.

B. The presence of streptococcal pharyngitis would be a supportive finding.

C. A skin biopsy of an established lesion may demonstrate classic histologic findings of psoriasis vulgaris.

Treatment

A. Guttate psoriasis is typically a self-limited eruption, although clearance can take weeks to months.

B. Remission can be hastened with the use of UV light treatments.

C. Antibiotics with antiinflammatory properties, such as erythromycin and tetracycline, can be additionally helpful for flares.

   1. There is an infectious trigger in many cases.

   2. Appropriate antibiotic treatment of any potentially causative infection should be administered.

D. Topical corticosteroids can be effective on individual lesions.

E. Systemic corticosteroids should be avoided in psoriasis because withdrawal may trigger flares.

F. Topical calcipotriene, a vitamin D derivative, is also effective.

MAKING A DIAGNOSIS

Based on the lesions' morphology, family history, and recent pharyngitis, guttate psoriasis was considered the likely diagnosis. A throat culture was sent. A skin biopsy was considered but not performed.

Have you crossed a diagnostic threshold for the leading hypothesis, guttate psoriasis? Have you ruled out the active alternatives? Do other tests need to be done to exclude the alternative diagnoses?

Alternative Diagnosis: Pityriasis Rosea

Textbook Presentation

Pityriasis rosea commonly presents as a "herald patch" and then multiple small, oval, scaly plaques develop over the trunk. The rash is mildly pruritic.

Disease Highlights

A. Description of lesion: oval or round plaque with central (trailing) scale (Figure 29-11).

B. Character of the lesion

   1. The primary eruption appears as a single oval or round, pink to brownish plaque with a collarette of scale around the inner margin of the lesion (the herald patch). This herald patch most often occurs on the trunk and is often misdiagnosed as tinea corporis.

   2. One to 2 weeks after the appearance of the herald patch, the secondary eruption emerges as generalized smaller but similar oval scaly plaques distributed along skin tension lines in a "fir tree" pattern.

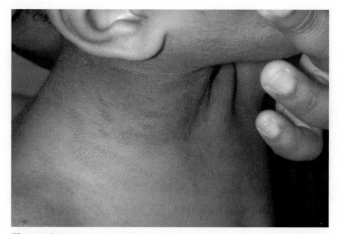
Figure 29-11. Pityriasis rosea.

   3. Variable degrees of pruritus

   4. Spontaneous resolution occurs over 8–12 weeks, often with subsequent postinflammatory hypopigmentation or hyperpigmentation.

C. A history of a mild prodrome of malaise, nausea, headache, and low-grade fever may be present.

D. Pityriasis rosea is a common worldwide disease without genetic or racial predilection, occurring sporadically throughout the year.

E. A viral cause is postulated; evidence suggests but does not confirm a role for human herpesvirus 7.

Evidence-Based Diagnosis

A. The diagnosis is clinical, based on morphology and distribution of the skin lesions.

B. Skin biopsy demonstrates many nonspecific findings of a subacute dermatitis but can provide supportive evidence for the diagnosis.

Treatment

A. No specific treatment is indicated or effective; the condition resolves over 8–12 weeks.

B. In cases with severe pruritus, symptomatic treatments, such as antihistamines and mild topical corticosteroids, may be beneficial.

C. UVB phototherapy has been advocated to decrease the severity, particularly when administered early in the course. This treatment may worsen the postinflammatory dyspigmentation.

Alternative Diagnosis: Tinea Corporis

Textbook Presentation

Tinea corporis commonly presents as round, pink plaques with small peripheral papules and a rim of scales. The neck and back are the most common locations (Figure 29-12).

Disease Highlights

A. Description of the lesion: multiple lesions are possible.

   1. Circular lesions with a sharply marginated raised border and central clearing, arising by centrifugal spread of the fungus from the initial site of infection

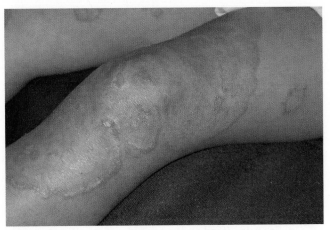

Figure 29-12. Tinea corporis.

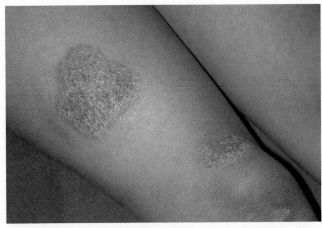

Figure 29-13. Nummular dermatitis.

2. Inflammatory lesions may demonstrate pustules or vesicles, especially around the margin.

3. Overlying scale is common, typically more prominent at the border of the lesion.

4. Solitary lesions may occur, or there may be multiple plaques that remain discrete or become confluent.

B. The degree of associated inflammatory change is variable, depending on the causative species of fungus.

C. The wide variation in clinical presentation depends on the species of fungus, size of the inoculum, body site infected, and immune status of the patient.

Evidence-Based Diagnosis

A. Identification of the fungus by microscopic examination of scales after application of 5–20% potassium hydroxide

B. Culture of tissue material (such as the scale)

C. Histopathology is rarely necessary to make the diagnosis of a superficial infection, but with the use of fungal stains the cell walls may be visible in fixed sections.

Treatment

A. Both topical and systemic antifungal agents are effective.

B. Decision of which to use is based on the extent and location of the infection.

C. Hair-bearing sites often require systemic therapy.

Alternative Diagnosis: Nummular Dermatitis

Textbook Presentation

Nummular dermatitis generally presents as an extremely pruritic rash of numerous, round, crusted lesions on a patient's legs.

Disease Highlights

A. Description of lesions: well-demarcated coin-shaped lesions composed of minute vesicles and papules on an erythematous base. The lesions have an overlying crust, frequently with a weeping exudate (Figure 29-13).

B. Nummular dermatitis is an acute eruption of numerous lesions predominantly on the extremities.

C. The lesions are severely pruritic.

D. The eruption runs a remitting and relapsing course.

E. Patients are often atopic.

F. Secondary infection is frequently present.

Evidence-Based Diagnosis

A. Microscopic examination of a scraping will rule out tinea.

B. Histopathology can assist in the diagnosis by demonstrating the features of an acute dermatitis.

Treatment

A. If present, secondary infections often require treatment with systemic antibiotics.

B. Antihistamines can help alleviate the pruritus.

C. Skin care, especially bathing practices and appropriate use of emollients, should be stressed.

D. Topical corticosteroids are useful for flares.

Alternative Diagnosis: Secondary Syphilis

Textbook Presentation

Secondary syphilis presents as oval macules in sexually active people. The lesions are present diffusely, including on the palms and soles. A history of a transient, painless, genital ulcer in the preceding weeks can often be obtained.

Disease Highlights

A. Description of lesion: papules and plaques distributed over the entire body. They are copper red to hyperpigmented in color.

B. Character of the lesion

1. There may be variable lesions at different stages of disease.

   a. A fleeting eruption of symmetric, coppery red, round and oval macules may be seen early in the secondary stage, about 8 weeks after the infecting exposure.

   b. The later, classic eruption includes involvement of mucosal surfaces and palms and soles.

   c. In the latest phases, thick scales may cover the plaques.

2. The rashes of secondary syphilis are nonpruritic.

3. The lesions are generally symmetrically distributed.

Evidence-Based Diagnosis

A. The Venereal Disease Research Laboratories (VDRL) and fluorescent treponemal antibody (FTA) tests are 100% sensitive for secondary syphilis.

B. FTA tests have specificities in the high 90% range.

Treatment

Penicillin is the treatment of choice for secondary syphilis.

CASE RESOLUTION

The patient's throat culture revealed group A streptococcus. A clinical diagnosis of guttate psoriasis was made. The patient was prescribed 10 days of penicillin as well as topical corticosteroids and topical calcipotriene. UVB treatments, 3 times weekly, were begun to induce remission of the psoriatic flare. She was counseled on her risk for future development of psoriasis vulgaris.

Guttate psoriasis affects those with a predisposition toward psoriasis. The guttate flares tend to remit quite reliably; however, affected individuals are at increased risk for the development of chronic psoriasis.

OTHER IMPORTANT CUTANEOUS DISORDERS

Urticaria

Textbook Presentation

Urticaria typically presents as an itchy rash with large or small, palpable, red areas over the entire body. The rash is transient, with no 1 lesion lasting very long. Both the rash and the pruritus respond to antihistamines.

Disease Highlights

A. Description of the lesion: transient pink to red gently elevated edematous papules and plaques that may coalesce into giant lesions. The lesions often leave purple discoloration or central clearing when they fade (Figure 29-14).

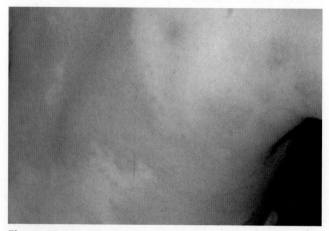

Figure 29-14. Urticaria.

B. Characteristics of the lesion

    1. Individual lesions should resolve within 24 hours while new lesions may continue to develop.

    2. The eruption is typically accompanied by itch, but excoriations are rare.

C. Mucous membranes, eyelids, hands, and feet may develop deeper subcutaneous swelling manifesting as angioedema.

D. Most urticaria is acute, lasting less than 6 weeks.

E. Urticaria is a hypersensitivity reaction to numerous insults.

    1. Etiologic factors can be remembered with the mnemonic *I-I-I-I-I*.

        a. Infection

        b. Infestation

        c. Ingestion (food or drug)

        d. Inhalation

        e. Injection

    2. Idiopathic should probably be added to this list because the etiologic agent may induce an immunologic cascade that persists in the absence of the inciting agent.

F. Chronic urticaria (lasting > 6 weeks) can also be seen in the setting of systemic disease such as collagen vascular disease, malignancy, parasitosis, and chronic infection.

Evidence-Based Diagnosis

A. Clinical findings of typical transient urticaria are diagnostic, and a skin biopsy is rarely indicated.

B. The morphologic differential diagnosis often includes the following:

    1. Erythema multiforme (because of the targetoid appearance of some urticaria)

    2. Insect bite reactions

    3. The early phases of bullous pemphigoid

C. Urticaria can be distinguished from all of the above disorders because it is the only one with lesions that last < 24 hours.

D. A careful history, including review of medications, recent exposures, and food ingestion, is the most important aspect of the evaluation to determine a cause.

E. Laboratory evaluation is sometimes undertaken in cases of chronic urticaria, but studies have shown that relevant results are so rarely found without other symptoms that this approach is discouraged.

Treatment

A. Identification of the inciting agent (medication, supplement, infection) is paramount and should be addressed as the first step in management.

B. Antihistamines are the mainstay of therapy. H_1-blockers should be given on a regular dosing schedule until the eruption is suppressed and then tapered gradually to prevent rebound flare.

C. Combinations of different H_1-blockers can be effective when a single agent is inadequate.

D. Addition of H_2-blockers may be helpful in refractory cases.

Purpura/Petechiae

Textbook Presentation

Purpura and petechiae are seen in patients with bleeding diatheses or vascular damage. Petechiae are capillary hemorrhages that

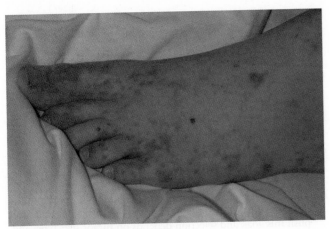

Figure 29-15. Purpura.

present as nonblanching, pinpoint, red spots over dependent body parts, most commonly the lower extremities. Purpura are larger hemorrhages into the skin.

Purpura are associated with a variety of life-threatening diseases such as vasculitis and sepsis.

Disease Highlights

A. Description of the lesion: petechiae are red, blue or purple, nonblanching, pinpoint spots. Purpura are larger (up to several centimeters) nonblanching macules, papules, or plaques that may or may not be palpable (Figure 29-15).

B. Both purpura and petechiae are, to some degree, nonblanching; (ie, the color cannot be compressed out of the lesion by pressure).

C. The shape of these lesions is variable, ranging from stellate to round or oval or targetoid to retiform (netlike).

D. The color, texture, and configuration of these lesions will be helpful in constructing a differential diagnosis of the cause.

E. The differential diagnosis of purpura/petechiae is vast, and many classification schemes have been proposed. The first step is to differentiate ecchymoses from purpura and petechiae.

F. Ecchymoses
   1. Ecchymoses are the most common form of hemorrhage in the skin.
   2. They are typically induced by trauma and, therefore, are seen on trauma-prone sites such as the dorsal hand, forearm, lateral thigh, and shin.
   3. The shape of ecchymoses tends to be geometric (rectangular) or linear because they are induced by an external force.
   4. Predisposing factors to ecchymoses include weakening of the dermal structure secondary to age, corticosteroid use, solar damage, and vitamin C deficiency (scurvy), as well as coagulation defects.

G. Petechiae are most commonly associated with thrombocytopenia.

H. Purpura
   1. Like petechiae, purpura signify hemorrhage into the skin.
   2. The hemorrhage may
      a. Be simple extravasation through leaky vessel walls.
      b. Be accompanied by inflammation that is damaging vessel walls. (These lesions are often partially blanching

because the inflammatory component blanches while the hemorrhagic component does not.)
      c. Be the result of occlusion of a vessel leading to ischemic damage to the skin.
   3. The degree to which purpuric lesions are palpable is helpful diagnostically.
      a. Nonpalpable hemorrhage in the skin is most concerning for thrombocytopenia or abnormal platelet function.
      b. Extravasation of blood alone into deep tissue layers can produce a nodule (such as occurs with a hematoma).
      c. Edema associated with the vessel injury (such as in cases of inflammatory vasculitis) may cause a palpable lesion.
         (1) Palpable purpura can be a sign of serious of illness.
         (2) Evaluation should include tests for vasculitis and, in the right setting, infectious causes (possibly including empiric treatment).

Evidence-Based Diagnosis

A. An evaluation of clotting (platelet number, function and measures of coagulation) is indicated to determine if purpura and petechiae are symptoms of a coagulopathy, thrombocytopenia, or vasculitis.

B. A skin biopsy can be helpful in determining
   1. The size and location of affected vessels within the dermal and subcutaneous tissues.
   2. The degree and character of associated inflammation.
   3. The type of vessel damage (leukocytoclastic or granulomatous).
   4. The presence and character of any occlusions within vessels (organisms, calcium, fibrin).

C. Immunofluorescence studies of histologic specimens can be helpful in identifying antibody and complement deposits on vessels walls.

Treatment

A. Treatment is directed toward management of the underlying cause of the vessel damage.

B. Supportive therapy includes local wound care and prevention of secondary infection.

Skin Cancer

There are innumerable specific forms of skin cancer, deriving from all of the structures of the skin and subcutaneous tissues. In addition, many cancers will metastasize to the skin. The three most common skin cancers are described.

1. Basal Cell Carcinoma

Textbook Presentation

Basal cell carcinoma most commonly presents as a flesh-colored, translucent, or slightly red papule or nodule, classically displaying a rolled border. Most commonly presents on the head or neck of older adults.

Disease Highlights

A. Description of lesion: the typical lesion is a flesh-colored, translucent, or slightly red papule or nodule, classically displaying a rolled border (Figure 29-16).
   1. Lesions are often friable, bleeding easily and developing crust. Telangiectasias on the surface can be a helpful sign.

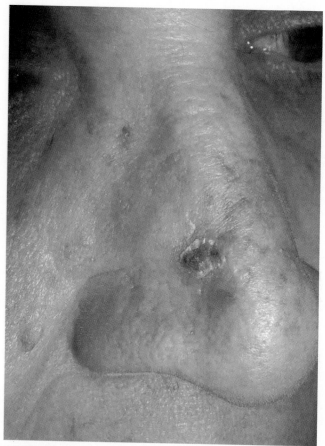

Figure 29-16. Basal cell carcinoma. (Used with permission from Dr. Anne E. Laumann.)

    2. Large tumors can be locally destructive.

B. Basal cell carcinoma is the most common malignant tumor in humans.

C. Lesions are typically asymptomatic except for the observation of easy bleeding from a site.

    1. Only rarely is pain associated.

    2. Metastasis from a basal cell carcinoma is rare.

D. Individuals at risk are adults with fair hair and eyes, easy freckling, and propensity for sunburn.

    1. Patients with skin of color are less likely to be affected.

    2. Men and women are about equally affected.

    3. Exposure to UV light has long been believed to play a causative role in the development of this tumor, although the exact mechanism is not clear. Several genetic mutations have been isolated in basal cell carcinoma and may serve as targets for therapeutics.

    4. Chronic wounds and sites of inflammation as well as immunosuppression can predispose to development of this tumor.

    5. Exposure to arsenic is another risk factor for basal cell carcinoma.

E. The head and neck are the most common sites affected with this tumor.

    1. Only 10–15% of tumors develop on sun-protected skin.

    2. The nose is the most common site, accounting for 20–30% of all cases.

F. Basal cell carcinoma is likely derived from the hair follicle. The name implies a resemblance of the tumor cells to the basal cells of the epidermis, although this is not believed to be their derivation.

G. Patients have up to a 45% risk of developing subsequent basal cell carcinomas in the 5 years after initial diagnosis.

Evidence-Based Diagnosis

Histologic evaluation of affected tissue is the gold standard for diagnosis.

Treatment

A. The goal of therapy is to eliminate the tumor and prevent local tissue destruction. Numerous methods are available to accomplish this goal, and selection depends on tumor size, type, and location, patient characteristics, and patient preferences.

B. 5-year recurrence rates vary by treatment modality. The lowest recurrence rate is achieved with Mohs micrographic surgery.

    1. This method involves excision of the visible tumor, followed by microscopic evaluation of frozen tissue sections to visualize tumor margins and repeat local excision until all margins are clear of tumor.

    2. The technique allows for maximal tissue sparing while ensuring complete eradication of tumor.

C. Follow-up of patients for recurrent or subsequent tumors is critical.

2. Squamous Cell Carcinoma

Textbook Presentation

Squamous cell carcinoma most commonly presents as a firm but somewhat indistinct nodule or plaque. It may evolve from actinic keratoses on the sun-exposed skin of middle-aged people.

Disease Highlights

A. Description of lesion: lesions are firm but somewhat indistinct nodules or plaques that may arise from an in situ carcinoma or in normal skin. Tumors may become ulcerated or bleed easily and become crusted (Figure 29-17).

    1. The surface may be smooth, verrucous, or papillomatous, with or without scaling.

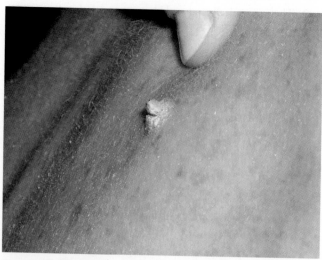

Figure 29-17. Squamous cell carcinoma. (Used with permission from Dr. Anne E. Laumann.)

2. Fixation to underlying structures develops as the lesion invades locally.

3. In situ lesions tend to be sharply demarcated erythematous scaling plaques.

B. This tumor most commonly affects fair-skinned individuals with excessive sun exposure.

1. May evolve from actinic keratoses on sun-exposed skin in these patients.

2. UV radiation is a major risk factor for the development of this tumor.

3. Additional predisposing factors include

   a. Radiation therapy

   b. Chronic scar formation

   c. Chemical carcinogens, such as hydrocarbons

   d. Viral exposures

   e. Thermal exposures

   f. Arsenic

   g. Long-term immunosuppression (such as in kidney transplant recipients).

C. Squamous cell carcinoma does carry a risk of local recurrence and metastasis.

1. The risk of local recurrence is around 3%.

2. Metastasis is less common but can reach 10% in patients with the thickest lesions.

3. Other factors, such as location (ears) and immunosuppression, are also associated with higher risk of metastasis.

D. Intraoral squamous cell carcinoma is predominantly a disease of adult men.

1. Risk factors are alcohol and tobacco use.

2. When detected in the early asymptomatic stage, these cancers are easily curable.

E. Incidence increases with age and varies with geographic location, ethnicity, and behavior patterns.

Evidence-Based Diagnosis

A. Histologic evaluation of affected tissue is the gold standard for diagnosis.

B. A high index of suspicion may be necessary to recognize a potential tumor when its appearance or location is unusual. For example, the verrucous form of squamous cell carcinoma can be mistaken for a wart.

Treatment

A. The goal of treatment is eradication of the tumor while producing the least disability and dysfunction for the patient.

B. Careful evaluation for the presence of metastatic disease is paramount. This may include lymph node dissection in some instances.

C. Multiple destruction modalities are available and are selected based on size, shape, and location of the tumor as well as patient preferences. These modalities include, but are not limited to

1. Excisional surgery

2. Mohs micrographic surgery

3. Electrosurgery

4. Radiation therapy

5. Local immunotherapy

D. Wide destruction of these tumors usually results in cure as squamous cell carcinomas grow by direct extension. However, residual tumor can invade and extend along peripheral nerves, allowing a deep recurrence on occasion.

E. A large percentage of squamous cell carcinomas could be prevented by avoidance of excessive solar exposure. Routine screening for tumors, especially in high-risk patients, is imperative.

3. Melanoma

Textbook Presentation

Melanoma typically presents as a dark brown or black macule or papule in a middle-aged person. The lesion has pigment variation throughout and irregular borders.

Disease Highlights

A. Description of lesion: the most common type of melanoma is superficial spreading (Figure 29-18).

1. These tumors may present as a dark brown to black macule or thin plaque, typically with pigment variation throughout and irregular borders.

2. With growth, the surface becomes glossy.

3. The most common location of superficial spreading melanomas is on the upper back in males and the leg in females.

B. These cancers are most commonly diagnosed in the fourth and fifth decades of life.

C. Melanoma may arise in a preexisting melanocytic nevus or de novo.

D. Multiple subtypes exist, including lentigo maligna melanoma, superficial spreading melanoma, nodular melanoma, acral lentiginous melanoma, and amelanotic melanoma among others.

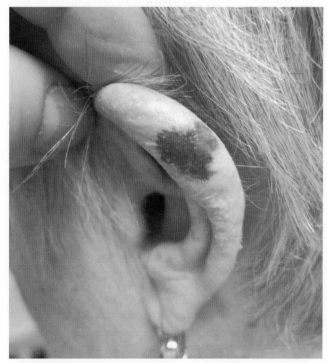

Figure 29-18. Malignant melanoma. (Used with permission from Dr. Anne E. Laumann.)

1. Nodular melanoma is the second most common type of melanoma.
   a. Presents most often on the head, neck, or trunk.
   b. These tumors evolve rapidly over months.
   c. They appear as a blue-black, reddish, purplish, or even a nonpigmented papule or nodule.
2. Acral lentiginous melanoma is the predominant type of melanoma seen in the more pigmented races, such as Africans, Asians, and Indians.
   a. Acral lentiginous melanoma occurs on the palms and soles and beneath the nail plate.
   b. Diagnosis of these lesions is often delayed; therefore, they are often of a more advanced stage at diagnosis.
   c. Affected individuals tend to be older.
3. Lentigo maligna melanoma is a rare type of melanoma found predominantly in the elderly on the sun-exposed portions of the head and neck.
   a. The tumor is usually flat, with irregular borders and a diameter of several centimeters.
   b. Color varies throughout from tan to brown to black and purple and blue.

E. Melanoma is a tumor of melanocytes.
   1. Benign pigmented nevi are composed of altered melanocytes, termed "nevomelanocytes."
   2. Malignant transformation of melanocytes and nevomelanocytes can result in melanoma, arising de novo from normal skin, or from a preexisting nevomelanocytic lesion (nevus or mole).

F. The incidence of cutaneous melanoma is increasing steadily in the United States. In 1935, the lifetime risk of an American developing melanoma was 1 in 1500 individuals, whereas in 2013 the risk was 1 in 50 for white Americans, 1 in 1000 for black Americans and 1 in 200 for Hispanic Americans.
   1. In 2013, it is estimated that melanoma will be diagnosed in 76,690 Americans, and 9480 will die of the disease.
   2. Melanoma will be the fifth most common cancer among males and the seventh most common cancer among females.

G. Epidemiologic studies strongly suggest that sun exposure is a major risk factor for the development of cutaneous melanoma in the light-skinned populations.
   1. Intense intermittent episodes of sun exposure before 18 years of age are thought to engender the highest risk in susceptible populations.
   2. Phenotypic features have been associated with increased risk for cutaneous melanoma: light skin pigmentation, ease of sunburning, blond or red hair, prominent freckling, and blue or green eyes.

H. Familial melanoma accounts for 8–12% of cases. Those with at least 2 first-degree relatives with a history of melanoma are at particularly high risk.

I. Dysplastic nevi (clinically atypical appearing nevi) are thought to be markers of an individual with an increased risk of developing cutaneous melanoma.
   1. The number of nevi on the body has been directly correlated with the magnitude of melanoma risk.
   2. About one-third of melanomas have been associated with an underlying nevus.

J. Recurrences of disease generally occur in a stepwise manner, first locally, then in regional lymph nodes, and lastly as distant metastases.

Evidence-Based Diagnosis

A. An excisional biopsy is the preferred method for obtaining tissue for diagnosis. This preserves the extent of the primary tumor and all associated histologic features without disrupting the lymphatic architecture.

B. Full-thickness incisional or punch biopsies of lesions too large to excise fully or in anatomically sensitive locations are satisfactory.

C. The histologic diagnosis of melanoma is based on a constellation of features; no single feature is diagnostic. Both cytologic and architectural features are evaluated.

D. The staging system for melanoma focuses on tumor thickness and presence of ulceration as the most important initial prognostic variables in localized disease (stages I and II). Stage III has regional nodal involvement, and stage IV has distant metastases.

Treatment

A. Management of cutaneous melanoma is guided by stage of disease. Wide excision of tumors is the general rule.

B. Sentinel lymph node mapping may be beneficial diagnostically in more advanced stages, decreasing the complications associated with full lymph node dissections.

C. Adjuvant treatment options for advanced stage disease include interferon alpha-2b, radiation of nodal basins, chemotherapy, and other novel strategies such as tumor vaccines and immunotherapies.

D. Follow-up of melanoma patients is critical to detect recurrences as well as new primary tumors and to provide ongoing education.

E. Melanoma prevention strategies focus on education about the risks of UV exposure via sunlight or tanning machines, sun protection guidelines, and the importance of routine self-skin exams.
   1. Early detection is important for improving outcomes.
   2. Patients should be instructed on the importance of their own skin examination and what constitutes a worrisome mole, easily remembered by the *ABCDE*s of mole evaluation.
      a. A: asymmetry
      b. B: borders that are irregular or changing
      c. C: color that is irregular or changing
      d. D: diameter > 6 mm (or larger than a pencil eraser)
      e. E: evolution of the lesion in general

REFERENCES

Brantsch KD, Meisner C, Schonfisch B et al. Analysis of risk factors determining prognosis of cutaneous squamous-cell carcinoma: a prospective study. Lancet Oncol. 2008; 9:713–20.

Gnann JW Jr, Whitley RJ. Clinical practice. Herpes zoster. N Engl J Med. 2002;347:340–6.

He L, Zhang D, Zhou M, Zhu C. Corticosteroids for preventing postherpetic neuralgia. Cochrane Database Syst Rev. 2008 Jan23;(1):CD005582.

Kotani N, Kushikata T, Hashimoto H et al. Intrathecal methylprednisolone for intractable postherpetic neuralgia. N Engl J Med. 2000;343:1514–9.

Kozel MM, Mekkes JR, Bossuyt PM, Bos JD. The effectiveness of a history-based diagnostic approach in chronic urticaria and angioedema. Arch Dermatol. 1998;134:1575–80.

Lens MB, Dawes M. Global perspectives of contemporary epidemiological trends of cutaneous malignant melanoma. Br J Dermatol. 2004;150:179–85.

Oxman MN, Levin MJ, Johnson GR et al; Shingles Prevention Study Group. A vaccine to prevent herpes zoster and postherpetic neuralgia in older adults. N Engl J Med. 2005;352(22):2271–84.

Roujeau JC, Kelly JP, Naldi L et al. Medication use and the risk of Stevens-Johnson syndrome or toxic epidermal necrolysis. N Engl J Med. 1995;333:1600–7.

Simor AE, Phillips E, McGeer A et al. Randomized controlled trial of chlorhexidine gluconate for washing, intranasal mupirocin, and rifampin and doxycycline versus no treatment for the eradication of methicillin-resistant *Staphylococcus aureus* colonization. Clin Infect Dis. 2007;44(2):178–85.

Viard I, Wehrli P, Bullani R et al. Inhibition of toxic epidermal necrolysis by blockade of CD95 with human intravenous immunoglobulin. Science. 1998;282:490–3.

Summary Table

Primary Lesion Morphology	Diagnosis	Clinical Clues	Distribution	Figure
Folliculopapular eruptions	Acne	Presents in adolescence Waxing and waning lesions Inflammatory papules, pustules, comedones, and nodulocysts	Face, chest, and back	29–2
	Rosacea	Presents in adults Telangiectasias and persistent centrofacial erythema, occasionally with inflammatory red papules and papulopustules	Face	29–3
Blistering disorders	Herpes zoster	Closely grouped vesicles on an erythematous base Over 2–3 days, the lesions become pustular and then crust over after 7–10 days Pain and paresthesias over involved dermatome may precede the rash	Single, unilateral dermatome	29–4
	Bullous impetigo	Presents as flaccid, transparent bullae that rupture easily and leave a rim of scale and shallow moist erosion Usually seen in children	Intertriginous areas	29–5
	Bullous arthropod bites	A cluster of large, tense blisters on exposed skin	Most common on the extremities	29–7
	Bullous pemphigoid	Seen in elderly patients Sudden onset of 1–2 cm tense blisters and bright, red, urticarial plaques	Begin on the lower extremities and progresses upward	29–8
	Stevens-Johnson syndrome	Targetoid or macular patches with dusky centers that subsequently blister and then erode The skin is usually excruciatingly tender The lips are typically eroded and become covered with hemorrhagic crust)	Begins on chest and face and then spreads Palms and soles often involved Mucosal surfaces (lips, conjunctiva, genitals) may be involved	29–9
Papulosquamous eruptions	Psoriasis	Well-demarcated erythematous plaques with silvery, adherent scales	Extensor surfaces, umbilicus, and scalp (Trunk and proximal extremities for guttate psoriasis)	29–10
	Pityriasis rosea	"Herald patch" progressing to small, oval, scaly plaques in a "fir tree pattern"	Trunk	29–11
	Tinea corporis	Round, pink plaques with small peripheral papules and an advancing scaling border	Anywhere	29–12
	Nummular dermatitis	Extremely pruritic rash of numerous, round, crusted lesions	Legs	29–13
	Secondary syphilis	Oval red/brown macules presenting diffusely, including palms and soles A history of a transient, painless, genital ulcer in the preceding weeks can often be obtained	Rash can be diffuse including palms and soles	
Skin cancers	Basal cell carcinoma	Flesh-colored, translucent, or slightly red papule or nodule, classically displaying a rolled border	Head, neck, or other sun-exposed skin	29–16
	Squamous cell carcinoma	Firm, but somewhat indistinct nodule or rough plaque	Sun-exposed skin	29–17
	Melanoma	Dark brown to black macule with pigment variation and irregular borders	Anywhere	29–18
Purpura and petechiae	Petechiae	Nonblanching, pinpoint, red spots	Dependent body parts, most commonly the lower extremities	29–15
	Purpura	Red, blue or purple nonblanching macules, papules or plaques, may or may not be palpable, up to several centimeters in diameter	Anywhere	

I have a patient with sore throat. How do I determine the cause?

CHIEF COMPLAINT

PATIENT 1

Mr. W is a 30-year-old man who complains of having a sore throat for 3 days.

 What is the differential diagnosis of a sore throat? How would you frame the differential?

CONSTRUCTING A DIFFERENTIAL DIAGNOSIS

Sore throat is a common condition seen in outpatient clinical practice. This chapter focuses on patients that present with the acute onset of sore throat. Infectious diseases are the cause of acute sore throat in the overwhelming majority of patients. Patients with chronic sore throat, those who do not have signs of infection, or those who do not respond to treatment should be evaluated for noninfectious causes of sore throat.

A useful framework for the differential diagnosis of acute sore throat is shown below. This framework divides the diagnoses into those caused by infection (bacterial and viral) and those caused by noninfectious processes. Viral respiratory infections are the most common cause of infectious pharyngitis with the common cold caused by rhinoviruses and coronaviruses accounting for at least 25% of cases. Group A beta-hemolytic *streptococcus* (GABHS) is the most common cause of acute bacterial pharyngitis, accounting for 5–15% of sore throats in adults. Approximately 30% of cases of pharyngitis have no identifiable cause. Table 30-1 shows the differential diagnosis with the estimated percentage of cases of sore throat and the associated clinical syndrome.

A. Infectious causes of sore throat
  1. Viruses
     a. Rhinovirus
     b. Coronavirus
     c. Adenovirus
     d. Herpes simplex virus (HSV)1 and 2
     e. Influenza A and B
     f. Parainfluenza virus
     g. Epstein-Barr virus (EBV)
     h. Cytomegalovirus (CMV)
     i. Human herpesvirus (HHV) 6
     j. HIV
  2. Bacteria
     a. GABHS
     b. Group C beta-hemolytic streptococci
     c. *Neisseria gonorrhoeae*

     d. *Corynebacterium diphtheriae*
     e. *Mycoplasma pneumoniae*
     f. *Chlamydophila pneumoniae*
     g. *Fusobacterium necrophorum*

B. Noninfectious causes of sore throat
  1. Persistent cough
  2. Postnasal drip
  3. Gastroesophageal reflux disease (GERD)
  4. Acute thyroiditis
  5. Neoplasm
  6. Allergies
  7. Smoking

Clinically, the primary goal when seeing a patient with acute, probably infectious sore throat is to identify and treat patients with GABHS pharyngitis in order to prevent complications of acute rheumatic fever, acute glomerulonephritis, and suppurative sequelae. The secondary goal is to diagnose the less common infections (peritonsillar abscess) as well as the bacterial pathogens (*N gonorrhoeae, F necrophorum*) that need to be treated. In addition, diagnosing the nonbacterial pathogens, such as primary HIV, influenza A and B, and mononucleosis is important for both therapeutic and prognostic reasons. Pivotal points in the evaluation of these patients therefore include the presence of unilateral symptoms (suggesting abscess formation or fusobacterium infection), the presence of exudate (suggestive of GABHS or risk factors for sexually transmitted infections or HIV, or signs and symptoms of influenza or mononucleosis.

Mr. W's symptoms started abruptly 3 days ago when sore throat, pain with swallowing, fever, and headaches developed. He denies symptoms of cough, coryza, or rhinorrhea.

 At this point, what is the leading hypothesis, what are the active alternatives, and is there a must not miss diagnosis? Given this differential diagnosis, what tests should be ordered?

PRIORITIZING THE DIFFERENTIAL DIAGNOSIS

The pivotal points in Mr. W's history include his sudden onset of sore throat, fever, and headache. These symptoms suggest an infectious cause of sore throat. The differential diagnosis includes bacterial pharyngitis, most commonly GABHS. The absence of cough, rhinorrhea, and coryza make the common viral causes

Table 30-1. Frequency and clinical syndrome for infectious causes of sore throat.

Class	Infection	Frequency[1]	Clinical Syndrome
Viruses	Rhinovirus	20%	Common cold
	Coronavirus	5%	Common cold
	Adenovirus	5%	Acute respiratory disease
	HSV1 and 2	4%	Stomatitis, pharyngitis
	Influenza A and B	2%	Influenza
	Parainfluenza virus	2%	Common cold, croup
	EBV	< 1%	Infectious mononucleosis
	CMV	< 1%	Infectious mononucleosis
	HIV	< 1%	Primary HIV infection
Bacteria	Group A beta-hemolytic streptococci	15–30%	Pharyngitis, tonsillitis
	Group C beta-hemolytic streptococci	5%	Pharyngitis, tonsillitis
	Neisseria gonorrhoeae	< 1%	Pharyngitis
	Corynebacterium diphtheriae	< 1%	Diphtheria
	Mycoplasma pneumoniae	< 1%	Pneumonia, bronchitis
	Chlamydophila pneumoniae	Unknown	Pneumonia, bronchitis
	Fusobacterium necrophorum	Rare	Lemierre syndrome, peritonsillar abscess

[1]Estimated percentage of cases in all ages.
CMV, cytomegalovirus; EBV, Epstein-Barr virus; HSV, herpes simplex virus.

of pharyngitis less likely. In general, patients with viral pharyngitis have cough, coryza, rhinorrhea, and hoarseness while those with bacterial pharyngitis or mononucleosis have fever, tender anterior cervical lymphadenopathy, tonsillar erythema with or without tonsillar swelling and exudates. They do not typically have rhinorrhea, cough, or conjunctivitis.

Influenza can cause fevers and throat pain but is usually associated with cough and myalgias. Infectious mononucleosis, which is most often caused by EBV, can also cause sore throat and fever but most often occurs in persons between the ages of 15 and 24 years and is associated with malaise and marked adenopathy. Primary HIV infection can present with nonspecific symptoms of pharyngitis, fever, adenopathy, and fatigue and should also be considered in high-risk persons. Table 30-2 lists the differential diagnosis for Mr. W.

Table 30-2. Diagnostic hypothesis for Mr. W.

Diagnostic Hypotheses	Demographics, Risk Factors, Symptoms and Signs	Important Tests
Leading Hypothesis		
GABHS pharyngitis	Sudden onset of symptoms, pain with swallowing, fever, tonsillar exudates, cervical lymphadenopathy, headache, abdominal pain	Throat swab using RADT Throat culture
Active Alternatives		
Influenza	Influenza season, fever, cough, myalgias, fatigue	Diagnosis is usually clinical, direct immunofluorescence or ELISA can be used
Infectious mononucleosis	Fever, malaise, sore throat, tonsillar exudates, lymphadenopathy (especially posterior cervical)	Heterophile antibody testing (Monospot test)
Primary HIV infection/ acute retroviral syndrome	Fever, nonexudative pharyngitis, mucocutaneous ulcers, lymphadenopathy, rash	Assays for HIV RNA; HIV antibodies are often negative during acute phase of infection

ELISA, enzyme-linked immunosorbent assay; GABHS, group A beta-hemolytic streptococci; RADT, rapid antigen detection test.

Mr. W is otherwise healthy. He has had no recent sick contacts and no recent travel. He is a heterosexual male, married, and monogamous with his wife. He has no history of blood transfusions or illicit drug use.

The physical exam is notable for temperature of 39.2°C, blood pressure is 130/70 mm Hg, pulse is 98 bpm, and respiratory rate is 12 breaths per minute. Sclera and conjunctiva are not injected. Oropharyngeal exam reveals bilateral tonsillar hypertrophy and exudates without ulcers. He has no cervical lymphadenopathy on exam. His abdominal is soft with normal bowel sounds. Skin exam is unremarkable.

 Is the clinical information sufficient to make a diagnosis, if not what other information do you need?

Leading Hypothesis: GABHS pharyngitis

Textbook Presentation

The presenting symptoms and signs of GABHS pharyngitis include rapid onset of severe throat pain, moderate fever (39–40.5°C), malaise, and headaches. Examination of the throat reveals edema and erythema of the posterior pharynx and tonsils are often covered with gray-white exudates. The anterior cervical lymph nodes are tender. Gastrointestinal symptoms of nausea, vomiting, and abdominal pain may also be present, especially in children.

Disease Highlights

A. GABHS is generally suspected when fever and throat pain are present and cough, coryza, and rhinorrhea are absent.

B. Untreated GABHS typically lasts 8–10 days. Patients are infectious during the acute illness and for up to 1 week afterward.

C. GABHS infection is associated with 2 important postinfectious syndromes.

   1. Acute rheumatic fever

      a. Presents 1–5 weeks after throat infection

      b. Important findings are pancarditis, rash, subcutaneous nodules, chorea, or migratory polyarthritis

      c. Due to aggressive treatment of GABHS, this complication is uncommon in the developed world (but still common in developing nations). Annual incidence in the United States is 1/1,000,000 population.

   2. Acute post-streptococcal glomerulonephritis

      a. Presents 1–2 weeks after GABHS pharyngitis

      b. Important findings are edema, hematuria, proteinuria, and hypertension

Evidence-Based Diagnosis

A. Clinical diagnosis of GABHS pharyngitis

   1. Pretest probability

      a. The pretest probability of a patient having GABHS pharyngitis is based primarily on the patient's age, clinical setting, and season.

      b. The pretest probability of strep throat in the adult clinic–based population is 5–10%.

      c. Because strep throat is more common in autumn and winter, it may be appropriate to adjust this estimate upward or downward according to season.

   2. Clinical findings and clinical decision rules

      a. Because individual clinical findings (such as the presence of fever or exudates) are not very predictive of GABHS, clinical prediction rules have been developed.

      b. These rules use the key features in the history and physical exam to predict the probability of strep throat.

      c. The Modified Centor score (one of the best validated clinical decision rules) assigns patients 1 point for each of the following findings: tonsillar exudates, swollen tender anterior cervical nodes, absence of cough, history of fever and age < 15 years. One point is subtracted for age over 45 and older.

      d. The likelihood ratios and posttest probabilities given a pretest probability of 10% in given in Table 30-3.

B. Laboratory diagnosis

   1. Throat culture

      a. A single swab throat culture has a sensitivity of approximately 90–95% and specificity of 95–99%.

      b. The major disadvantage of throat cultures is the 24- to 72-hour delay in obtaining results.

   2. Rapid antigen detection test (RADT)

      a. Results from RADTs are available within a few minutes

      b. Sensitivity ranges from 70% to 90% when compared with throat culture with sensitivities in actual practice being toward the lower end of this range.

Table 30-3. Likelihood ratios of modified Centor score and posttest probabilities.[1]

Centor Score	LR	Posttest Probability
−1–0	0.05	0.55%
1	0.52	5.46
2	0.95	9.55
3	2.5	21.74
4–5	4.9	35.25

[1]Assuming 10% pretest probability.

      c. Specificity for RADTs ranges from 90% to 100%.

C. Integrated use of clinical decision rules and laboratory methods

   1. Generally, clinicians use the results of a clinical decision rules to determine which patients require further testing.

   2. Patients at the lowest risk (low pretest probability and low Modified Centor Score) receive no testing.

   3. Patients at higher risk (posttest probability 5–50%) usually receive a RADT or throat culture.

   4. Those at the highest risk (> 50%) are often treated empirically but may be receive a RADT or throat culture.

   5. Given the sensitivity of RADT and the exceptionally low risk of acute rheumatic fever in adults, a throat culture is not necessary when an RADT is negative. (In children and adolescents, a negative RADT should be verified by throat culture.)

   6. Positive RADTs do not require back up with a culture because they are highly specific.

Treatment

A. Patients with GABHS pharyngitis should be treated with appropriate antibiotic therapy to prevent development of acute rheumatic fever.

   1. Penicillin and amoxicillin are the first-line antibiotics given their narrow spectrum of activity and modest cost.

   2. For patients with an allergy to penicillin, choices include first-generation cephalosporins, clindamycin, clarithromycin, or azithromycin.

B. Treatment decreases severity of symptoms, reduces risk of transmission, and reduces the likelihood of suppurative complications.

C. There is no evidence that antibiotic treatment can prevent the development of acute glomerulonephritis.

D. Clinical improvement within 48 hours is expected; patients who do not improve should be re-evaluated.

E. Tonsillectomy is only indicated for patients with 4 or more episodes of severe pharyngitis in a year.

Any patient with documented GABHS pharyngitis who does not improve within 48 hours of treatment with an appropriate course of antibiotics should be re-evaluated.

MAKING A DIAGNOSIS

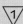

Mr. W has 3 points on the modified Centor Score (fever, exudate, and absence of cough). A RADT test is performed.

 Have you crossed a diagnostic threshold for the leading hypothesis? Have you ruled out the active alternatives? Do other tests need to be done to exclude the alternative diagnoses?

Given a modified Centor score of 3, the patient's risk of having GABHS is 28–35%. In this group of patients the results of a RADT will be very helpful, essentially ruling out or ruling in disease. Mr. W has no risk factors for HIV and tested negative for HIV when he donated blood 2 months ago. He has no symptoms of fatigue, malaise, or cough making influenza a less likely diagnosis. He reports no fatigue or lymphadenopathy and is older than the typical patient with mononucleosis, making this diagnosis less likely.

Alternative Diagnosis: Influenza

See discussion in Chapter 10, Cough, Fever, & Respiratory Infections.

Alternative Diagnosis: Infectious Mononucleosis

Textbook Presentation

Infectious mononucleosis typically presents with a prodrome of fever, malaise, chills, and sweats. The illness then progresses to the classic triad of severe sore throat, fever (38–40°C) and lymphadenopathy.

Disease Highlights

A. Infectious mononucleosis is most common in patients 15–24 years of age. It is uncommon in adults. (It accounts for < 2% of pharyngitis in patients over 40 years of age.)

B. Infectious mononucleosis is most often caused by EBV (the focus of this discussion) but can be caused by CMV or HHV 6.

C. EBV is spread in saliva.

   1. May be shed in salivary secretions for many weeks

   2. As many as 20% of healthy, previously infected adults intermittently shed virus for decades.

D. Most people are infected with EBV during childhood and the typical childhood infection is subclinical. Less than 10% of children exhibit symptoms.

E. Approximately 90% of adults are EBV seropositive.

Evidence-Based Diagnosis

A. History

   1. The earliest symptoms of EBV are fever, malaise, chills, and sweats.

   2. These symptoms then progress to the classic triad of severe sore throat, fever, and lymphadenopathy.

B. Physical exam

   1. Common findings include enlarged tonsils; pharyngeal erythema; thick, coating, pharyngeal exudate; palatal petechiae; and tender anterior and/or posterior cervical adenopathy.

   2. Table 30-4 lists test characteristics for findings suggestive of EBV.

   3. Rash is uncommon in infectious mononucleosis unless there is antibiotic exposure.

Table 30-4. Symptoms and clinical signs suggestive of infectious mononucleosis.

Symptom or Sign	Sensitivity	Specificity	LR+	LR−
Splenomegaly	7%	99%	7.0	0.94
Palatal petechiae	27%	95%	5.4	0.77
Posterior cervical adenopathy	40%	87%	3.1	0.69
Fatigue	93%	23%	1.2	0.3
Temperature > 37.5°C	27%	84%	1.7	0.87
Anterior cervical lymphadenopathy	70%	43%	1.2	0.7

   a. 5–10% of patients have a rash of varying morphology

   b. 27–69% of patients with infectious mononucleosis who are treated with amoxicillin or ampicillin develop a rash.

 Infectious mononucleosis is characterized by a triad of fever, sore throat, and lymphadenopathy.

C. Laboratory testing

   1. The heterophile antibody test (Monospot test) is highly specific for EBV.

      a. Specificity 99%

      b. Sensitivity

         (1) False-negative rate in first week is as high as 25%.

         (2) 5–10% in second week

         (3) 5% in third week of illness

   2. Serum IgM antibody to the EBV viral capsid antigen is accurate but the turn around time on the test is generally longer than the Monospot.

      a. This test is useful in patients with suspected infectious mononucleosis who have negative Monospot.

      b. Test characteristics

         (1) Sensitivity, 97%

         (2) Specificity, 94%

         (3) LR+, 16

         (4) LR−, 0.03

   3. Other tests

      a. Lymphocytosis and the presence of atypical lymphocytes are diagnostically useful.

         (1) Lymphocytosis of > 50% on peripheral smear; sensitivity 66%, specificity 84%

         (2) Atypical lymphocytes >10% of total lymphocytes; sensitivity 75%, specificity 92%

      b. Elevated aminotransferases are seen in the majority of patients.

Treatment

A. Infectious mononucleosis is a self-limited illness; most symptoms resolve within 3 weeks.

B. Symptomatic treatment, including hydration, antipyretics, analgesics, and rest, remains the mainstay of care.

C. Corticosteroids, acyclovir, and antihistamines are *not* recommended for routine treatment of infectious mononucleosis.

   1. Acyclovir does decrease viral shedding but does not alter the clinical course.

   2. Corticosteroids are indicated for patients with impending airway compromise.

D. Splenomegaly may persist after symptoms resolve. Patients should avoid heavy lifting and contact sports for 4 weeks.

E. Potential complications are rare but include the following:

   1. Splenic rupture

      a. Rare but potentially life-threatening complication

      b. Estimated incidence is 1–2 cases/1000

   2. Airway obstruction

   3. Pneumonitis

   4. Hematologic complications

      a. Hemolytic anemia

      b. Thrombocytopenia

      c. Neutropenia

      d. Aplastic anemia

   5. Neurologic

      a. Encephalitis

      b. Meningitis

      c. Cranial nerve palsies

      d. Seizures

      e. Myelitis

      f. Optic neuritis

      g. Guillain-Barré syndrome

Alternative Diagnosis: Primary HIV Infection - Acute Retroviral Syndrome (ARS)

Textbook Presentation

Symptoms of ARS are generally nonspecific and resolve spontaneously without treatment. The most common findings are fever, lymphadenopathy, sore throat, rash, myalgia/arthralgia, headache, and mucocutaneous ulcers. ARS may resemble EBV mononucleosis and can be distinguished by its more acute onset, absence of tonsillar exudate, rash (which is rare in mononucleosis except after treatment with amoxicillin), and mucocutaneous ulcers.

Disease Highlights

A. Transmission of HIV is common in the first 3 months.

   1. This is a period of high viral load.

   2. There are high levels of virus in blood and genital secretions.

   3. Patients often do not know they are infected.

   4. Early diagnosis is thus important to decrease rates of transmission.

B. The highest risk populations for HIV infection are:

   1. Men who have sex with men

   2. Injection drug users

   3. Healthcare workers with needle-stick exposure

Evidence-Based Diagnosis

A. Clinical presentation

   1. The usual lag between exposure to HIV and development of symptoms is 2–4 weeks.

   2. 40–90% patients with acute HIV infection experience symptoms of ARS.

   3. Symptoms seen in over 50% of patients with symptomatic ARS are:

      a. Fever

      b. Fatigue

      c. Rash

      d. Headache

      e. Lymphadenopathy

      f. Pharyngitis

      g. Myalgia or arthralgia

      h. Nausea, vomiting, or diarrhea

   4. Painful mucocutaneous ulcerations

      a. Less common but distinctive manifestation of the syndrome

      b. Often shallow and sharply demarcated

      c. Can involve the oral mucosa, anus, penis, or esophagus

B. Laboratory testing

   1. Laboratory testing is appropriate for patients in whom there is a clinical suspicion for ARS.

   2. Testing should include:

      a. HIV antibody test (ELISA and Western blot): Seroconversion usually occurs 3–7 weeks after infection.

      b. HIV viral load assay

         (1) HIV is typically detected 11 days after infection.

         (2) Patients with ARS typically have high viral loads of > 100,000 copies/mL.

         (3) False-positive result should be suspected if viral load < 10,000 copies/mL.

         (4) Sensitivity 95–98%

      c. Genotype resistance testing is recommended in all patients with primary HIV infection, since transmission of drug-resistant HIV strains has been documented.

 Because HIV antibody tests may be negative at the time of acute seroconversion, an HIV viral load assay should always be sent when this diagnosis is being considered.

Treatment

A. Acute HIV is infrequently diagnosed, and data about outcomes of early antiretroviral therapy are limited.

B. Antiretroviral therapy for acute infection remains controversial, and referral to HIV specialist for management is recommended.

CASE RESOLUTION

A RADT test is performed and is positive. Mr. W has no allergies to antibiotics and he is treated with penicillin 500 mg twice daily for 10 days. Two days after starting treatment, he reports improvement in symptoms.

CHIEF COMPLAINT

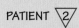

PATIENT

Ms. L is a 25-year-old woman with no significant past medical history in whom sore throat, fever, and malaise developed 7 days ago. She complains of severe throat pain, more pronounced on the right, and right ear pain. She reports severe pain with swallowing. She also reports that for the past day she has not been able to open her mouth widely.

At this point, what is the leading hypothesis, what are the active alternatives, and is there a must not miss diagnosis? Given this differential diagnosis, what tests should be ordered?

PRIORITIZING THE DIFFERENTIAL DIAGNOSIS

The pivotal points in this case are the unilateral nature of the throat pain as well as the odynophagia and trismus. This presentation suggests a peritonsillar abscess, classically referred to as quinsy. Peritonsillar abscesses generally form in the area of the soft palate, just above the superior pole of the tonsil.

Peritonsillar abscess is a must not miss diagnosis because if left untreated, it may progress to airway obstruction, abscess rupture, or septic necrosis. Other important diagnoses to consider in this case would be retropharyngeal abscess or epiglotittis. Lemierre disease, a rare disease caused by *F necrophorum*, must also be considered. Table 30-5 lists the differential diagnosis.

Table 30-5. Diagnostic hypothesis for Ms. L.

Diagnostic Hypotheses	Demographics, Risk Factors, Symptoms and Signs	Important Tests
Leading Hypothesis		
Peritonsillar abscess	Severe unilateral sore throat with fever and muffled voice, unilaterally enlarged, medially displaced tonsil and deviation of uvula to unaffected side	Diagnosis is usually clinical
Active Alternative—Must Not Miss		
Epiglottitis	Sore throat with muffled voice, stridor, drooling and anterior neck tenderness	Lateral neck radiograph Direct visualization with laryngoscopy
Retropharyngeal abscess	Similar to epiglottitis with more prominent neck symptoms (stiffness and pain)	Lateral neck radiograph or CT scan of the neck
Lemierre syndrome	Pain, swelling and induration at the angle of the mandible with persistent high fevers and trismus	CT scan of the neck

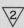

On physical exam she is breathing comfortably. Her vital signs are temperature, 39.0°C; pulse, 102 bpm; BP, 110/70 mm Hg; and RR, 15 breaths per minute. Examination of the oropharynx revealed a markedly enlarged right tonsil with associated swelling of the soft palate uvular deviation to the left. The right tympanic membrane is clear, with good light reflex and no bulging. There is tender anterior cervical lymphadenopathy bilaterally. The lung exam was normal and no stridor was noted.

Is the clinical information sufficient to make a diagnosis? If not, what other information do you need?

Leading Hypothesis: Peritonsillar Abscess

Textbook Presentation

The typical clinical presentation of peritonsillar abscess is a severe unilateral sore throat associated with fever and a muffled "hot potato" voice. Malaise, dysphagia, and otalgia are also often present. Swallowing is painful, which sometimes leads to pooling of saliva or drooling. Trismus, difficulty opening the mouth because of pain from the inflammation, may be present. The oropharyngeal exam reveals an extremely swollen tonsil with displacement of the uvula to the unaffected side and a bulging soft palate on the affected side. The patient may have markedly tender cervical lymphadenitis on the affected side.

Disease Highlights

A. A peritonsillar abscess usually begins as an acute exudative tonsillitis that progresses to cellulitis and eventually to abscess formation. The abscess may also occur without preceding infection via obstruction of the Weber glands, a group of salivary glands in the soft palate.

B. It is the most common deep infection of head and neck, accounting for approximately 30% of abscesses of the head and neck.

C. Occurs primarily in young adults between the ages of 20 and 40 years

D. Peritonsillar abscesses are polymicrobial. Common organisms include:

  1. Aerobic bacteria

    a. Group A streptococcus

    b. *Staphylococcus aureus*

    c. *Haemophilus influenzae*

  2. Anaerobic bacteria

    a. *Fusobacterium*

    b. *Peptostreptococcus*

    c. Pigmented prevotella

    d. *Veillonella*

Evidence-Based Diagnosis

A. Diagnosis of peritonsillar abscess can be made clinically without laboratory data or imaging in patients with a typical presentation

  1. Symptoms

    a. Fever

    b. Malaise

c. Severe sore throat (worse on 1 side)

d. Dysphagia

e. Ipsilateral otalgia

2. Signs

 a. Erythematous, swollen soft palate with uvula deviation and an enlarged tonsil

 b. Trismus

 c. Drooling

 d. Muffled "hot potato" voice

 e. Rancid or fetor breath

 f. Cervical lymphadenitis

B. Culture of pus from abscess drainage can confirm the diagnosis; however, the rate of positive cultures from peritonsillar abscess in the literature ranges from < 50% to 100%.

C. Trismus occurs in nearly 66% of patients with peritonsillar abscesses.

D. Laboratory evaluation

1. Laboratory evaluation is not necessary to make the diagnosis but may help gauge the level of illness and direct therapy.

2. Testing usually includes:

 a. Complete blood cell count

 b. Routine throat culture for group A streptococcus

 c. Gram stain, culture, and susceptibility testing of abscess fluid, especially in patients with persistent infection or diabetes or in those who are immunocompromised.

E. Imaging

1. Generally not necessary to make a diagnosis, but may be considered in the following cases:

 a. Suspected spread beyond peritonsillar space

 b. Inability to successfully examine the pharynx because of trismus

 c. Monitoring patients unresponsive to initial treatment with antibiotics and drainage

2. The preferred imaging modality is CT with IV contrast (sensitivity, 100%; specificity, 75%; LR+, 4; LR–, 0)

3. Intraoral ultrasonography may be used to distinguish peritonsillar abscess from cellulitis and guide needle aspiration.

Treatment

A. Drainage, antibiotic therapy, and supportive care are the mainstays of therapy.

1. Randomized, controlled trials have shown that needle aspiration and incision and drainage are equally effective.

2. Rates of re-collection and failed resolution in 1–2 days were comparable at 10% for both procedures.

3. Needle aspiration is generally less invasive, less painful, and better tolerated.

B. Antibiotics are recommended in conjunction to drainage to effectively treat the abscess and provide coverage for GABHS, *S aureus,* and respiratory anaerobic bacteria.

1. Drainage and antibiotic therapy resolves peritonsillar abscess in more than 90% of cases.

2. Evidence regarding the use of corticosteroids to treat edema and inflammation associated with peritonsillar abscess is inconsistent and is not routinely recommended.

C. Many patients can be treated as outpatients. These patients should be:

1. Observed after needle aspiration or I and D to ensure they can tolerate oral antibiotics, pain medication, and liquids.

2. Scheduled to be seen for follow up in 24–36 hours

3. Advised to return for reevaluation for:

 a. Dyspnea

 b. Worsening throat pain, neck pain, or trismus

 c. Enlarging mass

 d. Fever

 e. Neck stiffness

 f. Bleeding

D. Treatment failure should prompt broadening of antibiotics, reevaluation with CT scan to look for extension of infection, and tonsillectomy.

MAKING A DIAGNOSIS

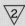

The patient's symptoms of a unilaterally enlarged, medially displaced tonsil with uvular deviation to contralateral side are sufficient to make the diagnosis of peritonsillar abscess. You arrange for ENT evaluation.

 Have you crossed a diagnostic threshold for the leading hypothesis? Have you ruled out the active alternatives? Do other tests need to be done to exclude the alternative diagnoses?

Alternative Diagnosis: Epiglottitis

See discussion of epiglotittis in Chapter 33.

Alternative Diagnosis: Retropharyngeal Abscess

See discussion of retropharyngeal abscess in Chapter 33.

Alternative Diagnosis: Lemierre Syndrome

Textbook Presentation

Lemierre syndrome is a septic thrombophlebitis of the internal jugular vein. Typically, presenting symptoms and signs include high fevers, rigors, respiratory distress, and neck or throat pain. Examination of the oropharynx may reveal ulceration, pseudomembrane, or erythema. Tenderness and swelling may be observed overlying the jugular vein. In some cases, no abnormal physical finings may be present.

Disease Highlights

A. Lemierre syndrome is a rare (3.6 cases/million/year) but potentially life-threatening cause of sore throat.

B. Approximately 81% of cases are caused by the anaerobic gram-negative rod *F necrophorum.*

C. Although widespread use of antibiotics in 1940s led to dramatic decline in its incidence, there has recently been an increase.

D. Symptoms

1. The most common symptoms of Lemierre syndrome are nonspecific (such as sore throat, neck tenderness or swelling or both, and fever).

2. Some findings seen in Lemierre syndrome that are not commonly seen in pharyngitis are dyspnea (23.8%), pleuritic chest pain (31.1%), abdominal pain (13.7%), and trismus (9.1%).

E. Septic emboli can arise from the septic thrombophlebitis. Potential complications include:

1. Lung lesions
   a. Septic emboli
   b. Infiltrates
   c. Lung abscess
   d. Pleural effusion
   e. Empyema
2. Bone and joint
   a. Septic arthritis
   b. Osteomyelitis
3. Liver abscess
4. Central nervous system complications
   a. Brain abscess
   b. Meningitis
   c. Cavernous sinus thrombosis

F. The symptoms of septic thrombophlebitis and septic emboli can mask the initial oropharyngeal symptoms.

In Lemierre syndrome, symptoms of thrombophlebitis and septic emboli can mask the initial oropharyngeal symptoms. The diagnosis should be considered in those patients with septic findings consistent with septic emboli.

Evidence-Based Diagnosis

A. A high clinical suspicion is necessary to make the diagnosis of Lemierre syndrome, since the signs and symptoms are often nonspecific.

B. Lemierre syndrome should be considered strongly in patients with chills, high fever, and unilateral neck swelling. Patients may also have antecedent pharyngitis, septic pulmonary emboli, and persistent fevers despite antimicrobial therapy.

C. It may take 5–8 days to microbiologically isolate *F necrophorum*.

D. The following criteria are accepted as strong evidence for the presence of Lemierre syndrome:

1. Anaerobic primary infection of the oropharynx
2. Subsequent septicemia (with at least 1 positive blood culture)
3. Metastatic infection of 1 or more distant site
4. Thrombophlebitis of the internal jugular vein

E. CT scan of neck with contrast is the best diagnostic modality.

Treatment

A. Antibiotics

1. *F necrophorum* is usually susceptible to beta-lactamase resistant beta-lactam antibiotics, clindamycin, metronidazole, and chloramphenicol.

2. There is variable response to second- and third-generation cephalosporins.

B. Surgical therapy maybe needed for patients with abscesses or those who do not respond to antibiotic therapy.

C. The role of anticoagulation in treatment of Lemierre syndrome is controversial. Due to low incidence of Lemierre syndrome, the risks and benefits of anticoagulation have not been addressed in controlled studies.

CASE RESOLUTION

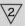

Consultation by ENT led to successful needle aspiration with drainage of 8 mL of purulent material. Peritonsillar abscess was the confirmed diagnosis. She was able to tolerate liquids and oral pain medication after the procedure and was discharged home with 14 days of clindamycin therapy. At follow-up in the ENT clinic 24 hours after needle aspiration she reports improvement in her sore throat and no fevers. She was advised to complete her 14-day course of antibiotics.

REFERENCES

Aronson MD, Komaroff AL, Pass TM, Ervin CT, Branch WT. Heterophile antibody in adults with sore throat. Ann Intern Med. 1982;96:505–8.

Bisno AL. Acute pharyngitis. N Engl J Med. 2001;344(3):205–11.

Brenner BG, Roger M, Routy JP et al. High rates of forward transmission events after acute/early HIV-1 infection. J Infect Dis. 2007;195(7):951–9.

Brook I. Microbiology and management of peritonsillar, retropharyngeal, and parapharyngeal abscesses. J Oral Maxillofacial Surg. 2005;62(12):1545–50.

Choby BA. Diagnosis and treatment of streptococcal pharyngitis. Am Fam Physician. 2009;79(5):383–90.

Chu C, Selwyn PA. Diagnosis and initial management of acute HIV infection. Am Fam Physician. 2010;81(10):1239–44.

Ebell MH. Epstein-Barr virus infectious mononucleosis. Am Fam Physician. 2004;70(7):1279–87.

Ebell MH, Smith MA, Barry HC, Ives K, Carey M. The rational clinical examination. Does this patient have strep throat? JAMA. 2000;284(22):2912–8.

Fox JW, Cohen DM, Marcon MJ, Cotton WH, Bonsu BK. Performance of rapid streptococcal antigen testing varies by personnel. J Clin Microbiol. 2006;44(11):3918–22.

Galioto NJ. Peritonsillar abscess. Am Fam Physician. 2008;77(2):199–202.

Hollingsworth TD, Anderson RM, Fraser C. HIV-1 transmission, by stage of infection. J Infect Dis. 2008;198(5):687–93.

Johnson RF, Stewart MG, Wright CC. An evidence-based review of the treatment of peritonsillar abscess. Otolaryngol Head Neck Surg. 2003;128(3):332–43.

McIsaac WJ, Goel V, To T, Low DE. The validity of a sore throat score in family practice. CMAJ. 2000;163(7):811–5.

Perlmutter BL, Glaser JB, Oyugi SO. How to recognize and treat acute HIV syndrome. Am Fam Physician. 1999;60(2):535–42, 545–6.

Renn CN, Straff W, Dorfmüller A, Al-Masaoudi T, Merk HF, Sachs B. Amoxicillin-induced exanthema in young adults with infectious mononucleosis: demonstration of drug-specific lymphocyte reactivity. Br J Dermatol. 2002;147(6):1166–70.

Shulman ST, Bisno AL, Clegg HW et al. Clinical practice guideline for the diagnosis and management of group A streptococcal pharyngitis: 2012 update by the Infectious Diseases Society of America. Clin Infect Dis. 2012;55(10):1279–82.

Vincent MT, Celestin N, Hussain AN. Pharyngitis. Am Fam Physician. 2004;69(6):1465–70.

31

I have a patient with syncope.
How do I determine the cause?

CHIEF COMPLAINT

PATIENT ⟍⟋1⟍

Mr. M is a 23-year-old medical student who had an episode of syncope this morning after entering his anatomy lab for the first time. He is quite alarmed (and embarrassed).

 What is the differential diagnosis of syncope? How would you frame the differential?

CONSTRUCTING A DIFFERENTIAL DIAGNOSIS

Transient loss of consciousness may be caused by trauma, intoxication, hypoglycemia, or true syncope. Syncope refers to the abrupt, transient complete loss of consciousness and postural tone due to transient global cerebral hypoperfusion, usually due to transient profound hypotension. Since such profound hypotension can be catastrophic or fatal if prolonged, syncope may portend sudden cardiac death; therefore, a careful evaluation is critical to identify and treat patients with potentially life- threatening etiologies of syncope.

 Patients with syncope should be carefully evaluated to determine if they are at risk for sudden cardiac death.

The differential diagnosis for syncope is best remembered by considering the 3 most common causes of syncope: reflex mediated syncope, cardiac syncope, and orthostatic hypotension (Figure 31-1).

Each of these categories of syncope is associated with specific diseases/entities that cause syncope. Cardiac syncope is usually due to bradyarrhythmias or tachyarrhythmias but occasionally due to outflow obstruction (eg, aortic stenosis, hypertrophic cardiomyopathy [HCM]) or inadequate filling (pulmonary embolism [PE], tamponade). Orthostatic hypotension is usually due to inadequate preload (from dehydration or hemorrhage), but may also be secondary to autonomic dysfunction or drugs. Reflex syncope refers to a group of disorders that cause syncope due to increased vagal tone causing bradycardia and vasodilation and includes vasovagal syncope, carotid sinus syncope, and situational syncope. The full differential is listed below.

Finally, cerebrovascular disease involving the posterior circulation is a rare cause of transient loss of consciousness but is almost invariably associated with other neurologic symptoms and is discussed briefly at the end of the chapter. On the other hand, seizures are easily confused with syncope and remain in the differential diagnosis of the patient who appears to have had syncope (see Figure 31-1).

The evaluation of all patients with syncope must include a thorough history, physical exam, ECG, and blood glucose. A detailed history of the event is critical including the setting (warm, standing, sitting, during exertion, pain, anxiety, etc.), associated symptoms (nausea, chest pain, palpitations), and any signs observed by bystanders. Any significant persistence of confusion beyond a minute or two is critical, as this would suggest a postictal period and seizure. The past medical history and the patient's medications should be carefully reviewed. The purpose of this evaluation is to uncover any findings that suggest cardiac disease, since patients with syncope and heart disease are at a markedly increased risk for ventricular tachycardia (VT) and sudden death. Such findings include syncope which occurs during sitting or exertion, associated symptoms of chest pain, palpitations, or dyspnea, a past medical history of heart disease (coronary artery disease [CAD], structural heart disease or heart failure [HF]), a family history of sudden cardiac death or significant murmurs, an S_3 gallop or jugular venous distention (JVD) (suggesting aortic stenosis and HF, respectively). On the other hand, syncope with prolonged standing or associated with abdominal discomfort increases the likelihood of vasovagal syncope whereas syncope immediately upon standing suggests orthostatic syncope. The physical exam should evaluate vital signs and orthostatic BPs in addition to a thorough cardiac and neurologic exam. Finally, an ECG should be obtained in every syncopal patient and scrutinized for signs of arrhythmia, conduction disease, ischemia, or structural heart disease. An echocardiogram may also be useful in patients with risk factors for heart disease but no known structural heart disease (eg, hypertension). Patients with any risk factors for cardiac syncope should be admitted for evaluation (Figure 31-2).

Differential Diagnosis of Transient Loss of Consciousness

A. Syncope
1. Reflex syncope
   a. Vasovagal syncope
   b. Situational syncope (cough, micturition, or defecation)
   c. Carotid sinus syndrome
2. Orthostatic syncope
   a. Inadequate left ventricular (LV) preload
      (1) Dehydration (nausea, vomiting, diarrhea, uncontrolled diabetes, over dialysis, adrenal insufficiency)
      (2) Hemorrhage
   b. Autonomic failure
      (1) Primary autonomic failure: multisystem atrophy, Parkinson disease
      (2) Secondary autonomic failure: diabetes mellitus, vitamin B_{12} deficiency, uremia

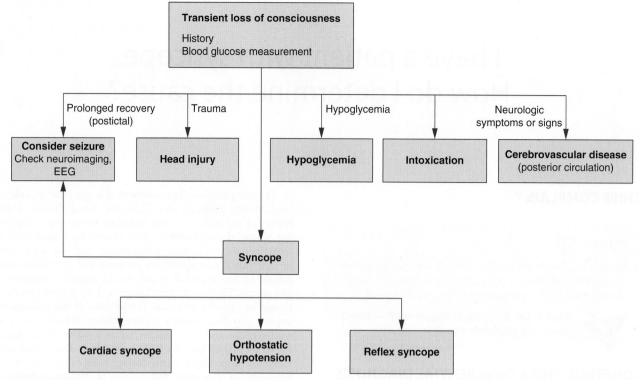

Figure 31-1. Conceptual framework of transient loss of consciousness and syncope.

c. Drug (alcohol, diuretics, alpha-blockers, vasodilators, nitrates)

3. Cardiac syncope

  a. Arrhythmias

    (1) Tachycardias

      (a) VT

        (i) Secondary to structural heart disease, eg, HF, ischemic heart disease, acute myocardial infarction (MI), valvular heart disease

        (ii) Congenital eg, long QT syndrome, Brugada syndrome

        (iii) Electrolyte derangements or hypoxia

        (iv) Medications (tricyclic antidepressants, antiarrhythmics, phenothiazines, macrolides, protease inhibitors, nonsedating antihistamines and diuretics (due to electrolyte abnormalities)

      (b) Supraventricular tachycardia associated with accessory pathway (Wolff-Parkinson-White [WPW] syndrome)

    (2) Bradycardias

      (a) Sinus node disorders

        (i) Sinus bradycardia (< 35 bpm)

        (ii) Sinus pauses (> 3 seconds or > 2 seconds with symptoms)

      (b) Atrioventricular (AV) block (second- or third-degree)

  b. Structural heart disease

    (1) Aortic stenosis

    (2) HCM

    (3) Rare causes: atrial myxoma, prosthetic valve dysfunction, aortic dissection

  c. Other: Inadequate filling

    (1) Cardiac tamponade

    (2) Pulmonary embolism

B. Generalized seizures

C. Cerebrovascular disorders

  1. Vertebrobasilar insufficiency

  2. Subclavian steal

Mr. M reports that he was in his usual state of health and felt perfectly well prior to entering the anatomy dissection room. Upon viewing the cadaver, he felt queasy and warm. He became diaphoretic and collapsed to the floor. When he regained consciousness, he was very embarrassed but not confused. The instructor told him that he was unconscious for only a few seconds.

At this point, what is the leading hypothesis, what are the active alternatives, and is there a must not miss diagnosis? Given this differential diagnosis, what tests should be ordered?

RANKING THE DIFFERENTIAL DIAGNOSIS

Mr. M's history clearly suggests syncope rather than trauma or intoxication. His rapid recovery without intervention argues against either seizure or hypoglycemia. The setting (associated with a strong emotional trigger) and associated symptoms of nausea and warmth are classic for vasovagal syncope, a form of reflex syncope. However, as mentioned above it is critical to also consider

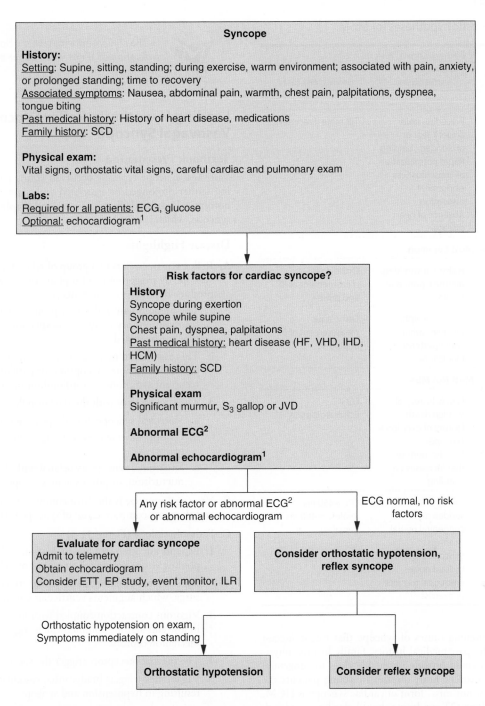

Figure 31-2. Distinguishing cardiac syncope.

The text inside the figure reads:

Syncope

History:
Setting: Supine, sitting, standing; during exercise, warm environment; associated with pain, anxiety, or prolonged standing; time to recovery
Associated symptoms: Nausea, abdominal pain, warmth, chest pain, palpitations, dyspnea, tongue biting
Past medical history: History of heart disease, medications
Family history: SCD

Physical exam:
Vital signs, orthostatic vital signs, careful cardiac and pulmonary exam

Labs:
Required for all patients: ECG, glucose
Optional: echocardiogram[1]

Risk factors for cardiac syncope?
History
Syncope during exertion
Syncope while supine
Chest pain, dyspnea, palpitations
Past medical history: heart disease (HF, VHD, IHD, HCM)
Family history: SCD

Physical exam
Significant murmur, S_3 gallop or JVD

Abnormal ECG[2]

Abnormal echocardiogram[1]

Any risk factor or abnormal ECG[2] or abnormal echocardiogram

ECG normal, no risk factors

Evaluate for cardiac syncope
Admit to telemetry
Obtain echocardiogram
Consider ETT, EP study, event monitor, ILR

Consider orthostatic hypotension, reflex syncope

Orthostatic hypotension on exam, Symptoms immediately on standing

Orthostatic hypotension

Consider reflex syncope

[1]Echocardiogram could be considered in patients with risk factors for heart disease such as CAD risk factors or long standing hypertension.
[2]Abnormal ECG defined as any non sinus rhythm or any abnormality which is new or of uncertain age. Would also include indications of underlying arrhythmia or heart disease, such as short PR interval, long QT interval, BBB or ischemic changes.

ECG, electrocardiogram; EP, electrophysiologic; ETT, exercise tolerance test; HCM, hypertrophic cardiomyopathy; HF, heart failure; IHD, ischemic heart disease; ILR, implantable loop recorder; JVD, jugular venous distention; SCD, sudden cardiac death; VHD, valvular heart disease

Table 31-1. Diagnostic hypotheses for Mr. M.

Diagnostic Hypotheses	Demographics, Risk Factors, Symptoms and Signs	Important Tests
Leading Hypothesis		
Reflex syncope: Vasovagal syncope	Preceding pain, anxiety, fear or prolonged standing Rapid normalization of consciousness Abdominal discomfort Absence of heart disease	Tilt table if recurrent
Active Alternatives—Most Common		
Orthostatic syncope: (Dehydration)	History of vomiting, diarrhea, poor oral intake	Orthostatic measurement of BP and pulse
Orthostatic syncope: (Medications)	History of alpha-blockers, other antihypertensive medication	Orthostatic measurement of BP and pulse
Active Alternatives—Must Not Miss		
Cardiac syncope: Hypertrophic cardiomyopathy	Family history of sudden death History of exertional syncope Systolic murmur that increases on standing	ECG Echocardiogram
Cardiac syncope: Long QT syndrome	Family history of sudden death, congenital neural deafness Syncope precipitated by loud noises, emotional triggers, or exercise	QTc > 450 ms (males), > 460 ms (females)

potentially life-threatening causes of syncope that might suggest cardiac syncope. The past medical history, family history, physical exam, and ECG could provide invaluable clues to congenital heart disease or preexistent heart disease. In young patients the most common "must not miss" form of cardiac syncope is HCM. Although rare, the long QT syndrome should also be considered. Patients with the long QT syndrome may have life-threatening arrhythmias triggered by emotional stress. Table 31-1 lists the differential diagnosis.

Mr. M reports no diarrhea or vomiting, and he is not taking any medications. He has no known heart disease and exercises vigorously without symptoms. There is no family history of sudden cardiac death. There is no history of confusion following the syncope, tonic-clonic activity, or incontinence. On physical exam, his BP and pulse are normal and do not change with standing. Cardiac exam reveals a regular rate and rhythm without a significant murmur, JVD, or S_3 gallop. His ECG is normal.

Is the clinical information sufficient to make a diagnosis? If not what other information do you need?

Leading Hypothesis: Reflex Syncope due to Vasovagal Syncope

Textbook Presentation

Vasovagal syncope typically occurs in young patients while standing (either prolonged or associated with pain or anxiety ie, phlebotomy). Lightheadedness, nausea, and diaphoresis may precede syncope, which is brief.

Disease Highlights

A. Reflex syncope refers to a group of related disorders that cause syncope by triggering inappropriate cardiovascular reflexes that produce hypotension and syncope.

  1. The predominant reflex may produce bradycardia (cardioinhibitory type), or vasodilatation (vasodepressor type) or be mixed.

  2. This distinction may affect the choice of therapy, with pacemakers a potential option for patients with severe, recurrent symptomatic cardioinhibitory reflex syncope.

  3. The triggers vary with the type of reflex syncope.

    a. Vasovagal syncope: upright posture with or without stress

    b. Carotid sinus hypersensitivity (Carotid pressure, see below)

    c. Situational syncope associated with defecation, micturition, or post exercise syncope).

B. Vasovagal syncope is the most common form of reflex syncope and the most common cause of syncope (20–33% of cases).

C. Pathophysiology (Figure 31-3)

  1. Patients are often in a low preload state due to venous pooling (from prolonged standing) or dehydration.

  2. Superimposed anxiety, pain, or fear triggers a sympathetic surge, which augments ventricular contraction.

  3. Vigorous contraction coupled with low preload results in low end-systolic volume, which triggers intracardiac mechanoreceptors.

  4. The mechanoreceptors trigger the vagal reflex.

  5. Vagal reflex triggers bradycardia, vasodilatation, or both, resulting in hypotension and syncope.

Evidence-Based Diagnosis

A. History

  1. Provocative circumstances include prolonged standing (37%), hot weather (42%), lack of food (23%), fear (21%), and acute pain (14%).

  2. No single finding is very sensitive for vasovagal syncope (14–40%).

  3. However, certain findings are fairly specific and increase the likelihood of vasovagal syncope when present.

    a. Prolonged standing (LR+ 9.0)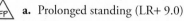

    b. Abdominal discomfort prior to syncope (LR+ 8)

    c. Occurring during injection/cannulation (LR+ 7)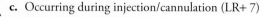

    d. Dehydration (LR+ 3.7)

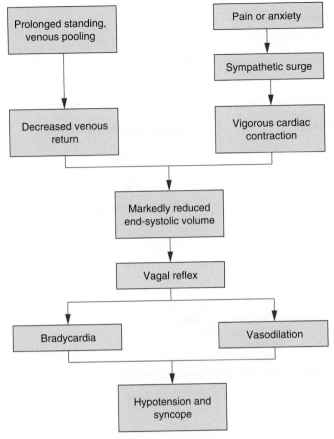

Figure 31-3. Pathophysiology of vasovagal syncope.

e. Nausea after syncope (LR+ 3.5)

f. Although vasovagal syncope can occur *after* exercise it is rare *during* exercise. Syncope during exercise should raise the suspicion of *cardiogenic* syncope.

B. Laboratory and radiologic tests

1. Patients with a typical history, a normal physical exam and ECG, and no evidence of heart disease or red flags do not require further testing.

2. Patients with an atypical history (ie, without a clear precipitant) and those with heart disease or red flags require an echocardiogram and tilt-table testing.

3. Tilt-table testing is particularly useful in patients with recurrent events in whom the diagnosis is unclear.

a. The patient is initially supine for 20–45 minutes.

b. The table is then tilted to 60–80 degrees and the patient kept upright for 30–45 minutes during which time the pulse and BP are continuously monitored.

c. Criteria for a positive test include the reproduction of the presyncopal or syncopal symptoms with hypotension, bradycardia, or both.

d. Sensitivity is 26–80% and specificity is about 90% for reflex syncope.

(1) Test characteristics are estimates because there is no real gold standard.

(2) Estimates vary depending on tilt-table angle, duration, and medications used.

(3) A variety of medications can increase sensitivity but may decrease specificity (eg, isoproterenol and nitrates).

e. Determining the mechanism of syncope (cardioinhibitory vs vasodepressor)

(1) Tilt-table testing does not reliably predict the mechanism of syncope in patients with reflex syncope and the potential utility of pacemaker therapy.

(2) Compared with implantable loop recorders (ILRs) (that documents rhythm disturbances during unprovoked syncope), tilt-table testing is specific but insensitive in detecting asystole or bradycardia (sensitivity 35%, specificity 90%, LR+ 3.5, LR– 0.72).

4. ILRs

a. ILRs are devices implanted into the left pectoral region that can record arrhythmias during syncope for up to 36 months.

b. Useful in patients with recurrent events that may not be captured with continuous loop event monitors and have not been reproduced using tilt table

c. Typically reserved for patients with severe recurrent events that are not amenable to standard therapies (see below) to determine whether the mechanism of vasovagal syncope is cardioinhibitory (and potentially amenable to pacemaker therapy) or vasodepressor

d. The diagnostic yield of ILR in undiagnosed but recurrent syncope in patients over age 40 without structural heart disease is 35% at 2 years. Importantly, 19% of such patients had severe symptomatic bradyarrhythmias (usually asystole). Another 11% of patients had no arrhythmia during syncope ruling out an arrhythmogenic cause.

5. An approach to reflex syncope is illustrated in Figure 31-4.

Treatment

A. Patients should be reassured, instructed to avoid triggers, and lie down if they notice the premonitory signs of an impending faint.

B. Vasodilators (eg, alpha-blockers), diuretics, and alcohol should be eliminated or decreased.

C. Hand grip, arm tensing, and leg crossing in which the muscles are tensed for 2 minutes significantly raises BP and can decrease vasovagal syncope (absolute risk reduction 19%, NNT 5).

D. Midodrine is an alpha-agonist that may be useful. However, compliance is limited due to its three times daily dosing requirements.

E. Fludrocortisone and beta-blockers have not been proven effective.

F. Pacemakers are useful for select patients with severe recurrent cardioinhibitory reflex syncope refractory to other treatments. Patients ≥ 40 years old (without structural heart disease) with asystole on ILR (≥ 3 seconds with syncope or ≥ 6 seconds without syncope) have fewer recurrences with pacemaker treatment (absolute risk reduction 32%, NNT 3).

MAKING A DIAGNOSIS

Mr. M's well-defined precipitant for vasovagal syncope and typical premonitory symptoms combined with the absence of red flags for serious cardiac syncope (such as HF, ischemic heart disease, advanced age, abnormal physical exam or ECG) makes neurocardiogenic syncope the most likely diagnosis. His normal ECG rules out the long QT syndrome. You still wonder if you need to consider HCM.

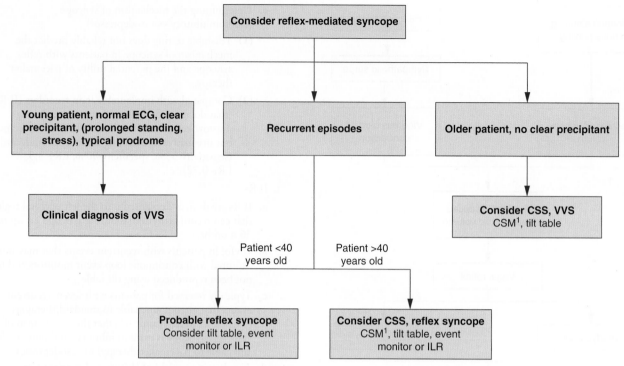

CSM, carotid sinus massage; CSS, carotid sinus syndrome; ECG, electrocardiogram; ILR, implantable loop recorder; VVS, vasovagal syncope.
[1]In patients without contraindications, see text.

Figure 31-4. Diagnostic approach to possible reflex syncope.

Have you crossed a diagnostic threshold for the leading hypothesis, neurocardiogenic syncope? Have you ruled out the active alternatives? Do other tests need to be done to exclude the alternative diagnoses?

Alternative Diagnosis: HCM

Textbook Presentation

Patients with HCM may be asymptomatic and discovered due to a family history of sudden cardiac death, during the evaluation of an asymptomatic systolic murmur, during preparticipation athletic screening, or when symptoms occur (syncope, HF, atrial fibrillation, or cardiac arrest).

Disease Highlights

A. The most common cause of cardiovascular death in young people and among young athletes

B. A large number of different autosomal dominant mutations in genes that encode sarcomere constituents result in myocyte hypertrophy with disarray, increased cardiac fibrosis, and diastolic dysfunction. Over 1400 variants in 11 genes have been reported.

C. Affects 1/500 adults in the general population

D. Left ventricular hypertrophy (LVH) in the absence of loading conditions (hypertension, aortic stenosis, etc.) is the hallmark of the disease.

  1. LVH may develop in childhood, adolescence, or adulthood.

  2. LVH can affect any part of the LV, although often preferentially affects the ventricular septum, which can cause outflow tract obstruction.

  3. Outflow tract obstruction increases the risk of progression to HF, stroke, and sudden cardiac death. The outflow obstruction can be fixed or variable.

  4. The obstruction may generate high velocities, which draw the mitral valve leaflet toward the septum (known as systolic anterior motion of the mitral valve). This further aggravates the outflow obstruction and simultaneously causes mitral regurgitation.

  5. Chamber size affects the magnitude of obstruction. A smaller chamber size (ie, from hypovolemia) brings the anterior leaflet of mitral valve closer to the hypertrophied septum and increases obstruction. This occurs when preload decreases (such as with standing), or when afterload decreases or contractility increases.

E. Most patients are asymptomatic or mildly symptomatic.

F. Complications include HF, angina, mitral regurgitation, atrial fibrillation, stroke, syncope, and sudden cardiac death.

  1. HF

    a. More common in patients with outflow obstruction

    b. Develops due to a combination of outflow obstruction and diastolic dysfunction

    c. Dyspnea on exertion is the most common symptom.

    d. Aggravated by concomitant mitral regurgitation when present

    e. Systolic dysfunction is unusual but may also develop.

  2. Angina

    a. May be typical or atypical in quality

    b. Develops in 25–30% of patients

    c. Ischemia is not primarily due to epicardial CAD, but results from a mismatch of oxygen supply and demand.

d. Aggravated by massive LVH and abnormal microvasculature

e. Concomitant CAD may be present.

3. Syncope

    a. Develops in 15–25% of patients with HCM

    b. May be due to ventricular arrhythmias, outflow tract obstruction, ischemia and, rarely, conduction blocks

4. Sudden cardiac death is the most dreaded complication.

    a. Often occurs in previously asymptomatic patients

    b. Secondary to ventricular tachyarrhythmias (which may be triggered by myocardial fibrosis and disarray, outflow tract obstruction, or ischemia)

    c. Annual risk among all patients with HCM: 0.6–1%

    d. *Major* risk factors include the following:

      (1) Prior events

        (a) Prior cardiac arrest

        (b) Spontaneous sustained VT

      (2) High-risk clinical factors

        (a) Family history of sudden cardiac death in first-degree relative

        (b) Unexplained syncope (particularly if repetitive, exercise-induced, or occurs in children)

        (c) Massive LVH (≥ 30 mm)

      (3) Other risk factors

        (a) Abnormal BP response to exercise

        (b) Nonsustained VT on Holter monitoring ≥ 3 beats at ≥ 120 bpm

      (4) Of note electrophysiologic (EP) studies are not recommended for routine risk stratification of sudden cardiac death.

5. Atrial fibrillation

    a. Left atrial enlargement may develop secondary to decreased LV compliance or mitral regurgitation and creates a substrate for the development of atrial fibrillation.

    b. Atrial fibrillation decreases LV filling and worsens the outflow tract obstruction.

6. Stroke is usually secondary to concomitant atrial fibrillation and subsequent embolization.

G. Annual evaluation

1. History and physical exam

2. Family history

3. Echocardiography

4. 48-hour Holter monitoring (to look for nonsustained VT)

5. Exercise stress testing (to assess BP response to exercise and evaluate ischemia)

Evidence-Based Diagnosis

A. The classic murmur of HCM is a harsh systolic murmur heard at the apex and lower left sternal border.

1. It is accentuated by maneuvers that decrease chamber size (resulting in an increased obstruction).

⚠️FP **2.** The murmur increases as a patient goes from a squatting to a standing position (sensitivity 95%, specificity 84%; LR+ 5.9, LR– 0.06).

⚠️FP **3.** Passive leg elevation decreases the murmur (sensitivity 85% specificity 91%; LR+ 9.4, LR– 0.16).

B. ECG findings

1. ECG abnormalities may *precede* echocardiographic abnormalities and may increase in frequency with age.

2. Abnormalities include repolarization changes (ST segment elevation, depression or T wave inversions) and voltage criteria for LVH. Other findings may include prominent Q waves, left atrial enlargement, and left axis deviation.

3. Abnormal in 86–90% of affected patients with echocardiographic LVH and 46% of affected patients (gene positive) without LVH.

4. Voltage criteria for LVH are present in 65% of patients with echocardiographic LVH and 32% of gene-positive patients without echocardiographic LVH.

C. Echocardiogram

1. May be normal until adolescence of later in life

2. Criteria for HCM include LV wall thickening (≥ 15 mm) in the absence of other conditions known to cause LVH (ie, hypertension or aortic stenosis).

    a. LVH can occur in any part of the LV and in an array of distributions but is often asymmetric in distribution.

    b. The classic pattern that has specific consequences is marked septal hypertrophy.

D. Cardiac MR can be used when echocardiography is suboptimal.

E. DNA analysis

1. DNA analysis can identify mutant genes but remains imprecise.

2. Less than 50% of affected patients have an identifiable mutation and many mutations are of uncertain significance.

3. Testing relatives of patients with HCM can be useful, especially when probands have a known pathogenic mutation. Testing can both identify affected relatives before the development of LVH and can also rule out the disease.

Treatment

A. Evaluation

1. Initial laboratory tests should include a 12-lead ECG, transthoracic echocardiography, Holter monitor and continuous loop event monitor (for patients with palpitations or light headedness).

2. Annual evaluation should include 12-lead ECG, echocardiogram and Holter monitoring.

3. Exercise transthoracic echocardiography can be used to evaluate dynamic obstruction in patients with a resting dynamic outflow obstruction of < 50 mm Hg.

B. Medical therapy

1. Asymptomatic patients

    a. Patients should avoid dehydration and strenuous exertion. Low intensity aerobic exercise is reasonable.

    b. Beta-blockers and calcium channel blockers are unproven in *asymptomatic* HCM with or without obstruction.

    c. Vasodilators and high-dose diuretics should be avoided in patients with HCM and obstruction.

    d. Septal reduction should not be performed in asymptomatic patients.

2. Symptomatic patients

    a. Beta-blockers

      (1) Decrease contractility and slow HR, augmenting diastolic filling and thereby decreasing dynamic outflow obstruction

      (2) Recommended in patients with dyspnea or angina

b. Verapamil

   (1) Can be used if beta-blockers are ineffective or not tolerated

   (2) Should not be used concurrently with beta-blockers due to a high frequency of heart block and HF associated with their combined use.

   (3) Other contraindications include advanced HF, high gradients, or sinus bradycardia.

c. Disopyramide has also been used.

d. Diuretics can be used if dyspnea persists despite treatment with beta-blockers or verapamil.

e. Many drugs are contraindicated (dihydropyridines, digoxin, positive inotropes, and others).

C. Surgery

  1. Septal reduction surgery can reduce LV outflow tract obstruction. Indications are complex but include drug refractory symptoms (chest pain, dyspnea, syncope or near syncope) in patients with significant (≥ 50 mm Hg) LV outflow tract obstruction.

  2. Alcohol septal ablation can induce septal infarction and is another option.

   a. However, compared with surgical myomectomy, there appears to be an increased risk of subsequent life-threatening arrhythmias, heart block, complications, and less reliable symptom relief.

   b. Reserved for nonsurgical candidates.

D. Implantable cardiac defibrillator (ICD)

  1. ICDs are the most effective strategy to prevent sudden cardiac death in patients with HCM.

  2. Recommended for high-risk HCM patients. The ACCF/AHA recommends an ICD for HCM patients with a history of a prior cardiac arrest, spontaneous sustained VT, a family history of sudden cardiac death in first-degree relative, massive LVH, or unexplained syncope.

  3. Some studies also suggest that an abnormal BP response to exercise (in patients' ≤ 40 years old), nonsustained VT, and gadolinium enhancement on cardiac MR also confer an increased risk of sudden cardiac death.

E. Screening

  1. First-degree relatives of affected patients should be screened for the specific mutation (if it is known).

  2. If the relative's screening results are normal, no further testing is required. If results are abnormal (or if the mutation is unknown), an ECG, transthoracic echocardiography, and clinical evaluation should be performed every 12–18 months in children and adolescents and every 5 years in adults.

  3. Preparticipation screening with a history (including family history), physical exam, and ECG of all young competitive athletes has been demonstrated to reduce the incidence of sudden cardiac death by 79% primarily due to a reduction in deaths from HCM.

CASE RESOLUTION

As noted above, Mr. M's history and physical exam and normal ECG suggest vasovagal syncope. There is no family history of sudden cardiac death, significant murmur, or ECG abnormality to suggest either the long QT syndrome or HCM. There is no history of dehydration or offending medications (eg, vasodilators). Tilt-table testing is not indicated in patients with isolated episodes of well-defined vasovagal syncope.

Mr. M is reassured, and although embarrassed, he feels much better. After explaining the pathophysiology of his disorder, you initiate standard recommendations for the prevention of further episodes.

CHIEF COMPLAINT

PATIENT 2

Mr. C is a 65-year-old man with diabetes who comes to see you with a chief complaint of losing consciousness. He reports that he was sitting at home watching television when he suddenly lost consciousness without any warning. His wife reports that he was unresponsive for approximately 30 seconds. There was no tonic-clonic activity or incontinence, and the patient was not confused after regaining consciousness. The patient's wife reports that she took Mr. C's blood glucose when he passed out and that the reading was 120 mg/dL.

At this point, what is the leading hypothesis, what are the active alternatives, and is there a must not miss diagnosis? Given this differential diagnosis, what tests should be ordered?

RANKING THE DIFFERENTIAL DIAGNOSIS

As illustrated in Figure 31-1 the first step in patients with loss of consciousness is to determine whether this was due to syncope, trauma, intoxication, hypoglycemia, or seizure. The patient was not intoxicated and did not experience any trauma. The spontaneous rapid recovery essentially rules out seizure and hypoglycemia (further substantiated by the normal blood glucose at the time). Thus, the history clearly suggests syncope. The second pivotal step in such patients is to determine whether the patient has cardiac syncope, orthostatic hypotension, or reflex syncope. As illustrated in Figure 31-2, this process is driven by a search for risk factors to determine whether the patient is at risk for cardiac syncope, which could be life-threatening. In particular, patients should be asked about a prior history of heart disease; syncope precipitated with exertion or while supine; and any associated chest pain, dyspnea, or palpitations.

Mr. C denies any history of exertion prior to his loss of consciousness. He denies any associated chest pain,

(continued)

palpitations, or dyspnea. Past medical history reveals that Mr. C has suffered 2 MIs. Subsequently, he has dyspnea upon walking more than 20 yards. Mr. C also has diabetes mellitus. His medications include atenolol, aspirin, atorvastatin, insulin, and lisinopril. On physical exam, his BP is 128/70 mm Hg with a pulse of 72 bpm, which is regular. There is no significant change upon standing. His lung exam is clear, and cardiac exam reveals prominent JVD and a loud S₃ gallop. There is no significant murmur. He has 2+ pretibial edema, and his rectal exam reveals guaiac-negative stool.

 Is the clinical information sufficient to make a diagnosis? If not, what other information do you need?

Mr. C's does not have exertional syncope, chest pain, palpitations, or dyspnea at the time of syncope. Nonetheless, his history of MIs substantially increases the likelihood of cardiac syncope, which becomes both the leading hypothesis and a must not miss hypothesis. Furthermore, his history of dyspnea on minimal exertion, JVD, and S₃ gallop all suggest HF. HF in turn markedly increases the likelihood of VT as a cause of cardiac syncope. Although he lacks chest pain, his prior history of CAD and MI increase the likelihood of syncope associated with an acute coronary syndrome, another must not miss hypothesis. Orthostatic syncope (secondary to dehydration, hemorrhage, or drugs) is unlikely given his lack of postural BP change with standing. Although hypoglycemia should be considered in diabetic patients taking insulin, sulfonylureas, or thiazolidinediones, it is essentially ruled out by the rapid recovery without intervention and documented normoglycemia at the time of syncope. Hypoglycemia-induced syncope is usually preceded by either confusion or sympathetic stimulation producing tremulousness, nervousness, or diaphoresis. Another "must not miss" alternative includes PE, which is an uncommon cause of syncope. Vasovagal syncope is unlikely because Mr. C.'s syncope occurred while sitting and was not preceded by any pain or anxiety. Table 31-2 lists the differential diagnosis.

Leading Hypothesis: Cardiac Syncope

Textbook Presentation

Cardiac syncope refers to syncope secondary to a disorder arising within the heart. Arrhythmias (either tachyarrhythmias or bradyarrhythmias) are the most common disorders. Less common disorders include acute coronary syndromes, severe valvular heart disease (eg, aortic stenosis), and PE. Rare causes include aortic dissection, cardiac tamponade, and atrial myxoma. Classically, patients with cardiac syncope are elderly patients with known heart disease (ie, HF or CAD) who experience sudden syncope, which may occur without warning. Patients may have palpitations.

Disease Highlights

A. Cardiac syncope is associated with increased mortality.

1. The 1-year mortality rate in patients with cardiac syncope is 18–33%, compared with 6% in patients with syncope of unknown cause.

2. Preexistent heart disease increases the likelihood of cardiac syncope.

3. Subsequent mortality in syncopal patients increases with the severity of heart disease.

    a. Class 1–2 HF, OR 7.7

    b. Class 3–4 HF, OR 13.5

Table 31-2. Diagnostic hypotheses for Mr. C.

Diagnostic Hypotheses	Demographics, Risk Factors, Symptoms and Signs	Important Tests
Leading Hypothesis		
Cardiac syncope: (Ventricular tachycardia)	History of CAD, HF, or valvular heart disease Syncope while supine or with exercise Palpitations, S₃ gallop, JVD, or significant murmur	ECG Echocardiogram Stress test Event monitor EP study
Active Alternatives—Must Not Miss		
Cardiac syncope (Myocardial infarction)	History of CAD or CAD risk factors, chest pain	ECG Troponin ETT Angiogram
PE	Risk factors for PE Pleuritic chest pain or dyspnea Loud S₂ Unexplained persistent hypotension Right heart strain on ECG (right bundle-branch block, right axis deviation) or right ventricular dilatation on echocardiogram	CT angiogram Ventilation-perfusion scan Leg venous duplex Angiogram

CAD, coronary artery disease; ECG, electrocardiogram; EP, electrophysiologic; ETT, exercise tolerance test; HF, heart failure; JVD, jugular venous distention; PE, pulmonary embolism.

4. Among patients with dilated cardiomyopathy, sudden cardiac death (presumably arrhythmogenic) accounts for 30% of the mortality.

5. Patients in whom cardiac syncope is suspected should be admitted for evaluation.

B. Although there are a large number of cardiac dysrhythmias, only a relative few produce syncope. Most supraventricular tachyarrhythmias will not cause syncope because the AV node limits the ventricular response rate. The most common arrhythmias associated with syncope include

1. Tachycardias

    a. VT

    b. Supraventricular tachycardias associated with an accessory pathway (ie, WPW syndrome [see end of chapter]).

2. Bradycardias

    a. Sinus node dysfunction

        (1) Sinus bradycardia (< 35 bpm)

        (2) Sinus pauses (defined as > 3 seconds or > 2 seconds with symptoms)

    b. AV heart block (second- or third-degree)

    c. Atrial fibrillation with a *slow* ventricular response

Evidence-Based Diagnosis

A. History

 1. Certain clinical findings are uncommon but substantially increase the likelihood of cardiac syncope when present including syncope associated with chest pain, syncope during exertion (LR+ 6.5–14), or syncope when supine (LR+ 4.0–∞).

 Syncope during exertion is unusual but worrisome and may suggest CAD, HCM, long QT syndrome, polymorphic VT, and WPW.

2. Other symptoms may suggest cardiac syncope but are less specific (palpitations, syncope of sudden onset, dyspnea associated with syncope).

3. Cardiac syncope is unlikely in patients without known or suspected cardiac disease on the basis of the initial history, physical exam, and ECG (LR 0.09–0.12).

4. Table 31-3 summarizes the sensitivity, specificity, and LR for symptoms in predicting cardiac syncope.

B. ECG

1. An abnormal ECG increases the OR of cardiac arrhythmias in patients without vasovagal syncope (OR, 23.5 [CI, 7 – 87]).

2. Certain ECG findings in syncopal patients may suggest particular cardiac etiologies.

   a. ECG evidence of prior MI or a long QT interval increases the likelihood of VT.

   b. ECG findings of significant bradycardia, second- or third-degree AV block increase the likelihood of syncope due to sick sinus syndrome (SSS) or AV block.

   c. Bundle branch block (BBB) on ECG increases the likelihood of both AV block and VT.

     (1) Mortality in syncopal patients with BBB is 28% at 40 months. 32% of the deaths were sudden death.

     (2) The increased mortality is attributed to a combination of VT or electromechanical dissociation in patients with underlying heart disease.

     (3) AV block develops in 17% of patients with BBB and syncope.

     (4) EP studies can document prolonged conduction through the His-Purkinje system and is highly specific but insensitive (67%). ILR recordings can also be useful.

     (5) Pacemaker therapy effectively prevents syncope in almost all such patients (but does not prevent sudden death).

Table 31-3. Sensitivity, specificity, and LRs for cardiac syncope.

Clinical Feature	Sensitivity	Specificity	LR+	LR–
Syncope with effort	13–14%	98–99%	6.5–14	0.87–0.89
Syncope while supine	4–14%	97–100%	4.0–∞	0.89–0.96
Suspected or certain cardiac disease	95%	53%	2.0	0.09

Table 31-4. Predicting cardiac syncope, EGSYS score.

Risk Factor	Points
Palpitations before syncope	+ 4
Abnormal ECG[1] and or heart disease[2]	+ 3
Syncope during effort	+ 3
Syncope while supine	+ 2
Autonomic prodrome[3]	– 1
Predisposing and or precipitating factors[4]	– 1

Total Score	2 Y Mortality
< 3	2%
≥ 3	21%

Total Score	Cardiac Syncope
< 3	2%
3	13%
4	33%
>4	77%

[1]Including sinus bradycardia, AV block greater than first degree, BBB, acute or old MI, SVT or VT, LVH or RVH, short PR or delta wave, long QT interval, and Brugada pattern.
[2]Including HF, ischemic, valvular or congenital heart disease or cardiomyopathy or signs of heart disease.
[3]Nausea/vomiting.
[4]Warm crowded environments, prolonged standing, fear, pain or anxiety.
AV, atrioventricular; BBB, bundle branch block; HF, heart failure; LVH, left ventricular hypertrophy; MI, myocardial infarction; RVH, right ventricular hypertrophy; SVT, supraventricular tachycardia; VT, ventricular tachycardia.

   d. Right ventricular strain (S1Q3T3) or right BBB suggests PE.

   e. Ischemic changes suggest MI.

   f. Delta wave or short PR interval suggests an accessory pathway (eg, WPW syndrome).

C. Clinical decision rules have been developed that combine the clinical risk factors and ECG to predict cardiac syncope and 2-year total mortality.

1. One such score is the EGSYS score (see Table 31-4).

2. A score of ≥ 3 predicted cardiac syncope (92% sensitive, 69% specific, LR+ 3, LR– 0.12).

3. Syncope while supine is uncommon and under-represented in studies. Patients with a score of 2 due to syncope while supine should be evaluated for cardiac syncope.

D. Other tests

1. Echocardiograms

   a. Rarely diagnostic of arrhythmia but useful for risk stratification because VT is much more common in presence of LV dysfunction.

   b. Used to assess LV function and valve function (eg, aortic stenosis)

   c. Should be obtained in patients with a history of CAD, HF, valvular disease, significant clinical findings (S_3 gallop, JVD, significant murmurs) or patients with risk factors for heart disease (eg, hypertension).

2. Exercise testing
   a. Particularly useful in patients with exertional syncope or chest pain
   b. Also obtained in patients with cardiac disease, ischemic changes on ECG
   c. May be useful in patients with dyspnea on exertion
3. Holter monitoring: External cardiac leads are applied to the patient and a 24- to 48-hour recording of the cardiac rhythm is made.
   a. Diagnostic only if
      (1) Arrhythmia captured *and* patient symptomatic during arrhythmia or
      (2) Rhythm normal during symptoms (excludes an arrhythmia)
   b. Often nondiagnostic due to
      (1) Absence of arrhythmia during study
      (2) Absence of symptoms during arrhythmia
4. External loop recorders
   a. External devices that can be worn for up to 1 month. A continuous recording is made.
   b. If symptoms occur, most recent 2–5 minutes can be frozen in memory and transmitted by telephone.
   c. Relative short duration of monitoring (1 month) still limits sensitivity.
   d. Often used in patients with nondiagnostic Holter monitoring, particularly when symptoms are infrequent. Sensitivity is 14%, compared with long-term ILR.
5. ILRs have been used successfully in some patients with recurrent unexplained syncope. The yield in such patients has been reported at 90%. This may be particularly useful at detecting bradycardias missed by EP studies.
6. EP studies require a right heart catheterization. During EP studies, stimuli are delivered in order to elicit tachyarrhythmias and detect accessory pathways. Bradyarrhythmias may be implied when patients have prolonged conduction times or when the sinus node responses to rapid pacing are abnormal.
   a. Sensitivity is 90% for VT.
   b. Sensitivity for bradyarrhythmias is low (33%).
   c. Overall diagnostic yield of EP studies
      (1) 36–70% in patients with heart disease
      (2) 22% in patients with abnormal ECGs
      (3) 14% in select patients with normal ECGs without heart disease
   d. Indications for EP studies in patients with unexplained syncope include
      (1) Prior MI
      (2) Structural heart disease
      (3) Impaired LV function
      (4) Bifascicular block
      (5) Monitoring suggests sinus node dysfunction or AV block
   e. Risk of EP studies include cardiac perforation, MI, AV fistulae (< 3%), deep venous thrombosis, and PE.

E. Figure 31-5 summarizes the clinical clues and diagnostic considerations in patients with possible cardiac syncope.

The ECG shows Q waves in leads V1–V4 and II, III and aVF consistent with prior anterior and inferior MI. These were present on his prior ECG 6 months previously. The PR interval is normal. There is no evidence of sinus bradycardia, sinus pause, or AV block. The QRS width is normal, excluding BBB. An echocardiogram reveals LV dysfunction with hypokinesis of the anterior and inferior walls. The ejection fraction is estimated to be 42%. The aortic valve is normal without evidence of aortic stenosis.

Reviewing Figure 31-5 for clues to potential cardiac syncope, Mr. C. dose not have any associated symptoms of palpitations, chest pain, or dyspnea with this acute event. His past medical history of CAD clearly raises the possibility of an acute coronary syndrome, which is an unusual cause of syncope. His echocardiogram confirms HF, markedly increasing his risk of VT. His ECG is consistent with his prior CAD and there are no additional ECG findings to suggest bradycardia (ie, heart block, BBB, sinus bradycardia). The leading hypothesis is revised to VT, but you wonder if this might be the presentation of an acute coronary syndrome.

Revised Leading Hypothesis: VT

Textbook Presentation

Patients with VT may be asymptomatic or have symptoms that range from palpitations to lightheadedness, near syncope, syncope, or sudden cardiac death.

VT occurs most commonly in patients with CAD and HF and should be seriously considered when patients with preexisting CAD, HF, or other heart disease present with syncope.

Disease Highlights

A. Etiology and associations
   1. Ischemic heart disease
      a. Associated with CAD in 80% of cases
      b. May be secondary to acute ischemia/MI or prior scar
   2. HF
   3. Other heart disease: HCM, valvular heart disease, infiltrative disorders
   4. Miscellaneous causes
      a. Electrolyte disorders (hypokalemia and hypomagnesemia)
      b. Hypoxia
      c. Drugs, particularly those that prolong the QT interval (eg, antiarrhythmics, antipsychotics, tricyclic antidepressants, macrolides, and some fluoroquinolones)
   5. Congenital disorders
      a. Congenital heart disease
         (1) Long QT syndrome
            (a) The ECG of affected families demonstrates long refractory periods (long QT intervals defined as a QTc of > 450 ms in males and 460 ms in females)
            (b) Affected patients are at risk for sudden cardiac death from a form of VT called torsades de pointes.

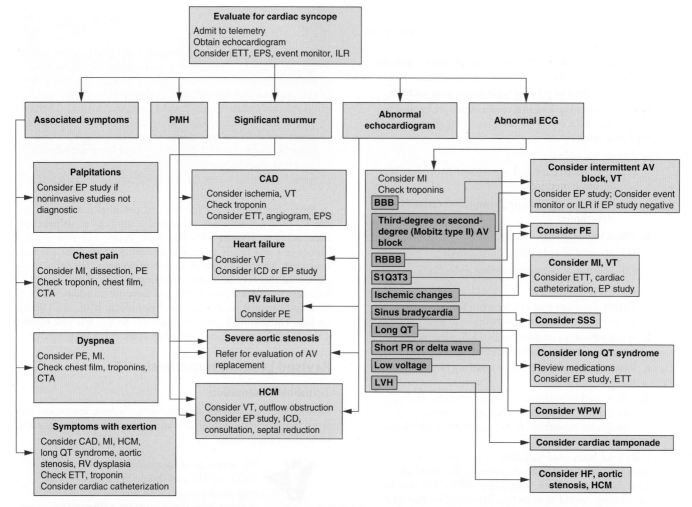

AV, aortic valve; BBB, bundle branch block; CAD, coronary artery disease; CTA, CT angiogram; EP, electrophysiologic; ETT, exercise tolerance test; HCM, hypertrophic cardiomyopathy; HF, heart failure; ICD, implantable cardiac defibrillator; ILR, implantable loop recorder; LVH, left ventricular hypertrophy; MI, myocardial infarction; PE, pulmonary embolism; RBBB, right bundle branch block; SSS, sick sinus syndrome; VT, ventricular tachycardia; WPW, Wolff Parkinson White.

Figure 31-5. Clinical clues and diagnostic considerations in patients with possible cardiac syncope.

(c) Arrhythmias may be precipitated by emotional stress, exercise, loud abrupt noises, or during sleep.

(d) Several symptoms typically associated with vasovagal syncope are also common in the long QT syndrome: triggered by emotional stress, pain, or noise (70%); sweating (67%); nausea (29%); situational (associated with micturition, defecation or coughing) (17%); abdominal discomfort (16%)

 Long QT syndrome may mimic vasovagal syncope. Even patients with symptoms typical of vasovagal syncope should have an ECG performed and QTc measured.

(e) A FH of sudden cardiac death is more common in the long QT syndrome than vasovagal syncope (66% vs. 17%)

(f) Associated with congenital neural deafness

(2) Brugada syndrome

(a) Unusual disorder secondary to mutation in the sodium channel gene, which predisposes

patients to polymorphic VT and sudden death.

(b) Suggestive baseline ECG abnormalities include a right BBB pattern with ST elevation in the right precordial leads.

B. Prognosis

1. VT is a potentially life-threatening arrhythmia.

2. Predictors of mortality in patients with VT include prior cardiac arrest, LV dysfunction, post MI, or inducible VT on EP studies.

Evidence-Based Diagnosis

A. ECG criteria for VT

1. ≥ 3 consecutive wide complex (QRS ≥ .12 seconds) beats (Figure 31-6) > 100 bpm constitutes a wide complex tachycardia

   a. 80–90% of wide complex tachycardias are due to VT

   b. However, supraventricular tachycardias can also occasionally manifest wide QRS complexes (> 0.12 s) due to conduction associated with a BBB or an accessory pathway, hyperkalemia or drug induced QRS changes (tricyclic antidepressants overdose and class 1a antiarrhythmics)

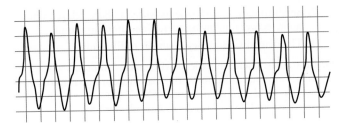

Figure 31-6. Ventricular tachycardia.

c. ECG criteria that increase the likelihood that the wide complex tachycardia is due to VT include:

(1) Fusion beats

(2) Capture beats

(3) AV dissociation

(4) Concordance of the precordial leads (all chest leads pointing either up or all pointing down.)

(5) The absence of these findings does not establish supraventricular tachycardia.

d. A history of CAD or HF increases the likelihood that the wide complex tachycardia is VT.

e. Hemodynamic stability does not rule out VT.

f. Review of prior ECGs can be helpful.

(1) A preexistent BBB on a prior ECG (during sinus rhythm) with the same QRS morphology as that during the arrhythmia favors supraventricular tachycardia with aberrancy.

(2) Evidence of WPW suggests supraventricular tachycardia with antidromic conduction down the accessory tract.

 All wide complex tachycardias should be assumed to be VT unless there is conclusive evidence of a supraventricular tachycardia (see above).

2. Sustained VT is defined as VT lasting longer than 30 seconds.

B. In patients with risk factors for VT (eg, ischemic heart disease, HF, HCM), (but without documented VT) EP studies can provoke sustained monomorphic VT and be diagnostic. This is particularly useful in patients in whom VT is suspected and who do not already have an indication for an ICD.

Treatment

A. Patients with ongoing VT

1. Unstable patients (with hypotension, angina, HF, or altered mental status) should receive immediate cardioversion. The management of *acute* VT evolves rapidly and is beyond the scope of this text. Please see appropriate ACLS guidelines.

2. Evaluation in stable patients with ongoing VT

a. Obtain baseline ECG and troponin to look for evidence of ischemia, long QT syndrome.

b. Check electrolytes (especially potassium, magnesium) and SaO_2.

c. Review of medications to search for drugs associated with QT prolongation

d. Consultation is advised regarding antiarrhythmic therapy.

B. Follow-up evaluation is directed at evaluating the etiologies of VT and risk for sudden death.

1. Stress testing (and coronary angiography in selected patients) can help uncover underlying ischemia

precipitating VT and is recommended for patients with exercise-induced syncope or chest pain or an intermediate or greater probability of CAD.

2. An echocardiogram should be obtained to evaluate LV function and rule out valvular heart disease and HF.

3. EP testing is recommended for selected patients (see above).

C. Prevention of recurrent VT and sudden cardiac death

1. Treat underlying conditions

a. Treat ischemic heart disease (including revascularization if necessary)

b. Treat HF (angiotensin-converting enzyme [ACE] inhibitors, beta-blockade, and spironolactone have all been shown to decrease mortality).

c. Optimize electrolytes, including magnesium.

2. Specific therapy for the treatment and prevention of VT includes antiarrhythmic drugs (especially beta-blockers and possibly amiodarone), catheter ablation, ICDs, and combinations of the above.

a. ICDs are implanted devices that monitor the cardiac rhythm and automatically detect and cardiovert patients in VT.

b. ICDs are used in selected patients at high risk for sudden death, including selected HF patients, survivors of sudden death, and patients in whom syncope was believed to have been caused by VT.

c. Precise indications for ICD therapy are complex and influenced by the cause of heart disease (ischemic or nonischemic), the ejection fraction, the type of arrhythmia (monomorphic VT, polymorphic VT or ventricular fibrillation), and in ischemic heart disease, plans for revascularization as well as the timing of the arrhythmia relative to the most recent MI. Appropriate use criteria have been published by the ACCF/AHA.

d. Consultation is advised.

Alternative Diagnosis: Acute Coronary Syndrome & Syncope

Acute coronary syndrome is an unusual cause of syncope and is covered extensively in Chapter 9, Chest Pain. This discussion will focus on patients who experience syncope due to an acute coronary syndrome. Briefly, acute coronary syndromes account for approximately 3% of patients presenting to emergency departments with syncope. The mechanism of syncope varies and includes reflex syncope (particularly in inferior MIs), advanced AV block (particularly in anterior MIs) and VT. Symptoms are often atypical in syncopal patients with acute MI; chest pain is present in only 17%, dyspnea in 30%, and a history of CAD in 54%. Lab abnormalities include troponin elevation on presentation (50%) and ST segment elevation (9%). Nonetheless, a normal ECG (defined as normal sinus rhythm without new or indeterminate changes) makes the diagnosis of acute MI unlikely, negative predictive value 99% (sensitivity 80%, specificity 64%, LR+ 2.2, LR– 0.31).

MAKING A DIAGNOSIS

 Mr. C's serum troponin levels are repeatedly undetectable (thus excluding acute MI.) The pretest probability of VT is very high. You elect to admit Mr. C for inpatient monitoring.

You still wonder if a significant bradyarrhythmia or a PE might be responsible for Mr. C's syncope.

Have you crossed a diagnostic threshold for the leading hypothesis, VT? Do other tests need to be done to exclude the alternative diagnoses?

Alternative Diagnosis: Bradycardia from SSS

Textbook Presentation

The presentation of SSS depends on the duration and severity of the bradyarrhythmia. When the bradyarrhythmia is severe and prolonged, patients may experience sudden syncope. With less severe bradycardia, patients may experience weakness, dyspnea on exertion, angina, transient ischemic attacks, or near syncope. Since the bradyarrhythmia may be short lived, patients may recover without intervention.

Disease Highlights

A. Episodic or persistent failure of sinus node

B. Most common indication for pacemaker placement

C. Often seen in the elderly (mean age 68) due to fibrosis and degeneration of sinus node

D. Underlying CAD is common and contributes to the pathogenesis of SSS in some patients.

E. A variety of medications can depress sinus node function and aggravate SSS, including beta-blockers, verapamil, diltiazem, digoxin, cimetidine, clonidine, lithium, methyldopa, and other antiarrhythmics.

F. Less common causes include hypothyroidism, infiltrative myocardial diseases, pericarditis, Lyme disease, and rheumatic fever.

G. Electrical manifestations may include
   1. Sinus bradycardia < 40 bpm
   2. Sinus pauses > 2 seconds
   3. Sinus arrest (with an escape junctional rhythm)
   4. Sinoatrial exit block (inability of the sinus impulse to exit the sinus node)

H. Concomitant AV conduction disturbances are present in over 50% of patients with SSS.

I. Associated with supraventricular *tachy*arrhythmias, in 40–60% of patients, particularly atrial fibrillation (tachy-brady syndrome). Such patients may complain of palpitations. The bradycardia often follows termination of the tachycardia. Tachy-brady syndrome markedly increases the risk of death or nonfatal stroke (2- to 3-fold) compared with SSS alone.

Evidence-Based Diagnosis

A. Simultaneous symptoms and ECG findings (sinus bradycardia, significant pauses or sinus exit block) establishes the diagnosis.

B. Holter monitoring may be used but is often nondiagnostic due to the intermittent nature of the arrhythmia.

C. External cardiac continuous loop event monitors allow for a longer period of monitoring and correlation with symptoms.

D. Carotid sinus massage may cause prolonged pauses in patients with SSS (> 3 seconds).

E. ILRs have also been used.

F. Pharmacologic studies
   1. Adenosine slows sinus node activity.

2. Small studies suggest patients with SSS have delayed sinus node recovery following adenosine administration.

3. The diagnostic accuracy is similar to EP studies.

G. EP studies: Useful in patients with severe symptoms when monitoring has failed to capture patients during symptoms (which could confirm or exclude SSS). However, sensitivity is imperfect and normal results to not rule out SSS.

Treatment

A. Discontinue any medications that may adversely affect sinus function (see above). (If beta-blockers or other drugs cannot be discontinued, patients may require pacemaker.)

B. Indications for pacemaker placement
   1. Documented **symptomatic** sinus node dysfunction
   2. Chronotropic incompetence: In this condition, the sinus rate does not increase appropriately with physical activity, leading to a relative bradycardia and symptoms.
   3. Pacemakers are used in certain situations when SSS is suspected but cannot be confirmed.
      a. Patients with HR < 40 bpm and prior symptoms
      b. EP study shows long sinus node recovery time following rapid atrial pacing in patients with prior unexplained syncope.
      c. Patients with a history of syncope and asymptomatic pauses ≥ 3 s (except when asleep or young trained persons)

C. Anticoagulation is indicated for patients with SSS and concurrent atrial fibrillation (persistent or intermittent).

Alternative Diagnosis: Bradycardia due to AV Heart Block

Textbook Presentation

Depending on the duration and severity of the heart block, patients with AV block may be asymptomatic or complain of syncope, near syncope, palpitations, angina or transient ischemic attacks.

Disease Highlights

A. Secondary to conduction abnormalities in the AV node, bundle of His, or bundle branches.

B. Classification (Table 31-5)
   1. In first-degree AV block *all* of the sinus impulses (P waves) are conducted (but the PR interval is prolonged)
   2. In second-degree block, *some* of the impulses are conducted.
   3. In third-degree AV block, *none* of the P waves are conducted (Figure 31-7).
   4. In second- or third-degree AV block, the ventricular rate slows and may depend on lower intrinsic pacemakers residing within the ventricle. The bradycardia can result in dyspnea, angina, hypotension, syncope, or death.

C. AV nodal disease should also be suspected in patients with atrial fibrillation who have a slow ventricular response and are not taking medications that slow AV conduction (eg, digoxin, beta-blockers, verapamil, or diltiazem).

D. Etiology
   1. Fibrosis of the conduction system
   2. Ischemic heart disease

Table 31-5. Classification of heart block.

Classification	Atrial ventricular Conduction	ECG Findings	Clinical Findings	Treatment
First-degree	1:1	PR interval > 0.2 seconds QRS width usually within normal limits	None	None
Second-degree Mobitz I	Intermittent	PR interval increases progressively until P wave is not conducted and QRS absent. PR interval after dropped QRS shorter than PR prior to dropped QRS QRS width < 0.12 sec	Associated with inferior MI Rarely progresses to third-degree AV block	Observation or atropine
Second-degree Mobitz II	Intermittent	Intermittent nonconduction of P waves QRS may be widened, BBB may be seen (due to more severe infranodal damage)	Associated with anterior MI Often progresses to third-degree AV block	Pacemaker
Third-degree	ϕ	P waves not conducted Complete AV disassociation Ventricular rate depends on escape pacemakers	Associated with CAD, drugs, degeneration, abnormal electrolytes, bradycardia, hypotension	Pacemaker

AV, atrioventricular; BBB, bundle branch block; CAD, coronary artery disease; MI, myocardial infarction.

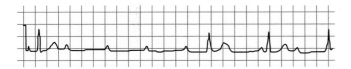

Figure 31-7. Third-degree atrioventricular block.

3. Medications (eg, beta-blockers, verapamil, diltiazem, digoxin, amiodarone)

 The combination of verapamil and beta-blockers should always be avoided. There is a high incidence of subsequent AV block and HF.

4. Hyperkalemia

5. Valvular heart disease (due to extension of calcification into the conduction system)

6. Increased vagal tone

7. Miscellaneous other causes (Lyme disease, sarcoidosis, etc)

Treatment

A. Discontinue medications that impair AV conduction.

B. Treat ischemia.

C. Correct electrolyte abnormalities.

D. Atropine can be useful in emergent situations.

E. Pacemakers

   1. Precise indications are complex. The ACC/AHA published guidelines in 2008.

   2. Pacing is recommended for patients with third-degree AV block and *symptomatic* second-degree AV block.

   3. Pacing is usually recommended for patients with Mobitz II second-degree AV block.

4. Pacing is also recommended for advanced second-degree AV block (defined as 2 consecutively blocked P waves) associated with any of the following: symptoms, pauses while awake ≥ 3 sec, HR < 40 bpm while awake, escape rhythms below the AV node or atrial fibrillation with ventricular pauses of ≥ 5 sec.

5. Pacing is not usually indicated in Mobitz I second-degree AV block.

6. Pacing is not indicated in asymptomatic first-degree AV block.

Alternative Diagnosis: PE

Textbook Presentation

PE is an unusual cause of syncope (about 1%) and is covered extensively in Chapter 15, Dyspnea. This discussion will focus on patients who experience syncope due to PE. Between 9% and 24% of patients with PE experience syncope (39% in patients with massive PE). Syncope in PE is usually secondary to massive embolization involving more than 50% of the pulmonary vascular bed, critically limiting blood return to the LV and cardiac output. This massive embolization increases the likelihood of findings consistent with more extensive PE including hypotension (ranging from 14% to 76% in various studies), cardiac arrest (24%), and ECG evidence of cor pulmonale (S1Q3T3 or new right BBB in 60%). Patients with PE who experience syncope are twice as likely to have right ventricular dysfunction as patients who do not experience syncope (17.4% vs 8.5%).

Despite this, the subset of patients with PE and syncope who survive to arrive at the hospital have often stabilized due to clot fragmentation and may be hemodynamically stable and relatively asymptomatic. Dyspnea has been reported in 50–90% of patients, hypoxia ($PaO_2 < 60$ mm Hg) in 91%.

PE should be considered in the differential diagnosis of patients with syncope who have symptoms of dyspnea, chest pain, or risk factors for PE; physical exam findings of unexplained hypotension, tachycardia, JVD, a loud S_2, or a right-sided S_3 gallop; hypoxia; ECG findings of a S1Q3T3 pattern, right axis deviation, or right

BBB; radiographic findings of an unexplained pleural effusion or infiltrate (that may suggest a pulmonary infarction); or echocardiographic findings of right atrial or right ventricular enlargement.

CASE RESOLUTION

After 24 hours, Mr. C is feeling well. He is anxious to go home. The telemetry reveals normal sinus rhythm without evidence of intermittent AV block or VT. Stress testing is performed and shows evidence of prior MI but no acute ischemia.

The sensitivity of telemetry is inadequate to exclude life-threatening arrhythmias such as VT. Furthermore, none of the alternative diagnoses are suggested by the history, physical exams, or laboratory test results (such as orthostatic hypotension, PE, SSS, or AV heart block). After careful discussion with Mr. C, you order an EP study.

The EP study demonstrates inducible sustained VT, placing the patient at high risk for spontaneous lethal ventricular arrhythmias. An ICD is placed. At follow-up 12 months later, Mr. C is doing well and has no subsequent syncopal events. His ICD has delivered 2 shocks.

CHIEF COMPLAINT

PATIENT

Mrs. S is a 60-year-old woman who arrives at the emergency department via ambulance after an episode of transient loss of consciousness. The patient reports that she was eating dinner, and the next thing she knew she was in the emergency department. Mr. S reports that he found his wife lying on the floor next to the dining room table when he came home. At that time, Mrs. S was conscious but lethargic. The food and plate were scattered on the floor. There was no evidence of incontinence. On physical exam, her vital signs are normal. HEENT exam reveals a contusion over the right eye and bruising along the right half of her tongue. Cardiac and pulmonary exams are normal. Abdominal exam is unremarkable. Stool is guaiac negative. Neurologic exam is nonfocal.

At this point, what is the leading hypothesis, what are the active alternatives, and is there a must not miss diagnosis? Given this differential diagnosis, what tests should be ordered?

RANKING THE DIFFERENTIAL DIAGNOSIS

The remarkable feature of Mrs. S's history is the prolonged period of lethargy and confusion that persisted until she reached the emergency department. As discussed at the beginning of the chapter, and illustrated in Figure 31-1, patients with *syncope* suffer from *transient* global cerebral hypoperfusion and rapid restoration of normal consciousness. Mr. S's prolonged confusion is a **pivotal clue** that suggests a non-syncopal etiology for her loss of consciousness. Diagnostic considerations include seizure, hypoglycemia, or another neurologic event (eg, an ischemic event involving the posterior circulation or trauma). The patient's bruised tongue is a diagnostic **fingerprint** that markedly increases the likelihood of a seizure. Hypoglycemia-induced syncope is usually preceded by either confusion or sympathetic stimulation producing tremulousness, nervousness, or diaphoresis and occurs almost exclusively in diabetic patients taking insulin, sulfonylureas, or thiazolidinediones. Table 31-6 lists the differential diagnosis.

Patients with syncope should be asked, "What was the next thing you remember?" Patients who do not remember the ambulance ride or suffer a period of amnesia **following the event** (> 5 minutes) should be evaluated for seizures.

The patient reports no prior history of epilepsy, CNS tumor, or stroke (which can increase the likelihood of seizures). She has no history of diabetes and is not taking

(continued)

Table 31-6. Diagnostic hypotheses for Mrs. S.

Diagnostic Hypotheses	Demographics, Risk Factors, Symptoms and Signs	Important Tests
Leading Hypothesis		
Seizure	Prolonged period of lethargy, confusion, amnesia suggesting postictal period Tonic-clonic activity Incontinence Prior stroke, CNS tumor, or neurologic disease Abnormal neurologic exam	EEG Contrast-enhanced CT or MRI scan
Active Alternatives—Most Common		
Hypoglycemia	Diabetes mellitus treated with either insulin, thiazolidinediones, or sulfonylureas	Glucose measurement at time of event
Cerebrovascular event (posterior circulation)	History of hypertension, atrial fibrillation, diabetes, tobacco use	CT scan MRI, MRA

CNS, central nervous system; EEG, electroencephalogram; MRA, magnetic resonance angiography.

any medications. She has no history of cerebrovascular disease, hypertension, or atrial fibrillation. She denies having any focal weakness, dysarthria, diplopia, or difficulty walking. She has no history of head trauma.

 Is the clinical information sufficient to make a diagnosis? If not, what other information do you need?

Leading Hypothesis: Seizures

Textbook Presentation

Generalized seizures classically present with tonic-clonic activity, loss of postural tone, incontinence, and a prolonged postictal period of lethargy. The purpose of this review is to focus on features that help distinguish seizures from syncope.

Disease Highlights

A. 3% of US population suffers a seizure in their lifetime

B. Seizures are the cause of syncope in 1–7% of patients.

C. Etiology of seizure and prevalence in patients over age 60

  1. Idiopathic, 35%

  2. Ischemic, 49%

  3. CNS tumor, 11%

    a. Primary, 35%

    b. Metastatic, 59%

  4. CNS trauma, 3%

  5. CNS infection, 2%

  6. Metabolic disturbances

    a. Hypoglycemia and hyperglycemia (marked)

    b. Hypoxia

    c. Hyponatremia

    d. Hypocalcemia

    e. Uremia

  7. Medications (Numerous medications have been implicated. Some commonly used medications that cause seizures (albeit rarely) include cyclosporine, fentanyl, meperidine, lidocaine, phenothiazines, quinolones, theophylline, tricyclic antidepressants, and bupropion.)

  8. Illicit drugs (ie, methylenedioxymethamphetamine [MDMA; Ecstasy], cocaine)

  9. Withdrawal states (ie, alcohol, baclofen, benzodiazepines, and opioids)

Evidence-Based Diagnosis

A. Postictal confusion is the most sensitive clinical feature (Table 31-7). The absence of a postictal period makes seizures an unlikely cause of syncope (sensitivity 94%, LR– 0.09).

 B. Tongue laceration, head turning, and unusual posturing are the most specific clinical features and substantially increase the likelihood of seizure (specificity 97%, LR+ 12–15).

C. Certain symptoms are unusual in patients with seizures and reduce the likelihood of seizure.

  1. Diaphoresis preceding spell, LR 0.17

  2. Chest pain preceding spell, LR 0.15

  3. Palpitations, LR 0.12

  4. Dyspnea prior to spell, LR 0.08

Table 31-7. Sensitivity, specificity, and LRs for seizures.

Clinical Feature	Sensitivity (%)	Specificity (%)	LR+	LR–
Cut tongue	45	97	15	0.57
Head turning	43	97	14	0.59
Unusual posturing	35	97	12	0.67
Bedwetting	24	96	6.4	0.79
Limb jerking noted by others	69	88	5.8	0.35
Prodromal trembling	29	94	4.8	0.76
Prodromal preoccupation	8	98	4.0	0.94
Prodromal hallucinations	8	98	4.0	0.94
Postictal confusion	94	69	3.0	0.09

Data from Sheldon Robert et al. Historical criteria that distinguish syncope from seizures. Journal of the American College of Cardiology 40:142–148. Copyright (c) 2002. With permission from American College of Cardiology Foundation

  5. CAD, LR 0.08

  6. Syncope with prolonged standing, LR 0.05

D. Convulsive syncope

  1. Limb jerking is not entirely specific for seizures.

  2. 15–90% of patients with syncope not related to seizures experience limb jerking, a phenomenon referred to as **convulsive syncope**. Limb jerking due to syncope is associated with myoclonic jerks, which should be distinguished from tonic-clonic activity.

    a. Myoclonic jerks tend to be arrhythmic and asymmetric, whereas the opposite is true of tonic-clonic activity.

    b. Myoclonic jerks tend to be briefer (average of 6.6 seconds) than tonic-clonic activity seen in seizures (≈ 1 minute)

    c. Myoclonic jerks never precede collapse, whereas tonic-clonic activity may precede collapse.

  3. Finally, unlike generalized seizures, which are usually associated with a significant postictal period, convulsive syncope is not associated with a significant postictal period (< 1 minute).

  4. Convulsive syncope has been reported in most diseases that cause syncope (cardiac arrhythmias (VT, WPW, heart block, long QT syndrome), aortic stenosis, carotid hypersensitivity, vasovagal syncope, and orthostatic hypotension.

  5. Patients who appear to have refractory "seizure disorders" and nonspecific abnormalities on electroencephalogram (EEG) should undergo a cardiac evaluation to rule out convulsive syncope with myoclonic jerks.

E. A point score to distinguish seizures from syncope has been developed (Table 31-8). Point scores of ≥ 1 suggest seizures (sensitivity, 94%; specificity, 94%; LR+, 16; LR–, 0.06).

F. Evaluation

  1. EEG

Table 31-8. A point score to distinguish seizures from syncope.[1]

Criteria	Points
Waking with cut tongue	2
Abnormal behavior (eg, limb jerking, prodromal trembling, preoccupation, hallucinations)	1
Lost consciousness with emotional stress	1
Postictal confusion	1
Head turning to 1 side	1
Prodromal déjà vu	1
Any presyncope	−2
Lost consciousness with prolonged standing	−2
Diaphoresis before a spell	−2

[1]Point scores of ≥ 1 suggest seizures.

  a. Indicated in the evaluation of patients with possible seizures
  b. Sensitivity (between episodes) of the spike and wave pattern is 35–50% (increased with sleep deprivation)
  c. Specificity 98%
2. Neuroimaging
  a. 37% of adults with new-onset seizures have structural lesions (eg, tumors, strokes)
  b. 15% of adults with new-onset seizures and nonfocal neurologic exams have structural lesions on neuroimaging.
  c. Indicated in all adults with new-onset seizures.
  d. In acute cases, a noncontrast CT is often performed to rule out an intracranial bleed. Follow-up MRI is recommended due to its increased sensitivity for both tumor and stroke.
3. Sodium, calcium, glucose, BUN, creatinine, and oxygen saturation should be measured.
4. Lumbar puncture
  a. A lumbar puncture should be considered if CNS infection is suspected (ie, patient is immunocompromised or has fever, meningismus, headache, or persistent confusion).
  b. Elevated intracranial pressure should be excluded prior to a lumbar puncture (usually with neuroimaging) in order to prevent lumbar puncture–induced herniation.
  c. Platelet count, prothrombin time, and partial thromboplastin time should be checked prior to lumbar puncture. (Thrombocytopenia and coagulopathies increase the risk of bleeding at the lumbar puncture site and subsequent spinal cord compression secondary to hemorrhage.)
5. Toxicology screen should be ordered if illicit drug use is suspected.
6. Elevated levels of serum neuron specific enolase can suggest generalized seizures versus other causes of syncope. Levels > 11.5 ng/mL had a sensitivity of 58%, specificity of 91%, an LR+ of 6.4, and LR– of 0.46.

7. Prolactin measurement: American Academy of Neurology concluded that serum prolactin levels cannot be used to distinguish seizures from syncope.

Treatment

Anticonvulsant therapy is complex and evolves rapidly (see neurology texts).

An EEG is ordered to evaluate the patient for possible seizures.

The patient's bruised tongue and postictal period strongly suggest seizures despite the lack of a previously known seizure disorder or witnesses to the event. You also wonder if an acute stroke is likely and if additional imaging of the extracranial or intracranial vessel is warranted.

Alternative Diagnosis: Cerebrovascular Disease & Syncope

Although physicians commonly consider carotid artery obstruction in the differential diagnosis of patients with syncope, unilateral obstruction of the carotid will not result in syncope. Therefore, *evaluation of the anterior circulation is not indicated in the patient with syncope.* On the other hand, obstruction of the posterior circulation may cause transient loss of consciousness by causing ischemia in the reticular activating system. This may occur in the subclavian steal syndrome, vertebrobasilar insufficiency, and basilar artery occlusion. These disorders are almost invariably associated with neurologic signs or symptoms and should be considered whenever patients have syncope and other symptoms referable to the brainstem (ie, diplopia, vertigo, ataxia, and weakness) (see Chapter 14, Dizziness). Finally, patients in whom subarachnoid hemorrhage develops can present with syncope. Such patients inevitably also complain of severe headache or confusion. Evaluation includes emergent noncontrast head CT scan.

MAKING A DIAGNOSIS

The patient's EEG revealed intermittent right temporal spike and wave pattern.

The EEG confirms new-onset seizures. Since structural lesions are common in adults with new-onset seizures, neuroimaging is required.

CASE RESOLUTION

An MRI scan revealed a solitary right temporal lobe mass. Subsequent biopsy demonstrated a glioblastoma multiforme. The patient underwent surgical resection and was treated with anticonvulsant therapy. She died approximately 6 months later.

CHIEF COMPLAINT

PATIENT 4

Mrs. P is a 39-year-old woman who arrives at the emergency department via ambulance with abdominal pain and syncope. She was in her usual state of health until the morning of admission when increasing left lower quadrant abdominal pain developed. The pain increased in intensity and became quite severe. Upon standing, she lost consciousness and collapsed to the floor. She recovered quickly and was helped to a chair by her husband. When she stood several minutes later, she briefly lost consciousness again. The patient reports that her abdominal pain is much better. She has no chest pain or dyspnea. Her vital signs are BP, 105/60 mm Hg; pulse, 85 bpm; temperature, 37.0°C; and RR, 18 breaths per minute. Her cardiac and pulmonary exams are normal, and abdominal exam reveals mild left lower quadrant tenderness. Her ECG is normal and her HCT is normal at 36.0%.

At this point, what is the leading hypothesis, what are the active alternatives, and is there a must not miss diagnosis? Given this differential diagnosis, what tests should be ordered?

RANKING THE DIFFERENTIAL DIAGNOSIS

As noted in Figure 31-1 the first step ascertains whether Mrs. P suffered from syncope or some other transient loss of consciousness. The history of rapid recovery without intervention, or history of trauma or intoxication, strongly suggests syncope. The next step considers whether this is likely due to reflex syncope, orthostatic syncope, or cardiac syncope. Several features of Mrs. P's syncope are noteworthy. First, her syncope occurred in association with abdominal pain raising the possibility of vasovagal syncope. Second, she had 2 episodes of syncope upon standing. This **pivotal clue** raises the possibility of orthostatic syncope from either dehydration, hemorrhage, medications, or autonomic dysfunction. Finally, cardiac syncope should be considered in all patients with syncope. Fortunately, Mrs. P has no prior history of heart disease that would increase the likelihood of cardiac syncope. Additionally, she has no suggestive symptoms (syncope with chest pain, syncope with exertion, syncope while supine, palpitations, or dyspnea), or risk factors (prior history of heart disease) or signs (significant murmur, gallop or JVD) to suggest cardiac syncope. Her ECG is also normal. The combination of the lack of underlying heart disease or suggestive symptoms of cardiac syncope, coupled with recurrent syncope immediately after standing makes orthostatic syncope likely and cardiac syncope unlikely. Table 31-9 lists the differential diagnosis.

4

Further history reveals that Mrs. P is not taking any medications. Your initial assessment is neurocardiogenic syncope secondary to transient abdominal pain.

As discussed in the first case presentation, vasovagal syncope is often precipitated by pain, is brief, and is followed by a rapid restoration of consciousness. Many of Mrs. P's features are consistent with this diagnosis. However, both episodes of syncope occurred

Table 31-9. Diagnostic hypotheses for Mrs. P.

Diagnostic Hypotheses	Demographics, Risk Factors, Symptoms and Signs	Important Tests
Leading Hypothesis		
Vasovagal syncope (faint)	Preceding pain, anxiety, fear or prolonged standing Rapid normalization of consciousness Absence of heart disease	Tilt table if recurrent
Active Alternatives—Most Common		
Orthostatic hypotension: (Dehydration)	History of vomiting, diarrhea, decreased oral intake	Orthostatic measurement of BP and pulse
Orthostatic hypotension: (Hemorrhage)	Melena, bright red blood per rectum or other blood loss Abdominal trauma, risk factors for AAA Unprotected intercourse in reproductive age women	Orthostatic measurement of BP and pulse CBC Beta HCG
Orthostatic hypotension: (Medications)	History of alpha-blockers, other antihypertensive medication	Orthostatic measurement of BP and pulse
Orthostatic hypotension: (autonomic dysfunction)	History of Parkinson disease, multisystem atrophy, diabetes mellitus, or advanced age	Orthostatic measurement of BP and pulse (hypotension frequently associated with inadequate rise in pulse)
Active Alternatives—Must Not Miss		
PE	Risk factors for PE Pleuritic chest pain or dyspnea Loud S_2 Unexplained persistent hypotension Right heart strain on ECG (right bundle-branch block, right axis deviation) or right ventricular dilatation on echocardiogram	CT angiogram Ventilation-perfusion scan Leg venous duplex Angiogram

AAA, abdominal aortic aneurysm; BP, blood pressure; CBC, complete blood cell; ECG, electrocardiogram; HCG, human chorionic gonadotropin; PE, pulmonary embolism.

immediately after standing providing a clue that her syncope was in fact orthostatic. In addition, although her abdominal pain is improved, it is still unexplained. You elect to check her BP and pulse for orthostatic change.

Mrs. P's BP while supine was 105/60 mm Hg with a pulse of 85 bpm, which changed when sitting to BP of 95/50 mm Hg with a pulse of 90 bpm. Upon standing her BP fell to 60/0, her pulse was 140 bpm, and she lost consciousness. She was quickly laid down and again rapidly regained consciousness.

The patient's volume status is always assessed utilizing clinical, **not just laboratory** findings. Orthostatic measurement of BP and pulse are critical. Life-threatening hypovolemia may be overlooked if the BP and pulse are not measured while the patient is standing.

Mrs. P's profound drop in BP upon standing and recurrent syncope is a key **pivotal clue** and clearly indicate that she is syncopal due to orthostatic hypotension. This is not consistent with reflex syncope. You revise the leading hypothesis to syncope due to orthostatic hypotension.

Is the clinical information sufficient to make a diagnosis? If not, what other information do you need?

Leading Hypothesis: Orthostatic Hypotension

Textbook Presentation

Orthostatic hypotension commonly presents with syncope or other symptoms (near syncope, visual blurring, weakness, leg buckling) when arising. Orthostatic hypotension should be distinguished from orthostatic dizziness, which describes *symptoms* on standing which may or may not be secondary to orthostatic hypotension. (Orthostatic dizziness may also be secondary to visual disturbances.) Patients with orthostatic hypotension often have obvious sources of fluid or blood loss. Common causes include vomiting, diarrhea, inadequate fluid intake, or GI bleeding (presenting as hematemesis, melena, or bright red blood per rectum). Importantly, orthostatic hypotension may develop secondary to massive but occult internal bleeding (rupture of abdominal aortic aneurysm, splenic rupture, retroperitoneal hemorrhage, or ruptured ectopic pregnancy). Finally, orthostatic hypotension may occur without volume loss, particularly in the elderly. Common causes include drugs and neurologic disorders.

Disease Highlights

A. Orthostatic hypotension occurs in 20% of patients over 75 and accounts for 12–30% of patients with syncope.

B. Etiology

   1. Hypovolemia

      a. Dehydration

         (1) Decreased oral intake

         (2) GI losses (vomiting, diarrhea)

         (3) Urinary losses

            (a) Uncontrolled diabetes mellitus

            (b) Salt losing nephropathy

            (c) Adrenal insufficiency

      b. Hemorrhage

         (1) GI

         (2) Ruptured abdominal aortic aneurysm

         (3) Ruptured spleen

         (4) Ruptured ectopic pregnancy

      c. Over-dialysis

      d. Postprandial hypotension, particularly common in the elderly and worse with large carbohydrate meals or alcohol ingestion. Splanchnic pooling decreases venous return.

      e. Hot environments (hot tubs, baths, saunas)

   2. Medications

      a. Alpha-blockers

      b. Diuretics

      c. Vasodilators (ie, nitrates, calcium channel blockers, hydralazine)

      d. ACE inhibitors and angiotensin receptor blockers (ARBs)

      e. Tricyclic antidepressants

      f. Phenothiazines and selective serotonin reuptake inhibitors

      g. Sildenafil and other phosphodiesterase inhibitors particularly when combined with nitrates

      h. Alcohol and opioids

   3. Autonomic insufficiency (characterized by a fall in BP upon standing *without* a concomitant increase in pulse)

      a. Central neurologic disorders (ie, Parkinson disease, multisystem atrophy, pure autonomic failure, multiple sclerosis, and numerous others)

      b. Peripheral neurologic disorders: Diabetes mellitus, vitamin B_{12} deficiency, uremia, and other causes of autonomic neuropathies

      c. Prolonged bed rest

Evidence-Based Diagnosis

A. Definition of orthostatic hypotension

   1. ≥ 20 mm Hg decrease in systolic BP within 3 minutes of standing; a decrease in systolic BP of ≥ 30 mm Hg may be a more appropriate criterion in patients with hypertension

   2. > 10 mm Hg decrease in diastolic BP within 3 minutes of standing

   3. Or > 30 bpm increase in pulse within 3 minutes of standing

B. The presence of orthostatic hypotension does not confirm that syncope was secondary to orthostatic hypotension. Syncope from orthostatic hypotension should be diagnosed in patients with orthostatic hypotension *and* syncope or presyncope on standing.

C. Orthostatic hypotension associated with volume loss (dehydration or hemorrhage)

   1. Several studies assessed the impact of phlebotomy on volunteers. Phlebotomy removed a moderate (450–630 mL) to large (630–1150 mL) volume of blood.

    a. An increase in pulse of > 30 bpm with standing is both highly sensitive for large volume blood loss (97%) and highly specific (98%, LR+ 48) (Table 31-10). The sensitivity falls dramatically if the patient sits instead of stands (39–78%).

      b. Simple supine measurements of BP and pulse were not sensitive for even large blood loss (sensitivity 12–33%).

Table 31-10. Accuracy of physical exam for *large* blood loss (630–1150 mL).

Clinical Finding	Sensitivity	Specificity	LR+	LR−
Postural increase in pulse > 30 bpm	97%	98%	48.0	0.03
Supine pulse > 100 bpm	12%	96%	3.0	0.9
Supine hypotension < 95 mm Hg	33%	97%	11.0	0.7

Data from McGee S, Abernethy WB 3rd, Simel DL. Is this patient hypovolemic? JAMA. 1999;281:1022–9.

c. Any abnormal finding on orthostatic maneuvers strongly suggested volume loss (specificity 94–98%; LR+, 3.0–48).

d. The sensitivity of orthostatic measurements is greatest if the supine and standing BPs are compared. If the supine BP is not measured, 67% of orthostatic patients may not be identified.

e. Patients should stand for 1 minute before the measurement of the upright BP.

f. No measure was very sensitive for moderate blood loss (0–27%).

2. Profound blood loss may occasionally paradoxically produce bradycardia. (The reduction in end-systolic volume may trigger the neurally mediated reflex.)

3. The admission HCT does not accurately reflect the severity of acute hemorrhage. A fall in HCT may take 24–72 hours.

4. A history of nausea, vomiting, diarrhea, or inadequate intake can suggest volume depletion that is supported by elevations in BUN, creatinine and/or low urinary Na+, FE_{Na+} or FE_{urea}.

Treatment

A. Acute blood loss: Blood transfusion is appropriate in the orthostatic patient with acute blood loss.

B. Dehydration (diarrhea, vomiting, or decreased oral intake)

1. Patients able to tolerate oral intake: oral rehydration

2. Patients unable to tolerate oral intake: IV hydration

a. Normal saline is preferred.

b. Usually 500 mL to 1 L boluses are given over 1 hour.

c. Smaller boluses may be given to fragile patients (ie, small elderly women or those with a history of kidney disease or HF).

d. Repeat orthostatic BP measurements are made following each bolus as well as a lung and cardiac exam to ensure the patient has not received excessive fluid.

e. Bolus therapy should be continued until orthostatic hypotension resolves.

C. Chronic orthostatic hypotension

1. Hydration (water, soup, or sports drinks)

2. Discontinue offending medications (diuretics, alpha-blockers, nitrates, tricyclic antidepressants, phenothiazines).

3. Patients are advised to arise slowly (sitting on the side of the bed, prior to standing), avoid large meals and excessive heat, and use waist high support hose.

4. Support stockings to the waist and exercise programs can be helpful.

5. Alpha-agonists (ie, midodrine) have also been used successfully. Side effects include urinary retention, hypertension, and worsening HF.

6. Other drugs that have been used with less conclusive evidence include fludrocortisone, nonsteroidal antiinflammatory drugs, caffeine, and erythropoietin in anemic patients.

MAKING A DIAGNOSIS

Mrs. P reports that she has not suffered from any diarrhea or vomiting and has taken in normal amounts of fluid. She denies any hematemesis, melena, or bright red blood per rectum.

It is important to remember that Mrs. P presented with syncope *and* abdominal pain. Although the pain has improved, it has not resolved; it may provide an important clue to the underlying etiology. Given the profound orthostatic hypotension and the lack of external blood or volume loss, or incriminating medication, internal bleeding must be considered as a source of her abdominal pain and syncope. In the differential diagnosis you consider splenic rupture, ruptured abdominal aortic aneurysm, and ruptured ectopic pregnancy. The lack of trauma argues against splenic rupture and the patient's age and gender are atypical for abdominal aortic aneurysm. You wonder if in fact she has suffered from a ruptured ectopic pregnancy.

It is important to remember the patient's chief complaint because it usually holds the most important clue to the diagnosis.

CASE RESOLUTION

Mrs. P reports that she missed her last menstrual period. An abdominal ultrasound is performed and reveals 750 mL of fluid (presumed to be blood) in the pelvis. A urine pregnancy test is positive.

Although the final diagnosis of ectopic pregnancy was not considered initially, a careful clinical exam confirmed orthostatic syncope. Once that pivotal clue was discovered, the differential diagnosis could be narrowed and the underlying cause determined. It is instructive to note that her initial HCT was normal because the remaining intravascular blood had not yet been diluted by any oral or IV fluids.

Initial HCT measurements will not accurately reflect the magnitude of blood loss in a patient with recent hemorrhage.

Mrs. P had 2 large bore IVs placed and was typed and crossed for RBC transfusions. CBC, prothrombin time, partial thromboplastin time, and platelet counts were measured and a 1 L bolus of normal saline was given while waiting for the packed RBCs. After volume and blood resuscitation, she underwent surgical exploration and removal of her ruptured fallopian tube.

REVIEW OF OTHER IMPORTANT DISEASES

Aortic Stenosis

Textbook Presentation

Aortic stenosis is usually diagnosed incidentally during routine exam rather than due to symptoms. Typically, aortic stenosis produces a loud crescendo-decrescendo systolic murmur at the right second intercostal space, which may radiate to the neck. When aortic stenosis becomes severe, patients may have any of the 3 cardinal symptoms: HF (dyspnea, typically with exertion), syncope, or angina.

Disease Highlights

A. Thickening and calcification of valve leaflets results in **progressive** obstruction to blood flow.

B. LVH develops to compensate for the obstruction.

C. Pathophysiology of symptoms is shown in Figure 31-8.

D. Prevalence is 3% in patients ≥ 75 years old.

E. Etiology
1. Degeneration of a previously normal valve
2. Congenital bicuspid valve
   a. 1–2% of population is born with congenital bicuspid valve.
   b. Severe aortic stenosis develops in 66% of patients and at an earlier age than in patients with tricuspid valves.
   c. Aortic root structure is usually abnormal and often associated with progressive dilation of the aortic root that may require repair to prevent rupture or dissection.
3. Rheumatic heart disease

F. Severe aortic stenosis is characterized by valve area < 1 cm or mean aortic valve gradient > 40 mm Hg. Gradients may be lower in patients with a low cardiac output.

G. Prognosis: Mortality increases markedly when symptoms develop (HF, angina, or syncope). The most common symptoms are decreased exercise tolerance and dyspnea on exertion. Mortality for symptomatic patients not undergoing valve replacement:
1. Aortic stenosis and angina: 50% 5-year mortality
2. Aortic stenosis and syncope: 50% 3-year mortality
3. Aortic stenosis and dyspnea: 50% 2-year mortality

H. Other late manifestations:
1. Atrial fibrillation may develop. This is often poorly tolerated because the LV is noncompliant and dependent on atrial contraction for filling.
2. An increased bleeding tendency secondary to disruption of large von Willebrand multimers by the abnormal aortic valve.

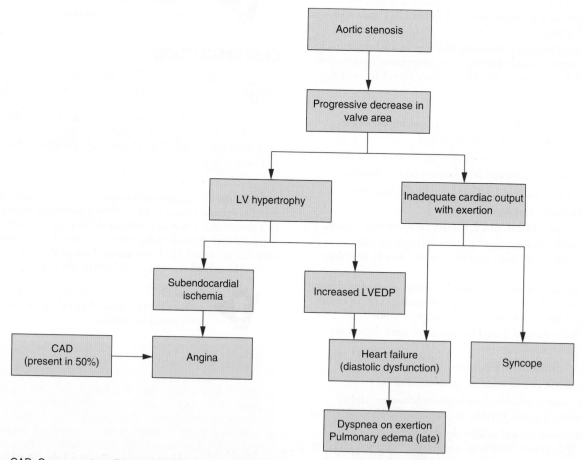

CAD, Coronary artery disease; LV, left ventricular; LVEDP, left ventricular end-diastolic pressure.

Figure 31-8. Pathophysiology of symptoms in aortic stenosis.

Evidence-Based Diagnosis

A. History and physical exam: Most studies demonstrate only a fair reproducibility between examiners.

1. Findings that help **rule in** aortic stenosis

    a. Effort syncope in patients with a systolic murmur (LR+ 1.3–∞, LR− 0.76)

    b. Slow carotid upstroke (sensitivity, 15–42%; specificity, 95–100%; LR+ 9.2–∞)

    c. Murmur radiating to right carotid (sensitivity, 71–73%; specificity, 90%; LR+ 7.5)

2. Findings that help **rule out** aortic stenosis

    a. Absence of any murmur (LR− 0.0)

    b. Absence of murmur below right clavicular head (LR− 0.1)

3. Murmurs may be less intense in patients with superimposed HF.

B. Doppler echocardiogram

1. The initial test of choice to assess for aortic stenosis

2. Recommended for patients with a systolic murmur ≥ grade III/VI

3. Aortic stenosis is graded as mild if the valve area is > 1.5 cm^2, moderate if the valve area is 1–1.5 cm^2, severe if the valve area < 1.0 cm^2 and critical if the valve area is < 0.8 cm^2.

4. Surveillance echocardiography is recommended to monitor progression (every 6 months for severe aortic stenosis, and every year for mild to moderate aortic stenosis associated with significant calcification). Echocardiography is also recommended for any change in symptoms or signs and during pregnancy.

5. Patients with bicuspid aortic valves and aortic stenosis or dilation of the aortic root (> 40 mm) should have annual echocardiography. In patients without stenosis or dilatation, echocardiography is recommended every 2 years.

Treatment

A. Since the prognosis changes markedly in symptomatic patients, patients with severe asymptomatic aortic stenosis should be reevaluated every 6 months and queried about HF symptoms, angina, or syncope. Patients should also be instructed to report new symptoms.

B. Symptomatic patients should undergo mechanical correction, not medical therapy.

C. While awaiting surgery, patients with HF symptoms may be treated cautiously with diuretics, ACE inhibitors, and digoxin (if there is systolic dysfunction).

D. Mechanical correction:

1. Valve replacement is guided almost exclusively by symptoms.

2. Definite indications for valve replacement

    a. Severe aortic stenosis in **symptomatic** patients

    b. Severe aortic stenosis in **asymptomatic** patients undergoing coronary artery bypass surgery, other valve surgery, or surgery on the ascending aorta.

    c. Severe aortic stenosis in asymptomatic patients with ejection fraction < 50%.

3. Standard preoperative evaluation includes angiography in many patients to determine whether the patient needs concomitant coronary artery bypass surgery. This includes patients with symptoms of CAD or CAD risk factors (including men ≥ 35, postmenopausal women, or premenopausal women ≥ 35 with CAD risk factors).

4. Mechanical and bioprosthetic valves have been used.

    a. Mechanical valves have greater durability and a significantly lower rate of failure and need for replacement. They are associated with a lower all-cause mortality than bioprosthetic valves.

    b. Mechanical valves are associated with an increased risk of thromboembolism and infection. Vitamin K antagonists (target INR 2.5) are recommended. In addition to warfarin, aspirin is recommended at 50–100 mg/day for patients at low risk for bleeding.

    c. Bioprosthetic valves

    (1) Reserved for patients who have a contraindication to warfarin therapy or who are noncompliant.

    (2) May be used in patients over 65 (whose life expectancy makes the need for a second replacement unlikely).

    (3) Aspirin 50–100 mg/day recommended.

    d. Another alternative is the Ross procedure in which the pulmonary valve is removed and used as the aortic valve. The pulmonary artery is reconstructed to create the pulmonary valve. The survival of these grafts is good and patients do not require anticoagulation therapy. In-hospital surgical mortality may be higher with this procedure.

5. Recent experience has increased with transcatheter aortic valve implantation (TAVI).

    a. An option for patients who are not surgical candidates (note that age alone is not a contraindication to aortic valve replacement).

    b. Superior to medical management in nonoperable patients with severe symptomatic aortic stenosis. Mortality was reduced (absolute risk reduction 20%, NNT 5) although strokes increased (absolute increased risk 5%, NNH 20)

    c. Comparable in mortality and stroke rate to aortic valve replacement in patients with a high surgical risk. TAVI is associated with higher rates of major vascular complications but lower rates of major bleeding and shorter hospital stays. Indications and patient selection are actively evolving.

6. Balloon valvotomy is a poor option.

    a. Provides only temporary relief (6–12 months) and does not improve survival.

    b. Complications occur in > 10%.

    c. Reserved for palliation in patients with other serious (or lethal) comorbidities and as a bridge to TAVI or aortic valve replacement in patients who are hemodynamically unstable or require urgent major noncardiac surgery.

    d. An exception to this may be the young adult with noncalcific aortic stenosis in whom balloon valvotomy is a viable option.

E. Vigorous exercise should be discouraged in patients with moderate to severe aortic stenosis.

Situational Syncope

A variant of reflex syncope, situational syncope occurs during or immediately after micturition, defecation, swallowing, or coughing which increase vagal tone.

Carotid Sinus Syndrome

Textbook Presentation

Carotid sinus syndrome (CSS) is another variant of reflex syncope. Patients typically complain of syncope or falls that may be precipitated by pressure applied to the carotid (eg, head turning, buttoning collar, shaving, or cervical motion) or occur spontaneously.

Disease Highlights

A. Carotid sinus hypersensitivity (CSH) represents a syndrome of increased carotid sensitivity with resultant bradycardia, hypotension, or both.

B. Increasingly common in the elderly in whom it may account for 15% of recurrent syncopal events. Unusual in patients < 40 years old.

C. 15–56% of affected patients complain of falls but deny syncope.

   1. May be due to retrograde amnesia or alternatively hypotension that is insufficient to maintain an upright posture but sufficient to avoid frank loss of consciousness.

   2. CSS present in 19–27% of patients with unexplained falls but 0% in patients with accidental falls.

 Consider CSS in elderly patients with unexplained falls.

Evidence-Based Diagnosis

A. CSH should be distinguished from CSS.

   1. CSH refers to a significant drop in pulse (≥ 3-second pause) or systolic BP (≥ 50 mm Hg drop in BP) accompanying pressure on the carotid artery. CSS is diagnosed in patients with CSH *and* spontaneous syncope.

   2. CSH occurs in 35% of asymptomatic elderly patients without prior falls, dizziness, or syncope.

   3. Given the frequency of CSH in an asymptomatic population, care must be taken before ascribing the cause of syncope to CSH.

   4. CSS occurs in only 5% of elderly patients without prior falls, dizziness, or syncope, suggesting it is a more specific finding than CSH alone.

B. 47% of patients report symptoms precipitated by head movement of looking upward.

C. Carotid sinus massage is used in the diagnosis of CSS.

   1. Carotid sinus massage is applied (unilaterally) for 5–10 seconds during continuous ECG and BP monitoring. Carotid sinus massage needs to be performed on each side separated in time by ≥ 1 minute and in the supine and then upright position.

   2. The inhibitory response is unilateral in 81% of patients.

   3. 30–50% of patients have findings only when upright.

D. Carotid sinus massage is contraindicated in patients with carotid bruits, recent cerebrovascular accident or transient ischemic attack within the last 3 months, MI (within 6 months), or severe dysrhythmias.

E. Carotid sinus massage has been complicated by transient and permanent neurologic symptoms in 0.3% and 0.05% of patients, respectively.

Treatment

Pacemakers are indicated in syncopal patients with cardioinhibitory CSS with documented symptomatic asystole of ≥ 3 sec with carotid sinus massage in whom they have been demonstrated to reduce the incidence of subsequent syncope and falls.

Wolff-Parkinson-White (WPW) Syndrome

Textbook Presentation

WPW syndrome may be asymptomatic or present with palpitations, near syncope, syncope, or sudden death. In asymptomatic cases, the diagnosis may only be made after typical findings are discovered on an ECG performed for some other reason.

Disease Highlights

A. A congenital disorder in which an accessory bundle directly connects the atria and ventricular muscle bypassing the AV node.

B. A variety of life-threatening arrhythmias may develop that may cause syncope or sudden cardiac death. These include

   1. Antidromic tachycardia in which an impulse spreads down the accessory pathway and then back up the His-Purkinje system in a retrograde fashion. This reentrant loop can result in rapid tachycardias, hypotension, syncope, and sudden death.

   2. The reentrant loop may run in the opposite direction (orthodromic tachycardia, Figure 31-9).

   3. Finally, atrial fibrillation or flutter can develop. In patients with atrial fibrillation or flutter, the accessory pathway facilitates rapid conduction of the atrial tachycardia into the ventricles allowing rapid ventricular depolarization and putting patients at risk for syncope or sudden death.

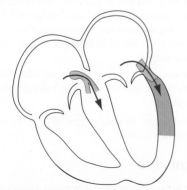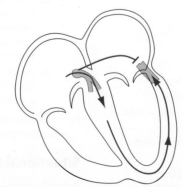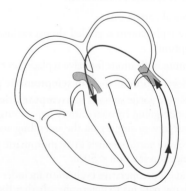

Figure 31-9. Orthodromic tachycardia in patients with the Wolff-Parkinson-White syndrome. Reproduced, with permission, from McPhee SJ. *Pathophysiology of Disease*, 5th edition. McGraw-Hill, 2006.

C. Syncope in patients with WPW is associated with a greater frequency (25%) of rapid, life-threatening, conduction over the accessory pathway.

Evidence-Based Diagnosis

A. Baseline ECG abnormalities during normal sinus rhythm may reveal a combination of a short PR interval and a delta wave.

1. Short PR interval

   a. In healthy persons, the normal PR interval is produced by a built-in delay at the AV node (designed to allow atrial emptying prior to ventricular systole).

   b. In WPW syndrome, the accessory pathway bypasses the AV node and initiates ventricular depolarization without such a delay; this results in a shortened PR interval in 75% of patients (Figure 31-10).

2. Delta wave

   a. In most patients with WPW syndrome, the accessory pathway inserts directly into ventricular muscle (rather than into the specialized His-Purkinje system).

   b. Ventricular depolarization spreads slowly from cell to cell through gap junctions, rather than rapidly through the specialized His-Purkinje conduction system.

   c. This results in slow ventricular depolarization and the slow initial upstroke of the QRS complex known as the delta wave (Figure 31-10).

   d. Finally, as this ventricular depolarization progresses, the AV node is also processing the supraventricular impulse. Eventually, the impulse passes through the AV node, activates the His-Purkinje system and causes rapid

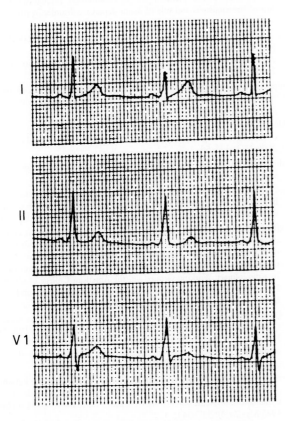

Figure 31-10. Electrocardiographic features of the Wolff-Parkinson White-syndrome. Reproduced, with permission, from Fuster V. *Hurst's The Heart,* 12th edition. McGraw-Hill, 2008.

depolarization. This results in a narrow *terminal* portion of the QRS complex.

Treatment

A. Risk stratification

1. Stress tests can provide prognostic information

   a. In certain patients, the accessory pathways cannot conduct at rapid heart rates (due to a long refractory period) and the patients are at low risk for life-threatening arrhythmia from WPW.

   b. Stress tests can monitor for loss of conduction during rapid heart rates. Patients whose surface ECG demonstrates clear loss of conduction down the bypass tract at rapid heart rates (normalization of the PR interval and loss of the delta wave) are unlikely to suffer from rapid WPW related arrhythmias.

   c. Patients whose bypass tract continues to conduct at rapid heart rates are at greater risk for rapid life-threatening arrhythmias and are candidates for more extensive evaluation with EP studies.

2. EP studies can be useful for diagnosis, prognosis, and therapy.

   a. EP studies can confirm the presence of a bypass tract.

   b. EP studies can measure the conduction characteristics of the bypass tract to determine if it can sustain rapid life-threatening arrhythmias.

   c. Radiofrequency ablation can obliterate the bypass tract in high-risk patients.

   d. An EP studies is typically offered to the following patients:

   (1) Symptomatic patients (eg, history of tachycardia, syncope, or sudden death)

   (2) Patients with structural heart disease who are at a higher risk for atrial fibrillation

   (3) Healthy patients whose stress test does not demonstrate loss of preexcitation at rapid heart rates.

B. Treatment

1. Immediate management: A variety of options exist for patients with acute WPW-related arrhythmias, including electrical cardioversion and pharmacotherapy. The choice of pharmacotherapy is dependent on the mechanism of the tachycardia. Consultation is recommended.

2. Long-term management

   a. Long-term therapeutic options include pharmacologic therapy and radiofrequency catheter ablation of the bypass tract.

   b. Radiofrequency ablation can be performed if the risk of rapid tachycardias is high.

   c. Consultation is recommended.

REFERENCES

Alboni P, Brignole M, Menozzi C et al. Diagnostic value of history in patients with syncope with or without heart disease. J Am Coll Cardiol. 2001;37(7):1921–8.

Anpalahan M, Gibson S. The prevalence of Neurally Medicated Syncope in older patients presenting with unexplained falls. Eur J Intern Med. 2012;23:e48–e52.

Bell WR, Simon TL, DeMets DL. The clinical features of submassive and massive pulmonary emboli. Am J Med. 1977;62(3):355–60.

Birnbaum A, Esses D, Bijur P, Wollowitz A, Gallagher EJ. Failure to validate the San Francisco Syncope Rule in an independent emergency department population. Ann Emerg Med. 2008;52:151–9.

Bonow RO, Carabello BA, Chatterjee K, et al; 2006 Writing Committee Members; American College of Cardiology/American Heart Association Task Force.

2008 Focused update incorporated into the ACC/AHA 2006 guidelines for the management of patients with valvular heart disease: a report of the American College of Cardiology/American Heart Association Task Force on Practice Guidelines (Writing Committee to Revise the 1998 Guidelines for the Management of Patients With Valvular Heart Disease): endorsed by the Society of Cardiovascular Anesthesiologists, Society for Cardiovascular Angiography and Interventions, and Society of Thoracic Surgeons. Circulation. 2008;118:e523–e661.

Calkins H, Shyr Y, Frumin H, Schork A, Morady F. The value of the clinical history in the differentiation of syncope due to ventricular tachycardia, atrioventricular block, and neurocardiogenic Syncope. Am J Med. 1995;98:365–73.

Calvo-Romero JM, Perez-Miranda M, Bureo-Dacal P. Syncope in acute pulmonary embolism. Eur J Emerg Med. 2004;11(4):208–9.

Castelli R, Tarsia P, Tantardini C, Pantaleo G, Guariglia A, Porro F. Syncope in patients with pulmonary embolism: comparison between patients with syncope as the presenting symptom of pulmonary embolism and patients with pulmonary embolism without syncope. Vasc Med. 2003;8(4):257–61.

Colman N, Nahm K, van Dijk JG, Reitsma JB, Wieling W, Kaufmann H. Diagnostic value of history taking in reflex syncope. Clin Auton Res. 2004;14 Suppl 1:37–44.

Colman N, Bakker A, Linzer M, Reitsma JB, Wieling W, Wilde AA. Value of history-taking in syncope patients: in whom to suspect long QT syndrome. Europace. 2009;11:937–43.

Davies AJ, Steen N, Kenny RA. Carotid sinus hypersensitivity is common in older patients presenting to an accident and emergency department with unexplained falls. Age Ageing. 2001;30:289–93.

Del Rosso A, Ungar A, Maggi R et al. Clinical predictors of cardiac syncope at initial evaluation in patients referred urgently to a general hospital: the EGSYS score. Heart. 2008;94:1620–6.

Elliott PM MW. Clinical manifestations of hypertrophic cardiomyopathy. In: UpToDate; 2006.

Epstein AE, DiMarco JP, Ellenbogen KA et al. ACC/AHA/HRS 2008 Guidelines for Device-Based Therapy of Cardiac Rhythm Abnormalities: a report of the American College of Cardiology/American Heart Association Task Force on Practice Guidelines (Writing Committee to Revise the ACC/AHA/NASPE 2002 Guideline Update for Implantation of Cardiac Pacemakers and Antiarrhythmia Devices): developed in collaboration with the American Association for Thoracic Surgery and Society of Thoracic Surgeons. Circulation. 2008;117(21):e350–408.

Etchells E, Bell C, Robb K. Does this patient have an abnormal systolic murmur? JAMA. 1997;277(7):564–71.

Etchells E, Glenns V, Shadowitz S, Bell C, Siu S. A bedside clinical prediction rule for detecting moderate or severe aortic stenosis. J Gen Intern Med. 1998;13(10):699–704.

European Heart Rhythm Association; Heart Rhythm Society, Zipes DP, Camm AJ, Borggrefe M et al; American College of Cardiology; American Heart Association Task Force; European Society of Cardiology Committee for Practice Guidelines. ACC/AHA/ESC 2006 guidelines for management of patients with ventricular arrhythmias and the prevention of sudden cardiac death: a report of the American College of Cardiology/American Heart Association Task Force and the European Society of Cardiology Committee for Practice Guidelines (Writing Committee to Develop Guidelines for Management of Patients With Ventricular Arrhythmias and the Prevention of Sudden Cardiac Death). J Am Coll Cardiol. 2006;48(5):e247–346.

Gersh BJ, Maron BJ, Bonow RO et al. 2011 ACCF/AHA Guideline for the Diagnosis and Treatment of Hypertrophic Cardiomyopathy: Executive Summary: A Report of the American College of Cardiology Foundation/American Heart Association Task Force on Practice Guidelines. Circulation. 2011;124:2761–96.

Goldberger ZD, Rho RW, Page L. Approach to the diagnosis and initial management of the stable adult patient with a wide complex tachycardia. Am J Cardiol. 2008;101:1456–66.

Graf D, Schlaepfer J, Gollut E et al. Predictive models of syncope causes in an outpatient clinic. Int J Cardiol. 2008;123:249–56.

Grubb BP. Clinical practice. Neurocardiogenic syncope. N Engl J Med. 2005;352(10):1004–10.

Joint Task Force on the Management of Valvular Heart Disease of the European Society of Cardiology (ESC); European Association for Cardio-Thoracic Surgery (EACTS), Vahanian A, Alfieri O, Andreotti F et al. Guidelines on the management of valvular heart diseases (version 2012). Eur Heart J. 2012;33:2451–96.

Kerr SR, Pearce MS, Brayne C, Davis RJ, Kenny RA. Carotid sinus hypersensitivity in asymptomatic older persons. Implications for diagnosis of syncope and falls. Arch Intern Med. 2006;166:515–20.

Lakdawala NK, Thune JJ, Maron BJ et al. Electrocardiographic features of sarcomere mutation carriers with and without clinically overt hypertrophic cardiomyopathy. Am J Cardiol. 2011;108:1606–13.

Lembo NJ, Dell'Italia LJ, Crawford MH, O'Rourke RA. Bedside diagnosis of systolic murmurs. N Engl J Med. 1988;318(24):1572–8.

Maron BJ, McKenna WJ, Danielson GK et al; American College of Cardiology/European Society of Cardiology clinical expert consensus document on hypertrophic cardiomyopathy. A report of the American College of Cardiology Foundation Task Force on Clinical Expert Consensus Documents and the European Society of Cardiology Committee for Practice Guidelines. J Am Coll Cardiol. 2003;42(9):1687–713.

McDermott D, Quinn JV, Murphy CE. Acute myocardial infarction in patients with syncope. CJEM. 2009;11(2):156–60.

McGee S, Abernethy WB 3rd, Simel DL. The rational clinical examination. Is this patient hypovolemic? JAMA. 1999;281(11):1022–9.

McKeon A, Vaughan C, Delanty N. Seizure versus syncope. Lancet Neurol. 2006;5(2):171–80.

Mitro P, Kirsch P, Valočik G, Murín P. Clinical history in the diagnosis of the cardiac syncope––the predictive scoring system. Pacing Clin Electrophysiol. 2011;34:1480–5.

Moya A, Brignole M, Menozzi C, et al; International Study on Syncope of Uncertain Etiology (ISSUE) Investigators. Mechanism of syncope in patients with isolated syncope and in patients with tilt-positive syncope. Circulation. 2001;104:1261–7.

Nishimura RA, Holmes DR Jr. Clinical practice. Hypertrophic obstructive cardiomyopathy. N Engl J Med. 2004;350(13):1320–7.

O'Mahony C, Tome-Esteban M et al. A validation study of the 2003 American College of Cardiology/European Society of Cardiology and 2011 American College of Cardiology Foundation/American Heart Association risk stratification and treatment algorithms for sudden cardiac death in patients with hypertrophic cardiomyopathy. Heart. 2013;99:534–41.

Pezawas T, Stix G, Kastner J, Schneider B, Wolzt M, Schmidinger H. Implantable loop recorder in unexplained syncope: classification, mechanism, transient loss of consciousness and role of major depressive disorder in patients with and without structural heart disease. Heart. 2008;94:e17.

Russo AM, Stainback RF, Bailey SR et al. ACCF/HRS/AHA/ASE/HFSA/SCAI/SCCT/SCMR 2013 appropriate use criteria for implantable cardioverter-defibrillators and cardiac resynchronization therapy. Heart Rhythm. 2013;10(4):1–48.

Schnipper J, Ackerman RH, Krier JB, Honour M. Diagnostic yield and utility of neurovascular ultrasonography in the evaluation of patients with syncope. Mayo Clin Proc. 2005;80(4):480–8.

Sheldon R, Rose S, Connolly S, Ritchie D, Koshman ML, Frenneaux M. Diagnostic criteria for vasovagal syncope based on a quantitative history. Eur Heart J. 2006;27(3):344–50.

Sheldon R, Rose S, Ritchie D et al. Historical criteria that distinguish syncope from seizures. J Am Coll Cardiol. 2002;40(1):142–8.

Solano A, Menozzi C, Maggi R et al. Incidence, diagnostic yield and safety of the implantable loop-recorder to detect the mechanism of syncope in patients with and without structural heart disease. Eur Heart J. 2004;25:1116–9.

Strickberger SA, Benson DW, Biaggioni I et al. AHA/ACCF Scientific Statement on the evaluation of syncope: from the American Heart Association Councils on Clinical Cardiology, Cardiovascular Nursing, Cardiovascular Disease in the Young, and Stroke, and the Quality of Care and Outcomes Research Interdisciplinary Working Group; and the American College of Cardiology Foundation: in collaboration with the Heart Rhythm Society: endorsed by the American Autonomic Society. Circulation. 2006;113(2):316–27.

Task Force for the Diagnosis and Management of Syncope; European Society of Cardiology (ESC); European Heart Rhythm Association (EHRA);Heart Failure Association (HFA); Heart Rhythm Society (HRS); Moya A, Sutton R, Ammirati F et al. Guidelines for the diagnosis and management of syncope (version 2009). Eur Heart J. 2009;30:2631–71.

Warren J. The Effect of Venesection and the Pooling of Blood in the Extremities on the Atrial Pressure and Cardiac Output in Normal Subjects with Observations on Acute Circulatory Collapse in Three Instances. J Clin Invest. 1945 May;24(3): 337–344.

I have a patient with unintentional weight loss. How do I determine the cause?

CHIEF COMPLAINT

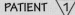

PATIENT 1

Mrs. M is an 85-year-old woman who comes to the office complaining of weight loss. She is quite concerned that she has something dreadful.

 What is the differential diagnosis of unintentional weight loss? How would you frame the differential?

CONSTRUCTING A DIFFERENTIAL DIAGNOSIS

Significant unintentional weight loss is defined as > 5% loss of usual body weight in the last 6–12 months. Significant unintentional weight loss can be a harbinger of serious underlying disease. One study documented significantly increased mortality in men with unintentional weight loss compared with men whose weight was stable or increased (36% vs ≈15%).

There are a large number of diseases that can cause unintentional weight loss, which are best organized by system (see below). The 4 most common causes of unintentional weight loss are cancer (most commonly gastrointestinal [GI] but also lung, lymphoma, and other malignancies), ≈29%; depression and alcoholism, 16%; nonmalignant GI diseases, 13%; and unknown, 22%. Endocrine disorders account for 7% of unintentional weight loss. Although cancer is the most common cause, it is not the cause in most patients. Dementia may also cause weight loss due to a combination of increased energy expenditure (due to agitation and pacing) and decreased caloric intake.

Three **pivotal points** are worth remembering when evaluating patients with unintentional weight loss (Figure 32-1). First, the weight loss should be documented, because 25–50% of patients that complain of unintentional weight loss, have not in fact lost weight (and do not need to be evaluated). Elderly adults often lose muscle mass and simply look like they lost weight. Weight loss should be documented by comparing prior weights or, if these are unavailable, by finding a significant decrease in a patient's clothing size.

 Clinicians should verify the weight loss or document significant changes in the patient's clothing or belt size.

Second, patients should be asked about diarrhea or other symptoms of malabsorption, including large, difficult to flush or malodorous stools. Such symptoms suggest small bowel or pancreatic disease and direct the diagnostic search.

Third, obtain a truly comprehensive history (including a psychosocial history and medication history) and perform a detailed head to toe physical exam and a baseline laboratory evaluation to search for any subtle diagnostic clues that may help focus the evaluation. Basic labs should include a CBC with differential, urinalysis, renal panel, calcium, liver panel, fasting glucose, fecal occult blood test (FOBT), erythrocyte sedimentation rate (ESR), thyroid-stimulating hormone (TSH), HIV and chest radiograph. Additionally, health examinations should be brought up to date (eg, mammogram, Papanicolaou exam, colonoscopy, and low-dose chest CT scan for smokers with ≥ 30 pack year smoking history unless they quit > 15 years previously.)

Abnormal findings discovered on history, physical exam, or initial labs are rarely diagnostic but often provide critical clues to the underlying diagnosis and should be thoroughly evaluated. Examples of such findings include anemia, which may be due to iron deficiency from an unsuspected carcinoma of the colon or stomach; an elevated alkaline phosphatase, which may be due to metastatic disease to the liver or bones; hematuria, which may be due to carcinoma of the kidney or bladder; or a markedly elevated ESR, which may be due to multiple myeloma, temporal arteritis, subacute bacterial endocarditis (SBE), or other chronic infection.

Patients without any such clues may benefit from an upper endoscopy and an abdominal ultrasound.

Differential Diagnosis of Involuntary Weight Loss

The differential diagnosis of weight loss is extensive and best organized by system.

A. Cardiovascular
   1. Heart failure (severe)
   2. SBE

B. Endocrine
   1. Adrenal insufficiency
   2. Diabetes mellitus
   3. Hyperthyroidism

C. GI (organized from mouth to rectum)
   1. Poor dentition (50% of patients edentulous by age 65)
   2. Anosmia
   3. Esophageal disorders
      a. Esophageal stricture or web
      b. Dysmotility
      c. Esophageal cancer
   4. Gastric disorders
      a. Peptic ulcer disease (PUD)
      b. Gastric cancer
      c. Gastroparesis
      d. Gastric outlet obstruction

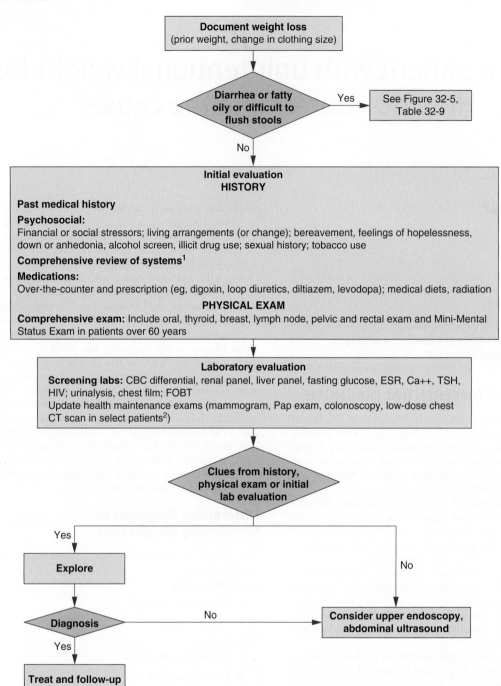

Document weight loss
(prior weight, change in clothing size)

Diarrhea or fatty
oily or difficult to
flush stools — Yes → See Figure 32-5,
Table 32-9

No

Initial evaluation
HISTORY

Past medical history

Psychosocial:
Financial or social stressors; living arrangements (or change); bereavement, feelings of hopelessness, down or anhedonia, alcohol screen, illicit drug use; sexual history; tobacco use

Comprehensive review of systems¹

Medications:
Over-the-counter and prescription (eg, digoxin, loop diuretics, diltiazem, levodopa); medical diets, radiation

PHYSICAL EXAM
Comprehensive exam: Include oral, thyroid, breast, lymph node, pelvic and rectal exam and Mini-Mental Status Exam in patients over 60 years

Laboratory evaluation
Screening labs: CBC differential, renal panel, liver panel, fasting glucose, ESR, Ca++, TSH, HIV; urinalysis, chest film; FOBT
Update health maintenance exams (mammogram, Pap exam, colonoscopy, low-dose chest CT scan in select patients²)

Clues from history,
physical exam or initial
lab evaluation

Yes — No

Explore

Diagnosis — No → **Consider upper endoscopy, abdominal ultrasound**

Yes

Treat and follow-up

¹Includes:
Cardiovascular: Shortness of breath, orthopnea, dyspnea on exertion, history of valvular heart disease or endocarditis
Endocrine: Heat intolerance, tremulousness, palpitations, polyuria, polydipsia
Gastrointestinal: Altered taste, smell, ill-fitting dentures, odynophagia, dysphagia, abdominal pain, NSAID use, early satiety, nausea, vomiting, diarrhea, difficult to flush stools, jaundice, dark urine, history of hepatitis, change in bowel habits, constipation, hematochezia, melena
Hematologic: Lymph node swelling, night sweats
Infectious: Fever, chills, rash
Neurologic: Impaired memory, headaches, resting tremor, history of stroke
Respiratory: Cough, hemoptysis, severe dyspnea, PPD or IGRA +, foreign born
Renal: History of renal disease, pruritus
Rheumatologic: Joint or muscle pain, rash, alopecia

²USPSTF 2013 recommends annual low-dose chest CT scans for patients 55–80 with ≥30-pack year smoking history who currently smoke or quit ≤15 years previously)

CBC, complete blood cell; ESR, erythrocyte sedimentation rate; FOBT, fecal occult blood test; Pap, Papanicolaou; TSH, thyroid-stimulating hormone.

Figure 32-1. Diagnostic approach: unintentional weight loss.

5. Small bowel diseases
   a. Mesenteric ischemia
   b. Crohn disease
   c. Celiac sprue
   d. Bacterial overgrowth syndromes
   e. Lactose intolerance
6. Pancreatic disease
   a. Acute pancreatitis
   b. Chronic pancreatitis
   c. Pancreatic insufficiency
   d. Pancreatic cancer
7. Hepatic disease
   a. Hepatitis
   b. Cholelithiasis
   c. Cirrhosis
   d. Hepatocellular carcinoma
8. Colonic diseases
   a. Chronic constipation
   b. Colon cancer
9. Chronic GI infections
   a. *Giardia lamblia*
   b. *Clostridium difficile*
   c. *Entamoeba histolytica*

D. Hematologic/oncologic
   1. Lung cancer
   2. Pancreatic cancer
   3. GI cancers
   4. Lymphoma
   5. Miscellaneous others

E. Infectious: HIV infection or complications

F. Neurologic
   1. Dementia
   2. Stroke
   3. Parkinson disease

G. Psychiatric
   1. Depression
   2. Anxiety
   3. Bipolar
   4. Schizophrenia

H. Psychosocial
   1. Poverty (15% of patients over age 65 live below the poverty line)
   2. Isolation
   3. Immobility or inadequate transportation
   4. Alcoholism

I. Renal/metabolic
   1. Uremia
   2. Hypercalcemia

J. Respiratory
   1. Chronic obstructive pulmonary disease (severe)
   2. Tuberculosis

K. Rheumatologic
   1. Polymyalgia rheumatica
   2. Temporal arteritis
   3. Rheumatoid arthritis
   4. Systemic lupus erythematosus

L. Miscellaneous
   1. Drugs (eg, digoxin, loop diuretics, diltiazem, levodopa, metformin, opiates, selective serotonin reuptake inhibitors [SSRIs], and many others)
   2. Medical diets
   3. Radiation
   4. Chronic pain

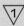

Mrs. M reports that she has lost weight over the last 6 months and notes that her appetite is not as good as previously. She does not weigh herself and is unsure of how many pounds she has lost.

 At this point, what is the leading hypothesis, what are the active alternatives, and is there a must not miss diagnosis? Given this differential diagnosis, what tests should be ordered?

RANKING THE DIFFERENTIAL DIAGNOSIS

The patient's history is typical of many patients complaining of weight loss. Patients report an unspecified amount of weight loss, associated with anorexia. The first pivotal step in the evaluation is to verify that weight loss did in fact occur.

Mrs. M is new to the clinic and prior weights are unavailable. While Mrs. M does not know how many pounds she has lost, she does report that her clothes are much too loose. Indeed, she has needed to buy clothes 2 sizes smaller.

Mrs. M's change in clothing size suggests true and significant weight loss. The second pivotal step in evaluating patients with documented weight loss determines whether the patient has symptoms suggestive of diarrhea or malabsorption.

Mrs. M does reports that she moves her bowels once every day or every other day. She notes no diarrhea, no difficult to flush stools, and no change in her bowel habits over the last several years.

Since the history does not suggest diarrhea or malabsorption, the third pivotal step in the evaluation of patients with unintentional weight loss is a comprehensive, system-based approach utilizing a thorough history, (including a past medical history, detailed psychosocial history, and review of systems), physical exam, basic laboratory exams and completion of her health maintenance examinations.

Mrs. M's past medical history is unremarkable. Her psychosocial history is also unrevealing. She lives with her husband and denies difficulty obtaining or cooking food. She never smoked tobacco and drinks alcohol rarely. The review of systems is negative in detail.

On physical exam, Mrs. M looks quite cachectic. She appears apathetic. Her vital signs are normal. HEENT exam reveals no oral lesions or adenopathy. Lungs are clear to percussion and auscultation. Cardiac exam reveals a regular rate and rhythm, with a grade I–II flow systolic murmur along the left sternal border. Her abdomen is scaphoid, without hepatosplenomegaly or mass. Rectal exam reveals guaiac-negative stool. Neurologic exam is normal, including a Mini-Mental State Exam.

Is the clinical information sufficient to make a diagnosis? If not what other information do you need?

Unfortunately, like many patients with unintentional weight loss, Mrs. M has no specific clues to suggest any particular diagnosis. Given her cachectic appearance and recognizing that cancer is the most common cause of unintentional weight loss and a must not miss hypothesis, it is the leading hypothesis. Her apathetic appearance also raises the possibility of depression. Finally, nonmalignant GI disease should also be considered since it is also a common cause of unintentional weight loss. Hyperthyroidism seems unlikely given her sluggish demeanor. Table 32-1 lists her differential diagnosis.

Leading Hypothesis: Cancer Cachexia

Textbook Presentation

Patients with cancer cachexia often have advanced disease. They suffer from anorexia, fatigue, and other symptoms specific to their particular malignancy. The cancer may have been diagnosed before the weight loss or the weight loss may lead to the diagnosis.

Disease Highlights

A. Cancer diagnoses account for ≈ 29% of cases of unexplained weight loss.

B. The most common malignancies associated with weight loss are GI, lung, and lymphoma.

C. Weight loss is 1 of the most common presenting symptoms in patients with lung cancer (comparable to cough). It is more frequent than dyspnea, hemoptysis, or chest pain.

D. Unintentional weight loss is common in cancer patients. At the time of diagnosis, 24% of patients with cancer have lost weight.

E. Patients with unintentional weight loss due to cancer have a higher 2-year mortality than patients with unintentional weight loss due to unknown causes (62% vs 18%).

F. Weight loss increases the risk of immobility, deconditioning, and adversely affects immunity. The risk of pulmonary embolism, pressure ulcers, and pneumonia are increased.

Evidence-Based Diagnosis

A. Patient estimation of weight loss

   1. In patients who overestimated their weight loss (by more than 0.5 kg), cancer was unlikely (6%) and no organic cause was found in 73%.

Table 32-1. Diagnostic hypotheses for Mrs. M.

Diagnostic Hypotheses	Demographics, Risk Factors, Symptoms and Signs	Important Tests
Leading Hypothesis		
Cancer		
Stomach	Early satiety	EGD or upper GI
Colon	Change in stools Hematochezia Positive FOBT, iron deficient anemia	Colonoscopy
Lung	Cough, hemoptysis Tobacco use	Chest radiograph, chest CT scan
Pancreas	Abdominal pain Jaundice, dark urine (bilirubinuria)	Abdominal ultrasound or CT scan
Active Alternatives—Most Common		
Depression	History of loss, personal or family history of depression, postpartum state, > 6 somatic symptoms, overestimation of weight loss	Complaints of feeling down or anhedonia
Nonmalignant GI disease		
Dental	New ill-fitting dentures	
Esophageal disease	Dysphagia	EGD or upper GI
PUD	Epigastric pain, early satiety, nausea, melena, NSAID or aspirin use	EGD H pylori breath test or stool antigen
Active Alternatives—Most Common		
Hyperthyroidism	Increased sweating Nervousness, goiter, tachycardia, atrial fibrillation, lid lag or stare, fine tremor, hyperactive reflexes, exophthalmos	TSH

EGD, esophagogastroduodenoscopy; FOBT, fecal occult blood test; GI, gastrointestinal; TSH, thyroid-stimulating hormone.

   2. In patients who underestimated their weight loss (by more than 1 kg), cancer was diagnosed in 52%.

B. Several studies have evaluated the history, physical exam, and initial laboratory studies to aid in the detection of cancer in patients with unintentional weight loss.

C. Laboratory studies usually included a CBC, chemical survey (including glucose, calcium, blood urea nitrogen [BUN], creatinine, and liver function tests), HIV when appropriate, ESR, TSH, urinalysis, and chest radiograph. Several of these studies also incorporated abdominal ultrasound.

D. Further work-up was dictated by abnormalities detected in the initial evaluation. (For instance, GI evaluation with endoscopy and colonoscopy would be initiated in patients with GI complaints or iron deficiency anemia; hepatobiliary and pancreatic imaging would be done in those with abdominal pain or abnormal liver function tests, etc).

1. Cancer was detected in 28% of patients in these studies.

2. The battery was 93% sensitive for the detection of cancer in patients with unintentional weight loss.

3. Only 2.6% of patients with a normal evaluation had occult cancer.

Treatment

A. Nutritional support

1. In many patients, artificial nutritional support is not effective.

2. Certain subgroups of patients may benefit from nutritional support.

   a. Head and neck cancer (after radiation therapy)

   b. Bowel obstruction

   c. Surgery patients (particularly upper GI tract cancer)

   d. Patients receiving high-dose chemotherapy

3. Enteral support is appropriate if the bowel is functional and always preferred if feasible

B. Treat underlying malignancy

C. Medroxyprogesterone and megestrol

1. Decreases nausea and anorexia and increases weight gain

2. May increase the risk of thromboembolic events

3. Other side effects include hyperglycemia, endometrial bleeding, edema, hypertension, and adrenal suppression and insufficiency

D. Corticosteroids

1. Decrease anorexia and nausea

2. Increase appetite, quality of life, and feeling of well-being

3. Because of the side effects, corticosteroids are often reserved for patients with terminal disease.

E. A variety of other medications have been tried with limited to no success.

1. Prokinetic drugs (metoclopramide) can decrease anorexia and nausea but did not increase appetite or caloric intake.

2. The cannabinoid dronabinol was less effective than progestins.

3. Other agents under study include gherlin, melatonin, ATP infusions, and oxandrolone.

MAKING A DIAGNOSIS

Clearly, a diagnosis is not yet apparent on history or physical exam. The data suggest that when the cause of unintentional weight loss is malignant, there are usually clues on history, physical exam, or on laboratory testing. You elect to check a CBC, liver panel, renal panel, urinalysis, chest radiograph, and screening mammogram. Finally, you elect to schedule Mrs. M for a colonoscopy, since she has never undergone colon cancer screening.

Surprisingly, Mrs. M's laboratory evaluation is strikingly normal. Her CBC is normal without evidence of iron deficiency anemia (which could have suggested gastric or colon cancer). The chest radiograph is also normal, making lung cancer unlikely, particularly in a patient who never smoked.

ALT (SGPT), AST (SGOT), alkaline phosphatase, and bilirubin were normal (an elevation can suggest hepatic metastasis or obstruction due to pancreatic cancer), and her renal panel is normal. Her HIV and FOBT are negative and there was no hematuria on urinalysis (which could suggest renal cell carcinoma or bladder cancer). Her mammogram and colonoscopy were normal.

Have you crossed a diagnostic threshold for the leading hypothesis, cancer cachexia? Have you ruled out the active alternatives? Do other tests need to be done to exclude the alternative diagnoses?

Alternative Diagnosis: Depression

Textbook Presentation

Depression may follow a recognizable loss or occur without a clear precipitant. Classically, patients complain of profound sadness, lack of interest in activities (anhedonia), sleep and appetite disturbances, impaired concentration, and other symptoms. Patients may lose or gain weight. Patients may experience suicidal or homicidal thoughts.

Disease Highlights

A. Point prevalence of major depressive disorder (MDD) is 5–13%. Lifetime prevalence 16.2%. Minor depression is twice as common.

B. Depression is the second most common condition seen in primary care practices and the fourth leading cause of disability.

C. Recurrences are common, up to 50% in 1 year. Many patients require lifelong therapy.

D. Risk factors for major depression

1. Prior episode of depression

2. Postpartum period

3. Comorbid medical illness

4. Older age (including concomitant neurologic disease)

5. Chronic pain

6. Absence of social support

7. Female sex (2–3 times more common than in males)

8. Family history (first-degree relative)

9. Stressful life events

10. Substance abuse

11. Unemployment and low socioeconomic status

E. Associated anxiety: 50% of patients have anxiety symptoms

1. 10–20% of patients with MDD have evidence of panic disorder and 30–40% have evidence of generalized anxiety disorder.

2. Patients with anxiety and MDD are at higher risk for suicide.

F. Minor depression

1. 10–18% progress to major depression within 1 year.

2. 20% have moderate to severe disability.

Evidence-Based Diagnosis

A. The DSM-V criteria for MDD requires 5 of the following 9 criteria (1 of which is depressed mood or anhedonia) for at least 2 weeks:

1. Depressed mood most of the day, nearly every day

2. Anhedonia with "marked diminished interest or pleasure in all or almost all activities"

3. Significant appetite or weight change (> 5% of body weight in 1 month not associated with dieting)

4. Sleep disturbance (insomnia or hypersomnia)

5. Psychomotor agitation or retardation

6. Fatigue

7. Feelings of worthlessness or excessive or inappropriate guilt

8. Impaired concentration

9. Suicidal ideation

B. These criteria must be associated with significant distress or impaired functioning and not be secondary to substance abuse or another medical condition; in addition, there should be no prior history of mania (which would be diagnostic of a bipolar disorder).

C. Minor depression requires 2–4 of the above symptoms, including anhedonia or depressed mood for > 2 weeks.

D. Severity can be estimated using the Hamilton Rating Depression Scale. Scores of ≤ 18 are classified as mild to moderate, 19–22 as severe, and ≥ 23 as very severe depression.

E. The sadness that accompanies major loss (grief), as in bereavement, may be difficult to distinguish from MDD and the 2 may coexist. Profound sadness, anorexia, insomnia, and weight loss may occur. Features that suggest grief (rather than MDD) include

1. The ability to have periods of happiness or pleasure in grief that is often absent in MDD.

2. Sadness in grief is often episodic rather than pervasive and constant.

3. In grief, the focus of sadness is typically on loss rather than self-loathing or worthlessness seen in MDD.

F. Screening

1. Depression is often missed on routine evaluation. In patients in whom depression was subsequently diagnosed, only 8.8% were found to be depressed during routine interview.

2. Screening tools increase identification of patients with depression by 2- to 3-fold (an absolute increase of 10–47%). Furthermore, screening coupled with treatment decreases clinical morbidity.

3. Screening is recommended by the US Preventive Services Task Force (USPSTF).

4. 2 screening questions perform as well as more complex tools (a positive response to either question is considered positive).

   a. "Over the past 2 weeks, have you felt down, depressed, or hopeless?"

   b. "Over the past 2 weeks, have you felt little interest or pleasure in doing things?"

   c. Sensitivity, 96–97%; specificity, 57–67%; LR+, 2.2–2.9; LR–, 0.04–0.07

   d. Patients with a positive response to either question should undergo a full diagnostic evaluation to determine if they meet diagnostic criteria for depression and to exclude a history of mania.

5. Clinical clues that might suggest a patient is depressed include

   a. Recent stress or loss

   b. Chronic medical illness, chronic pain syndromes

   c. > 6 physical symptoms

d. Higher patient ratings of symptom severity

e. Lower patient rating of overall health

f. Physician perception of encounter as difficult

g. Substance abuse (23% have MDD)

h. The patient appears more functionally restricted than explained by their medical illness.

i. The language used to describe their condition is extreme (terrible, unbearable, etc).

j. Sleep disturbances

k. Even in patients with depression, care must be taken before ascribing weight loss solely to depression. Many medical illnesses that cause weight loss are also associated with depression (eg, 20–45% of patients with cancer are depressed, and 40% of patients with Parkinson disease are depressed).

 The diagnosis of depression does not exclude other serious illnesses causing unintentional weight loss. Patients should be monitored to ensure weight gain following treatment of their depression.

Treatment

A. Work-up should include a full psychosocial history, including degree of functional impairment, history of domestic violence, and a drug history to look for agents that can worsen or precipitate depression (alcohol, interferon, L-dopa, corticosteroids, oral contraceptives, propranolol, cocaine).

B. Patients should be screened for a history of manic symptoms that suggest bipolar illness (periods of reduced need for sleep, impulsivity, euphoric mood, racing thoughts, increased sexual activity, and grandiosity).

C. Screening tests (ie, TSH, basic metabolic panel, liver function tests, CBC) are recommended to rule out medical conditions (eg, hypothyroidism) that can simulate or cause depression.

D. Assess suicide risk: Ideation, intent, or plan

1. Have you been having thoughts of dying?

2. Do you have a plan?

3. Does patient have the means (eg, weapons) to succeed?

4. Other risk factors include

   a. Older men

   b. Psychotic symptoms

   c. Alcohol or illicit substance abuse

   d. History of prior attempts

   e. Family history of suicide or recent exposure to suicide

5. Risk factors for suicide attempts in blacks included young age (OR 9.4), less than high school education (OR 3.6), mood disorder (OR 3.8), anxiety disorder (OR 6.0), and substance abuse (OR 4.5).

6. Emergent psychiatric evaluation should be performed in patients with risk factors for suicide, who appear intoxicated, who cannot contract for safety, or have poor social support.

E. Pharmacotherapy

1. Based on the number of symptoms *and* functional impairment

2. *Not* influenced by whether or not there is well-defined precipitant (ie, stress). Therapy should be strongly considered in grieving patients with persistent symptoms of MDD for more than 2 months after a loss.

3. Multiple classes of medications are effective: SSRIs, serotonin and norepinephrine reuptake inhibitors (SNRIs), tricyclic antidepressants (TCAs), and monoamine oxidase inhibitors (MAOIs).

4. A patient level meta-analysis reported that pharmacotherapy was more effective (compared with placebo) in patients with increasingly severe depression. The benefit is most marked in patients with very severe depression (Hamilton Depression Rating Scale ≥ 25). The numbers needed to treat are 16, 11, and 4 for patients with mild to moderate, severe, and very severe depression, respectively.

5. SSRIs are often used as first-line agents due to low frequency of adverse effects and safety in overdose. SSRIs and SNRIs may cause sexual dysfunction. Venlafaxine (an SNRI) can be lethal in overdose.

6. Caution is recommended in the use of SSRIs in certain age groups:
   a. The USPSTF concluded that fair evidence suggests that SSRIs increase suicidal behaviors in patients 18–29 years of age, especially those with MDD who receive paroxetine (OR 6.7; CI, 1.1–149.4). The risk was highest in the first month of treatment.
   b. The USPSTF also concluded that there is fair evidence that SSRIs increase the risk of upper GI bleeding, particularly in adults over 70.
   c. For those age groups, alternative medications or psychotherapy may be preferred.

7. Mirtazapine may be useful in patients with weight loss and insomnia and bupropion may be useful in patients with daytime lethargy and fatigue.

8. TCAs frequently cause troubling anticholinergic side effects, significant weight gain (> 20 lbs) and are dangerous in overdose, so they are used less often. High-dose TCAs may increase the risk of sudden cardiac death.

9. MAOIs interact with a variety of tyramine-containing foods and medications and may precipitate a hypertensive crisis. Typically, only psychiatrists prescribe these.

10. Patients with a prior history of manic symptoms should be referred for psychiatric evaluation prior to the institution of antidepressant therapy. Antidepressant therapy can trigger mania.

11. Continue treatment for 6–9 months *after* clinical recovery.

12. Patients with multiple recurrences (≥ 2–3) may require lifetime therapy.

F. Psychotherapy
   1. Equally effective as pharmacotherapy in patients with mild to moderate depression. Options include cognitive behavioral therapy, problem solving therapy, and interpersonal psychotherapy.
   2. Less effective than pharmacotherapy in patients with severe depression. Combined psychotherapy and pharmacotherapy may be the best option.

G. Exercise programs may be helpful in older adults with mild to moderate depression.

H. Electroconvulsive therapy (ECT) is an alternative therapy for patients with severe, refractory depression, particularly those with psychotic or suicidal features.

I. Indications for referral include psychotic features; substance abuse; panic disorder; agitated, severe, or relapsing depression; bipolar features; suicidality; and dysthymia.

Mrs. M reports no unusual stresses or losses. She lives with her husband, regularly sees her daughter and other family members, and remains actively involved in her church. She denies feeling down, depressed or hopeless in the last month and denies loss of interest or pleasure in doing things.

Mrs. M's answers to the screening questions make depression highly unlikely (LR– 0.07). Although her appearance seems antithetical to hyperthyroidism, you wonder if that possibility should be pursued.

Alternative Diagnosis: Hyperthyroidism

Textbook Presentation

Classically, patients with hyperthyroidism present with a myriad of symptoms and signs obvious to the experienced observer. Symptoms include palpitations, heat intolerance, increased sweating, insomnia, tremulousness, diarrhea, and *weight loss*. Signs of hyperthyroidism include sinus tachycardia, systolic hypertension, frightened stare, an enlarged goiter, a fine resting tremor, and exophthalmos (only if hyperthyroidism is secondary to Graves disease). Other manifestations may include hyperpigmentation, irregular menses, pruritus, and thinning of hair. Complications include osteoporosis, tracheal obstruction (from the goiter), tachyarrhythmias (particularly atrial fibrillation), high output heart failure, anemia, and proximal muscle weakness.

Disease Highlights

A. Prevalence, 0.3%.

B. Hyperthyroidism is actually an endocrine syndrome caused by several distinct pathophysiologic entities (Table 32-2).

Evidence-Based Diagnosis

A. History and physical exam

1. Certain findings of hyperthyroidism are quite specific (ie, lid lag and lid retraction) and help rule in the diagnosis (specificity, 99%; LR+, 17–32).

2. Clinical findings are not highly sensitive. Therefore, absent clinical findings do not rule out hyperthyroidism.
   a. Goiter is present in 70–93% of cases.
   b. Pulse > 90 bpm is present in 80% of cases.
   c. Lid lag is present in 19% of cases.
   d. Ophthalmopathy is present in 25–50% of patients with Graves disease.
   e. Hyperreflexia is variable depending on the age of the patient (see below).

B. Elderly patients
   1. Prevalence of hyperthyroidism in elderly is 2–3%.
   2. Hyperthyroidism often presents atypically in elderly patients. Expected adrenergic findings are often absent, whereas atrial fibrillation is more common, resulting in the phenomenon referred to as *apathetic hyperthyroidism of elderly*. Table 32-3 compares the findings in young and older patients with hyperthyroidism.

Consider hyperthyroidism in elderly patients with weight loss (OR 8.7), tachycardia (OR 11.2), atrial fibrillation, or apathy (OR 14.8). Hyperthyroidism was not even considered in 54% of admitted patients in whom hyperthyroidism was subsequently diagnosed.

Table 32-2. Distinguishing features of several hyperthyroid states.

Disease	Pathogenesis/Important features	TSH	T4, free T4 or T3	Thyroid Scan and Other Tests
Graves disease	Autoimmune production of antibody (TSI) binds and stimulates TSH receptor Exophthalmos (unilateral or bilateral) unique to Graves	↓	↑	Homogenously increased uptake Elevated TSI
Toxic multinodular goiter	Most common form in elderly	↓	↑	Patchy increased uptake
Painful subacute thyroiditis	Viral or immune inflammatory attack on thyroid resulting in neck pain, tenderness, fever and release of hormone	↓	↑	Decreased uptake Elevated ESR
Toxic adenoma	Autonomously functioning benign thyroid nodule	↓	↑	Hot nodule, uptake in rest of gland is suppressed
Iodine or amiodarone	Amiodarone[1] may cause the release of T4 and T3	↓	↑	Usually decreased uptake
TSH-producing pituitary adenoma	Autonomously functioning benign *pituitary* adenoma May cause bitemporal hemianopsia Galactorrhea develops in 33% of women	↑	↑	Diffusely increased uptake
Factitious or iatrogenic	Self or physician induced	↓	↑	Decreased uptake T4/FTI more elevated than T3 Thyroglobulin concentration low

[1]Amiodarone causes *hypothyroidism* in 20% of patients by impairing conversion of T4 to T3.
ESR, erythrocyte sedimentation rate; FTI, free thyroxine index; TSI, thyroid stimulating immunoglobulin.

C. Laboratory tests

1. TSH is the test of choice (in the absence of pituitary disease) (sensitivity > 99%, specificity > 99%, LR+ > 99, LR– < .01).

   a. Low TSH indicates hyperthyroidism.

   b. Normal TSH indicates euthyroidism.

   c. High TSH indicates hypothyroidism.

Table 32-3. Sensitivity of findings in patients with hyperthyroidism.

Signs and Symptoms	Patients Aged 70 Years or Older	Patients Aged 50 Years or Younger
Sinus tachycardia	41%	94%
Atrial fibrillation	35–54%	2%
Fatigue	56%	84%
Anorexia	32–50%	4%
Weight loss	50–85%	51–73%
Goiter	50%	94%
Ophthalmopathy	6%	46%
Tremor	44–71%	84–96%
Nervousness	31%	84%
Hyperactive reflexes	28%	96%
Increased sweating	24–66%	92–95%
Heat intolerance	15%	92%

2. Exception occurs when the pituitary itself is diseased (rare).

   a. Pituitary adenomas can produce TSH causing hyperthyroidism with increased TSH and free T4.

   b. Pituitary destruction (eg, sarcoidosis) results in hypothyroidism with decreased TSH and free T4.

3. T4 measurements

   a. The total T4 measures the total thyroid hormone in the serum, including both the free T4 and T4 bound to thyroid-binding globulin (TBG).

   b. Free T4 (FT4) is active and more accurately reflects thyroid activity than the total T4.

   c. The free T4 can be measured directly or estimated by the FTI.

   d. Many conditions alter the TBG and total T4. However, they do not affect the FTI level (or free T4), and patients remain euthyroid. (For example, pregnancy raises the TBG and total T4; however, the FTI and free T4 are normal and the patient is euthyroid.)

4. Occasionally, patients with hyperthyroidism have isolated elevations in T3, or T3 thyrotoxicosis. In such patients, the TSH is still suppressed.

5. An approach to thyroid function tests is shown in Figure 32-2.

6. Established hyperthyroidism

   a. Certain features can help distinguish the *etiology* of hyperthyroidism, including thyroid-stimulating immunoglobulin and radioactive iodine uptake scan (see Table 32-2).

   b. Doppler flow can be useful in patients unable to undergo the radioactive uptake scan. Increased flow correlates with increased uptake.

   c. Women of child-bearing years should have a pregnancy test performed prior to iodine scanning or instituting therapy.

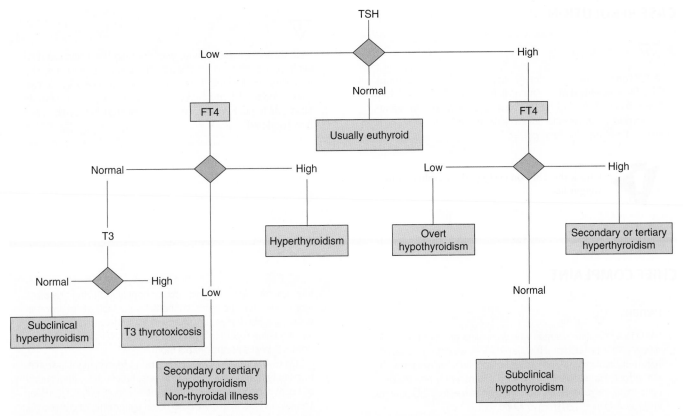

TSH, thyroid-stimulating hormone.

Figure 32-2. Diagnosis of thyroid function disorders. (Reproduced, with permission, from Muller AF. Thyroid function disorders. Neth J Med. 2008;66(3):134–42.)

d. Imaging with ultrasound or occasionally CT scan or MRI can be useful in patients with large goiters, particularly if there is a suggestion of airway obstruction.

Treatment

A. Beta-blockers can be used to decrease the sympathetic stimulation and the tremor, tachycardia, palpitations, and sweating.

B. Definitive treatment of hyperthyroidism depends on underlying etiology.

1. Graves disease or toxic multinodular goiter: Options include antithyroid drugs, radioactive iodine or surgery. Consultation is advised.

   a. Antithyroid drugs (methimazole, carbimazole and propylthiouracil)

      (1) Act rapidly

      (2) May cause agranulocytosis (0.1–0.3%)

      (3) ≈ 40% of patients relapse

      (4) Requires frequent monitoring

      (5) Methimazole is preferred over propylthiouracil due its more rapid onset of action and lower incidence of hepatotoxicity. However, propylthiouracil is preferred for women in their first trimester of pregnancy or patients in thyroid storm.

   b. Radioactive iodine

      (1) Used successfully for over 60 years.

      (2) ≈ 21% relapse rate

      (3) Pretreatment with antithyroid drugs is advised for some patients.

      (4) Contraindications include pregnancy, lactation, and severe ophthalmopathy.

      (5) Results in permanent hypothyroidism and the requirement for lifelong thyroid hormone replacement.

   c. Surgery

      (1) Occasionally used, particularly if the goiter is troublesome.

      (2) Pretreatment with antithyroid drugs is advised for some patients.

      (3) Results in permanent hypothyroidism and the requirement for lifelong thyroid hormone replacement.

      (4) Complications may include hypoparathyroidism, recurrent laryngeal nerve damage, and postoperative thyroid storm.

2. Subacute thyroiditis

   a. Aspirin or nonsteroidal antiinflammatory drugs (NSAIDs) decrease thyroid inflammation. Prednisone can be used in severe cases.

   b. Hyperthyroidism is usually transient and does not require antithyroid drugs. Beta-blockers are used to decrease symptoms of hyperthyroidism until inflammation subsides.

   c. Transient mild hypothyroidism may develop as the thyroiditis resolves. Occasionally, treatment with levothyroxine is required.

CASE RESOLUTION

A TSH on Mrs. M is completely suppressed (< 0.1 mcU/mL). The T4 is elevated at 20 mcg/dL (nl 5–11.6) and the free T4 is 3.6 (nl 0.0–1.8 ng/L). You diagnose hyperthyroidism. A thyroid scan reveals heterogeneous uptake consistent with a toxic multinodular goiter.

 Check the TSH on every patient evaluated for weight loss.

Due to her advanced age, you elect to have her treated with radioactive iodine. Six months later she returns; she is taking replacement levothyroxine for the radioactive iodine–induced hypothyroidism. Laboratory exam reveals that she is euthyroid. She complains that her clothes are now too tight.

CHIEF COMPLAINT

PATIENT 2

Mr. O is a 55-year-old man who complains of weight loss. He reports that he has tried for years to lose weight (unsuccessfully) but that recently he has lost more and more weight without effort. He was initially pleased but recently has become concerned. He reports that altogether he has lost 30 pounds in the last 6 months (from 200 lbs to 170 lbs).

 At this point, what is the leading hypothesis, what are the active alternatives, and is there a must not miss diagnosis? Given this differential diagnosis, what tests should be ordered?

RANKING THE DIFFERENTIAL DIAGNOSIS

As noted above the first pivotal step in the evaluation of unintentional weight loss is to verify the weight loss. Mr. O has clearly suffered from verifiable significant unintentional weight loss. The second pivotal step in the evaluation of patients with *documented* weight loss is to determine whether or not the patient is having symptoms that suggest diarrhea or malabsorption.

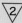

Mr. O reports no diarrhea, large foul-smelling stools, or difficult to flush stools. He reports that he previously moved his bowels once a day but lately only once every other day. He attributes this to his decreased appetite.

Since Mr. O's weight loss is not clearly secondary to malabsorption or diarrhea, the focus turns to the third pivotal step, which takes a system-based approach and uses a comprehensive history, physical exam, basic laboratory studies and updating his health maintenance screening exams to look for clues.

Mr. O notes that he has a decreased appetite and feels full quickly after starting to eat. His past medical history is unremarkable. On psychosocial history he reports that he

has not felt down, depressed, or hopeless during the past month nor has he been bothered by a lack of interest in activities. He denies any changes at home and has no trouble obtaining food. He has never been a tobacco smoker and drinks 2 beers about once a month.

On review of systems there are no fevers, night sweats, swollen lymph nodes, muscle aches, headaches, shortness of breath, unusual cough, heat intolerance, palpitations or tremulousness. There are also no GI symptoms of dysphagia, odynophagia, melena, hematochezia, abdominal pain, or jaundice.

His medications include 600 mg of ibuprofen 2–3 times a day for mild osteoarthritis of his left knee.

Physical exam reveals a thin but otherwise healthy appearing middle-aged man. Vital signs are normal. The remainder of his exam is completely normal. Laboratory tests, including CBC, differential, hepatic panel, renal panel, urinalysis, ESR, and TSH, are normal. HIV and FOBT are negative. A chest radiograph is normal without mass or adenopathy.

The cause of Mr. O's weight loss is not obvious. However, his early satiety and NSAID use are clues that suggest PUD or gastric cancer. You consider PUD your leading hypothesis. Gastric cancer is an alternative hypothesis, and colon cancer is a must not miss hypothesis given his change in bowel habits. Table 32-4 lists the differential diagnosis.

 All medications (prescription and over the counter) should be carefully scrutinized in patients complaining of unintentional weight loss. Some medications cause anorexia directly, others through various organ toxicities.

 Colon cancer causing subtotal obstruction may present as a change in bowel habits, either constipation *or* diarrhea.

 Is the clinical information sufficient to make a diagnosis? If not what other information do you need?

Table 32-4. Diagnostic hypotheses for Mr. O.

Diagnostic Hypotheses	Demographics, Risk Factors, Symptoms and Signs	Important Tests
Leading Hypothesis		
PUD	Epigastric pain, early satiety, nausea, melena, NSAID use	EGD *H pylori* breath test or stool antigen
Active Alternatives—Most Common		
Stomach cancer	Early satiety	EGD or upper GI
Active Alternatives—Must Not Miss		
Colon cancer	Change in stools Hematochezia Positive FOBT, iron deficient anemia	Colonoscopy

EGD, esophagogastroduodenoscopy; NSAID, nonsteroidal antiinflammatory drug; PUD, peptic ulcer disease;

Leading Hypothesis: PUD

Textbook Presentation

The pain of PUD is classically described as a dull or hunger-like pain in the epigastrium that is either exacerbated or improved by food intake. The pain is often worse on waking and may radiate to the back. Symptomatic periods often last for several weeks. Nausea and early satiety may be seen.

Disease Highlights

A. 250,000 cases per year in the United States

B. Etiology: Most ulcers are secondary to NSAID use, *Helicobacter pylori* infection or both.

   1. *H pylori* infection

   a. Present in 50% of world's population

   b. Asymptomatic in the majority of patients

   c. Peptic ulcer develops in 1–10% of infected patients.

   (1) May cause duodenal or gastric ulcers

   (2) Gastric ulcers caused directly by *H pylori*–mediated damage

   (3) Pathogenesis of *H pylori*–induced duodenal ulcers more complex (Figure 32-3)

   d. *H pylori* may also cause atrophic gastritis, intestinal metaplasia and rarely gastric cancer (0.1–3% of infected patients).

   2. NSAIDs

   a. Virtually all NSAIDs increase the risk of PUD, including over-the-counter NSAIDs and low-dose aspirin. The risk is lower with cyclooxygenase (COX)-2 inhibitors (see below).

   b. Ulcer disease develops in 25% of persons who take NSAIDs regularly.

   c. PUD-related bleeding or perforation is present in 2–4% of persons who take NSAIDs regularly.

   d. Results in 100,000 NSAID-associated hospitalizations in the United States annually, with 7000–10,000 deaths.

   e. Gastric ulcers are 5 times more common than duodenal ulcers.

   f. Ulcers are most likely to occur in the first 1–3 months of NSAID use.

   g. Risk factors for NSAID-associated PUD include the following:

   (1) History of prior PUD

   (2) Age > 65 years

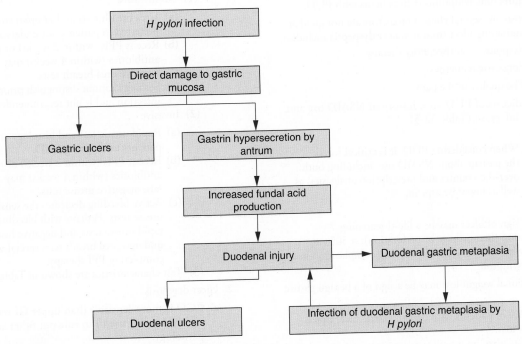

Figure 32-3. Pathogenesis of *H. pylori* associated PUD.

(3) High-dose NSAID therapy

(4) Concomitant use of aspirin (low or high dose), corticosteroids, or anticoagulants.

(5) Concurrent *H pylori* infection

h. NSAIDs may be nonselective, inhibiting both COX-1 and COX-2, or selective, inhibiting only COX-2.

(1) Selective COX-2 inhibitors have less GI toxicity.

(2) However, several selective COX-2 inhibitors *increase* the risk of myocardial infarction and several have been withdrawn from the market. Celecoxib is still available.

(3) Alternate strategies to decrease the risk of NSAID-related PUD include concurrent use of proton pump inhibitors (PPIs) or misoprostol with NSAIDs (see below).

3. Zollinger-Ellison syndrome is a rare cause of PUD.

C. Complications

1. Bleeding, which can vary from massive hemorrhage (with hematemesis and melena or hematochezia) to occult GI blood loss and iron deficiency anemia (see Chapter 19, GI Bleeding).

2. Perforation

3. Weight loss

Evidence-Based Diagnosis

A. History and physical exam

1. Pain is not a good predictor of PUD.

a. Ulcers are often asymptomatic.

(1) 60% of NSAID-associated ulcers are asymptomatic.

(2) 25% of non-NSAID ulcers are asymptomatic.

b. Pain often reflects nonulcer dyspepsia rather than PUD.

(1) Less than one-third of patients with epigastric discomfort have PUD.

(2) Among patients undergoing endoscopy, patients with nonulcer dyspepsia have more severe and more numerous symptoms than patients with PUD.

c. Surprisingly, several clinical predictors are not good at discriminating ulcer from nonulcer dyspepsia including

(1) Response to antisecretory therapy

(2) Epigastric tenderness

(3) The quality of the pain

2. Best predictors of PUD are a history of NSAID use and *H pylori* infection (Table 32-5).

 When considering PUD, it is critical to ask the patient about NSAID use, including both over-the-counter and prescription analgesics, as well as low-dose aspirin.

3. The first sign of ulcer may be a life-threatening complication (hemorrhage or perforation): > 50% of patients with serious to life-threatening complication had no prior symptom.

4. Unintentional weight loss may be a sign of a benign gastric ulcer.

a. 31–55% of patients with benign gastric ulcer noted weight loss.

b. ~50% lost 10–20 lbs; 21% lost > 20 lb

Table 32-5. Prevalence of PUD in patients with dyspepsia.

Age	Neither *H pylori* nor NSAIDs	Current NSAID use	*H pylori* infection
40 years	1%	5%	20%
75 years	3%	20%	30%

NSAID, nonsteroidal antiinflammatory drug; PUD, peptic ulcer disease.

c. PUD is found more often in patients undergoing esophagogastroduodenoscopy (EGD) for weight loss than for dyspepsia.

 A significant number of patients with NSAID-induced ulcers do not experience pain. Anemia, GI bleeding, early satiety, or weight loss can be the only symptom of PUD.

B. Laboratory studies

1. *H pylori* testing

a. Eradication markedly decreases recurrence of PUD from 60–100% to < 20%. All patients with documented PUD, whether or not they are taking NSAIDs, should be tested for *H pylori*.

b. Patients with a prior history of PUD who have not previously been treated for *H pylori* should also be tested.

c. Testing for *H pylori* is also recommended for patients with dyspepsia. Eradication of *H pylori* is recommended in symptomatic patients. (EGD is only recommended for those with "alarm" symptoms (see below) or those who do not respond to therapy.)

d. Options for diagnosing *H pylori* infection include invasive and noninvasive testing.

(1) Noninvasive

(a) Urea breath tests and *H pylori* stool antigen are preferred in patients not undergoing EGD.

(b) Recent PPIs (within 2 weeks) or recent antibiotics (within 4 weeks) may cause false-negative urea breath tests.

(c) Serology cannot distinguish prior from current infection and is not recommended.

(2) Invasive

(a) Rapid urease test and histology are preferred in patients undergoing EGD.

(b) Recent PPIs (within 2 weeks) or recent antibiotics (within 4 weeks) may also cause false-negative urease tests.

(c) Active bleeding decreases the sensitivity of rapid urease tests. Patients with bleeding and negative rapid urease tests and negative histology should undergo urea breath tests several weeks after completing PPI therapy.

(3) Test characteristics are shown in Table 32-6.

2. Ulcer diagnosis

a. EGD is more sensitive than upper GI series (92% vs 54%) and is useful to rule out other serious pathology.

b. Indications for EGD (Figure 32-4)

Table 32-6. Test characteristics for detecting *Helicobacter pylori* infection.

Test	Sensitivity	Specificity	LR+	LR-
Invasive tests				
Rapid urease test	90%	95%	18	0.11
Histology	70%	90%	7	0.33
Culture	45%	98%	22.5	0.56
Noninvasive tests				
Urea breath test	95%	95%	19	0.05
Stool antigen	95%	95%	19	0.05
Serology	85%	79%	4.0	0.19

(1) Bleeding

(2) Anemia

(3) Weight loss

(4) Early satiety

(5) Dysphagia

(6) Recurrent vomiting

(7) Prior esophagogastric malignancy or family history of GI cancer

(8) Patients who do not respond to initial therapy

(9) Age > 45–55 years (45 for patients from high gastric cancer incidence areas, eg, Latin America or Asia; 55 for patients from other lower incidence areas)

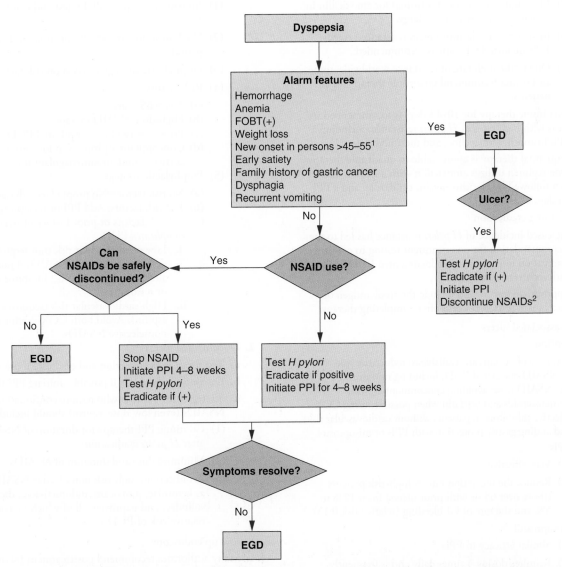

[1]The age cutoff varies dependent on the prevalence of gastric cancers. A cutoff of 45 is recommended for persons from high prevalence areas (e.g. Asia or Latin America) and 55 is recommended for patients from low prevalence areas

[2]See text

EGD, esophagogastroduodenoscopy; NSAIDs, nonsteroidal antiinflammatory drugs; PPI, proton pump inhibitor.

Figure 32-4. Workup of dyspepsia and indications for EGD.

Treatment

A. The 3 components of therapy for PUD include eradication of *H pylori*, if present; discontinuation of NSAIDs, if possible; and use of PPIs. In addition, gastric ulcers warrant biopsy to rule out adenocarcinoma.

B. Regardless of the cause of the ulcer, and the presence or absence of bleeding, PPIs dramatically suppress acid secretion and are the mainstay of therapy. For patients infected with *H pylori*, PPIs are given during the course of antibiotic therapy and longer for larger ulcers (> 1–2 cm) or patients with complications.

C. *H pylori* eradication

1. Multiple options: Ideal initial therapy is controversial and recommendations are likely to evolve due to changing resistance patterns.

   a. Standard triple therapy:

   (1) Includes a PPI, amoxicillin, and clarithromycin for 7–14 days.

   (2) Metronidazole can be substituted for amoxicillin in patients with a penicillin allergy.

   (3) In areas where clarithromycin resistance exceeds 15% quadruple therapy is recommended.

   (4) Due to the high rate of resistance worldwide, some authorities recommend quadruple therapy for all patients.

   b. Quadruple therapy for 10–14 days is recommended in areas with high rates of *H pylori* resistance, including a PPI, bismuth, tetracycline, and metronidazole.

   c. Sequential therapy is comparable to quadruple therapy. One regimen utilizes amoxicillin with a PPI on days 1–5 followed by clarithromycin, tinidazole, and a PPI on days 6–10.

2. Confirming eradication

   a. Increased incidence of *H pylori* resistance has led to the recommendation for posttreatment testing to confirm eradication in patients with documented PUD or those with recurrent dyspepsia.

   b. Appropriate tests would include the stool antigen or urea breath tests 4–6 weeks after completing therapy.

D. NSAID-associated ulcers

1. Prevention

   a. A variety of options are available to reduce the risk of NSAID-associated PUD, including minimizing the NSAID dose; avoiding concomitant aspirin, corticosteroids and warfarin when possible; using COX-2 selective inhibitors in patients without cardiovascular risk; and adding gastric protection with PPIs or misoprostol.

   b. PPIs

   (1) Very effective.

   (2) Reduce the ulceration rate in high-risk patients (those over 65 or with prior ulcers) from 17% to 5% and the rate of GI bleeding (relative risk 0.13).

   c. Misoprostol

   (1) Similar efficacy to PPIs

   (2) Requires dosing 4 times daily and is frequently associated with diarrhea, limiting its usefulness.

   d. H$_2$-receptor antagonists are less effective than PPIs.

   e. COX-2 inhibitors

   (1) Reduce the rate of ulcers compared with nonselective NSAIDs (relative risk 0.26) but appear less effective than PPIs (when combined with nonselective NSAIDs).

   (2) Increase the risk of cardiovascular events

   (3) The gastric protection of COX-2 inhibitors is eliminated in patients on concurrent low-dose aspirin.

   f. Ineffective strategies for preventing NSAID-associated gastric ulcers include sucralfate and enteric-coated aspirin.

   g. Patients with recent PUD-related bleeding.

   (1) Continuing NSAIDs (nonselective with a PPI or COX-2 selective) still results in high complication rates.

   (2) The combined use of PPIs with COX-2 inhibitors was safe in patients with documented ulcer bleeding who did not have *H pylori* infection.

   h. Current guidelines

   (1) All patients: If prior PUD, test and eradicate *H pylori*.

   (2) Use lowest dose of NSAID possible for briefest period.

   (3) Prophylactic strategy is based on risk factors.

   (4) Risk factors

   (a) Age > 65 years
   (b) High-dose NSAID therapy
   (c) Prior history of uncomplicated PUD
   (d) Concomitant aspirin (even low dose), corticosteroid, or anticoagulant use

   (5) Prophylactic strategy

   (a) No risk factors: No prophylaxis advised
   (b) 1–2 risk factors: Add PPI or misoprostol
   (c) > 2 risk factors or prior history of *recent* or *complicated* PUD

   i. Low cardiovascular risk (not requiring low-dose aspirin): Avoid NSAIDs if possible or alternatively use COX-2 inhibitor with PPI or misoprostol.

   ii. High cardiovascular risk (requiring low-dose aspirin): Avoid both COX-2 inhibitors and nonselective NSAIDs.

2. Documented ulcers

   a. Test for *H pylori* infection and eradicate if present.

   b. Discontinue NSAIDs if possible, initiate PPI therapy.

   c. Strategies for patients who require continuation of NSAIDs (even low-dose aspirin) should include:

   (1) Continue PPI therapy for duration of NSAID (even after *H pylori* eradication).

   (2) Minimize dose and duration of NSAIDs

   (3) Avoid certain high-risk nonselective NSAIDS, such as ketorolac, piroxicam, indomethacin, diclofenac, sulindac, and naproxen, all of which increase the relative risk of PUD.

E. Follow-up endoscopy

1. Many authorities recommend posttreatment follow-up endoscopy for patients with documented gastric ulcers to rule out an underlying gastric cancer missed on initial endoscopy.

2. This will have the greatest yield in high-risk groups (Asians, Hispanics, patients over 55, and those with a history of *H pylori* infection without recent NSAID use).

3. Follow-up endoscopy is particularly important in patients with gastric ulcers in whom adequate biopsies were not obtained during the initial endoscopy.

MAKING A DIAGNOSIS

Despite the absence of pain, Mr. O's history of NSAID use, the early satiety, and weight loss convinces you to order an EGD.

The EGD reveals 2 gastric ulcers 1.5 cm in size. Pathology reveals organisms consistent with *H pylori*.

Have you crossed a diagnostic threshold for the leading hypothesis, gastric ulcer? Have you ruled out the active alternatives? Do other tests need to be done to exclude the alternative diagnoses?

You conclude that the likely cause of Mr. O's weight loss is gastric ulcer. You elect to initiate therapy without further testing.

Altogether, malignant and nonmalignant GI diseases are the cause of unintentional weight loss in 28% of patients. The yield of EGD in patients with unintentional weight loss is 12–44%. EGD should be considered in the evaluation of patients with unexplained weight loss.

CASE RESOLUTION

Mr. O received eradication therapy, a PPI, and stopped the ibuprofen. Three months later, his appetite is excellent and his weight is approaching baseline. He is advised to use acetaminophen for his arthritis pain and to perform nonimpact physical activities.

CHIEF COMPLAINT

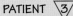 PATIENT

Mr. A. is a 62-year-old man who complains of recent weight loss. He reports that he has lost 15 pounds over the last 6–9 months, and that his clothes no longer fit. He denies diarrhea but admits to abdominal bloating and having several large stools a day that are difficult to flush. He reports that his appetite is not what it used to be but attributes that to his recent separation from his wife. He confides that they have not gotten along for years. She seemed to blame everything on his drinking, but he assures you that alcohol was definitely not a problem. Further, he reports that he is glad she is out of his life.

At this point, what is the leading hypothesis, what are the active alternatives, and is there a must not miss diagnosis? Given this differential diagnosis, what tests should be ordered?

RANKING THE DIFFERENTIAL DIAGNOSIS

The first step in unintentional weight loss is to verify Mr. A's weight loss. This is clearly established by his history and a review of his medical records. The second step looks for symptoms suggestive of malabsorption and although he denies frank diarrhea, his large frequent stools raise the possibility of GI diseases associated with malabsorption. The third pivotal step reviews the history, physical exam, and laboratory studies to look for other clues that might suggest a diagnosis. Mr. A's social history raises several possibilities. First, you suspect that his drinking is a problem and might be contributing to his weight loss. Alternatively, he may be more depressed than he acknowledges or simply adjusting to lifestyle changes precipitated by his separation. Table 32-7 lists the differential diagnosis.

On further questioning, Mr. A reports that he drinks 2 or so alcoholic beverages a night. He proudly states that he has never missed work due to a hangover and never drinks before noon. When you ask him how much alcohol he uses in each drink and whether anyone else has commented on his drinking, he gets defensive and reminds you he is here because he is losing weight.

Is the clinical information sufficient to make a diagnosis? If not, what other information do you need?

Mr. A's defensiveness increases your suspicion of alcoholism. You wonder how much alcohol consumption is normal and how to screen him more thoroughly for alcoholism.

Leading Hypothesis: Alcoholism

Textbook Presentation

Alcohol intake varies from low risk use to risky use, problem drinking, abuse, and finally alcohol dependence. Patients with alcoholism present along a continuum, from the functioning executive to the homeless alcoholic. Psychosocial complications include job loss, marital difficulties, loss of driving license, and violent behavior. Medical complications may include injury, pancreatitis, gastritis, cirrhosis, vitamin deficiency, cardiomyopathy, hypertension, malnutrition, weight loss, and death. Weight loss may be multifactorial secondary to decreased caloric intake during intoxication or due to alcohol-related illnesses (gastritis, pancreatitis, cirrhosis). Alcoholism is difficult to recognize early, when intervention may prevent progression.

Disease Highlights

A. Alcohol is responsible for 79,000 deaths per year in the United States and alcohol misuse disorders affects 9% of the US

Table 32-7. Diagnostic hypotheses for Mr. A.

Diagnostic Hypotheses	Demographics, Risk Factors, Symptoms and Signs	Important Tests
Leading Hypothesis		
Alcoholism	Quantity of alcohol use Family or work-related problems Injury Family history of alcoholism Resistant hypertension	Alcohol screen with Audit tool or single question Elevated AST or MCV
Active Alternatives—Most Common		
Depression	History of loss Personal or family history of depression Postpartum state > 6 somatic symptoms	Admission of feeling down or anhedonia
Chronic pancreatitis	Epigastric pain History of alcohol use or acute pancreatitis Diarrhea or large difficult to flush stools	Calcifications on radiograph and CT scan, ERCP
Crohn disease	Diarrhea Chronic abdominal pain Family history of IBD Jewish descent Vitamin B_{12} deficiency Uveitis, erythema nodosum Hematochezia, anemia, rectal abscess, aphthous ulcers Polymicrobial urinary tract infection	Colonoscopy Capsule endoscopy
Ulcerative colitis	Bloody diarrhea Family history of IBD Jewish descent Uveitis, erythema nodosum	Colonoscopy
Bacterial overgrowth	Diarrhea Prior bowel surgery, stricture, blind loop Chronic pancreatitis Small bowel diverticula	Quantitative jejunal aspirates D-xylose breath test
Celiac disease	Diarrhea Family history Iron deficiency anemia Dermatitis herpetiformis	IgA-tGT Ab IgA endomysial Ab

AST, aspartate aminotransferase; ERCP, endoscopic retrograde cholangiopancreatography; IBD, inflammatory bowel disease; MCV, mean corpuscular volume;

population. Causes of alcohol-related deaths include motor vehicle accidents, drownings, suicides, cirrhosis, and an increased risk of several cancers (esophageal, breast, pharyngeal, laryngeal, and hepatocellular cancer).

B. Women are more likely to deny alcohol-related problems and to have associated eating disorders, depression, and panic disorders.

C. 37% of adults with alcohol abuse or dependence have concomitant mood or personality disorders.

D. Categories and definitions of patterns of alcohol use (1 drink is defined as 12 g of alcohol or 1.5 oz of liquor, 5 oz of wine, or 12 oz of beer)

   1. Risky use: Prevalence 4–29%. Criteria:

   a. Men ≤ 65 years: > 14 drinks/wk or > 4 drinks per occasion

   b. Women (and men > 65 years): > 7 drinks/wk or > 3 drinks per occasion

   2. Hazardous drinking: At risk for consequences from alcohol

Evidence-Based Diagnosis

A. The USPSTF recommends screening all adults for alcohol misuse annually.

   1. The 3 recommended screening tools are the 10 question Audit tool, the 3 question Audit-C tool (found at http://www.integration.samhsa.gov/clinical-practice/screening-tools#drugs) or a single question "How many times in the past year have you had 5 or more drinks per day (for men) or 4 (for women and persons over 65 years).

   2. An Audit score of ≥ 4 in men (≥ 3 in women) has a sensitivity of 84–85%, specificity of 77–84%, LR+ 4.2, LR– 0.2.

   3. A single positive response to the 1 question tool has a sensitivity of 82%, specificity of 79% for unhealthy use; LR+ 3.9, LR– 0.23

B. The DSM-V defines alcohol use disorder as "a problematic pattern of alcohol use leading to clinically significant impairment or distress, as manifested by at least two of the following" over a 1 year period:

   1. Alcohol often consumed in larger amounts or over a longer period than was intended.

   2. Persistent desire or unsuccessful efforts to cut down or control alcohol use.

   3. A great deal of time spent obtaining, using, or recovering from alcohol.

   4. Craving, or strong desire to use alcohol.

   5. Recurrent use resulting in failure to fulfill major role or obligations.

   6. Continued use despite social or interpersonal problems caused by or exacerbated by alcohol.

   7. Important social, occupational, or recreational activities are given up or reduced because of alcohol use.

   8. Continued use despite knowledge of a physical or psychological problem caused by or exacerbated by alcohol.

   9. Tolerance

   10. Withdrawal

C. A variety of clinical clues can suggest alcohol misuse including: injury, resistant hypertension, family, work or legal problems, violence, depression, substance abuse, chronic pain, anemia, thrombocytopenia or a family history of alcoholism.

D. Laboratory abnormalities (Table 32-8)

   1. A variety of laboratory abnormalities may be seen in patients with heavy alcohol use, including an elevated GGT (gamma glutamyl transpeptidase) or macrocytosis.

Table 32-8. Accuracy of detecting unhealthy drinking using laboratory tests.

	Sensitivity	Specificity	LR+	LR−
Increased GGT	65%	80%	3.3	0.44
Macrocytosis	24%	96%	6	0.79

2. Elevated levels may increase the suspicion of alcoholism but are insensitive and should not be used to rule out the diagnosis.

3. The sensitivity increases in patients with alcohol dependency in whom the diagnosis is increasingly obvious.

E. Patients in whom risky drinking is suspected should be asked about symptoms that suggest the alcohol use disorder (see above), health problems related to alcohol use (gastritis, pancreatitis, liver disease, cirrhosis, resistant hypertension), readiness to change and their pattern of consumption (including average number of drinks per day, *maximum* number of drinks per day, and days per week that they consume alcohol).

Treatment

A. Brief (6–15 minute) multi-contact counseling interventions for persons identified with risky or hazardous drinking has been demonstrated to reduce weekly consumption, heavy drinking, traumatic injury, and death and is recommended by the USPSTF.

B. Components of effective interventions for hazardous drinkers include:
   1. Specialty referral
   2. Feedback on clinical and laboratory assessment
   3. Comparison to drinking norms
   4. Discussion of the adverse effects of alcohol
   5. Statement of the recommended drinking limits
   6. Prescription to "Cut down on your drinking"
   7. Patient educational material (www.niaaa.nih.gov)
   8. Drinking diary
   9. Follow-up office sessions and phone contact

C. Patients at moderate to high risk for alcohol withdrawal, a potentially fatal condition, and those with concomitant psychiatric disorders (especially suicidal ideation) or unstable home environments should be hospitalized in a detoxification unit (see Chapter 11, Delirium & Dementia).

D. Patients with alcohol use disorder should also receive a referral to a specialty treatment center, pharmacotherapy, and support groups (see below).

E. Relapse prevention: Several options
   1. Alcoholics Anonymous (AA), a 12-step program that has demonstrated effectiveness in increasing the rate of abstinence at 3 years from 43% to 62%
   2. Motivational enhancement therapy
   3. Therapy to develop cognitive-behavioral coping skills.
   4. Naltrexone, acamprosate, and disulfiram have reduced drinking in patients with alcohol dependence. Pharmacotherapy is most effective when combined with behavioral support.
   5. Treatment of depression, if present.

MAKING A DIAGNOSIS

Mr. A's history of "2 or so" drinks per night suggest at-risk drinking. Furthermore, his marital separation, while possibly multifactorial, raises the real possibility of alcohol abuse. You ask Mr. A the screening question if he has had 5 or more drinks on any day in the last year.

Mr. A reports that he probably drinks that much at least once a month when he is "partying."

Mr. A's intake raises your concern further. You elect to administer the Audit score questionnaire.

Mr. A scores 15 (out of a possible 40). He acknowledges that he tried to **cut** down while he was married but since his separation, he no longer feels that restraint. He acknowledges that occasionally he hears funny stories about himself from these parties that he cannot recollect (**amnesia**).

Mr. A also reluctantly reports that he received 2 tickets for driving while intoxicated within the past year. He feels mildly guilty about this but assures you he knows better than to make that mistake again. He reiterates that he has never missed work due to his drinking but did miss several family events because he was "partying."

Mr. A's Audit score, marital difficulties, blackouts, tickets for driving while intoxicated, missed social events, and continued use despite interpersonal difficulties is diagnostic of an alcohol use disorder. You elect to check a CBC and a liver panel. The CBC shows macrocytosis and the liver panel shows a mildly elevated AST and ALT. The elevation in AST is more marked than the elevation in ALT, a pattern commonly seen in alcoholic hepatitis.

Clearly, Mr. A suffers from alcohol abuse. This may be the sole cause or a contributing cause of his unintentional weight loss. You elect to initiate a treatment plan and reevaluate him once he is abstinent.

CASE RESOLUTION

You have a frank discussion of the issues with Mr. A. You acknowledge that his marital difficulties are complex but that many features of his alcohol use suggest an alcohol use disorder. The missed family gatherings, alcoholic blackouts, tolerance, tickets for driving while intoxicated, and abnormal blood test results all suggest this is a serious medical problem. Mr. A confides that he is frightened to go "cold turkey." He feels shaky and agitated whenever he stops drinking. You suggest admission to a detoxification unit. Mr. A listens carefully and agrees to be admitted.

FOLLOW-UP OF MR. A

Two months later, Mr. A returns to your office. His mood is clearly better. He proudly reports that he is "on the wagon" and feeling better. He attends AA meetings 5–7 nights per week. However, he remains concerned about his weight. He reports that his appetite is better and he is eating well but has not regained any weight.

At this point, what is the leading hypothesis, what are the active alternatives, and is there a must not miss diagnosis? Given this differential diagnosis, what tests should be ordered?

Mr. A's response to your intervention is rewarding. It is surprising that his weight is not improving particularly in light of his improved appetite. During his previous visit, he mentioned difficult to flush, large stools and you wonder if part of his weight loss is secondary to malabsorption. You revisit the common causes of malabsorption. (Table 32-9 and Figure 32-5).

RANKING THE DIFFERENTIAL DIAGNOSIS

Mr. A's history of difficult to flush stools but no diarrhea is more suggestive of chronic malabsorption than a chronic infectious diarrhea. You review those causes carefully and consider chronic small bowel disease (eg, inflammatory bowel disease [IBD], bacterial overgrowth, and celiac sprue) and chronic pancreatitis.

Mr. A denies ever being diagnosed with acute pancreatitis. He does remember multiple episodes of abdominal pain over the years following a night of binging. He did not seek medical care but remained at home drinking only clear fluids for several days until the pain subsided. He denies any history of bowel surgery, family history of IBD, or hematochezia.

Mr. A's history of alcohol abuse and recurrent pain leads you to suspect that he may have chronic pancreatitis. This becomes the leading hypothesis.

Is the clinical information sufficient to make a diagnosis? If not, what other information do you need?

Leading Hypothesis: Chronic Pancreatitis

Textbook Presentation

Patients typically seek medical attention for long-standing postprandial abdominal pain. Frequent, loose, malodorous bowel movements are common, and weight loss occurs. Patients may note that several flushes are required to clear the toilet. A prior history of alcoholism and acute pancreatitis are clues to the diagnosis.

Disease Highlights

A. Usually secondary to recurrent acute pancreatitis, primarily from alcohol abuse (70% of adult cases). Less common causes in adults include cystic fibrosis, hereditary pancreatitis, ductal

Table 32-9. Differential diagnosis of diarrhea organized by mechanism.

Most common causes: IBS, lactose intolerance, chronic infections, IBD, celiac disease

Osmotic diarrhea:
- Diagnostic clue: increased osmolar gap
- Lactose intolerance
- Mg++ laxatives, antacids

Fatty diarrhea:
- Diagnostic clue: Stool fecal fat
- Celiac disease
- Crohn disease
- Short bowel syndrome
- Bacterial overgrowth
- Pancreatic insufficiency

Inflammatory diarrhea:
- Diagnostic clue: Fecal calprotectin, fecal lactoferrin
- Inflammatory bowel disease
- Infectious
- Ischemic colitis
- Radiation colitis
- Neoplasia

Secretory diarrhea:
- Diagnostic clue: no osmolar gap
- Laxative abuse (nonosmotic laxative)
- Bacterial toxin
- Inflammatory bowel disease
- Collagenous colitis
- Ileal bile salt malabsorption
- Microscopic colitis
- Motility disorders: diabetic neuropathy, hyperthyroidism, IBS
- Neuroendocrine: Mastocytosis, carcinoid syndrome, VIPoma
- Neoplasia: Colon cancer, lymphoma, villous adenoma

Infections include invasive bacteria, *C difficile*, TB, HSV, CMV, amebiasis, giardiasis
Osmolar gap ≡ Measured fecal osmolarity – calculated fecal osmolarity Nl < 50 osm/L.
Calculated fecal osmolarity = 2 × (fecal Na⁺ + fecal K⁺)
CMV, cytomegalovirus; HSV, herpes simplex virus; IBD, inflammatory bowel disease; IBS, irritable bowel syndrome; TB, tuberculosis.

obstruction (ie, stones, tumor), autoimmune disease, hypercalcemia, and hypertriglyceridemia.

B. Progressive destruction results in both exocrine and endocrine insufficiency.

C. Manifestations include
1. Chronic, disabling, mid-epigastric postprandial pain is very common (80–100% of patients) and a major cause of morbidity. The pain may radiate to the back and be relieved by sitting forward.

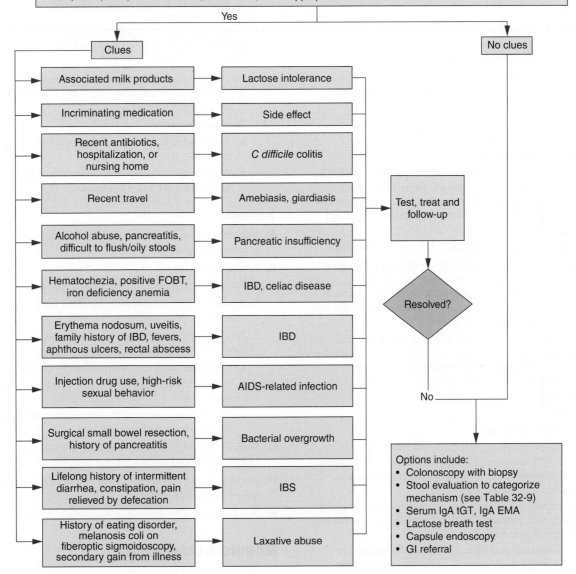

Figure 32-5. Diagnostic approach: malabsorption and diarrhea.

BMP, basic metabolic panel; FOBT, fecal occult blood test; IBD, inflammatory bowel disease; IBS, irritable bowel syndrome; LFTs, liver function tests; O & P, ova and parasite.

2. Weight loss secondary to anorexia and steatorrhea

3. Steatorrhea

    a. Defined as fat malabsorption ≥ 14 g/d (nl ≤ 7 g/d fecal fat on 75–100 g fat diet. Patients with primarily watery diarrhea may excrete up to 13 g/d of fecal fat).

    b. Manifestations include difficult to flush oily stools and weight loss. Elderly patients may not have diarrhea.

    c. Floating stools are not specific for steatorrhea (bacterial gas may also result in floating stools).

    d. Diarrhea may develop secondary to bacterial overgrowth, which develops in 40% of patients with chronic pancreatitis.

  4. Diabetes may develop due to the concomitant destruction of islet cells.

    a. Ketoacidosis is rare.

    b. Hypoglycemia is common due to loss of glucagon-producing pancreatic alpha cells.

  5. Complications include pseudocysts, obstruction of the common bile duct or duodenum, and pancreatic ascites. Splenic vein thrombosis may also develop, leading to gastric varices.

  6. Pancreatic cancer develops in 4% of patients.

Evidence-Based Diagnosis

A. One study reported unintentional weight loss and diarrhea in 68%, and bloating in 30%. Diabetes was found in 28%.

B. Laboratory tests

  1. Manifestations may be structural (pancreatic calcifications, atrophy and ductal dilatation) or functional (with pancreatic insufficiency).

  2. While patients with advanced disease typically have both structural and functional changes, patients with early disease may have either just structural changes (diagnosed on imaging) or just functional abnormalities (diagnosed with secretin testing [see below]).

  3. The gold standard is biopsy, which is rarely performed.

  4. Precise sensitivity and specificity are difficult to estimate due to the (1) infrequency of biopsy, (2) difficulty interpreting results in patients with discordant structural and functional changes, and (3) variation of sensitivity and specificity with stage of the disease.

  5. Structural changes are typically diagnosed with CT scan, endoscopic retrograde cholangiopancreatography (ERCP), endoscopic ultrasonography (EUS), or magnetic resonance cholangiopancreatography (MRCP).

  6. CT scan

    a. Initial test of choice.

    b. CT manifestations include ductal calcifications (74–90% sensitive, 85% specific), ductal dilatations, and pancreatic atrophy. Pancreatic pseudocysts or tumors can also be diagnosed.

    c. Pancreatic calcifications are often assumed to be specific for chronic pancreatitis but have also been reported in a variety of pancreatic tumors.

  7. ERCP is invasive and typically reserved for patients in whom it might be therapeutic (ie, stenting) (sensitivity, 75–95%; specificity ≈ 90%).

  8. Secreting stimulation functional assessment

    a. Typically the most sensitive tests in chronic pancreatitis

    b. Time consuming, labor intensive, invasive and not widely available

    c. Secretin is administered and the pancreatic juices collected in the duodenum. Peak bicarbonate concentration is measured.

    d. Cholecystokinin stimulation of the acini (to produce lipase) has also been used.

    e. Compared with an aggregate of historical data, follow-up data, and imaging studies (CT, MRI, and EUS),

secretin stimulation is 96% sensitive, 93% specific, LR+ 13.7, LR– 0.04

    f. Greatest utility may be in patients with early chronic pancreatitis in whom imaging studies may be normal.

  9. EUS: Using secretion as gold standard, 71% sensitive, 92% specific, LR+ 7.9, LR– 0.32

  10. Other less diagnostic tests

    a. Amylase and lipase are often normal or slightly elevated.

    b. Abdominal radiographs may reveal pancreatic calcifications. Sensitivity is only 30%.

    c. Routine abdominal ultrasound is 60–70% sensitive and 80–90% specific.

  11. MRCP with secretin (used to enhance visualization of the pancreatic ducts) is being evaluated for the diagnosis of chronic pancreatitis.

  12. Fecal elastase is low in patients with advanced chronic pancreatitis; 75% sensitive, 100% specific (cutoff < 200 mcg/g) LR+ ∞, LR– 0.25.

  13. Tests for steatorrhea

    a. Stool Sudan III stain (qualitative) is 90% sensitive for fecal fat ≥ 10 g/d.

    b. Acid steatocrit (performed on spot stool specimen) is 100% sensitive and 95% specific.

Treatment

A. Abstinence from drinking is vital (but not universally effective at halting progression).

B. Pain management

  1. Exclude other causes of increasing or persistent pain

  2. NSAIDs, TCAs, and opioids are often used. Opioid dependence is a common problem.

  3. Pancreatic enzymes can decrease pain and improve nutritional status.

    a. Give with meals and low fat diets (< 20 g/d).

    b. Nonenteric coated enzymes may provide superior pain relief.

    c. Coadministration of PPIs is recommended to prevent the inactivation of the enzymes.

C. Diabetes should be treated, with care to avoid hypoglycemia. Metformin should be avoided due to concomitant alcoholism.

D. ERCP, stenting, and surgery are useful in selected patients to relieve obstruction and pain.

E. Pseudocysts require surgical or endoscopic drainage.

MAKING A DIAGNOSIS

A CT scan of the abdomen reveals multiple areas of pancreatic calcifications consistent with chronic pancreatitis. A Sudan stain for fecal fat is positive consistent with fat malabsorption.

Have you crossed a diagnostic threshold for the leading hypothesis, chronic pancreatitis? Have you ruled out the active alternatives? Do other tests need to be done to exclude the alternative diagnoses?

Alternative Diagnosis: Bacterial Overgrowth

Textbook Presentation

Classically, patients have previously undergone GI surgery that resulted in some type of surgical blind loop that allows for bacterial multiplication. Patients may experience long-standing diarrhea, bloating, and weight loss.

Disease Highlights

A. Mechanism of diarrhea is multifactorial.

   1. Bacteria digest carbohydrates producing gas and osmotically active byproducts promoting an osmotic diarrhea.

   2. Bacteria and their fatty acid byproducts injure mucosa and contribute to diarrhea.

   3. Mucosal injury can create lactase deficiency.

   4. Bacterial deconjugation of bile salts interferes with fat absorption and the absorption of fat-soluble vitamins.

B. Etiologies

   1. Stasis

      a. Strictures (surgical, Crohn disease, radiation enteritis)

      b. Anatomic abnormalities (surgical blind loops or diverticula)

      c. Dysmotility (diabetic autonomic neuropathy, scleroderma)

      d. Chronic pancreatitis (obstruction or opioid therapy can promote stasis).

   2. Abnormal small to large intestine connections (ie, fistula or resection of ileocecal valve (allows retrograde colonization from heavily colonized colon into ileum)

   3. Achlorhydria (ie, PPI therapy or autoimmune)

   4. Miscellaneous (cirrhosis up to 60% of patients, end-stage renal disease)

C. Bacteria may utilize B_{12}, leading to B_{12} deficiency.

D. Unusual complications include tetany (due to hypocalcemia) and night blindness due to vitamin A deficiency.

Evidence-Based Diagnosis

A. Healthy older patients may also have bacterial overgrowth without any symptoms, making diagnosis difficult.

B. Gold standard is quantitative jejunal aspirates demonstrating $> 10^5$ bacteria/mL.

C. A variety of tests detect bacterial byproducts in exhaled breath as an aid to diagnosis. Since bacteria normally reside in the colon, but only in low levels in the small intestine, early peaks in the concentration of these byproducts suggests small intestinal bacterial overgrowth. False-positives and false-negatives occur when other conditions increase or decrease bowel transit time, respectively. Antibiotics can interfere with the breath tests.

   1. D xylose breath test is usually abnormal secondary to bacterial digestion of xylose-releasing radiolabeled C14.

      a. Sensitivity 30–95%, specificity 89–100%.

      b. Avoid in fertile women.

   2. Hydrogen breath tests measure exhaled bacterial hydrogen production after patients ingest sugar.

      a. Their accuracy is similar to the xylose tests and avoids radioactivity.

      b. Some bacteria produce methane, and this measurement may increase accuracy.

D. Consider bacterial overgrowth if upper GI series demonstrates hypomotility, obstruction, or diverticula.

E. Weight loss may occur without diarrhea.

F. Therapeutic trials of antibiotics may be necessary.

Treatment

A. Eliminate drugs that reduce intestinal motility or reduce gastric acidity.

B. A variety of oral antibiotics have been used for 7–10 days. Rotating courses of antibiotics have been used in some patients. Rifaximin is a nonabsorbable antibiotic that has been useful.

C. Correct calcium, vitamin A, D, K, and B_{12} deficiency.

D. Minimizing carbohydrates, especially lactose, can be helpful.

Alternative Diagnosis: IBD

IBD (Crohn disease and ulcerative colitis) are complex diseases. Genetic factors and commensal bacterial factors play a role. They are found most commonly in patients of Jewish descent and among patients with a family history of IBD. Crohn disease is a transmural process that may affect the entire GI tract whereas ulcerative colitis is a mucosal disease limited to the colon. Manifestations may be intestinal or extraintestinal (uveitis, erythema nodosum, pyoderma granulosum, large or small joint peripheral arthritis, ankylosing spondylitis, sclerosing cholangitis, secondary amyloidosis, and venous thromboembolism). Chronic colitis increases the risk of colon cancer in proportion to the amount of the colon involved and the duration of disease.

1. Crohn Disease

Textbook Presentation

Common complaints include chronic abdominal pain, diarrhea, fever, weight loss, enterocutaneous fistulas, and acute abdominal pain (which can mimic acute appendicitis).

Disease Highlights

A. Patchy, transmural inflammation can lead to fistula formation, phlegmon, strictures and obstruction, perforation, abscess formation, and peritonitis.

B. Manifestations

   1. The disease course is characterized by exacerbations and remissions.

   2. Typically presents with insidious onset of symptoms of weight loss, diarrhea, and abdominal pain, although occasionally acute symptoms (eg, acute toxic megacolon or acute ileitis mimicking acute appendicitis) are the presenting manifestations of Crohn disease.

   3. Can involve any part of GI tract with normal "skip areas" between involved areas. At presentation:

      a. ≈ 20% of patients had ileitis, 45% ileocolitis, and 33% colitis. Upper GI involvement can occur.

      b. ≈ 27% had strictures or perforation

   4. Perianal or rectal fistulas occurs in 14–37% of patients.

   5. Diarrhea (with or without gross bleeding), weight loss, abdominal pain, and fever are common.

   6. Diarrhea may occur due to

      a. Small bowel disease impairing absorption

      b. Ileal disease

         (1) May decrease bile salt absorption, allowing bile salts into the colon, which cause irritation and diarrhea.

(2) Severe bile salt malabsorption also causes bile salt deficiency and steatorrhea.

    c. Bacterial overgrowth secondary to strictures

7. Obstruction due to strictures

8. Fistulas may be enterocutaneous fistulas (most commonly perianal), enterovesicular (resulting in polymicrobial urinary tract infections), enterovaginal or enteroenteric (bowel to bowel).

9. B_{12} deficiency (secondary to ileal disease)

10. Calcium oxalate kidney stones

    a. Normal GI oxalate absorption is limited by intraluminal intestinal binding of oxalate to calcium.

    b. Malabsorption increases intraluminal fat. Intraluminal fat binds intraluminal calcium decreasing calcium's availability to oxalate.

    c. This leads to increased oxalate absorption.

    d. Increased oxalate absorption causes hyperoxaluria and promotes the formation of calcium oxalate kidney stones.

11. Osteoporosis due to vitamin D deficiency, calcium malabsorption, and corticosteroid therapy.

12. Gross bleeding is less frequent than in ulcerative colitis.

13. Aphthous ulcers

Evidence-Based Diagnosis

A. The history should include changes in weight, abdominal pain, fever, a personal history of recent antibiotic or NSAID use (to consider the likelihood of *C difficile*– or NSAID-associated colitis), symptoms or history of extraintestinal manifestations (uveitis, arthritis, or erythema nodosum) and family history of IBD.

B. The physical exam should include weight (and changes from prior), vital signs, the abdominal and rectal exam.

C. Initial labs studies should include a CBC, comprehensive metabolic panel, ESR, C-reactive protein, vitamin B_{12}, folate, and plain abdominal radiographs to rule out colonic dilatation.

D. Active infection with the following organisms should be excluded in patients with diarrhea: *Salmonella, Shigella, Campylobacter, Yersinia, Escherichia coli 0157:H7, Giardia, C difficile,* and *E histolytica*

E. Colonoscopy with ileoscopy and biopsy often diagnostic but may be contraindicated in acute severe colitis.

F. Upper endoscopy may be useful in patients with concurrent dyspepsia.

G. Diagnostic imaging

    1. A variety of imaging techniques are available to visualize the small bowel for diagnosis and are useful in the following situations:

        a. When colonoscopy/ileoscopy fails to establish the diagnosis

        b. Evaluation of complications (ie, strictures, abscesses) and disease extent

        c. Options include ultrasound, small bowel follow through, enteroclysis, CT enterography, CT enteroclysis, MR enterography, MR enteroclysis, and capsule endoscopy.

    2. The precise role of imaging studies is not yet defined. Local expertise and availability may guide choices.

        a. MR

        (1) Avoids radiation

        (2) Can detect abscesses

        (3) May distinguish fibrotic from inflammatory strictures

        (4) Recommended as the preferred technique

    b. CT

        (1) Widely available

        (2) Can detect abscesses

        (3) Associated with radiation risks (which may be of particular importance in young patients needing serial examinations)

        (4) Requires IV contrast

    c. Capsule endoscopy

        (1) Can visualize aphthous ulcers not visible on MRI or CT

        (2) Some studies suggest improved sensitivities over MR and CT

        (3) Capsules may get lodged in strictures.

        (4) Guidelines suggest ruling out strictures prior to capsule endoscopy with either small bowel follow through, CT enterography, or MR enterography.

        (5) A capsule that auto-dissolves has been developed.

    d. Ultrasound is inexpensive but operator dependent and cannot provide comprehensive evaluation of the bowel.

Treatment

A. Therapeutic goals include the induction and maintenance of remission. Options include 5-aminosalicylic acid (5-ASA), budesonide or conventional corticosteroids, 6 mercaptopurine (6MP), methotrexate, antitumor necrosis factor (TNF) therapy, cyclosporine, tacrolimus, and natalizumab. 5-ASA and corticosteroids may be given systemically or topically (as enemas or suppositories). Consultation is advised.

B. Antibiotics are often necessary for bacterial overgrowth, peritonitis, or abscesses (which may also require drainage).

C. Smoking cessation is associated with a 65% reduction in relapse.

D. Adjunctive therapy

    1. Treat lactose intolerance if present.

    2. Assess and replete as necessary vitamin B_{12}, folate, vitamin D, zinc, iron, and calcium.

    3. Total parenteral nutrition may be necessary in patients unable to maintain adequate nutrition.

    4. Bile acid resins for patients with watery diarrhea and ileal disease.

    5. Periodic colonoscopy to monitor for colon cancer in patients with colonic involvement.

    6. Surgery

        a. 50% of patients require surgery in the first 10 years.

        b. Not curative. High rate of recurrence following surgery (10–15%/y clinical recurrence, 80% endoscopic recurrence).

        c. Indications include the management of massive hemorrhage, fulminant colitis, abscesses, peritonitis, obstruction, or disease refractory to medical therapy.

    7. Avoid NSAIDs and opioids if possible.

8. Vaccinations
   a. Patients should receive influenza, pneumococcal, and human papillomavirus vaccines.
   b. Hepatitis B vaccination is recommended in the nonimmune patients prior to immunosuppressive or anti-TNF therapy.
   c. Live vaccines (BCG, MMR, oral polio, live typhoid, and varicella) should be avoided in patients taking immunosuppressants (including corticosteroids).

2. Ulcerative Colitis

Textbook Presentation

Typically, bloody diarrhea and fecal urgency are the presenting symptoms. The disease course is typically one of exacerbations and remissions.

Disease Highlights

A. Primarily mucosal disease. (Occasionally, severe inflammation may extend deeper, involving muscular layers resulting in dysmotility and toxic megacolon.)

B. Strictly limited to colon

C. Starts at rectum and proceeds proximally in a *continuous fashion;* may be limited to rectum or involve rectosigmoid or entire colon. Rectal sparing suggests another disease (ie, Crohn disease).

D. Decreased risk among smokers (opposite of Crohn disease)

E. Anemia, fever, and increasing diarrhea are seen with more extensive disease.

F. Complications
   1. Massive hemorrhage (rare)
   2. Toxic megacolon
   3. Stricture
   4. Colon cancer
      a. The cancer risk is increased except in patients with just proctitis or very distal colitis.
      b. Increased risk begins 7–8 years after onset of disease.

Evidence-Based Diagnosis

A. Sigmoidoscopy or colonoscopy demonstrates loss of vascular markings, erythema, friability, and exudates in a continuous fashion extending from the rectum proximally.

B. Biopsy specimen reveals crypt abscesses, branching crypts, and glandular atrophy.

C. Patients should be asked about travel history or recent antibiotic use that increases the likelihood of bacterial gastroenteritis or *C difficile* colitis. Stool samples should be sent to exclude acute infectious processes (*Salmonella, Shigella, Campylobacter, E coli 0157:H7, C difficile, E histolytica*).

D. The diagnosis is typically made in patients with characteristic endoscopic and pathologic findings in the absence of infection. Small bowel imaging can be also useful if Crohn disease is considered (small bowel involvement suggests Crohn disease since ulcerative colitis does not affect the small bowel).

E. NSAIDs may cause colitis and their use should also be excluded.

Treatment

A. Patients should be monitored for relapse regularly and asked about diarrhea, rectal bleeding, and systemic symptoms. The patient's weight and hemoglobin should be monitored.

B. Decisions regarding choice of therapy depend on a combination of disease location and severity.
   1. Distal disease (descending colon and beyond) can often be treated with topical preparations (suppositories or enemas). Options include topical preparations of 5-ASA or corticosteroids (suppositories, enemas, or foams) or oral 5–ASA preparations.
   2. More proximal disease requires systemic therapy.
   3. Therapy is also intensified in patients with severe disease manifested by greater stool frequency, increased bleeding, systemic symptoms (fever, tachycardia, anemia, and elevated ESR) or sigmioidoscopic appearance.

C. Oral or systemic corticosteroids can be added for more severe disease or nonresponders.

D. Cyclosporine, 6MP, and infliximab have been effective in some patients with severe, corticosteroid-refractory disease.

E. Antibiotics may be useful in select ill patients, particularly those with toxic megacolon or peritonitis.

F. 5-ASA preparations (but not topical corticosteroids) are effective at maintaining remission. 6MP and infliximab can also be effective.

G. Surgery (colectomy) is curative. Indications include:
   1. Patients with high-grade dysplasia, carcinoma in situ, or cancer on surveillance colonoscopy. Low-grade dysplasia should also prompt consideration for colectomy.
   2. Other severe complications including massive hemorrhage, perforation, and toxic megacolon.
   3. Intractable disease

H. Adjuvant therapy
   1. Persistent diarrhea
      a. Test for lactose intolerance
      b. Avoid fresh fruits, vegetables, and caffeine
   2. Surveillance colonoscopy for colon cancer for ulcerative colitis and Crohn disease begins 8 years after diagnosis and then every 1–2 years.
   3. Supplemental iron
   4. Fish oils and nicotine (transdermal) have been demonstrated to induce remission in some patients.
   5. Total parenteral nutrition if patients are unable to maintain adequate nutrition
   6. Antidiarrheals may *increase* the increased risk of toxic megacolon.
   7. Screen patients who have been taking corticosteroids for > 3 months for osteoporosis.

CASE RESOLUTION

Mr. A's history and CT scan point strongly toward chronic pancreatitis. IBD is possible but unlikely. Since bacterial overgrowth can complicate chronic pancreatitis, an empiric trial of antibiotics could be given if therapy for chronic pancreatitis is unsuccessful.

Mr. A is given pancreatic enzymes. He subsequently reports that his diarrhea and bloating are greatly improved. Six months later he is back to his baseline weight.

REVIEW OF OTHER IMPORTANT DISEASES

Celiac Disease

Textbook Presentation

Classically, chronic diarrhea, steatorrhea, and weight loss are present. Iron and vitamin deficiencies may be seen.

Disease Highlights

A. Occurs worldwide. Prevalence ≈ 0.5–1% in Northern Europeans; affects women 1.5 times more often than men.

B. Develops only in persons with either the HLA-DQ2 or HLA-DQ8 haplotype.

  1. Develops in only a subset of such patients

  2. Those haplotypes expressed on antigen presenting cell surfaces can bind the deaminated gluten peptide found in wheat, rye, and barley.

  3. This triggers an abnormal immune response within the intestinal mucosa with subsequent mucosal injury, atrophy, and malabsorption.

  4. Antibodies develop to gliadin, transglutaminase (tTG), and endomysin (EMA).

C. Clinical manifestations

  1. Usually presents between ages 10 and 40 years, although may be recognized in older patients.

  2. Symptoms precipitated by exposure to wheat, rye, or barley protein (gluten) and resolve within weeks to months on gluten-free diet.

  3. Diarrhea is seen in 27–50% of patients. Patients may also have weight loss (6 – 22%), unexplained iron deficiency anemia, osteoporosis, aphthous stomatitis, or abnormal liver function tests; however, they could be asymptomatic.

  4. Osteopenia and osteoporosis may develop due to vitamin D deficiency and subsequent secondary hyperparathyroidism.

  5. Strongly associated with dermatitis herpetiformis, which develops secondary to antibodies against epidermal transglutaminase.

  6. Far more common in patients with Down syndrome.

  7. Increase risk of other autoimmune disorders including thyroiditis and type 1 diabetes mellitus.

  8. Patients with celiac disease are at increased risk for intestinal adenocarcinoma and enteropathy-associated T cell lymphoma.

Evidence-Based Diagnosis

A. Diagnostic options include duodenal biopsy (the gold standard), serology, and clinical response to gluten-free diet.

B. Small bowel biopsy is the gold standard and useful but invasive. Strategies can help determine when biopsies are necessary (see below).

C. Serologic testing is highly accurate but not perfect.

  1. Tissue glutaminase antibody (IgA tGT)

    a. Very accurate: 87% sensitive, 97% specific, LR+ 29, LR– 0.12

    b. Simpler, cheaper, and less operator dependent than IgA EMA (below)

    c. Initial test of choice

  2. Endomysial antibody (IgA EMA) also very accurate: 87% sensitive, 99% specific, LR+ 850, LR– 0.13.

  3. There are several causes of false-negative serologies including

    a. IgA deficiency: IgG tGT antibodies or deaminated gliaden peptide antibodies can be tested when the suspicion is high and IgA levels are low or absent.

    b. Gluten-free diets: IgA tGT and IgA EMA levels fall (and may become negative) in patients on gluten-free diet. (Increasing titers in celiac patients suggest dietary noncompliance.)

D. HLA typing

  1. Virtually all patients with celiac disease express HLA-DQ2 or HLA-DQ8 heterodimers.

    a. 100% sensitive but only 57–75% specific

    b. LR+ 2.3, LR– 0

  2. Celiac disease can be virtually ruled out in patients who are negative for HLA-DQ2 or HAL-DQ8.

  3. May be useful in patients in patients who instituted a gluten-free diet before evaluation in whom IgA-tGT and IgA EMA antibody levels may be low due to decreased disease activity. If the patient expressed neither HLA-DQ haplotype, celiac disease could be excluded.

E. Due to the low prevalence of celiac disease, positive EMA and tGT serologies do not confirm the diagnosis, despite the high specificity.

  1. The positive predictive value ranges from 29% to 76% and small bowel biopsy is necessary to confirm the diagnosis.

  2. On the other hand, negative EMA and tGT serologies make the diagnosis very unlikely (negative predictive value ≈ 99%) and essentially rule out the disease.

  3. If concern remains despite a negative result, HLA typing could help completely exclude the disease.

  4. One approach is shown in Figure 32-6.

F. Certain patients complain of gluten-related symptoms and improvement on a gluten-free diet despite negative serologies and biopsy. Such patients may have an ill-defined gluten sensitivity or wheat allergy.

Treatment

A. Gluten-free diet (no wheat, rye, and barley)

B. Oats that are uncontaminated with gluten are usually tolerated in patients with celiac disease.

C. Lactose avoidance may be necessary due to concomitant lactase deficiency.

D. Correct iron, folic acid, vitamin B_{12}, and vitamin D deficiencies.

E. Pneumococcal vaccine is recommended by some experts.

F. Corticosteroids or other immunosuppressives have rarely been necessary in patients with refractory celiac sprue.

G. Osteoporosis screening is recommended.

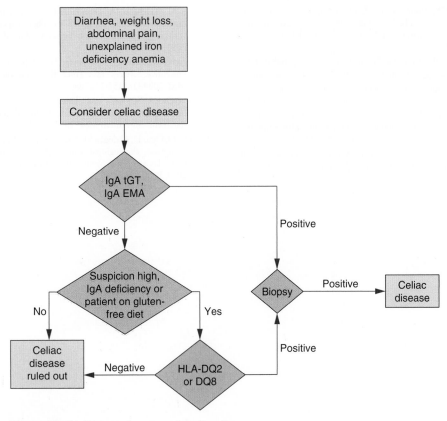

Figure 32-6. Diagnostic approach: celiac disease.

REFERENCES

American Psychiatric Association. *Diagnostic and Statistical Manual of Mental Disorders,* 5th ed. DSM-5. Arlington, VA: American Psychiatric Publishing. 2013.

Arroll B, Khin N, Kerse N. Screening for depression in primary care with two verbally asked questions: cross sectional study. BMJ. 2003;325:1144–6.

Bergstrom JP, Helander A. Clinical characteristics of carbohydrate-deficient transferrin (% disialotransferrin) measured by HPLC: sensitivity, specificity, gender effects, and relationship with other alcohol biomarkers. Alcohol Alcohol. 2008;43(4):436–41.

Bhatt DL, Scheiman J, Abraham NS. ACCF/ACG/AHA 2008 expert consensus document on reducing the gastrointestinal risks of antiplatelet therapy and NSAID use. Circulation. 2008;118:1894–909.

Bilbao-Garay J, Barba R, Losa-Garcia JE et al. Assessing clinical probability of organic disease in patients with involuntary weight loss: a simple score. Eur J Intern Med. 2002;13:240–5.

Bradley KA, Boyd-Wickizer J, Powell SH, Burman ML. Alcohol screening questionnaires in women: a critical review. JAMA. 1998;280(2):166–71.

Brent GA. Clinical practice. Graves' disease. N Engl J Med. 2008;358(24):2594–605.

Callery MP, Freedman SD. A 21-year-old man with chronic pancreatitis. JAMA. 2008;299(13):1588–94.

Fasano A, Catassi C. Celiac disease. N Engl J Med. 2012;367:2419–26.

Fournier JC, DeRubeis RJ, Hollon SD et al. Antidepressant drug effects and depression severity: a patient-level meta-analysis. JAMA. 2010;303:47–53.

Friedmann P. Alcohol use in adults. N Engl J Med. 2013;368:365–71.

Gisbert JP, Abraira V. Accuracy of *Helicobacter pylori* diagnostic tests in patients with bleeding peptic ulcer: a systematic review and meta-analysis. Am J Gastroenterol. 2006;101(4):848–63.

Gisbert JP, de la Morena F, Abraira V. Accuracy of monoclonal stool antigen test for the diagnosis of *H. pylori* infection: a systematic review and meta-analysis. Am J Gastroenterol. 2006;101(8):1921–30.

Hadithi M, von Blomberg BM, Crusius JB et al. Accuracy of serologic tests and HLA-DQ typing for diagnosing celiac disease. Ann Intern Med. 2007;147(5):294–302.

Hernandez JL, Riancho JA, Matorras P, Gonzalez-Macias J. Clinical evaluation for cancer in patients with involuntary weight loss without specific symptoms. Am J Med. 2003;114(8):631–7.

Hopper AD, Cross SS, Hurlstone DP et al. Pre-endoscopy serological testing for coeliac disease: evaluation of a clinical decision tool. BMJ. 2007;334(7596):729.

Lanza FL, Chan FK, Quigley EM; Practice Parameters Committee of the American College of Gastroenterology. Guidelines for prevention of NSAID-related ulcer complications. Am J Gastroenterol. 2009;104:728–38.

Lieb JG, Brensinger CM, Toskes PP. The significance of the volume of pancreatic juice measured at secretin stimulation testing: a single-center evaluation of 224 classical secretin stimulation tests. Pancreas. 2012;41:1073–9.

McColl K. *Helicobacter pylori* infection. N Engl J Med. 2010;362:1597–604.

McMinn J, Steel C, Bowman A. Investigation and management of unintentional weight loss in older adults. BMJ. 2011;342:d1732.

Metalidis C, Knockaert DC, Bobbaers H, Vanderschueren S. Involuntary weight loss. Does a negative baseline evaluation provide adequate reassurance? Eur J Intern Med. 2008;19(5):345–9.

Mowat C, Cole A, Windsor A et al. Guidelines for the management of inflammatory bowel disease in adults. Gut. 2011;60:571–607.

Moyer VA on behalf of the U.S. Preventive Services Task Force. Screening and Behavior Counseling Interventions in Primary Care to Reduce Alcohol Misuse. U.S. Preventive Services Task Force Recommendations Statement. Ann Intern Med. 2013 May 14;158.

Moyer VA on behalf of the U.S. Preventive Services Task Force. Screening for Lung Cancer: U.S. Preventive Services Task Force Recommendation Statement. Ann Intern Med. www.annals.org Dec 31, 2013.

Nakao H, Konishi H, Mitsufuji S et al. Comparison of clinical features and patient background in functional dyspepsia and peptic ulcer. Dig Dis Sci. 2007;52(9):2152–8.

Peyrin-Biroulet L, Loftus EV Jr, Colombel JF, Sandborn WJ. The natural history of adult Crohn's disease in population-based cohorts. Am J Gastroenterol. 2010;105:289–97.

Pignone MP, Gaynes BN, Rushton JL et al. Screening for depression in adults: a summary of the evidence for the U.S. Preventive Services Task Force. Ann Intern Med. 2002;136(10):765–76.

Reese GE, Constantinides VA, Simillis C et al. Diagnostic precision of anti-Saccharomyces cerevisiae antibodies and perinuclear antineutrophil cytoplasmic antibodies in inflammatory bowel disease. Am J Gastroenterol. 2006;101(10):2410–22.

Saitz R. Clinical practice. Unhealthy alcohol use. N Engl J Med. 2005;352(6):596–607.

Schoepfer AM, Trummler M, Seeholzer P, Seibold-Schmid B, Seibold F. Discriminating IBD from IBS: comparison of the test performance of fecal markers, blood leukocytes, CRP, and IBD antibodies. Inflamm Bowel Dis. 2008;14(1):32–9.

Stevens T, Dumot JA, Zuccaro G Jr et al. Evaluation of duct-cell and acinar-cell function and endosonographic abnormalities in patients with suspected chronic pancreatitis. Clin Gastroenterol Hepatol. 2009;7:114–9.

Talley NJ, American Gastroenterological Association. American Gastroenterological Association medical position statement: evaluation of dyspepsia. Gastroenterology. 2005;129(5):1753–5.

Triester SL, Leighton JA, Leontiadis GI et al. A meta-analysis of the yield of capsule endoscopy compared to other diagnostic modalities in patients with non-stricturing small bowel Crohn's disease. Am J Gastroenterol. 2006;101(5):954–64.

U.S. Preventive Services Task Force; Screening for Depression in Adults: U.S. Preventive Services Task Force Recommendation Statement. Ann Intern Med. 2009 Dec;151(11):784–92.

US Preventive Services Task Force. Screening and behavioral counseling interventions in primary care to reduce alcohol misuse: recommendation statement. Ann Intern Med. 2004;140(7):554–6.

Uskudar O, Oguz D, Akdogan M, Ahiparmak E, Sahin B. Comparison of endoscopic retrograde cholangiopancreatography, endoscopic ultrasonography, and fecal elastase 1 in chronic pancreatitis and clinical correlation. Pancreas. 2009;38:503–6.

I have a patient with wheezing or stridor. How do I determine the cause?

CHIEF COMPLAINT

PATIENT ▽1

Mr. C is a 32-year-old man with occasional wheezing.

What is the differential diagnosis of wheezing? How would you frame the differential?

CONSTRUCTING A DIFFERENTIAL DIAGNOSIS

Wheezing and stridor are symptoms of airflow obstruction caused by the vibration of the walls of pathologically narrow airways. **Wheezing** is a musical sound produced primarily during expiration by airways of any size. **Stridor** is a single pitch, inspiratory sound that is produced by large airways with severe narrowing; it may be caused by severe obstruction of any proximal airway (see A through D in the differential diagnosis outline below).

Stridor is often a sign of impending airway obstruction and should be considered an emergency.

Distinguishing between wheezing and stridor is essential. Typically, patients with either wheezing or stridor describe their symptoms simply as wheezing. The physical exam will determine whether the patient actually has wheezing or stridor. Because the differential diagnosis for airway obstruction is extensive, an anatomic approach is helpful.

A. Stridor
1. Nasopharynx and oropharynx
   a. Tonsillar hypertrophyb.
   b. Pharyngitisc.
   c. Peritonsillar abscessd.
   d. Retropharyngeal abscess
2. Laryngopharynx and larynx
   a. Epiglottitisb.
   b. Paradoxical vocal cord movement (PVCM)
   c. Anaphylaxis and laryngeal edemad.
   d. Postnasal dripe.
   e. Benign and malignant tumors of the larynx and upper airwayf.
   f. Vocal cord paralysis

3. Trachea
   a. Tracheal stenosis
   b. Tracheomalacia
   c. Goiter
4. Proximal airways
   a. Foreign-body aspiration
B. Wheezing
1. Proximal airways: Bronchitis
2. Distal airways
   a. Asthma
   b. Chronic obstructive pulmonary disease (COPD)
   c. Pulmonary edema
   d. Pulmonary embolism
   e. Bronchiectasis
   f. Bronchiolitis
   g. Heart failure
   h. Sarcoid

▽1

Mr. C has been having symptoms for 1–2 years. His symptoms have always been so mild that he has never sought care. Over the last month, he has been more symptomatic with wheezing, chest tightness, and shortness of breath. His symptoms are worse with exercise and worse at night. He notes that he often goes days without symptoms.

At this point, what is the leading hypothesis, what are the active alternatives, and is there a must not miss diagnosis? Given this differential diagnosis, what tests should be ordered?

RANKING THE DIFFERENTIAL DIAGNOSIS

The presence of wheezing, chest tightness, and shortness of breath are pivotal clues that place asthma at the top of the differential diagnosis. Although asthma is by far the most likely diagnosis, other diseases that could account for recurrent symptoms of airway obstruction should be considered (Table 33-1). Allergic rhinitis can cause cough and wheezing, but it would be very unusual for it to cause shortness of breath. Vocal cord dysfunction, such as PVCM, is frequently confused with asthma and can cause recurrent stridor. COPD can also cause chronic wheezing and pulmonary symptoms (Figure 33-1).

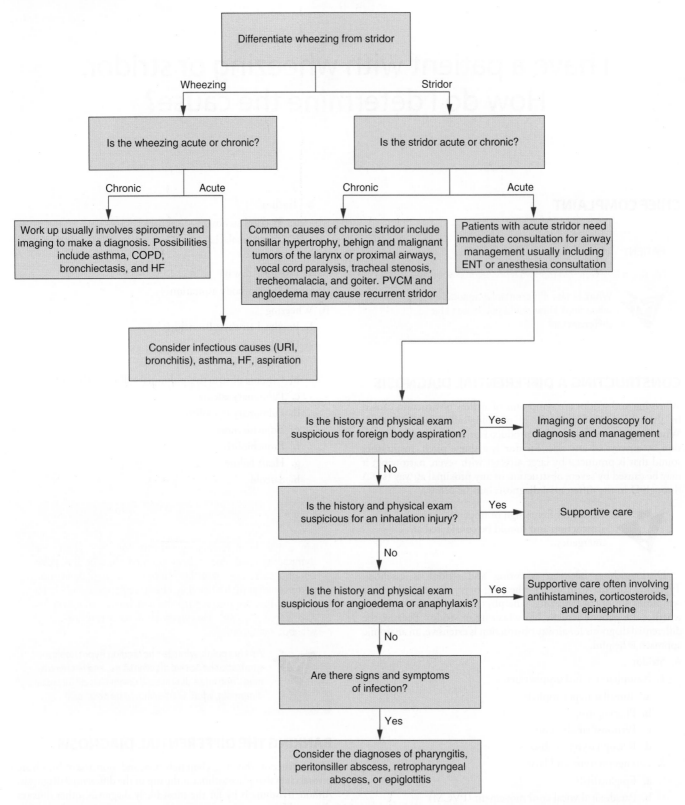

COPD, chronic obstructive pulmonary disease; ENT, ear, nose, and throat; HF, heart failure; PVCM, paradoxical vocal cord movement; URI, upper respiratory infection.

Figure 33-1. Evaluation of the patient with wheezing or stridor.

Table 33-1. Diagnostic hypotheses for Mr. C.

Diagnostic Hypotheses	Demographics, Risk Factors, Symptoms and Signs	Important Tests
Leading Hypothesis		
Asthma	Episodic and reversible airflow obstruction Intermittent wheezing, chest tightness, and shortness of breath are classic symptoms	Spirometry Methacholine challenge Response to treatment
Active Alternative		
Allergic rhinitis	Rhinitis with seasonal variation	Response to treatment
Vocal cord dysfunction	Voice pathology accompanies airflow obstruction	Abnormal vocal cord movement visualized
Active Alternative—Must Not Miss		
COPD	Presence of smoking history	Pulmonary function tests

On further history, Mr. C reports that he had asthma as a child and was treated for years with theophylline. He was without symptoms until he moved 2 years ago.

He reports that his symptoms are worst when he has a cold, when he jogs, and when he is around dogs or cats. His most common symptoms are chest tightness and dyspnea. Only when his symptoms are at their worst does he hear wheezing. He has never smoked cigarettes.

On physical exam he appears well. His vital signs are BP, 120/76 mm Hg; RR, 14 breaths per minute; pulse, 72 bpm; temperature, 36.9°C. His lung exam is normal without wheezes or prolonged expiratory phase. His peak flow is 550 L/min (87% of predicted).

 Is the clinical information sufficient to make a diagnosis? If not, what other information do you need?

Leading Hypothesis: Asthma

Textbook Presentation

Asthma commonly presents as recurrent episodes of dyspnea, often with chest tightness, cough, and wheezing. Patients usually report stereotypical triggers (eg, allergens, cold weather, exercise) and rapid response to beta-agonist inhalers.

 Asthma is a common cause of wheezing; however, the absence of wheezing by no means excludes the diagnosis of asthma.

Disease Highlights

A. Definition: The definition of asthma in the National Asthma Education and Prevention Program's Expert Panel Report is "A chronic inflammatory disease of the airways in which many cells and cellular elements play a role." "In susceptible individuals, this inflammation causes recurrent episodes of wheezing, breathlessness, chest tightness, and cough, particularly at night and/or in the early morning. These episodes are usually associated with widespread but variable airflow limitation that is often reversible either spontaneously or with treatment."

B. Clinical manifestations

1. Asthma is recurrent and intermittent.

   a. Most patients will have periods with no, or only mild, symptoms.

   b. Patients with severe disease will have persistent symptoms.

2. Asthma usually presents during childhood but presentation as an adult is not uncommon.

3. Airway function fluctuates in people with asthma more widely than in those without the diagnosis.

   a. Airway function is most commonly measured by peak expiratory flow (PEF).

   b. Values are generally lowest in the morning and highest at mid-day.

   c. PEF will vary by more than 20% in asthmatic patients over the course of the day.

4. Identifying exacerbating factors and timing of symptoms is important. It aids in the diagnosis of asthma (exacerbating factors are stereotypical) and in treatment (if the factors are reversible).

   a. Asthma frequently worsens at night (probably related to decreased mucociliary clearance, airway cooling, and low levels of endogenous catecholamines).

   b. Asthma frequently worsens with exercise (probably related to airway cooling and drying).

   c. Viral infections are a common cause of asthma exacerbations.

   d. A long list of occupational agents may cause or exacerbate asthma by a number of mechanisms:

      (1) Corrosive agents (ammonia)

      (2) Pharmacologic agents (organophosphates)

      (3) Reflex bronchoconstriction (ozone)

      (4) IgE-mediated (latex)

 Asthma should be in the differential diagnosis of any patient with intermittent respiratory symptoms.

C. Classification: The present classification scheme for asthma helps focus attention on the severity of the asthma and dovetails nicely with treatment considerations (Table 33-2). It should be noted, however, that by necessity this scheme simplifies asthma phenotypes and many patients do not fit well into a single category.

D. Exacerbations or "flares"

1. Asthma exacerbations are periods of increased disease activity identified by increased airflow obstruction, increased symptoms, and increased medication use.

2. Exacerbations may or may not be caused by an identifiable trigger.

3. Management of an exacerbation depends on an accurate assessment of the cause of the exacerbation and the risk to the patient.

Table 33-2. Classification of asthma severity.

Classification	Symptoms	Lung Function
Mild intermittent	Symptoms less than twice a week Asymptomatic between exacerbations and brief exacerbations Nighttime symptoms < twice monthly	PEF > 80% of predicted
Mild persistent	Symptoms between once a day and twice a week Asymptomatic between exacerbations but exacerbations may limit activity Nighttime symptoms > twice monthly	PEF > 80% of predicted
Moderate persistent	Daily symptoms Exacerbations limit activity Nighttime symptoms > weekly	PEF 60–80% of predicted
Severe persistent	Continual symptoms Symptoms chronically limit physical activity Frequent nighttime symptoms	PEF < 60% of predicted

PEF, peak expiratory flow.

Evidence-Based Diagnosis

A. There is no 1 test to diagnose asthma; the diagnosis is clinical, based on multiple findings in the history, physical exam, and spirometry.

B. Asthma is easily recognized when it presents with intermittent wheezing; in fact the diagnosis is often made by the patient.

C. Diagnosing asthma is challenging when it presents in atypical ways. Asthma should be high in the differential diagnosis when a patient has any of the following intermittent symptoms:

1. Wheezing
2. Dyspnea
3. Cough
4. Chest tightness

D. The key points in establishing the diagnosis of asthma are:

1. Episodic symptoms of airflow obstruction
2. Reversibility of the airflow obstruction
3. Exclusion of other likely diseases

E. There are not great data on the test characteristics of various symptoms of asthma.

4. One large study interviewed nearly 10,000 healthy, community-dwelling people regarding pulmonary symptoms in the preceding 12 months.

a. 225 of these people had asthma, defined as reporting that they had asthma and that a medical professional had confirmed the diagnosis.

b. The test characteristics of the most predictive historical features are shown in Table 33-3.

c. It is important to note that these test characteristics were derived in a healthy population. Specificities would be lower in a population containing patients with other cardiopulmonary diseases.

d. In another study, which used a methacholine challenge test to diagnose asthma, 90% specificity was achieved for making the diagnosis of asthma with the question, "Do you cough during or after exercise?"

F. Other clues that make the diagnosis more likely are outlined in the National Asthma Education and Prevention Program's Expert Panel Report:

1. Diurnal variability in PEF (> 20% variability between best and worst)

2. Symptoms occur or worsen in the presence of:

   a. Exercise
   b. Viral infections
   c. Animals with fur or hair
   d. House dust mites
   e. Mold
   f. Smoke
   g. Pollen
   h. Weather changes
   i. Laughing or hard crying
   j. Airborne chemicals or dust

3. Symptoms occur or worsen at night.

G. There is some evidence that persons with asthma describe their dyspnea differently from people with other cardiorespiratory diseases.

Table 33-3. Test characteristics of symptoms for the diagnosis of asthma.

Criteria	Sensitivity	Specificity	LR+	LR−
Wheezing	74.7%	87.3%	5.77	0.29
Dyspnea at rest	47.1%	94.9%	9.23	0.56
Wheezing without URI symptoms	59.8%	93.6%	9.34	0.43
Nocturnal dyspnea	46.2%	96%	11.55	0.56
Wheezing and exertional dyspnea	54.2%	95.7%	12.60	0.48
Wheezing and dyspnea	65.2%	95.1%	13.30	0.37
Wheezing and nocturnal chest tightness	40.9%	97.5%	16.44	0.61
Wheezing and nocturnal dyspnea	37.5%	98.6%	26.79	0.61
Wheezing and dyspnea at rest	38.4%	98.7%	29.54	0.62

LR, likelihood ratio; URI, upper respiratory infection.
Adapted, with permission, from Sistek D et al. Clinical diagnosis of current asthma: predictive value of respiratory symptoms in the SAPALDIA study. Swiss Study on Air Pollution and Lung Diseases in Adults. Eur Respir J. 2001;17:214–19.

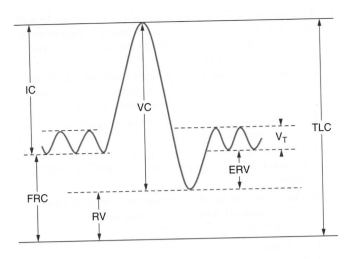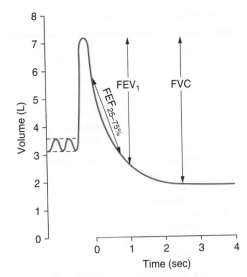

Figure 33-2. Pulmonary function tests. ERV, expiratory reserve volume; FEF 25–75%, forced expiratory flow measured during exhalation of 25–75% of the FVC; FEV$_1$, forced expiratory volume in 1 second; FRC, functional reserve capacity; FVC, forced vital capacity; IC, inspiratory capacity; RV, residual volume; TLC, total lung capacity; VC, vital capacity; V$_T$, tidal volume.

They are more likely to refer to symptoms of chest tightness or constriction.

H. Pulmonary function tests (PFTs)

1. Spirometry is recommended for patients with suspected asthma. The results are useful both as a diagnostic test and to provide objective data to be used in the assessment of management.

2. Figure 33-2 shows a schematic diagram of many of the lung volumes, capacities, and flows measured in PFTs.

3. The following all support the diagnosis of asthma:

   a. Decreased forced expiratory volume in 1 second (FEV$_1$)

   b. Decreased FEV$_1$/forced vital capacity (FVC) ratio

   c. Reversibility (defined as at least a 200 mL increase in FEV$_1$ and > 12% improvement with bronchodilators)

I. Other tests

1. Chest radiography is useful mainly in excluding other diseases.

2. Methacholine challenge

   a. Useful for diagnosing (or excluding) asthma in patients who have a suspicious history but normal PFTs

   b. A decrease in FEV$_1$ of < 20% has a 95% negative predictive value.

Treatment

A. The goals of asthma therapy are to

1. Prevent chronic symptoms (dyspnea, exercise intolerance, nighttime wakening)

2. Maintain normal pulmonary function (assessed by PEF and spirometry)

3. Maintain normal levels of physical activity.

   a. It can be challenging to achieve this goal.

   b. Many patients become accustomed to being limited by their breathing and thus may not report that their breathing limits their activity.

4. Prevent exacerbations

B. The National Asthma Education and Prevention Program's Expert Panel Report lists 4 components of asthma care.

1. Assessing and monitoring control of asthma severity and control. This entails accurately diagnosing the severity of patients' symptoms at baseline and during therapy.

2. Patient education

3. Control of environmental factors and comorbid conditions that affect asthma. This may include pharmacologic and nonpharmacologic interventions for, among others, the following:

   a. Tobacco use and secondhand smoke

   b. Air pollution (ozone, SO$_2$, NO$_2$)

   c. Gastroesophageal reflux disease (GERD)

   d. Common allergens

   e. Dander, dust, mold, insects

 It is critical to control diseases and factors that exacerbate asthma in order to achieve control with the least intensive regimen possible.

4. Medication use

   a. Medical therapy for asthma itself is aimed at treating the factors that cause the disease and its symptoms. The drugs are summarized in Table 33-4.

   b. The current guidelines advocate a stepwise approach to management. Step 1 is for patients with intermittent asthma and steps 2–6 build on one another for worsening levels of persistent asthma.

   (1) Step 1: Short-acting beta-2-agonists used as needed.

   (2) Step 2: Low-dose inhaled corticosteroids.

   (3) Step 3: Low-dose inhaled corticosteroids with long-acting beta-2-agonists. An alternative at this point is medium-dose inhaled corticosteroids.

   (4) Step 4. Medium-dose inhaled corticosteroids with long-acting beta-2-agonists.

Table 33-4. Pharmacotherapy of asthma.

Medication	Purpose	Common Adverse Effects
Short-acting beta-2-agonists	Immediate relief of symptoms	Tachycardia, jitteriness
Inhaled corticosteroids	Mainstay of long-term therapy	Thrush, dysphonia, potentially osteopenia at high doses
Long-acting beta-2-agonists	Long-term therapy when inhaled corticosteroids have not adequately controlled symptoms. Useful for nocturnal symptoms	Tachycardia, jitteriness
Omalizumab[1]	For patients with allergies and asthma not controlled by inhaled corticosteroids and long-acting beta-2-agonists	Injection site reactions and viral infections
Leukotriene antagonists	Another option for patients with allergies and poorly controlled asthma	No significant adverse effects
Systemic corticosteroids	Immediate therapy for exacerbations or long-term therapy in patients with refractory asthma	Traditional corticosteroid side effects (weight gain, hyperglycemia, bone loss)
Theophylline	Similar to long-acting beta-2-agonists but used less frequently	Dose-related tachycardia, nausea, jitteriness

[1]Monoclonal antibody that binds to IgE.

(5) Step 5. High-dose inhaled corticosteroids with long-acting beta-2-agonists with consideration of omalizumab for patients with allergies

(6) Step 6. High-dose inhaled corticosteroids with long-acting beta-2-agonists and oral corticosteroids with consideration of omalizumab for patients with allergies

c. Consideration should be given for escalating therapy whenever short-acting beta-2-agonists are being used more than twice a week.

d. Efforts should always be made to step down therapy when control is achieved.

e. Recent data suggest that inhaled tiotropium may be beneficial for patients whose asthma is poorly controlled with inhaled corticosteroids with long-acting beta-2-agonists.

 At each visit, review a patient's medications and symptoms and make an effort to step down therapy when possible.

C. Refractory asthma: Although most cases of asthma can be well controlled, there are patients whose asthma is refractory to the standard therapy. This may be due to the inherent severity of the disease or other factors:

1. Problem with adherence to prescribed regimen. This includes poor inhaler technique (common) and poor understanding of the use of maintenance and as-needed medications.

2. Precipitants that are unrecognized or untreated such as GERD, sinusitis, and allergies.

3. Incorrect diagnosis; consider other causes of chronic intermittent airway obstruction such as PVCM, COPD, or sarcoid.

4. The presence of rare diseases that can cause or worsen asthma (such as Churg-Strauss disease, allergic bronchopulmonary aspergillosis).

D. Exacerbations

1. History

   a. Duration of exacerbation

   (1) Exacerbations that are very recent (hours) and mild may improve with beta-agonists alone while more established and more severe exacerbations require corticosteroids.

   (2) Because early treatment leads to better outcomes, it is important that patients monitor their own disease and know how to initiate appropriate treatment and contact their physician when necessary.

   b. Precipitants

   (1) Consider if there is a clear precipitant of the exacerbation that needs to be addressed (eg, sinusitis, allergen exposure).

   (2) Consider if there is an exacerbating factor that hospital admission might alleviate (eg, house painting, recent insect extermination).

   c. Severity of disease. The following patients are at risk for asthma-related death. Any patient with an exacerbation and 1 of these factors require special attention with regards to education, monitoring, and care:

   (1) Previous severe exacerbations

   (2) Multiple, recent emergency department visits or hospitalizations

   (3) Use of more than 2 canisters of beta-agonist in the past month

   (4) Current use or recent discontinuation of systemic corticosteroids

   (5) Difficulty perceiving airflow obstruction

   (6) Low socioeconomic status or inner-city residence

   (7) Illicit drug use

   (8) Comorbid medical or psychiatric disease

 Any patient with risk factors for asthma-related death who presents with an asthma exacerbation requires special attention, beginning with serious consideration for hospitalization.

2. Physical exam

   a. The lung exam is generally a poor marker of the severity of disease.

   b. Lack of wheezing can either reflect improved or worsening airflow.

Patients whose decreased wheezing is accompanied by worsening distress or decreased mental status probably have worsening airflow obstruction. Conversely, a patient whose decreased wheezing is accompanied by lessened respiratory distress likely has improved airflow obstruction.

3. Other tests

   a. Spirometry is crucial in determining severity of exacerbation.

      (1) A mild exacerbation is defined by symptoms only with activity and a FEV_1 or PEF or $\geq 70\%$ of predicted.

      (2) A moderate exacerbation includes symptoms with usual activities and a FEV_1 or PEF 40–69% of predicted.

      (3) In a severe exacerbation, patients will have dyspnea at rest and dyspnea that interferes with conversation and a FEV_1 or PEF < 40% of predicted.

 Spirometry and the history of the patient's prior exacerbations are the most important pieces of information for making admission decisions.

   b. Arterial blood gases (ABGs) are useful in patients whose peak flows are not improving with treatment. ABGs during severe exacerbations should reveal a respiratory alkalosis. A respiratory acidosis (or even a normal PCO_2 during a severe exacerbation) is very worrisome because it suggests severe airway narrowing and respiratory fatigue.

   c. Chest radiograph is only helpful for identifying the uncommon concomitant infection or complication (eg, pneumothorax).

4. Treatment of exacerbations. Figure 33-3 is a guide to the management of asthma exacerbations.

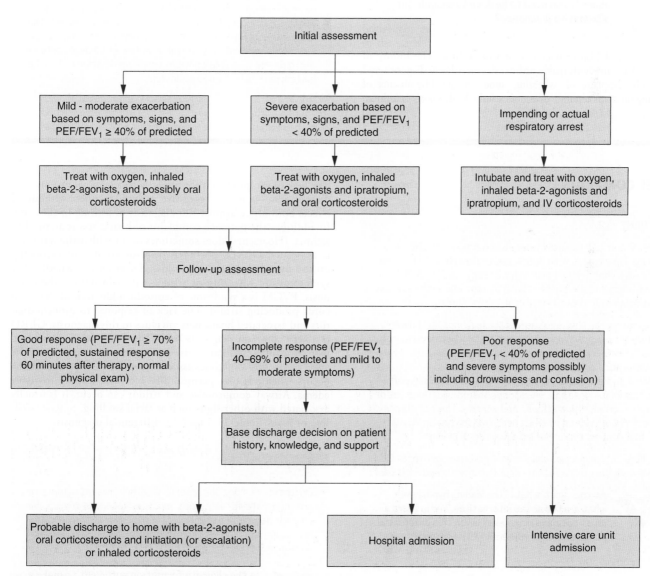

Figure 33-3. Management of asthma exacerbation. (Adapted, with permission, from National Heart, Lung, and Blood Institute, National Asthma Education and Prevention Program. Expert Panel Report 3: guidelines for the diagnosis and management of asthma: full report 2007.)

MAKING A DIAGNOSIS

Mr. C was scheduled for spirometry and prescribed an albuterol inhaler. He was told to use 2 puffs as needed as well as 30 minutes before exercise or expected animal exposure. On follow-up 6 weeks later, Mr. C reported improvement in his symptoms. He was able to exercise without difficulty as long as he was using his inhalers and could spend short amounts of time around friends' pets.

Spirometry revealed an FEV$_1$ of 70% of predicted that normalized with albuterol.

At follow up a few months later he reported that he was using his albuterol inhaler daily to maintain his asthma control.

 Have you crossed a diagnostic threshold for the leading hypothesis, asthma? Have you ruled out the active alternatives? Do other tests need to be done to exclude the alternative diagnoses?

Mr. C's clinical history is consistent with asthma. The history of childhood asthma both makes asthma the most likely diagnosis and makes his complaint of "wheezing" more reliable. The absence of wheezing on exam certainly does not exclude the diagnosis of asthma.

He has intermittent symptoms of wheezing, dyspnea, and chest tightness. The presence of exacerbating factors and the results of spirometry further raise the likelihood of asthma as the diagnosis.

 Because asthma is very common and the initial treatment is benign, the treatment threshold is low. A therapeutic trial of medication is nearly always appropriate.

CASE RESOLUTION

The patient's history and response to therapy confirms the diagnosis of asthma. The patient has no nasal symptoms that would suggest allergic rhinitis. COPD is unlikely without a smoking history. Vocal cord dysfunction will be discussed below and is also unlikely. Heart failure (HF) is unlikely given the patient's age, the absence of a history of heart disease, and his response to bronchodilators.

Given the frequency of his use of albuterol, the patient was given low-dose inhaled corticosteroids. His symptoms subsequently improved with only rare need for albuterol. The following year, Mr. C's symptoms worsened. His asthma was eventually controlled with higher doses of inhaled corticosteroids. He was able to wean these medications after he had carpets in his house removed.

CHIEF COMPLAINT

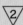
PATIENT 2

Mrs. P is a 62-year-old woman who arrives at the emergency department with shortness of breath and wheezing. She says that the symptoms have been present for 3 days. The symptoms are present both at rest and with exertion and have not improved with an albuterol inhaler.

She reports that she has had these symptoms intermittently for 6 years. When the symptoms occur, they generally last for hours to a few days. She had been diagnosed with asthma and took long- and short-acting beta-agonists and inhaled and systemic corticosteroids, before coming off all medications 1 year ago. She stopped her medications out of frustration with side effects and perceived lack of efficacy. She decided instead to treat herself with yoga and meditation. She reports no episodes since this decision.

Presently she denies cough, chest pain, fever, or rhinitis. She does report hoarseness that occurs when her breathing is bad.

 At this point, what is the leading hypothesis, what are the active alternatives, and is there a must not miss diagnosis? Given this differential diagnosis, what tests should be ordered?

RANKING THE DIFFERENTIAL DIAGNOSIS

As discussed above, asthma is very common and should be considered in anyone with intermittent pulmonary symptoms.

The lack of symptom improvement with a beta-agonist and the discontinuation of an aggressive asthma regimen without ill effects both argue against the diagnosis of asthma in this case. In addition, the patient's complaint of hoarseness is atypical in asthma. (Hoarseness does sometimes occur with asthma if there is associated GERD, postnasal drip, or vocal cord myopathy caused by inhaled corticosteroids.) Determining whether her symptoms are wheezing or stridor will help narrow the diagnosis. PVCM is a syndrome of episodic adduction of the vocal cords producing stridor. The lack of response to bronchodilators and associated hoarseness are clues to this diagnosis. GERD is a very common diagnosis (see Chapter 9). It can cause and worsen asthma and can cause hoarseness via irritation of the vocal cords. It is sometimes associated with PVCM. Angioedema occurs when vascular permeability increases leading to tissue edema. Airway compromise and stridor can occur. It is usually associated with other signs such as facial swelling, tongue swelling, or hives. Table 33-5 lists the differential diagnosis.

On further history, she reports that her present symptoms are moderate for her. Past medical history is remarkable only for depression and hypertension. Her only medication is enalapril. She has no known drug allergies. She does not smoke cigarettes.

 Is the clinical information sufficient to make a diagnosis? If not, what other information do you need?

Table 33-5. Diagnostic hypotheses for Mrs. P.

Diagnostic Hypotheses	Demographics, Risk Factors, Symptoms and Signs	Important Tests
Leading Hypothesis		
Paradoxical vocal cord movement	Episodic airflow obstruction associated with stridor	Laryngoscopy demonstrating abnormal vocal cord movement
Active Alternative—Most Common		
Asthma	Episodic and reversible airflow obstruction	Peak flow PFTs Methacholine challenge Response to treatment
Active Alternative		
Gastroesophageal reflux disease	May cause or worsen asthma and cause voice pathology	Identification of esophageal and laryngeal abnormalities on endoscopy
Active Alternative—Must Not Miss		
Angioedema	Often associated with hives and causative exposure	Clinical presentation with or without risk factors

PFTs, pulmonary function tests.

Leading Hypothesis: PVCM

Textbook Presentation

PVCM typically presents as episodic attacks of respiratory distress accompanied by wheezing or stridor or both. The respiratory distress is often accompanied by voice pathology and does not respond to traditional asthma therapy.

Disease Highlights

A. PVCM has gone by many names including vocal cord dysfunction, episodic laryngeal dyskinesia, Munchausen stridor, psychogenic stridor, and factitious asthma.

B. Most commonly occurs in younger patients (< 35 years) but can be seen in any age.

C. Female predominance

D. PVCM has been associated with a number of diseases including:

 1. Anxiety and other psychiatric conditions

 2. Exercise

 3. Airway injury (iatrogenic, inhalational)

 4. GERD

 5. Neurologic injury

E. The symptoms are not produced consciously.

F. During asymptomatic periods, there are no abnormalities of lung function:

 1. Spirometry is normal.

 2. There is none of the increased variability in airway function seen with asthma.

 3. Bronchial provocation tests are normal.

Evidence-Based Diagnosis

A. Given the prevalence of asthma and the similarity of the presentation, asthma needs to be excluded in any patient with PVCM. This is especially true as the 2 disorders may coexist.

B. Clues to the differentiation of the diseases are:

 1. The lack of exacerbating factors (eg, exercise, allergens) and diurnal variation seen with asthma.

 2. The lack of response to asthma medications.

 3. The occasional disappearance of symptoms during sleep.

 4. The striking voice pathology during attacks.

 5. The preponderance of auscultatory findings in the neck.

  a. PVCM should really produce inspiratory stridor, as opposed to the predominantly expiratory wheezing heard with asthma.

  b. In practice, these can be hard to differentiate.

 6. A flattened inspiratory limb on flow-volume loops suggesting variable extrathoracic airway obstruction.

C. The definitive diagnosis is made during laryngoscopy.

 1. There is adduction of the vocal cords during flares.

 2. There is generally normal vocal cord function between flares.

Treatment

A. There are no controlled trials of treatments for PVCM.

B. Speech therapy, concentrating on laryngeal relaxation seems to be the most effective therapy.

C. Psychiatric intervention is suggested for patients with psychiatric illness.

D. Acute attacks may be quite hard to manage.

 1. Helium/oxygen mixtures have been suggested to obtain better flow through the narrowed larynx though there is no evidence to support its utility.

 2. Instructing the patient to lay his tongue on the floor of the mouth and breathe through pursed lips may also help.

MAKING A DIAGNOSIS

On physical exam, the patient is in mild respiratory distress. Her voice is hoarse and "squeaky." Her vital signs are temperature, 37.1°C; pulse, 110 bpm; BP, 140/90 mm Hg; RR, 32 breaths per minute. There is inspiratory and expiratory stridor in the neck transmitted throughout the lungs.

The remainder of the physical exam was normal.

PEF is 300 L/min, 70% of predicted.

 Have you crossed a diagnostic threshold for the leading hypothesis, PVCM? Have you ruled out the active alternatives? Do other tests need to be done to exclude the alternative diagnoses?

The physical exam is consistent with stridor and the presence of recurrent stridor makes PVCM likely. The other important diagnosis to consider at this point is angioedema.

Alternative Diagnosis: Angioedema

Textbook Presentation

Angioedema presents with the acute swelling of soft tissues, especially the face, lips, tongue, larynx, or foreskin. Bowel edema can result in abdominal pain. Patients nearly always have a history of angioedema or a risk factor for it.

Disease Highlights

A. The onset of angioedema is usually rapid, over minutes to hours.

B. Angioedema may be caused by:

  1. Medications (angiotensin-converting enzyme [ACE] inhibitors and nonsteroidal antiinflammatory drugs [NSAIDs] being, by far, the most common culprits)

  2. Allergic reactions

  3. Hereditary and acquired forms of C1-inhibitor deficiency

C. The presentation can range from mild, only sensed by the patient; to disfiguring, obvious to the casual observer; to life-threatening.

D. The diverse causes of angioedema produce symptoms by different mechanisms, have different presentations, and different treatments.

  1. Histamine-related angioedema

  a. Almost always accompanied by pruritus and urticaria (hives).

  b. Usually related to an allergic exposure such as an insect bite or a food.

  c. Urticaria can also be chronic, caused by allergy, drug effect, autoimmune phenomena, or malignancy.

  2. Nonhistamine-related angioedema (caused by elevated levels of bradykinin)

  a. Most commonly the result of ACE inhibitor therapy

  b. Deficiency of C1-inhibitor also causes elevated bradykinin levels as well as elevated C2b levels, another cause of angioedema.

 If angioedema is associated with urticaria, it is not due to ACE inhibitor therapy.

Evidence-Based Diagnosis

A. A diagnosis of angioedema is clinical, based on the recognition of angioedema and associated symptoms.

B. Angioedema most commonly presents as swelling of the lips, tongue, or both.

C. Figure 33-4 presents a useful algorithm for considering the differential diagnosis and treatment of angioedema.

Treatment

A. The most critical aspect of the management of angioedema is airway stabilization.

B. All patients receive H_1- and H_2-blockers as well as corticosteroids.

C. Patients with airway compromise or any intraoral swelling should also receive epinephrine.

D. Patients need to be closely monitored because intubation is sometimes necessary.

E. Patients with C1-inhibitor deficiency can be treated with androgens, which increase the production of C1-inhibitor, or C1-inhibitor concentrate.

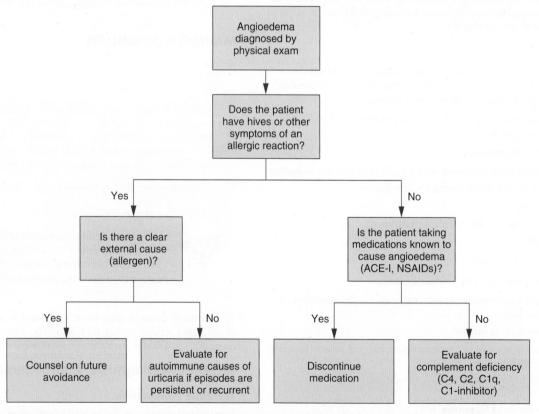

ACE-I, angiotensin-converting enzyme inhibitors; NSAIDs, nonsteroidal antiinflammatory drugs.

Figure 33-4. Differential diagnosis and treatment of angioedema.

CASE RESOLUTION

A helium oxygen mixture was given to the patient briefly before laryngoscopy was performed. The findings on laryngoscopy were consistent with PVCM. The patient was counseled in the emergency department on ways to

(continued)

improve her airflow and symptoms subsided over the next hour. The patient spent 2 days in the hospital, experiencing only 1 mild episode of dyspnea during the period of observation.

Laryngoscopic findings can make the diagnosis of PVCM. Except for her use of an ACE inhibitor, there is little evidence to support angioedema; the patient has no facial swelling, and there are no consistent findings on laryngoscopy.

CHIEF COMPLAINT

PATIENT

Mr. S is a 50-year-old man who arrives at the emergency department with sore throat, fever, and wheezing. He reports being well until 2 days ago when his sore throat started. Over the last 2 days, the sore throat became progressively more severe and he lost his voice. On the morning of admission, a fever of 38.0°C and wheezing developed. He was also unable to eat because of the pain. He has never had similar symptoms.

 At this point, what is the leading hypothesis, what are the active alternatives, and is there a must not miss diagnosis? Given this differential diagnosis, what tests should be ordered?

RANKING THE DIFFERENTIAL DIAGNOSIS

The pivotal points in Mr. S's presentation are the acuity of the illness and the fever. Both of these points make an infectious etiology likely. Because the symptoms are not recurrent, asthma (the most common cause of airway obstruction) is unlikely. Acute infectious causes need to be considered first. These include common conditions, such as pharyngitis, and rare but serious causes, such as epiglottitis and retropharyngeal abscess. Angioedema is possible, but the infectious symptoms (fever and pain) and the lack of visible swelling make this less likely. Aspiration of a foreign body could cause either a pneumonia or infection of the soft tissues of the neck resulting in fever. Table 33-6 lists the differential diagnosis.

On physical exam, Mr. S is in obvious distress. He is uncomfortable, is sitting upright, and speaks in a muffled-voice. His vitals signs are temperature, 38.3°C; pulse, 110 bpm; BP, 128/88 mm Hg; RR, 18 breaths per minute. Examination of the oropharynx is notable only for mild tonsillar edema without exudates. There is diffuse cervical lymphadenopathy and significant tenderness over the anterior neck. The neck is supple. Lungs are clear, but there is stridor transmitted from the neck.

Table 33-6. Diagnostic hypotheses for Mr. S.

Diagnostic Hypotheses	Demographics, Risk Factors, Symptoms and Signs	Important Tests
Leading Hypothesis		
Pharyngitis	Sore throat often with fever, exudates and lymphadenopathy	Clinical exam Throat culture
Active Alternative—Must Not Miss		
Epiglottitis	Sore throat with muffled voice, stridor, and anterior neck tenderness	Direct visualization with laryngoscopy
Retropharyngeal abscess	Similar to epiglottitis with more prominent neck symptoms (stiff, painful)	Lateral neck radiograph or CT scan of the neck
Other Alternative		
Foreign body aspiration	Usually history of acute-onset pain or airway obstruction	Documentation of foreign body directly or radiographically

 Is the clinical information sufficient to make a diagnosis? If not, what other information do you need?

The patient's physical exam clarifies the picture; Mr. S has stridor. In a patient with acute stridor and infectious symptoms, epiglottitis and retropharyngeal abscess must top the differential diagnosis.

Leading Hypothesis: Epiglottitis

Textbook Presentation

Fever and sore throat are usually the presenting symptoms. There can be evidence of varying degrees of airway obstruction including wheezing, stridor, and drooling. The disease has become significantly less common in children since the use of the *Haemophilus influenzae B* vaccine.

Disease Highlights

A. Epiglottitis is an infectious disease, classically caused by *H influenzae,* that causes swelling of the epiglottis and supraglottic structures.

B. Because epiglottitis can rapidly cause airway compromise, the diagnosis should always be considered an airway emergency.

C. The classic presentation is a patient with sore throat, muffled "hot potato" voice, drooling, and stridor.

D. *H influenzae* is cultured in only a small percentage of adult patients; respiratory viruses are the likely cause of most cases of epiglottitis.

E. Epiglottitis is a difficult diagnosis because, early in its course, it may resemble pharyngitis.

Evidence-Based Diagnosis

A. The gold standard for diagnosis is visual identification of swelling of the epiglottis.

   1. Otolaryngology consultation is thus mandatory if there is a high suspicion for the disease.

   2. Visualization can be achieved with direct or indirect laryngoscopy.

   3. In patients with signs of severe disease (eg, muffled voice, drooling, and stridor), an experienced physician should perform direct laryngoscopy and be prepared to intubate the patient or perform a tracheostomy (if airway control cannot be obtained).

B. The classic symptoms of muffled voice, drooling, and stridor are seen very rarely and signify imminent airway obstruction.

   1. Stridor and the patient sitting in an erect posture are independent predictors of subsequent airway intervention.

   2. The test characteristics of these signs for airway intervention are:

   a. Stridor: Sensitivity, 42%; specificity, 94%; LR+, 7; LR-, 0.61.

   b. Sitting erect at presentation: Sensitivity, 47%; specificity, 90%; LR+, 4.7; LR-. 0.59.

C. Common symptoms and signs of patients with epiglottitis; prevalence is given in parentheses

   1. Sore throat (95%)

   2. Odynophagia (94%)

   3. Muffled voice (54%)

   4. Pharyngitis (44%)

   5. Fever (42%)

   6. Cervical adenopathy (41%)

   7. Dyspnea (37%)

   8. Drooling (30%)

   9. Sitting erect (16%)

   10. Stridor (12%)

D. Lateral neck films, a commonly used diagnostic tool, have a sensitivity of about 90%. The classic finding is the "thumb sign" of a swollen epiglottis.

 A normal lateral neck film does not rule out epiglottitis. Laryngoscopy should be performed in a patient with a high clinical suspicion of epiglottitis, even if the neck film is normal.

Treatment

A. Airway control

   1. All patients should be admitted to the intensive care unit (ICU) for close monitoring.

   2. Patients with signs or symptoms of airway obstruction should be intubated electively.

   3. Elective intubation is preferred because intubation in a patient with epiglottitis can be very difficult.

   4. Some advocate prophylactic intubation of all patients.

B. Epiglottitis is an airway emergency. Patients need to be monitored extremely closely and not left alone until the airway is stable. Otolaryngology consultation is mandatory.

C. Antibiotics

   1. Necessary to cover *H influenzae.*

   2. Second- or third-generation cephalosporins are usually recommended.

MAKING A DIAGNOSIS

Mr. S's history is very concerning. His upright posture, voice changes, and stridor not only strongly suggest epiglottitis but also imminent airway closure. Foreign-body aspiration does not fit the history. Retropharyngeal abscess remains a possibility.

Given the concern for epiglottitis, lateral neck films were obtained, and an otolaryngologist was called to examine the patient's upper airway.

 Have you crossed a diagnostic threshold for the leading hypothesis, epiglottitis? Have you ruled out the active alternatives? Do other tests need to be done to exclude the alternative diagnoses?

Alternative Diagnosis: Retropharyngeal Abscess

Textbook Presentation

Retropharyngeal abscess can be seen in either children or adults. Patients usually have symptoms similar to those seen in epiglottitis but commonly have a history of a recent upper respiratory infection or trauma from recently ingested materials (bones), or procedures (pulmonary or gastrointestinal endoscopy).

Disease Highlights

D. Symptoms that suggest retropharyngeal abscess rather than epiglottitis are:

   1. Patients with retropharyngeal abscesses often will sense a lump in their throat.

   2. Patients are often most comfortable supine with neck extended (very different from epiglottitis).

Evidence-Based Diagnosis

A. The diagnosis of retropharyngeal abscess is made when a thickening of the retropharyngeal tissues is seen on lateral neck radiographs.

B. Radiographs are probably not 100% sensitive, so when radiographs are normal and clinical suspicion is high, CT scanning should be done to verify the diagnosis.

Treatment

A. Retropharyngeal abscesses are usually polymicrobial.

B. Treatment is both medical and surgical.

   1. Surgical drainage should be accomplished as soon as possible.

2. Many antibiotics have been suggested. Coverage of gram-positive organisms and anaerobes make clindamycin a common choice.

CASE RESOLUTION

The patient's lateral neck radiograph showed probable acute epiglottitis with a thumb sign. An otolaryngologist

(continued)

visualized the epiglottis and, given the patient's symptom-sand severity of the visualized airway obstruction, placed an endotracheal tube. Mr. S was admitted to the ICU and treated with a second-generation cephalosporin. Cultures of the blood and epiglottis were negative.

The patient's infection was diagnosed on the lateral neck radiographs. Intubation was necessary because the patient had signs and symptoms of airway obstruction. The obstruction was visualized on laryngoscopy.

CHIEF COMPLAINT

PATIENT 4

Mrs. A is 52-year-old woman who comes to your office with shortness of breath and wheezing. She reports that her symptoms have been present for about 2 years. She reports almost constant, mild dyspnea that is worst with exercise or when she has a cold. Only rarely does she feel "nearly normal." She also complains of a mild cough productive of clear sputum. She does not feel that her cough is much of a problem as it is significantly better since she stopped smoking 2 years ago.

 At this point, what is the leading hypothesis, and what are the active alternatives? What other tests should be ordered?

RANKING THE DIFFERENTIAL DIAGNOSIS

The pivotal points in this case are the patient's chronic dyspnea, wheezing, and smoking history. COPD and asthma should be high in the differential diagnosis. HF is also a possibility. The patient's smoking history is a risk factor for coronary disease, the most common cause of HF. As noted in Chapter 15, Dyspnea, HF frequently complicates COPD or is misdiagnosed as the pulmonary disease. Bronchiectasis could cause symptoms of dyspnea, cough, and sputum production, but the patient's sputum production seems to be a minor symptom, unlike what is usually seen in bronchiectasis. Tuberculosis (TB) should probably be considered in the differential, since it can cause chronic cough and dyspnea. Given the chronic nature of the symptoms, if TB were the cause, weight loss and other constitutional signs would be expected. Table 33-7 lists the differential diagnosis.

Mrs. A reports a 60 pack-year history of smoking. She stopped 2 years ago, after smoking 2 packs a day for 30 years, when her chronic cough began to worry her. She reports that she still coughs but only rarely brings up sputum.

She has not experienced fever, chills, weight loss, or peripheral edema. She does say that when her breathing is bad it is worse when lying down. She has never had symptoms consistent with paroxysmal nocturnal dyspnea.

Table 33-7. Diagnostic hypotheses for Mrs. A.

Diagnostic Hypotheses	Demographics, Risk Factors, Symptoms and Signs	Important Tests
Leading Hypothesis		
COPD	Chronic irreversible airway obstruction with a smoking history	Spirometry and sometimes imaging
Active Alternative—Most Common		
Asthma	Episodic and reversible airflow obstruction	Peak flow PFTs Methacholine Challenge Response to treatment
Active Alternative—Must Not Miss		
HF	Presence of risk factors and consistent physical exam findings	Echocardiography
Other Alternative		
Bronchiectasis	Chronic, heavy, purulent sputum production	CT scan of the chest

COPD, chronic obstructive pulmonary disease; HF, heart failure; PFTs, pulmonary function tests.

 Orthopnea is a very nonspecific symptom. It is found in many types of cardiopulmonary disease.

 Is the clinical information sufficient to make a diagnosis? If not, what other information do you need?

Leading Hypothesis: COPD

Textbook Presentation

Presenting symptoms of COPD include progressive dyspnea, decreased exercise tolerance, cough, and sputum production.

The onset is usually slow and progressive with occasional acute exacerbations. A long smoking history is present in almost all patients with COPD who live in industrialized countries.

Disease Highlights

A. COPD is defined in the WHO/NHLBI Global Strategy for the Diagnosis, Management, and Prevention of Chronic Obstructive Pulmonary Disease (GOLD) as a "disease state characterized by airflow limitation that is not fully reversible. The airflow limitation is usually both progressive and associated with an abnormal inflammatory response of the lungs to noxious particles or gases."

B. COPD should be considered in any patient with a smoking history who has pulmonary complaints. These complaints can be:

   1. Mild (smokers' cough or lingering colds)

   2. Moderate (chronic cough, sputum production, and dyspnea)

   3. Severe (activity-limiting dyspnea with life-threatening exacerbations)

C. COPD can also be seen in patients without a smoking history but with significant exposure to secondhand smoke, occupational dust and chemicals and, especially in less developed countries, indoor air pollution from cooking stoves.

D. Because of the wide variation in disease course, it is impossible to give an average amount of exposure necessary to cause disease.

   1. Pulmonary symptoms usually develop after about 10 years of exposure.

   2. Airflow obstruction may develop later.

E. Emphysema and chronic bronchitis are currently being used less as descriptors of types of COPD.

   1. Emphysema is a pathologic term not accurately correlating with its general clinical usage.

   2. Chronic bronchitis is the presence of mucus production for most days of the month, 3 months of a year, for 2 successive years. This symptom does not relate to the airflow obstruction that causes the morbidity in COPD.

   3. Due to the overlap and lack of specificity of these 2 terms, COPD should be used as the diagnostic term.

F. The Gold staging system is often used to classify patients based on their symptoms and level of risk of exacerbations. The system uses both spirometry and symptom data and incorporates them into a combined assessment of symptoms and risk of exacerbation:

   1. Spirometry

      a. Mild: FEV_1 ≥ 85% of predicted

      b. Moderate: FEV_1 > 50% to < 85% of predicted

      c. Severe: FEV_1 ≥ 30% to ≤ 50% of predicted

      d. Very Severe: FEV_1 < 30% of predicted

   2. Symptoms, based on the Modified Medical Research Council (MMRC) dyspnea scale

      a. Grade 0: "I only get breathless with strenuous exercise."

      b. Grade 1: "I get short of breath when hurrying on level ground or walking up a slight hill."

      c. Grade 2: "On level ground, I walk slower than people of the same age because of breathlessness, or have to stop for breath when walking at my own pace."

      d. Grade 3: "I stop for breath after walking about 100 yards or after a few minutes on level ground."

      e. Grade 4: "I am too breathless to leave the house or I am breathless when dressing."

   3. Combined Assessment

      a. Low risk, few symptoms: Mildly to moderately abnormal spirometry, and/or ≤ 1 exacerbation/year, and grade 0–1 symptoms.

      b. Low risk, more symptoms: Mildly to moderately abnormal spirometry, and/or ≤ 1 exacerbation/year, and ≥ grade 2 symptoms.

      c. High risk, few symptoms: Severely or very severely abnormal spirometry, and/or ≥ 2 exacerbations/year, and grade 0–1 symptoms.

      d. High risk, many symptoms: Severely or very severely abnormal spirometry, and/or ≥ 2 exacerbations/year and ≥ grade 2 symptoms.

G. The BODE index, a widely available clinical decision rule, takes into account other patient features, such as body mass index, and 6 minute walk distance, to give a 4-year mortality.

Evidence-Based Diagnosis

A. The diagnosis of COPD is based on history, physical exam, and ancillary tests (primarily PFTs).

B. History

   1. Important aspects of the history are:

      a. Chronic cough

      b. Lingering colds

      c. Sputum production

      d. Dyspnea

      e. Decreased exercise tolerance

   2. Other important historical features that argue for airflow limitation include:

      a. Smoking history ≥ 70 pack-years: sensitivity, 40%; specificity, 95%; LR+, 8.0; LR–, 0.63.

      b. Sputum production > ¼ cup: sensitivity, 20%; specificity, 95%; LR+, 4; LR–, 0.84.

C. Physical exam

   1. The physical exam is useful mainly in patients with more advanced disease.

   2. No findings are sensitive enough to exclude a diagnosis of COPD.

    3. The test characteristics for some of the physical exam findings are listed in Table 33-8.

 The absence of wheezing does not rule out, or even significantly decrease the likelihood of, COPD.

D. Combinations of historical features, signs and symptoms are most effective in diagnosing COPD.

   1. There are many decision rules that aid in the diagnosis of COPD.

   2. The combination of > 55 pack-year smoking history, wheezing on auscultation, and patient reported wheezing diagnoses airflow obstruction (LR+, 156).

   3. The absence of cigarette smoking is the most effective test to rule out airflow obstruction (LR–, 0.16)

E. Spirometry

   1. Spirometry should be used in all patients with suspected COPD and respiratory symptoms.

Table 33-8. Test characteristics for physical exam findings in COPD.

Criteria	Sensitivity	Specificity	LR+	LR−
Subxiphoid cardiac impulse	4–27%	97–99%	≈ 8	≈ 1
Absent cardiac dullness at the LLSB	15%	99%	15	≈ 1
Diaphragmatic excursion < 2 cm	13%	98%	6.5	≈ 1
Early inspiratory crackles	25–77%	97–98%	8–38.5	≈ 1
Any unforced wheeze	13–56%	86–99%	1–56	≈ 1

COPD, chronic obstructive pulmonary disease; LLSB, left lower sternal border LR, likelihood ratio.
Modified from McGee SR. Evidence-based physical diagnosis. Philadelphia, PA: Saunders, 2001:382. With permission from Elsevier.

2. Because the results of spirometry are part of the information required to make a diagnosis of COPD, test characteristics cannot be calculated.

3. For the diagnosis of COPD, the most important spirometric values are postbronchodilator, since COPD is defined by irreversible airway obstruction.

4. Typically PFTs in COPD reveal:

    a. Increased total lung capacity secondary to decreased elastic recoil

    b. Increased functional residual capacity and residual volume secondary to air trapping

    c. Decreased FEV_1 and FVC due to airflow obstruction

    d. Decreased DLCO secondary to destruction of the oxygen/Hgb interface.

F. Other tests

1. Spirometry with bronchodilator response is recommended to rule out asthma. Patients with completely reversible airflow obstruction likely have asthma.

2. Chest radiograph is generally not useful in diagnosing COPD.

    a. Some findings are suggestive

      (1) Upper lobe bullous disease (uncommon but nearly diagnostic)

      (2) Flattened diaphragm on the lateral chest radiograph

      (3) Large retrosternal air space

      (4) Hyperlucency of the lungs

      (5) Diminished distal vascular markings

    b. Chest radiography is always recommended to rule out other causes of symptoms.

G. ABG measurement is recommended in patients with FEV_1 < 40% predicted or right-sided heart failure.

H. Testing for alpha-1-antitrypsin deficiency (a rare cause of COPD) is recommended in patients:

1. In whom COPD develops before age 45 years

2. Who do not have a smoking history or suspicious exposure

In general, any patient with a smoking history who complains of chronic cough, sputum production, or dyspnea should be considered to have COPD if no other diagnosis can be made. Additional testing can be used to establish the diagnosis and assess severity.

Treatment

A. Management of stable disease

1. Nonpharmacologic and preventive therapy

    a. Smoking cessation and avoidance of other inhaled toxic agents

Smoking cessation is more effective than any pharmacotherapy at preserving lung function in patients with COPD.

    b. Exercise programs, if allowable from a cardiovascular standpoint

    c. Vaccination against influenza and pneumococcal pneumonia

2. Pharmacologic

    a. The patients who benefit the most from therapy are patients with symptoms and an FEV_1 < 60% of predicted. These patients should be prescribed bronchodilator inhalers such as long-acting beta-agonist or anticholinergic inhalers.

    b. Patients with less severe disease may benefit from treatment as well, especially as needed bronchodilators.

    c. Combination therapy with both long-acting beta-agonist and anticholinergic inhalers may improve outcomes in patients who do not get a sufficient response with monotherapy.

    d. Inhaled corticosteroids

      (1) Use remains somewhat controversial

      (2) There is some evidence that inhaled corticosteroids, used with long-acting beta-agonists or anticholinergics, decrease symptoms and reduce the frequency of exacerbations. This is probably most true in patients with some reversible airway obstruction on spirometry.

      (3) They do not seem to affect the rate of decline in pulmonary function and may increase rates of pneumonia.

    e. Home oxygen is recommended for persons with chronic hypoxia or cor pulmonale.

    f. Recent evidence suggests that long-term antibiotic therapy reduces the risk of exacerbations in patients with COPD.

B. Management of exacerbations

1. Evaluation

    a. Patients who are likely to have the worst outcomes have low baseline FEV_1, PaO_2, pH, and high PCO_2. Discharge of such patients from an emergency department should only be done with great care.

    b. Exacerbating factors

      (1) Factors that may have led to the COPD exacerbation should be sought and addressed during treatment.

      (2) Historical evidence of infection or exposure (air pollution, ozone) should be sought.

(3) All patients should have a chest radiograph to look for pneumonia.

(4) As discussed in Chapter 15, Dyspnea, if a cause of the exacerbation is not found, consideration should be given to pulmonary embolism and HF.

   c. Unlike in the assessment of asthma exacerbations, spirometry is of little value in making admission decisions.

2. Therapy

   a. Anticholinergic and beta-agonist inhalers should be given to all patients.

   b. Systemic corticosteroids are effective when given for up to 2 weeks. There is no evidence that inhaled corticosteroids are effective.

3. Antibiotics are effective for more severe exacerbations.

4. Oxygen therapy is beneficial.

   a. Oxygen does carry a risk of hypercapnia and respiratory failure.

   b. The development of respiratory failure is somewhat predictable.

   c. The following equation identifies patients who are at high risk for CO_2 retention and for requiring mechanical ventilation: $pH = 7.66 - 0.00919 \times PaO_2$. If the calculated pH is greater than the patient's true pH, he or she is at high risk for being intubated. Sensitivity is $\approx 80\%$.

If a patient with a COPD exacerbation requires oxygen, it should be provided and not withheld for fear of causing CO_2 retention. If respiratory failure does ensue, it is caused by COPD and not by the physician who administered the oxygen.

5. Noninvasive positive pressure ventilation (eg, bilevel positive airway pressure) decreases rates of intubation, length of stay, and in-hospital mortality in patients with severe exacerbation.

6. Mucolytics, theophylline, and chest physiotherapy have no role in the treatment of COPD exacerbations.

MAKING A DIAGNOSIS

On the physical exam, Mrs. A appears well. Her vital signs are normal. The only findings on lung exam are decreased breath sounds, a prolonged expiratory phase, and scant expiratory wheezing. Her chest radiograph is normal. Some of the results of her PFTs are shown in Table 33-9.

Have you crossed a diagnostic threshold for the leading hypothesis, COPD? Have you ruled out the active alternatives? Do other tests need to be done to exclude the alternative diagnoses?

The combination of her smoking history, reported wheezing, and wheezing on auscultation indicates airflow obstruction. The remainder of her history and physical exam support the diagnosis of COPD and the chest radiograph does not argue for another diagnosis.

Her PFTs also support the diagnosis. Most importantly, there is an irreversible decrease in airflow. The low DLCO (carbon

Table 33-9. Pulmonary function test results for Mrs. A.

Test	Prebronchodilator Result	Prebronchodilator % of Predicted	Postbronchodilator Result	Postbronchodilator % Change
Total lung capacity (L)	6.92	128		
Forced vital capacity (L)	3.03	91	2.90	−4.0
FEV₁ (L)	1.03	43	1.00	−4.0
FEV₁/FVC (%)	34	NA	34	0
DLCO (mL/min/mm Hg)		50		

DLCO, carbon monoxide diffusing capacity of the lungs; FEV_1/FVC, forced expiratory volume in 1 second/forced vital capacity.

monoxide diffusing capacity), suggests loss of a portion of the Hgb/air interface. She falls into the high risk, few symptoms category.

Asthma and HF, the alternative diagnoses, are very unlikely. The irreversibility of the airway disease excludes asthma as a potential cause. HF remains a much less likely possibility because it is not supported by the PFTs. The lack of purulent sputum essentially excludes the other remaining diagnosis bronchiectasis.

Alternative Diagnosis: Bronchiectasis

Textbook Presentation

Dyspnea and chronic, purulent sputum production are usually present in patients with bronchiectasis. There is usually a history of a chronic infection that has led to airway destruction.

Disease Highlights

A. Chronic sputum production is the hallmark of bronchiectasis.

B. The disease is caused by the combination of an airway infection and an inability to clear this infection because of impaired immunity or anatomic abnormality (congenital or acquired). Bronchiectasis can be the result of common (viral infection) or rare (Kartagener syndrome) diseases.

   1. Pertussis and TB were the classic causes of bronchiectasis.

   2. Some of the common causes now are:

      a. Postviral, often with lymphadenopathy causing airway obstruction

      b. *Aspergillus fumigatus,* mainly in association with allergic bronchopulmonary aspergillosis

      c. *Mycobacterium avium* complex infection, usually causing middle lobe disease

      d. Cystic fibrosis

      e. HIV

C. The most common bacteria isolated from the sputum of people with bronchiectasis are *H influenzae, Pseudomonas aeruginosa,* and *Streptococcus pneumoniae.*

D. Complications of the disease include hemoptysis and rarely amyloidosis due to the chronic inflammation.

Evidence-Based Diagnosis

A. The diagnosis of bronchiectasis depends on recognizing the clinical symptoms (chronic sputum production) and demonstrating airway destruction, usually by high-resolution CT scanning.

B. Symptoms and their prevalence

1. Dyspnea and wheezing, 75%

2. Pleuritic chest pain, 50%

C. Signs and their prevalence

1. Crackles, 70%

2. Wheezing, 34%

D. Differentiation of bronchiectasis from COPD can sometimes be difficult because both may present with cough, sputum production, dyspnea, and airflow limitation. Important points in the differentiation are as follows:

1. Sputum production is heavy and chronic in bronchiectasis, while it is only truly purulent in COPD during exacerbations.

2. There is usually a smoking history associated with COPD.

3. Spirometry is not helpful since bronchiectasis can cause both airflow limitation and airway hyperreactivity.

4. Imaging (CT scan) will show diagnostic airway changes in bronchiectasis. In COPD, imaging may or may not demonstrate parenchymal destruction.

Treatment

A. Antibiotics are used both to treat flares of disease and to suppress chronic infection.

B. Pulmonary hygiene

1. Chest physiotherapy

2. There may be a role for bronchodilators, mucolytics, and antiinflammatory medication.

C. Surgery is mainly used to treat airway obstruction, to remove destroyed and chronically infected lung tissue, and to treat life-threatening hemoptysis.

CASE RESOLUTION

Mrs. A is given a tiotropium inhaler, and she reports mild improvement in her symptoms. A month later, a long-acting agonist-agonist inhaler is added. This regimen produces better control of her symptoms. Four months later, she arrives at the emergency department with acute worsening of her symptoms at the time of an upper respiratory tract infection. She is admitted with an exacerbation of COPD.

REFERENCES

Aaron SD, Vandemheen KL, Fergusson D et al. Tiotropium in combination with placebo, salmeterol, or fluticasone-salmeterol for treatment of chronic obstructive pulmonary disease: a randomized trial. Ann Intern Med. 2007;146(8):545–55.

Bach PB, Brown C, Gelfand SE, McCrory DC. Management of acute exacerbations of chronic obstructive pulmonary disease: a summary and appraisal of published evidence. Ann Intern Med. 2001;134:600–20.

Barker AF. Bronchiectasis. N Engl J Med. 2002;346:1383–93.

Bingham CO. An Overview of Angioedema. UpToDate, accessed 4/2008.

Bone RC, Pierce AK, Johnson RL Jr. Controlled oxygen administration in acute respiratory failure in chronic obstructive pulmonary disease: a reappraisal. Am J Med. 1978;65:896–902.

Calverley PM, Anderson JA, Celli B et al. Salmeterol and fluticasone propionate and survival in chronic obstructive pulmonary disease. N Engl J Med. 2007;356(8):775–89.

Christopher KL, Wood RP 2nd, Eckert RC, Blager FB, Raney RA, Souhrada JF. Vocal-cord dysfunction presenting as asthma. N Engl J Med. 1983;308:1566–70.

Corren J, Newman KB. Vocal cord dysfunction mimicking bronchial asthma. Postgrad Med. 1992;92:153–6.

Frantz TD, Rasgon BM, Quesenberry CP Jr. Acute epiglottitis in adults. Analysis of 129 cases. JAMA. 1994;272:1358–60.

Kerstjens HA, Engel M, Dahl R et al. Tiotropium in asthma poorly controlled with standard combination therapy. N Engl J Med. 2012;367:1198–207.

Mahler DA, Harver A, Lentine T, Scott JA, Beck K, Schwartzstein RM. Descriptors of breathlessness in cardiorespiratory diseases. Am J Respir Crit Care Med. 1996;154:1357–63.

McGee SR. *Evidence-based physical diagnosis.* Philadelphia, PA: Saunders; 2001.

National Heart, Lung, and Blood Institute, National Asthma Education and Prevention Program. Expert Panel Report 3: guidelines for the diagnosis and management of asthma: full report 2007. (http://www.nhlbi.nih.gov/guidelines/asthma/asthgdln.pdf.)

Qaseem A, Wilt TJ, Weinberger SE et al. Diagnosis and management of stable chronic obstructive pulmonary disease: a clinical practice guideline update from the American College of Physicians, American College of Chest Physicians, American Thoracic Society, and European Respiratory Society. Ann Intern Med. 2011;155:179–91.

Turcotte H, Langdeau JB, Bowie DM, Boulet LP. Are questionnaires on respiratory symptoms reliable predictors of airway hyperresponsiveness in athletes and sedentary subjects? J Asthma. 2003;40:71–80.

Global Initiative for Chronic Obstructive Pulmonary Disease. http://www.goldcopd.com

Simel DL, Rennie D. *The Rational Clinical Examination: Evidence-Based Clinical Diagnosis.* New York: McGraw Hill; 2009.

Index

Page numbers followed by italic *f* or *t* denote figures or tables, respectively.